# Lovell and Winter's
# Pediatric Orthopaedics

**SIXTH**

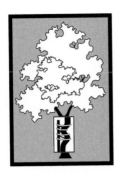

# Lovell and Winter's Pediatric Orthopaedics

### SIXTH EDITION

## VOLUME 2

**EDITORS**

### ▬ RAYMOND T. MORRISSY, MD

Clinical Professor of Orthopaedics
Department of Orthopaedics
Emory University

Orthopaedic Surgeon
Department of Orthopaedics
Children's Healthcare of Atlanta at Scottish Rite
Atlanta, Georgia

### ▬ STUART L. WEINSTEIN, MD

Ignacio V. Ponseti Chair and Professor of Orthopaedic Surgery
Department of Orthopaedic Surgery and Rehabilitation
University of Iowa Hospitals and Clinics
Iowa City, Iowa

## LIPPINCOTT WILLIAMS & WILKINS
### A **Wolters Kluwer** Company
Philadelphia • Baltimore • New York • London
Buenos Aires • Hong Kong • Sydney • Tokyo

*Acquisitions Editor*: Robert Hurley
*Managing Editor*: Jenny Kim
*Developmental Editor*: Grace R. Caputo, Dovetail Content Solutions
*Project Manager*: Nicole Walz
*Senior Manufacturing Manager*: Ben Rivera
*Marketing Director*: Sharon Zinner
*Design Coordinator*: Holly Reid McLaughlin
*Cover Designer*: Vasiliky Kiethas
*Production Services*: Laserwords Private Limited
*Printer*: Edwards Brothers

Sixth Edition

© 2006 by Lippincott Williams & Wilkins
© 2001 by Lippincott Williams & Wilkins
530 Walnut Street
Philadelphia, PA 19106
www.LWW.com

Printed in the United States

**Library of Congress Cataloging-in-Publication Data**

Lovell and Winter's pediatric orthopaedics / [edited by] Raymond T. Morrissy, Stuart L. Weinstein.-- 6th ed.
        p. ; cm.
   Includes bibliographical references and index.
   ISBN-10: 0-7817-5358-9
   ISBN-13: 978-0-7817-5358-6
   1.  Pediatric orthopedics.  I. Lovell, Wood W., 1915-  II. Winter, Robert B., 1932-  III. Morrissy, Raymond T.  IV. Weinstein, Stuart L.  V. Title: Pediatric orthopaedics.
   [DNLM: 1.  Orthopedics--Adolescent. 2.  Orthopedics--Child. 3.  Orthopedics--Infant.  WS 270 L911 2005]
   RD732.3.C48P43 2005
   618.92'7--dc22

                                                                            2005015788

Care has been taken to confirm the accuracy of the information presented and to describe generally accepted practices. However, the authors, editors, and publisher are not responsible for errors or omissions or for any consequences from application of the information in this book and make no warranty, expressed or implied, with respect to the currency, completeness, or accuracy of the contents of the publication. Application of this information in a particular situation remains the professional responsibility of the practitioner.

The authors, editors, and publisher have exerted every effort to ensure that drug selection and dosage set forth in this text are in accordance with current recommendations and practice at the time of publication. However, in view of ongoing research, changes in government regulations, and the constant flow of information relating to drug therapy and drug reactions, the reader is urged to check the package insert for each drug for any change in indications and dosage and for added warnings and precautions. This is particularly important when the recommended agent is a new or infrequently employed drug.

Some drugs and medical devices presented in this publication have Food and Drug Administration (FDA) clearance for limited use in restricted research settings. It is the responsibility of healthcare providers to ascertain the FDA status of each drug or device planned for use in their clinical practice.

The publisher has made every effort to trace copyright holders for borrowed material. If they have inadvertently overlooked any, they will be pleased to make the necessary arrangements at the first opportunity.

To purchase additional copies of this book, call our customer service department at (800) 638-3030 or fax orders to (301) 223-2320. International customers should call (301) 223-2300. Lippincott Williams & Wilkins customer service representatives are available from 8:30 am to 6:30 pm, EST, Monday through Friday, for telephone access. Visit Lippincott Williams & Wilkins on the Internet: http://www.lww.com.

10 9 8 7 6 5 4 3 2

To orthopaedic residents and fellows
that through continued inquiry and learning
they may find medicine to be fun for a lifetime

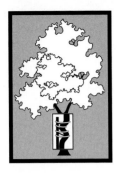

# Contents

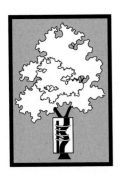

# Contributing Authors

**MICHAEL C. AIN, MD**   Assistant Professor of Orthopaedic and Neurosurgery, Director of Orthopaedics Residency Program, Department of Orthopaedic Surgery, Johns Hopkins University, Baltimore, Maryland

**BENJAMIN A. ALMAN, MD, FRCSC**   Canadian Research Chair, Professor and Vice Chair, Department of Surgery, University of Toronto; Head and Senior Scientist, Orthopaedics and Developmental Biology, Hospital for Sick Children, Toronto, Ontario, Canada

**DAVID D. ARONSSON, MD**   Professor, Departments of Orthopaedics and Rehabilitation and Pediatrics, University of Vermont College of Medicine; Chief, Pediatric Orthopaedics, Department of Orthopaedics and Re-habilitation and Pediatrics, Fletcher Allen Healthcare, Burlington, Vermont

**FRANK R. BERENSON, MD**   Vice Chair of Neurology, Department of Pediatrics, Children's Healthcare of Atlanta at Scottish Rite, Atlanta, Georgia

**WILLIAM G. COLE, MBBS, MSc, PhD, FRACS, FRCSC**   Professor, Department of Surgery, University of Toronto; Surgeon, Division of Orthopaedics, Hospital for Sick Children, Toronto, Ontario, Canada

**ROGER CORNWALL, MD**   Assistant Professor, Department of Orthopaedic Surgery, University of Pennsylvania; Attending Physician, Department of Orthopaedic Surgery, The Children's Hospital of Philadelphia, Philadelphia, Pennsylvania

**COLLEEN COULTER-O'BERRY, MS, PT, PCS**   Team Leader, Limb Deficiency Center, Children's Healthcare of Atlanta; Physical Therapist IV, Department of Orthotics and Prosthetics, Children's Healthcare of Atlanta at Scottish Rite, Atlanta, Georgia

**PETER A. DELUCA, MD**   Assistant Professor, Department of Orthopaedic Surgery, Yale University; Department of Orthopaedic Surgery, Yale–New Haven Hospital, New Haven, Connecticut

**FREDERICK R. DIETZ, MD**   Professor, Department of Ortho-paedic Surgery, University of Iowa and University of Iowa Hospitals and Clinics, Iowa City, Iowa

**ALAIN DIMÉGLIO, MD**   Professor, Department of Ortho-paediatric Surgery, University of Montpellier, True de l'ecole de Medecine; Chief, Department of Orthopaediatric Surgery, Hospital Lapeyroiuie, Montpellier, France

**MATTHEW B. DOBBS, MD**   Assistant Professor, Department of Orthopaedic Surgery, Washington University School of Medicine, St. Louis, Missouri

**JOHN P. DORMANS, MD**   Professor of Orthopaedic Surgery, University of Pennsylvania School of Medicine; Chief of Orthopaedic Surgery, The Children's Hospital of Philadelphia, Philadelphia, Pennsylvania

**GEORGES Y. EL-KHOURY, MD**   Professor, Department of Radiology and Orthopaedics, University of Iowa, Carver College of Medicine; Director, Musculoskeletal Section, Department of Radiology and Orthopaedics, University of Iowa Hospitals and Clinics, Iowa City, Iowa

**JOHN B. EMANS, MD**   Professor, Department of Orthopaedic Surgery, Harvard Medical School; Director, Division of Spine Surgery, Department of Orthopaedic Surgery, Children's Hospital, Boston, Massachusetts

**JOHN M. FLYNN, MD**   Associate Professor of Orthopaedics, University of Pennsylvania; Associate Chief of Orthopaedic Surgery, Division of Orthopaedic Surgery, The Children's Hospital of Philadelphia, Philadelphia, Pennsylvania

**PETER G. GABOS, MD**   Associate Professor, Department of Orthopaedic Surgery, Thomas Jefferson University Hospital, Philadelphia, Pennsylvania; Co-director, Spine and Scoliosis Center, Department of Orthopaedics, Alfred I. duPont Hospital for Children, Wilmington, Delaware

**MARK C. GEBHARDT, MD**   Frederick W. and Jane M. Ilfeld Professor of Orthopaedics, Department of Orthopaedic Surgery, Harvard Medical School; Orthopaedic Surgeon-in-Chief, Department of Orthopaedic Surgery, Beth Israel Deaconess Medical Center, Boston, Massachusetts

**BRIAN J. GIAVEDONI, MBA, CP(C), CP**   Clinical Supervisor of Prosthetics, Assistant Manager, Department of Orthotics and Prosthetics, Children's Healthcare of Atlanta at Scottish Rite, Atlanta, Georgia

**MICHAEL J. GOLDBERG, MD** Professor and Chairman, Department of Orthopaedics, Tufts University School of Medicine; Orthopaedist-in-Chief, Tufts–New England Medical Center, Boston, Massachusetts

**ANDREW W. HOWARD, MD, MSc, FRCSC** Associate Professor, Department of Surgery, University of Toronto; Orthopaedic Surgeon/Attending Staff, Division of Orthopaedic Surgery, The Hospital for Sick Children, Toronto, Ontario, Canada

**JAMES R. KASSER, MD** John E. Hall Professor, Department of Orthopaedic Surgery, Harvard Medical School; Orthopaedic Surgeon-in-Chief, Children's Hospital Boston, Boston, Massachusetts

**ROBERT M. KAY, MD** Associate Professor, Department of Orthopaedic Surgery, Keck–University of Southern California School of Medicine; Pediatric Orthopaedic Surgeon, Children's Orthopaedic Center, Children's Hospital Los Angeles, Los Angeles, California

**GEETIKA KHANNA, MD** Assistant Professor, Department of Radiology, University of Iowa Hospitals and Clinics, Iowa City, Iowa

**MININDER S. KOCHER, MD, MPH** Assistant Professor of Orthopaedic Surgery, Harvard School of Public Health, Harvard Medical School; Attending Physician, Department of Orthopaedic Surgery, Children's Hospital Boston, Boston, Massachusetts

**LAWRENCE G. LENKE, MD** The Serome S. G. Idea Professor of Orthopaedic Surgery, Department of Orthopaedic Surgery, Washington University Medical School; Co-Chief, Adult/Paediatric Spinal Service, Department of Orthopaedic Surgery, Barnes Hospital, St. Louis, Missouri

**RANDALL T. LODER, MD** Garcean Professor, Department of Orthopaedic Surgery, Indiana University; Chief of Orthopaedics, Riley Children's Hospital, Indianapolis, Indiana

**SCOTT J. LUHMANN, MD** Assistant Professor, Department of Orthopaedic Surgery, Washington University School of Medicine, St. Louis, Missouri

**WILLIAM G. MACKENZIE, MD** Associate Professor, Department of Orthopaedic Surgery, Thomas Jefferson University Hospital, Philadelphia, Pennsylvania; Acting Chairman, Department of Orthopaedics, Alfred I. duPont Hospital for Children, Wilmington, Delaware

**YUSUF MENDA, MD** Assistant Professor, Department of Radiology, University of Iowa College of Medicine, Iowa City, Iowa

**JOSÉ A. MORCUENDE, MD, PhD** Assistant Professor, Orthopaedic Surgery and Rehabilitation, University of Iowa, Iowa City, Iowa

**RAYMOND T. MORRISSY, MD** Clinical Professor of Orthopaedics, Department of Orthopaedics, Emory University; Orthopaedic Surgeon, Department of Orthopaedics, Children's Healthcare of Atlanta at Scottish Rite, Atlanta, Georgia

**COLIN F. MOSELEY, MD, CM** Clinical Professor, Department of Orthopaedics, University of California at Los Angeles; Chief of Staff, Shriners Hospitals for Children, Los Angeles, California

**PETER O. NEWTON, MD** Associate Clinical Professor, Department of Orthopaedic Surgery, University of California; Director of Scoliosis Service, Department of Orthopaedic Surgery, Children's Hospital, San Diego, California

**MICHAEL F. O'BRIEN, MD** Orthopedic Surgeon, Department of Orthopaedic Surgery, Miami Children's Hospital, Miami, Florida

**KENNETH J. NOONAN, MD** Associate Professor, Departments of Pediatrics and Orthopaedics, University of Wisconsin Medical School; American Family Children's Hospital, Orthopaedics and Rehabilitation, University of Wisconsin, Madison, Wisconsin

**TOM F. NOVACHECK, MD** Associate Professor, Department of Orthopaedic Surgery, University of Minnesota, Minneapolis, Minnesota; Director, Center for Gait and Motion Analysis, Gillette Children's Specialty Healthcare, St. Paul, Minnesota

**CHARLES T. PRICE, MD** Chief, Pediatric Orthopaedic Education and Research, Department of Orthopaedic Surgery, Nemours Children's Clinic; Chief of Pediatric Orthopaedics, Orlando Regional Medical Center's Arnold Palmer Hospital for Children and Women, Orlando, Florida

**THOMAS S. RENSHAW, MD** Professor of Orthopaedic Surgery, Residency Program Director, Department of Orthopaedics and Rehabilitation, Yale University; Chief of Pediatric Orthopaedic Surgery, Orthopaedic Surgery, Yale–New Haven Hospital, New Haven, Connecticut

**MARGARET M. RICH, MD, PhD** Assistant Chief of Staff, Shriners Hospitals for Children, St. Louis, Missouri

**PERRY L. SCHOENECKER, MD** Professor, Department of Orthopaedic Surgery, Washington University School of Medicine; Chief of Staff, Shriners Hospitals for Children; Interim Chairman, Department of Orthopaedic Surgery, St. Louis Children's Hospital, St. Louis, Missouri

**PAUL D. SPONSELLER MD, MBA** Professor, Department of Orthopaedic Surgery, Johns Hopkins University; Head, Division of Pediatrics Orthopaedics, Johns Hopkins Medical Institutions, Baltimore, Maryland

**DEMPSEY S. SPRINGFIELD, MD**  Professor and Chair, Leni and Peter W. May Department of Orthopaedics, Mount Sinai School of Medicine; Chief of Service, Department of Orthopaedics, Mount Sinai Hospital, New York, New York

**ANTHONY A. STANS, MD**  Assistant Professor, Department of Orthopaedic Surgery, Mayo Clinic, Rochester, Minnesota

**GEORGE H. THOMPSON, MD**  Professor, Departments of Orthopaedic Surgery, and Pediatrics, Case Western Reserve University; Director, Pediatric Orthopaedics, Rainbow Babies and Children's Hospital, Cleveland, Ohio

**WILLIAM C. WARNER, JR., MD**  Associate Professor, Department of Orthopaedics, University of Tennessee; Chief of Staff, LeBonheur Children's Hospital, Memphis, Tennessee

**PETER M. WATERS, MD**  Associate Professor, Department of Orthopaedic Surgery, Harvard Medical School; Associate Chief, Department of Orthopaedic Surgery, Children's Hospital Boston, Boston, Massachusetts

**STUART L. WEINSTEIN, MD**  Ignacio V. Ponseti Chair and Professor of Orthopaedic Surgery, Department of Orthopaedic Surgery and Rehabilitation, University of Iowa Hospitals and Clinics, Iowa City, Iowa

**DENNIS R. WENGER, MD**  Clinical Professor, Department of Orthopaedic Surgery, University of California; Director, Orthopaedic Training Program, Pediatric Orthopaedics, Children's Hospital, San Diego, California

**R. BAXTER WILLIS MD, FRCSC**  Professor, Department of Surgery, Faculty of Medicine, University of Ottawa; Chief, Department of Surgery, Children's Hospital of Eastern Ontario, Ottawa, Ontario, Canada

**DOWAIN A. WRIGHT, MD, PhD**  Clinical Assistant Professor, Department of Pediatrics, University of California School of Medicine; Medical Director, Division of Immunology, Rheumatology and Immunology, Children's Hospital Central California, Madera, California

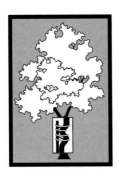

# Preface
# to the First Edition

The field of pediatric orthopaedics has changed significantly in recent years. In the main, textbooks have kept abreast of change, to the extent that there is now a broad and useful literature addressed to the techniques of treatment of the orthopaedic disorders of children. The editors believe, however, that their fellow surgeons will have increasingly shared the desire for a work focused especially upon the decision-making process that precedes and governs the selection of surgical technique. Basic research and clinical specialization have had a dual effect upon clinical decision making. They have broadened the field of choice, and at the same time have made judicious choice more difficult.

Chapters that will aid the reader at the critical junctures at which decisions must be made have been contributed by authorities of eminence, persons who have long and successful experience dealing with the conditions about which they have written. The reader will notice that each topic is covered in depth, and that the emphasis on decision making will facilitate his assessment of the indications and contraindications for a particular treatment approach.

Although we have attempted to match depth with breadth, children's fractures have not been included because the subject is well covered in other textbooks that have recently appeared.

We would like to state that our task has been made not only worthwhile but pleasurable by the continued thoughtful and kind cooperation of the contributors whose names appear in the pages of this book. They have our deepest thanks.

*Wood W. Lovell, MD*
*Robert B. Winter, MD*

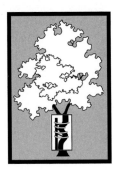

# Preface

This sixth edition of *Lovell and Winter's Pediatric Orthopaedics* is being published 30 years after the first edition. The difference between the knowledge in the first edition and this sixth edition is astounding and illustrates the tremendous progress in the understanding and treatment of orthopaedic conditions in infants, children, and adolescents. This edition is being published halfway through the Bone and Joint Decade, 5 years after the fifth edition, and it documents more progress than in any previous 5-year period.

The current editors have preserved the original intent of Dr. Lovell and Dr. Winter that the textbook should be "focused especially upon the decision-making process that precedes and governs the selection of surgical technique." To achieve this goal, the authors (including 17 new authors and additional new coauthors with expertise in certain areas) have been asked to cull, evaluate, and synthesize the latest literature for the orthopaedic surgeon who takes on the care of the child.

With the increasing emphasis on evidence-based medicine and the research that supports it, a new chapter is included on the evaluation of medical literature for the orthopaedic surgeon. With progress in scoliosis, a new chapter on congenital scoliosis has been added, permitting expansion of the chapter on idiopathic scoliosis to allow inclusion of several new treatments and techniques that were not ready for publication in the last edition.

The orthopaedic surgeon will find two things missing from this edition, as was true for the earlier editions. The first is the etiology of many common conditions, as well as the natural history of these conditions, as this has not yet been elucidated. However, the tremendous contribution already made in the last 5 years, especially in genetics, to our understanding of and ability to diagnose many of these conditions stands out. What will be in the next edition can only be speculated.

The second missing piece is how to perform the surgery, a very important part of orthopaedic care. This is covered in a separate specialized book, *Atlas of Pediatric Orthopaedic Surgery*. In this way, the special focus this text brings to the decision-making process can be preserved and the same focus can be applied to the description of surgical technique. To aid the reader, the table of contents of the *Atlas* is printed in this textbook on the inside front cover.

As with previous editions, the editors have engaged the authors in a spirited dialogue and often have requested more than one revision of their chapters to arrive at what we all hope will be a great help to orthopaedic surgeons, their patients, and their patients' families.

*Raymond T. Morrissy, MD*
*Stuart L. Weinstein, MD*

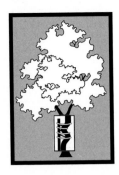

# Acknowledgments

The editors would like to acknowledge the great fortune that we have had to practice our profession in the finest medical system in the world during a period of unprecedented advances in research and innovation, combined with extraordinary cross-fertilization provided by our scientific societies and publishers. This text stands as a testimony to these advances and provides an information base for our colleagues that physicians of past generations would certainly envy.

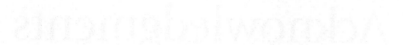

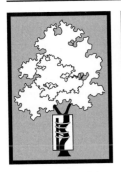

# 19 Congenital Scoliosis

*John B. Emans*

## INTRODUCTION

Congenital scoliosis presents a diverse spectrum of clinical deformity, functional significance, and natural history. Congenital spine deformities appear to result from disordered vertebral formation occurring early in embryogenesis, presumably during somitogenesis between the 5th and 8th week of gestation (1,2). The coexistence of vertebral malformations and nonspinal visceral and musculoskeletal malformations is common in congenital scoliosis and other congenital spine deformities (3). The broad range of congenital scoliosis originates from varied combinations of vertebral anomalies caused by failures of formation, failures of segmentation, and failures of midline fusion. Congenital spinal deformities are of significance not just for the spinal deformities themselves and the potential risk they pose to neurologic structures, but also because they are associated with thoracic deformity, loss of spinal mobility, and altered body shape; these may occur either without treatment or in spite of it. Each congenital spine deformity condition is associated with a specific deformity and natural history. Although some are discovered by fetal ultrasound (4–6) or are visible at birth, many instances of congenital scoliosis go unrecognized until a later age. Congenital vertebral deformity may be troublesome at birth or within the first 2 years of rapid growth, or it may remain quiescent until the preadolescent growth acceleration (7). Although generalizations and caveats are possible, the history of each congenital spinal deformity remains unique. For many congenital deformities early treatment is critical, because later on deformity correction is either not possible or entails greater risk. Generally, the goal of observation and treatment in congenital spinal deformity should be prevention of severe deformity rather than restoration of normal spinal contours. Nonsurgical treatment is of extremely limited value and early surgical treatment remains the most conservative treatment for progressive deformity (8,9).

## DEFINITIONS

By definition, congenital scoliosis is caused by failures of vertebral segmentation or formation, or a combination of the two (Fig. 19.1), producing a deformity in the coronal plane. The distinction between congenital scoliosis and congenital kyphosis or lordosis may be blurred, as many deformities are mixed, with aberrations both in the coronal and sagittal planes. A list of other spinal anomalies and syndromes in which congenital scoliosis is commonly present includes occipitocervical anomalies such as occipitalization of C1 with atlantal hypoplasia, Klippel-Feil deformity, Jarcho-Levin syndrome, spondylocostal or spondylothoracic dysplasia, spinal dysgenesis, and congenital spinal dislocation. Related anomalies that are generally considered distinct from congenital scoliosis include spinal dysraphisms and neural tube defects including spina bifida, myelodysplasia, lipomyelomeningocele, caudal regression syndromes, and other major disruptions of normal vertebral formation in which the natural history of the underlying neurologic deficit usually overshadows any associated congenital scoliosis.

Congenital scoliosis is in a diagnostic category distinct from scoliosis or kyphosis that occur in association with congenital bone dysplasias; it is also distinct from other multiple vertebral abnormalities associated with generalized anomalies in bone development. For example, although the vertebral deformities associated with spondyloepiphyseal or multiple-epiphyseal dysplasia or with mucopolysaccharidoses originate early in gestation, they are caused by a generalized failure of normal bone growth and development, and the failure of normal vertebral shape and spinal growth are secondary. They are not caused by early failures of vertebral segmentation or formation as in congenital scoliosis. A clear distinction is also made between congenital scoliosis or kyphosis and infantile idiopathic or early-onset idiopathic scoliosis. Infantile idiopathic scoliosis may be present *in utero*, but it originates from normally formed vertebral segments and has a natural history quite distinct from that of congenital scoliosis. The term *congenital scoliosis* is often mistakenly applied to infantile idiopathic scoliosis, but the two entities must be clearly separated for purposes of diagnosis and treatment.

Many features are shared within the range of congenital spinal deformities (Fig. 19.2A–C and Fig.19.3). All congenital vertebral anomalies share a common etiologic mechanism of failure of segmentation and/or formation, but may also exhibit a mutually shared association with exposure to teratogens, maternal diabetes (2,10–14) and other syndromes that involve vertebral anomalies. Any vertebral anomaly may be associated with malformations of other organ systems including auditory anomalies, renal and renal-collecting-system anomalies, congenital heart anomalies, visceral, uterine, and vaginal anomalies, and upper extremity anomalies such as radial hypoplasia (3,15–24). Likewise, any of the congenital vertebral anomalies may be identified with a syndrome such as Goldenhar; Poland; Noonan; Crouzon, basal cell nevus; vertebrae, anus, cardiovascular, trachea, esophagus, renal system, and limb buds (VACTERL); coloboma, heart, atresia, renal, genital, ear (CHARGE); and others (2,25–35).

## EPIDEMIOLOGY

### Incidence and Prevalence

Prevalence studies of scoliosis and spinal deformity do not distinguish congenital scoliosis from idiopathic scoliosis, and the true prevalence of congenital scoliosis is therefore unknown, partly because so many vertebral malformations go unrecognized. Assessment of a number of congenital scoliosis operations done at a large center suggests that as many as 20% of cases serious enough to require surgery among adolescents and children are congenital in etiology (36).

### Early Diagnosis of Congenital Scoliosis

Advances in fetal ultrasound (4–6,37–40) have permitted earlier and more comprehensive detection of fetal spinal anomalies. Families may wish to understand the outlook for the child's spinal deformity even at the prenatal stage.

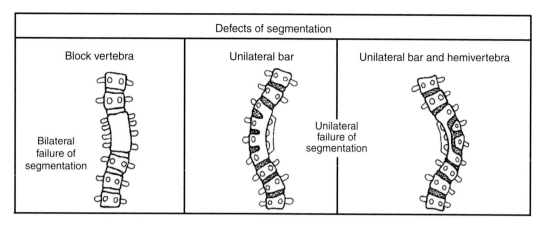

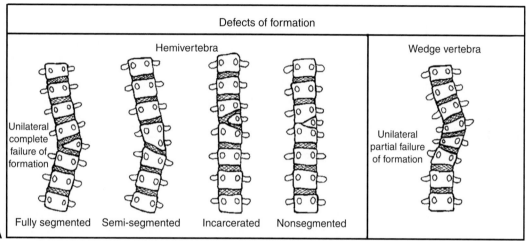

**Figure 19.1** **A:** Classification of congenital scoliosis. Failures of segmentation or formation, singly or in combination, describe nearly all congenital scoliosis. Hemivertebrae can be classified as fully segmented, semisegmented, or nonsegmented. When deficiencies of vertebrae above and below compensate for the hemivertebra, it is described as *incarcerated*. The growth potential of hemivertebrae can be estimated by the presence and thickness of superior and inferior endplates. A unilateral bar opposite a fully segmented hemivertebra is very likely to progress with growth. **B:** Classification of congenital kyphosis. Many instances of congenital scoliosis contain elements of congenital kyphosis. Nearly all congenital kyphotic deformities are progressive and are best treated by early *in situ* posterior fusion if the patient is less than 5 years and the curve is less than 50 degrees. If untreated, progressive kyphotic deformities with failure of formation may produce paraplegia. (**A:** From McMaster MJ, Ohtsuka K. The natural history of congenital scoliosis. A study of two hundred and fifty-one patients. *J Bone Joint Surg Am* 1982;64(8):1128–1147, with permission. **B:** From McMaster MJ, Singh H. Natural history of congenital kyphosis and kyphoscoliosis. A study of one hundred and twelve patients. *J Bone Joint Surg Am* 1999;81(10):1367–1383, with permission.)

Fetal screening is still an evolving field, and predictions of postnatal anomalies by prenatal screening continue to be imperfect. Multiple vertebral anomalies noted on prenatal screening may prove to have minimal significance postnatally, whereas apparently localized vertebral anomalies seen prenatally may result in more generalized defects and syndromic associations with profound postnatal effects. It is also difficult to accurately predict the postnatal course on the basis of prenatal neural tube defects. Caution is urged in prognosticating on the basis of prenatal ultrasound.

## Genetic Aspects, Family Incidence

The familial incidence of congenital vertebral anomalies is low (31,41). Winter et al. noted that only 13 of 1215

patients had first or second degree relatives with vertebral defects (34). It would be potentially valuable to provide genetic counseling to apprise the family of the exact risk of having a subsequent child with a similar anomaly, but it is difficult to achieve (42). Wynne-Davies (43) noted a risk of recurrence of 2% to 3% in siblings when multiple vertebral defects were present, and multiple occurrences have been documented in the same family (41). Some anomalies such as Klippel-Feil deformity have a clear risk of recurrence in other siblings (2,44). Purkiss et al. (45) noted a 20% overall incidence of spinal deformity and 17% incidence of idiopathic scoliosis in families of patients with congenital scoliosis. For many families there is a sense of guilt associated with the birth of a child with a congenital anomaly, because they are under the

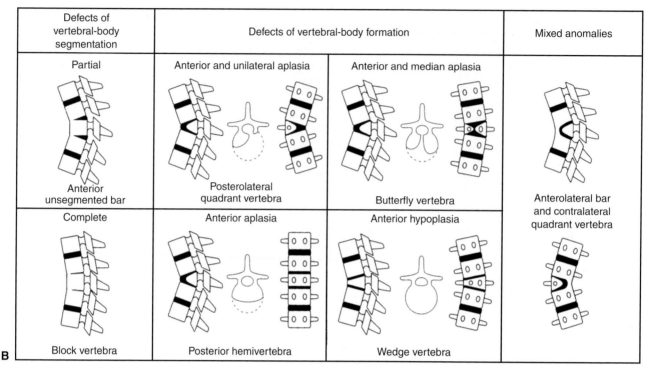

**Figure 19.1** *(continued)*

mistaken impression that environmental influences or parental factors have contributed to the congenital anomaly. Although this view may be correct for some teratogens (46) and for maternal diabetes (14), most congenital vertebral defects represent a spontaneous occurrence. Recent research has identified genetic associations for congenital vertebral anomalies in laboratory animals. In the mouse model, connections between the genes regulating somite formation and segmentation have been associated with genes in the "notch" family (2,47–49). Notch genes have been shown to regulate development of the somite and vertebral precursors in the mouse, and in humans they are associated with spondylocostal dysostosis and Alagille syndrome (48–50).

## Syndrome Associations

Associations between known genetic malformations (including genetic trisomies) and an increased incidence of congenital vertebral malformations are also well documented (2,19,25,44,45,51–60). A few recognized syndromes are associated with congenital scoliosis, and a knowledge of the genetic basis of these syndromes may help with planning and screening for future siblings. The genetic markers associated with some syndromes, such as spondylocostal dysostosis, have been identified and may be of significance to families (1,47–49). Continued elucidation of the control mechanisms of somitogenesis will likely lead to identification of other genetic abnormalities among patients with congenital vertebral anomalies.

## ETIOLOGY

### Embryology

All congenital scoliosis results from a failure of normal vertebral development in early embryogenesis. Early disruption of normal somitogenesis is presently agreed to be the source of the failures of segmentation and formation seen in congenital scoliosis (1). Failure to form normal pairs of somites is reflected in hemivertebrae and wedged vertebrae and in hemimetameric shifts (61), whereas failure in the temporal sequence of somitogenesis from cranial to caudal manifests as segmentation failures such as block vertebrae and multiple contiguous vertebral anomalies. Butterfly vertebrae are presumed to originate from failure of anterior midline fusion between somite pairs. Use of animal models and inspection of human embryos have determined that somitogenesis occurs between the 5th and 7th week of gestation. This is also the time of organogenesis for many organ systems, and therefore it is not surprising that there is a considerable association between malformations in the vertebral column and malformations in the auditory, renal, cardiac, and visceral systems. Signaling and formation of somite precursors for rib and limb development occur during a similar interval,

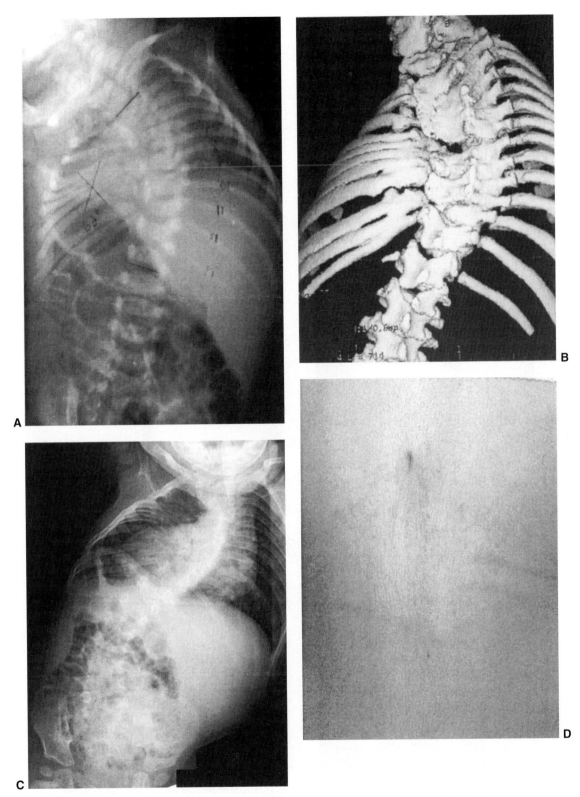

**Figure 19.2**  Anomalies associated with congenital scoliosis. **A:** One-week-old infant with congenital scoliosis. The multiple vertebral anomalies seen here include vertebral bony bars, hemivertebrae, and wedge vertebrae. Other anomalies included ear anomalies and deafness, solitary kidney, imperforate anus, tethered spinal cord, atrial septal defect, hypoplastic lung, and radial hypoplasia. **B:** Three-dimensional computed tomography (CT) scan of the same patient at 10 months. Fused ribs on the concavity of the thoracic scoliosis will act as a tether, producing more deformity with growth. **C:** Upright radiograph at 10 months. A new curvature in the more normal thoracolumbar spine is compensatory to the upright position, but should suggest the possibility of spinal cord tethering. **D:** Cutaneous abnormalities such as this skin dimple over the thoracolumbar spine may indicate an underlying intraspinal anomaly.

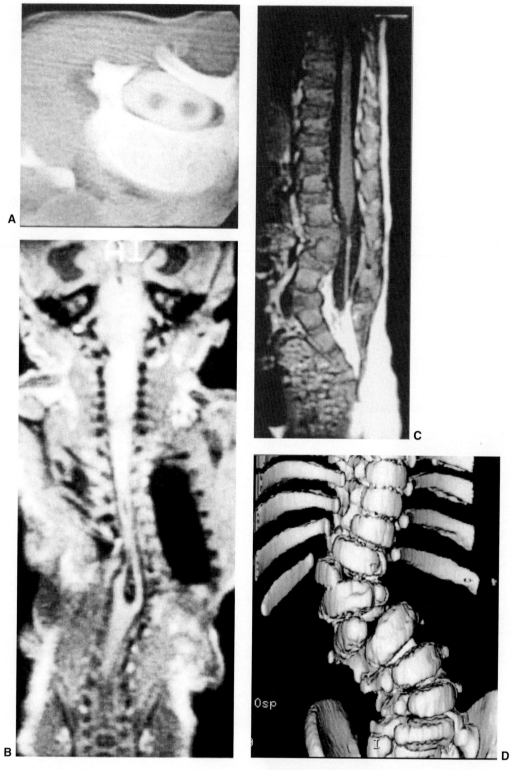

**Figure 19.3   A:** Intraspinal anomalies accompanying vertebral anomalies are common. Indications for magnetic resonance imaging (MRI) include planned surgical intervention, abnormalities found on neurologic examination, and progressive curvature in the unaffected section of the spine. Diplomyelia is visible in this computed tomography (CT) myelogram. **B:** Diastematomyelia, diplomyelia, tethered spinal cord, and other anomalies are present in this infant with multiple vertebral anomalies. Surprisingly, the lower extremity neurologic exam is normal (MRI scan image). **C:** Tethered spinal cord with thickened filum terminale (MRI scan image). **D:** A CT scan with sagittal, coronal, or three-dimensional reformatting is helpful for understanding details of congenital vertebral anomalies. Two lumbar hemivertebrae are readily visible here.

hence rib and limb anomalies are commonly found in association with congenital vertebral anomalies (Fig. 19.2A–C).

## Teratogens, Environmental Effects

The association between vertebral anomalies and teratogens such as carbamazine and valproic acid has long been noted (62), although the mechanism of action of these teratogens has not yet been determined. Likewise, the association between maternal diabetes (particularly type I diabetes) and fetal vertebral anomalies has been well documented (63).

Transient hypoxia has been shown to produce congenital vertebral anomalies in animal model gestation (10,64,65). Likewise, transient exposure to various toxic elements during the fetal period has produced vertebral anomalies (66); in these experiments vertebral anomalies and associated skeletal defects have been similar to those seen in more extensive instances of congenital scoliosis associated with anomalies of the ribs and extremities. These same animal experiments have demonstrated that the location and extent of skeletal malformations are partly dependent upon the timing of the toxic insult, presumably because of the temporal sequence of creation of somites from cranial to caudal. Oxygen deficiency and carbon monoxide exposure, studied in mice, produce considerable skeletal defects including vertebral malformations. Although there is no direct evidence linking hypoxia or carbon monoxide exposure in humans to congenital vertebral defects, there is an increased incidence of Klippel-Feil syndrome noted among patients with fetal alcohol syndrome (30,32,67). Hyperthermia may also be a cause of vertebral malformation and has been shown to disrupt normal vertebral development in animal models (12,68).

## CLINICAL FEATURES

The clinical presentation of congenital scoliosis varies greatly. Many instances are unrecognized until an incidental x-ray film shows an underlying vertebral anomaly. If balancing deformities are present (Fig. 19.4) (hemimetameric shift), the congenital scoliosis may be completely unapparent clinically except for diminished spinal motion. Some congenital scoliosis deformities are immediately apparent at birth, with major malformation of the spine and an associated deformity or shortening (Fig. 19.2A–C). Clinical features that may suggest congenital scoliosis or other vertebral

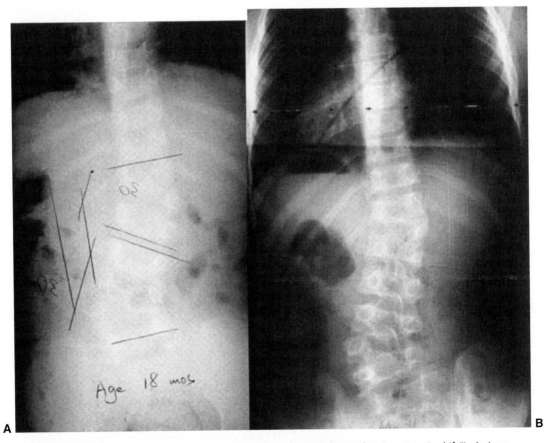

**A**    **B**

**Figure 19.4** Nonprogressive, balanced, double hemivertebrae ("hemimetameric shift"). **A:** In a child 18 months of age, two hemivertebrae balance each other well. **B:** At 11 years of age, there has been extensive growth but no worsening of the untreated, balanced deformity.

anomalies include signs of spinal dysraphism such as skin dimples (Fig. 19.2D) or hairy patches near the spine, limb paralysis (69) or atrophy, and signs of chronic neurologic abnormality including foot deformity, particularly if asymmetric. Spinal dysgenesis or congenital spinal dislocation may be manifest as early lower-extremity paralysis or dysfunction (70,71).

Multiple vertebral anomalies frequently result in a shorter-than-normal spine (72), and this shortness may be manifest as a relative limb–trunk disproportion. Most anomalies involving multiple vertebral levels are associated with loss of motion of the affected spinal segment. In Klippel-Feil deformity this may manifest as a torticollis with diminished motion of the cervico-thoracic junction or cervical spine. Likewise, vertebral anomalies involving the entire thoracic and lumbar spine may manifest not as deformity but as diminished mobility. Rarely, vertebral anomalies may present as a mass or bump near the spine rather than as a spinal deformity. Congenital lordosis caused by posterior failures of fusion may appear as an abnormally concave area of spine without scoliosis. Congenital anomalies at the cervicothoracic junction may present as a supraclavicular mass or may mimic Sprengel deformity, with a high-riding scapula. Congenital scoliosis centered at the cervicothoracic level may produce a profound cosmetic deformity with head tilt, shoulder elevation, and secondary spinal imbalance. Hemivertebrae at the thoracolumbar junction may manifest as trunk imbalance, whereas those at the lumbosacral junction may appear as pelvic tilt or apparent leg-length inequality.

Rotational thoracic deformity or "rib-hump" occurs predictably in thoracic idiopathic, neurogenic, and paralytic scoliosis, but is variable in congenital scoliosis. Some congenital thoracic scoliosis is associated with little if any rotational thoracic asymmetry, whereas other cases, particularly when many spinal segments are involved or the deformity is progressive, manifest as severe thoracic deformity (73). Rarely, well-balanced congenital scoliosis with rib fusions may first present with restrictive respiratory difficulty caused by a short, stiff thorax. Congenital scoliosis, when progressive, worsens during periods of rapid growth and may therefore first be noted during either early childhood or adolescence.

## RADIOGRAPHIC FEATURES

The diagnosis and classification of congenital scoliosis can generally be made from plain radiographs. Careful assessment of well-penetrated anteroposterior and lateral radiographs will usually reveal nearly all the salient details of a congenital vertebral anomaly. Absence of spinous processes, rib fusions, joined pedicles, or absent or narrowed disc spaces may suggest an underlying congenital anomaly. More extensive radiographic evaluation is needed preoperatively for surgical planning, but not usually for classification

or observation. MRI is helpful for assessment of spinal cord anatomy and will reveal vertebral body segmentation and formation anomalies with accuracy, but it can be confusing in the assessment of posterior elements.

## Classification

Classification of congenital scoliosis is generally done by modifications of the Nasca classification (74,75). This classification system is based on failure of formation, failure of segmentation, or combinations of the two (Fig. 19.1), and is helpful in describing anomalies and predicting which of them will be progressive (8,74–79). Sagittal plane anomalies are often important concomitant deformities that should be included in any description. If the failure of formation or of segmentation occurs only on the right or left side, a scoliosis results. If the failure occurs only anteriorly or posteriorly, then a congenital kyphosis or congenital lordosis will occur. Most cases are subtle combinations of both coronal and sagittal plane deformities, and a more three-dimensional classification system is needed. Recognizable patterns of failures of formation include wedge vertebrae and hemivertebrae in congenital scoliosis, and type I (Winter) failures of formation in congenital kyphosis (80,81) (Fig. 19.5). Wedged vertebrae result from a unilateral partial failure of

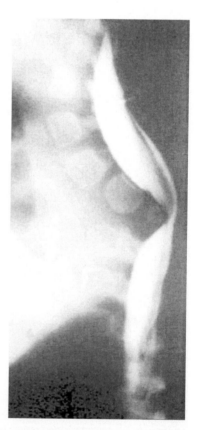

**Figure 19.5** Congenital kyphosis (type I by Winter classification) with posterior hemivertebra. Neurologic function has regressed from normal to paraplegic by 9 months of age, the time of this computed tomography (CT) myelogram image. Anterior decompression and stabilization were needed.

formation, and usually a pedicle is present bilaterally. Unilateral complete failure of formation manifests as a hemivertebra, recognizable by the absence of a contralateral paired pedicle. Hemivertebrae can be subclassified as fully segmented, semisegmented, or nonsegmented on the basis of the presence or absence of a full growth plate and disc remnants at the cephalad and caudad sides of the hemivertebra (Fig. 19.1). Hemivertebrae can be either paired or unilateral and can be offset with a "hemimetameric shift" (Fig. 19.4). Failures of segmentation can result in block vertebrae (Fig. 19.6), anterior or posterior unilateral bars, congenital lordosis, or type II congenital kyphosis. Complete bilateral failures of segmentation anteriorly result in a block vertebra. Unilateral anterior failure of segmentation produces an anterior unilateral bar. Partial failure of segmentation of the anterior portion of the disc and growth plate results in a type II congenital kyphosis (Fig. 19.7). Posterior failure of segmentation can be bilateral and symmetric, producing congenital lordosis, or unilateral, creating a posterior cartilaginous or bony bar. Complete anterior and posterior failure of segmentation creates a block vertebra, whereas unilateral anterior and posterior failure of segmentation causes a unilateral bar.

The standard classification system of failure of segmentation, failure of formation, and mixed failures of segmentation and formation assumes that anterior spinal anatomy is similar to posterior spinal anatomy. Clinical observation and CT scans (82,83) show that it is not rare for anomalies in the posterior elements to show no correspondence with the anomalous anterior elements. The anterior elements, best seen on plain x-ray film or MRI, guide the overall classification. Posterior elements are better seen by CT scan and CT reconstructions.

The lack of correspondence between anterior and posterior anomalies may explain some of the difficulty in accurately predicting which deformities will be progressive. If, for example, an anterior fully segmented hemivertebra is associated with a bilateral posterior failure of segmentation over the same levels, there may be slow progression rather than rapid progression, or the progression may occur more into lordosis than into scoliosis, the posterior failure of segmentation preventing or slowing the tendency of the fully segmented hemivertebra to progress. The availability of the three-dimensional reconstruction of CT scans makes it easier to understand and describe these anomalies. Radiographic findings may also include associated anomalies (Fig. 19.2). The presence of rib fusions or of distortion of the thoracic cavity should be noted. The presence of multiple rib fusions may act as a paraspinal tether creating thoracogenic scoliosis, or may enhance progressive deformity because of the vertebral bar that is commonly juxtaposed to rib fusions. Examination of the underlying vertebral anatomy and an attempt at classification is helpful for prognosis (Fig. 19.8). If certain patterns are identified, such as a fully segmented hemivertebra, the likelihood of rapid progression may be much higher. If a unilateral bar

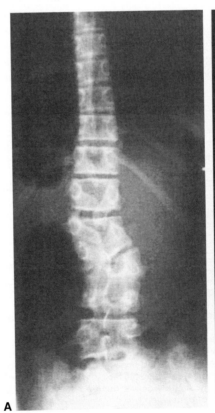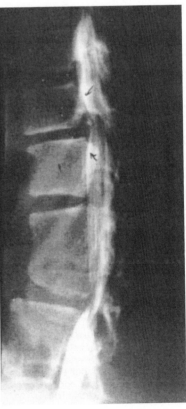

**Figure 19.6** Adjacent segment hypermobility, sometimes with instability or stenosis, may occur adjacent to naturally occurring congenital or surgically created rigid segments of spine. **A:** A well-balanced untreated congenital scoliosis with increasing spasticity of the lower extremities. **B:** Myelogram reveals hypertrophic discs and spinal stenosis. Treatment was by decompression and fusion of the hypermobile segments.

A

B

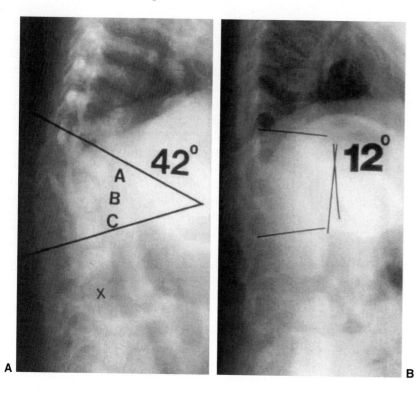

**A**  **B**

**Figure 19.7** Early *in situ* fusion is the standard treatment for progressive congenital curves. Early posterior *in situ* fusion with cast and/or instrumentation immobilization can produce progressive correction in patients younger than 5 years of age with moderate congenital kyphosis (less than 50 degrees) without neurologic involvement. **A:** Progressive type II congenital kyphosis at 13 months of age. At 14 months of age, the patient was treated with *in situ* posterior fusion and postoperative cast. **B:** At age 4 years, there is progressive correction of the kyphosis due to the posterior spinal fusion acting as a tether, while anterior growth continues.

is noticed, there is a great likelihood of continued progression of the deformity. The combined presence of one or more fully segmented hemivertebra as well as a cartilaginous bar and/or rib fusions is highly likely to lead to progressive deformity with growth (7–9,74–76,79,84,85).

## Measurement

Absolute Cobb angle magnitude is of much less significance than overall deformity and the change in that deformity over time with growth. Documentation of radiographic

change with growth is the mainstay of observation and surgical decision making. Comparison of current with early x-ray films is needed in order to ascertain whether there has been deformity progression. Radiographic change may be very gradual, and archiving of original x-ray films is useful for later comparison and remeasurement of Cobb angles.

Measurement of sequential radiographs is crucial for the assessment of deformity progression. Unlike idiopathic scoliosis, in which a standard measure, the Cobb angle, is fairly reproducible within and between observers, meaningful documentation of progression in congenital scoliosis

| Site of curvature | Type of congenital anomaly | | | | | |
|---|---|---|---|---|---|---|
| | Block vertebra | Wedge vertebra | Hemivertebra | | Unilateral unsegmented bar | Unilateral unsegmented bar and contralateral hemivertebrae |
| | | | Single | Double | | |
| **Upper thoracic** | <1°–1° | ★–2° | 1°–2° | 2°–2.5° | 2°–4° | 5°–6° |
| **Lower thoracic** | <1°–1° | 2°–3° | 2°–2.5° | 2°–3° | 5°–6.5° | 6°–7° |
| **Thoracolumbar** | <1°–1° | 1.5°–2° | 2°–3.5° | 5°–★ | 6°–9° | >10°–★ |
| **Lumbar** | <1°–★ | <1°–★ | <1°–1° | ★ | >5°–★ | ★ |
| **Lumbosacral** | ★ | ★ | <1°–1.5° | ★ | ★ | ★ |

▢ No treatment required ▪ May require spinal surgery □ Require spinal fusion ★ Too few or no curves

**Ranges represent the degree of derotation before and after 10 years of age**

**Figure 19.8** McMaster has compiled data about the likelihood of progression of congenital scoliosis associated with different vertebral anomalies, based on annual rate of progression. Double hemivertebrae, unsegmented bars, and unsegmented bars opposite hemivertebrae were noted to be rapidly progressive and to require spinal fusion. (From McMaster MJ, Ohtsuka K. The natural history of congenital scoliosis. A study of two hundred and fifty-one patients. *J Bone Joint Surg Am* 1982;64(8):1128–1147, with permission.)

requires measurement of reference points that are consistent over time. It is mandatory that congenital scoliosis be measured in a reproducible way on the basis of reference to prior radiographs. Reference to only the immediately prior radiograph may miss slow change and produce cumulative error in measurement. Because change may occur slowly over many years, families should be urged to archive original and intermediate films for later comparison. Of necessity, initial radiographs of an infant's spine will be taken in the supine position, but as the child grows older radiographs should be taken with the child in the upright position. Caution is needed in interpreting a change in deformity over this period of time if the comparison is between a supine-position film and an upright-position film (Fig. 19.2A,C). Generally, both posteroanterior and lateral films are necessary. Subtle worsening of congenital kyphosis or congenital lordosis may go unrecognized if only posteroanterior films are taken.

Measurement of the Cobb angle of curvature in the coronal and sagittal planes requires the consistent identification of end points (86,87). Identification of end points can be done easily in patients with idiopathic scoliosis, but requires innovation and consistency in those with congenital scoliosis. Cobb angle measurement of a pure coronal deformity may be made by using the vertebral body endplates or, commonly, the pedicles as endpoints. Measurement of a low lumbar spinal deformity may be more easily achieved by using the tops of the iliac crest as the lower end point, in essence measuring pelvic obliquity. The choice of measurement end points must be consistent between films, and usually it will be necessary to go back and remeasure films, starting from infancy, with the same end points in order to determine whether progression has occurred. It is appropriate to measure not only the anomalous congenital segment but also the entire curve associated with it. Attention to secondary curves is equally important, and all curves should be measured at all intervals. A change in a secondary curve may reflect an unrecognized change in the associated congenital "primary" curve. A change in the normally segmented part of the spine without any change in the congenital curve raises the possibility of the change being caused by spinal cord tethering, and should prompt an MRI examination of the intraspinal contents for anomalies (Fig. 19.3A–B) and tethered spinal cord (Fig. 19.3C) if not already done (3,21,88–90). Other indications of spinal deformity, including trunk imbalance, apical vertebral deviation, occipital or cervical spine imbalance relative to the pelvis, and appearance of sagittal plane posture and sagittal plane balance as seen on lateral radiographs, may be of even greater significance than the Cobb angle. Loder et al. (87) found that intra- and interobserver error in Cobb angle measurement in congenital scoliosis was as much as 13 degrees, thereby suggesting that Cobb angle alone may be a poor marker for documentation of progression in congenital scoliosis. Lonstein et al. (86), however, showed that if sequential radiographs were measured and care was taken to use the same end points, inter- and intraobserver error in Cobb measurement of congenital scoliosis was similar to or better than studies of measurement error in idiopathic scoliosis. Their observation that sequential radiographs and reproducibility of measurement end points over time enhance accuracy is of the utmost importance, and the clinician should follow their advice to re-examine multiple prior radiographs each time that the patient's new radiographs are measured.

## OTHER IMAGING STUDIES

As discussed later in this chapter, additional imaging, including screening for underlying renal anomalies, is mandatory. If the child is less than 6 to 8 weeks of age, spinal ultrasound (91) may be effective for the screening of intraspinal contents for such major anomalies as low-lying conus, diplomyelia, dermoid, diastematomyelia, syringomyelia, or tethered spinal cord. If there is a high suspicion of intraspinal anomaly, however, MRI is needed and in infants will usually require anesthesia or sedation.

The availability of MRI has greatly facilitated the detection of intraspinal anomalies in congenital scoliosis (Fig. 19.3A–C). Typically, a 20% incidence of intraspinal anomalies is reported in large series (3,19,21,88,90), with one series (3) reporting a rate of 37%. An MRI is clearly indicated prior to any surgical intervention. Even if the surgical intervention does not involve correction, a search for underlying intraspinal anomalies should be made before altering the spinal anatomy by fusion or instrumentation. Anomalies include associated syringomyelia with or without Chiari I malformation, fatty filum terminale, intradural lipoma, and occult split cord or diastematomyelia malformations. Major intraspinal malformations increase the likelihood of progressive deformity and progressive or acute neurologic loss if acute surgical correction of the deformity is attempted (92). Any tethering lesions should be considered for surgical release (17,21,93–95). Urodynamic testing may help establish the significance of a tethering lesion in a patient who otherwise does not have a progressive deformity or neurologic abnormalities of the extremities (96).

Experts agree on the need for MRI before surgical intervention or if progressive scoliosis is noted in a structurally normally segmented area of the spine. Whether MRI should be performed as a screening test in all individuals with congenital spinal anomalies is, however, controversial. Some series recommend a screening MRI in all individuals with vertebral malformations (3,88). In young children, an MRI requires sedation or general anesthesia, and thus other sources suggest that MRI screening needs to be done only preoperatively or if neurologic abnormalities are present (90). Subtle signs of root tension or root irritation such as limited neck flexion or tight hamstrings, an extended trunk and extremity posture, or asymmetric reflexes mandate a screening MRI. More obvious neurologic findings, including asymmetry in the girth or strength of the extremities, weakness in the extremities, or otherwise unexplained incontinence, should prompt an MRI of the intraspinal contents. MRI of the spinal cord done in infancy may not reveal anomalies that become visible later in childhood, and motion artifact may obscure underlying anomalies. Some anomalies such as intradural lipomas or syringomyelia may change over time. If a child has had a normal MRI study in infancy but there are clinical signs of intraspinal abnormalities at a later time, a subsequent MRI in later childhood is potentially useful. If progressive deformity is noted in the normal part of the spine, MRI is mandatory, as spinal cord tethering or some intraspinal anomaly may be responsible for the change in deformity.

If the congenital deformity extends into the cervical spine, consideration should be given to dynamic flexion/extension views periodically to assess instability.

## OTHER DIAGNOSTIC STUDIES WHEN INDICATED

Renal, cardiac, auditory, and intraspinal anomalies are associated with congenital scoliosis and other congenital spinal anomalies at rates as high as 61% (3,15), particularly in more extensive and mixed vertebral anomalies. Screening of the kidneys and renal collecting system should be done in every individual with congenital scoliosis. Asymptomatic obstructive uropathy can occur; in one series (3), one third of the patients noted to have renal anomalies required treatment. The orthopaedic surgeon may be the only medical provider to recognize the potential occurrence of renal anomalies in association with congenital vertebral anomalies. Screening renal ultrasounds can be performed on small children without sedation. If the kidneys and collecting system are visualized incidentally on an MRI, a screening ultrasound is not needed.

The incidence of auditory anomalies associated with congenital vertebral anomalies is high (97), particularly with cervical anomalies and Klippel-Feil syndrome, in which as many as one third of the patients may have hearing loss (29). Major hearing deficits can go unrecognized in infants, particularly if the child has other major health problems which distract from the diagnosis. Infant auditory screening is probably sufficient to rule out a major hearing deficit, but if it has not been performed, auditory testing should be considered.

Underlying cardiac anomalies are frequent with congenital scoliosis, but the spine in most scoliosis that is associated with severe congenital heart disease is normally segmented (98,99). A clinical examination will pick up manifestations of congenital heart disease such as abnormal heart sounds, abnormal rhythm, and abnormal oxygenation, but may not reveal significant underlying cardiac anomalies. An echocardiographic examination of the heart

is probably warranted in individuals with congenital spinal deformities who will be undergoing major surgical intervention, because the incidence of cardiac anomalies is reportedly as high as 26% with congenital scoliosis (3).

## PATHOANATOMY

The pathoanatomy of deformity in congenital scoliosis and congenital kyphosis is highly variable. Four mechanisms are probably responsible for the evolution of deformity in congenital vertebral anomalies.

The first such mechanism is failure of formation or failure of segmentation. Early fetal ultrasound of vertebral defects sometimes reveals a major deformity early in embryogenesis. Asymmetric growth of malformed vertebral elements is the presumed mechanism for worsening of the deformity during the remainder of embryogenesis after initial vertebral column formation. Asymmetric growth originates from the presence of asymmetric tissue with growth potential, including both vertebral cartilaginous endplates as well as vertebral cartilage destined for endochondral growth. Examination of coronal or sagittal cross sections of congenital vertebral pathologic specimens, or CT or MRI scans, readily reveal an asymmetry in growth-related tissue. The growth potential of any given area of tissue can be estimated from the thickness of the growth plate seen on imaging, which is also juxtaposed to disc material. If a thick, asymmetric disc space is seen on imaging, it may be presumed that the growth potential of that area is also asymmetric. Estimation of the growth potential of posterior elements is less well understood.

A second mechanism of deformity progression includes asymmetric tethering of spinal growth by a cartilaginous or bony bar, rib fusions, or even iatrogenic fusions. Tethering probably produces progressive deformity only if there is substantial growth on the side of the spine opposite the tethering structure. If an area with substantial growth is juxtaposed to an area of complete absence of growth or tethering, then progression will likely occur and may evolve quickly (Fig. 19.9). Associated rib fusions may produce a tether adjacent to the spine with or without vertebral anomalies (Fig. 19.10A), much like a thoracogenic scoliosis associated with burn scars. Relatively normal growth may occur in the spine but if an adjacent tethering structure is strong, the spine will be drawn into a progressively deformed position with the ribs acting as a concave tether. Campbell demonstrated growth in bony vertebral bars (100), but bony or cartilaginous bars will reliably act as a tether if there is considerable growth on the opposite side of the spine (79,85).

A third mechanism of spinal deformity is the presumed long-term action of gravity and posture. Just as idiopathic deformities can progress in the presence of what was initially a normally formed vertebral column, so also congenital scoliosis can deform over time through asymmetric

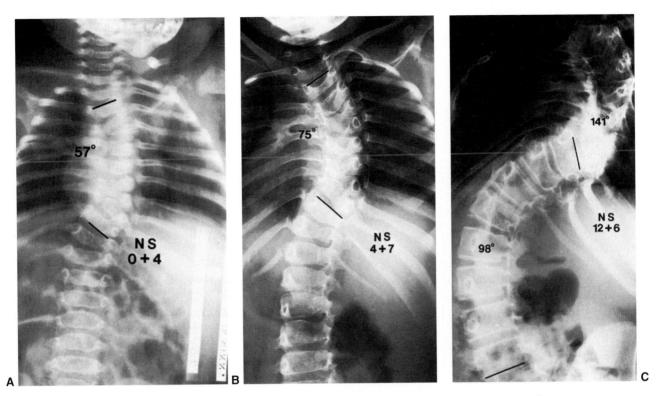

**Figure 19.9**   Relentless progression of untreated thoracic congenital scoliosis from 4 months of age (**A**) to 4 years of age (**B**) to 12 years of age (**C**). Progression has occurred in the area of an unsegmented bar (segmentation defect) opposite hemivertebrae, with fused ribs in the concavity of the curve.

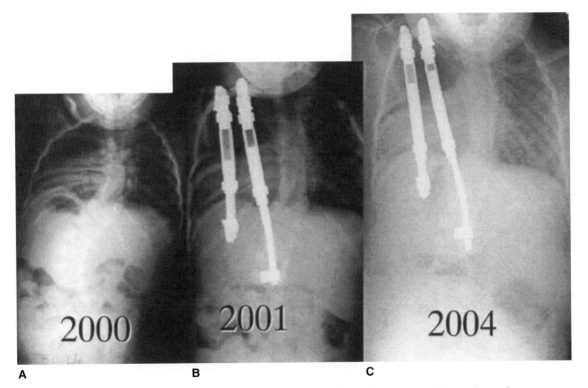

**Figure 19.10**   This two-and-a-half-year-old patient with vertebrae-anus-cardiovascular-trachea-esophagus-renal-limb-buds (VACTERL) syndrome underwent *in situ* fusion of progressive congenital thoracic scoliosis associated with concave fused ribs at 14 months of age. **A:** At $2\frac{1}{2}$ years thoracic curve progression has continued postoperatively. **B:** One year postoperatively, after expansion thoracostomies at two levels, insertion of rib-to-rib and rib-to-spine devices, and device lengthening. **C:** Three years postoperatively after vertical expandable prosthetic titanium rib (VEPTR) devices were outgrown and replaced with longer devices.

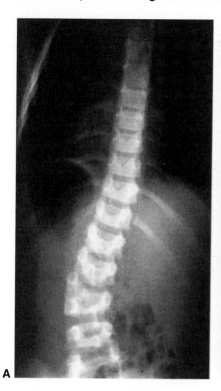

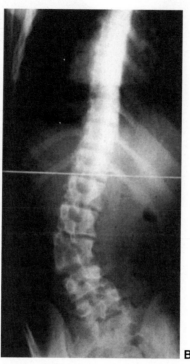

**Figure 19.11** Congenital scoliosis may be stable during childhood but then progress with the preadolescent growth acceleration. **A:** A 12-year-old boy with a semisegmented hemivertebra noted incidentally on screening exam. **B:** At 14 years of age, after 18 months of rapid growth, there has been a drastic increase in curvature. MRI was negative for tethering lesions.

growth of previously symmetric structures. This progression is presumably caused by the prolonged effect of gravity on an asymmetric or out-of-balance spine, which best explains the rapid worsening of previously stable congenital deformities seen during the preadolescent growth acceleration (Fig. 19.11), the same period when progression of idiopathic spinal deformity is commonly noted.

A fourth etiology of progressive deformity is associated with intraspinal anomaly or tethered spinal cord. The mechanism of deformity production is not clear in this instance, but the presence of abnormal intraspinal elements and growth can combine to produce progressive deformity either in a normally segmented spine or in congenital scoliosis. MRI investigation is mandated when a progression of deformity is noted in a part of the spine that was free from congenital deformity, or when a previously stable congenital deformity worsens rapidly.

## NATURAL HISTORY

Knowledge of the natural history of congenital scoliosis is hampered by the rarity of the condition and the extreme variability in severity of congenital spine deformities. The natural history of untreated congenital scoliosis ranges from relentless progression of deformity (Fig. 19.9) with severe consequences for pulmonary and neurologic function, to no progression and no functional deficit (Fig. 19.12). The natural history of congenital scoliosis is best seen as separate but interrelated problems of short- and long-term concern:

progression of spinal deformity, spinal instability and function, pulmonary function, and height.

## Progression of Spinal Deformity with Growth

The short-term natural history of congenital scoliosis during growth is well understood and documented. The natural history in the short term ranges from anomalies with dire short term neurologic consequences, such as spinal dysgenesis (55,70,71,101) or type I kyphosis (Fig. 19.5), to those with rapid deformity change during growth, such as fully segmented hemivertebrae opposite a bar (79,85) (Fig. 19.9), to those which are completely stable through growth and adulthood. If the congenital spine deformity is progressive, it generally mirrors growth velocity, changing rapidly during the first 2 years, slowly during childhood, and then rapidly again during the preadolescent rapid growth phase (7) (Fig. 19.11). Changes in deformity during childhood growth reflect anomalous, asymmetric, or tethered growth, whereas those seen during preadolescence may reflect these effects and the effects of gravity as well. Worsening deformity in congenital scoliosis, congenital lordosis, or congenital kyphosis may occur most rapidly during the first 2 years of growth. Progression of the deformity depends upon the balance of cross-sectional growth in the spine and the secondary effects of any tethering structures. The presence of intact growth plates unbalanced by similar growth forces on the opposite side of the spine, particularly if a tether is present, leads to progressive deformity.

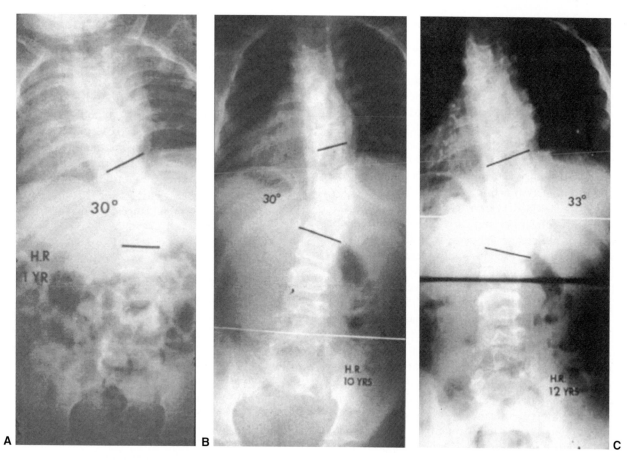

**Figure 19.12** Some extensive congenital anomalies are either not progressive or only minimally progressive. **A:** Fully segmented hemivertebrae with concave rib fusions and other anomalies are noted at 1 year of age. **B:** The patient was put under observation only, and no treatment was given. No significant progression has occurred by 10 years of age. **C:** At 12 years of age after preadolescent growth acceleration there has been slight progression. No treatment was needed.

McMaster, Winter, and others have documented the vertebral malformations most likely to demonstrate progression (7,74,76,78,79,102), noting that progression depends on the type of deformity, its location in the thoracolumbar spine, the length of spine involved, and the amount of growth remaining (Fig. 19.8). A unilateral bar opposite a contralateral hemivertebra is most likely to progress by as much as 10 degrees per year during rapid growth (Fig. 19.9). Unilateral bars or fully segmented hemivertebrae alone may also progress rapidly. Wedge and block vertebrae are less likely to show progression (Figs. 19.4 and 19.6). Early prophylactic fusion without waiting for progression may be justified for some deformities with a high likelihood of worsening such as congenital kyphosis (Fig. 19.7) or a fully segmented hemivertebrae opposite a bony or cartilaginous bar (79,85,103).

Progression may be more rapid in more mobile sections of the spine. Lumbosacral hemivertebrae and thoracolumbar hemivertebrae may show more rapid progression of deformity than congenital deformities contained within the thoracic spine and constrained by the secondary stability of the chest. Rib fusions may act as a tether, causing thoracogenic scoliosis that may either enhance or counteract the tendency of vertebral deformity to progress (104,105) (Fig. 19.10A). During adulthood larger deformities may continue to progress (106,107), presumably due to the forces of gravity and imbalance acting through vertebral remodeling.

## Spinal Instability and Neurologic Dysfunction

The short-term natural history of congenital spinal deformity during infancy rarely includes instability and neurologic change. Neurologic loss caused by spinal canal encroachment may occur in segmental spinal dysgenesis (11,55,70,71) or type I congenital kyphosis (102) (Fig. 19.5), but is uncommon otherwise in congenital scoliosis unless there is an associated intraspinal anomaly, stenosis, instability, or a major kyphotic component in the deformity (92). Spinal mobility is restricted in areas of marked congenital scoliosis, and the concentration of motion stress at the junction between stiff, abnormal congenital spine and mobile, normal spinal segments may produce junctional degenerative changes, instability, or stenosis (Fig. 19.6). Adjacent segment degeneration, instability, and late spinal stenosis are best documented in association with Klippel-Feil syndrome (2), but can also be seen with congenital scoliosis (106).

## Pulmonary Insufficiency and Trunk Height

Many patients with congenital vertebral anomalies suffer adverse effects in overall growth and health that are independent of any associated syndrome such as VACTERL or Klippel-Feil. Concomitant with abnormalities of vertebral shape, there are consistently observed deficiencies in spine size and height. Goldberg et al. (72) have brought attention to the short stature associated with congenital scoliosis, with and without treatment. One of the later consequences of disordered growth of the thoracic spine is the effect on pulmonary function (104,108). Campbell, Day, and others (104,108–111) have documented the associations of both congenital and early-onset scoliosis with pulmonary insufficiency. Pehrsson et al. have linked the diagnosis of early-onset scoliosis with decreased adult survival because of pulmonary insufficiency (111). It seems clear that if congenital scoliosis involves the thoracic spine, and if the thoracic spine is very short or the chest very distorted, then the likelihood of major pulmonary insufficiency during adulthood is increased (104). Campbell et al. have documented the combination of interrelated thoracic spinal deformity and chest cage distortion leading to compromise in respiratory function in progressive congenital and other early-onset spinal deformities (104), and has introduced the useful concept of *thoracic insufficiency syndrome* to describe the interdependence of chest wall, spinal growth, deformity, and lung function (Figs. 19.2A–C, 19.3, 19.10, 19.13, and 19.14). By definition, thoracic insufficiency syndrome is the inability of the spine and chest wall to support normal lung growth and function. In the series studied by Campbell et al. (104), thoracic insufficiency occurred in patients with fused ribs and congenital scoliosis as well as in those with extensive spinal and rib anomalies such as Jarcho-Levin, spondylocostal, and spondylothoracic dysplasias (104,112). Their description of thoracic insufficiency syndrome has led to a heightened awareness of the potential short- and long-term effects of early spinal deformity and associated chest wall deformity on pulmonary function. The inherent shortness of the thoracic spine, associated congenital rib fusions, distortion of the chest shape with progressive spinal deformity, and "penetration" of the chest by lordotic thoracic deformities all contribute to thoracic insufficiency by diminishing thoracic volume and compliance (Fig. 19.14). Deformity of the lumbar spine, or thoracolumbar or lumbar kyphosis, may also create "secondary" thoracic insufficiency (104) by diminishing the space between thorax and pelvis, thereby in terfering with normal diaphragmatic excursion and respiration (16).

## TREATMENT RECOMMENDATIONS

Defining goals of treatment depends upon understanding the natural history of the congenital scoliosis and the continuum of treatment options available. Treatment may be early and prophylactic for predicted progression of deformity or later and corrective for existing deformity. *In situ* fusion is commonly employed, and a choice must usually be made between simply arresting the deformity with a relatively safe predictable procedure or correcting the deformity with a more elaborate procedure. Overall a reasonable goal of treatment of congenital scoliosis is to prevent the development of a severe deformity. For many congenital deformities no treatment is needed (Fig. 19.12), and the best choice may be to perform as little surgery as possible. Generally, waiting for more growth leads to worse deformity (Figs. 19.14A and 19.15A,B) and exposes the patient to the risk of a more dangerous operation.

## Observation

Serial measurement of curvature is the basis for accurate observation in congenital scoliosis. Difficulty with radiographic measurement in congenital scoliosis has been well documented, with a high inter-observer variability noted by Loder et al. (87). In this frequently quoted study, intraobserver error for progression in congenital scoliosis was as high as 13 degrees. Facanha-Filho et al. (86) documented a much smaller, acceptable inter- and intraobserver error when care was taken to use the same measurement endpoints and expert measurers were employed. Observation of change is best done by reexamination and remeasurement of a range of radiographs begun at infancy and followed up through the most recent radiograph. Choosing endpoints for Cobb measurement is arbitrary, so the same endpoints, whether they be pedicles or vertebral endplates, should be used for each measurement. Archiving of films is crucial, and it may prove useful to ask families to retain copies of all the films for the purposes of repeat measurement. Change in congenital scoliosis may be rapid in infancy and preadolescence, whereas during middle childhood years the curve change can be very slow or subtle. Frequency of radiographic observation should reflect prior behavior of the curve and growth rate. Observation should include the Cobb angle for all curves, but also measures of trunk balance. Cobb angle itself may be very differently interpreted for the same curve. If the most congenitally distorted section of the curve is measured, it may yield a much higher Cobb angle than would the overall curve including the congenital deformity. Other elements of trunk balance, such as deviation of C7 with reference to the sacrum, trunk shift, apical vertebral displacement, and sagittal balance, should also be measured, and the results may be more important than the Cobb angle to treatment decisions. Secondary curves involving noncongenitally involved vertebrae should also be measured and may be the most accurate reflection of progression. The secondary curves may act as a marker or indicator of otherwise unrecognized progression in the congenitally deformed section of the spine. Films in infancy of necessity need to be in the supine posture. Upright view x-ray films should be taken

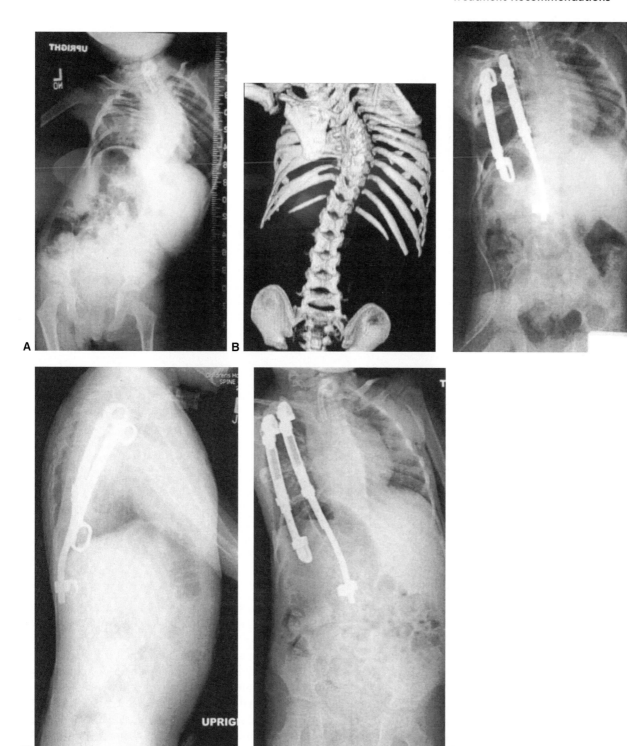

**Figure 19.13**   This 2-year-old boy has progressive congenital scoliosis, rib fusions, progressive thoracic deformity, and thoracic insufficiency syndrome. Tracheotomy was needed after birth. Ventilator dependence persists. **A:** Preoperative posteroanterior view. Note the disparity in space available for the left lung as compared to the right lung. **B:** Preoperative computed tomography (CT) scan with three-dimensional reformatting shows the block vertebrae and fused ribs. **C:** Postoperative posteroanterior view after two expansion thoracostomies through fused ribs, and insertion of one rib-to-rib and one rib-to-spine vertical expandable prosthetic titanium rib (VEPTR) device (Titanium Ribs). Space available for the previously constricted left lung is now increased, and shortly after the surgery ventilator requirements diminished. **D:** Postoperative lateral view after expansion thoracostomy and placement of two VEPTR devices. **E:** Two years after the initial procedure. VEPTR devices were lengthened every 6 to 9 months. Ventilator dependence diminished postoperatively, and 2 years postoperatively he is ventilator free. Space available for the left lung continues to be nearly that of the right. The thoracic spine continues to lengthen. The central portion of the devices will need to be substituted with longer ones after several more lengthenings. Fusion will be necessary near maturity.

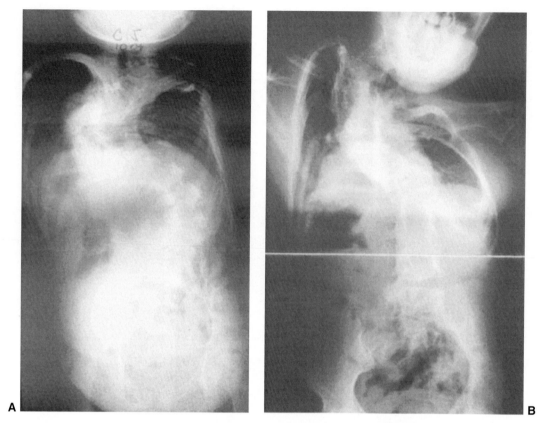

**Figure 19.14** The natural history of congenital scoliosis can include severe respiratory insufficiency, either with or without treatment. **A:** A patient 10 years of age with severe congenital scoliosis. Misguided, ineffective orthotic treatment of congenital scoliosis while waiting for "maturity" for surgical intervention led to this severe deformity. The vital capacity of the lung is only 20% of normal and was not helped by subsequent surgical intervention. Earlier surgical intervention would have been preferable. **B:** Another patient at maturity after several spinal fusions for severe congenital scoliosis. Although there are reasonable overall spinal contours, there is also severe distortion of the thorax, which occurred early in the progression of deformity. Lung fields are small, and there is severe three-dimensional rotational deformity of the thorax, which inhibits thoracic movement on respiration. This patient's restrictive lung disease necessitates full-time oxygen supplementation.

when practical. The interval of observation with x-rays depends upon growth rate, curve severity, and prior curve behavior. Growth is most rapid during the first 2 or 3 years of life, and during this time radiography as frequent as every 3 or 4 months may be appropriate. If a curve has remained stable for an interval of observation, it is reasonable to extend the interval between subsequent observations. The need for early detection of curve progression must be balanced against the theoretical risks of repetitive diagnostic radiographs in patients with early-onset scoliosis (113).

## Nonsurgical Treatment

There are few indications for active nonoperative treatment of congenital spine deformities, there being little evidence of its efficacy. At times treatment of the noncongenital part of the spinal deformity with spinal orthoses can be effective. If there is progression of a deformity within the noncongenital part of the spine, however, the possibility

of spinal cord tethering should be investigated with MRI; likewise, conditions such as thickened filum terminale, syringomyelia, or intradural lipoma may be responsible for curve progression, rather than the actual congenital deformity itself. There is minimal documentation, and that only in limited circumstances, about the efficacy of bracing in congenital spinal deformity. There is no evidence for the efficacy of exercises or chiropractic in slowing the progression of congenital spine deformities. James noted that the curve progressed in more than 50% of cases of infantile scoliosis treated with the advocated casts and Milwaukee braces (114). Winter et al., however, reported that the Milwaukee brace was useful for compensatory curves above and below a congenital curve, for long flexible curves containing congenital elements, and for maintaining trunk and spine balance following localized fusion during growth (115). The potential negative long-term effect of casting and thoracic-lumbar sacral orthosis (TLSO) treatment on the shape of the chest has caused concern but is not well documented. If long-term bracing is utilized in the child with congenital scoliosis, it should be nonrestrictive to the chest, as is the Milwaukee brace technique, which carefully applies pressure in localized areas rather than globally over the chest wall. One should be sure that the nonsurgical treatment is providing some meaningful effect rather than just taking up time and permitting development of a more severe deformity (Fig. 19.14A).

## Surgical Treatment

Surgical treatment remains the mainstay of treatment in congenital spinal deformity. Because the deformity associated with congenital scoliosis is difficult to correct, early treatment is preferable to late treatment of a deformity that has become severe. Allowing the progression of a deformity will inevitably result in greater risks and a more difficult final surgical procedure (Fig. 19.15).

## Preoperative Assessment

Preoperative screening tests should include an MRI for assessment of intraspinal anomalies. The MRI should be used not just to seek the presence or absence of congenital anomalies but to determine whether a significant spinal stenosis or disc protrusion exists. Because segment instability and degeneration with secondary stenosis with hypertrophy of discs and ligamentum flavum may be present adjacent to congenital cervical, thoracolumbar, or lumbar scoliosis, there may be a relative stenosis at either end of a block of congenital deformity. Dynamic flexion/extension radiographs may be helpful. Awareness of a relative spinal stenosis preoperatively may be crucial for planning operative fixation devices or osteotomies. Surgical planning may include CT assessment using two- or three-dimensional image reconstruction where possible (Figs. 19.2B, 19.3D, 19.13B, and 19.15D). Newton et al. and Hedequist and Emans (82,83) have demonstrated the efficacy of three-dimensional CT scan in surgical planning. Although the congenital anomaly may be readily visible on preoperative plain x-ray film, the posterior anatomical anomalies may not correspond to the anterior anomalies seen on plain radiographs. If surgical correction is planned, and particularly if instrumentation is planned, it is helpful to have adequate three-dimensional imaging. Initial preoperative screening tests should also include an assessment of renal anatomy if one has not already been done. If not already investigated, a cardiac evaluation including cardiac echocardiography may be helpful in ruling out substantial underlying congenital heart disease

## Preoperative Spinal Cord Detethering

If an underlying spinal cord anomaly is found, consideration should be given to correcting the anomaly prior to surgical correction of the deformity. Simple deformities such as tight filum terminale (Fig. 19.3C) or a small intradural lipoma may be effectively dealt with at the time of the operation, prior to actual deformity correction. An argument can be made that more major deformities such as diastematomyelia or major intradural anomalies should be corrected well in advance of a surgical correction of the deformity itself (17,21,88,93,94) in order to prevent the possibly additive adverse effects of deformity surgery and intradural deformity. The group led by Transfeldt reported that 3 of 38 patients (8%) experienced worsened neurologic symptoms when scoliosis fusion surgery was done without previous syrinx decompression (94). Detethering well in advance allows one to distinguish neurologic deficits caused by the detethering from those caused by the surgical procedure itself. Disadvantages of detethering as a separate procedure include the need for a repeated surgery on the same area and resultant increased difficulty of the second procedure because of operative scarring.

## Choosing Surgical Options

Choosing among surgical options for progressive deformity is complex. In trying to determine guidelines for how to deal surgically with a progressive congenital spinal deformity, several factors may help define an appropriate treatment. It is helpful to assess how severe the deformity is. If the deformity itself is minor but progressive, a simple *in situ* fusion may suffice. If the deformity is severe and causes secondary distortion of the remainder of the spine, then deformity correction, with its increased risk, may be justified. Whether the deformity, and hence the corrective procedure, involves a long or short section of spine can influence the choice of treatment. Is there impingement by the deformity on the intraspinal contents? Has the deformity primarily or secondarily affected respiratory function (thoracic insufficiency syndrome), and will the proposed treatment create or worsen thoracic insufficiency? The decision to simply arrest rather than correct progressive deformity assumes that the existing deformity is acceptable. The acceptability of an existing deformity is relative. If correction is very dangerous, then a more severe deformity can be accepted. If correction is relatively safe, correction with the goal of improving the deformity may be justified. Therefore, knowledge of all techniques and an understanding of how much risk is involved are necessary. Another factor to consider is the effect of the operation on overall spinal growth (116). If a large segment of the spine is fused in a small child, the overall height of the child may be adversely affected (116) and thoracic insufficiency syndrome rendered more likely. The consequences of any fusion on the stability of adjacent segments must also be considered. Arthrodesis for progressive deformity will make more of the spine stiff, possibly creating or worsening functional stiffness and degeneration or instability of adjacent segments. This dichotomy between extending fusion and creating more junctional stress is frequently encountered in Klippel-Feil deformity and cervico-thoracic

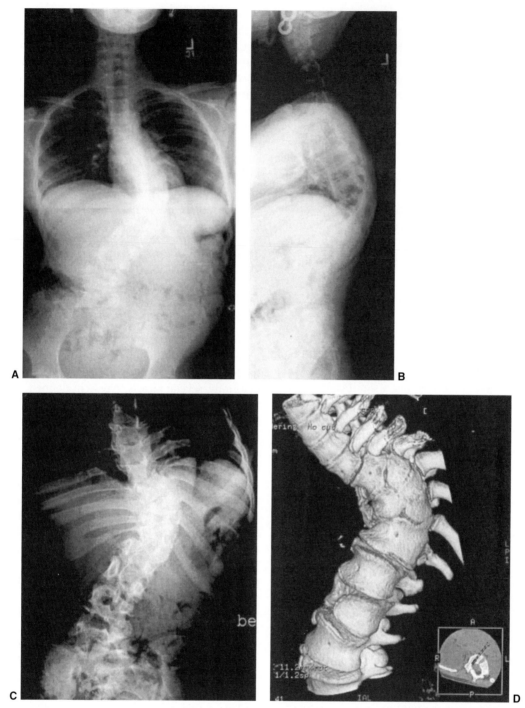

**Figure 19.15** A 12-year-old patient with progressive congenital scoliosis treated with anterior and posterior osteotomy and fusion. Drastic progression of the curve occurred because of a mistaken decision to place the patient under observation and delay surgery until "maturity." **A:** Preoperative posteroanterior upright view shows a rigid mid-thoracic congenital scoliosis. **B:** Preoperative lateral view shows substantial congenital kyphosis. Congenital kyphosis is thought to be strongly associated with postoperative neurologic deficit. **C:** Preoperative bending view shows rigid nature of curve. **D:** Three-dimensional computed tomography (CT) scan helps evaluate rigid thoracolumbar anatomy. **E:** Preoperative angiography of the spinal cord was performed because of the need for extensive anterior vertebrectomies. Angiography revealed major segmental feeding vessels at T8 and L3 (L3 vessel shown). Wedge resections and vertebrectomy were performed well away from L3 and T8 segmental vessels. Anterior and posterior procedures were staged. **F:** Postoperative posteroanterior radiograph with restoration of balance, and preservation of some low lumbar motion segments. **G:** Postoperative lateral radiograph with reduction in kyphosis. Resected wedges were larger posteriorly in order to improve kyphosis. The instrumentation exaggerated the shortening. An easier, less risky procedure could have been performed years earlier at the first presentation of progression.

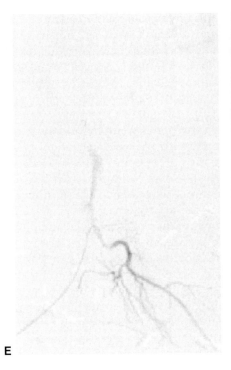

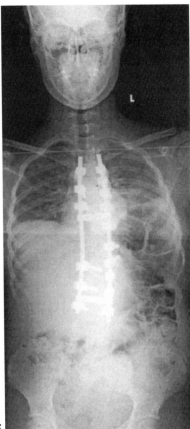

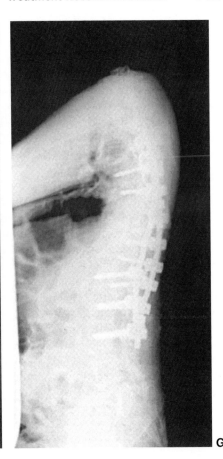

E

**Figure 19.15**   *(continued)*                                          F                                                         G

deformity. Extending the fusion to include more vertebrae may help arrest progressive deformity or instability, but it also concentrates stresses on a more localized section of spine. Finally, the dangers inherent in the operation must be examined. The risks of neurologic loss and intraoperative bleeding are increased by the need for a large degree of correction or lengthening of the spinal canal, the presence of spinal stenosis or neurologic deficits, older age of the patient, the need for circumferential procedures, and other factors (92).

## Hemiepiphyseodesis

Hemiepiphyseodesis for congenital scoliosis is an established technique and has been documented in groups led by Winter, Lonstein, Lindseth, Dubousset, and Thompson (117–119) who report a variable epiphyseodesis effect (120–122). Hemiepiphyseodesis can be done posteriorly, or both anteriorly and posteriorly. When kyphosis is present hemiepiphyseodesis should be done posteriorly, and when lordosis is present, anteriorly and posteriorly. Hemiepiphyseodesis can be done as an "eggshell" transpedicular procedure (119,123). The anterior portion of an anterior and posterior hemiepiphyseodesis can also be done thoracoscopically. Immobilization and passive

correction associated with the epiphyseodesis is a critical part of the procedure, and is best done with a cast. All surgeons document that a substantial portion of the correction is achieved at the time of the initial casting and correction (117–119,123,124). The optimal patient for hemiepiphyseodesis is 5 years or less in age, with a curve that is moderate (50 degrees or less). Compared with a localized wedge resection for hemivertebra, hemiepiphyseodesis involves more of the spine, and to some extent builds in an existing deformity. Further correction of the curves is slow after the initial cast correction, and some surgeons report the unpredictability of results following hemiepiphyseodesis (125). The major advantage of epiphyseodesis is that it is very safe and is unlikely to cause new neurologic problems. Posterior *in situ* fusion (in effect, posterior hemiepiphyseodesis) works well for early moderate kyphosis (Fig. 19.7).

### In Situ Fusion

*In situ* fusion remains the standard treatment for progressive deformity (17,103,107,126,127). *In situ* fusion can be performed anteriorly, posteriorly, or both as dictated by the direction of the deformity and extent of growth remaining. In a lordotic deformity an anterior fusion is mandatory. In a kyphotic deformity posterior fusion alone may help correct the kyphosis by acting as a tether while continued anterior growth produces some correction of the kyphosis. *In situ* fusion, as classically described, is performed without instrumentation; however, the availability of modern down-sized instrumentation makes their use feasible (128), probably diminishing the incidence of pseudarthrosis and length of time the patient must spend in a cast (129).

## Fusion with Correction

Spinal fusion with partial or complete correction of deformity is a commonly selected surgical option (Fig. 19.16). Correction of congenital vertebral deformity can be much more difficult than correction of idiopathic deformity. Any correction of a congenital vertebral anomaly carries with it some serious risk of neurologic injury (92,128). Where possible, early arrest of progressive deformity is the preferable option. The underlying congenital vertebral deformities are unyielding and, if correction is desired, much more than simple instrumentation may be required. Bending, traction, or supine view x-ray films (that remove the effect of gravity) may indicate the stiffness of the congenital vertebral anomaly. Correction beyond that suggested by bending

position radiographs can be achieved by several means. Releases through discs and facet joints, as with any severe idiopathic deformity, will permit more correction only if the congenital deformity is relatively normally segmented. Osteotomy of anterior vertebral bars or posterior vertebral fusions may be necessary over areas of block vertebrae or prior fusions (Figs. 19.15 and 19.17). A decision as to whether deformity correction is worth the additional risk must take into account the effects of correction on the remaining mobile parts of the spine. Other risks associated with osteotomy or releases include excessive bleeding and direct cord injury. Corpectomy, vertebrectomy, or vertebral column resection may be necessary for achieving any improvement of the most deformed sections of the spine (130,131). Traction alone after release or osteotomy remains an option for slow correction of deformity. Caution should be exercised in using traction after vertebrectomy, osteotomy, or extensive release, as the segmental instability of the spine created by the vertebrectomy or osteotomy may be severe enough to make traction dangerous. In the case of a preexisting neurologic deficit, traction (halo-gravity, halo-pelvic, or halo-femoral) (132–134) may be either helpful or disastrous, depending upon the spinal anatomy and cause of the paralysis.

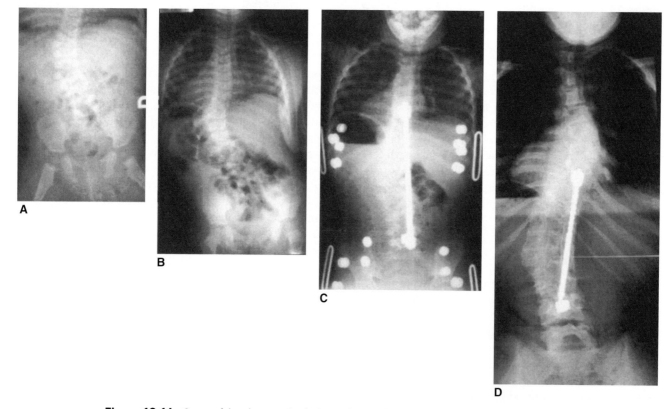

**Figure 19.16** Successful early posterior fusion at 21 months of age in a patient with a slowly progressing curve since infancy. **A:** Infancy. **B:** Twenty-one months of age, showing progression. Myelogram was negative for tethering lesions. **C:** Thirty months of age after fusion and Harrington rod. **D:** Twelve years of age. At maturity the patient is active, asymptomatic, and has normal pulmonary function. Early fusion for congenital scoliosis can be well tolerated. Excision of two hemivertebra might also have been successful.

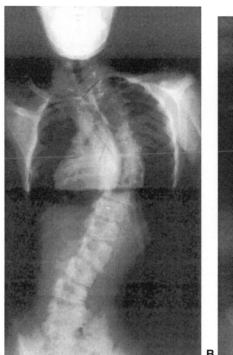 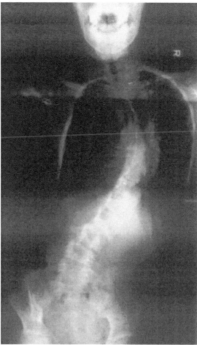 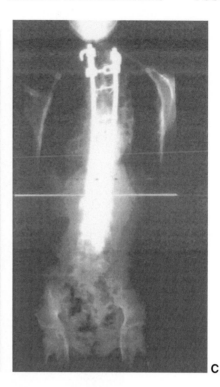

A                                    B                                    C

**Figure 19.17** This girl with progressive thoracic congenital scoliosis underwent thoracic *in situ*, posterior-only fusion at 3 years of age with cast immobilization. Steady continued progression and increasing thoracic lordosis occurred postoperatively. Anterior and posterior fusion might have prevented the progression. **A:** At 11 years of age, after 8 years of progression, she declined further surgery. **B:** At 14 years of age before anterior and posterior osteotomies, further trunk imbalance was caused by fixed thoracic deformity. **C:** After anterior and posterior osteotomies at 15 years of age, balance has been restored. If the initial procedure had included an anterior fusion and more correction, the later procedure and osteotomies might not have been needed.

Particular care should be exercised if the deformity involves kyphosis, because elongation of the spine with traction may draw the compromised spinal cord more tightly against the kyphotic deformity before the deformity itself improves (81).

## Hemivertebra Excision

Hemivertebra excision has been well documented (19,135–145). The ideal indication for hemivertebra excision is an isolated, fully segmented hemivertebra, at the thoracolumbar junction or below, that has produced a single deformity (Fig. 19.18). The rationale for early hemivertebra excision includes correction of the deformity and presumed prevention of subsequent secondary deformity in the remaining relatively normal spine. Excision of anterior and posterior hemivertebra elements or "wedge resection" can be performed through staged or simultaneous anterior and posterior approaches or through a posterior approach alone. The choice of approach should depend upon the experience of the surgeon and the location and direction of the deformity. Anterior hemivertebrectomy followed by a separate posterior hemivertebrectomy and posterior instrumentation is the standard practice. The anterior and posterior incisions can be performed at the same time

if desired, although this makes the posterior instrumentation more awkward to fit. Positioning of the patient in a manner to permit this procedure has been described (143).

The utility of simultaneous anterior and posterior approaches includes the ability to readjust the amount of resection either anteriorly or posteriorly in order to ensure satisfactory correction. It is also feasible to perform a single posterior or posterolateral approach for hemivertebra excision. A posterior-only approach is easier in kyphotic than in lordotic deformities. When performed on the thoracic spine, the posterior approach may be combined with costotransversectomy for added exposure. Difficulty in controlling vertebral body bleeding may be encountered in any hemivertebra excision but is probably greatest in a purely posterior approach.

Hemivertebrectomy performed from any approach should be planned so as to include enough of the convex hemivertebra and adjacent cartilage and disc and to extend far enough toward the concavity so that complete correction can be achieved. Excising the hemivertebra just to the midline where the bony hemivertebra may end will usually be insufficient for substantial curve correction. A wedge resection including the hemivertebra, hinged on the concave edge of the curve, is generally necessary. Without extensive correction of the deformity associated with the hemivertebra, the

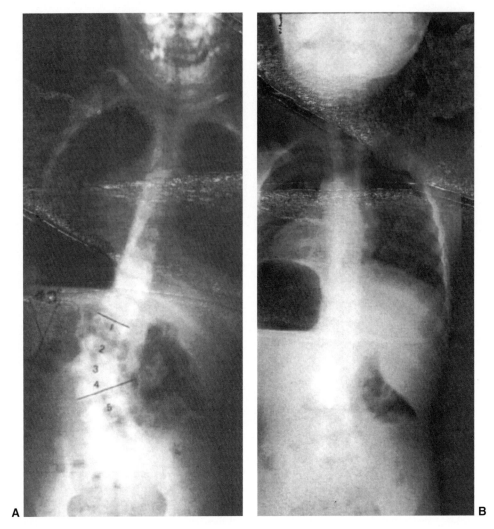

**A**  **B**

**Figure 19.18**  Hemivertebra excision or wedge resection can correct substantial localized deformity, while not affecting the growth of the remainder of the spine. **A:** A 3-year-old with an isolated lumbar hemivertebra and a slowly progressing deformity. MRI is negative for tethering lesions. **B:** After simultaneous anterior and posterior excision and wedge resection of the hemivertebra and fusion of adjacent vertebrae, the patient was placed in cast immobilization for 2 months. The global spinal deformity remains corrected, although the operation was confined to a localized region.

major advantage of early hemivertebra excision is not achieved. Contraindications to hemivertebrectomy probably include the inability to maintain the correction with a cast or instrumentation; the presence of rigid curves above or below the excision, which will cause spine imbalance; a major intraspinal anomaly in the area; and, probably, location of the hemivertebra in the cervical spine, where the vertebral artery complicates excision. Early hemivertebra excision is advocated because, if allowed to progress, a deformity associated with the hemivertebra may produce more structural deformity over a longer section of the spine, eventually requiring longer fusion and more growth arrest. By doing a hemivertebra excision early, one may restrict the growth arrest to a short section of spine. The timing of hemivertebra excision depends upon several factors. The longer the child remains in an upright position with a severe deformity from a hemivertebra, the more likely the secondary curves are to

become structural. On the other hand, hemivertebra excision in the very small child, younger than 1 year, is made more difficult by the need for very small instrumentation.

The neurocentral synchondrosis closes at 3 to 6 years of age (146,147), but it is probably safe to perform fusion or instrumentation before that age without fear of creating spinal stenosis, as the canal diameter at birth is already approximately two-thirds of the adult dimension (148). Kim et al. (129) found no instances of permanent neurologic deficit in wedge resections done before the age of 5 years; in general, the earlier the procedure was performed, the less likely neurologic injury was (92,129). Other series of hemivertebra excisions have also indicated that early excision makes neurologic injury less likely (141,144). Injury may come from direct contusion of cord or roots or may come from stretching of the concave roots as a new position is achieved. Some hemivertebrae are nonprogressive (Figs. 19.4 and 19.12) and do not produce a deformity. Indications for hemivertebra excision must therefore include either progressive deformity or an existing deformity that has a considerable effect on the overall configuration of the spine above and below. In the absence of specific contraindications, lumbosacral, lumbar, or thoracolumbar locations are optimal for hemivertebra excision, whereas deformity correction with hemivertebra excision in the mid- and upper thoracic spine is limited by the inflexible thorax, and probably entails greater neurologic risk because of the presence of thoracic spinal cord at the level of the operation. For an isolated hemivertebra in the midthoracic spine, *in situ* fusion or hemiepiphyseodesis may be a better choice than excision.

## Osteotomy of Prior Fusion Masses

When a block deformity or previous iatrogenic fusion exists and contributes to congenital spinal deformity, osteotomy may be required for achieving correction of deformity and balance (Figs. 19.15 and 19.17). Generally both anterior and posterior osteotomies and/or release will be needed, and can be staged or done sequentially. Vertebral column resection (131) may be done in a similar fashion. Anterior procedures can be osteotomies at each vertebral level in the area of deformity or can be restricted to a limited number of osteotomies if localized correction is planned. Posterior osteotomies also can be done at multiple levels or locally. Pedicle subtraction osteotomy has gained currency for treatment of adult spinal deformity (149) and has similar application in children's congenital deformities. Transpedicular eggshell procedures may be carried out (150) for previously fused pediatric congenital spine deformities. With any vertebral osteotomy, the risk of neurologic injury is considerable, and substantial bleeding can be anticipated. Osteotomy technique is well described in the literature, but each procedure should include careful localization and preoperative planning. Three-dimensional CT scans (Fig. 19.15D) will help rationalize the decisions regarding an osteotomy and help the surgeon localize the site of osteotomy. Inner edges of osteotomies should be tapered and undercut so that there is no impingement on the spinal canal at the time of closure. Correction after osteotomy should emphasize avoidance of spinal column elongation (Fig. 19.15F,G).

## Instrumentation, Casting

Immobilization is necessary after surgery for correction of a deformity. Traditional immobilization has included cast fixation either with or without instrumentation. Cast immobilization has obvious disadvantages but is entirely feasible in children. Maintenance of correction with cast immobilization alone requires attention to details relating to the cast. Many of the instrumentations used in small children are not strong enough to permit immediate mobilization, and therefore backup immobilization of instrumentation may be needed for several months after the operation. Instrumentations used in fusion with correction can be of various kinds. Preoperative evaluation of the congenital vertebral anomaly, usually by CT scan, should include an assessment of available anatomic anchor points for fixation (82,83). Pedicles may be very distorted or absent and laminae may be distorted, oblique, absent, bifid, or very thin. Canal diameters may be restricted. Individualization of fixation, balancing risk against stability, is needed. The increasing availability of downsized instrumentation, either intended specifically for smaller children or adapted from adult cervical applications, has made instrumentation of deformity in smaller children more feasible and permitted a reduction in the use of cast and brace immobilization postoperatively (128). However, the posterior and especially anterior osseous elements in small children are much less dense than the equivalent structures in adults and do not permit the application of corrective forces via anchor points as they would in adults. Where possible, correction and instrumentation of congenital scoliosis should not involve elongation of the spinal column, because the spinal cord in congenital deformity is likely to tolerate elongation poorly.

## Growing Rods (Instrumentation without Fusion) or Expansion Thoracostomy and Vertical Expandable Prosthetic Titanium Rib Procedure

Traditional approaches to severe early congenital spinal deformity have included early fusion. The rationale behind this approach has been to avoid the development of more severe deformities that would necessitate more extensive and dangerous procedures later in childhood or adulthood. The use of early fusion to prevent further progression of deformity assumes that the loss of growth associated with early fusion is well tolerated. In general, this is true, and the principle of early arrest of progressive deformity remains the mainstay of surgical treatment. Some patients, however, particularly those with an already shortened spine whose deformity would necessitate fusion of a long portion of spine at an early age, and especially those with associated chest wall anomalies, may be better treated by techniques that permit some continued growth of the abnormal spinal elements while still controlling the deformity. Expandable posterior rods and instrumentation without fusion have been employed in children with infantile and juvenile idiopathic deformities, but also in small series of those with congenital deformity (132,151,152) (Fig. 19.19). A major disadvantage of this treatment is the need for repetitive lengthening procedures, but it may be an appropriate temporary choice in the very young child with a deformity involving a large portion of the spine.

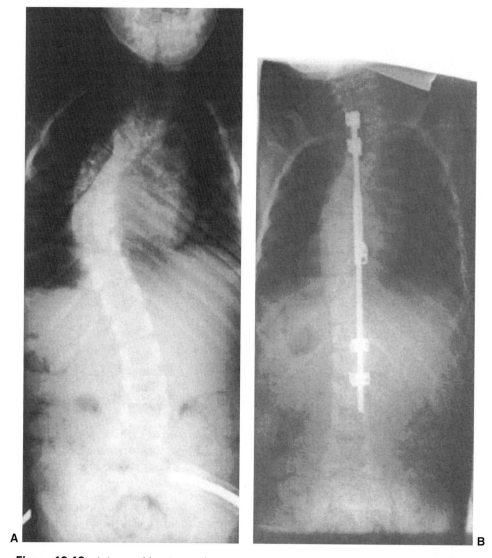

**Figure 19.19**    A 6-year-old patient with progressive congenital cervicothoracic scoliosis and non-congenital structural thoracic scoliosis. Both conditions are progressive. MRI is negative for tethering lesion. **A:** Preoperative posteroanterior view. **B:** Immediate postoperative posteroanterior view. Treatment consisted of *in situ* fusion of the cervicothoracic congenital scoliosis and instrumentation without fusion of the thoracic curve, and later included periodic rod lengthening. Fusion is planned later in growth. Dual extensible rods might be preferred now. [Currently, extensible rods are not approved by the U.S. Food and Drug Administration (FDA) for use without complete fusion.]

The group headed by Campbell has pioneered the use of expansion thoracostomy and a VEPTR (153) for the treatment of thoracic insufficiency syndrome (104) in growing children (Figs. 19.10 and 19.13). Combined spine and thoracic deformity caused by congenital vertebral deformities associated with multiple rib fusions is particularly amenable to the use of this technique during growth, and is the indication best documented by Campbell et al. (112). By performing one or more expansion thoracostomies through the constricted chest wall, either between ribs or through the rib fusion mass, expansion of the chest and secondary control of the spinal deformity without fusion is possible. The expandable devices attach rib to rib, rib to spine, or rib to pelvis and are periodically expanded to permit growth. Eventual fusion near the end of growth is anticipated, but by expanding and controlling the shape of the chest while permitting longitudinal growth of the spine, the chance of thoracic insufficiency syndrome is minimized. Growth of the spine and growth of concave bony bars has been demonstrated in association with this technique (100). It was Campbell who brought attention to thoracic insufficiency syndrome, pointing out that growth of the spine and chest are intricately intertwined. Primary chest wall deformity, such as massive areas of fused ribs, associated with congenital spinal deformity acts as a powerful deforming force on the spine. Treatment of the spine alone will often be defeated by the tethering effect of rib fusions or rib abnormalities. In young children, a primary chest wall deformity usually creates a secondary spine deformity, and conversely, severe progressive spinal deformity usually creates a chest deformity. While considering treatment of any early-onset spinal deformity, one should keep in mind the need to prevent irreversible chest wall deformity and thoracic insufficiency syndrome (104).

## AUTHOR'S RECOMMENDATIONS

I believe that a contemporary approach to the observation and surgical treatment of congenital scoliosis requires that orthopedists acknowledge the impossibility of accurately predicting progressive deformity in many instances of congenital scoliosis, while at the same time considering potential long-term problems, including the creation of thoracic insufficiency syndrome. Traditional attitudes toward congenital scoliosis are outlined in this chapter. Early fusion or early epiphyseodesis of progressive deformity is strongly advocated. Prophylactic fusion for deformities that can be accurately predicted to be progressive are similarly advocated. In my experience, however, those deformities that are predicted to be progressive do not necessarily prove to be so if observation is continued, and in some instances early prophylactic fusion or hemiepiphyseodesis are not successful in halting the progression of deformity (Fig. 19.10A) and may in fact contribute to long-term difficulties such as short stature, stiffness, and thoracic insufficiency. This attitude is probably colored by a referral practice, which includes many failures. Although it has been the author's practice to prophylactically fuse congenital kyphosis, a more contemporary attitude toward congenital scoliosis has been to conduct close observation and employ prophylactic procedures only for congenital kyphosis or for hemivertebrae, which cause considerable trunk imbalance. If multiple areas of the spine are involved in progressive deformity, or if the procedure necessary to halt the deformity would require a long segment of fusion in a small child, I have chosen procedures that offer some preservation of spine length, such as growing rods or expansion thoracostomy with titanium rib insertion, instead of fusion.

### Observations at Variance with General Practice

Several observations are at variance with general practice. In my experience, many congenital anomalies predicted to be progressive are not progressive or are not progressive until the preadolescent growth spurt. Although most congenital kyphosis is indeed progressive, and early posterior *in situ* fusion is usually the best choice, some instances of nonprogressive congenital kyphosis have been observed. Three-dimensional CT scan visualization of posterior elements may explain why some anomalies are not progressive; fully segmented hemivertebrae seen on plain x-ray film may include nonsegmented posterior elements on the convex side of the curve. Therefore the underlying posterior congenital anomaly acts as its own "tether" on the convex side, preventing progression. This phenomenon may also be the reason why occasionally congenital kyphosis does not progress, with a spontaneous fusion of posterior elements acting as a tether opposite the congenital kyphosis.

It is also my observation that the hemiepiphyseodesis effect, at least in my hands, is much less effective than is suggested by the literature, and that the hemiepiphyseodesis effect of further correction after cast correction is infrequent in spite of careful cast correction and immobilization. Hemiepiphyseodesis was developed as a technique in an era when instrumentation was not available for the congenital spine deformities in very young children and when intraspinal imaging of anomalies was less advanced. With the availability of small pediatric instrumentation (128), it now seems more effective to achieve correction over an area of deformity by instrumentation rather than by casting alone.

Transpedicular eggshell vertebrectomies and/or transpedicular hemiepiphyseodesis have, in my experience, been more difficult than anticipated and less satisfactory. In very small children, nearly complete obliteration of the pedicle is necessary in order to achieve enough access to the endplates to assure growth arrest. Destruction of the pedicles and further disruption of posterior elements in some instances seems counterproductive to the goal of achieving a solid fusion.

Congenital rib fusions are often ignored in the planning for surgical correction or the execution of epiphyseodesis or fusion. If major rib fusions exist in the concavity of a curvature, it has been the author's observation that the rib fusions will usually continue to deform the affected spine in spite of *in situ* fusion, instrumented fusion, or osteotomy. With the present availability of expansion thoracostomy, rib fusions should be taken into consideration in surgical planning.

Congenital scoliosis is a potential problem very early in growth, and severe instances of congenital scoliosis are rapidly progressive during infancy and early childhood. As a result, there is a focus on early progression of congenital scoliosis, and a false sense of security often results if the deformity has not progressed by mid-childhood. Families and caregivers alike are falsely assured that if the deformity is nonprogressive during early childhood, it will remain nonprogressive through the remainder of growth. Late, considerable progression during the preadolescent growth spurt is often unanticipated and can be devastating. Continued observational vigilance is needed all through growth.

### Preferred Procedures

In my experience, early posterior *in situ* fusion for congenital kyphosis or congenital scoliosis with a major kyphotic component has been highly successful (Fig. 19.7). Supplementation of posterior *in situ* fusion with instrumentation lessens the need for cast immobilization. The principle of early creation of a posterior tether opposite an anterior congenital kyphosis with anticipated continued anterior growth and later kyphosis correction is valid and effective. Because the incidence of perioperative paralysis associated with congenital kyphosis is high in late reconstructive procedures, particularly circumferential procedures, early *in situ* posterior fusion seems warranted and is easily accomplished.

Likewise, hemivertebra excision or global wedge resection for localized deformity has been highly successful. If the deformity involves a short section of spine, and particularly if this short deformed section causes a compensatory deformity above or below in a relatively normally structured region of spine, hemivertebra excision or wedge resection should be strongly considered. Usually fusion can be restricted to the segment just above and below the hemivertebra, not involving any normal spine above or below with fusion or instrumentation. Preoperative planning requires the demonstration by CT scan of posterior elements suitable for fixation and corresponding to what is seen in the anterior elements on plain x-ray film. Complete correction of the deformity is necessary in this procedure, and enough of the hemivertebra and associated disc must be excised to provide correction. The excision must traverse to the concave corner of the wedge in order to provide mobility for correction. Simply excising the bony hemivertebra results in undercorrection and defeats the goal of complete correction involving a short segment of spine. The use of growing rod constructs in congenital scoliosis is poorly documented.

It has been my experience that *in situ* fusion or *in situ* instrumented fusion of a short congenital segment of spine and growing rod construct treatment of the longer, normally segmented section of spine has worked well for large deformities involving normally segmented spinal curves adjacent to congenital curves (Fig. 19.19). Likewise, very long, relatively mobile sections of congenital spinal anomaly in young children seem to be amenable to growing rod treatment, provided the curve is relatively flexible and sufficient anchor points are present. If a chest wall anomaly is present or there is severe chest distortion in a young child, and thoracic insufficiency syndrome is a consideration, then expansion thoracostomy with VEPTR treatment is my preferred choice (Figs. 19.10 and 19.13). If there is no considerable thoracic deformity and if the problem is restricted to the spine, it is my preference to use a growing rod construct. However, if the chest deformity is advanced, then expansion thoracostomy, as described by Campbell et al., may be the preferable way to control spinal deformity while still permitting growth and improving chest volume and shape. The clearest indication for expansion thoracostomy and VEPTR, in my opinion, is the combination of congenital vertebral anomalies over a substantial section of spine and concave fused ribs. If a spine operation alone is performed, the fused ribs will continue to tether the spine, causing the deformity to worsen (Fig. 19.10A). Combined treatment of concave fused ribs and extensive vertebral anomalies by expansion thoracostomy and an expandable rib-to-spine and rib-to-rib prosthesis has been highly effective in the experience of Campbell et al. (112) and also in my practice. Presumably most patients treated with expansion thoracostomy will need a definitive spinal fusion at the end of growth.

The current popularity of growth-preserving procedures such as growing rods and expansion thoracostomy makes the choice between traditional fusion-based treatment and growth-sparing procedures more complex. Several factors can be considered in choosing a treatment: the age of the patient, and therefore the amount of growth remaining; the length of the spine involved; and the availability of a satisfactory, traditional, early fusion, hemiepiphyseodesis, or hemivertebra excision procedure for that area of spine. Essentially, if the deformity is easily treatable with a localized procedure such as hemivertebra excision or wedge excision involving a short section of the spine, then this sort of one-time, traditional, fusion-based procedure is preferable to repetitive surgeries associated with growing rod techniques or expansion thoracostomy. However, if the child is very young and a long section of the spine is involved, early fusion-based techniques will result in growth arrest over a longer, more significant section of spine. In such an instance, where a lot of growth remains, the choice of growing rods or expansion thoracostomy in the VEPTR procedure may be preferable even though it involves multiple procedures and multiple hospitalizations. Finally, if major rib fusions are present, the child is very young, and a long section of thoracic spine is involved in the curvature, then expansion thoracostomy with VEPTR procedure is preferable.

In making choices regarding surgical treatment of congenital scoliosis it is of paramount importance to have specific goals in mind. Treatment should maximize the length of the spine at the end of growth and should minimize thoracic deformity; it should leave as many segments of the spine mobile as is possible, and should place the patient at as little risk as possible. Hospitalizations and repetitive procedures should be kept to a minimum. For example, a procedure such as hemivertebra excision for an isolated thoracolumbar hemivertebra can be expected to diminish total spine height very little, and calls for a single, brief hospitalization. A more complex procedure such as expansion thoracostomy and VEPTR insertion will require multiple procedures and likely be associated with some surgical problems or complications, but will maximize the available spine length at the end of growth. Early *in situ* fusion for congenital kyphosis, although it may possibly result in less trunk height than an anterior release and strut grafting, is a less complex procedure, exposes the patient to a minimum risk of paralysis, and is therefore preferable.

# COMPLICATIONS

Complications occur frequently with congenital spinal deformity both with and without treatment. It may be difficult to separate the long-term complications of treatment from the natural history of the underlying congenital spinal deformity itself. Failure to recognize a progressive deformity or the potential significance of congenital spinal deformity and to act in a timely fashion may be as common a complication as those related to surgical treatment. Allowing extensive progression of congenital spine deformity (Figs. 19.14 and 19.15A) may necessitate more complex, complication-prone treatment. As an example, early *in situ* posterior fusion for moderate congenital kyphosis (103) is safe and reliably produces subsequent spontaneous correction with further growth, whereas permitting extensive deformity progression may necessitate later complex surgical procedures with a higher risk of neurologic complications. Recognized complications associated with treatment of congenital spine deformity include recurrent or progressive deformity, neurologic injury, further loss of spinal height, thoracic insufficiency syndrome, and deterioration of adjacent segments.

## Recurrent Deformity

In spite of surgical treatment (hemiepiphyseodesis, *in situ* fusion or fusion with correction), progressive deformity occurs with variable frequency as the patient grows (9,103,107,117–119,121,137,154). Deformity can recur within the fusion mass through bending, through the crankshaft phenomenon (155–158), or by "adding on" to the curvature above or below the prior surgical treatment. Recurrent deformity can be addressed by extension of fusion and instrumentation and osteotomy of prior fusions.

## Neurologic Injury

Neurologic loss is commonly associated with surgical treatment of congenital spine deformity, notably congenital kyphotic deformity (9,92,159–161). Early morbidity reports from the Scoliosis Research Society (160) and other reports (9,92) note the considerable risk of neurologic complications associated with surgery of congenital spine deformity, particularly congenital kyphosis. Neurologic problems are associated with progression of the deformity (159) as well as with surgical treatment. Although type I congenital kyphosis may be associated with paralysis if untreated, it is uncommon for untreated progressive congenital scoliosis to cause neurologic loss unless there is a very severe deformity, associated kyphotic deformity, lateral translocation or dislocation (162), a spinal cord anomaly, or spinal cord tethering.

Several possible etiologies of neurologic injury in congenital spinal deformity explain the relatively high incidence of neurologic injury associated with treatment. The final common pathway for most perioperative neurologic complications is probably vascular insufficiency of the spinal cord. The combination of an inherently anomalous or insufficient vascular supply to the spinal cord (Fig. 19.15E) coupled with corrective forces and change in position or shape of the spinal canal may result in neurologic compromise more commonly in surgeries for congenital deformities than in surgical correction of idiopathic deformities. Apel documented changes in somatosensory evoked potential (SSEP) monitoring with anterior segmental vessel ligation in congenital scoliosis (163). This has also been the author's experience in several instances. The vascular supply of the spinal cord associated with congenital scoliosis can be anomalous, and wherever possible surgical procedures should consider the possible effect of interruption of spinal cord blood supply during anterior surgical procedures. Distraction of the spinal cord in an animal model has been shown to be associated with diminished vascular flow, which precedes the appearance of neurologic dysfunction (164,165).

A similar mechanism probably occurs in neurologic injuries associated with correction of congenital spine deformity. Wherever possible, acute surgical correction should shorten the spinal column rather than distract the spinal cord. There may be value in staging corrections or producing the correction slowly in traction in order to allow monitoring of neurologic function when the patient is conscious (134). Neurologic injury may also occur from direct mechanical impingement on the spinal canal. Translation or angulation of the canal associated with spinal column correction may result in a new spinal stenosis or angular impingement on the spinal cord.

The risk of mechanical impingement can be lessened by preoperative imaging assessment of canal anatomy and dimension, and adequate control, observation, and decompression of the spinal canal during corrective maneuvers. Undercutting of lamina and procedures that shorten the area of deformity may make impingement less likely. Neurologic injuries associated with surgical treatment of congenital spinal deformity may occur without obvious cause (preoperative stenosis or spinal cord anomaly or tethering), and may be delayed (81).

The presence of a preexisting neurologic deficit should be cause for thorough preoperative evaluation, and probably signifies an increased risk of postoperative neurologic deficit. Early treatment is preferred where possible, while the deformity is less severe. Also, during early childhood the spinal cord appears more resistant to injury, and there is a lower incidence of neurologic injury (129). However, surgeons should realize that even with the most cautious approach, there is still a risk associated with manipulation of the congenitally anomalous vertebral column and spinal cord, and that the incidence of neurologic injury is still much higher than with idiopathic deformity. Standard treatment measures for neurologic loss following surgery for congenital scoliosis include maximizing spinal cord perfusion and oxygenation, considering diminishing correction or removing instrumentation, and evaluation for direct mechanical compression of the cord by appropriate imaging such as CT myelogram.

## Loss of Spinal Height, Thoracic Insufficiency Syndrome

Treatment of congenital scoliosis may lead to a worsening of deficiencies in existing trunk height. Generally the loss of trunk height is well tolerated (103,166,167) and is not considerable compared with the deformity that would have resulted if the condition had been allowed to progress. Goldberg et al. have brought attention to the shortened spine height associated with congenital spinal deformity and diminished trunk and spinal dimensions after spinal arthrodesis (72,107). Campbell et al. have described thoracic insufficiency following spinal arthrodesis for congenital scoliosis (104) associated with fused ribs. Patients with a preexisting short trunk, chest wall anomalies, or other causes of restrictive lung disease may not tolerate the further shortening associated with an extensive spinal arthrodesis. In this select group, procedures such as instrumentation without fusion or expansion thoracostomy with VEPTR insertion may be preferable to an early extensive arthrodesis, acknowledging that eventual arthrodesis will be needed at a later stage of growth. Diminished height of the spine, thoracic insufficiency syndrome, and the effects of early fusion (168) may not become apparent until the adolescent period, when the normal thoracic volume increases greatly.

## Adjacent Segment Degeneration

Degeneration of adjacent segments and difficulties with the transition zone between spinal fusion and the mobile unfused spine are acknowledged and documented phenomena associated with spinal fusions in all ages (169–171). A similar phenomenon of increased instability and degeneration of adjacent segments occurs adjacent to congenital fusions that extend into the cervical spine in the Klippel-Feil association (27,29,106,172). Adjacent segment degeneration or transition zone instability can be seen after fusion for congenital scoliosis; they may manifest as pain or neurologic deficit associated with spinal cord compression at the degenerated level caused by hypertrophy of the hypermobile disc, ligamentum flavum, or associated osteophytes. A consideration of the possible occurrence of adjacent segment degeneration should be factored into the choice of surgical options in congenital scoliosis.

## REFERENCES

### Indtroduction

1. Erol B, Tracy MR, Dormans JP, et al. Congenital scoliosis and vertebral malformations: characterization of segmental defects for genetic analysis. *J Pediatr Orthop* 2004;24(6):674–682.
2. Tracy MR, Dormans JP, Kusumi K. Klippel-Feil syndrome: clinical features and current understanding of etiology. *Clin Orthop Relat Res* 2004(424):183-190.
3. Basu PS, Elsebaie H, Noordeen MH. Congenital spinal deformity: a comprehensive assessment at presentation. *Spine* 2002;27(20):2255–2259.
4. Dyson RL, Pretorius DH, Budorick NE, et al. Three-dimensional ultrasound in the evaluation of fetal anomalies. *Ultrasound Obstet Gynecol* 2000;16(4):321–328.
5. Song TB, Kim YH, Oh ST, et al. Prenatal ultrasonographic diagnosis of congenital kyphosis due to anterior segmentation failure. *Asia Oceania J Obstet Gynaecol* 1994;20(1):31–33.
6. Barnewolt CE, Estroff JA. Sonography of the fetal central nervous system. *Neuroimaging Clin N Am* 2004;14(2):255–271.
7. Shahcheraghi GH, Hobbi MH. Patterns and progression in congenital scoliosis. *J Pediatr Orthop* 1999;19(6):766–775.
8. Winter RB, Moe JH, Lonstein JE. Posterior spinal arthrodesis for congenital scoliosis. An analysis of the cases of two hundred and ninety patients, five to nineteen years old. *J Bone Joint Surg Am* 1984;66(8):1188–1197.
9. McMaster MJ, Singh H. The surgical management of congenital kyphosis and kyphoscoliosis. *Spine* 2001;26(19):2146–2154.

### Definitions

10. Alexander PG, Tuan RS. Carbon monoxide-induced axial skeletal dysmorphogenesis in the chick embryo. *Birth Defects Res Part A Clin Mol Teratol* 2003;67(4):219–230.
11. Dias MS, Li V, Landi M, et al. The embryogenesis of congenital vertebral dislocation: early embryonic buckling? *Pediatr Neurosurg* 1998;29(6):281–289.
12. Edwards MJ. Hyperthermia as a teratogen: a review of experimental studies and their clinical significance. *Teratog Carcinog Mutagen* 1986;6(6):563–582.
13. Adra A, Cordero D, Mejides A, et al. Caudal regression syndrome: etiopathogenesis, prenatal diagnosis, and perinatal management. *Obstet Gynecol Surv* 1994;49(7):508–516.
14. Aberg A, Westbom L, Kallen B. Congenital malformations among infants whose mothers had gestational diabetes or preexisting diabetes. *Early Human Development* 2001;61(2):85–95.
15. Beals RK, Robbins JR, Rolfe B. Anomalies associated with vertebral malformations. *Spine* 1993;18(10):1329–1332.
16. Belmont PJ Jr, Kuklo TR, Taylor KF, et al. Intraspinal anomalies associated with isolated congenital hemivertebra: the role of routine magnetic resonance imaging. *J Bone Joint Surg Am* 2004;86-A(8):1704–1710.
17. Bernard TN Jr, Burke SW, Johnston CE, et al. Congenital spine deformities. A review of 47 cases. *Orthopedics (Thorofare, NJ)* 1985;8(6):777–783.
18. Eckford SD, Westgate J. Solitary crossed renal ectopia associated with unicornuate uterus, imperforate anus and congenital scoliosis. *J Urol* 1996;156(1):221.
19. McMaster MJ. Occult intraspinal anomalies and congenital scoliosis. *J Bone Joint Surg Am* 1984;66(4):588–601.
20. Milerad J, Larson O, Ph DD, et al. Associated malformations in infants with cleft lip and palate: a prospective, population-based study. *Pediatrics* 1997;100(2 Pt 1):180–186.
21. Prahinski JR, Polly DW Jr, McHale KA, et al. Occult intraspinal anomalies in congenital scoliosis. *J Pediatr Orthop* 2000;20(1):59–63.
22. Pravda J, Ghelman B, Levine DB. Syringomyelia associated with congenital scoliosis. A case report. *Spine* 1992;17(3):372–374.
23. Rai AS, Taylor TK, Smith GH, et al. Congenital abnormalities of the urogenital tract in association with congenital vertebral malformations. *J Bone Joint Surg Br* 2002;84(6):891–895.
24. Rivard DJ, Milner WA, Garlick WB. Solitary crossed renal ectopia and its associated congenital anomalies. *J Urol* 1978;120(2):241–242.
25. Anderson PJ, Hall C, Evans RD, et al. The cervical spine in Crouzon syndrome. *Spine* 1997;22(4):402–405.
26. Berker N, Acaroglu G, Soykan E. Goldenhar's syndrome (oculo-auriculo-vertebral dysplasia) with congenital facial nerve palsy. *Yonsei Med J* 2004;45(1):157–160.
27. Clarke RA, Catalan G, Diwan AD, et al. Heterogeneity in Klippel-Feil syndrome: a new classification. *Pediatr Radiol* 1998;28(12):967–974.
28. Cornier AS, Ramirez N, Carlo S, et al. Controversies surrounding Jarcho-Levin syndrome. *Curr Opin Pediatr* 2003;15(6):614–620.

29. Dubey SP, Ghosh LM. Klippel-Feil syndrome with congenital conductive deafness: report of a case and review of literature. *Int J Pediatr Otorhinolaryngol* 1993;25(1–3):201–208.
30. Schilgen M, Loeser H. Klippel-Feil anomaly combined with fetal alcohol syndrome. *Eur Spine J* 1994;3(5):289–290.
31. Thomsen MN, Schneider U, Weber M, et al. Scoliosis and congenital anomalies associated with Klippel-Feil syndrome types I-III. *Spine* 1997;22(4):396–401.
32. Tredwell SJ, Smith DF, Macleod PJ, et al. Cervical spine anomalies in fetal alcohol syndrome. *Spine* 1982;7(4):331–334.
33. Viljoen D. Congenital contractural arachnodactyly (Beals syndrome). *J Med Genet* 1994;31(8):640–643.
34. Winter RB, Moe JH, Lonstein JE. The incidence of Klippel-Feil syndrome in patients with congenital scoliosis and kyphosis. *Spine* 1984;9(4):363–366.
35. Whiteford ML, Coutts J, al-Roomi L, et al. Uniparental isodisomy for chromosome 16 in a growth-retarded infant with congenital heart disease. *Prenat Diagn* 1995;15(6):579–584.

## Epidemiology

36. Liu SL, Huang DS. Scoliosis in China. A general review. *Clin Orthop Rel Res* 1996(323):113–118.
37. Carvalho MH, Brizot ML, Lopes LM, et al. Detection of fetal structural abnormalities at the 11–14 week ultrasound scan. *Prenat Diagn* 2002;22(1):1–4.
38. Sales de Gauzy J, Accadbled F, Sarramon MF, et al. Prenatal sonographic diagnosis of the congenital dislocated spine: a case report. *Spine* 2003;28(2):E41–E44.
39. Weisz B, Achiron R, Schindler A, et al. Prenatal sonographic diagnosis of hemivertebra. *J Ultrasound Med* 2004;23(6):853–857.
40. Hubbard AM. Ultrafast fetal MRI and prenatal diagnosis. *Semin Pediatr Surg* 2003;12(3):143–153.
41. Temple IK, Thomas TG, Baraitser M. Congenital spinal deformity in a three generation family. *J Med Genet* 1988;25(12):831–834.
42. Connor JM, Conner AN, Connor RA, et al. Genetic aspects of early childhood scoliosis. *Am J Med Genet* 1987;27(2):419–424.
43. Wynne-Davies R. Congenital vertebral anomalies: aetiology and relationship to spina bifida cystica. *J Med Genet* 1975;12(3):280–288.
44. Lowry RB, Jabs EW, Graham GE, et al. Syndrome of coronal craniosynostosis, Klippel-Feil anomaly, and Sprengel shoulder with and without Pro250Arg mutation in the FGFR3 gene. *Am J Med Genet* 2001;104(2):112–119..
45. Purkiss SB, Driscoll B, Cole WG, et al. Idiopathic scoliosis in families of children with congenital scoliosis. *Clin Orthop Rel Res* 2002(401):27–31.
46. Dean JC, Hailey H, Moore SJ, et al. Long term health and neurodevelopment in children exposed to antiepileptic drugs before birth. *J Med Genet* 2002;39(4):251–259.
47. Turnpenny PD, Whittock N, Duncan J, et al. Novel mutations in DLL3, a somitogenesis gene encoding a ligand for the Notch signalling pathway, cause a consistent pattern of abnormal vertebral segmentation in spondylocostal dysostosis. *J Med Genet* 2003;40(5):333–339.
48. Whittock NV, Ellard S, Duncan J, et al. Pseudodominant inheritance of spondylocostal dysostosis type 1 caused by two familial delta-like 3 mutations. *Clin Genet* 2004;66(1):67–72.
49. Whittock NV, Sparrow DB, Wouters MA, et al. Mutated MESP2 causes spondylocostal dysostosis in humans. *Am J Hum Genet* 2004;74(6):1249–1254.
50. Cornier AS, Ramirez N, Arroyo S, et al. Phenotype characterization and natural history of spondylothoracic dysplasia syndrome: a series of 27 new cases. *Am J Med Genet* 2004;128A(2):120–126.
51. Chen CP, Lee CC, Pan CW, et al. Partial trisomy 8q and partial monosomy 15q associated with congenital hydrocephalus, diaphragmatic hernia, urinary tract anomalies, congenital heart defect and kyphoscoliosis. *Prenat Diagn* 1998;18(12):1289–1293.
52. Denton JR. The association of congenital spinal anomalies with imperforate anus. *Clin Orthop Rel Res* 1982(162):91–98.
53. Geormaneanu M, Iagaru N, Popescu-Miclosanu S, et al. Congenital hemihypertrophy. Tendency to association with other abnormalities and/or tumors. *Morphol Embryol (Bucur)* 1983;29(1):39–45.
54. Healey D, Letts M, Jarvis JG. Cervical spine instability in children with Goldenhar's syndrome. *Can J Surg* 2002;45(5):341–344.

55. Hughes LO, McCarthy RE, Glasier CM. Segmental spinal dysgenesis: a report of three cases. *Journal J Pediatr Orthop* 1998;18(2):227–232.
56. Kishore K, Kumar H. Congenital ocular fibrosis with musculoskeletal abnormality: a new association. *J Pediatr Ophthalmol Strabismus* 1991;28(5):283–286.
57. Reckles LN, Peterson HA Jr, Weidman WH, et al. The association of scoliosis and congenital heart defects. *J Bone Joint Surg Am* 1975;57(4):449–455.
58. Schey WL. Vertebral malformations and associated somaticovisceral abnormalities. *Clin Radiol* 1976;27(3):341–353.
59. Tori JA, Dickson JH. Association of congenital anomalies of the spine and kidneys. *Clin Orthop Rel Res* 1980(148):259–262.
60. Wynne-Davies R, Littlejohn A, Gormley J. Aetiology and interrelationship of some common skeletal deformities. (Talipes equinovarus and calcaneovalgus, metatarsus varus, congenital dislocation of the hip, and infantile idiopathic scoliosis.) *J Med Genet* 1982;19(5):321–328.

## Etiology

61. Shawen SB, Belmont PJ Jr, Kuklo TR, et al. Hemimetameric segmental shift: a case series and review. *Spine* 2002;27(24):E539–E544.
62. Wide K, Winbladh B, Kallen B. Major malformations in infants exposed to antiepileptic drugs in utero, with emphasis on carbamazepine and valproic acid: a nation-wide, population-based register study. *Acta Paediatr* 2004;93(2):174–176.
63. Lowy C, Beard RW, Goldschmidt J. Congenital malformations in babies of diabetic mothers. *Diabet Med* 1986;3(5):458–462.
64. Loder RT, Hernandez MJ, Lerner AL, et al. The induction of congenital spinal deformities in mice by maternal carbon monoxide exposure. *J Pediatr Orthop* 2000;20(5):662–666.
65. Farley FA, Loder RT, Nolan BT, et al. Mouse model for thoracic congenital scoliosis. *J Pediatr Orthop* 2001;21(4):537–540.
66. Giavini E, Menegola E. Gene-teratogen interactions in chemically induced congenital malformations. *Biol Neonate* 2004;85(2):73–81.
67. Smith DF, Sandor GG, MacLeod PM, et al. Intrinsic defects in the fetal alcohol syndrome: studies on 76 cases from British Columbia and the Yukon Territory. *Neurobehav Toxicol Teratol* 1981;3(2):145–152.
68. Edwards MJ, Saunders RD, Shiota K. Effects of heat on embryos and foetuses. *Int J Hyperthermia* 2003;19(3):295–324.

## Clinical Features

69. Winter RB, House JH. Congenital cervical scoliosis with unilateral congenital nerve deficit in the upper extremity. Report of two cases. *Spine* 1981;6(4):341–346.
70. Flynn JM, Otsuka NY, Emans JB, et al. Segmental spinal dysgenesis: early neurologic deterioration and treatment. *J Pediatr Orthop* 1997;17(1):100–104.
71. Faciszewski T, Winter RB, Lonstein JE, et al. Segmental spinal dysgenesis. A disorder different from spinal agenesis. *J Bone Joint Surg Am* 1995;77(4):530–537.
72. Goldberg CJ, Moore DP, Fogarty EE, et al. Growth patterns in patients with unoperated congenital vertebral anomaly. *Stud Health Technol Inform* 2002;91:101–103.
73. Lopez-Sosa F, Guille JT, Bowen JR. Rotation of the spine in congenital scoliosis. *J Pediatr Orthop* 1995;15(4):528–534.

## Radiographic Features

74. Birnbaum K, Weber M, Lorani A, et al. Prognostic significance of the Nasca classification for the long-term course of congenital scoliosis. *Arch Orthop Trauma Surg* 2002;122(7):383–389.
75. Nasca RJ, Stilling FH III, Stell HH. Progression of congenital scoliosis due to hemivertebrae and hemivertebrae with bars. *J Bone Joint Surg Am* 1975;57(4):456–466.
76. Tanaka T. A study of the progression of congenital scoliosis in non-operated cases. *Nippon Seikeigeka Gakkai Zasshi—J Jpn Orthop Assoc* 1988;62(1):9–22.
77. Winter RB. Congenital scoliosis. *Orthop Clin North Am* 1988;19(2):395–408.
78. McMaster MJ, Ohtsuka K. The natural history of congenital scoliosis. A study of two hundred and fifty-one patients. *J Bone Joint Surg Am* 1982;64(8):1128–1147.

79. McMaster MJ, Singh H. Natural history of congenital kyphosis and kyphoscoliosis. A study of one hundred and twelve patients. *J Bone Joint Surg Am* 1999;81(10):1367–1383.

80. Winter RB. Congenital kyphosis. *Clin Orthop Rel Res* 1977(128): 26–32.

81. Winter RB, Moe JH, Lonstein JE. The surgical treatment of congenital kyphosis. A review of 94 patients age 5 years or older, with 2 years or more follow-up in 77 patients. *Spine* 1985;10(3):224–231.

82. Hedequist DJ, Emans JB. The correlation of preoperative three-dimensional computed tomography reconstructions with operative findings in congenital scoliosis. *Spine* 2003;28(22): 2531–2534.

83. Newton PO, Hahn GW, Fricka KB, et al. Utility of three-dimensional and multiplanar reformatted computed tomography for evaluation of pediatric congenital spine abnormalities. *Spine* 2002;27(8):844–850.

84. Cil A, Yazici M, Alanay A, et al. The course of sagittal plane abnormality in the patients with congenital scoliosis managed with convex growth arrest. *Spine* 2004;29(5):547–552.

85. McMaster MJ. Congenital scoliosis caused by a unilateral failure of vertebral segmentation with contralateral hemivertebrae. *Spine* 1998;23(9):998–1005.

86. Facanha-Filho FA, Winter RB, Lonstein JE, et al. Measurement accuracy in congenital scoliosis. *J Bone Joint Surg Am* 2001;83-A(1):42–45.

87. Loder RT, Urquhart A, Steen H, et al. Variability in Cobb angle measurements in children with congenital scoliosis. *J Bone Joint Surg Br* 1995;77(5):768–770.

88. Bradford DS, Heithoff KB, Cohen M. Intraspinal abnormalities and congenital spine deformities: a radiographic and MRI study. *J Pediatr Orthop* 1991;11(1):36–41.

89. Fribourg D, Delgado E. Occult spinal cord abnormalities in children referred for orthopedic complaints. *Am J Orthop* 2004;33(1):18–25.

90. Suh SW, Sarwark JF, Vora A, et al. Evaluating congenital spine deformities for intraspinal anomalies with magnetic resonance imaging. *J Pediatr Orthop* 2001;21(4):525–531.

## Other Imaging Studies

91. Unsinn KM, Geley T, Freund MC, et al. US of the spinal cord in newborns: spectrum of normal findings, variants, congenital anomalies, and acquired diseases. *Radiographics* 2000;20(4): 923–938.

92. Carlioz H, Ouaknine M. Neurologic complications of surgery of the spine in children. *Chirurgie* 1994;120(11):26–30.

93. Acaroglu E, Alanay A, Akalan N, et al. Risk factors associated with corrective surgery in congenital scoliosis with tethered cord. *Turk J Pediatr* 1997;39(3):373–378.

94. Ozerdemoglu RA, Transfeldt EE, Denis F. Value of treating primary causes of syrinx in scoliosis associated with syringomyelia. *Spine* 2003;28(8):806–814.

95. Sato T, Kokubun S, Tanaka Y, et al. Paraparesis associated with mild congenital kyphoscoliosis in an adult. *Tohoku J Exp Med* 1997;183(4):303–308.

96. Scott JE. Bladder function in congenital non-cystic spinal abnormalities. *Chir Pediatr* 1982;23(5):348–352.

## Other Diagnostic Studies When Indicated

97. Mayer B, Lenarz T, Haels J. Cervically-induced symptoms of the Klippel-Feil syndrome. *Laryngol Rhinol Otol (Stuttg)* 1984;63(7): 364–370.

98. Farley FA, Phillips WA, Herzenberg JE, et al. Natural history of scoliosis in congenital heart disease. *J Pediatr Orthop* 1991;11(1):42–47.

99. Coran DL, Rodgers WB, Keane JF, et al. Spinal fusion in patients with congenital heart disease. Predictors of outcome. *Clin Orthop Rel Res* 1999(364):99–107.

## Pathoanatomy

100. Campbell RM Jr, Hell-Vocke AK. Growth of the thoracic spine in congenital scoliosis after expansion thoracoplasty. *J Bone Joint Surg Am* 2003;85-A(3):409–420.

## Natural History

101. Ford EG, Jaufmann BA, Kaste SC, et al. Successful staged surgical correction of congenital segmental spinal dysgenesis and complete rotary subluxation of the thoracolumbar spine in an infant. *J Pediatr Surg* 1996;31(7):960–964.

102. Winter RB, Moe JH, Wang JF. Congenital kyphosis. Its natural history and treatment as observed in a study of one hundred and thirty patients. *J Bone Joint Surg Am* 1973;55(2):223–256.

103. Winter RB, Moe JH. The results of spinal arthrodesis for congenital spinal deformity in patients younger than five years old. *J Bone Joint Surg Am* 1982;64(3):419–432.

104. Campbell RM, Jr., Smith MD, Mayes TC, et al. The characteristics of thoracic insufficiency syndrome associated with fused ribs and congenital scoliosis. *J Bone Joint Surg Am* 2003;85-A(3):399–408.

105. Damsin JP, Cazeau C, Carlioz H. Scoliosis and fused ribs. A case report. *Spine* 1997;22(9):1030–1032.

106. Theiss SM, Smith MD, Winter RB. The long-term follow-up of patients with Klippel-Feil syndrome and congenital scoliosis. *Spine* 1997;22(11):1219–1222.

107. Goldberg CJ, Moore DP, Fogarty EE, et al. Long-term results from in situ fusion for congenital vertebral deformity. *Spine* 2002;27(6):619–628.

108. Day GA, Upadhyay SS, Ho EK, et al. Pulmonary functions in congenital scoliosis. *Spine* 1994;19(9):1027–1031.

109. Appierto L, Cori M, Bianchi R, et al. Home care for chronic respiratory failure in children: 15 years experience. *Paediatr Anaesth* 2002;12(4):345–350.

110. Noble JS, Davidson JA. Cor pulmonale presenting in a patient with congenital kyphoscoliosis following intercontinental air travel. *Anaesthesia* 1999;54(4):361–363.

111. Pehrsson K, Larsson S, Oden A, et al. Long-term follow-up of patients with untreated scoliosis. A study of mortality, causes of death, and symptoms. *Spine* 1992;17(9):1091–1096.

112. Campbell RM, Jr., Smith MD, Mayes TC, et al. The effect of opening wedge thoracostomy on thoracic insufficiency syndrome associated with fused ribs and congenital scoliosis. *J Bone Joint Surg Am* 2004;86-A(8):1659–1674.

## Treatment Recommendations

113. Morin Doody M, Lonstein JE, Stovall M, et al. Breast cancer mortality after diagnostic radiography: findings from the U.S. Scoliosis Cohort Study. *Spine* 2000;25(16):2052–2063.

114. James JI. The management of infants with scoliosis. *J Bone Joint Surg Br* 1975;57(4):422–429.

115. Winter RBMJ, MacEwen GD, Peon Vidales H. The Milwaukee brace in the nonoperative treatment of congenital scoliosis. *Spine* 1976;1(1):85–96.

116. Dimeglio A. Growth of the spine before age 5 years. *J Pediatr Orthop B* 1993;1(2):102–107.

117. Winter RB. Convex anterior and posterior hemiarthrodesis and hemiepiphyseodesis in young children with progressive congenital scoliosis. *J Pediatr Orthop* 1981;1(4):361–366.

118. Winter RB, Lonstein JE, Denis F, et al. Convex growth arrest for progressive congenital scoliosis due to hemivertebrae. *J Pediatr Orthop* 1988;8(6):633–638.

119. Keller PM, Lindseth RE, DeRosa GP. Progressive congenital scoliosis treatment using a transpedicular anterior and posterior convex hemiepiphyseodesis and hemiarthrodesis. A preliminary report. *Spine* 1994;19(17):1933–1939.

120. Thompson AG, Marks DS, Sayampanathan SR, et al. Long-term results of combined anterior and posterior convex epiphysiodesis for congenital scoliosis due to hemivertebrae. *Spine* 1995;20(12):1380–1385.

121. Kieffer J, Dubousset J. Combined anterior and posterior convex epiphysiodesis for progressive congenital scoliosis in children aged < or = 5 years. *Eur Spine J* 1994;3(2):120–125.

122. Dubousset J, Katti E, Seringe R. Epiphysiodesis of the spine in young children for congenital spinal deformations. *J Pediatr Orthop B* 1993;1(292):123–130.

123. King AG, MacEwen GD, Bose WJ. Transpedicular convex anterior hemiepiphysiodesis and posterior arthrodesis for progressive congenital scoliosis. *Spine* 1992;17(Suppl 8):S291–S294.

124. Uzumcugil AA, Cil AA, Yazici MM, et al. The efficacy of convex hemiepiphysiodesis in patients with iatrogenic posterior element deficiency resulting from diastematomyelia excision. *Spine* 2003;28(8):799–805.

125. Marks DS, Sayampanathan SR, Thompson AG, et al. Long-term results of convex epiphysiodesis for congenital scoliosis. *Eur Spine J* 1995;4(5):296–301.

126. Arlet V, Odent T, Aebi M. Congenital scoliosis. *Eur Spine J* 2003; 12(5):456–463.

127. Benli IT, Duman E, Akalin S, et al. [An evaluation of the types and the results of surgical treatment for congenital scoliosis]. *Acta Orthop Traumatol Turc* 2003;37(4):284–298.

128. Hedequist DJ, Hall JE, Emans JB, et al. The safety and efficacy of spinal instrumentation in children with congenital spine deformities. *Spine* 2004;29(18):2081–2086.

129. Kim YJ, Otsuka NY, Flynn JM, et al. Surgical treatment of congenital kyphosis. *Spine* 2001;26(20):2251–2257.

130. Leatherman KD, Dickson RA. Two-stage corrective surgery for congenital deformities of the spine. *J Bone Joint Surg Br* 1979;61-B(3):324–328.

131. Boachie-Adjei O, Bradford DS. Vertebral column resection and arthrodesis for complex spinal deformities. *J Spinal Disord* 1991; 4(2):193–202.

132. Arlet V, Papin P, Marchesi D. Halo femoral traction and sliding rods in the treatment of a neurologically compromised congenital scoliosis: technique. *Eur Spine J* 1999;8(4): 329–331.

133. Kopits SE, Steingass MH. Experience with the "halo-cast" in small children. *Surg Clin North Am* 1970;50(4):935–943.

134. Sink EL, Karol LA, Sanders J, et al. Efficacy of perioperative halo-gravity traction in the treatment of severe scoliosis in children. *J Pediatr Orthop* 2001;21(4):519–524.

135. Bergoin M, Bollini G, Taibi L, et al. Excision of hemivertebrae in children with congenital scoliosis. *Ital J Orthop Traumatol* 1986; 12(2):179–184.

136. Callahan BC, Georgopoulos G, Eilert RE. Hemivertebral excision for congenital scoliosis. *J Pediatr Orthop* 1997;17(1):96–99.

137. Holte DC, Winter RB, Lonstein JE, et al. Excision of hemivertebrae and wedge resection in the treatment of congenital scoliosis. *J Bone Joint Surg Am* 1995;77(2):159–171.

138. King JD, Lowery GL. Results of lumbar hemivertebral excision for congenital scoliosis. *Spine* 1991;16(7):778–782.

139. Mehlman CT, Wall EJ. Re: Klemme WR et al. Hemivertebral excision for congenital scoliosis in very young children. *J Pediatr Orthop* 2001;21:761–764.

140. Freeman BJ, Oullet JA, Webb JK. Excision of hemivertebrae in the management of congenital scoliosis. *J Bone Joint Surg Br* 2002;84(2):305.

141. Klemme WR, Polly DW Jr, Orchowski JR. Hemivertebral excision for congenital scoliosis in very young children. *J Pediatr Orthop* 2001;21(6):761–764.

142. Nakamura HH, Matsuda HH, Konishi SS, et al. Single-stage excision of hemivertebrae via the posterior approach alone for congenital spine deformity: follow-up period longer than ten years. *Spine* 2002;27(1):110–115.

143. Hedequist DJ, Hall JE, Emans JB, et al. Hemivertebra excision in children via simultaneous anterior and posterior exposures. *J Pediatr Orthop* 2005;25(1):60–63.

144. Ruf M, Harms J. Hemivertebra resection by a posterior approach: innovative operative technique and first results. *Spine* 2002; 27(10):1116–1123.

145. Ruf M, Harms J. Posterior hemivertebra resection with transpedicular instrumentation: early correction in children aged 1 to 6 years. *Spine* 2003;28(18):2132–2138.

146. Maat GJ, Matricali B, van Persijn van Meerten EL. Postnatal development and structure of the neurocentral junction. Its relevance for spinal surgery. *Spine* 1996;21(6):661–666.

147. Wang JC, Nuccion SL, Feighan JE, et al. Growth and development of the pediatric cervical spine documented radiographically. *J Bone Joint Surg Am* 2001;83-A(8):1212–1218.

148. Jeffrey JE, Campbell DM, Golden MH, et al. Antenatal factors in the development of the lumbar vertebral canal: a magnetic resonance imaging study. *Spine* 2003;28(13):1418–1423.

149. Bridwell KH, Lewis SJ, Rinella A, et al. Pedicle subtraction osteotomy for the treatment of fixed sagittal imbalance. Surgical technique. *J Bone Joint Surg Am* 2004;86-A (Suppl 1): 44–50.

150. Mikles MR, Graziano GP, Hensinger AR, et al. Transpedicular eggshell osteotomies for congenital scoliosis using frameless stereotactic guidance. *Spine* 2001;26:2289–2296.

151. Grass PJ, Soto AV, Araya HP. Intermittent distracting rod for correction of high neurologic risk congenital scoliosis. *Spine* 1997; 22(16):1922–1927.

152. Schmitz A, Schulze Bertelsbeck D, Schmitt O. Five-year follow-up of intermittent distracting rod correction in congenital scoliosis. *Eur J Pediatr Surg* 2002;12(6):416–418.

153. Campbell RM Jr, Smith MD, Hell-Vocke AK. Expansion thoracoplasty: the surgical technique of opening-wedge thoracostomy. Surgical technique. *J Bone Joint Surg Am* 2004;86-A (Suppl 1):51–64.

## Complications

154. Hall JE, Herndon WA, Levine CR. Surgical treatment of congenital scoliosis with or without Harrington instrumentation. *J Bone Joint Surg Am* 1981;63(4):608–619.

155. Dubousset J, Herring JA, Shufflebarger H. The crankshaft phenomenon. *J Pediatr Orthop* 1989;9(5):541–550.

156. Terek RM, Wehner J, Lubicky JP. Crankshaft phenomenon in congenital scoliosis: a preliminary report. *J Pediatr Orthop* 1991; 11(4):527–532.

157. Hamill CL, Bridwell KH, Lenke LG, et al. Posterior arthrodesis in the skeletally immature patient. Assessing the risk for crankshaft: is an open triradiate cartilage the answer? *Spine* 1997; 22(12):1343–1351.

158. Kesling KL, Lonstein JE, Denis F, et al. The crankshaft phenomenon after posterior spinal arthrodesis for congenital scoliosis: a review of 54 patients. *Spine* 2003;28(3):267–271.

159. Lonstein JE, Winter RB, Moe JH, et al. Neurologic deficits secondary to spinal deformity. A review of the literature and report of 43 cases. *Spine* 1980;5(4):331–355.

160. MacEwen GD, Bunnell WP, Sriram K, et al. Acute neurological complications in the treatment of scoliosis. A report of the Scoliosis Research Society. *J Bone Joint Surg Am* 1975;57(3):404–408.

161. Winter RB. Congenital kyphoscoliosis with paralysis following hemivertebra excision. *Clin Orthop Rel Res* 1976(119):116–125.

162. Zeller RD, Dubousset J. Progressive rotational dislocation in kyphoscoliotic deformities: presentation and treatment. *Spine* 2000;25(9):1092–1097.

163. Apel DM, Marrero G, King J, et al. Avoiding paraplegia during anterior spinal surgery. The role of somatosensory evoked potential monitoring with temporary occlusion of segmental spinal arteries. *Spine* 1991;16(Suppl 8):S365–S370.

164. Kai Y, Owen JH, Lenke LG, et al. Use of sciatic neurogenic motor evoked potentials versus spinal potentials to predict early-onset neurologic deficits when intervention is still possible during overdistraction. *Spine* 1993;18(9):1134–1139.

165. Naito M, Owen JH, Bridwell KH, et al. Effects of distraction on physiologic integrity of the spinal cord, spinal cord blood flow, and clinical status. *Spine* 1992;17(10): 1154–1158.

166. Winter RB, Smith MD, Lonstein JE, et al. Congenital scoliosis due to unilateral unsegmented bar: posterior spine fusion at age 12 months with 44-year follow-up. *Spine* 2004;29(3): E52–E55.

167. Winter RB, Lonstein JE. Congenital scoliosis with posterior spinal arthrodesis T2–L3 at age 3 years with 41-year follow-up. A case report. *Spine* 1999;24(2):194–197.

168. Emans J, Kassab F, Caubet JF, et al. Earlier and more extensive thoracic fusion is associated with diminished pulmonary function. Outcome after spinal fusion of 4 or more thoracic spinal segments before age 5. *Paper presentation 101, Scoliosis Research Society Annual Meeting*, Buenos Aires, Argentina, Sept. 6–9, 2004.

169. Seitsalo S, Schlenzka D, Poussa M, et al. Disc degeneration in young patients with isthmic spondylolisthesis treated operatively or conservatively: a long-term follow-up. *Eur Spine J* 1997;6(6):393–397.

170. Hilibrand AS, Robbins M. Adjacent segment degeneration and adjacent segment disease: the consequences of spinal fusion? *Spine J: Official journal of the North American Spine Society* 2004; 4(Suppl 6):190S–194S.

171. Park P, Garton HJ, Gala VC, et al. Adjacent segment disease after lumbar or lumbosacral fusion: review of the literature. *Spine* 2004;29(17):1938–1944.

172. Ulmer JL, Elster AD, Ginsberg LE, et al. Klippel-Feil syndrome: CT and MR of acquired and congenital abnormalities of cervical spine and cord. *J Comput Assist Tomogr* 1993;17(2): 215–224.

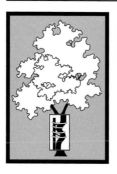

# 20

# Kyphosis

*William C. Warner, Jr.*

Kyphosis is a curvature of the spine in the sagittal plane in which the convexity of the curve is directed posteriorly. Lordosis is a curvature of the spine in the sagittal plane in which the convexity of the curve is directed anteriorly. The thoracic spine and the sacrum are normally kyphotic, and the cervical spine and the lumbar spine normally are lordotic (1). Although several authors have tried to define normal kyphosis of the thoracic spine and normal lordosis of the lumbar spine, these studies have shown much variability in what is considered normal (2–8). The ranges of normal kyphosis and lordosis change with increasing age, and vary according to gender and the area of the spine involved (2–5). The degree of kyphosis or lordosis that is considered normal or abnormal depends on the location of the curvature and the age of the patient. For example, 30 degrees of kyphosis is normal in the thoracic spine, but abnormal at the thoracolumbar junction.

The normal range of thoracic kyphosis was considered to be 20 to 40 degrees, and that of lumbar lordosis, 30 to 60 degrees (9). The Terminology Committee of the Scoliosis Research Society has expanded the normal range for thoracic kyphosis to 20 to 50 degrees, and lumbar lordosis to 31 to 79 degrees. The measurement of thoracic kyphosis from a lateral radiograph is the angle between the superior endplate of the highest measurable thoracic vertebra, usually T2 or T3, and the inferior endplate of T12. The thoracolumbar junction should have no kyphosis or lordosis (10). Lumbar lordosis begins at L1-2 and increases gradually until the L3-4 disc space. The apex of normal thoracic kyphosis is the T6-7 disc space (10,11).

Initially, during fetal and intrauterine development, the entire spine is kyphotic. During the neonatal period the thoracic, lumbar, and sacral portions of the spine remain in a kyphotic posture. Cervical lordosis begins to develop when a child starts holding his or her head up. When an upright posture is assumed, the primary and secondary curves begin to develop. The primary curves are thoracic and sacral kyphosis, and the secondary or compensatory curves in the sagittal plane are cervical and lumbar lordosis. These curves balance each other so that the head is centered over the pelvis (2,12,13).

Cutler et al. (14) and Fon et al. (15) showed that the ranges of normal thoracic kyphosis and lumbar lordosis are dynamic, progressing gradually with growth. During the juvenile and adolescent growth periods thoracic kyphosis and lumbar lordosis become more pronounced and take on a more adult appearance. Differences also exist between male and female spines (6). Thoracic kyphosis and spine mobility are different in boys and girls. Mellin and others (3,11) have shown that during the juvenile and adolescent periods (ages 8 to 16 years), girls have less thoracic kyphosis and thoracic spinal mobility than do boys of the same age. Thoracic kyphosis also tends to progress with age. Fon et al. (15) showed that from 30 to 70 years of age women have a progressive increase in kyphosis, from a mean of 25 degrees to a mean of 40 degrees. Men also show a definite progression with age, but at a lower rate.

Normal sagittal balance is defined as a plumb line dropping from C7 and intersecting the posterosuperior corner of the S1 vertebral body (Fig. 20.1). Positive sagittal balance occurs when the plumb line falls in front of the sacrum, and negative sagittal balance occurs when the plumb line falls behind the sacrum (16).

Different forces are exerted on the spine, depending on the presence of kyphosis or lordosis. In the upright position the spine is subjected to the forces of gravity, and several structures maintain its stability: the disc complex (nucleus pulposus and annulus), the ligaments (anterior longitudinal ligament, posterior longitudinal ligament, ligamentum flavum, apophyseal joint ligaments, and interspinous ligament), and the muscles (the long spinal muscles, the short

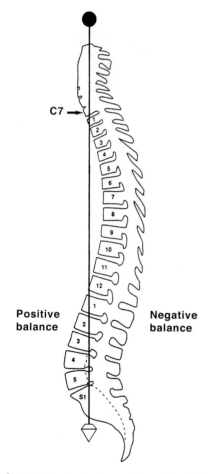

**Figure 20.1** A plumb line is dropped from the middle of the C7 vertebral body to the posterosuperior corner of the S1 vertebral body. (From Bernhardt M. Normal spinal anatomy: normal sagittal plane alignment. In: Bridwell KH, DeWald RL, eds. *The textbook of spinal surgery*, 2nd ed. Philadelphia, PA: Lippincott-Raven, 1997:185.)

intrinsic spinal muscles, and the abdominal muscles). Alteration in function resulting from paralysis, surgery, tumor, infection, or alteration in growth potentials can cause a progressive kyphotic deformity in a child (17). Both compressive and tensile forces are produced by the action of gravity on an upright spine (Fig. 20.2). In normal thoracic kyphosis, the compressive forces borne by the anterior elements are balanced by the tensile forces borne by the posterior elements. In a lordotic spine, the compressive forces are posterior and the tensile forces are anterior. These forces of compression and tension on the spinal physes can cause changes in normal growth, and a growth deformity can be added to a biomechanical deformity to cause a pathologic kyphosis (17,18).

Voutsinas and MacEwen (19) believe that relative differences in forces applied to the spine are reflected more accurately by the length and width of a kyphotic curve than by just the degree of the curve. For example, curves that are longer and wider (farther from the center of gravity) are more likely to cause deformity in an immature spine (Fig. 20.3). Winter and Hall (20) classified disorders that result in kyphosis of the spine. Only the more common causes are

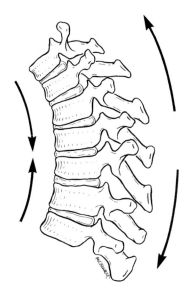

**Figure 20.2** Forces that contribute to kyphotic deformity of the thoracic spine. The anterior vertebral bodies are in compression, and the posterior vertebral elements are in tension. (From White AA III, Panjabi MM. Practical biomechanics of scoliosis and kyphosis. In: White AA, Panjabi MM, eds. *Clinical biomechanics of the spine.* Philadelphia, PA: JB Lippincott, 1990:127.)

presented in this chapter; the other causes are discussed elsewhere in this book (Table 20.1).

## POSTURAL KYPHOSIS

Postural kyphosis is a flexible deformity of the spine, and is a common complaint seen in juvenile and adolescent patients. Usually, the parents are more concerned about the postural roundback deformity than the adolescent is, and

these parental concerns typically are what bring the patient to the physician's office. The physician's role in this situation is to rule out more serious causes of kyphosis. Postural kyphosis should be differentiated from pathologic types of kyphosis, such as Scheuermann disease, and from congenital kyphosis. When observed from the side, patients with postural roundback have a gentle rounding of the back while bending forward (Fig. 20.4). Patients with Scheuermann disease and congenital kyphosis have a sharp angular kyphosis or gibbus on forward bending when observed from the side. Radiographs are usually necessary in order to rule out pathologic types of kyphosis. Patients with postural kyphosis do not have radiographic vertebral body changes, and the deformity is completely correctable by changes in position or posture. This deformity is common in patients who are taller than their peers, and in young adolescent girls undergoing early breast development who tend to stoop because they are self-conscious about their bodies (21).

No active medical treatment is necessary. Bracing is not indicated. Exercises have been suggested and may help maintain better posture, but adherence to such a therapy program is difficult for juveniles and young adolescents. This problem is best treated by educating the patient and, more important, the parents, and by observation (22).

## CONGENITAL KYPHOSIS

Congenital kyphosis is an uncommon deformity but, despite its rare occurrence, neurologic deficits resulting from this deformity are frequent.

**Figure 20.3** The two spinal curvatures represented by these drawings are different in magnitude; however, using Cobb's method to measure the deformities, the degrees of curvature are identical. The differences in the curves are more accurately reflected when the length of the curves (*L*) and their respective widths (*W* and *W*¹) are taken into consideration. (From Voutsinas SA, MacEwen GD. Sagittal profiles of the spine. *Clin Orthop* 1986;210:235.)

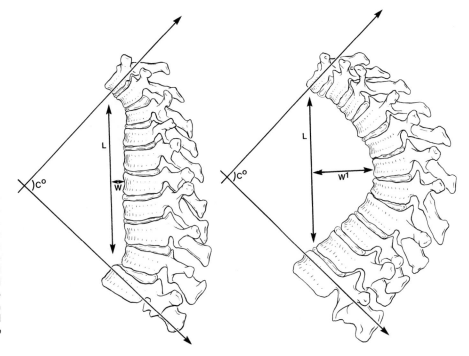

**TABLE 20.1**

**DISORDERS AFFECTING THE SPINE AND RESULTING IN KYPHOSIS**

| | |
|---|---|
| I. Postural disorders | IX. Inadequate fusion |
| II. Scheuermann kyphosis |   a. Too short |
| III. Congenital disorders |   b. Pseudoarthrosis |
|   a. Defect of formation | X. Postirradiation |
|   b. Defect of segmentation |   a. Neuroblastoma |
| IV. Paralytic disorders |   b. Wilms tumor |
|   a. Poliomyelitis | XI. Metabolic |
|   b. Anterior horn cell disease |   a. Osteoporosis |
| V. Myelomeningocele |     1. Senile |
| VI. Posttraumatic |     2. Juvenile |
|   a. Acute |   b. Osteogenesis imperfecta |
|   b. Chronic | XII. Developmental |
|   c. With/without cord damage |   a. Achondroplasia |
| VII. Inflammatory |   b. Mucopolysaccharidosis |
|   a. Tuberculosis |   c. Other |
|   b. Other infection | XIII. Collagen disease (e.g., Marie-Strumpell) |
| VIII. Postsurgical | XIV. Tumor |
|   a. Postlaminectomy |   a. Benign |
|   b. Postbody (tumor) excision |   b. Malignant |
| | XV. Neurofibromatosis |

From Winter RB, Hall JE. Kyphosis in childhood and adolescence. *Spine* 1978;3:285.

Congenital kyphosis occurs because of abnormal development of the vertebrae, including a failure of developing segments of the spine to form or to separate properly (23). The spine may be either stable or unstable, or it may become unstable with growth (24). Spinal deformity in congenital kyphosis usually progresses with growth, and the amount of progression is directly proportional to the number of vertebrae involved, the type of involvement, and the amount of remaining normal growth in the affected vertebrae (24,25).

Van Schrick in 1932 (26) and Lombard and LeGenissel in 1938 (27) initially described two basic types of congenital

kyphosis: a failure of formation of part or all of the vertebral body, and a failure of segmentation of part or all of the vertebral body. Winter et al. (23,28) developed the most useful classification of congenital kyphosis, which divides the deformity into three types (Table 20.2). Type I is failure of formation of all or part of the vertebral body (Fig. 20.5A); type II is failure of segmentation of one or multiple vertebral levels (Fig. 20.5B); and type III is a mixed form, with elements of both failure of formation and failure of segmentation.

McMaster and Singh further subdivided this classification into types of vertebral body deformity. Defects of

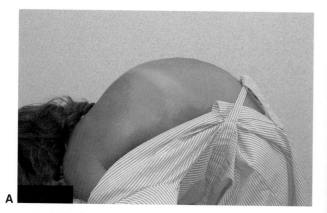

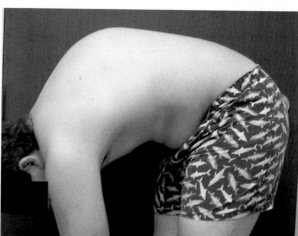

**Figure 20.4  A:** Lateral view of normal spinal contour on forward bending. **B:** Lateral view of a patient with Scheuermann disease on forward bending. Note the break in the normal contour and sharp angular nature of the spine.

## TABLE 20.2

### WINTER'S CLASSIFICATION OF CONGENITAL DEFORMITY

| Type | Description |
|------|-------------|
| I | Failure of formation of all or part of the vertebral body |
| II | Failure of segmentation of one or multiple vertebral levels |
| III | Mixed form, with elements of both failure of formation and failure of segmentation |

vertebral body segmentation consist of a partial (anterior unsegmented bar) or a complete (block vertebrae) failure of segmentation. Defects of vertebral body formation are divided into four types; (a) posterolateral quadrant vertebrae, (b) butterfly vertebrae, (c) posterior hemivertebrae, and (d) wedged vertebrae (Fig. 20.6) (29). A classification by Dubousset (30) and Zeller et al. (31) includes a rotary dislocation of the spine. Shapiro and Herring (32) also described a type III congenital kyphosis, but further divided the displacement into type A (sagittal plane only) and type B (rotary, transverse, and sagittal planes). Any classification can be subdivided further into deformities with or without neurologic compromise; this is useful for making treatment decisions, because each type of congenital kyphosis has a distinct natural history and risk of progression.

Most of the vertebral malformations that cause spinal deformity occur between the 20th and 30th days of fetal development (24,28,33). The somatic mesoderm, which is devoted to the formation of the vertebral column and rib cage, undergoes segmentation into 38 to 44 pairs of discrete, bilateral somites. The formation of a vertebra depends on contributions of cells from two separate and successive

pairs of sclerotomes. This condensation of the paired sclerotomes occurs at approximately 5 weeks of gestation. If one side of the pair of sclerotomes fails to develop, this will cause a hemivertebra to be formed, resulting in congenital scoliosis (34,35).

Tsou (36) concluded that congenital kyphosis and congenital scoliosis occur during different periods of spinal development. He divided the development of the spine into an embryonic period (the first 56 days) and a fetal period (from 57 days to birth). During the embryonic period, failure of segmentation and aplasia of part of the vertebrae, resulting in hemivertebra formation, cause scoliosis. He believes that the causes of congenital kyphosis occur in the fetal period, during the cartilaginous phase of development. Failure of formation occurs in this phase when the cartilaginous centrum of the vertebral body forms a functionally inadequate growth cartilage.

Failure of formation varies from complete aplasia (which involves the pars and the facet joints and makes the spine unstable) to involvement of only the anterior one third to one half of the vertebral body. This abnormal development is thought to be the result of inadequate vascularization of the vertebral body during the fetal period, leading to hypoplasia or aplasia of the anterior vertebral body. If one side of the vertebra is involved more than the other side, scoliosis also may occur (Fig. 20.7). Unlike hemivertebral anomalies that occur in the embryonic period because of maldevelopment of corresponding pairs of somites causing congenital scoliosis, posterior arch anomalies are almost universally absent in pure congenital kyphosis.

Failure of segmentation is believed by Tsou (36) to be an osseous metaplasia of the annulus fibrosus (36,37), acting as a tether against normal growth and causing spinal deformity. The height of the vertebral bodies is relatively normal, but the depth of the ossification of the annulus fibrosus varies. Ossification may be delayed, with a period of normal growth followed by spontaneous ossification. Morin et al. (38) believe that kyphosis caused by a "segmentation defect" represents a developmental defect of the perivertebral structures (the annulus fibrosis, the ring apophysis, and the anterior longitudinal ligament) rather than a true intervertebral bar.

The natural history of congenital kyphosis is well known and based on the type of kyphosis: failure of formation (type I), failure of segmentation (type II), or mixed anomalies (type III). Congenital kyphosis tends to be progressive, with the greatest rate of progression occurring during the time of most rapid growth of the spine (birth to 3 years of age) and during the adolescent growth spurt. Winter et al. found that failure of formation (type I deformity) produces a much more severe kyphosis, with a rate of progression that averages 7 degrees per year, whereas type II deformities progress an average of 5 degrees per year (28). McMaster and Singh found the most rapid progression in type III kyphosis, followed by type I, because of

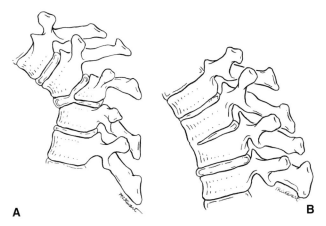

**A**          **B**

**Figure 20.5** **A:** Congenital kyphosis caused by failure of formation of the vertebral body (type I). **B:** Congenital kyphosis caused by failure of segmentation (type II). (Courtesy of Robert Winter, MD, Minneapolis.)

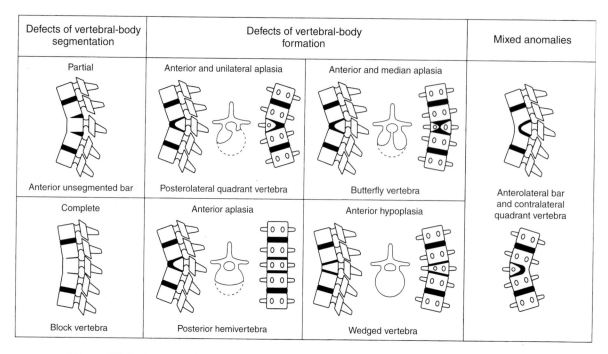

| Defects of vertebral-body segmentation | Defects of vertebral-body formation | | Mixed anomalies |
|---|---|---|---|
| Partial | Anterior and unilateral aplasia | Anterior and median aplasia | |
| Anterior unsegmented bar | Posterolateral quadrant vertebra | Butterfly vertebra | Anterolateral bar and contralateral quadrant vertebra |
| Complete | Anterior aplasia | Anterior hypoplasia | |
| Block vertebra | Posterior hemivertebra | Wedged vertebra | |

**Figure 20.6**  Drawings showing the different types of vertebral anomalies that produce congenital kyphosis or kyphoscoliosis. (From McMaster MJ, Singh H. Natural history of congenital kyphosis and kyphoscoliosis. *J Bone Joint Surg* 1999;81A:1367–1383.)

involvement of posterolateral quadrant vertebrae. In their study, a type III kyphosis progressed at a rate of 5 degrees per year before 10 years of age and 8 degrees per year thereafter until the end of growth. Type I (failure of formation) kyphosis progressed 2.5 degrees per year before 10 years of age and 5 degrees per year thereafter (29). Type I and type III deformities are associated with a much higher incidence of neurologic involvement and paraplegia than type II deformities are. Neurologic problems occur more frequently in patients with type I and type III deformities because they tend to have an acute angular kyphosis over a short segment, which places the spinal cord at higher risk for compression at the level of acute angulation. Type II deformities (failure of segmentation) rarely result in neurologic problems because involvement of several segments produces a more gradual kyphosis, and vertebral body height is usually maintained with little or no vertebral body wedging. The most frequent location of congenital kyphosis is T10–L1 (28).

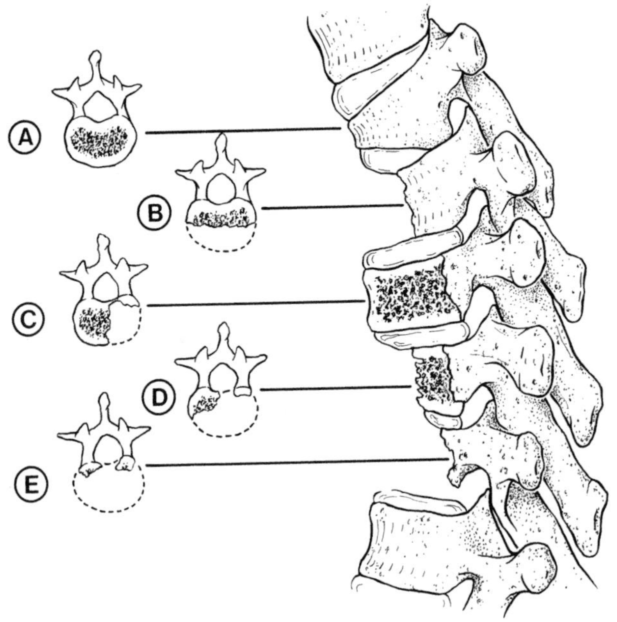

Patients with congenital kyphosis may have other anomalies. Intraspinal abnormalities have been reported to occur in 5% to 37% of patients with congenital kyphosis and congenital scoliosis (39–42). A study by Bradford et al. (43) indicates that this incidence may be even greater. They found that six of eight patients with congenital kyphosis had spinal cord abnormalities visible on magnetic resonance imaging (MRI). Although the proposed time of development of the deformity may be different from that of congenital scoliosis, other nonskeletal anomalies such as cardiac, pulmonary, renal, and auditory disorders or Klippel-Feil syndrome (44,45) can be associated with congenital kyphosis.

**Figure 20.7**  The five most common patterns of congenital vertebral hypoplasia and aplasia are illustrated in lateral and transverse views. Types *B* and *E* tend to produce pure congenital kyphosis. (From Tsou PM. Embryology of congenital kyphosis. *Clin Orthop* 1977;128:18.)

## Patient Presentation

The diagnosis of a congenital spine problem is usually made by a pediatrician before the patient is seen by an orthopaedist. The deformity may be detected before birth on prenatal ultrasonography (46) or noted as a clinical deformity in the newborn. If the deformity is mild, congenital kyphosis can be overlooked until a rapid growth spurt makes the condition more obvious. Some mild deformities are found by chance on radiographs that are obtained for other reasons. Clinical deformities seen in the newborn tend to have a worse prognosis than those discovered as incidental findings on plain radiographs. Physical examination usually reveals a kyphotic deformity at the thoracolumbar junction or in the lower thoracic spine. An attempt should be made to determine the rigidity of the deformity by flexion and extension of the spine. A detailed neurologic examination should be done, looking for any subtle signs of neurologic compromise. Associated musculoskeletal and nonmusculoskeletal anomalies should be sought on physical examination.

High-quality, detailed anteroposterior and lateral radiographs provide the most information in the evaluation of congenital kyphosis (Fig. 20.8). Failure of segmentation and the true extent of failure of formation may be difficult to detect on early films because of incomplete ossification. Flexion and extension lateral radiographs are helpful in determining the rigidity of the kyphosis and possible instability of the spine. Computerized tomography (CT) with three-dimensional reconstructions can identify the amount of vertebral body involvement and can determine whether more kyphosis or scoliosis might be expected (Fig. 20.9). CT scans can only identify the nature of the bony deformity and the size of the cartilage anlage. They do not show the amount of growth potential in the cartilage anlage, and therefore only an estimate of possible progression can be made. MRI should be obtained in most cases because of the significant incidence of intraspinal abnormalities. In addition, the location of the spinal cord and any areas of spinal cord compression caused by the kyphosis can be seen on MRI. The cartilage anlage will be well defined by MRI in patients with failure of formation (Fig. 20.10); however, as with CT scans and plain radiographs, MRI cannot reveal how much growth potential is present in the cartilage anlage, and can only help one to estimate the probability of a progressive deformity.

Congenital kyphosis, as well as associated renal problems, can be seen on routine prenatal ultrasonography at as early as 20 weeks of gestation (46). Myelograms have been used for documenting spinal cord compression but have been mostly replaced by MRI. If myelography is used, images should be taken in the prone and supine positions. Myelograms obtained in only the prone position may miss information about spinal cord compression because of pooling of dye around the apex of the deformity. Myelography can be used in conjunction with CT scanning to add to the diagnostic information obtained.

## Treatment

Because the natural history of this condition is usually one of continued progression with an increased risk of neurologic compromise, surgery is usually the preferred method of treatment (23). If the deformity is mild or if the diagnosis is uncertain, close observation may be a treatment option. However, observation of a congenital kyphotic deformity must be used with caution, and the physician must not be lulled into a false sense of security if the deformity progresses only 3 to 5 degrees over a 6-month period. If the deformity is observed over 2 to 3 years, it will have progressed 20 to 30 degrees and cannot thereafter be easily corrected. Bracing has no role in the treatment of congenital kyphosis, unless compensatory curves are being treated above or below the congenital kyphosis (23,44,47). Bracing a rigid structural deformity, such as congenital kyphosis, neither corrects the deformity nor stops the progression of kyphosis. To document that there has been a significant change in kyphosis, the radiographs should be taken by a standardized method, and the same end vertebral bodies should be measured. This will ensure that any change that has occurred since the previous radiograph is accurately measured.

Surgery is the recommended treatment for congenital kyphosis. The type of surgery depends on the type and size

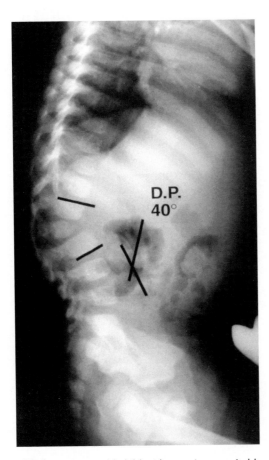

**Figure 20.8** A 2-year-old child with type I congenital kyphosis measuring 40 degrees. Radiograph demonstrates failure of formation of the anterior portion of the first lumbar vertebra.

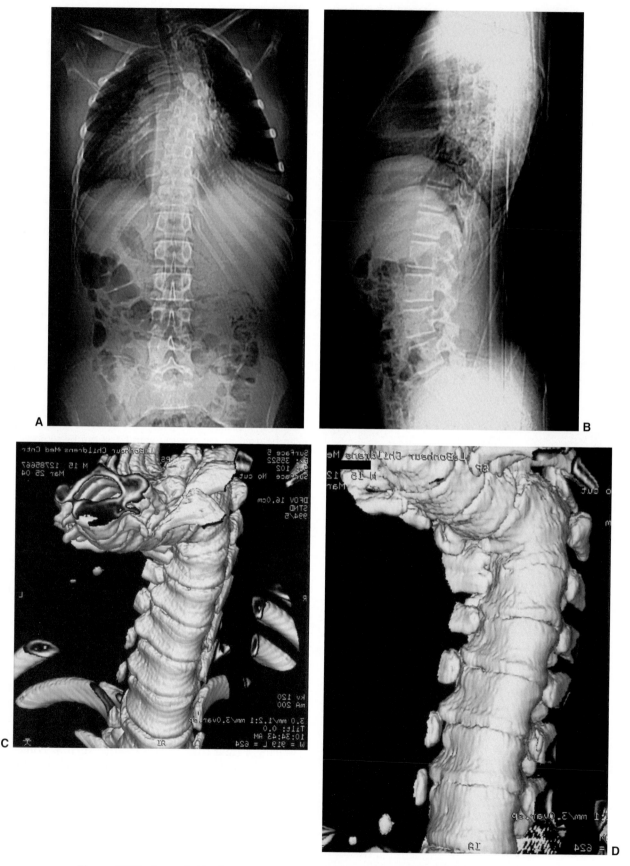

**Figure 20.9** Congenital kyphosis. **A** and **B:** Anteroposterior and lateral radiographs. Note inadequate detail of kyphosis on lateral radiograph of spine. **C** to **E:** Computerized tomography (CT) three-dimensional reconstruction views that clearly demonstrate the bony anatomy of congenital kyphosis.

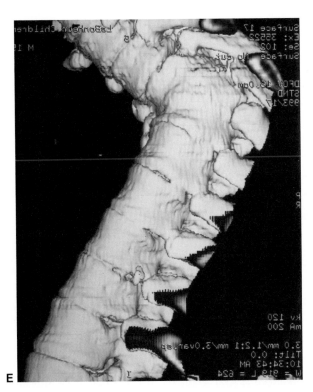

**Figure 20.9** *(continued)*

*Late Treatment of Moderate to Severe Deformities.* In older patients with type I kyphotic deformities, posterior arthrodesis alone may be successful if the kyphosis is less than 50 to 55 degrees (28,50). If the deformity is more than 55 degrees (which usually is the case in deformities detected late), anterior and posterior fusion produces more reliable results (28,50). Anterior arthrodesis alone will not correct the deformity. Any correction of the deformity requires anterior strut grafting with temporary distraction and posterior fusion, with or without posterior compression instrumentation. The posterior instrumentation may allow for some correction of the kyphosis but should be regarded more as an internal stabilizer than as a correction device (23). Correction by instrumentation should be used with caution in rigid, angular curves because of the high incidence of neurologic complications. If anterior strut grafting is performed, the strut graft should be placed anteriorly under compression. If no correction is attempted and the goal of surgery is just to stop progression of the kyphosis, a simple anterior interbody fusion combined with a posterior fusion can be performed. The use of skeletal traction (halo-pelvic, halo-femoral, or halo-gravity) to correct the deformity is tempting, but is not recommended because of the risk of paraplegia (51). In a patient with a

of the deformity, the age of the patient, and the presence of neurologic deficits. Procedures can include posterior fusion, anterior fusion, both anterior and posterior fusions, and anterior osteotomy with posterior fusion. Fusion can be performed with or without instrumentation.

### Treatment of Type I Deformities

The treatment of type I deformities depends on the stage of the disease: early with mild deformity, late with moderate or severe deformity, and late with severe deformity and spinal cord compression.

*Early Treatment of Mild Deformities.* For type I deformities the best treatment is early posterior fusion. If the deformity is less than 50 or 55 degrees and the patient is younger than 5 years of age, posterior fusion alone, extending from one level above the kyphotic deformity to one level below, is recommended (23,28,44,48). This may allow for some improvement in the kyphotic deformity because of continued growth anteriorly from the anterior end plates of the vertebrae one level above and one level below the congenital kyphotic vertebrae that are included in the posterior fusion. Anterior and posterior spinal fusions at least one level above and one level below the congenital kyphosis are indicated in curves greater than 60 degrees (49). Anterior and posterior fusion predictably halts the progression of the kyphotic deformity but, because of ablation of the anterior physes (31,48,49), it does not allow for the possibility of some correction of the deformity with growth.

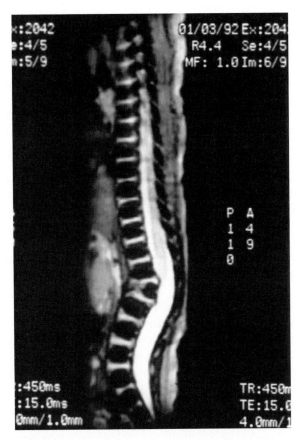

**Figure 20.10** Magnetic resonance image (MRI) of type I congenital kyphosis. Failure of formation of the anterior vertebral body is demonstrated, but the growth potential of the involved vertebra cannot be determined. Note the pressure on the dural sac.

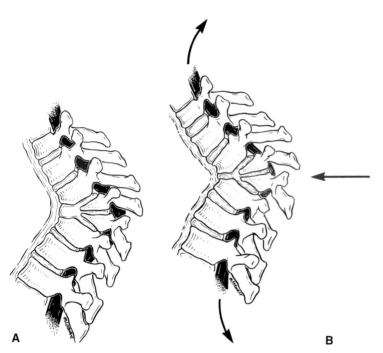

**A**

**B**

**Figure 20.11** The effect of traction on a rigid congenital kyphosis. **A:** The apical area does not change with traction, but the adjacent spine is lengthened. **B:** As the spine lengthens, so does the spinal cord, producing increased tension in the cord and aggravating existing neurologic deficits. (From Lonstein JE, Winter RB, Moe JH, et al. Neurologic deficit secondary to spinal deformity. *Spine* 1980;5:331.)

rigid gibbus deformity, traction pulls the spinal cord against the apex of the rigid kyphosis and can lead to neurologic compromise (Fig. 20.11).

***Late Treatment of Severe Deformities with Cord Compression.*** It is difficult to attempt late treatment of a severe congenital kyphotic deformity that is accompanied by spinal cord compression. If congenital kyphosis causes spinal cord compression, anterior decompression is indicated. The compression is created by bone or disc material pressing into the front of the spinal cord, and this can be decompressed only by an anterior procedure; laminectomy has no role in the treatment of this condition (20). If associated with scoliosis, the anterior approach for decompression should be on the concavity of the scoliosis to allow the spinal cord to move both forward and into the midline after decompression. After adequate decompression has been achieved, the vertebrae involved are fused with an anterior strut graft. This is followed by a posterior fusion, with or without posterior stabilizing instrumentation. Postoperative support with a cast, brace, or halo cast may be required.

### Treatment of Type II Deformities

Treatment of type II deformities can be divided into early treatment of mild deformities and late treatment of severe deformities as outlined by Mayfield et al. (52). If a type II kyphosis is mild and detected early, posterior fusion with compression instrumentation can be performed. The kyphosis should be less than 50 degrees for a posterior fusion alone to have a good chance of success. The posterior fusion should include all the involved vertebrae, plus one vertebra above and one vertebra below the congenital kyphosis.

Compression instrumentation can be used more safely in type II deformities, because the kyphosis is more rounded and affects several segments, instead of being sharply angular as in type I deformities. If the deformity is severe and detected late, correction can be obtained only by performing anterior osteotomies and fusion, followed by posterior fusion and compression instrumentation (52).

## Complications of Treatment

Some of the more frequent complications of treatment of congenital kyphosis are pseudarthrosis, progression of kyphosis, and paralysis. Pseudarthrosis and progression of the kyphotic deformity can be minimized by performing anterior and posterior fusions for deformities of more than 50 degrees. The posterior fusion should extend from one level above to one level below the involved vertebrae. This may allow for some correction with growth.

Paralysis is perhaps the most feared complication of spinal surgery. The risk of this complication can be lessened by not attempting to maximally correct the deformity with instrumentation. Instrumentation should be used only for stabilization of rigid deformities. The use of halo traction in rigid congenital kyphotic deformities has been associated with an increased risk of neurologic compromise (51). Another long-term problem, occurring in approximately 38% of patients with kyphosis, is low back pain caused by increased lumbar lordosis, which is needed to compensate for the kyphotic deformity (53).

## SEGMENTAL SPINAL DYSGENESIS

Segmental spinal dysgenesis is a congenital anomaly of the lumbar or thoracolumbar spine, consisting of focal agenesis

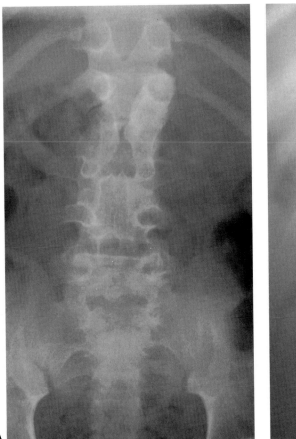
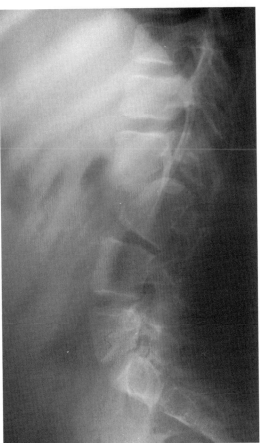

A
B

**Figure 20.12** Segmental spinal dysgenesis. Anteroposterior **(A)** and lateral **(B)** radiographs show narrowing of spinal canal and absence of L1 and part of L2 vertebral bodies.

or dysgenesis of the spine, and resulting in severe spinal stenosis and instability (54). A progressive kyphosis occurs at the site of segmental spinal dysgenesis. This condition is often confused with other spinal anomalies such as type I congenital kyphosis, sacral agenesis, lumbosacral agenesis, and lumbar agenesis. Faciszewski et al. (55) have given detailed radiographic and clinical definitions of this condition. Segmental spinal dysgenesis is characterized by severe focal stenosis of the spinal canal at the involved segment, and is associated with significant narrowing of the thecal sac and absence of adjacent nerve roots. At the involved level, a ring of bone encircles the posteriorly positioned spinal canal, causing stenosis. The spinal canal is hourglass-shaped with no neurocentral junctions. There is limited potential for enlargement with growth because of the absence of neurocentral junctions, where growth occurs (Fig. 20.12). No pedicles or spinous or transverse processes are present at this level. Anterior to the bony ring is a fat-filled space. The distal bony anatomy and spinal canal are usually normal, although spina bifida has been noted in a few cases (56). Neurologic function can range from normal to complete paraplegia. Associated anomalies are common, and there is a high incidence of neurogenic bladder.

The etiology of segmental spinal dysgenesis is unknown. The diagnosis can be made on the basis of plain radiographs, but MRI and CT scans and three-dimensional reconstructions are usually needed in order to fully show the extent of this condition. A progressive kyphosis will occur with this condition. Progressive neurologic deterioration has been noted by Flynn et al. (57) and Faciszewski et al. (55). Early anterior and posterior fusion, with or without decompression, is recommended. The use of spinal instrumentation is controversial because of the small size of the patient. Hughes et al. (56) believe that treatment should be directed toward the establishment and maintenance of spinal stability first, and toward decompression of the cord secondarily.

## SACRAL AGENESIS

Sacral agenesis consists of a complete or partial absence of the sacrum (58–61). Rarely is it associated with absence of the most caudal segment of the lumbar spine. The association with maternal diabetes has been well documented (58–61). Kyphosis may occur with this condition, although it is usually not progressive and does not require treatment (62,63).

## PROGRESSIVE ANTERIOR VERTEBRAL FUSION

Progressive anterior vertebral fusion (PAVF) is rare and an uncommon cause of kyphosis in pediatric patients; however, if discovered late it may be confused with type II congenital kyphosis. Knutsson (64), in 1949, was the first to describe PAVF in the English-language literature, and a total of 80 cases have since been reported. This condition is distinguishable from type II congenital kyphosis because the disc spaces and vertebral bodies are normal at birth and later become affected with an anterior fusion. Although the etiology is unknown, PAVF is probably a distinct clinical condition; however, consideration has been given to the possibility that it may represent a delayed type II congenital kyphosis. Dubousset (30) suggested that certain forms of type II congenital kyphosis (failure of segmentation) may be inherited. The patients have a failure of segmentation, with delayed fusion of the anterior vertebral elements, which is not visible on radiographs until 8 or 10 years of age. He described one family in which three individuals had delayed ossification and congenital kyphosis, and another family in which the grandmother, mother, and two sisters had the deformity. Kharrat and Dubousset (65) also found this condition to be familial in 6 of 15 patients, and Van Buskirk et al. (66) reported associated anomalies in 46% of 15 patients, including heart defects, tibial agenesis, foot deformities, Klippel-Feil syndrome, Ito syndrome, pulmonary artery stenosis, and hemisacralization of L5.

Neurologic deficits are usually not seen in PAVF, but Smith (67) reported one case of spinal cord compression resulting from an acutely angled kyphosis. Van Buskirk et al. (66) and Dubousset (24,30) described five stages of PAVF: stage 1 is disc space narrowing, which occurs to a greater extent anteriorly than posteriorly; stage 2 is increased sclerosis of the vertebral end plates of the anterior and middle columns; stage 3 is fragmentation of the anterior vertebral end plates; stage 4 is fusion of the anterior and sometimes the middle columns; and stage 5 is development of a kyphotic deformity.

Kyphosis is the last stage in PAVF and is caused by the anterior disc space fusing while part of the posterior disc space remains open, allowing for continued growth in the posterior disc space and the posterior column. Bollini et al. (68) found that patients with thoracic PAVF had a relatively good prognosis, whereas those with lumbar involvement had a poor prognosis. Involvement of the thoracic spine is better tolerated by patients than is involvement of the lumbar area because of the normal kyphotic posture of the thoracic spine. Therefore, nonoperative treatment is recommended for most thoracic PAVF deformities. For PAVF in the lumbar spine, a posterior spinal fusion is indicated in stages 1, 2, and 3. In stages 4 and 5, the kyphotic deformity has already occurred in a normally lordotic lumbar spine. Posterior fusion will only stop progression of kyphotic deformity. If normal sagittal alignment is to be obtained, an anterior osteotomy followed by posterior fusion and instrumentation is recommended (64–71).

## SCHEUERMANN DISEASE

Scheuermann disease is a common cause of structural kyphosis in the thoracic, thoracolumbar, and lumbar spine. Scheuermann originally described this rigid juvenile kyphosis in 1920; it is characterized by vertebral body wedging that is believed to be caused by a growth disturbance of the vertebral end plates (72,73) (Fig. 20.13).

### Classification

Scheuermann disease can be divided into two distinct groups: a typical form and an atypical form. These two types are determined by the location and natural history of the kyphosis, including symptoms occurring during adolescence and after growth is completed. Typical Scheuermann disease usually involves the thoracic spine, with a well-established natural history during adolescence and after skeletal maturity (74). This classic form of Scheuermann kyphosis will have three or more consecutive vertebrae,

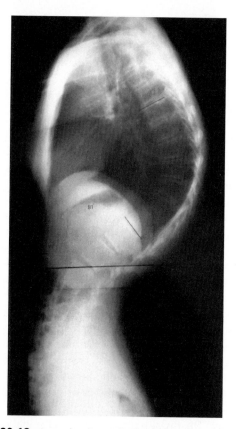

**Figure 20.13** Lateral radiograph of a patient with Scheuermann disease and an 81-degree kyphotic deformity. Note the narrowing of the intervertebral disc spaces and the irregularity of the vertebral end plates. There is an associated increase in lumbar lordosis below the kyphotic deformity.

each wedged 5 degrees or more (Sorensen criteria), producing a structural kyphosis. In contrast, atypical Scheuermann disease is usually located in the thoracolumbar junction or in the lumbar spine, and its natural history is well defined. The atypical type is characterized by vertebral end-plate changes, disc space narrowing, and anterior Schmorl nodes, but does not necessarily fulfill Sorensen's criteria of three consecutively wedged vertebrae of 5 degrees. Thoracic Scheuermann is the most common form, with the atypical form less frequently seen.

## Epidemiology

Typical Scheuermann disease consists of a rigid thoracic kyphosis in a juvenile or adolescent spine. The apex of kyphosis is located between T7 and T9 (10). The reported incidence of Scheuermann deformities in the general population ranges from 0.4% to 10% (75–79). Reported male-to-female ratios vary in the literature. Scheuermann originally reported a male preponderance of 88% (72). Most reports in the literature note either a slight male preponderance or an equal male-to-female ratio (35,77–82). Bradford et al. (76) has been the only one to report an increased incidence of Scheuermann disease in women.

The age at onset of Scheuermann kyphosis is during the prepubertal growth spurt, between 10 and 12 years of age. Sorensen (78) described a Scheuermann prodrome in patients who had a lax, asthenic posture from the age of approximately 4 to 8 years, and in whom, within a few years, a fixed kyphosis developed. The clinical detection of Scheuermann disease occurs at approximately 10 to 12 years of age. Wedging of apical vertebrae has not been reported before 10 years of age (83). Radiographic evidence of Scheuermann disease is usually not detectable in patients younger than 10 years of age because the ring apophysis is not yet ossified. Until the ring apophysis ossifies, vertebral body wedging and irregularity of the end plate are difficult to measure on radiographs.

## Etiology

Many possible etiologies have been suggested for Scheuermann disease, but the true cause remains unknown. Genetic, vascular, hormonal, metabolic, and mechanical factors have been suggested as causes of Scheuermann kyphosis. Sorensen (78) noted a high familial predilection, and Halal et al. (84), in a study of five families, and McKenzie and Sillence (85), in a study of 12 families, suggested that the disease may be inherited in an autosomal dominant fashion with a high degree of penetrance. Additional support for a genetic basis for this condition is provided by Carr et al. (86,87) in a report of Scheuermann disease occurring in identical twins. Halal et al. (84), McKenzie and Sillence (85), and Carr et al. (87) have reported possible autosomal dominant inheritance of Scheuermann kyphosis.

Scheuermann believed that the kyphosis was caused by a form of avascular necrosis of the ring apophysis, which led to a growth disturbance resulting in a progressive kyphosis with growth (72,73). The problem with this theory is that the ring apophysis contributes little, if at all, to the longitudinal growth of the vertebrae (87,88). Bick and Copel (89) demonstrated that the ring apophysis lies outside the true cartilaginous physis and contributes nothing to the longitudinal growth of the vertebral body. Therefore, a disturbance in the ring apophysis should not affect growth of the vertebrae or cause vertebral wedging.

Schmorl (90) described a herniation of disc material through the cartilaginous end plate, known as *Schmorl nodes*. He believed that the herniation of disc material occurred because of a weakened end plate. The disc herniation was thought to damage the anterior end plate, resulting in abnormal growth, which in turn caused the kyphosis. There is a definite increased incidence of Schmorl nodes in patients with Scheuermann kyphosis, but the problem with this theory is that Schmorl nodes are found outside the area of kyphosis, and are also present in individuals who have asymptomatic, normal spines and do not have a kyphotic deformity.

Ferguson (91) suggested that persistence of an anterior vascular groove altered the anterior growth of the vertebral body, but Aufdermaur and Spycher (92,93) and Ippolito and Ponseti (94) were unable to document growth disturbances around the anterior vascular groove, and concluded that persistence of an anterior vascular groove is a sign of immaturity of the spine. Lambrinudi (95) postulated that Scheuermann disease resulted from upright posture and a tight anterior longitudinal ligament. The fact that no cases of Scheuermann disease have been found in quadruped animals lends support to this theory (96). This has led to the more popular belief that the anterior end-plate changes are caused by mechanical forces in response to Wolff's law or the Hueter-Volkmann principle. Compression forces in the anterior growth plate cause a decrease in growth in the area of the kyphosis. Indirect support for this argument can be found in the changes in the wedging of the involved vertebral bodies and the reversal of these changes when bracing or casting is used in the immature spine. Scoles et al. (96) also support this theory by demonstrating disorganized endochondral ossification in the involved vertebrae, similar to that seen in Blount disease. They conclude that the changes in endochondral ossification are the result of increased pressure on the vertebral growth plate.

Ascani et al. (97,98) found that patients who have Scheuermann disease tend to be taller than normal for their chronologic and skeletal ages, and that their bone age tends to be more advanced than their chronologic age. Because they found increased growth hormone levels in these patients, they suggested that the increased height and the advanced skeletal age could be caused by the increased growth hormone (97,98). The increased height and more rapid growth may make the vertebral end plates more susceptible to increased pressure and result in the changes seen in Scheuermann disease. The increased growth hormone levels noted by Ascani et al. may also lead to a relative osteoporosis of the spine, which, in turn, may predispose the spine to the development of Scheuermann disease.

Bradford et al. (75,99), Burner et al. (100), and Lopez et al. (101) reported in the 1980s that Scheuermann kyphosis may be caused by a form of juvenile osteoporosis. However, using quantitative CT scans, Gilsanz et al. (102) found no evidence of osteoporosis in patients with Scheuermann kyphosis compared with normal research subjects. The authors suggested that the technique used to determine osteoporosis might account for the differences between their report and those that show osteoporosis. In a study using single-photon absorptiometric analysis of cadaver vertebrae from patients with Scheuermann kyphosis, Scoles et al. (96) also found no evidence of osteoporosis.

What is shown by the histologic studies of Ascani et al. (97), Ippolito et al. (94,103), and Scoles et al. (96) is that an alteration in endochondral ossification occurs. Whether this altered endochondral ossification is the cause or result of kyphosis is not known. Ippolito and Ponseti (94) found a decrease in the number of collagen fibers, which were thinner than normal, and an increase in proteoglycan content. Some areas of the altered end plate showed direct bone formation from cartilage instead of the normal growth-plate sequences for ossification. These studies help support the belief that Scheuermann kyphosis is an underlying growth problem of the anterior vertebral end plates.

Atypical Scheuermann kyphosis, or thoracolumbar and lumbar kyphosis, is believed to be caused by trauma to the immature spine, resulting in irregularities of the end plate (104).

## Natural History

Many early studies suggested an unfavorable natural history for Scheuermann disease and recommended early treatment to prevent severe deformity, pain, impaired social functioning, embarrassment about physical appearance, myelopathy, degeneration of the disc spaces, spondylolisthesis, and cardiopulmonary failure. Despite these reports, few long-term follow-up studies of Scheuermann disease were performed until that of Murray et al. (77). Findings by Travaglini and Conti (35,105), Murray et al. (77), and Lowe (106) suggest that the natural history of the disease tends to be benign.

The kyphotic deformity progresses rapidly during the adolescent growth spurt. Bradford et al. (107) noted that, among the patients who required brace treatment, more than half had progression of their deformities during this growth spurt before brace treatment was begun. Little is known about progression of the kyphosis after growth is completed, and whether it is similar to that in scoliosis. It is not well documented whether the kyphosis will continue to progress beyond a certain degree during adulthood.

Tragvaglini and Conte (35) found that the kyphosis did progress during adulthood, but few patients developed severe deformities. What is known is that patients with Scheuermann kyphosis have more intense back pain, jobs that require relatively little physical activity, less range of motion of the trunk in extension, and different localization of back pain than the general population that does not have Scheuermann kyphosis (77). Even with these findings, when compared with normal individuals, patients with Scheuermann kyphosis have no significant differences in self-esteem, social limitations, or level of recreational activities. The number of days they miss from work because of back pain is also similar.

The data regarding the natural history of Scheuermann disease suggest that, although patients may have some functional limitations, their lives are not seriously restricted, and they have few clinical or functional problems. Pulmonary function actually increases in these patients, probably because of the increased diameter of the chest cavity, until their kyphosis is more than 100 degrees. Patients with kyphosis of more than 100 degrees have restrictive pulmonary function. Another finding in patients with Scheuermann kyphosis was that disc degeneration was five times more likely to be seen on MRI in patients with Scheuermann compared with controls (108). The clinical significance of this finding is not known (77).

## Associated Conditions

Mild to moderate scoliosis is present in about one third of patients with Scheuermann disease (106), but the curves tend to be small, approximately 10 to 20 degrees. Scoliosis associated with Scheuermann disease usually has a benign natural history. The scoliotic curve is rarely progressive, and usually does not require treatment. Deacon et al. (109,110) divided scoliotic curves found in patients with Scheuermann disease into two types, based on the location of the curve and the rotation of the vertebrae into or away from the concavity of the scoliotic curve. In the first type of curves, the apices of scoliosis and kyphosis are the same, and the curve is rotated toward the convexity. The rotation of the scoliotic curve is opposite to that normally seen in idiopathic scoliosis. Deacon et al. (109,110) suggested that the difference in direction of rotation is caused by scoliosis occurring in a kyphotic spine, instead of the hypokyphotic or lordotic spine that is common in idiopathic scoliosis. In the second type of curves, the apex of the scoliosis is above or below the apex of the kyphosis, and the scoliotic curve is rotated into the concavity of the scoliosis, more like idiopathic scoliosis. This type of scoliosis seen with Scheuermann kyphosis is the more common, and it rarely progresses or requires treatment.

Lumbar spondylolysis is a frequently associated finding in Scheuermann kyphosis (Fig. 20.14). The suggested reason for the increased incidence of spondylolysis is that increased stress is placed on the pars interarticularis because of the associated compensatory hyperlordosis of

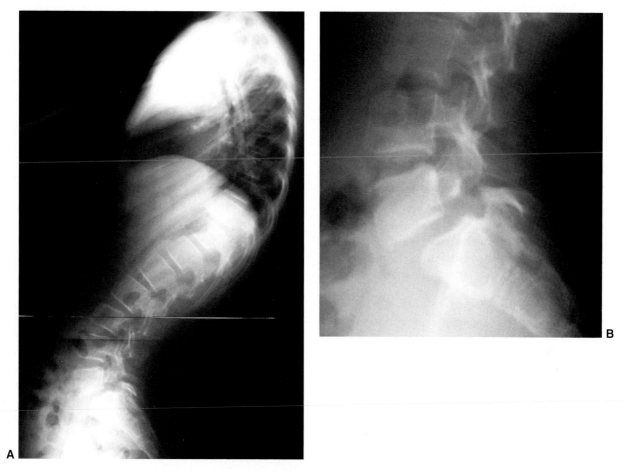

**Figure 20.14** **A** and **B:** Lateral radiographs demonstrating spondylolisthesis with kyphosis.

the lumbar spine in Scheuermann disease. This increased stress causes a fatigue fracture at the pars interarticularis, resulting in spondylolysis. Ogilvie and Sherman (111) found a 50% incidence of spondylolysis in the 18 patients they reviewed. Stoddard and Osborn reported a 54% incidence of spondylolysis in their patients with Scheuermann kyphosis (112).

Other conditions reported in patients with Scheuermann disease include endocrine abnormalities (113), hypovitaminosis (114), inflammatory disorders (112,113), and dural cysts (96,115).

## Clinical Presentation

Clinical signs of Scheuermann disease occur around the time of puberty. The clinical feature that distinguishes postural kyphosis from Scheuermann kyphosis is rigidity. Often, mild Scheuermann disease is believed to be postural because the kyphosis may be more flexible in the early stages than in later stages. Usually, the patient seeks treatment because of a parent's concern about poor posture. Sometimes the poor posture has been present for several months or longer, or the parents may have noticed a recent change during a growth spurt. Attributing kyphotic

deformity in a child to poor posture often causes a delay in diagnosis and treatment.

Pain may be the predominant clinical complaint rather than deformity. The pain is generally located over the area of the kyphotic deformity, but also occurs in the lower lumbar spine if compensatory lumbar lordosis is severe. Back pain is usually aggravated by standing, sitting, or physical activity. The distribution and intensity of the pain vary according to the age of the patient, the stage of the disease, the site of the kyphosis, and the severity of the deformity. Pain usually subsides with the cessation of growth, although pain in the thoracic spine can sometimes continue even after the patient is skeletally mature (77,116). More commonly, after growth is completed patients complain of low back pain caused by the compensatory or exaggerated lumbar lordosis.

Most symptoms relating to Scheuermann disease occur during the rapid growth phase. During the growth spurt, pain is reported by 22% of patients, but as the end of the adolescent growth spurt approaches, this figure reaches 60%. Some authors believe that when growth is complete the pain recedes completely, except for well-circumscribed paraspinal discomfort (117–119). In adult patients with Scheuermann disease, pain may be located in and around the posterior iliac crest. This pain is thought to result from arthritic changes at T11 and T12, because the posterior crest is supplied by this dermatome. Stagnara (120) believes that the mobile areas above and below the rigid segment are the source of pain.

Symptoms also depend on the apex of kyphosis. Murray et al. (77) noted that if the apex of kyphosis is in the upper thoracic spine, patients have more pain with everyday activities. The degree of kyphosis has also been correlated with symptoms. It seems logical that the larger the kyphosis, the more likely it is to be symptomatic, but Murray et al. (77) found that curves between 65 and 85 degrees produced the most symptoms, whereas curves of more than 85 degrees and less than 65 degrees produced fewer symptoms. However, in patients with thoracolumbar or lumbar kyphosis (atypical Scheuermann disease), activity decreased as the degree of kyphosis increased.

### Lumbar Scheuermann Disease

Patients with lumbar Scheuermann disease differ from those with thoracic deformity. These patients usually have low back pain but, unlike patients with the more common form of Scheuermann disease, their kyphotic deformity is not as noticeable. Pain is associated with spinal movement. Lumbar Scheuermann is especially common in men involved in competitive sports and in farm laborers, suggesting that the cause may be an injury to the vertebral physes from repeated trauma (121).

## Physical Examination

In a patient with Scheuermann disease, a thorough examination of the back and a complete neurologic evaluation are essential. With the patient standing, the shoulders appear to be rounded and the head protrudes forward. The anterior bowing of the shoulders is caused by tight pectoralis muscles. Angular kyphosis is seen most clearly when the patient is viewed from a lateral position and is asked to bend forward. Normally, the back exhibits a gradual rounding with forward bending, but in patients with Scheuermann disease an acute increase is evident in the kyphosis of the thoracic spine or at the thoracolumbar junction. Stagnara et al. (122) found cutaneous pigmentation to be common at the most protruding spinous process at the apex of the kyphosis, probably the result of friction exerted by the backs of chairs and clothing. Compensatory lumbar and cervical lordosis, with forward protrusion of the head, further increases the anterior flexion of the trunk. Associated hamstring and hip flexor muscle tightness are often present.

The kyphotic deformity has some rigidity and will not correct completely with hyperextension. Larger degrees of kyphosis are not necessarily more rigid, and the amount of rigidity will vary with the age of the patient (77).

The neurologic evaluation is usually normal but must not be overlooked. Spinal cord compression has been reported occasionally in patients with Scheuermann disease (123–127). Three types of neural compression have been reported: ruptured thoracic disc (128), intraspinal extradural cyst, and mechanical cord compression at the apex of kyphosis. However, spinal cord compression and neurologic compromise are rare (129). Bouchez et al. (70) found that only 1% of patients with a paralyzing disc herniation had Scheuermann disease. Ryan and Taylor (126) suggest that the factors influencing the onset of cord compression in patients whose cord compression is caused by the kyphosis alone are the angle of kyphosis, the number of segments involved, and the rate of change of the angle of kyphosis. This may be why neurologic findings are rare in Scheuermann kyphosis: the kyphosis occurs gradually, over several segments, and without acute angulation.

## Radiographic Examination

The most important radiographic views are anteroposterior and lateral views of the spine with the patient standing. The amount of kyphosis present is determined by the Cobb method on a lateral radiograph of the spine. This is accomplished by selecting the cranial- and caudal-most tilted vertebrae in the kyphotic deformity. A line is drawn along the superior end plate of the most cranial vertebra and the inferior end plate of the most caudal vertebra. Lines are drawn perpendicular to the lines along the end plates, and the angle they form where they meet is the degree of kyphosis (130).

The criterion for diagnosis of Scheuermann disease on a lateral radiograph is more than 5 degrees of wedging of at least three adjacent vertebrae (78). The degree of wedging is determined by drawing one line parallel to the superior end plate and another line parallel to the inferior end plate of the vertebra, and measuring the angle formed by their intersection. Bradford believes that three wedged vertebrae are not necessary for the diagnosis, but rather an abnormal, rigid kyphosis is indicative of Scheuermann disease (131).

The vertebral end plates are irregular, and the disc spaces are narrowed. The anteroposterior diameter of the apical vertebra is frequently increased (96) (Fig. 20.15). Associated Schmorl nodes are often seen in the vertebrae in the kyphosis. Flexibility is determined by taking a lateral radiograph with the patient lying over a bolster placed at the apex of the deformity, to hyperextend the spine and maximize the amount of correction seen on a hyperextension radiograph. On the lateral radiographs, most patients will be in negative sagittal balance (132). Sagittal balance is measured on the radiographs by dropping a plumb line from the center of the C7 vertebral body and measuring the distance from this line to the sacral promontory; a positive value indicates that the plumb line lies anterior to the promontory of the sacrum. Normal sagittal balance values are ± 2 cm to the sacral promontory. On a lateral radiograph of lumbar Scheuermann kyphosis, irregular

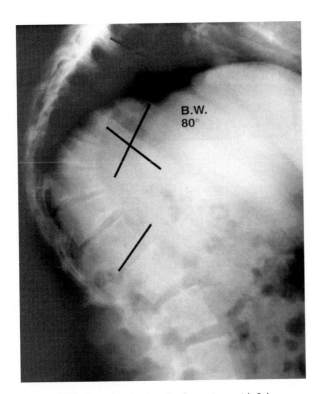

**Figure 20.15**   Lateral radiograph of a patient with Scheuermann disease demonstrates the kyphotic deformity seen in this disorder. Note the irregularity of the vertebral end plates and the anterior vertebral wedging.

end plates, Schmorl nodes, and disc-space narrowing will be seen, but vertebral-body wedging is not as common. MRI and CT scans are necessary only if the patient has unusual symptoms or positive neurologic findings. An anteroposterior or posteroanterior radiograph of the spine should be obtained to look for associated scoliosis or vertebral anomalies. The patient's skeletal maturity can be estimated from a radiograph of the left hand and wrist, or from the Risser sign on the anteroposterior radiograph of the spine.

### Treatment

The indications for the treatment of patients with Scheuermann kyphosis can be grouped into five general categories: pain, progression of deformity, neurologic compromise, cardiopulmonary compromise, and cosmesis.

Treatment options include observation, nonoperative methods, and surgery. Observation is an active form of treatment. If the deformity is mild and nonprogressive, the kyphosis can be observed every 4 to 6 months with lateral radiographs. The parents and patient must understand the need for regular follow-up visits. If the deformity begins to progress, another form of treatment, such as bracing, casting, or surgery, may be indicated.

Nonoperative methods of treatment include exercise, physical therapy, bracing, and casting. Exercise and physical therapy alone will not permanently improve kyphosis that is caused by skeletal changes. The improvement seen with these methods is due to improved muscle tone and correction of bad posture. The goals of physical therapy are to increase flexibility of the spine, correct lumbar hyperlordosis, strengthen extensor muscles of the spine, and stretch tight hamstring and pectoralis muscles. The efficacy of this treatment method has not been proven, and although it may improve the postural component of Scheuermann disease, its effect on a rigid kyphosis is questionable.

Other nonoperative treatment methods can be divided into active correction systems (braces) and passive correction systems (casts). For either a brace or a cast to be effective, the kyphotic curve must be flexible enough to allow correction of at least 40% to 50% (83,98,133).

The Milwaukee brace is the brace recommended for the treatment of Scheuermann disease (134) (Fig. 20.16). The

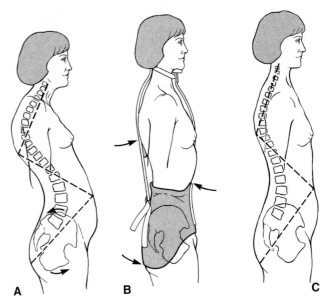

**Figure 20.16**   **A:** Patient with Scheuermann kyphosis has thoracic kyphosis, compensatory lumbar lordosis, anterior protrusion of the head, and rotation of the pelvis. **B:** Patient with Scheuermann kyphosis in a Milwaukee brace. The placement of the pelvic girdle, posterior thoracic pads, occipital pads, and neck ring encourage correction of the kyphosis. **C:** Correction of kyphosis after Milwaukee brace treatment. (Courtesy of Robert Winter, MD, Minneapolis.)

**A**          **B**          **C**

Milwaukee brace functions as a dynamic three-point orthosis that promotes extension of the thoracic spine. The neck ring maintains proper alignment of the upper thoracic spine, and the padded poster uprights apply pressure over the apex of the kyphosis. The pelvic girdle stabilizes the lumbar spine by flattening the lumbar lordosis. A low-profile brace, without a chin ring and with anterior shoulder pads, can be used for curves with an apex at the level of T9 or lower. The indications for brace treatment are an immature spine (at least 1 year of growth remaining in spine), some flexibility of the curve, and kyphosis of more than 50 degrees. The brace is initially worn full-time for an average of 12 to 18 months. If the curve is stabilized and no progression is noted after this time, a part-time brace program can be used until skeletal maturity is reached. Gutowski and Renshaw (135) reported that part-time bracing (16 hours per day) is as effective as full-time bracing, and is associated with improved patient compliance. In this study, a Boston lumbar orthosis was used to treat the kyphosis. The rationale for correction with this orthosis is that reduction of the lumbar lordosis causes the patient to dynamically straighten the thoracic kyphosis to maintain an upright posture. This presupposes a flexible thoracic kyphosis, a normal neurovestibular axis, and the absence of hip-flexion contractures.

Several orthopaedists have noted that, after initial improvement, there is a significant loss of correction after the discontinuation of brace treatment (50,136). Montgomery and Erwin (82) believe that if permanent correction of kyphosis is possible, a change in vertebral body wedging should be seen before bracing is discontinued. Although some loss of correction can occur after bracing is discontinued, it is still effective in obtaining some correction of the kyphosis, and possibly in reversing vertebral body wedging, or at least preventing progression of the kyphotic deformity (82) (Fig. 20.17). Poor results with brace treatment have been reported in patients in whom the kyphosis exceeded 75 degrees; in cases when the wedging of the vertebral bodies was more than 10 degrees; or when the patient was near or past skeletal maturity (131).

Antigravity and localizer casts have been used extensively in Europe for nonoperative treatment of Scheuermann kyphosis, with good results (120,137–139). De Mauroy and

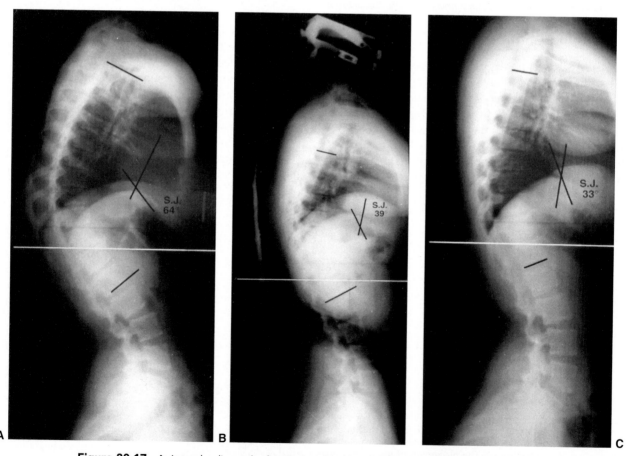

**Figure 20.17**   **A:** Lateral radiograph of a 15-year-old girl with a 64-degree thoracic kyphosis secondary to Scheuermann disease. **B:** Lateral radiograph of the patient in a Milwaukee brace with the kyphotic deformity improved to 39 degrees. **C:** Lateral radiograph obtained after the patient completed brace treatment; the kyphotic deformity has improved to 33 degrees.

Stagnara (137) developed a therapeutic regimen that uses serial casts for correction. This method consists of three stages. First, a physical therapy program is started in preparation for the casts. Next, three sequential antigravity casts, changed at 45-day intervals, are applied in order to obtain gradual correction of the deformity. The third stage involves the use of a plastic maintenance brace that is worn until skeletal maturity is reached. With this regimen the deformity was reported to improve by 40%, and there was less loss of correction after this form of nonoperative treatment was discontinued (120,138,139).

The indications for surgical correction remain unclear because of various opinions about pain, disability, trunk deformity, and importance of cosmesis. Therefore, the decision for surgery must be made on an individual basis. The current indications for surgery are a progressive kyphosis of more than 75 degrees, or significant kyphosis associated with pain that is not alleviated by nonoperative treatment methods. The biomechanical principles of correction of kyphosis secondary to Scheuermann disease include lengthening the anterior column (anterior release), providing anterior support (interbody fusion), and shortening and stabilizing the posterior column (compression instrumentation and arthrodesis) (140). Surgical correction of kyphosis can be achieved by a posterior approach, an anterior approach, or a combined anterior and posterior approach. The combined anterior and posterior approach has been the most frequently recommended and reliable procedure (141–144) (Fig. 20.18). A posterior procedure alone can be considered if the kyphosis can be corrected to, and maintained at, less than 50 degrees while a posterior fusion occurs (136–138,145,146). The spine can be instrumented with Harrington compression rods (77,147) or a posterior segmental hook-and-screw type of instrumentation system (148). If Harrington compression rods are used for posterior instrumentation, $\frac{1}{4}$-inch rods are used. Even when $\frac{1}{4}$-inch Harrington compression rods are used, a brace or cast should be applied after surgery to prevent rod breakage until a solid fusion is obtained. Prolonged immobilization is necessary, however, and there are potential complications. With posterior segmental instrumentation systems and the use of pedicle screws, posterior-only surgery for flexible curves has become more popular, but long-term outcome studies have yet to be published. When this type of instrumentation system is used, postoperative immobilization may not be required. Anterior instrumentation for Scheuermann disease has been reported by Kostuik (149); it consists of anterior interbody fusion and anterior instrumentation with a Harrington distraction system augmented by postoperative bracing. The single or dual rods and multiple bone screws that are available in the present-day spine instrumentation systems may be used instead of the Harrington distraction system. Although Kostuik has reported good results with this technique, the anterior instrumentation approach for treatment of Scheuermann kyphosis is not widely used (149).

When anterior and posterior surgery together are performed for Scheuermann disease, the anterior release and fusion are performed first. The anterior release can be done by an open anterior exposure or by thoracoscopy. The posterior fusion and instrumentation can be done on the same day as the anterior release and fusion, or they can be done as a staged procedure. Harrington compression rods can be used for posterior instrumentation, but usually a segmental instrumentation system using multiple hooks or pedicle screws is used. Lowe (143) and Coscia et al. (150) have reported a high complication rate after using Luque rods and wires for posterior fixation, because this system does not allow for any compression. The posterior instrumentation should include at least three fixation points above the apex and at least two fixation points below the apex of the kyphosis. The fusion and instrumentation should include the proximal vertebra in the measured kyphotic deformity and the first lordotic disc distally (104,132,140,151). If the fusion and instrumentation end in the kyphotic deformity, a junctional kyphosis at the end of the instrumentation is likely to develop.

Lowe emphasized that overcorrection of the deformity should be avoided in order to prevent junctional kyphosis (140,143). He recommended that no more than 50% of the preoperative kyphosis be corrected and that the final kyphosis should never be less than 40 degrees. He also found that patients with Scheuermann disease tend to be in negative sagittal balance and become further negatively balanced after surgery, which may predispose them to the development of junctional kyphosis (132). Reinhardt and Bassett (152) recommended fusion to the first square vertebra distally if the end vertebra distally is wedged, so as to prevent junctional kyphosis. The type of instrumentation used will determine whether postoperative immobilization is needed. This immobilization can consist of a brace or a Risser body cast. The patient's activity is restricted for 6 to 9 months until a solid fusion is obtained.

## POSTLAMINECTOMY KYPHOSIS

A laminectomy or multiple laminectomies are needed most often in children for the diagnosis and treatment of spinal cord tumors, but may also be needed for other conditions such as neurofibromatosis, Arnold-Chiari malformation, and syringomyelia (153,154). Although deformity after laminectomy is unusual in adults, it is common in children because of the unique and dynamic nature of the growing spine (128,155–159). Postlaminectomy deformities usually result in kyphotic deformity, but a scoliotic deformity may also occur (156).

The pathophysiology of postlaminectomy kyphotic deformity can be multifactorial. Deformity of the spine after multiple laminectomies can be caused by (a) skeletal deficiencies (facet joint, laminae, and associated anterior column defects), (b) ligamentous deficiencies,

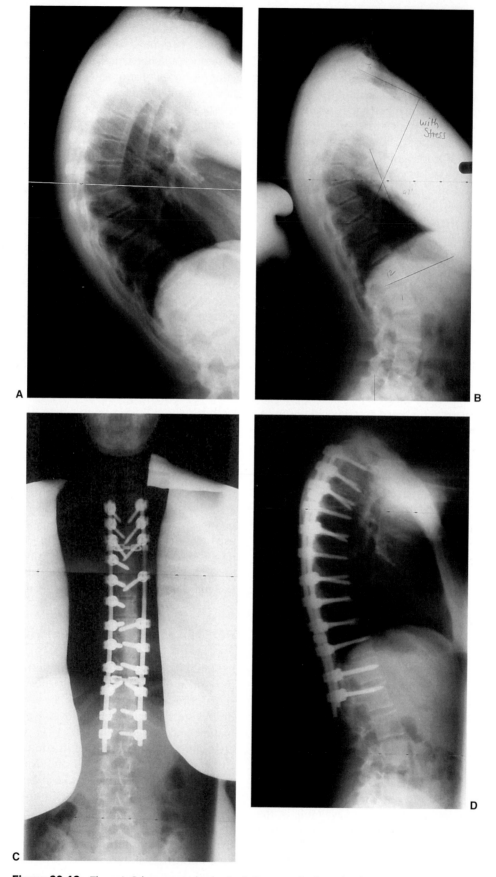

**Figure 20.18** Thoracic Scheuermann kyphosis. **A:** Preoperative lateral radiograph. **B:** Stress lateral radiograph. **C** and **D:** Postoperative status of posterior instrumentation and fusion with pedicle screws. (Courtesy of Dr. Anant Kumar.)

(c) neuromuscular imbalance, (d) effects of gravity, and (e) progressive osseous deformity resulting from growth disturbances (153,160). Panjabi et al. (161) showed that with loss of posterior stabilizing structures caused by removal of the interspinous ligaments, spinous processes, and laminae, the normal flexion forces placed on the spine will produce kyphosis. Gravity places a flexion moment on the spine, producing compression force on the anterior vertebrae and discs, and a tensile force on the remaining posterior structures. This may explain why postlaminectomy deformities occur most often in the cervical and thoracic spine and less often in the lumbar spine. Gravity tends to cause a kyphosis in the cervical and thoracic spine, whereas it accentuates the usual lordosis of the lumbar spine.

Skeletal deficiencies can also produce deformity. The factor noted as the most important one influencing the development of postlaminectomy deformity is the integrity of the facet joint (156,161–163). If the facet joint is removed or damaged during surgery, deformity is likely to develop. In addition, any secondary involvement of the anterior column, by tumor or surgical resection, adds to the risk of instability and deformity after laminectomy. Also, multiple laminectomies increase the risk of deformity when compared to single-level laminectomies (164,165).

Insufficient soft tissue restraints and paralysis of muscles that help stabilize the spine can also add to a postlaminectomy deformity. The spine is unable to resist the normal flexion forces placed on it by gravity and by the normal flexor muscles (166). Yasuoka et al. (167) noted increased wedging of the vertebrae and excessive motion after laminectomy in children, but not in adults. This increased wedging is caused by increased pressure on the cartilaginous end plates of the vertebral bodies. With time, the increased pressure will cause a decrease in growth of the anterior portion of the vertebrae, according to the Hueter-Volkmann principle (Fig. 20.19). Excessive spinal motion in children after laminectomy can be attributed to the facet joint anatomy in the cervical spine and the greater ligamentous laxity of growing children. The orientation of the cervical joint in a child is more horizontal than that seen in an adult. This horizontal orientation offers less resistance to forces that tend to cause kyphosis in the cervical spine.

Kyphosis is the most common deformity, although scoliosis may also occur, either as the primary deformity or in association with kyphosis. The incidence of postlaminectomy kyphotic deformity ranges from 33% to 100% (168), and depends on the age of the patient and the level of the laminectomy. Generally, the deformity is more likely in younger patients, and after more cephalad laminectomy. For example, Yasuoka et al. (167) found that spinal deformity occurred in 46% of patients younger than 15 years of age, but in only 6% of patients 15 to 24 years of age. All the patients between 15 and 24 years of age in whom deformity developed were 18 years of age or younger. Yasuoka et al. (167)

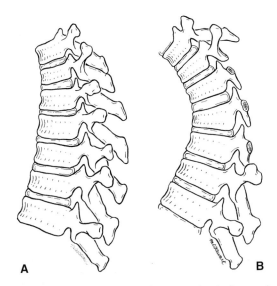

**A**                    **B**

**Figure 20.19** Drawings of the thoracic spine before and after repeated laminectomy demonstrate the effects on growth of the vertebral bodies. **A:** Before laminectomy, the anterior vertebral bodies are rectangular in configuration. **B:** The spine that has had multiple laminectomies will have increased compression anteriorly because of loss of posterior supporting structures. This compression results in less growth in the anterior portion of the vertebral body than in the posterior portion. In time, this will result in wedging of the vertebral bodies, causing a kyphotic deformity. (From Peterson HA. Iatrogenic spinal deformities. In: Weinstein SL, ed. *The pediatric spine: principles and practice.* New York: Raven, 1994:651.)

and Fraser et al. (169) found that higher levels of laminectomy were associated with a greater chance of deformity. In their studies, deformity occurred after 100% of cervical spine laminectomies, after 36% of thoracic laminectomies, and in none of the lumbar laminectomies. Hockley found that the greater the number of laminae removed, the greater the risk is for developing kyphosis (165,170).

Kyphosis in the cervical and thoracic spine is the most common postlaminectomy deformity. The lumbar spine is normally in lordosis, and this may protect it from developing kyphosis after multiple lumbar laminectomies. Papagelopoulos et al. (170) reported that hyperlordosis occurred in children who had lumbar laminectomies for intraspinal tumors. If the laminectomies extended into the thoracolumbar junction, kyphosis at the thoracolumbar junction occurred in 33% of his patients. Peter et al. (171) found that most of his patients did not develop a significant deformity after multiple lumbar laminectomies for selective posterior dorsal root rhizotomy; however, 9% developed spondylolysis. This may be the result of increased lordosis in this patient population (172).

Postlaminectomy deformity can occur early in the postoperative period or gradually over time. Kyphotic deformities have been reported to occur as late as 6 years after surgery (155,172). Progression can be either sudden or gradual, or the deformity may progress significantly only during the adolescent growth spurt.

The natural history of postlaminectomy spinal deformity is varied and depends on the age of the patient at the time of surgery, the location of the laminectomy or laminectomies, and the integrity of the facet joint. Three types of postlaminectomy kyphosis have been described in children: (a) instability after facetectomy, (b) hypermobility between vertebral bodies associated with gradual rounding of the spine, and (c) wedging of vertebral bodies caused by growth disturbances (168).

Kyphosis from instability after facetectomy tends to be sharp and angular and usually occurs in the immediate or early postoperative period, causing associated loss of neurologic function (Fig. 20.20). Gradual rounding of the kyphotic deformity is seen more often when the facet

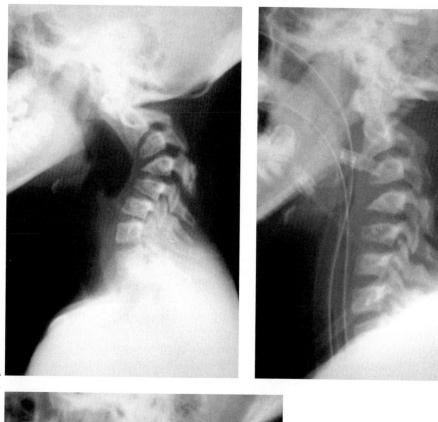

**Figure 20.20** Radiographs of a 13-year-old girl treated for a low-grade astrocytoma. She underwent resection of the tumor, a portion of the occiput, and the laminae of C1-C4, followed by radiotherapy at a dose of 5400 cGy. **A:** A progressive cervical kyphosis developed. Note wedging of the anterior vertebral body. **B:** Radiograph in halo traction demonstrates partial reduction of the kyphosis. **C:** Postoperative radiograph after anterior and posterior fusion.

joints are preserved. Kyphosis increases gradually over time because of the stress placed on the remaining posterior structures. If the spine is immature when the laminectomy is performed, the resulting kyphosis can inhibit the growth of the anterior growth plates of the involved vertebrae. Unequal growth results in wedge-shaped vertebrae and a progressive kyphotic deformity that is accelerated during the adolescent growth spurt.

Other associated conditions that also may add to or cause kyphotic deformities include persistent spinal cord tumors, neurologic deficits, intraspinal pathology (hydromyelia), and radiation therapy (173,174).

## Evaluation

The evaluation of a postlaminectomy deformity should focus on (a) the flexibility of the deformity, (b) loss of spinal structures, and (c) determination of future deformity with growth. The flexibility of a deformity can be estimated by flexion and extension lateral radiographs. If these cannot be obtained, a lateral traction film may be used. CT scans and three-dimensional reconstruction views may better delineate which bony elements are missing. MRI may be used but gives more information about the spinal cord, disc, and surrounding soft tissue than about the bony elements. To aid in preoperative planning, Lonstein recommends drawing the spine preoperatively (153). The lines should represent the spinous processes and intact laminae and facet joints. This may aid in predicting progression of a postlaminectomy deformity.

## Treatment

Treatment of postlaminectomy kyphosis is difficult, and it is best to prevent the deformity from occurring (175). The facet joints should be preserved whenever possible during laminectomy. Localized fusion at the time of facetectomy or laminectomy may help prevent progressive deformity (176). Because of the loss of bone mass posteriorly, however, localized fusion may not produce a large enough fusion mass to prevent kyphosis. Even so, this approach is advocated because it may produce enough bone mass posteriorly to stabilize what otherwise would be a severe progressive deformity.

The surgical technique of laminoplasty to expose the spinal cord may lessen the chance of progressive deformity. This approach involves suturing the laminae back in place after removal, or removing just one side of the laminae and allowing them to hinge open like a book to expose the spinal cord, then suturing that side of the laminae back in place (177–179). This procedure may provide only a fibrous tether connecting the laminae to the spine, but studies have shown a decreased incidence of postlaminectomy kyphosis when it has been used (180,181). Another technique is to hinge the laminae open in a lateral direction after dividing the laminae in the midline. This provides a lateral trough for the placement of bone graft for a lateral

fusion (182,183). The use of these techniques has been reported to decrease the incidence of postlaminectomy deformity (165,184).

After surgery in which the laminae have been removed, bracing has been suggested to prevent deformity (185,186), although no studies have documented the efficacy of this form of treatment. After the deformity has occurred and started to progress, bracing is ineffective in preventing further progression (153,156).

For progressive or marked deformity, spinal fusion is recommended, although the patient's long-term prognosis should be considered before making definitive treatment plans. If the prognosis for survival is poor, spinal fusion may not be appropriate. However, given the availability of effective treatment protocols for tumors and the improved survival rates, fusion is usually indicated for progressive deformity. Combined anterior and posterior spinal fusion is preferred in most patients (187) because the frequency of pseudarthrosis is greater if either procedure is done alone.

Lonstein (153) reported pseudarthrosis in 57% of patients after posterior fusion and in 15% of patients after anterior fusion. Anterior and posterior fusion can be performed on the same day, or as staged procedures. When the anterior procedure is performed, care must be taken to remove all the physes back to the posterior longitudinal ligament. Leaving some of the physes in the vertebral body can cause an increase in the deformity. When the posterior procedure is performed, instrumentation of the involved spine is desirable, but not always possible, because of the absence of posterior elements. The development of pedicle screw fixation has been helpful in allowing the use of posterior instrumentation for postlaminectomy kyphosis. When it can be performed safely, this procedure provides secure fixation while the spinal fusion is maturing. Torpey et al. (188) recommend a posterior fusion using titanium rod instrumentation at the time of laminectomy. The instrumentation provides stability postoperatively, and the titanium rods allow for postoperative MRI to evaluate spinal cord tumors. In certain cases, anterior instrumentation with rod and bone screws or plates may be used in order to obtain stability and correction of the deformity (188). If the deformity is severe or long-standing, anterior release followed by halo traction, or a halo cast with an Ilizarov device, can be used for obtaining gradual correction (189,190).

## RADIATION KYPHOSIS

The relative radiosensitivity of growing cartilage was discovered by investigators during the 1940s. Animal studies by Engel (191,192), Gall et al. (193), Hinkel (194), Barr et al. (195), and Reidy et al. (196) documented radiation-induced growth inhibition in growing cartilage and bone. The longitudinal growth of a vertebral body takes place through normal endochondral ossification, similar to the longitudinal growth of the metaphyses of long bones. Bick and Copel (88,89) demonstrated this on histologic sections in fresh autopsy specimens of vertebral bodies, taken from research subjects ranging in age from 14 weeks of fetal development to 23 years. This endochondral ossification at the physeal growth plate is radiosensitive (88,89,191,192,194,196,197). Engel (191,192) and Arkin and Simon (198) were able to produce spinal deformities in experimental animals using radiation. Arkin et al. (199) were the first to report a case of spinal deformity in humans that was caused by radiation. After these reports, it has become clear that exposing an immature spine to radiation can produce spinal deformity, including scoliosis, kyphoscoliosis, lordoscoliosis, and kyphosis.

The three most common solid tumors of childhood for which radiation therapy is part of the treatment regimen, and in which the vertebral column is included in the radiation fields, are neuroblastoma, Wilms tumor, and medulloblastoma. Early in the history of radiation therapy, survival rates were poor and spinal deformities were not as prevalent. With improved treatment protocols and survival rates, the incidence of spinal deformities has increased. The degree of growth inhibition of the spine is related to the accumulated radiation dose and the age of the child when the spine is irradiated. Progression is directly dependent on the remaining growth potential in the irradiated vertebrae. The younger the child and the greater the accumulated radiation dose, the greater the chance of deformity (200–205). The most severe growth changes occur in patients who are 2 years of age or younger at the time of irradiation. Initial vertebral changes usually occur 6 months to 2 years after radiation exposure (206), but the deformity may not become apparent until years later, after a period of growth (201,204).

Reports of radiation involving the spinal column show that an accumulated dose of less than 1000 cGy does not produce a detectable inhibition of vertebral growth, whereas a dose of 1000 to 2000 cGy causes a temporary inhibiting effect on growth. Sometimes this is manifested as a transverse growth arrest line in the vertebra, which gives the appearance of a bone within a bone. A dose of radiation between 2000 and 3000 cGy causes irregularity or scalloping of vertebral end plates and diminution of axial height and sometimes leads to a flattened, beaked vertebra (201,202,204,206–210). A dose of 5000 cGy causes bone necrosis (202). The effect that radiation has on soft tissue also affects the progression of spinal deformity. The soft tissue anterior to the spine and the abdominal muscle can become fibrotic and act as a tether with growth, adding to the deformity of the spine as the child grows (211).

The incidence of spinal deformity after irradiation of the spine has been reported to range from 10% to 100% (201,204,205,207,212–215). These rates are decreasing because of shielding of growth centers, symmetric field selection, and decreased total accumulated radiation doses. The last of these changes has resulted from an increase in the use and effectiveness of chemotherapeutic regimens that reduce the need for large doses of radiation. Early reports showed an increased incidence of scoliotic deformities with the use of asymmetric radiation fields, and the incidence of kyphotic postirradiation deformities has increased with the use of symmetric radiation fields (216).

Any child who has received irradiation of the spine should be observed carefully for the development of spinal deformity. Because the development of deformity is related to the amount of disordered growth in the vertebral bodies that were affected by irradiation, it depends to a large extent on the amount of growth left in the spine when the irradiation was started, and the amount of damage to the physes caused by irradiation (which correlates directly with the accumulated radiation dose). If the dose of radiation is large enough to cause permanent damage to the physes, the deformity will be progressive. Postirradiation scoliosis and kyphosis both progress more rapidly during times of rapid growth such as the adolescent growth period (204,205,208,216). Before the adolescent growth spurt, the deformity may remain relatively stable or progress at a steady rate. Severe curves can continue to progress even after skeletal maturity, and these patients may require continued observation.

Radiographic evaluation of a postirradiation deformity should include standard posteroanterior and lateral radiographs of the spine. Occasionally, CT scans with sagittal or coronal reconstruction are needed for better delineation of the vertebral body deformities. The spinal cord and surrounding soft tissue are evaluated best with MRI. Neuhauser et al. (202) described the radiographic changes seen in irradiated spines. The earliest changes were alterations in the vertebral bodies within the irradiated section of the spine caused by impairment of endochondral growth at the vertebral end plates. Growth arrest lines produced a bone-within-a-bone picture. This occurred in 28% of the 81 patients in the study by Riseborough et al. (204). Other radiographic changes were end-plate irregularity with an altered trabecular pattern, and decreased vertebral body height. This pattern was the most common radiographic change reported by Riseborough et al. (83%) (204). Contour abnormalities causing anterior narrowing and beaking of the vertebral bodies, much like those seen in patients with conditions that affect endochondral ossification (e.g., Morquio syndrome, achondroplasia), were the third type of radiographic change noted by Neuhauser et al. (202).

## Treatment

Milwaukee brace treatment has been recommended for progressive curves, but generally has been ineffective for postirradiation kyphosis (204,216), especially in patients with soft tissue contractures contributing to the deformity. The irradiated skin may also be of poor quality, making long-term brace wear difficult. If progression occurs, spinal fusion, with or without instrumentation, should be performed regardless of the age of the patient. Because bone quality is poor, fusion can be difficult to obtain after a single attempt. Anterior and posterior fusion are recommended, and should extend at least one or two levels above and below the end of the kyphosis (168,188,204,216–218). The posterior fusion mass may require reexploration and repeated bone grafting after 6 months, and immobilization may need to be prolonged for 6 to 12 months. Posterior instrumentation should be used whenever feasible, because it adds increased stability while the fusion mass is maturing and may allow for some limited correction of the kyphotic deformity (Fig. 20.21). Anterior instrumentation can be used in certain cases. However, because of the radiation, the vertebral bodies usually remain in an infantile form, and instrumentation with bone screws may be difficult.

Correction of postirradiation kyphosis is difficult. Typically, these curves are rigid, and soft tissue scarring and contractures often further hamper correction. Healing can be prolonged, and pseudarthrosis is common. Infection is a frequent complication in these patients because of poor vascularity of the irradiated tissue (204). Riseborough et al. (204) reported a pseudarthrosis rate of 37% and an infection rate of 23% in his patients after surgery. King and Stowe (216) also reported a high complication rate in patients who were treated surgically. Because viscera also can be damaged by irradiation, bowel obstruction, perforation, and fistula formation may occur after spinal fusion. This can be difficult to differentiate from postoperative cast syndrome, and the treating physician should be aware of this complication (219). Radiation myelopathy may also occur in this patient population (220). King and Stowe (216) reported postoperative paraplegia in 2 of 7 patients who had undergone radiation treatment for neuroblastoma and surgery for correction of their kyphotic spine deformity. King and Stowe believed that these two patients had a subclinical form of radiation myelopathy and that spinal correction compromised what little vascular supply there was to the cord. Therefore, the surgeon should be aware of this possibility and try to avoid overcorrection.

# MISCELLANEOUS CAUSES OF KYPHOTIC DEFORMITIES

Spinal deformity in the sagittal plane can occur in patients with skeletal dysplasia (221,222). The natural history of spinal deformity varies with the type of deformity and the type of dysplasia. Some sagittal plane deformities that appear severe at birth or in infancy improve spontaneously with growth, whereas others continue to progress and eventually can cause paraplegia. A knowledge of the various skeletal dysplasias and the natural history of sagittal plane deformities in each is necessary to prevent overtreatment and undertreatment.

## Achondroplasia

Treatment of spinal problems is required most often in patients with achondroplasia. The most common sagittal plane deformity in achondroplastic dwarfs is thoracolumbar kyphosis (223–225). The kyphosis is usually detected at birth, and is accentuated when the child is sitting because of the associated hypotonia in these infants (226). Ambulation is delayed until approximately 18 months of age, but after ambulation begins, the thoracolumbar kyphosis tends to improve. The kyphosis usually does not resolve in children who have more hypotonia. According to Lonstein (227), thoracolumbar kyphosis resolves in 70% of achondroplastic dwarfs, and persists in 30%. In one third of these patients, or 10% of achondroplastic dwarfs, the thoracolumbar kyphosis is progressive (227) (Fig. 20.22).

A lateral radiograph of the thoracolumbar spine during infancy shows anterior wedging of the vertebrae at the apex of the kyphosis (225). In patients whose thoracolumbar kyphosis resolves, the anterior vertebral body wedging also improves. When the kyphosis is progressive, anterior vertebral body wedging persists.

Sponseller has reported three reasons why thoracolumbar kyphosis should be corrected: (a) it may cause pressure on the conus and result in neurologic symptoms; (b) it results in an increase in the compensatory lumbar lordosis, which can increase problems from an already stenotic lumbar spine; (c) it may increase significantly if decompressive laminectomies are needed for lumbar stenosis in the future (226).

If no improvement in the thoracolumbar kyphosis is evident once a child begins walking, a thoracolumbosacral orthosis (TLSO) is recommended in order to try to prevent progression of the kyphosis (228–231). Early treatment to prevent the development of a progressive kyphosis has been recommended by Pauli et al. (232). They developed an algorithm for treatment of the young achondroplastic patient, first counseling the parents against unsupported sitting and continuing with close follow-up. If kyphosis develops and is greater than 30 degrees, TLSO bracing is begun and continued until the child is walking independently and there is evidence of improvement in vertebral body wedging and kyphosis. Using this form of early intervention, Pauli et al. (232) reported no occurrences of progressive kyphosis. Sponseller recommends serial hyperextension casting if the kyphosis does not respond to bracing. If there is a satisfactory response to serial casting (50% or more correction in 3 to 4 months), brace treatment can be resumed (226).

Indications for surgery are documented progression of a kyphotic deformity, kyphosis of more than 40 degrees in a child older than 5 or 6 years of age, and neurologic deficits relating to the spinal deformity (224,226,233). Distinguishing between neurologic deficits that result from a kyphotic deformity and those associated with lumbar stenosis (which is common in achondroplastic dwarfs) can

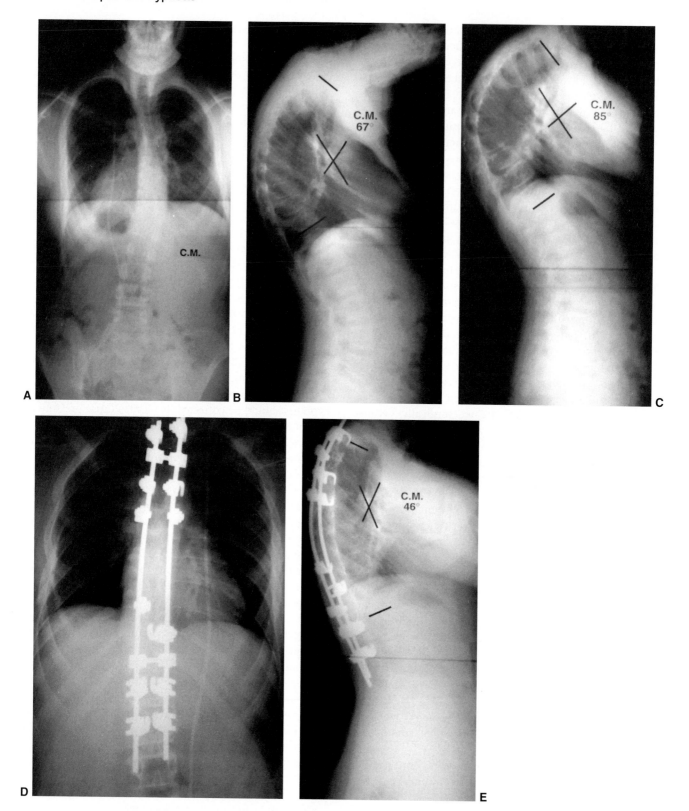

**Figure 20.21** **A** and **B:** Anteroposterior and lateral radiographs of a 16-year-old child with a suprasellar germinoma treated with resection and 3400 cGy of radiation to the base of the skull and the entire spine. Radiographs demonstrate a 67-degree kyphosis with associated scoliosis. **C:** The kyphosis progressed to 85 degrees over 18 months despite bracing. **D** and **E:** Anteroposterior and lateral radiographs after anterior and posterior fusion with posterior instrumentation. The kyphosis has been corrected to 46 degrees.

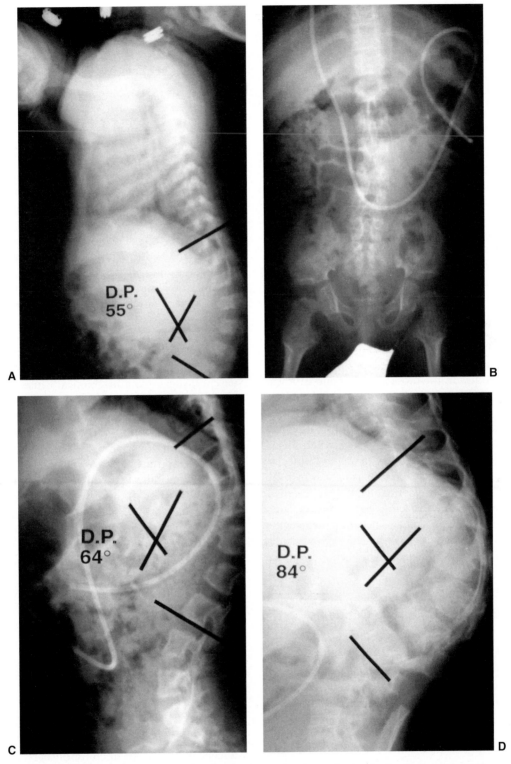

**Figure 20.22**  Achondroplastic dwarf with progressive thoracolumbar kyphosis. **A:** Lateral radiograph at 1 year of age shows a 55-degree thoracolumbar kyphosis. **B:** Anteroposterior radiograph at 5 years of age shows narrowing of the lumbar interpedicular distance characteristic of achondroplasia. **C:** Lateral radiograph at 5 years of age reveals a 64-degree kyphosis. **D:** Lateral radiograph at 9 years of age shows an 84-degree thoracolumbar kyphotic deformity.

be difficult. A thorough physical examination and diagnostic studies such as CT scan and MRI may be necessary in order to determine appropriate treatment. The infant should be evaluated for foramen magnum stenosis, because this may be the underlying cause for the hypotonia and delayed ambulation in achondroplastic patients with kyphosis. If present, the stenosis should be treated by decompression of the foramen magnum (234). Most patients with progressive thoracolumbar kyphosis require combined anterior and posterior fusion. Instrumentation that uses hooks or wires that go into the spinal canal is not recommended in these patients because the small size of the spinal canal and the lack of epidural fat make instrumentation hazardous. Ain has reported good results with anterior fusion and instrumentation combined with posterior fusion. This has the advantage of not entering an already stenotic spinal canal and giving secure fixation to aid in spinal fusion (235).

## Pseudoachondroplasia

Kyphotic deformities can also occur in children with pseudoachondroplasia and are caused by wedging of multiple vertebral bodies in the thoracolumbar and thoracic spine. The kyphotic deformity in patients with pseudoachondroplasia differs from that in patients with achondroplasia. In patients with pseudoachondroplasia, the kyphosis involves multiple levels, and is less acutely angular than the deformity in patients with achondroplasia, which involves only one or two levels. Bracing may prevent progression of this deformity, but surgery is indicated if progression occurs despite bracing. Spinal fusion with instrumentation can be performed safely in patients with pseudoachondroplasia because there is no associated stenosis of the spinal canal as in patients with achondroplasia (236,237).

## Spondyloepiphyseal Dysplasia Congenita

Thoracolumbar kyphotic deformities occur in approximately half of the patients with congenital spondyloepiphyseal dysplasia; these deformities usually respond to a modified TLSO (226). If surgery is needed for a progressive kyphosis, anterior and posterior fusions are recommended (237).

## Diastrophic Dwarfism

Spinal deformity is a common finding in diastrophic dysplasia (238). These spinal deformities consist of cervical kyphosis, thoracic kyphoscoliosis, and lumbar hyperlordosis. Midcervical kyphosis occurs in 15% to 33% of patients with diastrophic dwarfism (226,239,240). However, Remes et al. and Herring have reported spontaneous improvement (239–241). Progressive cervical kyphosis (>60 degrees) can be stabilized with a spinal fusion (210,220,221). If a posterior fusion is to be performed, the increased incidence

of cervical spina bifida in diastrophic dwarfism must be considered during dissection (239,240,242).

## Mucopolysaccharidosis

Mucopolysaccharidoses are inherited lysosomal storage disorders caused by deficiency of the enzymes that are necessary for the degradation of glycosaminoglycans. There are at least 13 types of mucopolysaccharidoses. The more common names of this condition are Hurler, Hunter, Sanfilippo, Morquio, and Moroteux-Lamy syndromes. Bone marrow transplantation has increased the life expectancy of these patients. Before this treatment method became available, most children did not survive long enough to require intervention for spinal deformities. With increased survival, progressive kyphotic deformities of the spine with neurologic compromise are being reported (243–245). Despite bone marrow transplantation, the deposition of metabolites in bone is not reversed to the same extent as that in soft tissue (246).

Children with mucopolysaccharidosis develop thoracolumbar kyphosis, with anterior beaking and flattening of the vertebral bodies at the level of the kyphotic deformity. Swischuk suggested a mechanical cause for the anterior beaking (247). He postulated that hypotonia results in thoracolumbar kyphosis, resulting in herniation of the nucleus pulposus into the anterior vertebral body, which causes the anterior beaking of the vertebral body. Field, however, examined two specimens at postmortem and found that the end-plate formation was normal, but there was a failure of ossification in the anterosuperior part of the vertebral body (246).

Bracing may be used in order to prevent progression of the kyphotic deformity, but the effectiveness of this form of treatment has not been documented. Spinal fusion is recommended for a progressive kyphosis in patients with mucopolysaccharidosis. Tandon reported good results with posterior spinal fusion, and Dalvie has reported good results with anterior fusion and instrumentation (243,244). Further studies will be needed to determine which approach is best, but the goal of surgery is to obtain a stable fusion of the involved area to prevent any further progression of the kyphosis (226,237,248).

## Gaucher Disease

Gaucher disease is an uncommon hereditary glycolipid storage disorder characterized by the accumulation of glucocerebroside in the lysosomes of macrophages of the reticuloendothelial system. Splenomegaly with associated pancytopenia is the most common clinical manifestation. The skeletal manifestations are caused by infiltration of the bone marrow by Gaucher cells; they include bone crisis, pathologic fracture, osteopenia, osteonecrosis, and osteomyelitis. Progressive kyphosis of the spine has been reported in these patients. The proposed etiology of the kyphosis is infiltration of the bone marrow by Gaucher cells, resulting in bone crisis, osteopenia, and osteonecrosis that lead to vertebral body collapse, often on multiple levels. Kyphosis can be progressive because of continued vertebral body collapse or growth abnormalities secondary to vertebral body collapse. If a progressive kyphosis develops, surgical intervention is recommended. If the spine is still flexible, posterior fusion and instrumentation are adequate, but if the deformity is rigid, anterior and posterior fusion and instrumentation are needed (Fig. 20.23) (249,250).

## Marfan Syndrome

Marfan syndrome is a generalized disorder of connective tissue that affects the supporting structures of the body, especially those in the musculoskeletal system. This syndrome is caused by mutations in coding of the genes for the glycoprotein fibrillin (251,252). Spinal deformity is the most common skeletal abnormality in Marfan syndrome, and scoliosis is the most common of these spinal deformities (227,253–258). Thoracic lordosis has been traditionally reported as the most common sagittal plane deformity (259,260). In some patients, the thoracic lordosis becomes severe enough to compromise respiration. With the lordotic posture of the thoracic spine, an associated kyphosis or relative kyphosis may develop in the lumbar spine. A third common spinal deformity associated with Marfan syndrome is thoracolumbar kyphosis, which affects approximately 10% of patients (Fig. 20.24). These spinal deformities usually occur during the juvenile growth period, before the adolescent growth spurt (260). Sponseller et al. found that 41% of their patients with Marfan syndrome had a kyphotic deformity of more than 50 degrees, with a tendency toward longer kyphoses extending through the thoracolumbar junction (261).

Brace treatment has been recommended to try to halt the progression of spinal deformity but has been found to be ineffective (262,263). Correction of kyphotic deformities requires anterior and posterior spinal fusion with segmental instrumentation (262). Thoracic lordosis is corrected by posterior segmental instrumentation to correct the lordotic deformity, followed by posterior fusion (264). Because dural ectasia corrodes pedicles, a CT scan of the pedicles should be obtained to plan fixation. In addition, fusion should be extended. Complications are more frequent after surgical correction of spinal deformity in patients with Marfan syndrome than after spinal surgery in other patients (262).

Cervical spine abnormalities are also common in patients with Marfan syndrome, but clinical problems from these

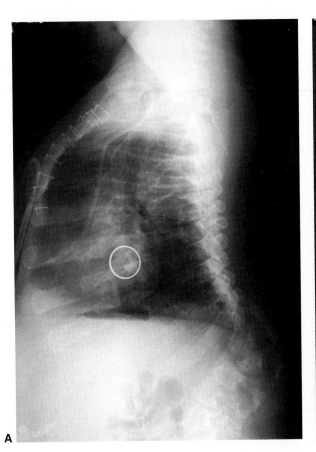
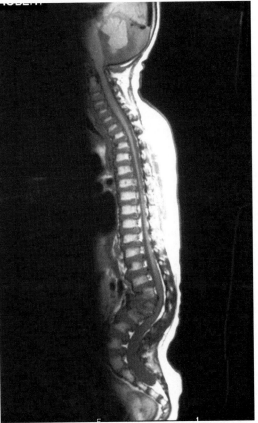

**Figure 20.23** Lateral radiograph **(A)** and magnetic resonance imaging (MRI) **(B)** demonstrate progressive thoracolumbar kyphosis in a patient with Gaucher disease.

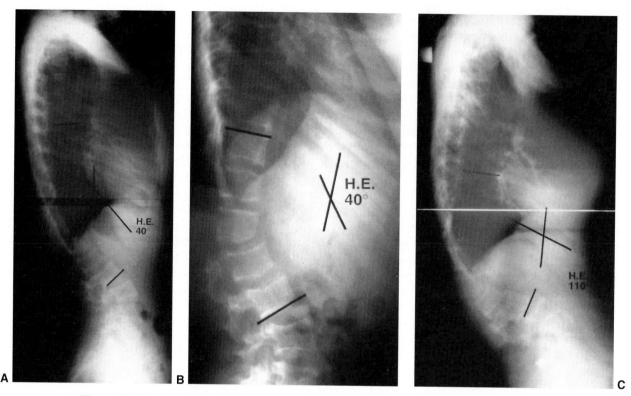

**Figure 20.24**   **A** and **B:** Lateral radiographs of a 17-year-old child with Marfan syndrome and a 40-degree progressive thoracolumbar kyphosis. **C:** Lateral radiograph of the same patient 3 years later shows that the thoracolumbar kyphosis has progressed to 110 degrees.

abnormalities are rare. Basilar impression and focal cervical kyphosis are the most frequently reported cervical spine abnormalities. Focal cervical kyphosis is usually associated with a lordotic thoracic spine (265).

Because of the increased incidence of cervical spine abnormalities, Hobbs et al. (265) have recommended that patients with Marfan syndrome should avoid sports that involve risks of high-impact loading of the cervical spine.

## Larsen Syndrome

In 1950, Larsen et al. (266) described a congenital malformation syndrome (267) consisting of facial dysmorphism and hyperelasticity of the joints, with congenital dislocation of the knees and frequent dislocation of the hips and elbows (119,268–271). Equinovarus or valgus foot deformities and ancillary calcaneal nuclei are also characteristic features of this syndrome. Abnormalities of the cervical spine, specifically cervical kyphosis, were not emphasized in the original description, and often this life-threatening finding is overlooked (189,268,272). Johnston et al. (267) reported cervical kyphosis and vertebral body anomalies in five of nine patients with Larsen syndrome. The apex of the kyphosis usually occurs at the fourth or fifth cervical vertebra, with marked hypoplasia of one or two of the vertebral bodies (Fig. 20.25). Cervical kyphosis is present in infants with Larsen syndrome. Developmental delay may be attributed to hypotonia and dislocation of the knees or hips, but the underlying cause for

developmental delay may be a chronic myelopathy from the cervical kyphosis. Cervical kyphosis and vertebral hypoplasia are easily demonstrated on lateral C-spine radiographs. Flexion and extension views are usually not needed and may be difficult to obtain safely in an infant. MRI scans will demonstrate spinal cord compression or compromise.

The treatment recommendation for cervical kyphosis in Larsen syndrome is the use of an early posterior arthrodesis to stabilize the spine. An *in situ* posterior arthrodesis with autogenous iliac crest bone graft, followed by immobilization in either a halo or Minerva cast or custom orthosis, is recommended. Reduction of the kyphosis is obtained only in the postoperative halo or Minerva cast or orthosis stage of the treatment. Johnston et al. (267) found that, over a period of time following a solid posterior arthrodesis, a gradual correction of the kyphosis occurs because of continued anterior vertebral body growth. Because the posterior arthrodesis is performed at a young age, the patient must be followed for potential complications from continued anterior growth, which would result in lordosis. Johnston and Schoenecker (273) described a patient who developed neurologic symptoms from this growth-related lordosis.

## Posttraumatic Deformities

Kyphosis can occur as a direct result of trauma to the spinal column or the spinal cord. Deformity can occur at a

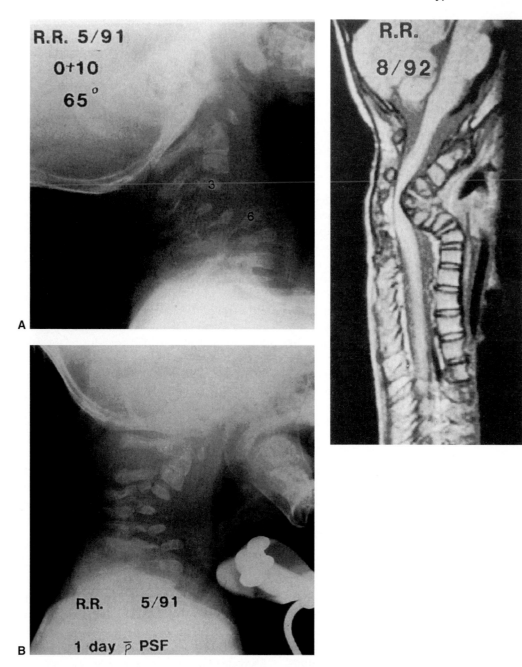

**Figure 20.25** Larsen syndrome. **A:** Lateral radiograph of a 10-month-old patient showing kyphosis of 65 degrees, with correction to only 48 degrees in extension. **B:** Lateral radiograph immediately after posterior arthrodesis, showing the patient with orthosis and correction of kyphosis to 39 degrees. **C:** T2-weighted magnetic resonance image 15 months postoperatively shows severe impingement on spinal cord. Kyphosis had progressed to 110 degrees, and the patient was quadriplegic after a fall. (From Johnston CE, Birch JG, Daniels JL. Cervical kyphosis in patients who have Larsen syndrome. *J Bone Joint Surg Am* 1996;78:538.)

fracture site from a malunion, chronic instability leading to progressive deformity, paralysis after spinal cord injury, or from anterior growth arrest (274–278). Kyphosis at the fracture site is acute and spans a short segment of vertebrae. Paralytic kyphosis is a long, C-shaped deformity that spans many vertebral segments. Progressive kyphosis may also occur after development of a posttraumatic syrinx (279).

Kyphosis at a fracture site requires surgical intervention for correction. Anterior, posterior, and combined anterior

and posterior procedures have been described for correction of posttraumatic kyphosis (280–284). Brace treatment has been ineffective for progressive paralytic kyphosis (274), and surgery is indicated for paralytic kyphosis of more than 60 degrees. If the kyphosis is flexible and can be reduced to less than 50 degrees, posterior fusion with segmental instrumentation can be performed. If the kyphosis is rigid and cannot be reduced to less than 50 degrees on preoperative bending view x-ray films, anterior release and fusion should be followed by posterior fusion and segmental instrumentation (274,278).

## Neurofibromatosis

Kyphoscoliosis is common in patients with neurofibromatosis, although kyphosis may be the predominant deformity (285). Funasaki et al. (286) found that 50% of their patients with neurofibromatosis and spinal deformity had an abnormal sagittal curve. The vertebral bodies are frequently deformed and attenuated at the apex of the kyphosis. Dystrophic vertebral body changes may develop over time (287,288). Crawford (287,289) described this as modulation of the deformity, from a nondystrophic curve to a dystrophic curve. The kyphosis is typically sharp and angular over a relatively small number of vertebral segments. Severely angular kyphosis can cause neurologic compromise (290,291). Lonstein et al. (292) found that cord compression due to spinal curvature from neurofibromatosis was second only to congenital kyphosis as a cause of spinal cord compression. The kyphosis in patients with neurofibromatosis typically involves the thoracic spine or upper thoracic spine. Involvement of the cervical and cervicothoracic vertebrae has also been reported (290,293–297).

Kyphotic deformities with dystrophic changes tend to be progressive, and they more commonly lead to neurologic compromise.

Treatment of kyphoscoliosis in patients with neurofibromatosis begins with a thorough physical examination for neurologic abnormalities. MRI scans should be obtained to demonstrate any intraspinal lesions, such as pseudomeningocele, dural ectasia, or neurofibroma, which may cause impingement on the spinal cord (298). Any intraspinal lesions should be treated appropriately before spinal fusion and instrumentation are undertaken. Because posterior fusion done alone has resulted in a high rate of pseudarthrosis (65%) (299), combined anterior and posterior spinal fusion combined with posterior instrumentation is recommended (300). Titanium instrumentation is preferred so as to allow for future MRI studies of the spine. Abundant autogenous bone grafts and prolonged immobilization may be required in order to obtain a solid fusion in these patients, and repeated bone grafting may be required 6 months after the initial surgery. Vascularized fibular or rib grafts may also be used for anterior fusion and structural support (99,287,293, 296,301–303).

## Tuberculosis

There is spine involvement in 50% of patients with skeletal tuberculosis (304). Spinal tuberculosis is the most dangerous form of skeletal tuberculosis because of its ability to cause bone destruction, deformity, and paraplegia. In childhood spinal tuberculosis, the extent and degree of abscess formation is greater than that seen in adult tuberculosis, but paraplegia is less common in children than in adults with spinal tuberculosis (305). The most frequent site of spinal tuberculosis in children is the thoracolumbar junction and its adjacent segments. Tuberculosis infection usually destroys the anterior elements of the spine and results in a significant angular kyphosis at the infected site. The involved anterior vertebral bodies usually fuse once the infection is adequately treated. In young children, continued growth of the intact posterior element can cause a late increase in kyphosis in an already kyphotic spine (305).

All forms of active spinal tuberculosis are treated with a complete course of chemotherapy. First-line drugs are streptomycin, isoniazid, and rifampicin, and second-line drugs are ethambutol and pyrazinamide (306). Medical therapies for spinal tuberculosis will adequately treat the tuberculum infection in most cases (304,307–310). Bracing or casting has been used along with medical therapy to try to prevent progression of kyphosis during therapy. Rajasekaran found an average increase of 15 degrees in deformity in all patients who were treated nonsurgically (311). The greatest increase in deformity occurred during the first 6 months of treatment.

Indications for surgery in spinal tuberculosis are spinal instability, neurologic involvement, prevention or correction of spinal deformity, drainage of significant abscesses, or diagnostic biopsy (307). Neurologic involvement and present or impending paraplegia are more obvious indications for surgical intervention than the other indications. Rajasekaran described four prognostic signs to predict spinal instability and late increase in deformity. When more than two signs are present, this is a reliable predictor of progressive deformity and spinal instability. These prognostic signs include: (a) dislocation of the facets, (b) posterior retropulsion of the diseased fragments, (c) lateral translation of the vertebrae in the anteroposterior view, and (d) toppling of the superior vertebra (Figs. 20.26 and 20.27) (312). Other factors that lead to a significant increase in kyphosis in children who are not treated surgically are involvement of three or more vertebral bodies, initial kyphosis of more than 30 degrees, and age younger than 15 years (313–315).

Several different surgical approaches have been used in the treatment of spinal tuberculosis (316–320). Anterior debridement and strut grafting, with or without a posterior fusion and instrumentation, has the most consistent long-term results (306,321–332). Good results have been reported with the use of allografts for structural support anteriorly (333–335). Anterior debridement and fusion with anterior instrumentation of the spine has also had positive results in the treatment of spinal tuberculosis (336,337). Some correction of the kyphosis may be obtained at the time of surgery. Kyphosis can also be a problem in patients with healed spinal tuberculosis (338). The infected area of the anterior spine usually fuses, and continued growth posteriorly causes progressive kyphosis that can result in paraplegia. The presence of neurologic symptoms is an indication for anterior decompression and

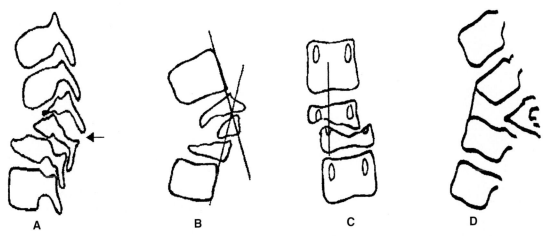

**A**          **B**          **C**          **D**

**Figure 20.26**  Radiologic signs for the spine at risk. **A:** *Separation of the facet joint.* The facet joint dislocates at the level of the apex of the curve, causing instability and loss of alignment. In severe cases the separation can occur at two levels. **B:** *Posterior retropulsion.* This is identified by drawing two lines along the posterior surface of the first normal vertebrae above and below the curve. The diseased segments are found to be posterior to the intersection of the lines. **C:** *Lateral translation.* This is confirmed when a vertical line drawn through the middle of the pedicle of the first lower normal vertebra does not touch the pedicle of the first upper normal vertebra. **D:** *Toppling sign.* In the initial stages of collapse, a line drawn along the anterior surface of the first lower normal vertebra intersects the inferior surface of the first upper normal vertebra. "Tilt" or "toppling" occurs when the line intersects higher than the middle of the anterior surface of the first normal upper vertebra. (Reproduced with permission and copyright of the British Editorial Society of Bone and Joint Surgery. Rajasekaran S. The natural history of post-tubercular kyphosis in children. *J Bone Joint Surg* 2001;83B:954.)

fusion, which can be followed by posterior fusion and instrumentation.

## Juvenile Osteoporosis

Idiopathic juvenile osteoporosis is an acquired systemic condition that consists of generalized osteoporosis in otherwise normal prepubertal children (339). Although idiopathic juvenile osteoporosis is uncommon, associated kyphosis and back pain are common in patients with this condition.

Schippers (340) first described this condition in 1939 and, since that time, other authors have described its clinical findings and natural history (143,341–347). The etiology of idiopathic juvenile osteoporosis is unknown. Laboratory values of serum calcium, phosphorus, alkaline phosphatase, parathyroid hormone, and osteocalcin are normal. The collagen type and ratios from skin biopsy samples are also normal. There have been some reports of a slight decrease in 1,25-dihydroxyvitamin D (345,348,349), but the significance of this finding is not known. Low serum calcitonin levels have also been reported, but treatment with calcitonin has not proven to be beneficial (343,350). In contrast, Saggese et al. (346) noted normal serum calcitonin levels in their patients. Green (351) believes that a mild deficiency of 1,25-dihydroxyvitamin D can explain most of the findings in idiopathic juvenile osteoporosis. During rapid growth phases the deficiency is discovered because growth requirements cannot keep pace, causing a relative osteoporosis. When puberty occurs, the increase in sex hormone overcomes the deficit in 1,25-dihydroxyvitamin D, and the relative osteoporosis improves. This theory has yet to be proved.

Clinically, these patients complain of insidious onset of back pain (352), lower-extremity pain or fractures, and difficulty in walking (67,251,353,354). Difficulty in walking may sometimes be the only finding. This condition occurs during the prepubertal period, and is slightly more common in boys than in girls. Vertebral collapse or wedging, with resulting kyphosis, is common. Brenton and Dent (350) classified idiopathic juvenile osteoporosis as mild, moderate, and severe types. Patients with the mild type have only back pain and vertebral fractures; those with the moderate type have back and lower-extremity pain and fractures, with some limitation of activities but eventual return to normal function; and those with the severe form have back and lower-extremity pain and fractures. Both metaphyseal and diaphyseal fractures can occur in the lower extremities. Patients with severe disease improve clinically but do not return to normal activity after puberty.

Plain radiographs show wedging or collapse of the vertebral bodies. A "codfish" appearance of the vertebral bodies can occur, with the superior and inferior borders of the vertebrae becoming biconcave (Fig. 20.28). Other studies that can be useful for following the progress of this disease are single-photon absorptiometry, dual-photon absorptiometry, and quantitative CT scanning (343,345,346). The problem with these tests is that normal ranges for adolescents and children are variable and have not been standardized.

Idiopathic juvenile osteoporosis is a diagnosis of exclusion. Other diseases that must be considered include metabolic bone diseases, leukemia, Cushing syndrome, lysinuric protein intolerance, type I homocystinuria, and

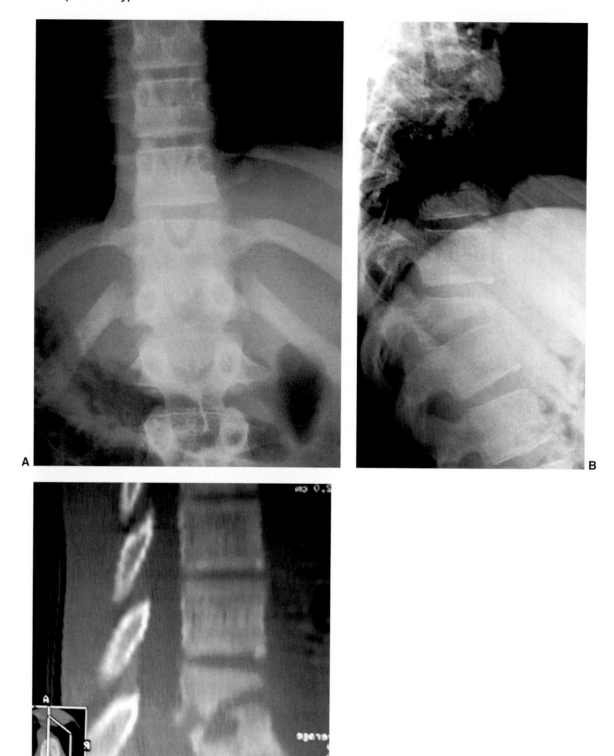

**Figure 20.27** Anteroposterior and lateral radiographs **(A** and **B)** and a computed tomography (CT) scan **(C)** demonstrating vertebral body collapse secondary to tuberculosis.

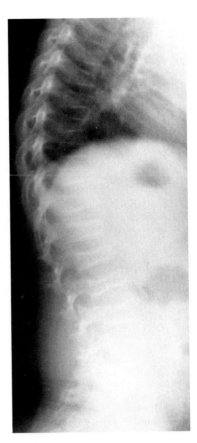

**Figure 20.28** Lateral radiograph taken of a standing 10-year-old girl with idiopathic juvenile osteoporosis shows diffuse osteopenia, multiple "codfish" vertebrae in the thoracic and lumbar spine, and "coin" vertebrae in the upper thoracic spine secondary to extreme collapse. (From Green WB. *Idiopathic juvenile osteoporosis.* New York: Raven, 1994.)

osteogenesis imperfecta. The natural history of this condition is spontaneous improvement or remission at the onset of puberty. Associated kyphosis tends to improve after the onset of puberty.

Treatment of idiopathic juvenile osteoporosis involves modification of activities, possible calcium and vitamin D supplementation, and supportive treatment of spinal deformities. It must be ensured that there is sufficient restriction of activities in order to prevent fractures, but not so much restriction as to cause an increase in osteoporosis. If a significant progressive kyphosis develops, the Milwaukee brace is the treatment of choice (344). The brace is to be worn until there is evidence of improvement of the osteoporosis. Operative therapy for this condition has been associated with a high complication rate because the poor bone quality makes instrumentation and fusion difficult (355).

## REFERENCES

1. O'Rahilly R, Benson D. The development of the vertebral column. In: Bradford DS, Hensinger RN, eds. *The pediatric spine.* New York: Thieme, 1985:3.
2. DiMeglio A, Bonnel F. Growth of the spine. In: Raimondi AJ, Choux M, Di Rocco C, eds. *The pediatric spine,* Vol. 1. New York: Springer-Verlag, 1989:39.
3. Mellin G, Harkonen H, Poussa M. Spinal mobility and posture and their correlations with growth velocity in structurally normal boys and girls aged 13 to 14. *Spine* 1988;3:152.
4. Mellin G, Poussa M. Spinal mobility and posture in 8- to 16-year-old children. *J Orthop Res* 1992;10:211.
5. Propst-Proctor SL, Bleck EE. Radiographic determination of lordosis and kyphosis in normal and scoliotic children. *J Pediatr Orthop* 1983;3:344.
6. Schultz AB, Sorensen SE, Andersson GBJ. Measurements of spine morphology in children, ages 10–16. *Spine* 1984;9:70.
7. Stagnara P, DeMauroy JC, Dran G, et al. Reciprocal angulation of vertebral bodies in the sagittal plane: approach to references in the evaluation of kyphosis and lordosis. *Spine* 1982;7:335.
8. Willner S, Johnson B. Thoracic kyphosis and lumbar lordosis during the growth period in children. *Acta Paediatr Scand* 1983;72:873.
9. Lowe T. *Mortality-morbidity committee report.* Vancouver, WA: Scoliosis Research Society, 1987.
10. Bernhardt M, Bridwell KH. Segmental analysis of the sagittal plane alignment of the normal thoracic and lumbar spines and the thoracolumbar junction. *Spine* 1989;14:717.
11. Hammerberg KW. Kyphosis. In: Bridwell KH, DeWald RL, eds. *The textbook of spinal surgery.* Philadelphia, PA: JB Lippincott, 1991:501.
12. LeMire RJ. Intrauterine development of the vertebrae and spinal cord. In: Raimondi AJ, Choux M, DiRocco C, eds. *The pediatric spine,* Vol. 1. New York: Springer-Verlag, 1989:20.
13. Schijman E. Comparative anatomy of the spine in the newborn infant and toddler. In: Raimondi AJ, Choux M, Di Rocco C, eds. *The pediatric spine,* Vol. 1. New York: Springer-Verlag, 1989:1.
14. Cutler WB, Friedman E, Genovese-Stone E. Prevalence of kyphosis in a healthy sample of pre- and postmenopausal women. *Am J Phys Med Rehabil* 1993;72:219.
15. Fon GT, Pitt MJ, Thies AC Jr. Thoracic kyphosis: range in normal subjects. *Am J Roentgenol* 1980;134:979.
16. Bernhardt M. Normal spinal anatomy: normal sagittal plane alignment. In: Bridwell KH, DeWald RL, eds. *The textbook of spinal surgery,* 2nd ed. Philadelphia, PA: Lippincott-Raven, 1997:185.
17. White AA III, Panjabi MM. Practical biomechanics of scoliosis and kyphosis. In: White AA, Panjabi MM, eds. *Clinical biomechanics of the spine.* Philadelphia, PA: JB Lippincott, 1990:127.
18. Roaf R. Vertebral growth and its mechanical control. *J Bone Joint Surg* 1960;42B:40.
19. Voutsinas SA, MacEwen GD. Sagittal profiles of the spine. *Clin Orthop* 1986;210:235.
20. Winter RB, Hall JE. Kyphosis in childhood and adolescence. *Spine* 1978;3:285.

### Postural Kyphosis

21. Wenger DR. Roundback. In: Wenger DR, Rang M, eds. *The art and practice of children's orthopaedics.* New York: Raven, 1993:422.
22. Winter RB. Spinal problems in pediatric orthopaedics. In: Morrissy RT, ed. *Lovell & Winter's pediatric orthopaedics,* 3rd ed. Philadelphia, PA: JB Lippincott, 1990:673.

### Congenital Kyphosis

23. Winter R. Congenital kyphosis. *Clin Orthop* 1977;128:26.
24. Dubousset J. Congenital kyphosis and lordosis. In: Weinstein SL, ed. *The pediatric spine: principles and practice.* New York: Lippincott Williams & Wilkins, 2000:179.
25. McMaster MJ, Ohtsuk AK. The natural history of congenital scoliosis: a study of two hundred and fifty-one patients. *J Bone Joint Surg Am* 1982;64:1128.
26. Van Schrick FG. Dir angeborene kyphose. *Zietr Orthop Chir* 1932;56:238.
27. Lombard P, LeGenissel M. Cyphoses congenitales. *Rev Orthop* 1938;22:532.
28. Winter RB, Moe JH, Wang JF. Congenital kyphosis: its natural history and treatment as observed in a study of one hundred and thirty patients. *J Bone Joint Surg Am* 1973;55:223.
29. McMaster MJ, Singh H. Natural history of congenital kyphosis and kyphoscoliosis. *J Bone Joint Surg* 1999;81A:1367–1383.
30. Dubousset J. Congenital kyphosis. In: Bradford DS, Hensinger RM, eds. *The pediatric spine.* New York: Thieme, 1985:196.

31. Zeller RD, Ghanem I, Dubousset J. The congenital dislocated spine. *Spine* 1996;21:1235.

32. Shapiro J, Herring J. Congenital vertebral displacement. *J Bone Joint Surg Am* 1993;75:656.

33. Rivard CH, Narbaitz R, Uhthoff HK. Congenital vertebral malformations: time of induction in human and mouse embryo. *Orthop Rev* 1979;8:135.

34. Philips MF, Dormans J, Drummond D. Progressive congenital kyphosis: report of five cases and review of the literature. *Pediatr Neurosurg* 1997;26:130.

35. Travaglini F, Conte M. Cifosi 25 anni. Progressi in patologia vertebrate. In: Goggia A, ed. *Le cifosi*, Vol. 5. Bologna: Goggia, 1982:163.

36. Tsou PM. Embryology of congenital kyphosis. *Clin Orthop* 1977;128:18.

37. Tsou PM, Yau A, Hodgson AR. Embryogenesis and prenatal development of congenital vertebral anomalies and their classification. *Clin Orthop* 1980;152:211.

38. Morin B, Poitras B, Duhaime M, et al. Congenital kyphosis by segmentation defect: etiologic and pathogenic studies. *J Pediatr Orthop* 1985;5:309.

39. Blake NS, Lynch AS, Dowling FE. Spinal cord abnormalities in congenital scoliosis. *Ann Radiol (Paris)* 1986;29:377.

40. Basu PS, Elsebaie H, Noordeen ChM. Congenital spinal deformity. A comprehensive assessment at presentation. *Spine* 2002;27:2255–2259.

41. Prahinski JR, Polly DW Jr, Mchale KA, et al. Occult intraspinal anomalies in congenital scoliosis. *J Pediatr Orthop* 2000;20:59–63.

42. Suh S-W, Sarwark JF, Vora A, et al. Evaluating congenital spine deformities for intraspinal anomalies with magnetic resonance imaging. *J Pediatr Orthop* 2001;21:525–531.

43. Bradford DS, Heithoff KB, Cohen M. Intraspinal abnormalities and congenital spine deformities: a radiographic and MRI study. *J Pediatr Orthop* 1991;11:36.

44. Guille JT, Forlin E, Bowen JR. Congenital kyphosis. *Orthop Rev* 1993;22:235.

45. Winter RB, Moe JH, Lonstein JE. The incidence of Klippel-Feil syndrome in patients with congenital scoliosis and kyphosis. *Spine* 1984;9:363.

46. Broekman BA, Dorr JP. Congenital kyphosis due to absence of two lumbar vertebral bodies. *J Clin Ultrasound* 1991;19:303.

47. Lubicky JP, Shook JE. Congenital spinal deformity. In: Bridwell HK, DeWald RL, eds. *The textbook of spinal surgery*. Philadelphia, PA: JB Lippincott, 1991:365.

48. Winter RB, Moe JH. The results of spinal arthrodesis for congenital spinal deformity in patients younger than five years old. *J Bone Joint Surg Am* 1982;64:419.

49. Kin Y-J, Otsuka NY, Flynn JM, et al. Surgical treatment of congenital kyphosis. *Spine* 2001;26:2251–2257.

50. Montgomery SP, Hall JE. Congenital kyphosis. *Spine* 1982;7:360.

51. Winter RB, Moe JH, Lonstein JE. The surgical treatment of congenital kyphosis: a review of 94 patients age 5 years or older, with 2 years or more followup in 77 patients. *Spine* 1985;10:224.

52. Mayfield JK, Winter RB, Bradford DS, et al. Congenital kyphosis due to defects of anterior segmentation. *J Bone Joint Surg Am* 1980;62:1291.

53. Winter RB. Congenital kyphosis. In: Bridwell KH, DeWald RL, eds. *The textbook of spinal surgery*, 2nd ed. Philadelphia, PA: Lippincott-Raven, 1997:1077.

## Segmental Spinal Dysgenesis

54. Scott RM, Wolpert SM, Bartoshesky LE, et al. Segmental spinal dysgenesis. *Neurosurgery* 1988;22:739.

55. Faciszewski T, Winter RB, Lonstein JE. Segmental spinal dysgenesis. A disorder different from spinal agenesis. *J Bone Joint Surg Am* 1995;77:530.

56. Hughes LO, McCarthy RE, Glasier CM. Segmental spinal dysgenesis: a report of three cases. *J Pediatr Orthop* 1998;18:227.

57. Flynn JM, Otsuka NY, Emans JB, et al. Segmental spinal dysgenesis: early neurologic deterioration and treatment. *J Pediatr Orthop* 1997;17:100.

## Sacral Agenesis

58. Andrish J, Kalamchi A, MacEwen GD. Sacral agenesis: a clinical evaluation of its management, heredity, and associated anomalies. *Clin Orthop* 1979;139:52.

59. Blumel J, Evans ER, Eggers GWN. Partial and complete agenesis or malformation of the sacrum with associated anomalies. Etiologic and clinical study with special reference to heredity. A preliminary report. *J Bone Joint Surg Am* 1959;41:497.

60. Rusnak SL, Driscoll SG. Congenital spinal anomalies in infants of diabetic mothers. *Pediatrics* 1965;35:989.

61. Banta JV, Nichols O. Sacral agenesis. *J Bone Joint Surg Am* 1969; 51:693.

62. Pang D. Sacral agenesis and caudal spinal cord malformations. *Neurosurgery* 1993;32:755.

63. Phillips WA, Cooperman DR, Lindquist TC, et al. Orthopaedic management of lumbosacral agenesis. *J Bone Joint Surg Am* 1964;64:1282.

## Progressive Anterior Vertebral Fusion

64. Knutsson F. Fusion of vertebrae following noninfectious disturbance in the zone of growth. *Acta Radiol* 1949;32:404.

65. Kharrat K, Dubousset J. Bloc vertebral anterieur progress if ches l'enfant. *Rev Chir Orthop* 1980;66:485.

66. Van Buskirk CS, Zeller RD, Dubousset JF. *Progressive anterior vertebral fusion; a frequently missed diagnosis*. Presented at Scoliosis Research Society, New York, 1998.

67. Smith R. Idiopathic juvenile osteoporosis: experience of twenty-one patients. *Br J Rheumatol* 1995;34:68.

68. Bollini G, Jowe JL, Zeller R. Progressive spontaneous anterior fusion of the spine. A study of seventeen patients. Presented at *15th Meeting of the European Pediatric Orthopaedic Society*, Prague, 1996.

69. Andersen J, Rostgaard-Christensen E. Progressive noninfectious anterior vertebral fusion. *J Bone Joint Surg Br* 1991;73:859.

70. Bouchez B, Arnott G, Combelles G, et al. Compression medullaire par hernie kiscale dorsale. *Rev Neural (Paris)* 1986;142:154.

71. Smith JRG, Martin IR, Shaw DG, et al. Progressive noninfectious anterior vertebral fusion. *Skeletal Radiol* 1986;15:599.

## Scheuermann Disease

72. Scheuermann HW. Kyphosis dorsalis juvenilis. *Zietr Orthop Chir* 1921;41:305.

73. Scheuermann HW. Kyphosis dorsalis juvenilis. *Ugeskr Laeger* 1920;82:385.

74. Bradford DS. Juvenile kyphosis. *Clin Orthop* 1977;128:45.

75. Bradford DS, Ahmed KB, Moe JH, et al. The surgical management of patients with Scheuermann's disease: a review of twenty-four cases managed by combined anterior and posterior spine fusion. *J Bone Joint Surg Am* 1980;62:705.

76. Bradford DS, Moe JH, Winter RB. Kyphosis and postural round-back deformity in children and adolescents. *Minn Med* 1973; 56:114.

77. Murray PM, Weinstein SL, Spratt KF. The natural history and long-term followup of Scheuermann kyphosis. *J Bone Joint Surg Am* 1993;75:236.

78. Sorensen KH. *Scheuermann's juvenile kyphosis. Clinical appearances, radiography, aetiology and prognosis.* Copenhagen: Munksgaard, 1964.

79. Robin GC. The etiology of Scheuermann's disease. In: Bridwell KH, DeWald RL, eds. *The textbook of spinal surgery*, 2nd ed. Philadelphia, PA: Lippincott-Raven, 1997.

80. Fisk JW, Raigent ML, Hill PD. Incidence of Scheuermann's disease. Preliminary report. *Am J Phys Med Rehabil* 1982;61:32.

81. Fisk JW, Baigent ML, Hill PD. Scheuermann's disease. Clinical and radiological survey of 17 and 18 year olds. *Am J Phys Med Rehabil* 1984;63:18.

82. Montgomery SP, Erwin WE. Scheuermann's kyphosis: long-term results of Milwaukee brace treatment. *Spine* 1981;6:5.

83. Ascani E, La Rosa G, Ascani C. Scheuermann kyphosis. In: Weinstein SL, ed. *The pediatric spine: principles and practice*, 2nd ed. Philadelphia, PA: Lippincott Williams & Wilkins, 2001.

84. Halal F, Gledhill RB, Fraser FC. Dominant inheritance of Scheuermann's juvenile kyphosis. *Am J Dis Child* 1978;132:1105.

85. McKenzie L, Sillence D. Familial Scheuermann disease: a genetic and linkage study. *J Med Genet* 1992;29:41.

86. Carr AJ. Idiopathic thoracic kyphosis in identical twins. *J Bone Joint Surg Br* 1990;72:144.

87. Carr AJ, Jefferson RJ, Turner-Smith AR, et al. Surface stereophotogrammetry of thoracic kyphosis. *Acta Orthop Scand* 1989;60:177.

88. Bick EM, Coepl JW, Spector S. Longitudinal growth of the human vertebra. A contribution to human osteogeny. *J Bone Joint Surg Am* 1950;32:803.

89. Bick EM, Copel JW. The ring apophysis of the human vertebra. Contribution to human osteogeny II. *J Bone Joint Surg Am* 1951;33:783.

90. Schmorl G. The pathogenese der juvenilen kyphose. *Fortschr Roentgen* 1930;41:359.

91. Ferguson AB Jr. The etiology of preadolescent kyphosis. *J Bone Joint Surg Am* 1956;38:149.

92. Aufdermaur M. Juvenile kyphosis (Scheuermann's disease): radiology, histology and pathogenesis. *Clin Orthop* 1981;154:166.

93. Aufdermaur M, Spycher M. Pathogenesis of osteochondrosis juvenilis Scheuermann. *J Orthop Res* 1986;4:452.

94. Ippolito E, Ponseti IV. Juvenile kyphosis: histological and histochemical studies. *J Bone Joint Surg Am* 1981;63:175.

95. Lambrinudi L. Adolescent and senile kyphosis. *BMJ* 1934;2:800.

96. Scoles PV, Latimer BM, Diglovanni BF, et al. Vertebral alterations in Scheuermann's kyphosis. *Spine* 1991;16:509.

97. Ascani E, Borelli P, Larosa G, et al. Malattia di Scheuermann. I: studio ormonale. In: Gaggia A, ed. *Progresi in patologia vertebrale*, Vol. 5. Bologna: Le Cifosi, 1982:97.

98. Ascani E, LaRossa G. *Scheuermann's kyphosis*. New York: Raven, 1994.

99. Bradford DS, Daher YH. Vascularized rib grafts for stabilisation of kyphosis. *J Bone Joint Surg Br* 1986;68:357.

100. Burner WL, Badger VM, Shermann FC. Osteoporosis and acquired back deformities. *J Pediatr Orthop* 1982;2:383.

101. Lopez RA, Burke SW, Levine DB, et al. Osteoporosis in Scheuermann's disease. *Spine* 1988;13:1099.

102. Gilsanz V, Gibbens DT, Carlson M, et al. Vertebral bone density in Scheuermann disease. *J Bone Joint Surg Am* 1989;71:894.

103. Ippolito E, Bellocci M, Montanaro A, et al. Juvenile kyphosis: an ultrastructural study. *J Pediatr Othop* 1985;5:315.

104. Wenger DR, Frick S. Scheuermann kyphosis. *Spine* 1999;29:2630.

105. Travaglini F, Conte M. Untreated kyphosis: 25 years later. In: Gaggi A. ed. *Kyphosis*. Bologna: Italian Scoliosis Research Group, 1984:21.

106. Lowe TG. Current concepts review, Scheuermann disease. *J Bone Joint Surg Am* 1990;72:940.

107. Bradford DS, Moe JH, Montalvo FJ, et al. Scheuermann's kyphosis. Results of surgical treatment by posterior spine arthrodesis in twenty-two patients. *J Bone Joint Surg Am* 1975;57:439.

108. Paajanen H, Alanen A, Erkintalo BM, et al. Disc degeneration in Scheuermann disease. *Skeletal Radiol* 1989;18:523.

109. Deacon P, Berkin C, Dickson R. Combined idiopathic kyphosis and scoliosis. An analysis of the lateral spinal curvature associated with Scheuermann's disease. *J Bone Joint Surg Br* 1985;67:189.

110. Deacon P, Flood BM, Dickson RA. Idiopathic scoliosis in three dimensions: a radiographic and morphometric analysis. *J Bone Joint Surg Br* 1984;66:509.

111. Ogilvie JW, Sherman J. Spondylolysis in Scheuermann's disease. *Spine* 1987;12:251.

112. Stoddard A, Osborn JF. Scheuermann's disease or spinal osteochondrosis. Its frequency and relationship with spondylosis. *J Bone Joint Surg Br* 1979;61:56.

113. Muller R, Gschwend N. Endokrine störungen und morbus Scheuermann. *Acta Med Scand* 1969;65:357.

114. Kemp FH, Wilson DC. Some factors in the aetiology of osteochondritis of the spine. *Br J Radiol* 1947;20:410.

115. Cloward RB, Bucy PC. Spinal extradural cyst and kyphosis dorsalis juvenilis. *Am J Roentgenol* 1937;38:681.

116. Roland M, Morris R. A study of the natural history of back pain. Part I: development of a reliable and sensitive measure of disability in low-back pain. *Spine* 1983;8:141.

117. Greene TL, Hensinger RN, Hunter LY. Back pain and vertebral changes simulating Scheuermann's disease. *J Pediatr Orthop* 1985;5:1.

118. Huskisson EC. Measurement of pain. *Lancet* 1974;9:1127.

119. Kaijser R. Obert kongenitale kniegelenksluxationen. *Acta Orthop Scand* 1935;6:120.

120. Stagnara P. Cyphoses thoraciques regulieres pathologiques. In: Gaggi A, ed. *Modern trends in orthopaedics*. Bologna, A Gaggi, 1982.

121. Blumenthal SL, Roach J, Herring JA. Lumbar Scheuermann's. A clinical series and classification. *Spine* 1987;12:929.

122. Stagnara P, Fauchet R, Dupeloux J, et al. Maladie des Scheuermann. *Pediatrics* 1966;21:361.

123. Bhojraj SY, Dandawate AV. Progressive cord compression secondary to thoracic disc lesions in Scheuermann's kyphosis managed by posterolateral decompression, interbody fusion, and pedicular fixation. A new approach to management of a rare clinical entity. *Eur Spine J* 1994;3:66.

124. Klein DM, Weiss RL, Allen JE. Scheuermann's dorsal kyphosis and spinal cord compression: case report. *Neurosurgery* 1986;18:628.

125. Lesoin F, Leys D, Rousseaux M, et al. Thoracic disk herniation and Scheuermann's disease. *Eur Neurol* 1987;26:145.

126. Ryan MD, Taylor TKF. Acute spinal cord compression in Scheuermann's disease. *J Bone Joint Surg Br* 1982;64:409.

127. Yablon JD, Kasdon DL, Levine H. Thoracic cord compression in Scheuermann's disease. *Spine* 1988;13:896.

128. Chiu KY, Luk KDK. Cord compression caused by multiple disc herniations and intraspinal cyst in Scheuermann's disease. *Spine* 1995;20:1075.

129. Bradford DS, Garcia A. Neurological complications in Scheuermann's disease. *J Bone Joint Surg Am* 1969;51:567.

130. Cobb J. Outline for the study of scoliosis. *Instr Course Lect* 1948;5:261.

131. Bradford DS. Vertebral osteochondrosis (Scheuermann's kyphosis). *Clin Orthop* 1981;158:83.

132. Lowe TG, Kasten MD. An analysis of sagittal curves and balance after Cotrel-Dubousset instrumentation for kyphosis secondary to Scheuermann's disease. A review of 32 patients. *Spine* 1994; 19:1680.

133. Sachs B, Bradford D, Winter R, et al. Scheuermann kyphosis: followup of Milwaukee brace treatment. *J Bone Joint Surg Am* 1987;69:50.

134. Bradford DS, Moe JH, Montalvo FJ, et al. Scheuermann's kyphosis and roundback deformity: results of Milwaukee brace treatment. *J Bone Joint Surg Am* 1974;56:740.

135. Gutowski WT, Renshaw TS. Orthotic results in adolescent kyphosis. *Spine* 1988;13:485.

136. Farsetti P, Tudisco C, Caterini R, et al. Juvenile and idiopathic kyphosis. Long-term followup of 20 cases. *Arch Orthop Trauma Surg* 1991;110:165.

137. De Mauroy JC, Stagnara P. *Resultats a long terme du traitment orthopedique*. Aix en Provence, 1978:60.

138. Michel CR, Caton J. Etude des resultants a long term d'une seie de cyphoses regulieeres traitees pariorset de Livet a charniers. Presented at *The Reunion of the Group d'Etude de la Scoliose*, Aix-en-Provence, 1978.

139. Ponte A, Gebbia F, Eliseo F. Nonoperative treatment of adolescent hyperkyphosis: a 30 years experience in over 3000 treated patients. *Orthop Trans* 1990;14:766.

140. Lowe TG. Scheuermann's disease. *Orthop Clin North Am* 1999; 30:475.

141. Bradford DS, Brown DM, Moe JH, et al. Scheuermann's kyphosis. A form of osteoporosis? *Clin Orthop* 1976;118:10.

142. Herndon WA, Emans JB, Micheli LG, et al. Combined anterior and posterior fusion for Scheuermann's kyphosis. *Spine* 1981;6:125.

143. Lowe TG. Double L-rod instrumentation in the treatment of severe kyphosis secondary to Scheuermann's disease. *Spine* 1987;12:336.

144. Nerubay J, Katznelson A. Dual approach in the surgical treatment of juvenile kyphosis. *Spine* 1986;11:101.

145. Speck GR, Chopin DC. The surgical treatment of Scheuermann's kyphosis. *J Bone Joint Surg Br* 1986;68:189.

146. Sturm PF, Dobson JC, Armstrong GWD. The surgical management of Scheuermann's disease. *Spine* 1993;18:685.

147. Johnston CE II. *TSRH instrumentation update*, Vol. 1. Texas Scottish Rite Hospital, 1997.

148. Shufflebarger HL. Cotrel-Dubousset instrumentation for Scheuermann's kyphosis. *Orthop Trans* 1989;13:90.

149. Kostuik JP. Anterior Kostuik-Harrington distraction systems. *Orthopedics* 1985;11:1379.

150. Coscia MF, Bradford DS, Ogilvie JW. Scheuermann's kyphosis: results in 19 cases treated by spinal arthrodesis and L-rod instrumentation. *Orthop Trans* 1988;12:255.

151. Otsuka NY, Hall JE, Mah JY. Posterior fusion for Scheuermann's kyphosis. *Clin Orthop* 1990;251:134.

152. Reinhardt P, Bassett GS. Short segmental kyphosis following fusion for Scheuermann's disease. *J Spinal Disord* 1990;3:162.

## Postlaminectomy Kyphosis

153. Lonstein JE. Post-laminectomy kyphosis. *Clin Orthop* 1977; 128:93.
154. McLaughlin MR, Wahlig JB, Pollack IF. Incidence of post-laminectomy kyphosis after Chiari decompression. *Spine* 1997; 22:613.
155. Haft H, Ransohoff J, Carter S. Spinal cord tumors in children. *Pediatrics* 1959;23:1152.
156. Lonstein JE, Winter RB, Moe JH, et al. Post-laminectomy spine deformity. *J Bone Joint Surg Am* 1976;58:727.
157. Mikawa Y, Shikata J, Yamamuro T. Spinal deformity and instability after multilevel cervical laminectomy. *Spine* 1987;12:6.
158. Tachdijian MO, Matson DD. Orthopaedic aspects of intraspinal tumors in infants and children. *J Bone Joint Surg Am* 1965;47:223.
159. Katsumi Y, Honma T, Nakamura T. Analysis of cervical instability resulting from laminectomies for removal of spinal cord tumor. *Spine* 1989;14:1171.
160. Cattell HS, Clark GL. Jr. Cervical kyphosis and instability following multiple laminectomies in children. *J Bone Joint Surg Am* 1967;49:713.
161. Panjabi MN, White AAI, Johnson RM. Cervical spine mechanics as a function of transection of components. *J Biomech* 1975;8:327.
162. Butler MS, Robertson WW Jr, Rate W, et al. Skeletal sequelae of radiation therapy for malignant childhood tumors. *Clin Orthop* 1990;251:235.
163. Saito T, Yamamuro T, Shikata J, et al. Analysis and prevention of spinal column deformity following cervical laminectomy I. Pathogenetic analysis of postlaminectomy deformities. *Spine* 1991;16:494.
164. Bell DF, Walker JL, O'Connor G, et al. Spinal deformity after multiple-level cervical laminectomy in children. *Spine* 1994; 19:406.
165. Yeh JS, Sgouros S, Walsh AR, et al. Spinal sagittal malalignment following surgery for primary intramedullary tumours in children. *Pediatr Neurosurg* 2001;35:318.
166. Albert TJ, Vacarro A. Postlaminectomy kyphosis. *Spine* 1998; 23:2738.
167. Yasuoka S, Peterson HA, Laws ER Jr, et al. Pathogenesis and prophylaxis of postlaminectomy deformity of the spine after multiple level laminectomy: difference between children and adults. *Neurosurgery* 1981;9:145.
168. Perra JH. Iatrogenic spinal deformities. In: Weinstein SL, ed. *The pediatric spine: principles and practice*, 2nd ed. New York: Lippincott Williams & Wilkins, 2000:491.
169. Fraser RD, Paterson DC, Simpson DA. Orthopaedic aspects of spinal tumours in children. *J Bone Joint Surg Br* 1977;59:143.
170. Papagelopoulos PJ, Peterson HA, Ebersold MJ, et al. Spinal column deformity and instability after lumbar or thoracolumbar laminectomy for intraspinal tumors in children and young adults. *Spine* 1997;22:442.
171. Peter JC, Hoffman EB, Arens LJ, et al. Incidence of spinal deformity in children after multiple level laminectomy for selective posterior rhizotomy. *Childs Nerv Syst* 1990;6:30.
172. Yasuoka S, Peterson HA, MacCarty CS. Incidence of spinal column deformity after multilevel laminectomy in children and adults. *J Neurosurg* 1982;57:441.
173. Donaldson DH. Scoliosis secondary to radiation. In: Bridwell HK, DeWald RL, eds. *The textbook of spinal surgery*. Philadelphia, PA: JB Lippincott, 1991:485.
174. Whitehouse WM, Lampe I. Osseous damage in irradiation of renal tumors in infancy and childhood. *Am J Roentgenol* 1953; 70:721.
175. Butler JC, Whitecloud TS. Postlaminectomy kyphosis: causes and surgical management. *Orthop Clin North Am* 1992;23:505.
176. Callahan RA, Johnson RM, Margolis RN, et al. Cervical facet fusion for control of instability following laminectomy. *J Bone Joint Surg Am* 1977;59:991.
177. Ishida Y, Suzuki K, Ohmori K, et al. Critical analysis of extensive cervical laminectomy. *Neurosurgery* 1989;24:215.
178. Raimondi AJ, Gutierrez FA, Di Rocco C. Laminotomy and total reconstruction of the posterior spinal arch for spinal canal surgery in childhood. *J Neurosurg* 1976;45:555.
179. Rama B, Markakis E, Kolenda H, et al. Reconstruction instead of resection: laminotomy and laminoplasty. *Neurochirurgia (Stung)* 1990;33(Suppl. 1):36.
180. Kehrli P, Bergamaschi R, Maitrot D. Open-door laminoplasty in pediatric spinal neurosurgery. *Childs Nerv Syst* 1996;12:551.
181. Mimatsu K. New laminoplasty after thoracic and lumbar laminectomy. *J Spinal Disord* 1997;10:20.
182. Shikata J, Yamamuro T, Shimizu K, et al. Combined laminoplasty and posterolateral fusion for spinal canal surgery in children and adolescents. *Clin Orthop* 1990;259:92.
183. Shimamura T, Kato S, Toba T, et al. Sagittal splitting laminoplasty for spinal canal enlargement for ossification of the spinal ligaments (OPLL and OLF). *Semin Musculoskelet Radiol* 2001;5:203.
184. Inoue A, Ikata T, Katoh S. Spinal deformity following surgery for spinal cord tumors and tumorous lesions: analysis based on an assessment of spinal functional curve. *Spinal Cord* 1996;34:536.
185. Sim FH, Svien HJ, Bickel WH, et al. Swan-neck deformity following extensive cervical laminectomy: a review of twenty one cases. *J Bone Joint Surg Am* 1974;56:564.
186. Steinbok P, Boyd M, Cochrane D. Cervical spinal deformity following craniotomy and upper cervical laminectomy for posterior fossa tumors in children. *Childs Nerv Syst* 1989;5:25.
187. Otsuka NY, Hey L, Hall JE. Postlaminectomy and postirradiation kyphosis in children and adolescents. *Clin Orthop Relat Res* 1998;354:189.
188. Torpey BM, Dormans JP, Drummond DS. The use of MRI-compatible titanium segmental spinal instrumentation in pediatric patients with intraspinal tumor. *J Spinal Disord* 1995;8:76.
189. Francis WR Jr, Noble DP. Treatment of cervical kyphosis in children. *Spine* 1988;13:883.
190. Graziano GP, Herzenberg JE, Hensinger RN. The halo-Ilizarov distraction cast for correction of cervical deformity. *J Bone Joint Surg Am* 1993;75:996.

## Radiation Kyphosis

191. Engel D. An experimental study on the action of radium on developing bones. *Br J Radiol* 1938;11:779.
192. Engel D. Experiments on the production of spinal deformities by radium. *Am J Roentgenol* 1939;42:217.
193. Gall EA, Luigley JR, Hilken JA. Comparative experimental studies of 200 kilovolt and 1000 kilovolt roentgen rays. I. The biological effects on the epiphyses of the albino rat. *Am J Pathol* 1940;16:605.
194. Hinkel CL. The effect of roentgen rays upon the growing long bones of albino rats. Quantitative studies of the growth limitation following irradiation. *Am J Roentgenol* 1942;47:439.
195. Barr JS, Lingley JR, Gall EA. The effect of roentgen irradiation on epiphyseal growth. I. Experimental studies upon the albino rat. *Am J Roentgenol* 1943;49:104.
196. Reidy JA, Lingley JR, Gall EA, et al. The effect of roentgen irradiation on epiphyseal growth. II. Experimental studies upon the dog. *J Bone Joint Surg* 1947;29:853.
197. Hinkel CL. The effect of roentgen rays upon the growing long bones of albino rats II. Histopathological changes involving endochondral growth centers. *Am J Roentgenol* 1943;49:321.
198. Arkin AM, Simon N. Radiation scoliosis: an experimental study. *J Bone Joint Surg Am* 1950;32:396.
199. Arkin AM, Pack GT, Ransohoff NS, et al. Radiation-induced scoliosis: a case report. *J Bone Joint Surg Am* 1950;32:401.
200. Katz LD, Lawson JP. Radiation-induced growth abnormalities. *Skeletal Radiol* 1990;19:50.
201. Katzman H, Waugh T, Berdon W. Skeletal changes following irradiation of childhood tumors. *J Bone Joint Surg Am* 1969;51:825.
202. Neuhauser EBD, Wittenborg MH, Berman CZ, et al. Irradiation effects of roentgen therapy on the growing spine. *Radiology* 1952;59:637.
203. Rate WR, Butler MS, Robertson WWJ, et al. Late orthopaedic effects in children with Wilms' tumor treated with abdominal irradiation. *Med Pediatr Oncol* 1991;19:265.
204. Riseborough EH, Grabias SL, Burton RI, et al. Skeletal alterations following irradiation for Wilms' tumor: with particular reference to scoliosis and kyphosis. *J Bone Joint Surg Am* 1976; 58:526.
205. Wallace WHB, Shalet SM, Morris-Jones PH, et al. Effect of abdominal irradiation on growth in boys treated for a Wilms tumor. *Med Pediatr Oncol* 1990;18:441.
206. Rutherford H, Dodd GD. Complications of radiation therapy: growing bone. *Semin Roentgenol* 1974;9:15.

207. Riseborough EJ. Irradiation induced kyphosis. *Clin Orthop* 1977;128:101.

208. Smith R, Daviddson JK, Flatman GE. Skeletal effects of ortho-voltage and megavoltage therapy following treatment of nephroblastoma. *Clin Radiol* 1982;33:601.

209. Vaeth JM, Levitt SH, Jones MD, et al. Effects of radiation therapy in survivors of Wilms' tumor. *Radiology* 1962;79:560.

210. Paulino AC, Wen B-C, Brown CK, et al. Late effects in children treated with radiation therapy for Wilms' tumor. *Int J Radiat Oncol Biol* 2000;46:1239.

211. Makipernaa A, Heikkila JT, Merikanto J, et al. Spinal deformity induced by radiotherapy for solid tumors in childhood: a long-term followup study. *Eur J Pediatr* 1993;152:197.

212. Barrera M, Roy LP, Stevens M. Long-term followup after unilateral nephrectomy and radiotherapy for Wilms' tumour. *Pediatr Nephrol* 1989;3:430.

213. Butler RW. The nature and significance of vertebral osteochondritis. *Proc R Soc Med* 1955;48:895.

214. Pastore G, Antonelli R, Fine W, et al. Late effects of treatment of cancer in infancy. *Med Pediatr Oncol* 1982;10:369.

215. Rubin P, Duthie RB, Young LW. The significance of scoliosis in postirradiated Wilms' tumor and neuroblastoma. *Radiology* 1962;79:539.

216. King J, Stowe S. Results of spinal fusion for radiation scoliosis. *Spine* 1982;7:574.

217. Donaldson WF, Wissinger HA. Axial skeletal changes following tumor dose radiation therapy. *J Bone Joint Surg Am* 1967;49:1469.

218. Mayfield JK. Post-radiation spinal deformity. *Orthop Clin North Am* 1979;10:829.

219. Shah M, Eng K, Engler GL. Radiation enteritis and radiation scoliosis. *N Y State J Med* 1980;80:1611.

220. Eyster EF, Wilsin CB. Radiation myelopathy. *J Neurosurg* 1970; 32:414.

## Miscellaneous Causes of Kyphotic Deformities

221. Hensinger RN. Kyphosis secondary to skeletal dysplasias and metabolic disease. *Clin Orthop Relat Res* 1977;128:113.

222. Tolo VT. Spinal deformity in short-stature syndromes. *Instr Course Lect* 1990;39:399.

223. Herring JA. Kyphosis in an achondroplastic dwarf. *J Pediatr Orthop* 1983;3:250.

224. Tolo VT. Surgical treatment of kyphosis in achondroplasia. In: Nicoletti B, Kopits SE, Ascani E et al., eds. *Human achondroplasia: a multidisciplinary approach*, New York: Plenum, 1988:257.

225. Eulert J. Scoliosis and kyphosis in dwarfing conditions. *Arch Orthop Trauma Surg* 1983;102:45.

226. Sponseller PD. Spinal deformity in skeletal dysplasia. In: Weinstein SL, ed. *The pediatric spine: principles and practice*, 2nd ed. New York: Lippincott Williams & Wilkins, 2000:279.

227. Lonstein JE. Treatment of kyphosis and lumbar stenosis in achondroplasia. *Basic Life Sci* 1986;48:283.

228. Kopits SE. Thoracolumbar kyphosis and lumbosacral hyperlordosis in achondroplastic children. In: Nicoletti B, Kopits SE, Ascani E et al., eds. *Human achondroplasia: a multidisciplinary approach*. New York: Plenum, 1988:241.

229. Siebens AA, Hungerford DS, Kirby NA. Achondroplasia: effectiveness of an orthosis in reducing deformity of the spine. *Arch Phys Med Rehabil* 1987;68:384.

230. Siebens AA, Kirby N, Hungerford DS. Orthotic correction of sitting abnormality in achondroplastic children. In: Nicoletti B, Kopits SE, Acsani E et al., eds. *Human achondroplasia: a multidisciplinary approach*. New York: Plenum, 1988:313.

231. Winter RB, Hall JE. Kyphosis in an achondroplastic dwarf. *J Pediatr Orthop* 1983;3:250.

232. Pauli RM, Breed A, Horton VK, et al. Prevention of fixed, angular kyphosis in achondroplasia. *J Pediatr Orthop* 1997;17:726.

233. Shikata J, Yamamuro T, Iida H, et al. Surgical treatment of achondroplastic dwarfs with paraplegia. *Surg Neurol* 1988;29:125.

234. Pauli RM, Horton VK, Glinski LP, et al. Prospective assessment of risks for cervicomedullary-junction compression in infants with achondroplasia. *Am J Hum Genet* 1995;56:732.

235. Ain MC, Shirley ED. Spinal fusion for kyphosis in achondroplasia. *J Pediatr Orthop* 2004;24:541.

236. Cooper RR, Ponseti IV, Maynard JA. Pseudoachondroplastic dwarfism. *J Bone Joint Surg Am* 1973;55:475.

237. Jones ET, Hensinger RN. Spinal deformity in individuals with short stature. *Orthop Clin North Am* 1979;10:877.

238. Matsuyama Y, Winter RB, Lonstein JE. The spine in diastrophic dysplasia. The surgical arthrodesis of thoracic and lumbar deformities in 21 patients. *Spine* 1999;24:2325.

239. Remes V, Tervahartiala P, Poussa M, et al. Cervical spine in diastrophic dysplasia: an MRI analysis. *J Pediatr Orthop* 2000;20:48.

240. Remes V, Marttinen E, Poussa M, et al. Cervical kyphosis in diastrophic dysplasia. *Spine* 1999;24:1990.

241. Herring JA. The spinal disorders in diastrophic dwarfism. *J Bone Joint Surg Am* 1978;60:177.

242. Poussa M, Merikanto J, Ryoppy S, et al. The spine in diastrophic dysplasia. *Spine* 1991;16:881.

243. Dalvie SS, Noordeen MHH, Vellodi A. Anterior instrumented fusion for thoracolumbar kyphosis in mucopolysaccharidosis. *Spine* 2001;26:E539.

244. Tandon V, Williamson JB, Cowie RA, et al. Spinal problems in mucopolysaccharidosis I (Hurler syndrome). *J Bone Joint Surg* 1996;78B:938.

245. Levin TL, Berdon WE, Lachman RS, et al. Lumbar gibbus in storage diseases and bone dysplasias. *Pediatr Radiol* 1997;27:289.

246. Field RE, Buchanan JAF, Copplemans MGJ, et al. Bone marrow transplantation in Hurler's syndrome: effect on skeletal development. *J Bone Joint Surg* 1994;76B:975.

247. Swischuk LE. The beaked, notched or hooked vertebra: its significance in infants and young children. *Radiology* 1970;95:661.

248. Benson PF, Button LR, Fensom AH, et al. Lumbar kyphosis in Hunter's disease (MPS II). *Clin Genet* 1979;16:317.

249. Kocher MS, Hall JE. Surgical management of spinal involvement in children and adolescents with Gaucher's disease. *J Pediatr Orthop* 2000;20:383.

250. Wiesner L, Niggemeyer O, Kothe R, et al. Severe pathologic compression of three consecutive vertebrae in Gaucher's disease: a case report and review of the literature. *Eur Spine J* 2003;12:97.

251. Dietz HC, Cutting GR, Pyeritz RE, et al. Marfan syndrome caused by a recurrent de novo missense mutation in the fibrillin gene. *Nature* 1991;352:337.

252. Dietz HC, Pyeritz RE, Hall BD, et al. The Marfan syndrome locus: confirmation of assignment to chromosome 15 and identification of tightly-linked markers at 15 q 15-921.3. *Genomics* 1991;9:355.

253. Amis J, Herring JA. Iatrogenic kyphosis: a complication of Harrington instrumentation in Marfan syndrome. *J Bone Joint Surg Am* 1984;66:460.

254. Beneux J, Rigault P, Poliquen JC. Les deviations rachidiennes de la maladie de Marfan chez 1'enfant. Etude de 10 cas. *Rev Chir Orthop Reparatrice Appar Mot* 1978;64:471.

255. Joseph KN, Kane HA, Milner RS, et al. Orthopaedic aspects of the Marfan phenotype. *Clin Orthop* 1992;277:251.

256. Robins PR, Moe JH, Winter RB. Scoliosis in Marfan syndrome: its characteristics and results of treatment in thirty-five patients. *J Bone Joint Surg Am* 1975;57:358.

257. Savini R, Cervellato S, Beroaldo E. Spinal deformities in Marfan syndrome. *Ital J Orthop Traumatol* 1980;6:19.

258. Taneja DK, Manning CW. Scoliosis in Marfan syndrome and arachnodactyly. In: Zorab PA, ed. *Scoliosis*. London: Academic. 1977:261.

259. Goldberg MJ. Marfan and the marfanoid habitus. In: Goldberg MJ, ed. *The dysmorphic child: an orthopaedic perspective*. New York: Raven, 1987:83.

260. Kumar SJ, Guille JT. Marfan syndrome. In: Weinstein SL, ed. *The pediatric spine: principles and practice*. 2nd ed. New York: Lippincott Williams & Wilkins, 2000:505.

261. Sponseller PD, Hobbs W, Riley LE, et al. The thoracolumbar spine in Marfan syndrome. *J Bone Joint Surg Am* 1995;77:867.

262. Birch JG, Herring JA. Spinal deformity in Marfan syndrome. *J Pediatr Orthop* 1987;7:546.

263. Jones KB, Drkula G, Sponseller PD, et al. Spine deformity correction in Marfan syndrome. *Spine* 2002;18:2003.

264. Winter RB. Thoracic lordoscoliosis in Marfan syndrome: report of two patients with surgical correction using rods and sublaminar wires. *Spine* 1990;15:233.

265. Hobbs WR, Sponseller PD, Weiss A-PC, et al. The cervical spine in Marfan syndrome. *Spine* 1997;22:983.

266. Larsen LJ, Schottstaedt ER, Bost FC. Multiple congenital dislocations associated with characteristic facial abnormality. *J Pediatr* 1950;37:574.

267. Johnston CE, Birch JG, Daniels JL. Cervical kyphosis in patients who have Larsen syndrome. *J Bone Joint Surg Am* 1996;78:538.

268. Muzumdar AS, Lowry RB, Robinson CE. Quadriplegia in Larsen syndrome. *Birth Defects* 1977;13:202.

269. Harris R, Cullen CH. Autosomal dominant inheritance in Larsen's syndrome. *Clin Genet* 1971;2:87.

270. Dudding BA, Gorlin RJ, Langer LD. The oto-palato-digital syndrome. A new symptom-complex consisting of deafness, dwarfism, cleft palate, characteristic facies, and generalized bone dysplasia. *Am J Dis Child* 1967;113:214.

271. McKusick VA. *Mendelian inheritance in man*, 4th ed. Baltimore, MD: Johns Hopkins University Press, 1975.

272. Micheli LJ, Hall JE, Watts HG. Spinal instability in Larsen's syndrome. Report of three cases. *J Bone Joint Surg Am* 1976;58:562.

273. Johnston CE II, Schoenecker PL. Correspondence to the editor. *J Bone Joint Surg Am* 1997;79:1590.

274. Renshaw TS. Spinal cord injury and posttraumatic deformities. In: Weinstein SL, ed. *The pediatric spine: principles and practice*, 2nd ed. New York: Lippincott Williams & Wilkins, 2000:585.

275. Dearolf WWI, Betz RR, Vogel LC, et al. Scoliosis in pediatric spinal cord–injured patients. *J Pediatr Orthop* 1990;10:214.

276. Malcolm BW. Spinal deformity secondary to spinal injury. *Orthop Clin North Am* 1979;10:943.

277. Mayfield JK, Erkkila JC, Winter RB. Spine deformity subsequent to acquired childhood spinal cord injury. *J Bone Joint Surg Am* 1981;63:1401.

278. Renshaw TS. Paralysis in the child: orthopaedic management. In: Bradford DS, Hensinger RM, eds. *The pediatric spine.* New York: Thieme, 1985:118.

279. Griffiths EF, McCormick CC. Post-traumatic syringomyelia (cystic myelopathy). *Paraplegia* 1981;19:81.

280. Bohm H, Harms J, Donk R, et al. Correction and stabilization of angular kyphosis. *Clin Orthop Relat Res* 1990;258:56.

281. Gertzbein SD, Harris MB. Wedge osteotomy for the correction of posttraumatic kyphosis. *Spine* 1992;17:374.

282. McAfee PC, Bohlman HH, Yuan HA. Anterior decompression of traumatic thoracolumbar fractures with incomplete neurological deficit using a retroperitoneal approach. *J Bone Joint Surg Am* 1985;67:89.

283. Roberson JR, Whitesides TF Jr. Surgical reconstruction of late post-traumatic thoracolumbar kyphosis. *Spine* 1985;10:307.

284. Wu SS, Hwa SY, Lin LC, et al. Management of rigid post-traumatic kyphosis. *Spine* 1996;21:2260.

285. Craig JB, Govender S. Neurofibromatosis of the cervical spine. A report of eight cases. *J Bone Joint Surg Br* 1992;74:575.

286. Funasaki H, Winter RB, Lonstein JB, et al. Pathophysiology of spinal deformities in neurofibromatosis. *J Bone Joint Surg Am* 1994;76:692.

287. Crawford AH. Pitfalls of spinal deformities associated with neurofibromatosis in children. *Clin Orthop* 1989;245:29.

288. Hsu LCS, Lee PC, Leong JCY. Dystrophic spinal deformities in neurofibromatosis, treated by anterior and posterior fusion. *J Bone Joint Surg Br* 1984;66:495.

289. Durrani AA, Crawford AH, Chouhdry SN, et al. Modulation of spinal deformities in patients with neurofibromatosis type I. *Spine* 2000;25:69.

290. Crawford AH. Neurofibromatosis. In: Weinstein SL, ed. *The pediatric spine: principles and practice.* New York: Raven, 1994:619.

291. Curtis BH, Fisher RL, Butterfield WL, et al. Neurofibromatosis with paraplegia: report of 8 cases. *J Bone Joint Surg Am* 1969;51:843.

292. Lonstein JE, Winter RB, Moe JH, et al. Neurologic deficit secondary to spinal deformity. *Spine* 1980;5:331.

293. Asazuma T, Yamagishi M, Nemoto K, et al. Spinal fusion using a vascularized fibular bone graft for a patient with cervical kyphosis due to neurofibromatosis. *J Spinal Disord* 1997;10:537.

294. Gioia G, Mandelli D, Capaccioni B, et al. Postlaminectomy cervical dislocation in von Recklinghausen's disease. *Spine* 1998; 23:273.

295. Kokubun S, Ozawa H, Sakurai M, et al. One-stage anterior and posterior correction of severe kyphosis of the cervical spine in neurofibromatosis. A case report. *Spine* 1993;18:2332.

296. Nijland EA, van den Berg MP, Wuisman PIJM, et al. Correction of a dystrophic cervicothoracic spine deformity in Recklinghausen's disease. *Clin Orthop Relat Res* 1998;349:149.

297. Ward BA, Harkey L, Parent AD, et al. Severe cervical kyphotic deformities in patients with plexiform neurofibromas: case report. *Neurosurgery* 1994;35:960.

298. Schorry EK, Stowens DW, Crawford AH, et al. Summary of patient data from a multidisciplinary neurofibromatosis clinic. *Neurofibromatosis* 1989;2:129.

299. Winter RB, Moe JH, Bradford DS, et al. Spine deformities in neurofibromatosis. *J Bone Joint Surg Am* 1979;61:677.

300. Halmai V, Doman I, de Jonge T, et al. Surgical treatment of spinal deformities associated with neurofibromatosis type I. Report of 12 cases. *J Neurosurg Spine* 2002;97:310.

301. Bradford DS. Anterior vascular pedicle bone grafting for the treatment of kyphosis. *Spine* 1980;5:318.

302. Bradford DS, Ganjavian S, Antonious D, et al. Anterior strut-grafting for the treatment of kyphosis. *J Bone Joint Surg Am* 1982;64:680.

303. Rose GK, Sanderson JM. Transposition of rib with blood supply for the stabilisation of a spinal kyphos. *J Bone Joint Surg Br* 1975;57:112.

304. Moon M-S. Tuberculosis of the spine. *Spine* 1977;22:1791.

305. Ho EKW, Leong JCY. Tuberculosis of the spine. In: Weinstein SL, ed. *The pediatric spine: principles and practice.* New York: Raven, 1994:837.

306. Antituberculosis Regimens of Chemotherapy. Recommendations from the Committee on Treatment of the International Union against Tuberculosis and Lung Disease. *Bull Int Union Tuberc Lung Dis* 1988;63:60.

307. Khoo LT, Mikawa K, Fessler RG. A surgical revisitation of Pott distemper of the spine. *Spine J* 2003;3:130.

308. Moon M-S, Moon Y-W, Moon J-L, et al. Conservative treatment of tuberculosis of the lumbar and lumbosacral spine. *Clin Orthop* 2002;398:40.

309. Moon MS, Kim I, Woo YK, et al. Conservative treatment of tuberculosis of the thoracic and lumbar spine in adults and children. *Int Orthop* 1987;11:315.

310. Wimmer C, Ogon M, Sterzinger W, et al. Conservative treatment of tuberculous spondylitis: a long-term follow-up study. *J Spinal Disord* 1997;10:417.

311. Rajasekaran S. The problem of deformity in spinal tuberculosis. *Clin Orthop* 2002;398:85.

312. Rajasekaran S. The natural history of post-tubercular kyphosis in children. *J Bone Joint Surg* 2001;83B:954.

313. Mushkin AY, Kovalenko KN. Neurological complications of spinal tuberculosis in children. *Int Orthop (SICOT)* 1999;23:210.

314. Klöckner C, Valencia R. Sagittal alignment after anterior debridement and fusion with or without additional posterior instrumentation in the treatment of pyogenic and tuberculous spondylodiscitis. *Spine* 2003;28:1036.

315. Parthasarathy R, Sriram K, Santha T, et al. Short-course chemotherapy for tuberculosis of the spine. *J Bone Joint Surg* 1999;81B:464.

316. Schulitz KP, Kothe R, Leong JC, et al. Growth changes of solidly fused kyphotic block after surgery for tuberculosis. Comparison of four procedures. *Spine* 1997;22:1150.

317. Medical Research Council Working Party on Tuberculosis of the Spine. A controlled trial of anterior spinal fusion and debridement in the surgical management of tuberculosis of the spine in patients on standard chemotherapy: studies in Hong Kong. *Br J Surg* 1974;61:853.

318. Medical Research Council Working Party on Tuberculosis of the Spine. A controlled trial of debridement and ambulatory treatment in the management of tuberculosis of the spine in patients on standard chemotherapy. *J Trap Med Hyg* 1974;77:72.

319. Medical Research Council Working Party on Tuberculosis of the Spine. Five-year assessments of controlled trials of ambulatory treatment, debridement and anterior spinal fusion in the management of tuberculosis of the spine: studies in Bulaway (Rhodesia) and in Hong Kong. *J Bone Joint Surg Br* 1978; 60:163.

320. Medical Research Council Working Party on Tuberculosis of the Spine. A ten-year assessment of a controlled trial comparing debridement and anterior spinal fusion in the management of tuberculosis of the spine in patients on standard chemotherapy in Hong Kong. *J Bone Joint Surg Br* 1982;64:393.

321. Altman GT, Altman DT, Frankovitch KF. Anterior and posterior fusion for children with tuberculosis of the spine. *Clin Orthop Relat Res* 1996;325:225.

322. Bailey HL, Gabriel M, Hodgson AR, et al. Tuberculosis of the spine in children: operative findings and results in one hundred consecutive patients treated by removal of the lesion and anterior grafting. *J Bone Joint Surg Am* 1972;54:1633.

323. Hsu LCS, Leong JCY. Tuberculosis of the lower cervical spine (C2-7): a report on forty cases. *J Bone Joint Surg Br* 1984;66:1.

324. Ito H, Tsuchiya J, Asami G. A new radical operation for Pott's disease. *J Bone Joint Surg* 1934;16:499.

325. Moon M-S. Spine update. Tuberculosis of the spine. Controversies and a new challenge. *Spine* 1997;22:1791.

326. Moon M-S, Woo Y-K, Lee K-S. Posterior instrumentation and anterior interbody fusion for tuberculous kyphosis of dorsal and lumbar spines. *Spine* 1995;20:1910.

327. Medical Research Council Working Party on Tuberculosis of the Spine. A controlled trial of ambulant outpatient treatment and inpatient rest in bed in the management of tuberculosis of the spine in young Korean patients on standard chemotherapy: a study in Masan, Korea. *J Bone Joint Surg Br* 1973;55:678.

328. Medical Research Council Working Party on Tuberculosis of the Spine. A ten-year assessment of controlled trials of inpatient and outpatient treatment and plaster-of-Paris jackets for tuberculosis of the spine in children on standard chemotherapy: studies in Masan and Pusan, Korea. *J Bone Joint Surg Br* 1985;67:103.

329. Upadhyay SS, Saji MJ, Sell P, et al. The effect of age on the change in deformity after anterior debridement surgery for tuberculosis of the spine. *Spine* 1996;21:2356.

330. Upadhyay SS, Saji MJ, Sell P, et al. Spinal deformity after childhood surgery for tuberculosis of the spine. A comparison of radical surgery and debridement. *J Bone Joint Surg Br* 1994;76:91.

331. Upadhyay SS, Saji MJ, Sell P, et al. The effect of age on the change in deformity after radical resection and anterior arthrodesis for tuberculosis of the spine. *J Bone Joint Surg Am* 1994;76:701.

332. Upadhyay SS, Sell P, Saji MJ, et al. 17-year prospective study of surgical management of spinal tuberculosis in children. Hong Kong operation compared with debridement surgery for short- and long-term outcome of deformity. *Spine* 1993;18:1704.

333. Govender S. The outcome of allografts and anterior instrumentation in spinal tuberculosis. *Clin Orthop* 2002;398:60.

334. Govender S, Kumar KPS. Cortical allografts in spinal tuberculosis. *Int Orthop (SICOT)* 2003;27:244.

335. Govender S, Parbhoo AH. Support of the anterior column with allografts in tuberculosis of the spine. *J Bone Joint Surg* 1999;81B:106.

336. Yilmaz C, Selek HY, Gürkan I, et al. Anterior instrumentation for the treatment of spinal tuberculosis. *J Bone Joint Surg* 1999;81A:1261.

337. Benli I, Acaroglu E, Akalin S, et al. Anterior radical debridement and anterior instrumentation in tuberculosis spondylitis. *Eur Spine J* 2003;12:224.

338. Hsu LCS, Cheng CL, Leong JCY. Pott's paraplegia of late onset: the cause of compression and results after anterior decompression. *J Bone Joint Surg Br* 1988;70:534.

339. Dent CE, Friedman M. Idiopathic juvenile osteoporosis. *Q J Med* 1965;134:177.

340. Schippers JC. Over een geval van "spontane" algemeene osteoporose bij een klein meisje. *Maandschr Kindergeneeskd* 1939; 8:108.

341. Evans BA, Dunstan CR, Hills E. Bone metabolism in idiopathic juvenile osteoporosis: a case report. *Calcif Tissue Int* 1983;35:5.

342. Hoekman K, Papapoulos SE, Peters ACB, et al. Characteristics and bisphosphonate treatment of a patient with juvenile osteoporosis. *J Clin Endocrinol Metab* 1985;61:952.

343. Jackson EC, Strife CF, Tsang RC, et al. Effect of calcitonin replacement therapy in idiopathic juvenile osteoporosis. *Am J Dis Child* 1988;142:1237.

344. Jones ET, Hensinger RN. Spinal deformity in idiopathic juvenile osteoporosis. *Spine* 1981;6:1.

345. Marder HK, Tsang RC, Hug G, et al. Calcitriol deficiency in idiopathic juvenile osteoporosis. *Am J Dis Child* 1982;136:914.

346. Saggese G, Bartelloni S, Baroncelli GI, et al. Mineral metabolism and calcitriol therapy in idiopathic juvenile osteoporosis. *Am J Dis Child* 1991;145:457.

347. Smith R. Idiopathic osteoporosis in the young. *Bone Joint Surg Br* 1980;62:417.

348. Rosskamp R, Sell G, Emmons D, et al. Idiopathische juvenile osteoporose—Bericht aber zwei Falle. *Klin Padiatr* 1987;199:457.

349. Samuda GM, Cheng MY, Yeung CY. Back pain and vertebral compression: an uncommon presentation of childhood acute lymphoblastic leukemia. *J Pediatr Orthop* 1987;7:175.

350. Brenton DP, Dent CE. Idiopathic juvenile osteoporosis. In: Bickel H, Stern J, eds. *Inborn errors of calcium and bone metabolism*, Baltimore, MD: University Park Press. 1976:222.

351. Green WB. *Idiopathic juvenile osteoporosis*. New York: Raven, 1994.

352. Dimar JRII, Campbell M, Glassman SD. Idiopathic juvenile osteoporosis. An unusual cause of back pain in an adolescent. *Am J Orthop* 1995;11:865.

353. Marhaug G. Idiopathic juvenile osteoporosis. *Scand J Rheumatol* 1993;22:45.

354. Villaverde V, De Inocencio J, Merino R, et al. Difficulty walking. A presentation of idiopathic juvenile osteoporosis. *J Rheumatol* 1998;25:173.

355. Bartal E, Gage J. Idiopathic juvenile osteoporosis and scoliosis. *J Pediatr Orthop* 1982;2:295.

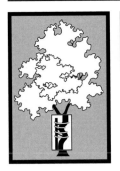

# 21

# Spondylolysis and Spondylolisthesis

*Scott J. Luhmann    Michael F. O'Brien    Lawrence G. Lenke*

In 1782, the Belgian obstetrician Herbinaux was the first to discuss the clinical significance of spondylolisthesis in a report detailing a difficult delivery in a woman with slippage of the 5th lumbar vertebra on the sacrum (1). He described spondylolisthesis as a lumbosacral dislocation. The actual term *spondylolisthesis* was not coined until 1854 by Kilian (2). The word *spondylolisthesis* arises from the Greek roots *spondylos,* which means "vertebra," and *listhesis,* meaning "slippage" or "movement," referring to the forward slipping of one vertebra on the adjacent caudal vertebra. *Spondylolysis* is a term used to refer to an isolated defect in the posterior elements of the vertebra, specifically the pars interarticularis. The term originates from the Greek roots *spondylos,* which means "vertebra," and *lysis,* meaning "break" or "defect." The spondylotic defect is most common at the L-5 vertebra in the pediatric and adolescent patient, and it can secondarily result in spondylolisthesis, with L-5 slipping anteriorly on S1.

## CLASSIFICATION

In 1962, Newman and Stone reported a long-term follow-up of 319 patients with spondylolisthesis (Fig. 21.1) (3). By describing spondylolisthesis both in terms of radiographic

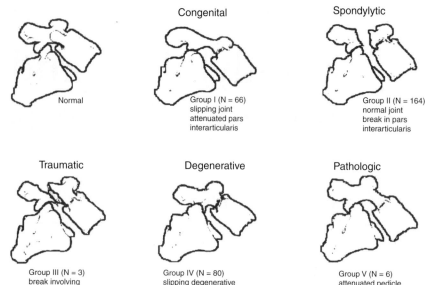

**Figure 21.1** Newman and Stone classification of spondylolisthesis in 319 patients.

appearance and potential causality, they created a five-part classification scheme. The slippage in group I, termed the "congenital" type, was attributed to the attenuation of the pars interarticularis with more transverse orientation of the facets than is normal, allowing slippage of one vertebra on the next caudal level with an intact neural arch. Patients in group II, termed "spondylitic," were believed to have morphologically normal L-5–S1 articulations, but a lytic lesion at the pars interarticularis, permitting L-5 to slip forward on S1. Patients in group III, the "traumatic" type, were also believed to have morphologically normal L-5–S1 facet joints, with a discontinuity of the pars interarticularis caused by an acute fracture creating the instability. The condition of patients in group IV was classified as "degenerative." The authors hypothesized that arthritic changes in the facet joints allowed slippage of the degenerative facet joint, resulting in a spondylolisthesis. The condition of patients in group V was labeled as "pathologic," and they were believed to have attenuated pedicles caused by a generalized or localized bone disease resulting in the development of spondylolisthesis. Wiltse et al. later refined and reorganized Newman and Stone's classification, and at present this is the best-known classification system (Table 21.1) (4–6). Both of these classification systems rely on the radiographic appearance of the anatomy to classify the spondylolisthesis, making no attempt to be predictive of the likelihood of progression of the condition. Only two of these types, specifically Wiltse Types I and II, occur in children and adolescents and are the focus of this chapter.

In 1982, Marchetti and Bartolozzi proposed a new classification that relied primarily on identification of developmental characteristics rather than the observed radiographic pathology (Table 21.2) (7). The initial version of their classification divided spondylolisthesis into "developmental" and "acquired" pathology. Developmental pathology included lytic lesions, spondylolisthesis caused by elongation of the pars interarticularis, and spondylolisthesis secondary to traumatic events such as acute fractures or stress fractures. The acquired pathology group consisted of iatrogenic, pathologic, and degenerative conditions. In 1994, Marchetti and Bartolozzi restructured and refined their classification system (8). In the updated scheme, the developmental category was further subclassified into high and low dysplastic groups, and within each of these dysplastic groups the par interarticularis could be further described as osteolytic or elongated. The acquired pathology group was further expanded to include postsurgical (previously named *iatrogenic*), pathologic, and degenerative conditions; traumatic lesions were moved from the developmental to the acquired pathology category. The classification scheme of Marchetti and Bartolozzi stresses the importance of the developmental aspect of the pathology, highlighting dysplasia of the posterior elements as a significant factor in the development and progression of spondylolisthesis.

## PREVALENCE AND NATURAL HISTORY

Of the two types of spondylolisthesis reported in children and adolescents, the congenital or dysplastic group is the less common. This type of spondylolisthesis occurs in a 2:1 ratio of girls to boys (9,10) and accounts for between 14% and 21% of the overall cases, according to several published reports (9,11). Most congenital/dysplastic spondylolistheses do not progress beyond 50% slippage, mainly on account of

**TABLE 21.1**

**CLASSIFICATION OF SPONDYLOLISTHESIS BY WILTSE ET AL.**

| Type | Description |
| --- | --- |
| I | Congenital (dysplastic) |
| II | Isthmic—defect in the pars interarticularis |
| IIA | Spondylolytic—stress fracture of the pars interarticularis region |
| IIB | Pars interarticularis—elongation of pars interarticularis |
| IIC | Acute pars interarticularis—traumatic fracture of pars interarticularis |
| III | Degenerative—due to a longstanding intersegmental instability |
| IV | Posttraumatic—acute fractures in the posterior elements beside the pars interarticularis region |
| V | Pathologic—destruction of the posterior elements from generalized or localized bone pathology |

From Wiltse LL, Newman PH, Macnab I. Classification of spondylolysis and spondylolisthesis. *Clin Orthop Relat Res* 1976;117:23–29.

the severe symptoms created by the intact posterior bony neural arch compressing the neural elements against the posterior margin of the next caudal vertebral body. The children with congenital/dysplastic spondylolistheses are at higher risk for neurologic injury (e.g., cauda equina syndrome) than are those with isthmic spondylolisthesis.

Isthmic spondylolisthesis is the more common type. Although most published series combine both types of spondylolisthesis (isthmic and congenital/dysplastic) with spondylolysis, most data in the literature refer to the isthmic type of spondylolisthesis. Some have suggested that the isthmic spondylytic defect may be caused by congenital factors. With one exception (12), a defect in the

pars interarticularis has never been found at birth (13–18). In fact, the pathology seems to be rare in patients younger than 5 years, with only a few cases reported in children younger than 2 years (15,16,18,19). Fredrickson et al. reported on the natural history of spondylolysis and spondylolisthesis in a review of 500 children in the first grade. The prevalence of spondylolysis was 4.4% at 6 years of age, increasing to the adult rate of 6% at 14 years of age (13). In addition, they documented and associated spondylolisthesis in 68% of the 5-year-old children, which increased to 74% in adulthood; the authors also implied that the development of spondylolisthesis after the age of 6 years in children with spondylolysis is infrequent. Only 7 patients in

**TABLE 21.2**

**CLASSIFICATION OF SPONDYLOLISTHESIS BY MARCHETTI AND BARTOLOZZI**

| 1982 Group | Pathology | 1994 Type | Form | Condition |
| --- | --- | --- | --- | --- |
| Developmental | | Developmental | | |
| | Lysis | | High dysplastic | Interarticular lysis |
| | Elongation of the pars interarticularis | | | Elongation of the pars interarticularis |
| | Trauma | | Low dysplastic | Interarticular lysis |
| | Acute fracture | | | Elongation of the pars interarticularis |
| | Stress fracture | | | |
| Acquired | | Acquired | | |
| | Iatrogenesis | | Traumatic | Acute fracture |
| | Pathology | | | Stress fracture |
| | Degeneration | | Postsurgical | Direct effect of surgery |
| | | | | Indirect effect of surgery |
| | | | Pathologic | Local pathology |
| | | | | Systemic pathology |
| | | | Degenerative | Primary |
| | | | | Secondary |

From Marchetti PC, Bartolozzi P. Classification of spondylolisthesis as a guideline for treatment. In: Bridwell KH, DeWald RL, Hammerberg KW et al., eds. *The textbook of spinal surgery*, 2nd ed., Vol. 2. Philadelphia, PA: Lippincott–Raven Publishers, 1997:1211–1254.

this series developed further slippage; all slippages were minimal, and none of the patients complained of pain. Virta et al. identified a 2:1 ratio of occurrence in boys and girls (20). In their review of 1,100 individuals in Finland ranging in age from 45 to 64 years, Virta et al. reported a 7% incidence of spondylolisthesis in a population of individuals who had radiographic evaluation for back pain.

The prevalence of spondylolisthesis appears to be influenced by the racial or genetic background of the population studied. African Americans have the lowest rate of spondylolisthesis, 1.8%, whereas Inuit Eskimos have a prevalence of 50%. South Africans and whites fall in an intermediate range, 3.5% and 5.6%, respectively (21–23). Rowe and Roche report a difference in the incidence of spondylolisthesis depending on sex and race: for the male sex, the incidence is 6.4% in whites and 2.8% in African Americans, and in the female sex, it is 2.3% in whites and 1.1% in African Americans (24). The role that gender plays in the natural history of spondylolisthesis is illustrated by the fact that, despite the twofold higher number of men the high-grade slips are four times more common in women. (For grading of spondylolisthesis, see the Meyerding measurements presented in Fig. 21.9 and the section in this chapter entitled "Slip Percentage.") Osterman et al. noted in their report that the lower grades of spondylolisthesis are far more common at the time of presentation: grade I, 79%; grade II, 20%; grade III, 1% (22). A slightly higher incidence of more severe slips has been reported by other authors (25).

In lytic spondylolisthesis, the osteolysis occurs at L-5 in 87% of the patients, at L-4 in 10%, and at L-3 in 3% (26,27). There is also an increasing prevalence of spondylolisthesis in individuals who participate in active sports, especially in physical activities that accentuate lumbar lordosis. Gymnasts have long been identified as an at-risk group for development of spondylolisthesis. Jackson et al. noted an 11% incidence of bilateral pars interarticularis defects in 100 female gymnasts (28). An even higher rate of spondylolysis or spondylolisthesis has been identified in a similar population of Asian female gymnasts. Other sports involving chronic repetitive hyperextension, including college football (specifically, linemen), weight lifting, and rugby also have been implicated in the development of spondylolysis (29–31). Other sports implicated in the development of spondylolisthesis include pole vaulting and volleyball (5,32–34). Generally, the course of this pathology is relatively benign (35).

The natural history of spondylolisthesis was reported by Saraste in a 20-year follow-up study of 255 patients with spondylolysis and spondylolisthesis (35). In this study, 40% of adults showed no progression of the slip, and 40% showed an additional 1- to 5-mm slip. Spondylolisthesis was much more common than spondylolysis, with approximately 22% of patients initially presenting with only spondylolysis. Significant progression of the slip occurs in

a low percentage of cases, occurring in 4% of patients in the series studied by Frennered et al., in 5% of the cases studied by Saraste, and in 3% of the 311 patients in the series studied by Danielson et al. (35–37). In the series of Fredrickson et al., progression was shown to be unlikely (1.4%) after adolescence (13), whereas other authors have reported progression, attributed to disc degeneration, during adolescence (23,38,39). Beutler reported a long-term follow-up of patients with spondylolisthesis and documented that the progression of the slippage declined with each decade (40). Various studies in the literature have reported that women are more likely to present at a younger age, and are at greater risk of slip progression in higher-grade spondylolisthesis, and of having posterior element dysplasia and lumbosacral kyphosis of more than 45 degrees (11,13,41–44). In patients with pre-existing lumbar spondylolisthesis, traumatic injuries usually do not aggravate the condition. Floman et al. reported on 200 patients with thoracolumbar trauma and documented that major axial skeletal trauma had little or no effect on pre-existing lumbar spondylolisthesis (45).

Several radiographic features have been associated with the likelihood of progression of the spondylolisthesis. Some researchers have associated the degree of slip at presentation with a greater chance of slip progression (46–48), but others have not (35,36). In the growing child, the amount of spondylolisthetic kyphosis or of the slip angle, especially when severe, is associated with progression. Other morphologic changes found with high-grade slips, for example, dome-shaped sacrum and trapezoidal L-5, are secondary or adaptive changes to the slip and have not been prognostic for slip progression (36).

# ETIOLOGY

The etiology of spondylolysis and spondylolisthesis remains unclear. A truly congenital etiology seems unlikely because, with one exception (12), no evidence exists for the presence of the lytic pars interarticularis defect in the newborn (13–17). Studies by Vaz et al., Legaye et al., and Labelle et al. suggest that the intrinsic architecture of the pelvis may be an important parameter, modulating the mechanical stresses experienced by the lumbosacral junction (49–51). This is confirmed by the higher incidence of spondylolysis in certain sports, previously mentioned, and in Scheuermann disease (52). In addition, spondylolysis has not been reported in adults (average age of 27 years) who have never walked (53), suggesting that mechanical factors associated with upright posture may play a role.

The absence of pars interarticularis defects at birth, along with the increased prevalence of spondylolysis and spondylolisthesis among athletes who participate in sports involving hyperextension, strongly suggest a mechanical etiology to the development of spondylolisthesis

(3,33,34,54–56). Several authors have postulated that a fracture is the underlying pathomechanical event in the development of a lytic spondylolisthesis (34,57–61). This may be either an acute traumatic event or secondary to an insidious fatigue failure during repetitive stress (62). Wiltse et al. theorized that spondylolysis is a stress fracture in the pars interarticularis, specifically due to repetitive microtrauma or microstresses, with inadequate healing (63). Although an acute fracture is the obvious cause of the acute traumatic type of spondylolysis, more commonly patients present after a traumatic episode. The impact of a traumatic event can be difficult to assess in some patients.

Biomechanical studies have suggested that the pars interarticularis is the weakest part of the posterior neural arch (28,58–60). During flexion and extension, the pars interarticularis is cycled through alternating compressive and tensile loads. During extension, the pars interarticularis experiences posterior compressive forces and anterior tensile forces (Fig. 21.2) (64). The ability of the pars interarticularis to resist the compressive and tensile forces during flexion and extension depends on the thickness of the cortical bone (65). The overall resilience of the pars interarticularis is undoubtedly high, as evidenced by the generally low prevalence of spondylolisthesis in the population. However, Hutton et al. have shown that fatigue fractures can be precipitated during biomechanical testing (60,66). Using 507 N of force at 100 cycles per minute, pars interarticularis fractures could be created with as few as 1,500 cycles. Other cadaveric specimens were able to tolerate 54,000 cycles before developing a fracture.

The importance of the pars interarticularis and its ability to resist shear stress has been well-documented; in contrast, the role of the intervertebral disc is less well understood. In the intact, morphologically normal spinal motion segment, the intervertebral disc contributes 60% of the total shear resistance (67). A skeletally immature animal model of shear load forces demonstrated that, in spines with pars interarticularis defects, the end-plate (apophyseal ring) most likely was responsible for the anterior listhesis (66,67). Kajiura et al. confirmed these findings and demonstrated that the increasing strength of the growth plate during skeletal maturity is the likely reason for the infrequent occurrence of further slippage after the completion of growth (68). In addition, the slippage through the ring apophysis, causing a growth disturbance, can lead to the development of a trapezoidal olisthetic vertebral body or sacral rounding.

Once the pars interarticularis defect has been created, anatomic and biomechanical forces conspire to prevent spontaneous healing of the fracture (Fig. 21.3). The shear forces created by the body's center of gravity tend to cause anterior displacement of L-5 on the sacrum because of the effects of gravity, muscular activity, and body movement. The posterior muscular forces tend to extend the posterior elements, thereby tending to open the spondylolytic defect and create the spondylolisthesis. These initial events tend to precipitate a cascade of worsening biomechanics as the center of gravity moves progressively anterior, causing a vector that increases the shear forces at the lumbosacral junction. This situation may be exacerbated by a low intercrestal line and small transverse processes of L-5, resulting in muscular and ligamentous connections between the pelvis and the spine that are not robust enough to resist the forward slippage of the rostral vertebrae on the caudal vertebrae. Loder has demonstrated in children with higher grades of lumbosacral spondylolisthesis that the sacrum becomes more vertical as the slip worsens (69). When the sacrum becomes more vertical there is an increase in the thoracic lordosis; this is likely an adaptive mechanism to maintain the normal upright posture.

Although mechanical considerations probably are the most significant factors in the development of lytic spondylolisthesis, genetic considerations have been discussed by some researchers (70). Familial studies have documented a high incidence (19% to 69%) of spondylolysis and spondylolisthesis in first-degree relatives of children with spondylolysis and dysplastic or isthmic spondylolisthesis

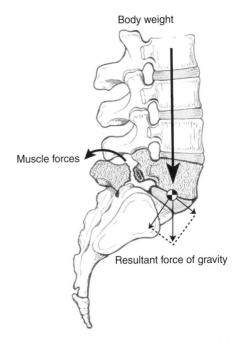

**Figure 21.3** Forces that affect distraction of spondylolytic defect at L-5.

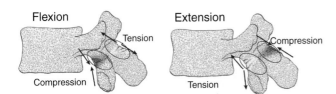

**Figure 21.2** Compressive and tensile forces experienced in the region of the pars interarticularis during flexion and extension.

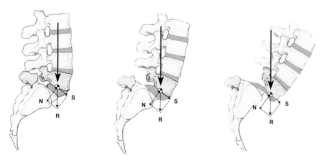

**Figure 21.4** The alteration in pathomechanics as a spondylolysis proceeds from a low-grade spondylolisthesis to a high-grade slip.

(16,71–74). Wynne-Davies and Scott noted an increased incidence of dysplastic lesions in affected relatives (74). First-degree relatives of patients with the dysplastic form of spondylolisthesis had a prevalence of 33%, compared to 15% for isthmic spondylolisthesis. These authors have suggested an autosomal dominant genetic predisposition, multifactorial and with reduced penetrance. Wiltse, on the other hand, suggested that a cartilaginous defect in the vertebral analogue may be an autosomal recessive characteristic with varying expressivity (56).

Whether mechanical or genetic, the underlying predisposition to develop spondylolysis or spondylolisthesis may be exacerbated by functional anatomic factors. The human bipedal gait causes L-5 to be precariously balanced on the sacrum. In the "best case" scenario, the anterior and posterior opposing forces are neutralized so that L-5 remains solidly atop the sacrum in spite of its inclined position; however, anything that unbalances these opposing forces may precipitate a spondylolisthesis (Fig. 21.4). Posterior elements already compromised by spina bifida or dysplastic lumbosacral facet joints may not withstand even normal daily activities. A low intercrestal line in a patient with short L-5 transverse processes may provide less robust muscular and ligamentous attachments between the spine and the pelvis, predisposing the patient to a spondylolisthesis. Undoubtedly, the etiology of spondylolisthesis is multifactorial. However, mechanical forces are highly implicated both in the development of lytic pars interarticularis defects and in the development and progression of spondylolisthesis.

## EVALUATION OF THE PATIENT

### History

There are many possible causes for low back pain, and these must be distinguished from pain secondary to a spondylolisthesis. Although back pain is often a presenting symptom in spondylolisthesis, many asymptomatic spondylolytic defects are identified incidentally on spine or pelvic radiographs. Spondylolisthesis incidentally discovered during screening for low back pain after trauma is typically a stable, chronic entity, probably not a result of the trauma and presenting little, if any, risk of a catastrophic structural instability that would result in neurologic sequela (45). Mild-to-moderate spondylolisthesis does not necessarily predispose to low back pain (75). In spite of this, spondylolisthesis is found to be two to five times more frequent in patients with low back pain. Patients with symptomatic low back pain have a spondylolisthesis rate of 5.3% to 11%, whereas in asymptomatic patients occult spondylolisthesis may occur in 2.2% (76). Libson et al. have documented a twofold increase in the incidence of spondylolisthesis in patients with symptomatic low back pain, compared to asymptomatic patients (77). Wiltse and Rothman identified 11% of 1,124 patients undergoing lumbosacral radiographic examination for back pain as having either unilateral or bilateral pars interarticularis defects (6). Saraste described radiographic features that correlated with low back symptoms: slip of greater than 25%, L-4 spondylolysis or spondylolisthesis, and early disc degeneration at the level of the slip (35). The most common period for the spondylolysis and spondylolisthesis to become symptomatic is during the adolescent growth spurt, between the ages of 10 and 15 years. However, the degree of the deformity does not always match the degree of pain (35).

The history of the patient is a crucial element in the diagnostic and therapeutic process; although radiographic investigations are important in defining the pathoanatomy, treatment is typically based on the patient's symptoms, history, and physical examination. The presence of a spondylolisthesis should not be presumed to be the cause of the patient's back and/or leg symptoms. Muscular strain induced by poor sagittal alignment and poor muscular tone could also be the cause (78). Symptomatic spondylolisthesis typically presents with back pain and/or neurologic symptoms. Knowledge of the location and duration of the symptoms and their association with various activities can be useful in developing a causal relation between the radiographic pathology and the patient's symptoms. It is important to determine whether the pain is acute, chronic, or an acute exacerbation superimposed on a chronic condition. Progression of low-grade non-dysplastic slips in older adolescents is uncommon, and it can be difficult to decide whether the symptoms are a direct result of the spondylolysis or spondylolisthesis. The patient's exercise and activity history, as well as the quality and severity of pain provoked by that activity, should be defined. The pain is usually a dull, aching, low back discomfort and is localized to the low back with occasional radiation into the gluteal region and posterior thighs. This pain is most likely due to the instability caused by the pars interarticularis defect, and is generally exacerbated by participation in athletic or other physical activity, and relieved by rest or restriction of activities. In a few cases, the pain may also follow an acute traumatic episode, usually involving hyperextension during athletic participation.

The presenting symptoms may also include a change in the child's posture or gait, usually noted by his or her parents, with or without accompanying pain. This can be present in mild degrees of spondylolisthesis, but is much more common in more marked degrees of slip. Additionally, these patients may present with scoliosis. As the degree of slip increases, the corresponding pain may cause a muscle-spasm-induced atypical scoliosis. Concomitant rotatory displacement of the spondylolisthetic segment can also create an olisthetic curve. Conversely, the presenting symptoms may be adolescent idiopathic scoliosis, with the spondylolysis or spondylolisthesis detected incidentally on the radiographic evaluation of the scoliosis.

It is important to clearly differentiate low back pain from radiculopathy. Radicular pain is atypical in the pediatric patient, being more common in the adolescent and adult (44,79). If present, aggressive treatment of the radiculopathy should be undertaken along with management of the low back pain. The neurologic symptoms that accompany spondylolisthesis may be either unilateral or bilateral radiculopathy, and may be either intermittent or chronic. In patients with spondylolisthesis and significant degenerative disease, the resulting neuroforaminal compression may cause chronic radiculopathy or neurogenic claudication. In addition, even in patients with low-grade slips that are hypermobile, radiculopathy may be a presenting complaint. Posterior to the nerve roots, the fibrocartilaginous scar or hypertrophic callus that forms around the lytic defect may be responsible for much of the neuroforaminal compression. Anterior to the nerve roots, annular bulging of the disc that results from the vertical collapse of the disc space and the anterior translation of the rostral vertebral body may cause a significant compression of the nerve root against the caudal surface of the pedicle. Although the radiculopathy is usually caused by either central or neuroforaminal stenosis at the level of the lytic defect and impingement of the nerve roots exiting at the level of the defect, compression of traversing nerve roots may cause radiculopathy in more distal roots/dermatomes. Because spondylolysis and spondylolisthesis are most common at L-5, the nerve roots most typically involved are at L-5 and S1. In spite of this, the presence of radiculopathy in a patient with radiographically documented spondylolysis or spondylolisthesis should not cause the clinician to exclude other possible etiologies for the radiculopathy, such as a disc herniation, especially far lateral disc herniations. In patients who have central stenosis with or without neuroforaminal narrowing, neurogenic claudication may be the presenting neurologic symptom. This is also common in patients with larger slips or slips that are hypermobile and worsen with extended periods of standing. Although uncommon, high-grade slips may be accompanied by acute or chronic cauda equina syndromes. Hypermobile, high-grade slips may present as intermittent neurologic symptoms.

## Physical Examination

History and physical examination are essential in determining the etiology of the back pain or radiculopathy. The mere presence of a spondylolisthesis does implicate it in the patient's symptoms. Important physical examination parameters include body habitus, coronal and sagittal alignment, and spinal mobility. The physical examination findings depend on whether pain is present, as well as on the degree of spondylolisthesis. In patients with spondylolysis and mild spondylolisthesis, the back and gait examinations may be completely normal, with no hamstring tightness. With increasing degrees of spondylolisthesis there is usually some degree of hamstring tightness. This may significantly restrict straight-leg raising and forward bending, and may create postural and gait changes. The compensatory increased lumbar lordosis caused by the spondylolisthetic kyphosis creates a flattening of the buttocks ("heart-shaped"), shortening of the waistline, a protuberant abdomen, and a waddling-type gait pattern or Phalen-Dickson sign (11,47,80). Some have attributed the hamstring tightness to signs of nerve root irritation; in any case, the exact mechanism remains unclear but typically resolves after solid bony fusion (80,81).

Palpation of the lumbosacral area may reveal a step-off with a prominent L-5 spinous process. Palpation of the lumbosacral region may also elicit a localized area of tenderness. In addition, the child with a severe slip tends to stand with the hips and knees flexed because of the anterior rotation of the pelvis, with the gait examination demonstrating a shortened stride length caused by the patient's inability to extend the hips. Both static and dynamic examinations are important for eliciting pertinent symptoms. Pain on flexion and extension, with limitation of these motions, may suggest hypermobility as the cause of the pain.

Neurologic examination is typically completely normal, but on occasion may reveal a diminished or absent ankle deep-tendon reflex or weakness of the extensor hallucis longus. Sphincter dysfunction is very rare (82). Provocation of neurologic symptoms during dynamic assessment, particularly radiculopathy in a particular position, may also imply the presence of hypermobility. Neurologic symptoms that correlate dermatome and myotome levels with the level of stenosis or lytic instability are also corroborative of the contribution of the spondylolisthesis to the development of symptoms. Scoliosis, which may be seen at the time of the presentation, is of the typical idiopathic type or, where there are more advanced grades of decompensation, may be caused by reflexive pain or spasm ("olisthetic scoliosis"). A thorough evaluation is essential to rule out other causations of the individual's pain and/or neurologic findings, such as tumors of bone, spinal cord, conus or cauda equina, disc herniation, and disc-space infection.

## RADIOLOGIC EVALUATION

### Routine Views

Numerous imaging modalities are required in order to completely document the three-dimensional pathoanatomy of spondylolysis and spondylolisthesis (83). Each modality contributes a unique view of the various aspects of the pathology. Typically, plain radiographs are obtained as the initial imaging modality. These films should be obtained with the patient in an upright, preferably standing position. Films of the patient supine may not show subtle instability (84). A complete plain radiographic investigation of a potential pars interarticularis defect or spondylolisthesis includes the following views: routine posteroanterior, spot lateral, right and left oblique, Ferguson anteroposterior, and flexion-extension lateral. In addition, long-cassette (14″×36″) anteroposterior and lateral thoracolumbar scoliosis radiographs may be useful for documenting overall coronal and sagittal alignments (Fig. 21.5).

Each of these radiographic views is useful in identifying certain aspects of the pathology. The routine posteroanterior and Ferguson anteroposterior projections may show spina bifida occulta, pars interarticularis defects, lumbar scoliosis, or dysplastic posterior elements (85). The lateral views often allow identification of a pars interarticularis defect even when a spondylolisthesis is not present. Oblique views will often better define the pars interarticularis defect, also known as the *collar* on the well-known "Scotty dog" (Fig. 21.6). The diagnosis of spondylolysis may be missed in 30% of symptomatic young patients if a lateral radiograph alone is obtained (86). The Ferguson

anteroposterior provides an *en face* view of L-5 that may improve the visualization of the transverse process and the sacrum and may more clearly identify a high-riding L-5 vertebral body. Flexion-extension views may uncover subtle instabilities that are not apparent on static standing views. Instability will almost certainly be underappreciated if only supine views are obtained. Other important anatomic features that can be identified on plain radiographs are rounding off of the anterior corner of the sacrum, wedging or erosion of L-5 in higher-grade spondylolisthesis, flexion at the S1-S2 disc, and bending of the sacrum (87) (Fig. 21.14A). In cases of a unilateral defect, the only finding may be sclerosis of the facet, lamina, or pars interarticularis on the intact side opposite the defect, secondary to increased bony stresses.

### Bone Scan

In the context of recent onset of pain, or when there is a distinct history of trauma, a bone scan may be useful for detecting an acute fracture of the pars interarticularis or for excluding a bony tumor. Bone scans may also provide information about the metabolic activity, enabling the evaluation of whether the lytic defect will heal. The most sensitive technique is a single-photon emission computed tomography (SPECT) scan because of the improved detail that it provides (88). An intensely "hot" SPECT scan suggests that the defect is metabolically active and could benefit from a period of immobilization or, failing this, direct osteosynthesis. A "cold" SPECT scan, on the other hand, implies that the lytic defect is chronic and metabolically inactive. These defects, when symptomatic, are not amenable to nonsurgical treatment such as immobilization. Symptomatic lytic lesions of the pars interarticularis that respond to local anesthetic injections may be amenable to fusion or repair (89).

### Computed Tomography Scan

A computed tomography (CT) scan can also be utilized in situations in which, although a pars interarticularis defect is strongly suspected on clinical evaluation, it is not identifiable on the lateral or oblique radiographs. The imaging of the pars interarticularis defect will be optimal if the cuts are no greater than 1.5 mm apart; otherwise the defect may be missed. CT scans are useful in order to clearly define the bony architecture of the posterior elements (90). They can delineate the pars interarticularis defects in the axial plane even when no spondylolisthesis is present (Fig. 21.11C, D). On the axial images, the spondylolytic defect is identified as a linear lesion of varying width with sclerotic osseous margins and hypertrophic osteophytes. The lytic defect is usually identified in the axial image either at, or immediately inferior to, the axial image containing the pedicles of the involved vertebrae. CT scans can also provide excellent visualization of complex anatomy in the

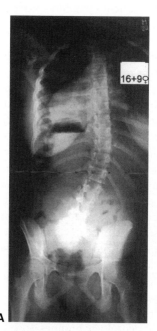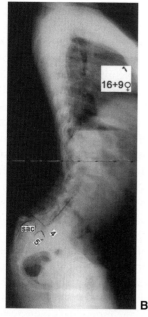

**A**                                                                                   **B**

**Figure 21.5**  Long-cassette upright posteroanterior **(A)** and lateral **(B)** radiographs show olisthetic scoliosis and also marked forward sagittal vertical axis (SVA).

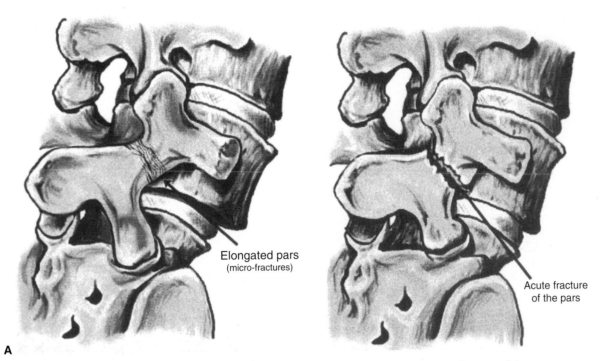

**Figure 21.6** Sketches of an elongated pars interarticularis **(A)** and an acute fracture of the pars interarticularis **(B)** across the neck of the "Scotty dog."

coronal and sagittal planes when reformatted images are obtained. When combined with myelography, CT scans provide excellent definition of even subtle neurologic compression and are particularly useful for visualizing high-grade slips and for patients with complex deformities. If a CT myelogram is anticipated, then plain myelogram films should be obtained at the time the CT scan is done in order to maximize the information garnered. Plain myelography is useful in identifying the longitudinal effect of either the spondylolisthesis or the intercanal compromise, which may be secondary to hypertrophic bone and the fibrous cicatrix formed as a result of the instability at the level of the pars interarticularis defect.

## Magnetic Resonance Imaging Scan

Magnetic resonance imaging (MRI) is an excellent imaging modality for the evaluation of the soft-tissue component of the spondylolisthesis and can also help define the degree of associated degenerative disc disease (39,91). Degenerative disc disease at, above, or below the slip level may be the cause of the patient's pain because of nuclear degeneration or annular injury. The MRI excels at visualizing the neural elements and the surrounding soft tissue, and it is the optimal modality when there is a neurologic deficit or the symptoms suggest a diagnosis other than spondylolysis or spondylolisthesis. MRI may not be as precise as CT myelography in distinguishing these soft tissues from the osseous elements of the pathology in high-grade slips; however, this small drawback is offset by the fact that MRI studies do not involve ionizing radiation,

myelographic dye that could precipitate an anaphylactic reaction, or invasive techniques. MRI studies can identify both central and foraminal stenosis (on parasagittal views) and provide a good indication of the degree of neural compression (Fig. 21.7). A consistent finding on MRI, especially in moderate- to high-grade slips, is a large, bulging disc at the level of the spondylolisthesis, trapping the exiting nerve root between the bulging anulus fibrosus and the pedicle above. In addition, the MRI can document the degree of encroachment on the neural elements by often

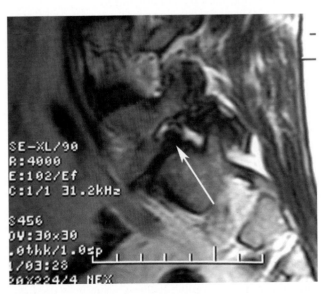

**Figure 21.7** Parasagittal reconstructed magnetic resonance imaging (MRI) view of lytic spondylolysis at L-5.

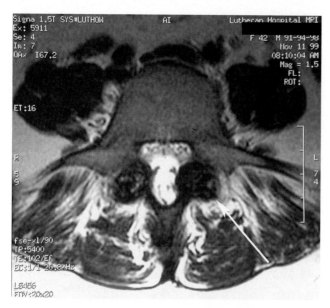

**Figure 21.8**   Axial magnetic resonance imaging (MRI) of bilateral pars interarticularis overgrowth (*arrow*) with foraminal narrowing.

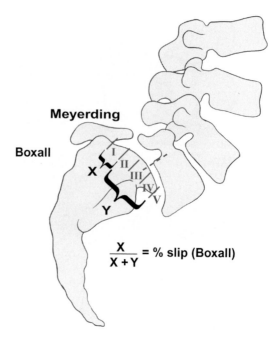

$$\frac{X}{X + Y} = \% \text{ slip (Boxall)}$$

**Figure 21.9**   Meyerding and Boxall measurement techniques for grading spondylolisthesis.

exuberant hypertrophic scar tissue which forms at the spondylolytic defect (Fig. 21.8). The degeneration of adjacent discs can also be discerned by reviewing the MRI. Often, in spite of the relatively normal appearance on plain radiographs or CT scans, the MRI may document premature degeneration of adjacent discs. The significance and the etiology of the degeneration of these adjacent discs are unclear. It is likely that abnormal biomechanics at the spondylolytic level probably result in increased biomechanical stress at adjacent levels, which may, in turn, precipitate degenerative disc disease at an accelerated rate. The MRI and CT scans are also useful in identifying facet joint hypertrophy and degeneration at the level of the slip and adjacent levels, as these factors may also contribute to the patient's low back pain or discomfort.

## Discography

Discography may be helpful when considering surgical intervention. When a pars interarticularis repair is contemplated and the health of the involved disc is not certain, discography may provide useful information about its functional quality. If a segmental fusion is required because of severe disc degeneration at the level of a pars interarticularis defect, and MRI shows degenerative changes at the adjacent level, discography may be helpful in deciding whether the fusion should include the adjacent degenerative level. Practically, however, we rarely carry out discography in pediatric patients.

## Measurement

The deformity in spondylolisthesis, usually at the lumbosacral junction, consists of anterior translation of L-5

on S1, with obligatory forward rotation of L-5 on S1 into lumbosacral kyphosis. The degree of slip can be quantified using the Meyerding classification, the percentage of slip described by Boxall et al. (Fig. 21.9), or the Newman classification which also describes angular slippage (Fig. 21.10A) (3,11,89,92,93). Sagittal rotation, slip angle, and sacral inclination are all direct measurements of the amount of lumbosacral kyphosis, and are assessed on spot lateral radiographs of the lumbosacral area taken with the patient in standing position (94).

### Slip Percentage

The Meyerding classification, which grades the slip from grade 0 (spondylolysis) through grades I–IV (spondylolisthesis) and V (spondyloptosis), is probably the most functional and widely used technique (92) (Fig. 21.9). The amount of anterior translation of the olisthetic vertebra on the caudal level is measured at the posterior vertebral body line. This classifies the spondylolisthesis into five grades: grade I (slip of 1% to 25%), grade II (slip of 26% to 50%), grade III (slip of 51% to 75%), grade IV (slip of 76% to 100%), and grade V (spondyloptosis). Higher-grade spondylolistheses have been shown to be predictive of spondylolisthetic progression (95). Boxall et al. describes a slip percentage which is more precise but requires exact measurements (96). On the radiograph, a line is drawn along the posterior border of the sacrum, and a perpendicular line is drawn at the upper end of the sacrum. The anterior displacement of the posteroinferior corner of L-5 from the line along the posterior border of the sacrum is quantified as the numerator. The width of S1 forms the

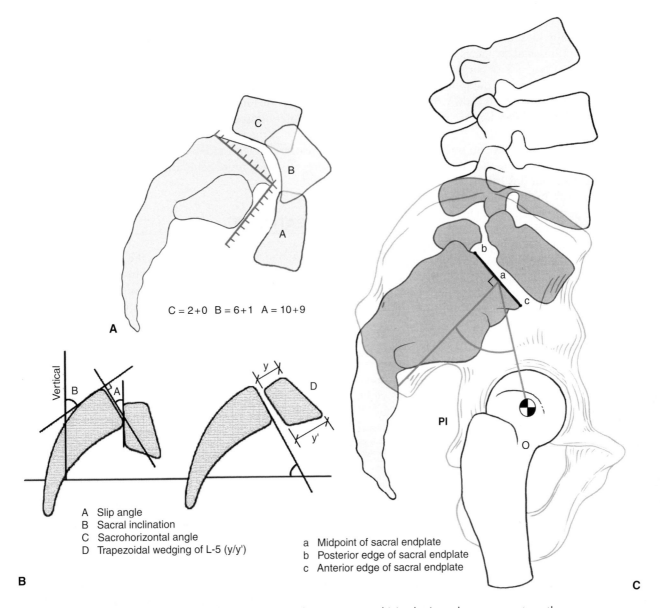

C = 2+0   B = 6+1   A = 10+9

**A**

Vertical

A   Slip angle
B   Sacral inclination
C   Sacrohorizontal angle
D   Trapezoidal wedging of L-5 (y/y')

a   Midpoint of sacral endplate
b   Posterior edge of sacral endplate
c   Anterior edge of sacral endplate

**B**

PI

O

**C**

**Figure 21.10  A:** Modified Newman grading system, combining horizontal measurements as the first number with vertical measurements as the second number. **B:** Radiographic parameters for angular measurements in the description of spondylolisthesis. **C:** Radiographic parameters and pelvic incidence (posterior instrumentation).

denominator, and the slip is expressed as a percentage. In the situation of a rounded superior end plate of S1, the anteroposterior width of L-5 is used instead.

A limitation of the Meyerding classification is its inability to describe the important rotational component in the sagittal plane of the subluxing rostral vertebrae. The modified Newman classification takes this into account (Fig. 21.10A). In this classification system, measurements are taken of both the anterior displacement (first number) and the vertical/downward displacement of the vertebral body in relation to the sacrum (second number). The superior end plate and the anterior face of the sacrum are divided into 10 equal segments. The first

number is the position of the posteroinferior corner of the L-5 vertebra with respect to the superior end plate of S1, and the second is the position of the anteroinferior corner of L-5 relative to the anterior surface of S1. A score by this method utilizes both numbers, for example; 7 + 5, with the "7" indicating the amount of sagittal slip and the "5" indicating the amount of angular roll of L-5 over the sacrum.

Although somewhat tedious, this classification allows a continuous scale of 0 to 20 to be applied to each spondylolisthesis, uniquely describing anterolisthesis and the degree of caudal migration of the rostral vertebrae (3,89,93).

### Slip Angle

The slip angle is the most commonly described measurement of the lumbosacral kyphosis of L-5 on S1 (Fig. 21.10B). On the radiograph, a perpendicular to the line drawn at the posterior cortex of the sacrum forms the sacral measuring line. A second line is drawn along the inferior end plate of L-5, and the angle formed by these two lines is the slip angle which, in the normal condition, is in lordosis and is expressed by a negative number (94). Boxall et al. (11) have used the line along the inferior edge of L-5 for their measurement, but this edge is often difficult to visualize accurately, and when slippage is considerable, the vertebral body is often trapezoidal in shape. In such a situation, use of the inferior end plate as reference may increase the measured slip angle by erroneously adding the measurement of the kyphosis and the wedging of olisthetic vertebra. Slip angles of greater than +45 degrees (kyphosis) correlate with an increased risk of slip progression (11,36,48,95).

### Sagittal Rotation

The amount of sagittal rotation can also be measured, and is the angle between the posterior cortex of the sacrum and the posterior cortex of the L-5 vertebral body. This sagittal rotation angle (SRA) should approximately equal the slip angle measured as described previously. In higher degrees of slip (translation or angulation), L-4 may show retrolisthesis on L-5. In severe slips of greater than 50%, the slip angle of L-4 in relation to the sacrum should also be measured, as this will be the new lumbosacral slip angle if surgical management is to be an L-4 to S1 fusion.

### Sacral Inclination

The inclination of the sacrum is determined by drawing a line along the posterior cortex of the sacrum and measuring the angle between that line and a vertical line from the floor (a line drawn parallel to the edge of the x-ray film) (Fig. 21.10B). Normal sacral inclination is greater than 30 degrees; however, with higher-degree slips, the sacrum usually becomes more vertical and sacral inclination decreases.

### Pelvic Incidence

This measurement assesses the relation between the sacropelvic and hip joints. Pelvic incidence is the angle between a perpendicular-to-superior end plate of S1 and a line from the center of the superior end plate of S1 to the center of the femoral head (Fig. 21.10C). In normally aligned individuals, the gravity line should pass through the hip joints. Increased pelvic incidence has been shown to correlate with the degree of slippage (51,96,97).

### Anatomic Changes

Bony adaptive changes occur at the spondylolisthetic level and are more common in high-grade slips. In L-5-S1 spondylolisthesis, the superior end plate of S1 undergoes bony remodeling with resorption of the anterior lip of S1, creating a rounded, dome-shaped surface. The cephalic level, usually the fifth lumbar vertebra, becomes trapezoidal, specifically more narrow posteriorly and wider anteriorly. The amount of L-5 wedging can be measured in terms of the lumbar index, with references to the height of the anterior aspect of the L-5 vertebra expressed as a percentage of the height of the posterior aspect (Fig. 21.10B). Greater slips tend to have lower lumbar indices, and slip progression is more common with lower indices (13,35).

## TREATMENT

The myriad treatment choices for the patient with spondylolysis or spondylolisthesis fall into two main groups: nonsurgical and surgical. The nonsurgical options include observation, activity modification, physiotherapy, bracing or casting, and oral medications. Surgical options include repair of a pars interarticularis defect, fusion, decompression, reduction of the slip, or a combination of these. The challenge lies in selecting the appropriate treatment for each patient. In making this choice, one must consider the patient's symptoms, age, slip angle and grade, causation, and physical findings (especially neurologic signs). The recommendations of Wiltse are still generally accepted for treatment of children with spondylolysis or spondylolisthesis (98) (Table 21.3).

- Asymptomatic grades I and II: If the child is less than 10 years old, follow up with radiographs every 6 months through 15 years, then annually until end of growth. No limitations on activity are necessary in grade I. Patients with grade II slips should avoid contact sports and activities requiring repetitive lumbar hyperextension.
- Symptomatic grades I and II: Nonoperative therapies should be tried. Contact sports and those calling for hyperextension should be avoided. Fusion is indicated for patients who are unresponsive to all nonoperative interventions.
- Grades III/IV: Surgical intervention is indicated regardless of symptoms.

**TABLE 21.3**

**TRADITIONAL RECOMMENDATIONS OF TREATMENT**

| Grade Slip | Symptoms? | Treatment |
|---|---|---|
| I/II | No | Follow-up radiograph |
| I/II | Yes | Conservative; fusion for unresponsive patients |
| III/IV | No | Fusion |
| III/IV | Yes | Fusion |

# Spondylolysis

## Nonoperative

***Observation.*** As previously mentioned, most patients with spondylolysis are asymptomatic. In the patient with minimal to no symptoms, the follow-up will depend upon the child's age and growth potential. In the adolescent who has completed growth, no follow-up is necessary. In the growing child, however, lumbar radiographs should be obtained at the end of growth to monitor any potential for slip formation. The child with an asymptomatic spondylolysis can be allowed to participate in all sporting activities without restriction. In the long term, most young patients with spondylolysis, nonoperatively managed, maintain good functional outcome up to 11 years after diagnosis (99). In fact, the unilateral defects can undergo bony healing which may take up to 12 weeks; however, the bilateral defects may undergo degeneration, with mild slip over time (100). Beutler et al. reported on a 45-year follow-up of patients with spondylosis and spondylolisthesis. Patients with unilateral pars interarticularis defects never experienced slippage over the 45-year period (40).

## Reduction of Activities

In general, when the child has a symptomatic spondylolysis there is typically a long history of low back pain associated with activity. Restriction of activity is recommended along with physiotherapy emphasizing abdominal muscle and spinal extensor muscle strengthening, with short-term bedrest reserved for only the most exceptionally symptomatic patient. When the patient is asymptomatic, physical activities are gradually resumed.

A common dilemma that faces the orthopaedist is determining the duration of the child's symptoms. Patients with increased radiotracer uptake at the pars interarticularis during a SPECT bone scan are typically classified as having undergone an acute injury or fracture. In cases in which the scan is positive at the pars interarticularis in a patient with more acute onset of symptoms, immobilization in a cast or brace can be used for symptom abatement, and to hasten healing at the pars interarticularis defect. The ideal method is to immobilize this area with a body cast including one thigh/leg in order to appropriately control the pelvis. Another less onerous option is to use a thoracolumbar sacral orthosis (TLSO) with thigh cuff extension. The use of a removable brace is better accepted by the patient and family and will allow the individual to perform strengthening exercises out of the brace. The downside to a removable orthosis is the uncertainty of the patient's compliance with wearing the brace. Regarding healing of the pars interarticularis defect, varying levels of success have been described, with "healing" occurring in 3 to 4 months and typically being documented with oblique plain radiographic views or repeat bone scans (100–103). In the patient with a cold SPECT scan the use of a TLSO can be an option if the back pain is bothersome; however, the goal in this situation is not healing of the pars interarticularis defect, but rather, the elimination or diminution of symptoms. Bracing for approximately 3 months along with marked activity modification usually results in complete resolution of symptoms. Once the patient is asymptomatic, regardless of the status of the pars interarticularis defect, gradual resumption of athletic activities can be initiated without restriction. In cases that do not respond to nonoperative treatment, surgery can be offered as a possible alternative.

## Operative

***Repair of Defect.*** Pars interarticularis repairs are particularly useful in young adults and adolescents. The ideal candidate has a spondylolysis of less than a full grade I slip and no degenerative disc disease at the olisthetic level, and has failed a full course of nonoperative treatment of the symptoms, including immobilization. Given such restrictive criteria of selection, this technique should be used cautiously in patients beyond the adolescent years. The use of pars interarticularis injections preoperatively can assist verifying that the defect is the sole cause of the back pain. An MRI is necessary to assess the involved intervertebral disc and vertebral end-plate in order to identify any degree of disc degeneration or end-plate destruction which would preclude a successful outcome (23,104).

In 1970, Buck described a translaminar screw osteosynthesis technique for direct repair (105,106). He reported on 16 patients, out of whom 15 underwent fusion with this technique. One patient required salvage with a posterolateral fusion following failure of the pars interarticularis repair. Several other surgical techniques have also been described (107–110). Pedersen and Hagen reviewed 18 patients treated with Buck's technique and reported 83% satisfactory results (111). Like Buck, they recommend pars interarticularis repair only in young patients with no degenerative disc disease. Bradford and Iza presented a technique of transverse process wiring bilaterally to fix the loose posterior element and to facilitate pars interarticularis osteosynthesis (112,113). This technique has been modified with placement of pedicle screws as anchor points for the wiring, rather than the transverse processes. Of the 21 (of 22) cases available for follow-up, 90% obtained solid fusion of the pars interarticularis defect, and 80% had a good or excellent result. Bradford and Iza were also of the opinion that the technique is best suited for patients younger than 30 years without degenerative disc disease (113). This construct facilitates a compressive osteosynthesis across the laminar defect. A sublaminar hook/pedicle screw technique has been demonstrated to achieve improved control over the fracture fragments, compared to the less predictable laminar or spinous process wiring technique (Fig. 21.11). This improved technique includes replacing the posterior wire with bilateral, sublaminar hooks connected to the pedicle screws by a short rod. This facilitates direct compression across the lytic defect and provides improved control of the loose

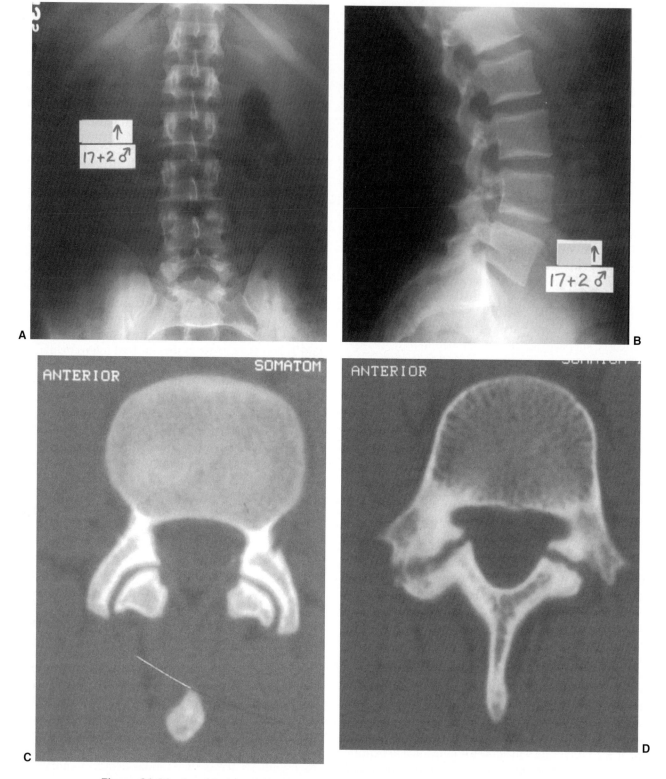

**Figure 21.11** **A** and **B:** A boy 17 years and 2 months old with a history of lumbosacral back pain and an associated L-4 bilateral spondylolysis. Normal facet joints at L-3–L-4 **(C)** contrast with the pars interarticularis defects of L-4 situated immediately caudal to the pedicles **(D)**. **E,F:** Following the failure of conservative treatment, and because the magnetic resonance imaging (MRI) showed absence of disc degeneration at L-4–L-5, he underwent an instrumented pars interarticularis repair at L-4. This was performed with bilateral L-4 pedicle screws connected to infralaminar hooks at L-4, with compression forces applied across the pars interarticularis defects that were grafted with auto-genous iliac crest bone. He experienced marked relief of lumbosacral pain postoperatively.

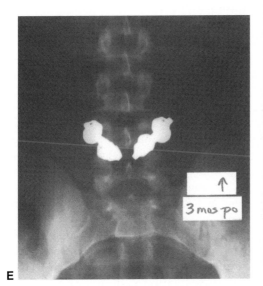 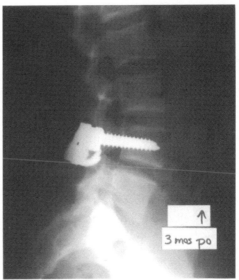

**Figure 21.11** (*continued*)

posterior element. In two small series of patients treated with sublaminar hook/pedicle screw constructs, 70% to 100% demonstrated clinical pain relief (107,108,114). The direct pars interarticularis repair is ideal for spondylolysis at the L-4 level and above, because it preserves lumbar motion segments.

A one-level L-5 to S1 posterolateral fusion is performed in patients who are unresponsive to nonoperative treatment and who are not candidates for direct pars interarticularis repair. Traditionally, this has been performed through a midline skin incision with an intertransverse process to sacrum fusion, utilizing autologous iliac crest bone graft as described by Wiltse and Jackson (10). Postoperative immobilization is dependent upon the surgeon's preference and various parameters relating to the patient. Spica casting for 3 months has been advocated on the basis of reports documenting high levels of good and excellent outcomes (11,115–120). However, others report good results with no immobilization (103), or immobilization in a corset (121) or Boston brace (122). The use of posterior spinal instrumentation (i.e., pedicle screw) is gaining acceptance, because it usually obviates the need for external immobilization and can rigidly maintain intraoperative correction. Overall, though, it is extremely rare for patients to require a fusion for a spondylolysis that fails conservative treatment.

## Spondylolisthesis

The treatment options for symptomatic spondylolisthesis fall into two categories: nonsurgical and surgical. The nonsurgical options consist primarily of observation, activity modification, bracing, and physiotherapy, and intervention in the form of medications or injections (123).

The natural history of mild spondylolisthesis is generally benign (5,13,36). Progression is atypical in patients whose growth has been completed and in those who have less than a 30% slippage (13,22). Nonoperative management regimens have generally included observation, activity modification, bracing, and physiotherapy, and several reports have documented good short-term and long-term results (13,16,36,44,124–127). Optimal candidates for successful nonoperative management appear to be those with spondylolysis and low-grade spondylolistheses (128).

An asymptomatic spondylolisthesis grade I or II in a skeletally immature child is kept under observation for progression with lateral lumbosacral radiographs taken with the patient in the standing position. A slip of less than 50% in an asymptomatic mature adolescent is also placed under observation. Observation is continued if there is no change in the slip angle or the amount of the slip; however, if there is progression of the spondylolisthesis or persistent symptoms, surgical stabilization is indicated.

Activity modification may involve the institution of proper bending and lifting activities and development of a sustained aerobic activities program. This program should aim at decreasing recumbent and sitting activities in favor of aerobic activities in order to facilitate achieving ideal body weight. A growing child who presents with low back pain and a spondylolisthesis grade I or II is advised to limit all physical activities which exacerbate the low back pain. Resumption of almost all activities is possible after symptoms have resolved.

If the pain does not resolve with restriction of activity, the use of a TLSO may be beneficial (102,118,128). This usually requires a period of 6 to 12 weeks in the brace. Once the symptoms are relieved, activities can gradually be resumed.

Physical therapy activities may be active or passive. Although passive modalities may be useful initially, when there is acute pain, active physical therapy techniques are probably more important in the long term. Examples of passive techniques are thermal therapy, massage, phonophoresis, ultrasound, immobilization, acupuncture, traction, and transcutaneous electrical nerve stimulation. These may facilitate the patient's acceptance of an active physical therapy program by ameliorating acute symptoms. Active physical therapy includes spinal flexibility exercises and muscle strengthening, especially abdominal and posterior lumbar muscles. Pelvic stabilization techniques are also important; these may involve isometric and isokinetic exercises as well as aerobic conditioning.

In the early phases of pain management, medications may be important. Nonsteroidal antiinflammatory drugs should be instituted early and are the mainstay of drug therapy. Because the use of muscle relaxants and narcotics remains controversial, we tend to avoid prescription medication in children and teens, if at all possible. If medications are to be used, the patient must be informed that narcotics will not be prescribed beyond a week or two, and their purpose is to facilitate the transition to physical therapy for managing the low back pain. Muscle relaxants may likewise be useful in the early, acute period to deal with muscle spasms secondary to injury.

Surgical intervention should be considered for persistently symptomatic spondylolisthesis which does not respond to nonoperative management, and which causes pain that prevents normal participation in daily and desirable physical activities. Additionally, the skeletally immature patient with slippage greater than grade II or the mature adolescent with a slip of more than 75% should be treated surgically even in the absence of symptoms (42,47,124,129). Surgical treatment options for symptomatic spondylolisthesis include decompression, fusion, or a combination of these techniques. In grade I and early grade II isthmic spondylolisthesis, the use of *in situ* posterolateral fusion is well established. However, for higher grades of spondylolisthesis, the decision-making process becomes more complex, involving decisions about the number of levels that should be fused, whether to aim for partial or complete slip reduction, whether to include anterior fusion, and whether to use instrumentation and postoperative immobilization.

For spondylolisthesis of grade I or higher in adolescents and perhaps also in young adults, pars interarticularis repair is a reasonable option if the caveats previously mentioned are followed. In particular, the disc at the slip level should be lordotic and without degenerative changes. Any degree of spondylolisthesis indicates the likelihood of disc degeneration or end-plate destruction, making MRI a necessity if a direct pars interarticularis repair is being considered.

Nerve root compression is documented by radicular pain, motor weakness, and a sensory deficit, and is confirmed with further imaging studies. No correlation has been found between tight hamstrings and the objective neurologic findings of weakness, sensory deficit, or changes in reflexes (11). In an L-5–S1 spondylolisthesis, the L-5 root is usually implicated; the compression occurs at the foraminal level, between the proximal part of the pars interarticularis as it slips forward with the vertebral body, or is caused by the fibrocartilaginous tissue at the pars interarticularis defect. True nerve root compression is an indication for formal nerve decompression. However, the presence of hamstring tightness is not by itself necessarily a sign of nerve root compression.

Decompression, alone or in combination with fusion, may be necessary if radicular or neurogenic claudication symptoms are present. Decompression alone may be a useful technique in patients with spondylolysis or a low-grade (grade II or less) spondylolisthesis when the symptoms are primarily neurologic and there is little evidence of instability. This situation is more common in adults than in children or adolescents. However, even patients with presumed stability and little back pain must be informed that decompression in the presence of a lytic defect or a low-grade spondylolisthesis may increase instability, causing low back pain. Intuitively, one would consider foraminotomies either unilaterally or bilaterally rather than a significant midline decompression in such a case. In 1955, Gill et al. reviewed 18 patients treated with complete removal of the loose posterior element (Gill laminectomy), and reported good results (130,131). A long-term follow-up study of 43 patients, published in 1965, revealed an increased slip in 14% of patients, but a 90% satisfactory result in the group overall (132). These results, however, have not been universally observed. Osterman et al. reported on 75 patients with long-term follow-up averaging 12 years, and although the initial results at the end of 1 year showed fair, good, or excellent results in 83% of the patients, these results did not hold up over time (133). When these same patients were evaluated 5 years postoperatively, satisfaction ratings had dropped to 75%, and the spondylolisthesis had progressed in 27% of patients. Marmor and Bechtol described a patient who progressed from a grade II slip to a spondyloptosis after a Gill laminectomy (134). In a more dismal review of 33 patients with a 7-year follow-up, Amuso et al. reported 36% poor results with Gill laminectomy (135). These authors did not observe any significant progression of the spondylolisthesis and do not believe there is any correlation between the progression of spondylolisthesis and poor results.

With the currently available options for stabilization, the Gill laminectomy as a stand-alone intervention is not a reasonable procedure, especially in a growing child, and should always be accompanied by a spinal fusion (130,131). However, decompression is often an important part of the surgical treatment of spondylolisthesis, and in patients with lytic defects a Gill laminectomy is an efficient start for achieving a wide decompression. It also often results in sufficient autologous bone for fusion of that level. It should be noted that the Gill laminectomy alone does not decompress the involved foraminal nerve root; to achieve this, an additional dissection and formal nerve root decompression is necessary. Wiltse and Jackson proposed that root decompression is rarely necessary and that the tight hamstrings, abnormal reflexes, and motor weakness will recover after posterior fusion alone (10). Formal decompression of the nerve is assumed to give the affected nerve root the optimal chance of recovery; however, this must be weighed against the chance of increased slip, if one is considering a decompression and fusion without instrumentation. In such a situation, nerve root decompression with an instrumented fusion will permit an adequate decompression of the affected nerve roots while stabilizing the fusion segment in the desired position.

Fusion is the standard surgical technique for treatment of symptomatic spondylolisthesis and is necessary when instability (documented on lateral flexion and extension radiographs) and low back pain exist. Fusion is probably also reasonable when performing primarily decompressive surgery on patients whose main symptom is lower extremity radiculopathy, but whose spondylolisthesis is grade III or greater, especially in the presence of degenerative disc disease. Available techniques include anterior and posterior procedures, either alone or in combination. Posterior techniques include posterior lumbar interbody fusions (PLIF) and posterolateral fusions with or without instrumentation.

### Instrumentation

Numerous historical studies extol the benefits of posterolateral uninstrumented fusions. In these studies, fusion rates have ranged from 67% to 96%, with 60% to 100% of the patients showing good results (25,41,122,136–139). Although the outcomes of these multiple studies have been excellent, the actual pseudarthrosis rate may be much higher than reported. Lenke et al. critically evaluated 56 patients with isthmic spondylolisthesis treated with *in situ* posterolateral fusions (140). When strict grading criteria were used, only 50% of the patients had bilateral solid fusions, 18% had unilateral solid fusions, and 21% had pseudarthrosis (Fig. 21.12). Despite the high rate of pseudarthrosis, overall clinical improvement was noted in more than 80% of patients who had presented with preoperative symptoms of back or leg pain or hamstring tightness.

Recent studies by Bridwell et al. highlight the benefit of instrumentation in achieving improved fusion rates and improved outcomes (141). Other groups have reported high fusion rates (90% to 95%) and 90% excellent or good outcomes with instrumented fusions for spondylolisthesis (142–144). External immobilization postoperatively is typically not necessary, because the spinal fixation of transpedicular instrumentation provides sufficient rigidity; however, in cases with poor bone quality, an adjunctive postoperative cast or brace may be helpful. *In situ* posterolateral fusion continues to offer satisfactory results for

patients with grade I and some grade II spondylolistheses; the risks are within reasonable limits, and this technique remains a good approach for this category of patients. However, if the surgeon is comfortable placing pedicle screws in children, the procedure can provide definitive stabilization with less reliance on postoperative immobilization in most circumstances (Fig. 21.13).

### Fusion Levels

For the prototypical low-grade L-5-S1 spondylolisthesis the customary procedure is a posterolateral one-level L-5-S1 fusion. Extension of the uninstrumented fusion to L-4 may be indicated for greater degrees of slip (i.e., more than 50%) for two main reasons (Fig. 21.14): (a) in high-grade slips the transverse process of L-5 is displaced anterior to the sacral ala, making it difficult to expose the transverse process of L-5 without exposing the L-4–L-5 facet and L-4 transverse process; and (b) the fusion mass placed from L-5 to the ala will be horizontal and under shear forces, whereas graft from the ala to the L-4 transverse process will lie in a more biomechanically sound, vertical direction. A two-level uninstrumented arthrodesis may also be necessary in a slip of less than 50% if the transverse process of L-5 is very small and provides an insufficient posterior bed for the fusion. With the advent of posterior instrumentation (i.e., pedicle screws) and anterior structural support (i.e., cages), the need for two-level fusion is decreasing, because of the high probability of creating a stable, solid bony union of the one-level fusion, even for high-grade slips. In addition, even a two-level L-4–sacrum uninstrumented fusion is not guaranteed to heal in a grade III or IV spondylolisthesis (Fig. 21.15). When pseudarthrosis and slip progression are noted postoperatively, revision fusion with instrumentation is indicated.

### Reduction of Spondylolisthesis

Minor degrees of slip (less than 25%) usually do not have a pathologic slip angle; therefore, surgeons prefer to treat such patients with fusion *in situ*, unless there is demonstrable instability on flexion-extension lateral radiographs. However, with a more marked deformity in higher-grade spondylolisthesis, especially in the presence of increased lumbosacral kyphosis and extreme spondyloptosis, some degree of reduction is necessary in order to realign the lumbar spine over the sacrum in a position that will permit a solid fusion with acceptable sagittal alignment (Fig. 21.16). Studies on *in situ* fusions for higher-grade slips have reported pseudarthrosis rates from 0% to 60% and slip progression rates of as much as 25%, gait disturbances, and persistent cosmetic deformity. These data have led many to advocate reduction of high-grade slips, not only to address these issues but also to save motion segments (14,25,118,121,143,145–153). Although there is some concern regarding the neurologic risk at the time of reduction, *in situ* fusions for high-grade slips have also been associated with adverse neurologic outcomes (125). Schoenecker et al. reported on 12 patients who developed

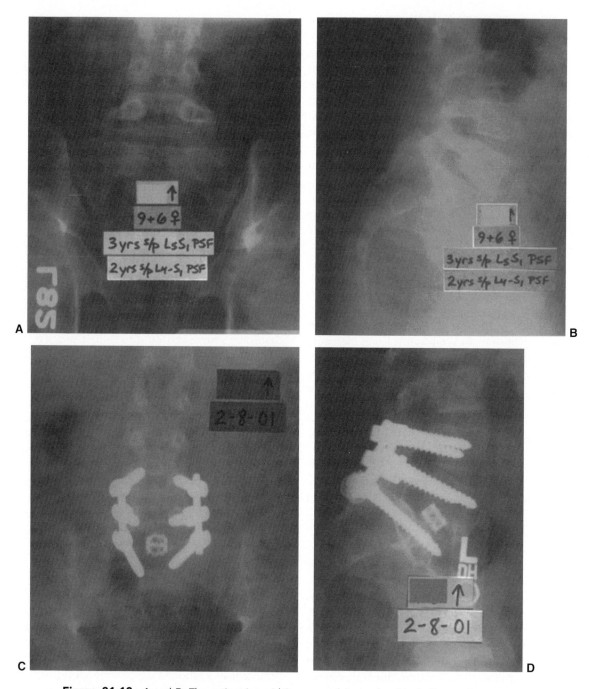

**Figure 21.12** **A** and **B:** The patient is a girl 9 years and 6 months old who has undergone two prior *in situ* fusions for a low-grade isthmic dysplastic spondylolisthesis at L-5–S1. She ultimately developed a solid fusion at L-4–L-5, and pseudarthrosis at L-5–S1, with continued lumbosacral pain. **C** and **D:** She then underwent a posterior instrumented revision fusion from L-4 to the sacrum as well as an anterior interbody fusion with a structural cage and bone graft at L-5–S1 in an attempt to alleviate the pain caused by her pseudarthrosis.

cauda equina syndrome after *in situ* arthrodesis for high-grade spondylolisthesis. Seven of the 12 patients had permanent neurologic injuries, which were attributed to the prone positioning during surgery and the postural reduction of the deformity during surgery (126).

In order to minimize complications associated with reduction procedures, a sound surgical technique and adherence to simple mechanical principles are important,

including wide laminectomy and complete bilateral nerve root decompression. Often nerve root decompression must be performed beyond the vertebral column. This is because of soft tissue constriction of the nerve roots within the paraspinal muscles and iliolumbar ligaments, which may result in neuropraxia caused by nerve root stretch during reduction of high-grade slips. Complete discectomy is necessary in order to release the olisthetic segment. Further

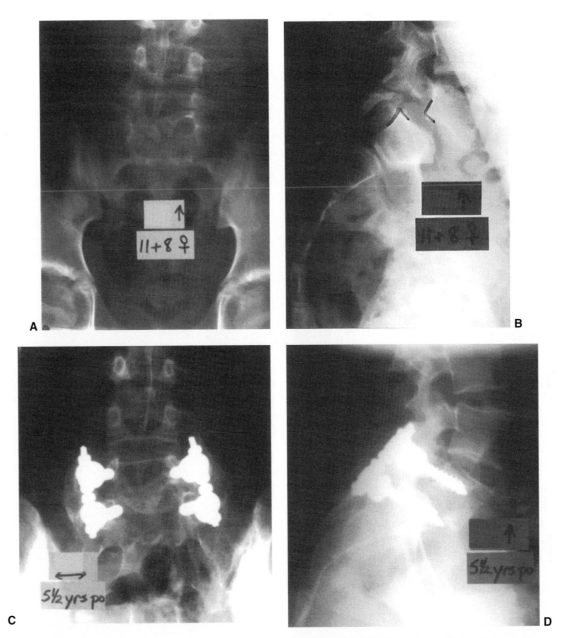

**Figure 21.13** **A** and **B:** This patient, a girl 11 years and 8 months old, had 50% back pain and 50% leg pain from a low-grade L-5 spondylolisthesis. Following failure of conservative treatment, she underwent a posterior decompression and instrumented posterolateral fusion from L-5 to the sacrum with autogenous iliac crest graft laterally. **C:** At 5 years 6 months postoperatively, she had an excellent solid arthrodesis seen on this Ferguson posteroanterior view. **D:** The lateral view, showing a stable L-5–S1.

release and mobilization of the olisthetic segment can be achieved by sacral dome osteotomy, which facilitates reduction without necessitating excessive vertebral distraction. Although excessive distraction may be dangerous, judicious distraction is a useful maneuver to help achieve reduction by lifting the L-5 body out and away from the pelvis. Various techniques for achieving distraction have been reported since its initial description by Jenkins in 1936 (154). External traction, that is, halo-femoral (83,137,155), passive positional reduction (151), temporary casting (152), temporary intraoperative hook

and rod constructs, and distraction using pedicle screw instrumentation as a staged part of the surgical procedure can all be useful (31,126,143,150,156–158). If distraction is used across segments that are not to be included in the final levels to be instrumented and fused, careful attention must be given to the intervening soft tissue to make sure that the uninstrumented facet joints are not injured. Overdistraction may result in iatrogenic instability of those uninstrumented levels. If excessive distraction is placed across the final instrumentation, the pedicle screws may loosen, resulting in the loss of fixation postoperatively.

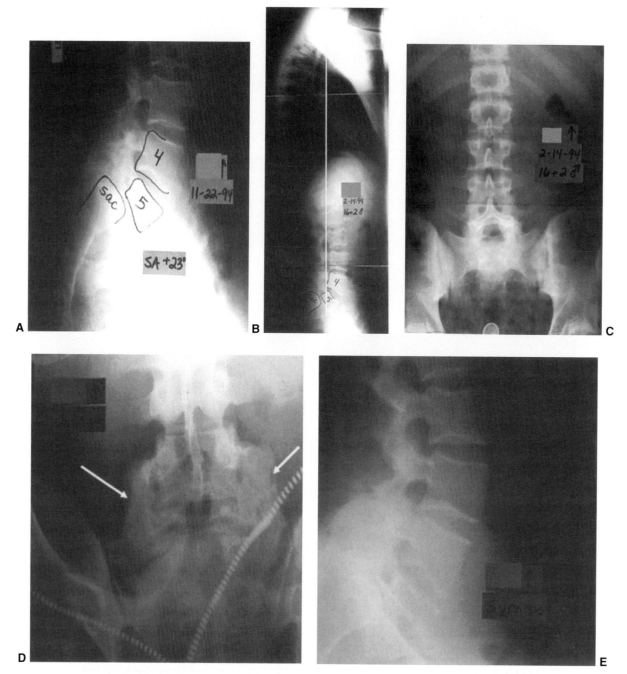

**Figure 21.14** This 16-year-old boy had a grade III isthmic spondylolisthesis at L-5–S1. He had chronic lumbosacral back pain without radicular pain. He was treated with a bilateral Wiltse paraspinal approach, with autogenous iliac crest bone graft placement following decortication from L-4 to the sacral ala. Postoperatively, he was maintained in a bilateral pantaloon cast for 3 months, and then in a lumbar-sacral orthosis for an additional 3 months. **A:** Preoperative lateral x-rays of a Grade III slip with a +25° angle. **B:** Upright long cassette lateral x-ray showing good overall sagittal balance. **C:** Preoperative frontal x-ray showing large lumbar transverse processess. **D** and **E:** At 5 years postoperatively, he had a rock-solid fusion from L-4 to the sacrum, with stable alignment in his lateral view radiograph. His pain was totally relieved postoperatively.

Posterior translation using reduction pedicle screws is a newly available technique. This instrumentation, used in conjunction with appropriate distraction, can constitute a powerful reduction method. However, it must be stressed that without first achieving appropriate soft tissue release through a combination of sacral dome osteotomy, discectomy, and distraction to provide room to allow posterior translation of the olisthetic segment, any attempt at translation with reduction pedicle screws is likely to result only in the fracture of the pedicles and dislodgement of the pedicle screws. The possible complications associated with the reduction procedure, both intraoperatively and postoperatively

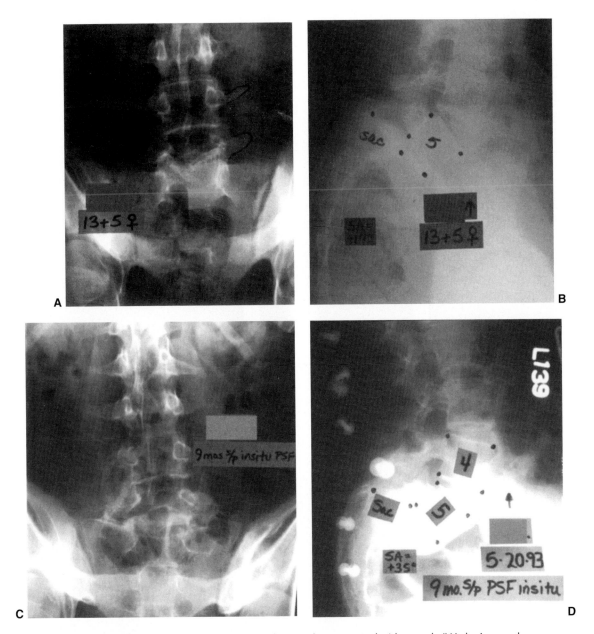

**Figure 21.15**  This girl, aged 13 years and 5 months, presented with a grade IV isthmic spondylolisthesis at L-5–S1. She had pain only in the back, and no symptoms in the legs. She underwent an *in situ* L-4–to–sacrum posterolateral fusion followed by 3 months of postoperative casting and 3 months of bracing. **A** and **B:** Preoperative AP and lateral radiographs of a Grade IV slip. **C** and **D:** Nine months postoperative AP and lateral radiographs showing increased slipage and a pseudarthrosis. She had, at that point, not only lumbosacral pain but also radicular leg pain caused by L-5 symptomatology. She then underwent a revision posterior decompression, partial reduction, instrumentation and fusion from L-4 to the sacrum and ilium. This was followed, at an early postoperative stage, by an anterior fibular strut graft placed between L-5 and the sacrum. At $1\frac{1}{2}$ years after her revision surgery, she has a solid fusion with elimination of her preoperative symptoms.

(159,160), raises questions about whether reduction is necessary or even desirable. Petraco et al. have suggested that complete reduction causes excessive stretch of the L-5 nerve root and should therefore not be performed (161). However, this study did not consider the effect that an adequate discectomy and sacral dome osteotomy have on shortening the spine, thereby making full reduction safer.

Proponents for full but judicious and safe reduction point to the improved weight bearing, decreased shear stress, and the improved bed for fusion provided by a full reduction (143,162–164). The improved biomechanical stability provided by full reduction with anterior column support may allow us to perform a shorter instrumentation and fusion because of the inherent stability found in the fully

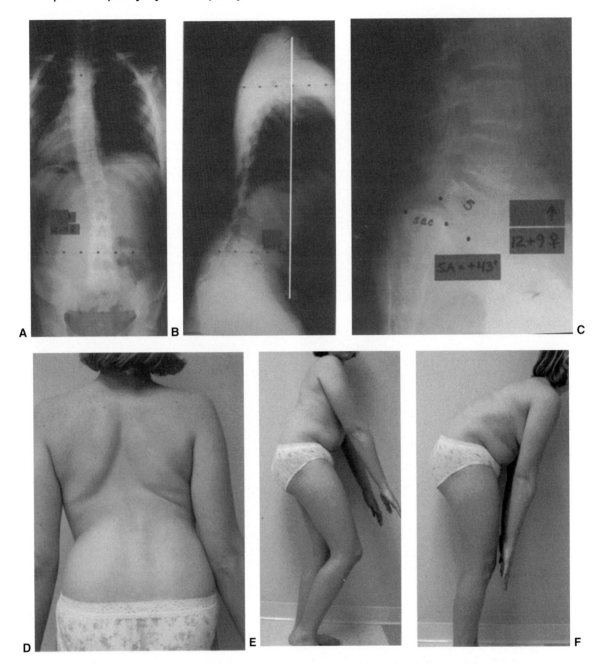

**Figure 21.16** The patient, a girl 12 years and 9 months of age, had a grade IV dysplastic isthmic spondylolisthesis with a 43-degree kyphotic slip angle. Her anteroposterior radiograph shows mild olisthetic scoliosis **(A)**, and her lateral radiographs show marked sagittal imbalance with a vertical sacrum **(B,C)**. Preoperative clinical photos show her clinical deformity **(D)**, with thoracic hyperextension, flattened buttocks, and flexed knees and hips, because of her significantly tight right and left L-5 nerve roots **(E)**, and marked limitation on forward flexion **(F)**. She was taken to surgery where she was positioned prone with her hips and knees flexed initially prior to her decompression. She had a dysplastic L-5 arch, and a spina bifida occulta just caudal to this. Following thorough decompression of the L-5 nerve roots, the right L-5 root was stimulated directly to obtain an electromyographic (EMG) distal recording corresponding to the innervation in the anterior tibialis of the L-5 root. On the left side, L-5–S1 disc excision and sacral dome osteotomy were performed to allow access into the disc and reduction of the spondylolisthesis. Spondylolisthesis was reduced in part by flexing the S1–iliac screw construct to meet the L-5 screw on the right side. Postoperative radiographs show the L-5–S1 instrumented posterolateral fusion **(G,H)** with partial reduction followed by a reamed anterior fibular graft (*arrow*) from L-5 to the sacrum **(I)**. Note the improved coronal alignment as well as the excellent sagittal realignment following the reconstruction **(G,H)**. Postoperatively, the clinical posture is normalized, with excellent ankle and toe dorsiflexion function noted bilaterally **(J–L)**.

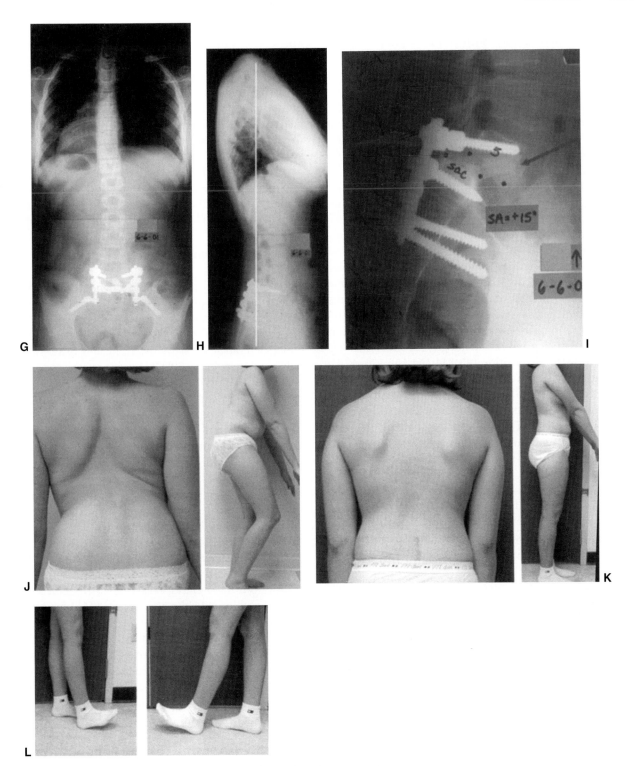

**Figure 21.16** (continued)

reduced construct. Once acceptable alignment is obtained after reduction, posterior instrumentation and anterior reconstruction with an intradisc graft or cage are typically necessary for maintaining the rigidity of the new lumbosacral alignment (143,157,162–165). As one would expect with these complex spinal realignment or reduction techniques, there is a risk of iatrogenic radiculopathy, and this must be borne in mind during the decision-making process (79,160,164,165). Perhaps a good compromise is a partial reduction of the translation and kyphotic angle component of the slip to an acceptable level, which usually entails less neurologic risk. As long as the L-5–S1 disc space has been repositioned adequately to allow placement of an intradiscal support device, such as an Allograft wedge or cage, then the new lumbosacral alignment should be biomechanically stable for fusion.

### Anterior Fusion

At present, the role of anterior fusion in the treatment of spondylolisthesis is reserved for cases in which it is necessary to reestablish segmental lordosis, to increase the size of the available fusion bed, or to increase the stability of the posterior instrumentation. Multiple studies on anterior fusion alone have reported overall good results when compared to posterior and circumferential fusions (166–169). Issues such as increased pseudarthrosis rate, and lesser correction of slip angle, slip grade, sacral inclination, and sacral rotation raise questions about the use of anterior fusion as a stand-alone procedure (166–169). Some authors have advocated combining anterior structural grafts with posterior pedicle screw constructs and posterolateral fusion; this approach would theoretically improve fusion rates while reducing and maintaining the spondylolisthesis in a more anatomic position (43,144,164,166,170–172). La Rosa reported on 35 patients who underwent an instrumented posterolateral fusion, out of whom 17 had an additional PLIF. At 2-year follow-up the PLIF group had better correction of subluxation, disc height, and maintenance of foraminal area; however, the clinical outcomes for patients in the two groups were statistically equivalent (173).

Bohlman and his associates have reported a single-stage technique for interbody fusion and posterior decompression for high-grade spondylolisthesis. Along with posterior decompression and fusion, this procedure additionally stabilizes the spondylolisthesis *in situ* by placing a fibular strut graft through the body of S1 and into the displaced body of L-5 through a posterior approach (174,175). This technique has been shown to be effective in primary and revision surgeries, and is associated with a low incidence of transient neurologic deficits (142,164,176). Hanson et al. reported on 17 patients who underwent combined partial slip reduction with dowel fibular strut grafts for high-grade dysplastic isthmic spondylolisthesis. Solid fusion was achieved in 16 of the 17 patients, and there were no cases of neurologic deficits (97).

PLIF has its attractions as a surgical technique for the treatment of high-grade spondylolisthesis. The wide exposure of the spinal canal at the time of decompression provides ideal access for performing a unilateral or bilateral PLIF, thereby permitting a biomechanically sound fusion of all three columns of the spine (164). The intervertebral structural grafts increase the surface area available for fusion, and permit compressive load-sharing through normal spinal biomechanics while opening up the narrowed neuroforamen. Several series have reported excellent results on combining PLIF with an instrumented posterior reduction and fusion (144,164,173).

### Immobilization and Bed Rest

The kind of postoperative immobilization recommended after fusion varies from no immobilization at all (17,177) or a brace to a single or bilateral spica cast (16,118), with the patient ambulatory or in bed rest. The decision to use immobilization will depend upon several factors such as the patient's body habitus, likelihood of compliance, preoperative slip grade and angle, whether the surgery was primary or a revision, and the adequacy of reduction and instrumentation purchase. If a TLSO is used, the thigh must be included into the brace without a hinge joint, in order to adequately control the pelvis. Brace use is continued for 3 to 4 months postoperatively until solid fusion is noted radiographically.

### Recommendations for Spondylolisthesis
#### Grade I

Direct pars interarticularis repair is an option in patients with spondylolysis or minimal spondylolisthesis, with L-5 in a lordotic position, and no degenerative changes at the olisthetic level. A "hot" SPECT scan at the pars interarticularis implies a biologically active defect, making osteosynthesis a viable option. A "cold" SPECT scan is a relative contraindication to a direct pars interarticularis repair, because the lack of biologic activity indicates little inherent ability to create a bony union. In addition, the absence of neurologic findings is essential, because the technique of direct pars interarticularis repair is not amenable to a nerve root decompression.

For low-grade slips in patients requiring fusions, pedicle screw and rod constructs provide ample support, particularly when anterior interbody support is used. In the case of a mild or moderately degenerated disc without significant collapse, a posterolateral instrumented fusion alone may not be sufficient, even if a wide decompression is not necessary and a large posterolateral surface area exists for fusion. We prefer to always stabilize even grade I slips so as to enhance our fusion rates. Posterior instrumented fusions without abdominal subcutaneous fat (ASF) may be sufficient in patients with significant disc-space collapse at the olisthetic level. The inherent stability provided by the collapsed disc will decrease the stress on the construct and the interface between the screws and the vertebrae. However, in patients with a large or hypermobile disc, anterior column support may be necessary for an effective reconstruction.

#### Grade II

In patients with grade II spondylolisthesis, instrumentation and fusion along with decompression will likely be required. Anterior column support in the form of intradiscal cages or Allograft wedges should be provided in order to ensure long-term stability of the construct and to allow for maximum correction of segmental sagittal alignment. The anterior column support can be achieved by either an anterior lumbar interbody fusion (ALIF) or a posterior lumbar interbody fusion/transforaminal lumbar interbody fusion (PLIF/TLIF) technique. Another attractive option is to perform a transperitoneal approach, which permits quick and easy access to the disc space, allowing complete disc removal and placement of a large footprint interbody spacer while reestablishing lordosis. Reestablishing or maintaining segmental alignment of the olisthetic level will theoretically protect adjacent levels.

### Grade III/IV

For slips of grade III or greater, the surgical technique can be extremely demanding. Because each high-grade slip presents with a unique combination of pathologic anatomy, biomechanics, and clinical symptoms, all surgical techniques should be considered and may be useful during any reduction and subsequent stabilization of the vertebral column (164,170,174). Slip angle reduction, anterior interbody support, and reconstruction of the anterior column are important components of the reconstruction for high-grade slips. With appropriate release, a complete discectomy, and possible sacral dome osteotomy, anterior column reconstruction may provide enough segmental stability to allow monosegmental fixation with a high degree of success. This has been advocated by Harms et al. for many years (159). Wide nerve root decompression is an essential component in minimizing the development of iatrogenic nerve root injury at the time of reduction of the slip, as has been mentioned earlier in the Reduction of Spondylothesis.

In patients with slips greater than or equal to grade III, in whom significant effort is required in order to achieve reduction of the olisthetic segment, fixation distal to S1 (i.e., iliac screws) should be provided for stability of the reconstruction. For these higher-grade slips, a posterior approach for achieving an anterior column reconstruction (i.e., PLIF/TLIF technique) is more practical than an ALIF procedure, for several reasons. Because of the forward flexion of the rostral vertebra, access into the disc space anteriorly may be difficult or impossible. Because these higher-grade slips often have significant posterior element dysplasia and neuroforaminal narrowing, the nerve roots should be identified and decompressed before vertebral reduction maneuvers are attempted. Failure to achieve an adequate decompression before reduction may result in severe irreversible nerve root injury. Usually by the time the wide laminectomy and foraminal decompression are carried out for bilateral nerve root decompression, the posterior aspect of the disc is clearly exposed. This facilitates the PLIF/TLIF technique. Sacral dome osteotomy, which is another useful technique for achieving release of the deformity and facilitating reduction of high-grade slips, can be performed through the posterior approach. The posterior approach is also an advantage because of the expansive posterior decompression that is accomplished with the Gill laminectomy.

### Grade V

In patients with grade V slips (i.e., spondyloptosis) options include L-4-sacrum fusion *in situ*, augmented with fibular dowel grafts; posterior reduction as previously discussed; or an L-5 spondylectomy. The posterior approach with sacral

dome osteotomy can be used effectively in many of these cases (Fig. 21.17). However, we occasionally prefer to treat this pathology with a Gaines procedure, which is a complete L-5 vertebrectomy (Fig. 21.18) (178,179). The first stage of this procedure is an anterior L-5 corpectomy, followed by a posterior approach to resect the posterior elements. This technique is followed by the reduction of L-4 to the sacrum and stabilization with pedicle screw instrumentation. Fusion is performed anteriorly and posteriorly. The L-5 nerve roots are in extreme jeopardy during anterior vertebral resection because they are usually trapped and tethered under the pedicles of L-5, the posterior aspect of the vertebral body of L-5, and the anterior cortex of the sacrum.

## COMPLICATIONS

### Pseudarthrosis

The reported pseudarthrosis rate after fusion varies from 0% to 39% (11,25,44,115,116,118,170,180), with most of the sources reporting less than 15%. Higher pseudarthritic complication rates have been associated with higher-grade spondylolisthesis and fusion *in situ* of these deformities (11,171).

### Progression of Slip

The magnitude of the slip, as measured by the amount of displacement or kyphosis, can increase even in the presence of a solid fusion (10,11,23,47,119,180). However, it should be noted that the fusions reported on were uninstrumented and were assessed with plain radiographs. CT scans may have been able to demonstrate that some of the instances of increased slippage were actually caused by the lack of adequate fusion. Further slippage following an uninstrumented surgery is more common because the removal of midline-stabilizing structures at the time of decompression increases lumbosacral instability. This is also more common in higher grades of spondylolisthesis, in patients with a greater degree of anterior displacement, and in slip kyphosis.

### Neurologic Complications

Radiculopathy is the most common complication after reduction of spondylolisthesis; it is usually an L-5 nerve root lesion and has varying recovery rates (79,160,164,165). One series on partial slip reduction with the use of a dowel fibular strut graft for high-grade slips reported no permanent neurologic complications (97). In contrast, acute postoperative cauda equina syndrome has been reported after a simple posterolateral fusion without decompression or reduction (125,126). This complication can occur through a midline or lateral muscle-splitting incision when the patient is prone or laterally positioned (115,126). The cause of this significant complication is not definitely known. However, in high-grade slips, the MRI scan can

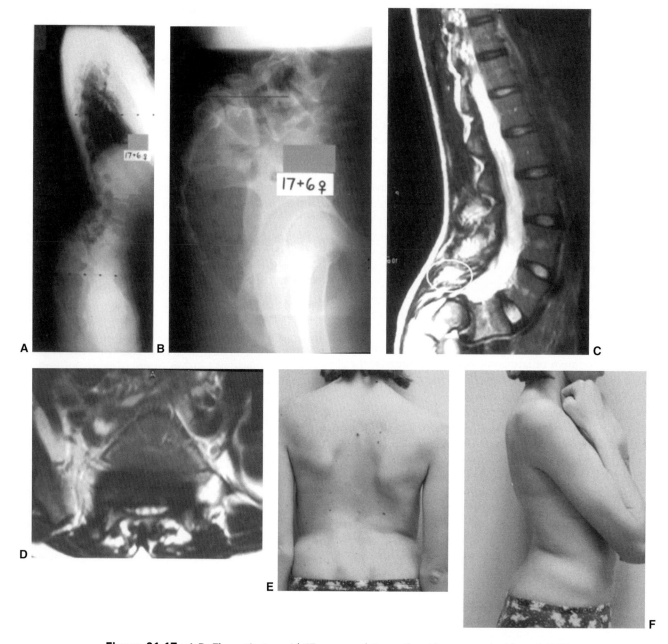

**Figure 21.17** **A,B:** The patient, a girl 17 years and 6 months old, presented with an L-5–S1 spondyloptosis as well as L-4 bilateral spondylolysis. **C,D:** Her preoperative sagittal and axial magnetic resonance imaging scans at L-5–S1 demonstrate a tight spinal canal with a pincer effect behind the posterior edge of the sacrum and the lumbosacral disc. **E–G:** Her preoperative clinical photos demonstrate prominent L-5 arch visible on the coronal as well as lateral clinical views. In forward flexion, she had limited flexion in her waist. **H–J:** She underwent a wide decompression and an instrumention of posterolateral fusion of L-4 to the sacrum and ilium which, aided by a proximal sacroplasty, resulted in marked reduction of her deformity. She also had transforaminal lumbar interbody fusions (TLIFs) at L-4–L-5 and L-5–S1 for anterior structural support and grafting. One year postoperatively, radiographs show excellent maintenance of alignment. **K–M:** Her postoperative clinical photos demonstrate her clinical alignment as well as excellent plantar and dorsal flexion of her feet bilaterally.

demonstrate a cleaved intervertebral disc at the spondylolisthetic segment, with the posterior half indenting the dural sac. The development of cauda equina syndrome is likely secondary to acute neural compression caused by this posterior disc fragment in a patient with a marked slip, which partially reduces at the time of surgery, causing further compression of the already at-risk neural elements. Patients with high-grade slips and the congenital types of

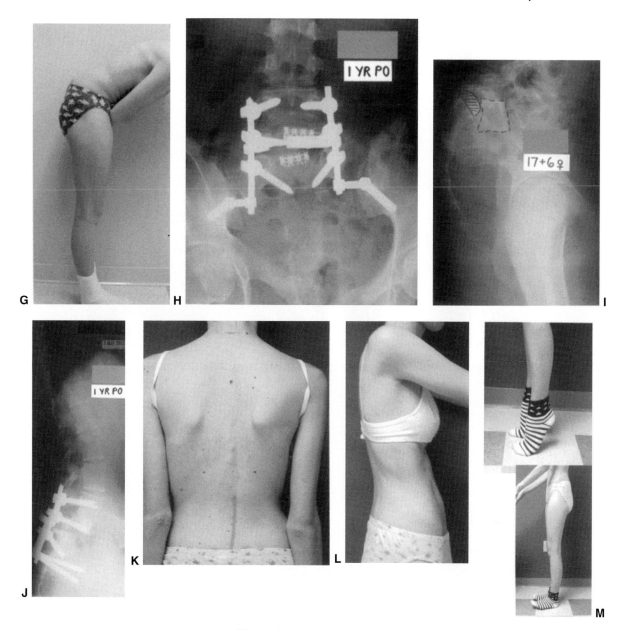

**Figure 21.17** (continued)

deformities are at an increased risk for neural compression at the time of surgery. MRI can be helpful in these situations by permitting visualization of the intervertebral disc pathology and neural compression, since such neurologic deficits can occur in the absence of any preoperative neurologic signs or symptoms (125,126).

Prevention of postoperative neurologic deficits is optimal, because permanent neurologic deficits can occur postoperatively, even after immediate decompression of iatrogenic neurologic deficits. Patients with spondylolisthesis who experience postoperative neurologic deficits should undergo MRI or CT myelogram imaging of the neural elements in order to elucidate the causes of the deficits. Any preoperative nerve root compression, irrespective of the grade of the spondylolisthesis, should be decompressed. Adequate decompression typically destabilizes the spine, however, increasing the risk of slip progression, neurologic deficit, and pseudarthrosis and making posterior stabilization with pedicle screw constructs an ideal option. Intraoperative neuromonitoring can be useful at the time of decompression and, if necessary, reduction, so as to minimize iatrogenic neurologic deficits. However, somatosensory and elecromyographic monitoring may not predict L-5 nerve root deficits, and therefore intraoperative wake-up test(s) are strongly recommended. Direct L-5 and S1 nerve stimulation is another technique for monitoring nerve integrity more closely during various stages of the surgery. Careful neurologic follow-up postoperatively is essential in all cases.

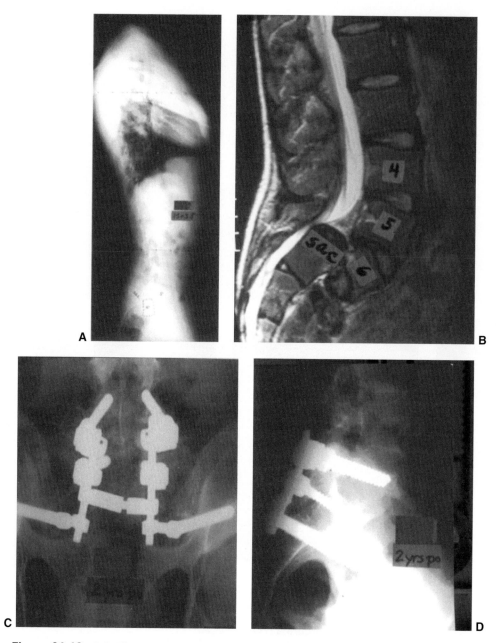

**Figure 21.18   A,B:** The patient is a 15-year-old boy who presented with a severe L-6 spondyloptosis. The magnetic resonance imaging shows the complete anterior and distal position of the L-6 vertebral body below the sacrum. He had lumbosacral back pain and bilateral L-5 radicular pain. **C,D:** He underwent an L-6 spondylectomy with anterior and posterior fusion, and posterior instrumentation of L-5 to the sacrum. Two years postoperatively, he has an excellent circumferential fusion, with chronic dorsiflexion weakness to his feet and ankles bilaterally, but there is no need for any ankle-foot orthotics (AFO) or ambulatory aids. Although he had an excellent result as seen radiographically, his case demonstrates the high risk to the L-5 roots associated with the spondylectomy procedure in the treatment of severe spondyloptosis.

## CONCLUSION

The treatment of pediatric patients with varying degrees and types of spondylolisthesis is a challenge for the pediatric spinal specialist. Most patients with the more common low-grade slips will be managed successfully with nonoperative treatment. Complete preoperative workup, detailed planning for intraoperative contingencies, technical execution, and common-sense postoperative adjunctive immobilization and activity restriction are all requirements for success. Severe cases of spondylolisthesis are some of the most challenging pediatric spinal problems encountered, and should be operatively treated only by those with expertise in the pathoanatomy of the condition and with the technical skills necessary for surgical success.

# REFERENCES

1. Herbiniaux G. *Traite sur divers accouchemens labprieux, et sur polypes de la matrice.* Bruxelles: JL DeBoubers, 1782.
2. Kilian HF. Schilderungen neuer beckenformen and ihres verhaltens im leben. Mannheim; Verlag von Bassermann & Mathy, 1854.

## Classification

3. Newman PH, Stone KH. The etiology of spondylolisthesis: with a special investigation. *J Bone Joint Surg Br* 1963;45:39–59.
4. Wiltse LL, Newman PH, Macnab I. Classification of spondylolysis and spondylolisthesis. *Clin Orthop Relat Res* 1976;117:23–29.
5. Wiltse LL, Rothman LG. Spondylolisthesis: classification, diagnosis, and natural history. *Semin Spine Surg* 1989;1:78.
6. Wiltse LL, Rothman SLG. Spondylolisthesis: classification, diagnosis, and natural history. *Semin Spine Surg* 1993;5:264–280.
7. Marchetti PG, Bartolozzi P. Classification of Spondylolisthesis as a guideline for treatment. In: Bridwell KH, DeWald RL, eds. *The textbook of spinal surgery,* Vol. 1. Lippincott, Wilkens and Williams, 1997:1211–1254.
8. Marchetti PC, Bartolozzi P. Classification of spondylolisthesis as a guideline for treatment. In: Bridwell KH, DeWald RL, Hammerberg KW et al., eds. *The textbook of spinal surgery,* 2nd ed., Vol. 2. Philadelphia, PA: Lippincott–Raven Publishers, 1997:1211–1254.

## Prevalence and Natural History

9. Newman PH. Surgical treatment for spondylolisthesis in the adult. *Clin Orthop Relat Res* 1976;117:106–111.
10. Wiltse LL, Jackson DW. Treatment of spondylolisthesis and spondylolysis in children. *Clin Orthop Relat Res* 1976;117:92–100.
11. Boxall D, Bradford DS, Winter RB, et al. Management of severe spondylolisthesis in children and adolescents. *J Bone Joint Surg Am* 1979;61:479–495.
12. Borkow SE, Kleiger B. Spondylolisthesis in the newborn. A case report. *Clin Orthop Relat Res* 1971;81:73–76.
13. Fredrickson BE, Baker D, McHolick WJ, et al. The natural history of spondylolysis and spondylolisthesis. *J Bone Joint Surg Am* 1984;66:699–707.
14. Newnan PH. The etiology of spondylolisthesis. *J Bone Joint Surg Br* 1963;45:39.
15. Taillard WF. Etiology of spondylolisthesis. *Clin Orthop Relat Res* 1976;117:30–39.
16. Turner RH, Bianco AJ Jr. Spondylolysis and spondylolisthesis in children and teen-agers. *J Bone Joint Surg Am* 1971;53:1298–1306.
17. Wiltse LL. Spondylolisthesis in children. *Clin Orthop Relat Res* 1961;21:156.
18. Beguiristain JL, Diaz-de-Rada P. Spondylolisthesis in pre-school children. *J Pediatr Orthop B* 2004;13:225–230.
19. Wiltse LL. Spondylolisthesis, classification and etiology: symposium on the spine. *American Academy of Orthopedic Surgeons.* St. Louis, MO: CV Mosby Company, 1969:143–147.
20. Virta L, Ronnemaa T, Osterman K, et al. Prevalence of isthmic lumbar spondylolisthesis in middle-aged subjects from eastern and western Finland. *J Clin Epidemiol* 1992;45:917–922.
21. Stewart T. The age incidence of neural arch defects in Alaskan natives, considered from the standpoint of etiology. *J Bone Joint Surg Am* 1953;35:937.
22. Osterman K, Schlenzka D, Poussa M, et al. Isthmic spondylolisthesis in symptomatic and asymptomatic subjects, epidemiology, and natural history with special reference to disk abnormality and mode of treatment. *Clin Orthop Relat Res* 1993;297:65–70.
23. Henson J, McCall IW, O'Brien JP. Disc damage above a spondylolisthesis. *Br J Radiol* 1987;60(709):69–72.
24. Roche M, Rowe C. The incidence of separate neural arch and coincident bone variations. *J Bone Joint Surg Am* 1952;34:491.
25. Velikas EP, Blackburne JS. Surgical treatment of spondylolisthesis in children and adolescents. *J Bone Joint Surg Br* 1981;63-B:67–70.
26. Rowe G, Roache M. Etiology of the separate neural arch. *J Bone Joint Surg Am* 1953;35:102.
27. Eisenstein S. Spondylolysis. A skeletal investigation of two population groups. *J Bone Joint Surg Br* 1978;60-B:488–494.
28. Jackson DW, Wiltse LL, Cirincoine RJ. Spondylolysis in the female gymnast. *Clin Orthop Relat Res* 1976;117:68–73.
29. Ferguson RJ, McMaster JH, Stanitski CL. Low back pain in college football linemen. *J Sports Med* 1975;2:63–69.
30. Semon RL, Spengler D. Significance of lumbar spondylolysis in college football players. *Spine* 1981;6:172–174.
31. Bradford D. Management of spondylolysis and spondylolisthesis. In: Evarts C, ed. *Instructional course lectures, American Academy of Orthopedic Surgeons,* Vol. 32. St. Louis, MO: CV Mosby Company, 1983:151.
32. Monticelli G, Ascani E. Spondylolysis and spondylolisthesis. *Acta Orthop Scand* 1975;46:498–506.
33. Troup JD. Mechanical factors in spondylolisthesis and spondylolysis. *Clin Orthop Relat Res* 1976;117:59–67.
34. Wiltse LL, Widell EH Jr, Jackson DW. Fatigue fracture: the basic lesion in isthmic spondylolisthesis. *J Bone Joint Surg Am* 1975;57:17–22.
35. Saraste H. Long-term clinical and radiological follow-up of spondylolysis and spondylolisthesis. *J Pediatr Orthop* 1987;7:631–638.
36. Frennered AK, Danielson BI, Nachemson AL. Natural history of symptomatic isthmic low-grade spondylolisthesis in children and adolescents: a seven-year follow-up study. *J Pediatr Orthop* 1991;11:209–213.
37. Danielson B, Frennerd K, Selvik G, et al. Roentgenologic assessment of spondylolisthesis: an evaluation of progression. *Acta Radiol* 1989;30:65–68.
38. Schlenzka D, Poussa M, Seitsalo S, et al. Intervertebral disc changes in adolescents with isthmic spondylolisthesis. *J Spinal Disord* 1991;4:344–352.
39. Szypryt EP, Twining P, Mulholland RC, et al. The prevalence of disc degeneration associated with neural arch defects of the lumbar spine assessed by magnetic resonance imaging. *Spine* 1989;14:977–981.
40. Beutler WJ, Fredrickson BE, Murtland A, et al. The natural history of spondylolysis and spondylolisthesis: 45-year follow-up evaluation. *Spine* 2003;28:1027–1035.
41. Dandy DJ, Shannon MJ. Lumbo-sacral subluxation. (Group I spondylolisthesis). *J Bone Joint Surg Br* 1971;53:578–595.
42. Harris IE, Weinstein SL. Long-term follow-up of patients with grade-III and IV spondylolisthesis: treatment with and without posterior fusion. *J Bone Joint Surg Am* 1987;69:960–969.
43. Bradford DS. Treatment of severe spondylolisthesis. A combined approach for reduction and stabilization. *Spine* 1979;4:423–429.
44. Sherman FC, Rosenthal RK, Hall JE. Spine fusion for spondylolysis and spondylolisthesis in children. *Spine* 1979;4:59–66.
45. Floman Y, Margulies JY, Nyska M, et al. Effect of major axial skeleton trauma on preexisting lumbosacral spondylolisthesis. *J Spinal Disord* 1991;4:353–358.
46. Baker D, Mc Hollick W. Spondylolysis and spondylolisthesis in children. *J Bone Joint Surg Am* 1956;38:933.
47. Hensinger RN. Spondylolysis and spondylolisthesis in children and adolescents (review). *J Bone Joint Surg Am* 1989;71:1098–1107.
48. Seitsalo S, Osterman K, Hyvarinen H, et al. Progression of spondylolisthesis in children and adolescents. A long-term follow-up of 272 patients. *Spine* 1991;16:417–421.

## Etiology

49. Vaz G, Roussouly P, Berthonnaud E, et al. Sagittal morphology and balance of the spine and pelvis. *Eur Spine J* 2002;1:80–88.
50. Legaye J, Duval-Beaupere C, Hecquet J, et al. Pelvic incidence: a fundamental pelvic parameter for three-dimensional regulation of spinal sagittal curves. *Eur Spine J* 1998;7:99–103.
51. Labelle HH, Roussouly P, Berthonnaud E, et al. Spondylolisthesis, pelvic incidence, and spinopelvic balance: a correlation study. *Spine* 2004;29:2049–2054.
52. Ogilvie JW, Sherman J. Spondylolysis in Scheuermann's disease. *Spine* 1987;12:251–253.
53. Rosenberg NJ, Bargar WL, Friedman B. The incidence of spondylolysis and spondylolisthesis in nonambulatory patients. *Spine* 1981;6:35–38.
54. Dietrich M, Kurowski P. The importance of mechanical factors in the etiology of spondylolysis: a model analysis of loads and stresses in human lumbar spine. *Spine* 1985;10:532–542.

55. Wiltse LL. Etiology of spondylolisthesis. *Clin Orthop Relat Res* 1957;10:48–60.
56. Wiltse LL. The etiology of spondylolisthesis. *J Bone Joint Surg Am* 1962;44:539–560.
57. Chandler FA. Lesions of the isthmus (pars interarticularis) of the laminae of the lower lumbar vertebrae and their relation to spondylolisthesis. *Surg Gynecol Obstet* 1931;53:273–306.
58. Farfan HF, Osteria V, Lamy C. The mechanical etiology of spondylolysis and spondylolisthesis. *Clin Orthop Relat Res* 1976;117:40–55.
59. Lafferty JF, Winter WG, Gambaro SA. Fatigue characteristics of posterior elements of vertebrae. *J Bone Joint Surg Am* 1977; 59:154–158.
60. Hutton WC, Stott JRR, Cyron BM. Is spondylolysis a fatigue fracture? *Spine* 1977;2:202–209.
61. O'Neill DB, Micheli LJ. Postoperative radiographic evidence for fatigue fracture as the etiology in spondylolysis. *Spine* 1989;14:1342–1355.
62. Pennell RG, Maurer AH, Bonakdarpour A. Stress injuries of the pars interarticularis: radiologic classification and indications for scintigraphy. *Am J Roentgenol* 1985;145:763–766.
63. Wiltse LL, Widell E Jr, Jackson DW. Fatigue fracture: the basic lesion is isthmic spondylolisthesis. *J Bone Joint Surg Am* 1975; 57:17–22.
64. Cyron BM, Hutton WC. Variations in the amount and distribution of cortical bone across the partes interarticularis of L-5: A predisposing factor in spondylolysis? *Spine* 1979;4:163–167.
65. Krenz J, Troup JD. The structure of the pars interarticularis of the lower lumbar vertebrae and its relation to the etiology of spondylolysis: with a report of a healing fracture in the neural arch of a fourth lumbar vertebra. *J Bone Joint Surg Br* 1973;55:735–741.
66. Hutton WC, Cyron BM. Spondylolysis: the role of the posterior elements in resisting the intervertebral compressive force. *Acta Orthop Scand* 1978;49:604–609.
67. Sairyo K, Katoh S, Sakamaki T, et al. Vertebral forward slippage in immature lumbar spine occurs following epiphyseal separation and its occurrence is unrelated to disc degeneration: is the pediatric spondylolisthesis a physis stress fracture of vertebral body? *Spine* 2004;29:524–527.
68. Kajiura K, Katoh S, Sairyo K, et al. Slippage mechanism of pediatric spondylolysis: biomechanical study using immature calf spines. *Spine* 2001;26:2208–2212.
69. Loder RT. Profiles of the cervical, thoracic, and lumbosacral spine in children and adolescents with lumbosacral spondylolisthesis. *J Spinal Disord* 2001;14:465–471.
70. Miki T, Tamura T, Senzoku F, et al. Congenital laminar defect of the upper lumbar spine associated with pars interarticularis defect: a report of eleven cases. *Spine* 1991;16:353–355.
71. Albanese M, Pizzutillo PD. Family study of spondylolysis and spondylolisthesis. *J Pediatr Orthop* 1982;2:496–499.
72. Friberg S. Studies on spondylolisthesis. Acta Chir Scand 1939;82(Suppl. 55):56.
73. Laurent L, Einola S. Spondylolisthesis in children and adolescents. *Acta Orthop Scand* 1961;31:45.
74. Wynne-Davies R, Scott JH. Inheritance and spondylolisthesis: a radiographic family survey. *J Bone Joint Surg Br* 1979;61-B:301–305.

## Evaluation of the Patient

75. Iwamoto J, Abe H, Tsukimura Y, et al. Relationships between radiographic abnormalities of the lumbar spine and incidence of low back pain in high school and college football players: a prospective study. *Am J Sports Med* 2004;32:781–786.
76. Stewart TD. The age incidence of neural-arch defects in Alaskan natives, considered from the standpoint of etiology. *J Bone Joint Surg Am* 1953;35:937–950.
77. Libson E, Bloom RA, Dinari G. Symptomatic and asymptomatic spondylolysis and spondylolisthesis in young adults. *Int Orthop* 1982;6:259–261.
78. Virta L, Ronnemaa T. The association of mild-moderate isthmic lumbar spondylolisthesis and low back pain in middle-aged patients is weak and it only occurs in women. *Spine* 1993; 18:1496–1503.

79. Amundson G, Edwards C, Garfin S. Spondylolisthesis. In: Rothman R, Simeone F, eds. *The spine*, 3rd ed. Philadelphia, PA: WB Saunders, 1992:913.
80. Phalen G, Dickson J. Spondylolisthesis and tight hamstrings. *J Bone Joint Surg Am* 1961;43:505–512.
81. Barash H, Galante JO, Lambert CN, et al. Spondylolisthesis and tight hamstrings. *J Bone Joint Surg Am* 1970;52:1319–1328.
82. Harris R. Spondylolisthesis. *Ann R Coll Surg Engl* 1951;8:259–297.

## Radiologic Evaluation

83. Saraste H, Brostrom LA, Aparisi T. Prognostic radiographic aspects of spondylolisthesis. *Acta Radiol Diagn (Stockh)* 1984;25:427–432.
84. Lowe RW, Hayes TD, Kaye J, et al. Standing roentgenograms in spondylolisthesis. *Clin Orthop Relat Res* 1976;117:80–84.
85. Burkus JK. Unilateral spondylolysis associated with spina bifida occulta and nerve root compression. *Spine* 1990;15:555–559.
86. Libson E, Bloom RA, Dinari G, et al. Oblique lumbar spine radiographs: importance in young patients. *Radiology* 1984; 151:89–90.
87. Antoniades SB, Hammerberg KW, DeWald RL. Sagittal plane configuration of the sacrum in spondylolisthesis. *Spine* 2000; 25:1085–1091.
88. Bellah RD, Summerville DA, Treves ST, et al. Low back pain in adolescent athletes: detection of stress injury to the pars interarticularis with SPECT. *Radiology* 1991;180:509–512.
89. Suh PB, Esses SI, Kostuik JP. Repair of pars interarticularis defect: the prognostic value of pars interarticularis infiltration. Spine 1991;16(Suppl. 8):S445–S448.
90. Grogan JP, Hemminghytt S, Williams AL, et al. Spondylolysis studied with computed tomography. *Radiology* 1982; 145:737–742.
91. Gibson MJ, Buckley J, Mawhinney R, et al. Magnetic resonance imaging and discography in the diagnosis of disc degeneration: a comparative study of 50 discs. *J Bone Joint Surg Br* 1986; 68:369–373.
92. Meyerding HW. Spondylolisthesis. *Surg Gynecol Obstet* 1932; 54:371–377.
93. Newman PH. A clinical syndrome associated with severe lumbosacral subluxation. *J Bone Joint Surg Br* 1965;47:472–481.
94. Wiltse LL, Winter RB. Terminology and measurement of spondylolisthesis. *J Bone Joint Surg Am* 1983;65:768–772.
95. Huang RP, Bohlman HH, Thompson GH, et al. Predictive value of pelvic incidence in progression of spondylolisthesis. *Spine* 2003;28:2381–2385.
96. Rajnics P, Templier A, Skalli W, et al. The association of sagittal spinal and pelvic parameters with isthmic spondylolisthesis. *J Spinal Disord* 2002;15:24–30.
97. Hanson DS, Bridwell KH, Rhee JM, et al. Dowel fibular strut grafts for high-grade dysplastic isthmic spondylolisthesis. *Spine* 2002;27:1982–1988.

## Treatment

98. Lonstein JE. Spondylolisthesis in children. Cause, natural history, and management. *Spine* 1999;24:2640–2680.
99. Miller SF, Congeni J, Swanson K. Long-term functional and anatomical follow-up of early detected spondylolysis in young athletes. *Am J Sports Med* 2004;32:928–933.
100. Blanda J, Bethem D, Moats W, et al. Defects of pars interarticularis in athletes: a protocol for nonoperative treatment. *J Spinal Disord* 1993;6:406–411.
101. Morita T, Ikata T, Katoh S, et al. Lumbar spondylolysis in children and adolescents. *J Bone Joint Surg Br* 1985;77:620–625.
102. Steiner ME, Micheli LJ. Treatment of symptomatic spondylolysis and spondylolisthesis with the modified Boston brace. *Spine* 1985;10:937–943.
103. Wiltse LL. Proceedings: lumbar spine: posterolateral fusion. *J Bone Joint Surg Br* 1975;57:261.
104. van Dam B. Nonoperative treatment and surgical repair of lumbar spondylolisthesis. In: Bridwell KH, DeWald RL, eds. *The textbook of spinal surgery*, 2nd ed. Philadelphia, PA: Lippincott–Raven Publishers, 1997:1263–1269.
105. Buck JE. Direct repair of the defect in spondylolisthesis. Preliminary report. *J Bone Joint Surg Br* 1970;52:432–437.
106. Buck JE. Abstract: further thoughts on direct repair of the defect in spondylolysis. *J Bone Joint Surg Br* 1979;61:123.

107. Gillet P, Petit M. Direct repair of spondylolysis without spondylolisthesis, using a rod-screw construct and bone grafting of the pars interarticularis defect. *Spine* 1999;24:1252–1256.

108. Kakiuchi M. Repair of the defect in spondylolysis. Durable fixation with pedicle screws and laminar hooks. *J Bone Joint Surg Am* 1997;79:818–825.

109. Morscher E, Gerber B, Fasel J. Surgical treatment of spondylolisthesis by bone grafting and direct stabilization of spondylolysis by means of a hook screw. *Arch Orthop Trauma Surg* 1984;103:175–178.

110. Songer MN, Rovin R. Repair of the pars interarticularis defect with a cable-screw construct. A preliminary report. *Spine* 1998;23:263–269.

111. Pedersen AK, Hagen R. Spondylolysis and spondylolisthesis: treatment by internal fixation and bone-grafting of the defect. *J Bone Joint Surg Am* 1988;70:15–24.

112. Bradford DS. Treatment of severe spondylolisthesis: a combined approach for reduction and stabilization. *Spine* 1979;4:423–429.

113. Bradford DS, Iza J. Repair of the defect in spondylolysis or minimal degrees of spondylolisthesis by segmental wire fixation and bone grafting. *Spine* 1985;10:673–679.

114. Tokuhashi Y, Matsuzaki H. Repair of defects in spondylolysis by segmental pedicle screw hook fixation: a preliminary report. *Spine* 1996;21:2041–2045.

115. Newton PO, Johnston CE II. Analysis and treatment of poor outcomes following in situ arthrodesis in adolescent spondylolisthesis. *J Pediatr Orthop* 1997;17:754–761.

116. Burkus JK, Lonstein JE, Winter RB, et al. Long-term evaluation of adolescents treated operatively for spondylolisthesis. A comparison of in situ arthrodesis only with in situ arthrodesis and reduction followed by immobilization in a cast. *J Bone Joint Surg Am* 1992;74:693–704.

117. Freeman BL III, Donati NL. Spinal arthrodesis for severe spondylolisthesis in children and adolescents. A long-term follow-up study. *J Bone Joint Surg Am* 1989;71:594–598.

118. Hensinger RN, Lang LE, MacEwen GD. Surgical management of the spondylolisthesis in children and adolescents. *Spine* 1976;1:207–216.

119. Pizzutillo PD, Mirenda W, MacEwen GD. Posterolateral fusion for spondylolisthesis in adolescence. *J Pediatr Orthop* 1986;6:311–316.

120. Dubousset J. Treatment of spondylolysis in children and adolescents. *Clin Orthop Relat Res* 1997;337:77.

121. Bosworth D, Fielding J, Demarest L, et al. Spondylolisthesis: a critical review of a consecutive series of cases treated by arthrodesis. *J Bone Joint Surg Am* 1955;37:767.

122. Frennered AK, Danielson BI, Nachemson AL, et al. Midterm follow-up of young patients fused in situ for spondylolisthesis. *Spine* 1991;16:409–416.

123. Daniel JN, Polly DW Jr, Van Dam BE. A study of the efficacy of nonoperative treatment of presumed traumatic spondylolysis in a young patient population. *Mil Med* 1995;160:553–555.

124. Hensinger RN. Spondylolysis and spondylolisthesis in children. *Instr Course Lect* 1983;32:132–151.

125. Maurice HD, Morley TR. Cauda equina lesions following fusion in situ and decompressive laminectomy for severe spondylolisthesis. Four case reports. *Spine* 1989;14:214–216.

126. Schoenecker PL, Cole HO, Herring JA, et al. Cauda equina syndrome after in situ arthrodesis for severe spondylolisthesis at the lumbosacral junction. *J Bone Joint Surg Am* 1990;72:369–377.

127. Steiner ME, Micheli LJ. Treatment of symptomatic spondylolysis and spondylolisthesis with the modified brace. *Spine* 1985;10:937–943.

128. Pizzutillo PD, Hummer CD. Nonoperative treatment of pain adolescent spondylosis and spondylolisthesis. *J Pediatr Orthop* 1989;9:538–540.

129. Bell DF, Ehrlich MG, Zaleske DJ. Brace treatment for symptomatic spondylolisthesis. *Clin Orthop Relat Res* 1988;236:192–198.

130. Gill GG. Long-term follow-up evaluation of a few patients with spondylolisthesis treated by excision of the loose lamina with decompression of the nerve roots without spinal fusion. *Clin Orthop Relat Res* 1984;182:215–219.

131. Gill GG, Manning JG, White HL. Surgical treatment of spondylolisthesis without spine fusion: excision of the loose lamina with decompression of the nerve roots. *J Bone Joint Surg Am* 1955;37:493–520.

132. Gill GG, White HL. Surgical treatment of spondylolisthesis without spine fusion. A long-term follow-up of operated cases. *Acta Orthop Scand Suppl* 1965;85:5–99.

133. Osterman K, Lindholm TS, Laurent LE. Late results of removal of the loose posterior element (Gill's operation) in the treatment of lytic lumbar spondylolisthesis. *Clin Orthop Relat Res* 1976;117:121–128.

134. Marmor L, Bechtol CO. Spondylolisthesis: complete slip following the Gill procedure: a case report. *J Bone Joint Surg Am* 1961;43:1068–1069.

135. O'Brien M7. Low and high grade spondylothesis in the pediatric and adult population. In: Lenke LG, Newton PO. *Semin Spine Surg* 2003;15(3):291–314.

136. Johnson LP, Nasca RJ, Dunham WK. Surgical management of isthmic spondylolisthesis. *Spine* 1988;13:93–97.

137. Rombold C. Treatment of spondylolisthesis by posterolateral fusion, resection of the pars interarticularis, and prompt mobilization of the patient. An end-result study of seventy-three patients. *J Bone Joint Surg Am* 1966;48:1282–1300.

138. Stauffer RN, Coventry MB. Anterior interbody lumbar spine fusion. Analysis of Mayo Clinic series. *J Bone Joint Surg Am* 1972;54:756–768.

139. Hanley EN Jr, Levy JA. Surgical treatment of isthmic lumbosacral spondylolisthesis. Analysis of variables influencing results. *Spine* 1989;14:48–50.

140. Lenke LG, Bridwell KH, Bullis D, et al. Results of *in situ* fusion for isthmic spondylolisthesis. *J Spinal Disord* 1992;5:433–442.

141. Bridwell KH, Sedgewick TA, O'Brien MF, et al. The role of fusion and instrumentation in the treatment of degenerative spondylolisthesis with spinal stenosis. *J Spinal Disord* 1993;6:461–472.

142. Roca J, Moretta D, Fuster S, et al. Direct repair of spondylolysis. *Clin Orthop Relat Res* 1989;246:86–91.

143. DeWald RL, Faut MM, Taddonio RF, et al. Severe lumbosacral spondylolisthesis in adolescents and children. Reduction and staged circumferential fusion. *J Bone Joint Surg Am* 1981;63:619–626.

144. Kai Y, Oyama M, Morooka M. Posterior lumbar interbody fusion using local facet joint autograft and pedicle screw fixation. *Spine* 2004;29:41–46.

145. DeWald RL. Spondylolisthesis. In: Bridwell KH, DeWald RL, Hammerberg KW et al. eds. *The textbook of spinal surgery*, 2nd ed. Philadelphia, PA: Lippincott–Raven Publishers, 1997:1201–1210.

146. Johnson JR, Kirwan EO. The long-term results of fusion *in situ* for severe spondylolisthesis. *J Bone Joint Surg Br* 1983;65:43–46.

147. Laurent LE, Osterman K. Operative treatment of spondylolisthesis in young patients. *Clin Orthop Relat Res* 1976;117:85–91.

148. Bradford D. Controversies: instrumented reduction of spondylisthesis (con). *Spine* 1994;14:1536–1537.

149. Dick WT, Schnebel B. Severe spondylolisthesis: reduction and internal fixation. *Clin Orthop Relat Res* 1988;232:70–79.

150. Edwards C. Reduction of spondylolisthesis: biomechanics and fixation. *Orthop Trans* 1986;10:543.

151. Emans JB, Waters PM, Hall JE. Technique for maintenance of reduction of severe spondylolisthesis using L-4–S4 posterior segmental hyperextension fixation. *Orthop Trans* 1987;11:113.

152. Scaglietti O, Frontino G, Bartolozzi P. Technique of anatomical reduction of lumbar spondylolisthesis and its surgical stabilization. *Clin Orthop Relat Res* 1976;117:165–175.

153. Shufflebarger HL. High grade isthmic spondylolisthesis: monosegmental surgical treatment. *Scoliosis research society annual meeting*, New York: 1998.

154. Jenkins J. Spondylolisthesis. *Br J Surg* 1936;24:80.

155. Harrington PR, Dickson JH. Spinal instrumentation in the treatment of severe progressive spondylolisthesis. *Clin Orthop Relat Res* 1976;117:157–163.

156. Wiesel SW, Garfin SR, Boden SD, et al. Spondylolisthesis. *Semin Spine Surg* 1994;6.

157. Ohki I, Inoue S, Murata T, et al. Reduction and fusion of severe spondylolisthesis using halo-pelvic traction with a wire reduction device. *Int Orthop* 1980;4:107–113.

158. Sijbrandij S. Reduction and stabilization of severe spondylolisthesis. A report of three cases. *J Bone Joint Surg Br* 1983;65:40–42.

159. Harms J, Jeszenszky D, Stoltze D, et al. True spondylolisthesis reduction and monosegmental fusion in spondylolisthesis. In: Bridwell KH, DeWald RL, Hammerberg KW et al., eds. *The textbook of spinal surgery*, 2nd ed., Vol. 2. Philadelphia, PA: Lippincott–Raven Publishers, 1997:1337–1347.

160. Transfeldt EE, Dendrinos GK, Bradford DS. Paresis of proximal lumbar roots after reduction of L-5-S1 spondylolisthesis. *Spine* 1989;14:884–887.

161. Petraco DM, Spivak JM, Cappadona JG, et al. An anatomic evaluation of L-5 nerve stretch in spondylolisthesis reduction. *Spine* 1996;21:1133–1138; discussion 1139.

162. Balderston RA, Bradford DS. Technique for achievement and maintenance of reduction for severe spondylolisthesis using spinous process traction wiring and external fixation of the pelvis. *Spine* 1985;10:376–372.

163. Bradford DS, Boachie-Adjei O. Treatment of severe spondylolisthesis by anterior and posterior reduction and stabilization. A long-term follow-up study. *J Bone Joint Surg Am* 1990;72: 1060–1066.

164. Molinari RW, Bridwell KH, Lenke LG, et al. Anterior column support in surgery for high-grade isthmic spondylolisthesis. *Clin Orthop Relat Res* 2002;394:109–120.

165. Matthiass HH, Heine J. The surgical reduction of spondylolisthesis. *Clin Orthop Relat Res* 1986;203:34–44.

166. Sevastikoglou JA, Spangfort E, Aaro S. Operative treatment of spondylolisthesis in children and adolescents with tight hamstrings syndrome. *Clin Orthop Relat Res* 1980;147:192–199.

167. Muschik M, Zippel H, Perka C. Surgical management of severe spondylolisthesis in children and adolescents. Anterior fusion in-situ versus anterior spondylodesis with posterior transpedicular instrumentation and reduction. *Spine* 1997;22:2036–2042.

168. Lindholm TS, Ragni P, Ylikoski M, et al. Lumbar isthmic spondylolisthesis in children and adolescents. Radiologic evaluation and results of operative treatment. *Spine* 1990;15:1350–1355.

169. van Rens TJ, van Horn JR. Long-term results in lumbosacral interbody fusion for spondylolisthesis. *Acta Orthop Scand* 1982; 53:383–392.

170. Molinari RW, Bridwell KH, Lenke LG, et al. Complications in the surgical treatment of pediatric high-grade, isthmic dysplastic spondylolisthesis: a comparison of three surgical approaches. *Spine* 1999;24:1701–1711.

171. Freebody D, Bendall R, Taylor RD. Anterior transperitoneal lumbar fusion. *J Bone Joint Surg Br* 1971;53:617–627.

172. Verbiest H. The treatment of lumbar spondyloptosis or impending lumbar spondyloptosis accompanied by neurologic deficit and/or neurogenic intermittent claudication. *Spine* 1979;4:68–77.

173. La Rosa G, Conti A, Cacciola F, et al. Pedicle screw fixation for isthmic spondylolisthesis: does posterior lumbar interbody fusion improve the outcome over posterolateral fusion? *J Neurosurg Spine* 2003;99:143–150.

174. Bohlman HH, Cook SS. One-stage decompression and posterolateral and interbody fusion for lumbosacral spondyloptosis through a posterior approach. Report of two cases. *J Bone Joint Surg Am* 1982;64:415–418.

175. Smith MD, Bohlman HH. Spondylolisthesis treated by a single-stage operation combining decompression with in situ posterolateral and anterior fusion. An analysis of eleven patients who had long-term follow-up. *J Bone Joint Surg Am* 1990;72:415–421.

176. Esses SI, Natout N, Kip P. Posterior interbody arthrodesis with a fibular strut graft in spondylolisthesis. *J Bone Joint Surg Am* 1995;77:172–176.

177. Nachemson A. Repair of the spondylolisthetic defect and intertransverse fusion for young patients. *Clin Orthop Relat Res* 1976; 117:101–105.

178. Gaines RW, Nichols WK. Treatment of spondyloptosis by two stage L-5 vertebrectomy and reduction of L-4 onto S1. *Spine* 1985;10:680–686.

179. Huizenga B. Reduction of spondyloptosis with two-stage vertebrectomy. *Orthop Trans* 1983;7:21.

## Complications

180. Seitsalo S, Osterman K, Poussa M. Scoliosis associated with lumbar spondylolisthesis. A clinical survey of 190 young patients. *Spine* 1988;13:899–904.

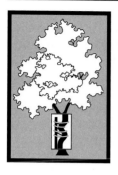

# 22

# The Cervical Spine

### *Randall T. Loder*

Many of the diseases and congenital anomalies affecting the pediatric cervical spine are simply a reflection of aberrant growth and developmental processes. This chapter discusses these diseases and anomalies in this framework. A basic knowledge of the normal embryology, growth, and development of the pediatric cervical spine is necessary in order to understand these conditions. Most of the anomalies and diseases involving the pediatric cervical spine are easily divided into those of the upper (occiput, C1, C2) and lower (C3-C7) segments.

# NORMAL EMBRYOLOGY, GROWTH, AND DEVELOPMENT

## Embryology

### Occipitoaxioatlas Complex

The occiput is formed from at least four or five somites. All definitive vertebrae develop from the caudal sclerotome half of one segment and the cranial sclerotome half of the succeeding segment (1). These areas of primitive mesenchyme separate from each other during fetal growth, then undergo chondrification and subsequent ossification. Chondrification and ossification are passive processes that follow the blueprint laid down by the mesenchymal anlage. Because of this sequencing, the cranial half of the first cervical sclerotome remains as a half segment between the occipital and the atlantal rudiments and is known as the *proatlas*. The primitive centrum of this proatlas becomes the tip of the odontoid process, and its arch rudiments assist in the formation of the occipital condyles (2). The vertebral arch of the atlas separates from its centrum, becoming the ring of C1; the separated

centrum fuses with the proatlas above and the centrum of C2 below to become the odontoid process and body of C2. The axis forms from the second definitive cervical vertebral mesenchymal segment. The odontoid process is the fusion of the primitive centra of the atlas and the proatlas half-segment. The posterior arches of C2 form only from the second definitive cervical segment.

Thus the atlas comprises three main components: the body and the two neural arches. The axis comprises four main components: the body, two neural arches, and the odontoid (or five components, if the proatlas rudiment is also considered) (Figs. 22.1 and 22.2).

### Vertebrae C3-C7

These vertebrae follow the normal formation schema of all vertebrae (3). A portion of the mesenchyme from the sclerotomal centrum creates two neural arches that migrate posteriorly and around the neural tube. This eventually forms the pedicles, the laminae, the spinous processes, and a very small portion of the body. Most of the body is formed by the centrum. An ossification center develops in each of the two neural arches and in the vertebral center, with a synchondrosis formed by the cartilage between the ossification centers.

## Basic Science, Embryology, and Gene Expression

In the past decade there has been an explosion of knowledge regarding the human genome, and how it relates to normal developmental processes and pathologic conditions. Vertebral segmentation begins with clustering segments of the paraxial mesoderm, the somites. Segmentation of the mesoderm into somites is an important and fundamental

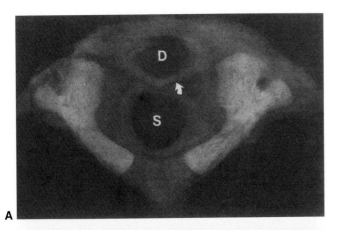

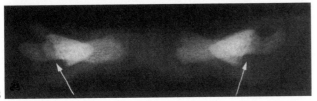

**Figure 22.1** **A:** Cross-sectional radiograph of C1 in a full-term neonate. The posterior ossification centers are present. No ossification is present in the anterior cartilage. The transverse ligament (*arrow*) separates the dens (*D*) from the spinal canal (*S*). **B:** Anteroposterior radiograph of C1 in a full-term neonate. (From Ogden JA. Radiology of postnatal skeletal development. XI. The first cervical vertebrae. *Skeletal Radiol* 1984;12:12–20.)

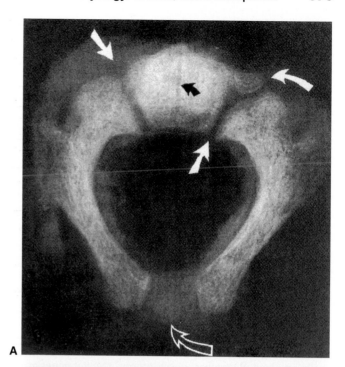

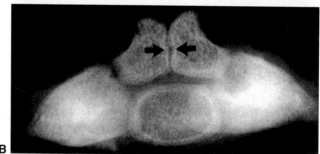

**Figure 22.2   A:** Cross-sectional radiograph of C2 in a neonate. The neurocentral (*solid white arrows*) and posterior (*open arrow*) synchondroses are evident. A small area of accessory ossification is present in the right neurocentral synchondrosis anteriorly (*curved arrow* at top right). Also note the central linear radiolucency (*black arrow*) indicating the synchondrosis between the dens ossification centers. The posterior ossification centers extend into the eventual vertebral body. **B:** Anteroposterior radiograph of C2 in a neonate. In this specimen, the dens ossification centers have not fused, leaving a midline synchondrosis (*arrows*) that extends from the chondrum terminale to the dentocentral synchondrosis. The superior margin of the eventual vertebral body is above the lower level of the dens. The neurocentral synchondroses are continuous with the "ring apophyseal" cartilage inferiorly, the facet cartilage inferiorly, and the dentocentral synchondrosis superiorly. (Ogden JA. Radiology of postnatal skeletal development. XI. The first cervical vertebrae. *Skeletal Radiol* 1984;12:12–20.)

process that allows for spatial specialization in the organism and is under genetic control.

The homeobox is a highly conserved 160 base-pair sequence found in the homeobox genes, termed *Hox* genes for short. These *Hox* genes encode a highly conserved family of transcription factors that play fundamental roles in morphogenesis during embryonic development. Vertebrate *Hox* genes help control developmental patterning in the embryo along the primary (head to tail) and secondary (genital and limb bud) axes. There are 39 *Hox* genes in vertebrates, organized into four clusters located on different chromosomes. In humans these clusters are named *HOXA*, *HOXB*, *HOXC*, and *HOXD*, located on chromosomes 7p14, 17q21, 12q13, and 2q31, respectively (4). When referring to animals, the names of the genes are written in title case (e.g., *Hoxc*); when referring to humans they are written in all caps (e.g., *HOXC*). Each cluster contains 9 to 11 genes, all oriented in the same 5′ to 3′ direction of transcription. There are 13 possible subsets of genes; no single cluster contains a representative from all 13 known numbered subsets (paralogous groups). The numbering of the genes in each cluster is based on their sequence similarity and relative positions, starting from the end of the complex that is expressed most anteriorly (cranially). The equivalent genes in each complex are called a *paralogous* group.

The expression domains of the *HOX* clusters display a nested arrangement. Along the body axis, the *Hox* genes are generally expressed with discrete rostral cutoffs that coincide with either existing or emergent anatomic landmarks. *Hox* genes at the end of the 3′ cluster (e.g., *HOXA1*) are generally expressed early, in anterior and proximal regions; *Hox* genes at the 5′ end (e.g., *HOXA13*) are generally expressed later, in more posterior and distal regions. Therefore, the lower numbered *Hox* genes are involved in the development of the axial skeleton, and the higher numbered *Hox* genes are involved in the development of the limbs. There has been an explosion of knowledge regarding defects in the *Hox* genes and resultant congenital spinal anomalies in experimental animals, and to a much lesser extent in humans (Table 22.1). The defect can be either a distinct *Hox* gene mutation intentionally produced by the investigator, or more random hits by teratogens (methanol, boric acid, retinoic acid, and maternal hyperthermia) (5–8).

## TABLE 22.1

### AXIAL SKELETAL MALFORMATIONS CAUSED BY GENETIC ABNORMALITIES

| Involved Gene | Gene Abnormality | Phenotypic Expression | Animal | Reference |
|---|---|---|---|---|
| *Hoxb4* | Knockout | C2 becomes C1 | Mouse | 9 |
| *Hoxd3* | Homozygous | Atlas fused to occiput, C2 becomes more like C1 | Mouse | 10 |
| *Hoxa4* | Homozygous | Development of ribs on C7 | Mouse | 11 |
| *Bapx1* | Knockout | Malformed basioccipital bone. Absence of anterior arch of atlas | Mouse | 12 |
| *Uncx4.1* | Homozygous | Absence of pedicles and transverse processes, cervical vertebrae | Mouse | 13 |
| *Cdx1* | Homozygous | Cranial transformations of cervical spine—absence of anterior arch of C1. C2 becomes like C1. C3 becomes like C2. Development of ribs on C7 | Mouse | 14,15 |
| *PAX1* | Sequence changes | Klippel-Feil syndrome | Human | 16 |

Another group of genes, the *Pax* genes, are also integrally involved in vertebral development. The *Pax* genes are a highly conserved family of developmental control genes that encode transcription factors containing a 128-amino acid DNA-binding domain (17,18) called the *paired box* (19). To date, there are nine known *Pax* genes (16,20). The *Pax* gene family is broken down into four subgroups (*Pax1* and *Pax9*; *Pax2*, *Pax5*, and *Pax8*; *Pax3* and *Pax7*; *Pax4* and *Pax6*). *Pax1* and *Pax9* induce chondrogenic differentiation in the paraxial mesenchymal mesoderm of the sclerotome (18,19,21). They are therefore critically involved in vertebral formation. Abnormalities in the *PAX1* sequence in humans have been associated with Klippel-Feil syndrome in some patients (16).

The Hedgehog family of proteins has also become increasingly recognized as being crucial in axial skeletal development. The best known of these proteins is the sonic hedgehog (*shh*), which is expressed in the notochord (22,23); *shh* is believed to be the signal for induction of the ventral somite to differentiate into the sclerotome (23). In *shh* knockout mice, most sclerotomal derivatives are absent, in conjunction with reduced expression of *Pax1* (23). Therefore, absence of *shh* leads to absence of *Pax1* expression and subsequent failure of the mesenchymal cells to chondrify. Defective *shh* signaling during embryogenesis in mice results in anomalies similar to those seen in association with the human (VACTERL) (24).

## Growth and Development

### Atlas

Ossification is present only in the two neural arches at birth (25). These ossification centers extend posteriorly toward the rudimentary spinous process to form the posterior synchondrosis and anteriorly into the articular facet region to form all of the bone present in the facets. Anteromedial to each facet the neurocentral synchondroses form, joining the neural arches and the body; this occurs on each side of the expanding anterior ossification center. The body starts to ossify between 6 months and 2 years of age, usually in a single center. By 4 to 6 years of age the posterior synchondrosis fuses, followed by the anterior ones slightly thereafter. The final internal diameter of the pediatric C1 spinal canal is determined by 6 to 7 years of age. Further growth is obtained only by periosteal appositional growth on the external surface, which leads to thickening and an increased height, but without changing the size of the spinal canal. Therefore, a spinal fusion after the age of 6 or 7 years has minimal impact on the internal canal diameter; when possible, surgical fusion should not be performed before this age because of the potential for later cervical stenosis.

### Axis

The odontoid develops two primary ossification centers that usually coalesce within the first 3 months of life; these centers are separated from the C2 centrum by the dentocentral synchondrosis (26,27). This synchondrosis is below the level of the C1 and C2 facets and contributes to the overall height of the odontoid, as well as to the body of C2. It is continuous with the vertebral body and facets, and it coalesces with the anterior neurocentral synchondroses and finally at the dentocentral synchondrosis. This closure occurs between 3 and 6 years of age. The tip of the dens is composed of a cartilaginous region similar to an epiphysis, known as the *chondrum terminale*. In patients between 5 and 8 years of age, this develops an ossification center, becoming the *ossiculum terminale*. The ossiculum terminale fuses to the remainder of the odontoid between 10 and 13 years of age.

The posterior neural arches are partially ossified at birth, and are joined by the posterior synchondrosis. By 3 months of age these arches, growing more posteriorly, form the rudimentary spinous process. By 1 year of age, ossification fills the spinous process, and by 3 years of age, the posterior synchondrosis has fused. Therefore, both the posterior and the anterior synchondroses are closed by 6 years of age, and there is no further increase in spinal canal size after this age.

### C3-C7

At birth, all three ossification centers are present. The anterior synchondrosis (i.e., neurocentral synchondrosis) is slightly anterior to the base of the pedicles; it usually closes between 3 and 6 years of age. The posterior synchondrosis is at the junction of the two neural arches; it usually closes by 2 to 4 years of age. In the neonate and young child the articular facets are horizontal but become more vertically oriented as the child grows older and reaches the normal adult configuration. They are also more horizontal in the upper cervical spine than in the lower cervical spine. The vertebral bodies enlarge circumferentially by periosteal appositional growth, whereas their vertical growth is by endochondral ossification. Secondary ossification centers develop at the tips of the spinous processes and the cartilaginous ring apophyses of the bodies around the time of puberty. These ring apophyses are involved in the vertical growth of the body. These secondary ossification centers fuse with the vertebral body by 25 years of age.

### Vertebral Body and Canal Diameter Changes with Growth

Because the immature vertebrae are more cartilaginous than the mature adult vertebrae, there are significant differences between normal vertebral measurements in the child compared to the adult (28). As the child grows older, the vertebral body height increases relative to the vertebral body depth. This is because the activity of the apophyseal end plates contributes proportionately more growth to the height of the vertebral body than the appositional growth contributes to the depth of the vertebral body. The height-to-depth ratio of the vertebral body increases from approximately 0.5 in children less than 1 year of age to 0.8 to 0.9 in adults. This ratio remains relatively constant for all vertebral bodies from C3 to C7. With these changes in the vertebral body height relative to depth, there are also changes in the sagittal diameter of the canal relative to vertebral body depth. The ratio of the sagittal diameter of the canal to vertebral body depth is stable at 1.4 in children from birth to 7 to 8 years of age, and then gradually decreases to the normal 1.0 adult value (28). Knowledge of these normal growth parameters is important when determining the possibility of occurrence of platyspondyly or spinal stenosis.

## Normal Radiographic Parameters

Certain radiographic parameters that indicate pathology of the cervical spine in adults represent normal developmental processes in children. These parameters are the atlantooccipital motion and atlantodens interval (ADI), pseudosubluxation and pseudoinstability, variations in the curvature of the cervical spine that may resemble spasm and ligamentous injury, variations in the presence of skeletal growth and growth centers that may resemble fractures, and anterior soft tissue widening. Normal cervical spine motion in children is also discussed.

### Atlantodens Interval and Atlantooccipital Motion

These intervals are determined on lateral flexion and extension radiographic views, with the movements performed voluntarily by the patient while awake. The ADI is the space between the anterior aspect of the dens and the posterior aspect of the anterior ring of the atlas (Fig. 22.3). An ADI of more than 5 mm on flexion and extension lateral radiographs indicates instability (29,30). This is more than the 3-mm adult value because there is increased cartilage in the odontoid and ring of the atlas in children, as well as increased ligamentous laxity. In extension, overriding of the anterior arch of the atlas on top of the odontoid can be seen in up to 20% of children (31).

A mild increase in the ADI may indicate a subtle disruption of the transverse atlantal ligament. In adults an ADI greater than 5 mm indicates ligament rupture (32). In chronic atlantoaxial conditions (e.g., rheumatoid arthritis, Down syndrome, congenital anomalies) the ADI is less useful. In children with these disorders who are frequently hypermobile but do not have ruptured transverse atlantal ligaments, the ADI is increased beyond the 3 to 5 mm

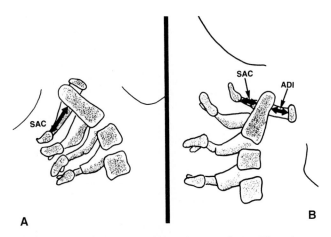

**Figure 22.3** Lateral view of the atlantoaxial joint. The atlantodens interval (ADI) is the distance between the anterior aspect of the dens and the posterior aspect of the anterior portion of the ring of the atlas. The space available for the cord (SAC) is the distance between the posterior aspect of the dens and the anterior aspect of the posterior portion of the ring of the atlas. In children, an ADI of 5 mm or larger is abnormal. In teenagers and adults, a SAC of 13 mm or smaller can be associated with canal compromise. In younger children, spinal cord impingement is imminent if the SAC is equal to or less than the transverse diameter of the odontoid. **A:** The relations in extension. **B:** The relations in flexion.

range. The complement of the ADI, the SAC, is a more useful measure in this situation. This space is the distance between the posterior aspect of the dens and the anterior aspect of the posterior ring of the atlas or the foramen magnum. A SAC of less than 13 mm may be associated with neurologic problems (33).

In patients in whom there is an attenuation of the transverse atlantal ligament without rupture, the alar ligament provides some stability. It acts like a checkrein (34), first tightening up in rotation, then becoming completely taut as the odontoid process continues to move posteriorly for a distance equivalent to its full transverse diameter. This safety zone between the anterior wall of the spinal canal of the atlas, the axis, and the neural structures is an anatomic constant equal to the transverse diameter of the odontoid. This constant defines Steel's rule of thirds: one third cord, one third odontoid, and one third space. This rule remains constant throughout the growth of the cervical spine (35). The cord can move into this space (safe zone) when the odontoid moves posteriorly because of an attenuated transverse atlantal ligament. It is here that the alar ligament

becomes taut, acting as a checkrein and secondary restraint, preventing further movement of the odontoid into the cord. In the chronic situation, it is important to recognize when this safe zone has been exceeded and the child is entering the stage of impending spinal cord compression. The alar ligament will be insufficient to prevent a fatal cord injury in the event of another neck injury similar to the one that caused the initial interruption of the transverse atlantal ligament.

Normal ranges of motion at the atlantooccipital joint are not well defined. In a series of 40 healthy college freshmen, the tip of the odontoid remained directly below the basion of the skull in both flexion and extension (36). That is, the joint should not normally allow any horizontal translation during flexion and extension. Tredwell et al. (37) believe that a posterior subluxation of the atlantooccipital relation of more than 4 mm in extension position indicates instability (Fig. 22.4). This subluxation can be measured as the distance between the anterior margin of the condyles at the base of the skull and the sharp contour of the anterior aspect of the concave joint of the atlas

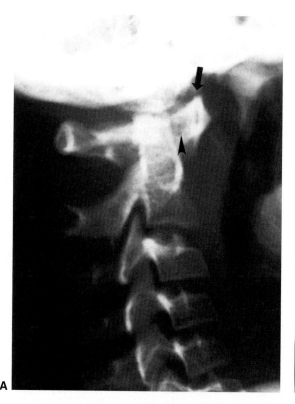

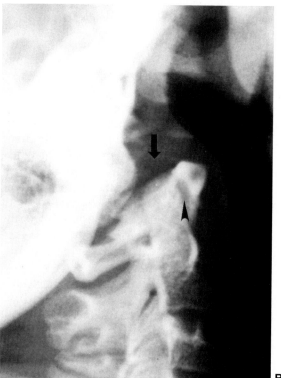

**A**

**B**

**Figure 22.4**  Lateral flexion (**A** and extension) **B** radiographs of an 11-year-old boy with Down syndrome. The child presented with loss of hand control when flexing his neck. Using the method of Tredwell et al. (37), the atlantooccipital distance is measured as the distance between the anterior margin of the condyles at the base of the skull and the sharp contour of the anterior aspect of the concave joint of the atlas. More than 4 mm of posterior translation is abnormal. The atlantooccipital distance (*arrows*) measures 10 mm in extension and 1 mm in flexion. The atlantodens interval is 1 mm in extension and 6 mm in flexion, for a total of 5 mm of motion (*arrowheads*). The space available for the cord is 17 mm in flexion and 20 mm in extension. Both occipitoatlantal instability (more than 4 mm posterior translation) and atlantodens hypermobility (5 mm atlantodens interval in flexion) are present.

of the anterior cortex of the posterior arch of C2. In pathologic dislocation of C2 on C3, the posterior cervical line misses the posterior arch of C2 by 2 mm or more.

The planes of the articular facets change with growth. The facets of the lower cervical spine change from 55 to 70 degrees, whereas the upper facets (i.e., C2-C4) may have initial angles as low as 30 degrees, gradually increasing to 60 to 70 degrees. This variation in facet angulation, together with normal looseness of the soft tissues and the relative increase in size and weight of the skull compared with the trunk, are the major factors responsible for this pseudosubluxation. No treatment is needed for this normal physiologic subluxation.

### Variations in the Curvature and Growth of the Cervical Spine that Can Resemble Injury

In the classic study of Cattell and Filtzer (31), 16% of normal children showed a marked angulation at a single interspace, suggestive of injury to the interspinous or posterior longitudinal ligament; 14% showed an absence of the normal lordosis in the neutral position; and 16% showed an absence of the flexion curvature between the 2nd and 7th cervical vertebrae, which could be erroneously interpreted as splinting secondary to injury. These findings may occur in children up to 16 years of age.

Spina bifida of the posterior arch, or multiple ossification centers of the ring of C1, may mimic fractures. They can be distinguished from fractures by their smooth cortical margins. In some children the posterior ring of C1 remains cartilaginous, and this is usually of no clinical significance (42). Spina bifida may also occur at other cervical levels and, on anteroposterior radiographs, the overlapping lucent areas crossing a vertebral body may mimic a vertical fracture of the body.

The dentocentral synchondrosis of C2 begins to close between 5 and 7 years of age (26). However, it may be visible in vestigial forms up to 11 years of age (31), and may be erroneously interpreted as an undisplaced fracture. Similarly, the apical odontoid epiphysis (i.e., ossiculum terminale) may appear by 5 years of age, although it most typically appears at approximately 8 years of age. This may be misinterpreted as an odontoid tip fracture.

Wedging of the C3 vertebral body is found radiographically in 7% of normal younger children (Fig. 22.6B, C); the wedging corrects as the child matures and is very rarely present after 13 years of age (43). If there is a history of trauma, and if it is unclear whether the wedging is a normal variation or a true compression fracture, a computerized tomography (CT) scan will demonstrate fracture lines through the body if a fracture is present. In the lower cervical levels, secondary centers of ossification of the spinous processes may resemble avulsion fractures (31).

### Normal Lower Cervical Spine Motion

Generally, the interspinous distances increase with increasing age, being the smallest at C4-C5 and the largest at C6-C7

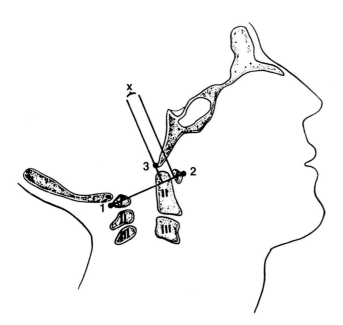

**Figure 22.5** The method of measuring atlantooccipital instability according to Weisel and Rothman (38). The atlantal line joins points 1 and 2. A perpendicular to the atlantal line is drawn at the posterior margin of the anterior arch of the atlas. The distance (x) from the basion (3) to the perpendicular line is measured in flexion and extension. The difference between flexion and extension represents the anteroposterior translation at the occipitoatlantal joint; in normal adults, this translation should be no more than 1 mm. [From Gabriel KR, Mason DE, Carango P. Occipito-atlantal translation in Down's syndrome. *Spine* 1990;15:996–1002, with permission (39).]

anteriorly, or as the distance between the occipital protuberance and the superior arch of the atlas posteriorly. Another method of measuring posterior subluxation of the atlantooccipital joint is that of Wiesel and Rothman (38) (Fig. 22.5). With this technique, occiput-C1 translation from maximum flexion to maximum extension should measure no more than 1 mm in normal adults. The corresponding norms in children have not yet been established.

### Pseudosubluxation

The C2-3 and, to a lesser extent, the C3-4 interspaces in children have a normal physiologic displacement. In a study of 161 children (31), marked anterior displacement of C2 on C3 was observed in 9% of the subjects between 1 and 7 years of age. In a more recent study, 22% of 108 polytrauma children demonstrated pseudosubluxation that had no association with intubation status or severity of the injury (40). In some children, the anterior physiologic displacement of C2 on C3 is so pronounced that it appears pathologic (pseudosubluxation). In order to differentiate physiologic from pathologic subluxation, Swischuk (41) has proposed using, as a reference line, the posterior cervical line drawn from the anterior cortex of the posterior arch of C1 to the anterior cortex of the posterior arch of C3 (Fig. 22.6). In physiologic displacement of C2 on C3, the posterior cervical line may pass through the cortex of the posterior arch of C2, touch the anterior aspect of the cortex of the posterior arch of C2, or come within 1 mm

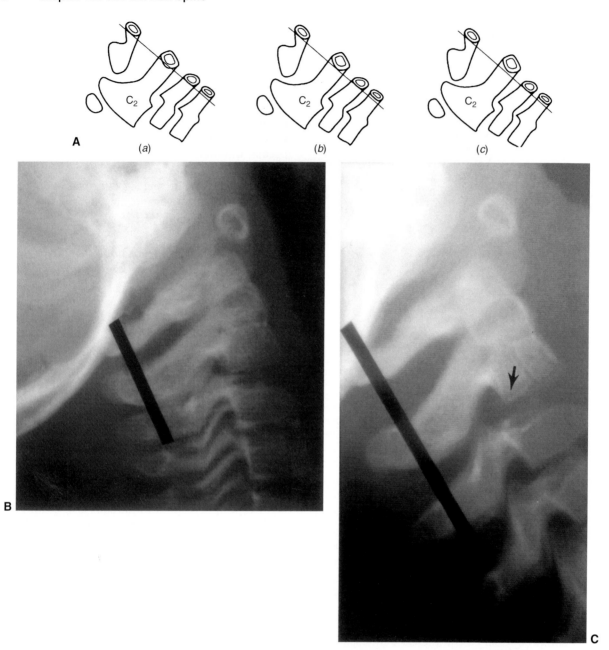

**Figure 22.6** **A:** The posterior cervical line referred to by Swischuk. In C2-C3 pseudosubluxation, the posterior cervical line may pass through (a), touch (b), or lie 1 mm in front of (c) the cortex of the posterior arch of C2. **B** and **C:** Lateral cervical radiographs of a child 2 years and 6 months of age with pseudosubluxation at C2-C3. The radiograph in extension **(B)** demonstrates no step-off at C2-C3, whereas the radiograph in flexion **(C)** demonstrates a step-off at C2-C3 (*arrow*), but with a normal posterior cervical line (*solid line*). Also note the anterior wedging of the C3 vertebral body, and the overriding of the anterior arch of the atlas on the tip of the odontoid in extension. (**A** from Shaw M, Burnett H, Wilson A, et al. Pseudosubluxation of C2 on C3 in polytraumatized children—prevalence and significance. *Clin Radiol* 1999;54:377–380, with permission.)

until 15 years of age, at which stage this distance is largest at C5-C6 (30). The anteroposterior displacement, from hyperflexion to hyperextension, decreases from C2-C3 to C6-C7. The angular displacement is greatest (15 degrees) at C3-C4 and C4-C5 in children 3 to 8 years of age, is greatest (17 degrees) at C4-C5 in children 9 to 11 years of age, and is greatest (15 degrees) at C5-C6 in children 12 to 15 years of age.

# CONGENITAL AND DEVELOPMENTAL PROBLEMS

## Torticollis

Torticollis is a combined head tilt and rotatory deformity. Torticollis indicates a problem at C1-C2, because 50% of the cervical spine rotation occurs at this joint. A head tilt alone indicates a more generalized problem in the cervical spine. The differential diagnosis of torticollis is large and can be divided into osseous and nonosseous types. In a recent large series from a tertiary care pediatric orthopaedic center (44), a nonmuscular etiology of torticollis was found in 18% of the patients, most frequently Klippel-Feil syndrome or a neurologic disorder (ocular pathology, or central nervous system lesion).

### Osseous Types

Occipitocervical synostosis, basilar impression, and odontoid anomalies are the most common congenital and developmental malformations of the occipitovertebral junction, with an incidence of 1.4 to 2.5 per 100 children (45). These lesions arise from a malformation of the mesenchymal anlages at the occipitovertebral junction.

*Basilar Impression.* Basilar impression is an indentation of the skull floor by the upper cervical spine. The tip of the dens is more cephalad and sometimes protrudes into the opening of the foramen magnum. This may encroach on the brain stem, risking neurologic damage from direct injury, vascular compromise, or alterations in cerebrospinal fluid flow (46).

Basilar impression can be primary or secondary. Primary basilar impression, the most common type, is a congenital abnormality often associated with other vertebral defects (e.g., Klippel-Feil syndrome, odontoid abnormalities, atlantooccipital fusion, and atlas hypoplasia). The incidence of primary basilar impression in the general population is 1% (47).

Secondary basilar impression is a developmental condition attributed to softening of the osseous structures at the base of the skull. Any disorder of osseous softening can lead to secondary basilar impression. These include: metabolic bone diseases [e.g., Paget disease (48), renal osteodystrophy, rickets, and osteomalacia (49)], bone dysplasias and mesenchymal syndromes [e.g., osteogenesis imperfecta (50–54), achondroplasia (55), hypochondroplasia (56), and neurofibromatosis (57)], and rheumatologic disorders (e.g., rheumatoid arthritis and ankylosing spondylitis). The softening allows the odontoid to migrate cephalad and into the foramen magnum.

These patients typically have short necks (78% in one series) (58). This shortening is only an apparent deformity because of the basilar impression. Asymmetry of the skull and face (68%), painful cervical motion (53%), and torticollis (15%) can also occur. Neurologic signs and symptoms are often present (59). Many children will have acute onset of symptoms precipitated by minor trauma (60). In cases of isolated basilar impression, the neurologic involvement is primarily a pyramidal syndrome associated with proprioceptive sensory disturbances (motor weakness, 85%; limb paresthesias, 85%). In cases of basilar impression associated with Arnold-Chiari malformations, the neurologic involvement is usually cerebellar, and

symptoms include motor incoordination with ataxia, dizziness, and nystagmus. In both types, the patients may complain of neck pain and headache from the distribution of the greater occipital nerve and of cranial nerves, particularly those that emerge from the medulla oblongata [trigeminal (V), glossopharyngeal (IX), vagus (X), and hypoglossal (XII)]. Ataxia is a very common finding in children with basilar impression (60). Hydrocephalus may develop because of obstruction of the cerebrospinal fluid flow caused by obstruction of the foramen magnum from the odontoid.

Basilar impression is difficult to assess radiographically. The most commonly used lines are Chamberlain's (61), McRae's (62), and McGregor's (63) (Fig. 22.7). McGregor's line is the best line for screening because the landmarks can be clearly defined at all ages on a routine lateral radiograph. McRae's line is helpful in assessing the clinical significance of basilar impression because it defines the opening of the foramen magnum; in patients who are symptomatic, the odontoid projects above this line. Nowadays, CT scans with sagittal plane reconstructions can show the osseous relations at the occipitocervical junction more clearly, and magnetic resonance imaging (MRI) clearly delineates the neural anatomy. Occasionally, vertebral angiography is needed (64).

Treatment of basilar impression can be difficult and requires a multidisciplinary approach (orthopaedic, neurosurgical, and neuroradiologic) (53,54,65,66). The symptoms can rarely be relieved with customized orthoses (67); the primary treatment is surgical. If the symptoms are caused by a hypermobile odontoid, surgical stabilization in extension at the occipitocervical junction is needed. Anterior excision of the odontoid is needed if it cannot be reduced (68), but this should be preceded by

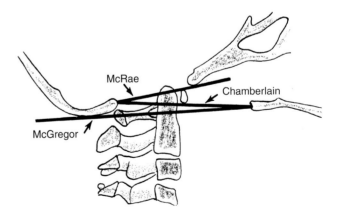

**Figure 22.7**  The landmarks used on a lateral radiograph of the skull and upper cervical spine used to assess basilar impression. McRae's line defines the opening of the foramen magnum. Chamberlain's line is drawn from the posterior lip of the foramen magnum to the dorsal margin of the hard palate. McGregor's line is drawn from the upper surface of the posterior edge of the hard palate to the most caudal point of the occipital curve of the skull. McGregor's line is the best for screening because of the clarity of the radiographic landmarks in children of all ages.

posterior stabilization and fusion. If the symptoms result from posterior impingement, suboccipital decompression and, often, upper cervical laminectomy are needed. The dura often needs to be opened so that the surgeon can look for a tight posterior band (58,69). Posterior stabilization should also be performed. In a recent series of 190 cases, decompression of the foramen magnum was found to be appropriate for those without an Arnold-Chiari malformation; transoral anterior decompression was reserved for those with an associated Arnold-Chiari malformation (70). These are general statements, and each case must be considered individually. Secondary basilar impression tends to progress despite arthrodesis (54).

*Atlantooccipital Anomalies.* Children with congenital bony anomalies of the atlantooccipital junction present with a wide spectrum of deformities. In these patients, the anterior arch of C1 is commonly assimilated to the occiput, usually in association with a hypoplastic ring posteriorly (Fig. 22.8) as well as condylar hypoplasia. The height of C1 is variably decreased, allowing the odontoid to project upward into the foramen magnum (i.e., primary basilar impression). More distal cervical anomalies can also occur in association with the atlantooccipital anomaly. The odontoid may be misshapen, or directed more posteriorly than normal. Up to 70% of children with this condition have a congenital fusion of C2 and C3 (Fig. 22.8). (Posterior congenital fusion of C2 and C3 is a clue that occiput–C1 anomalies, or other more distal cervical fusions, may be present. These may be cartilaginous initially, and may not appear on plain radiographs until the child becomes more mature.)

Clinically, these children resemble those with the Klippel-Feil syndrome: short, broad necks; restricted neck motion; low hairline; high scapula; and torticollis (69,71). Recently hemifacial microsomia has been noted to have associated atlantooccipital anomalies (72). The skull may demonstrate a positional deformational plagiocephaly. These patients may also have other associated anomalies, including dwarfism, funnel chest, jaw anomalies, cleft palate, congenital ear deformities, hypospadias, genitourinary tract defects, and syndactyly. They can present with neurologic symptoms during childhood, but more often present at between 40 and 50 years of age. These symptoms can be initiated by traumatic or inflammatory processes, and they progress slowly and relentlessly. Rarely do they present suddenly or dramatically, although they have been reported as a cause of sudden death. The most common signs and symptoms, in decreasing order of frequency, are neck and occipital pain, vertigo, ataxia, limb paresis, paresthesias, speech disturbances, hoarseness, diplopia, syncope, auditory malfunction, and dysphagia (73,74).

Standard radiographs are difficult to obtain because of fixed bony deformities and overlapping shadows from the mandible, occiput, and foramen magnum. An x-ray beam directed 90 degrees perpendicular to the skull (rather than to the cervical spine) usually gives a satisfactory view of the occipitocervical junction. The anomaly is usually studied further with a CT scan. In young children, the head-wag autotomography technique can be quite useful (75). This technique involves side-to-side rotation of the child's head while a slow anteroposterior radiographic exposure of the upper cervical spine is performed. This rotation blurs the overlying head and mandibular structures, allowing for improved visualization of the occiput–C1-C2 complex.

The position of the odontoid relative to the opening of the foramen magnum has been described as the distance measured from the posterior aspect of the odontoid to the posterior ring of C1 or the posterior lip of the foramen magnum, whichever is closer (71,76). This should be determined in flexion, because this position maximizes the reduction in the SAC. If this distance is less than 19 mm, a neurologic deficit is usually present. Lateral flexion and extension views of the upper cervical spine often show up to 12 mm of space between the odontoid and the C1 ring anteriorly (71); associated C1-C2 instability has been reported to develop eventually in 50% of these patients.

MRI is used for imaging the neural structures. Flexion-extension MRI is often necessary to fully evaluate the pathology (77). Compression of the brain stem or upper cervical cord anteriorly occurs because of the backward-projecting odontoid. This produces a range of findings and symptoms, depending on the location and degree of compression. Pyramidal tract signs and symptoms (e.g., spasticity, hyperreflexia, muscle weakness, and gait disturbances) are most common, although signs of cranial nerve involvement (e.g., diplopia, tinnitus, dysphagia, and auditory disturbances) can also be seen. Compression from the posterior lip of the foramen magnum or dural constricting band can disturb the posterior columns, leading to a loss of proprioception as well as vibration and tactile sensation. Nystagmus also occurs frequently because of posterior cerebellar compression. Vascular disturbances from vertebral artery involvement can result in brain stem ischemia, manifested by syncope, seizures, vertigo, and unsteady gait. Cerebellar tonsil herniation can occur. The altered mechanics of the cervical spine may result in a dull, aching pain in the posterior occiput and neck with intermittent stiffness and torticollis. Irritation of the greater occipital nerve may cause tenderness in the posterior scalp.

The natural history of atlantooccipital anomalies is unknown. The neurologic symptoms may develop so late and progress so slowly because the frequently associated C1-C2 instability progresses slowly with age, and the increased demands placed on the C1-C2 interval only gradually produce spinal cord or vertebral artery compromise.

Treatment is difficult. Surgery for atlantooccipital anomalies is more risky than with isolated anomalies of the odontoid (69,74). For this reason nonoperative methods should be initially attempted. Cervical collars, braces, and traction often help patients with persistent head and neck pain, especially after minor trauma or infection.

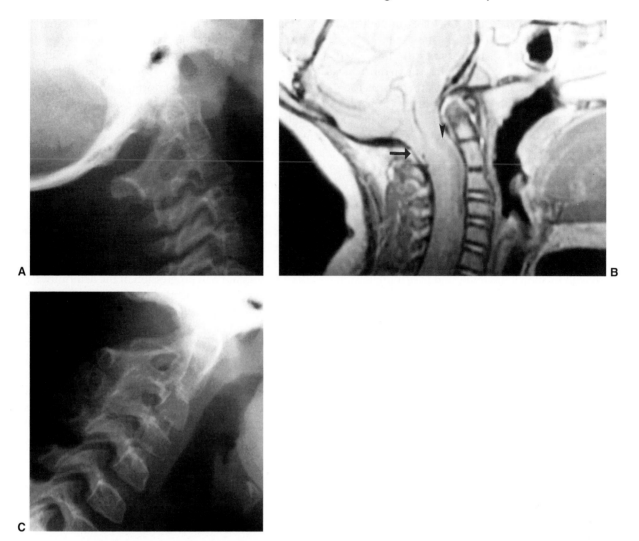

**Figure 22.8**   This girl, 3 years and 9 months of age, had a history of vertex headaches for 1 year. One month prior to presentation, she developed a painful, left-sided torticollis. **A:** Plain lateral radiograph shows fusion of C2 and C3 and absence of the ring of C1 with occipitalization. **B:** Magnetic resonance image (MRI) shows an Arnold-Chiari malformation, with herniation of the cerebellar tonsils into the foramen magnum (*arrow*). Also note the cordal edema (*arrowhead*). **C:** The child underwent an occipital decompression and laminectomy to C3, posterior cervical fusion from the occiput to C4, and halo cast immobilization for 4 months. Flexion and extension lateral radiographs 1 year after treatment show solid incorporation of the fusion from C2 to C4, with dissolution of the graft from the occiput to C2. However, there is no atlantooccipital instability. The child's symptoms resolved.

Immobilization may achieve only temporary relief if neurologic deficits are present. Patients with evidence of a compromised upper cervical area should take precautions not to expose themselves to undue trauma.

When symptoms and signs of C1-C2 instability are present, a posterior C1-C2 fusion is indicated. Preliminary traction to attempt reduction is used if necessary. If a reduction is possible and there are no neurologic signs, surgery has an improved prognosis (69,73,74). Posterior signs and symptoms may be an indication for posterior decompression depending on the evidence of dural or osseous compression. Results vary from complete resolution to increased deficits or death (69,78). In situations where there is no instability but only compressive pathology, the role of concomitant posterior fusion has not yet been determined. However, if decompression (whether anterior or posterior) could lead to a destabilized spine, then concomitant posterior fusion should be considered.

***Unilateral Absence of C1.*** This congenital malformation of the first cervical vertebra is, in essence, a hemiatlas or a congenital scoliosis of C1. Doubousset (79) described 17 patients with this condition. No definite population incidence is known. The problem is often associated with other anomalies common to children with congenital spine deformities (e.g., tracheoesophageal fistula).

Two thirds of the children with the condition present at birth; in others the condition is noticed later, when torticollis develops. A lateral translation of the head on the trunk, with variable degrees of lateral tilt and rotation (best appreciated from the back), is the typical finding. There also may be severe tilting of the eye line. The sternocleidomastoid muscle is not tight, although there is regional aplasia of the muscles in the nuchal concavity of the tilted side. Neck flexibility is variable and decreases with age. The condition is not painful. Plagiocephaly can occur, and increases as the deformity increases. Neurologic signs (e.g., headache, vertigo, myelopathy) are present in about one-fourth of the patients. The natural history is unknown.

Standard anteroposterior and lateral radiographs rarely give the diagnosis, although the open-mouth odontoid view may suggest it. Tomograms or CT scans usually are needed in order to see the anomaly (Fig. 22.9). The defect can range from a hypoplasia of the lateral mass to a complete hemiatlas with rotational instability and basilar impression. Occasionally the atlas is occipitalized. Doubousset classifies this disorder as one of the three types (71). Type I is an isolated hemiatlas. Type II is a partial or complete aplasia of one hemiatlas, with other associated anomalies of the cervical spine (e.g., fusion of C3-C4 and congenital bars in the lower cervical vertebrae). Type III is a partial or complete atlantooccipital fusion and symmetric or asymmetric hemiatlas aplasia, with or without anomalies of the odontoid and the lower cervical vertebrae.

Once this malformation is diagnosed, radiographs of the entire spine should be taken in order to rule out other congenital vertebral anomalies. Other imaging studies that may be needed are vertebral angiography and MRI. Angiography should be performed if operative intervention is to be undertaken, because arterial anomalies (e.g., multiple loops, vessels smaller than normal, and abnormal routes between C1 and C2) are often found on the aplastic side. MRI also should be performed if operative intervention is undertaken, because many of these children will have stenosis of the foramen magnum, and a few may have an Arnold-Chiari malformation.

The deformity should be observed in order to document the presence or absence of progression. This observation is primarily clinical (e.g., photographs) because radiographic measurements are difficult if not impossible to obtain. Bracing does not halt progression of the deformity. Surgical intervention is recommended in patients with severe deformities. A preoperative halo is used for gradual traction correction over 6 to 8 days. An ambulatory method of gradual correction of cervical spine deformity has been described using the halo-Ilizarov technique (80). A posterior fusion from the occiput to C2 or C3 is then performed, depending on the extent of the anomaly. Decompression of the spinal canal is necessary if the canal size is not ample or if projections show that it will not be able to fully accommodate the

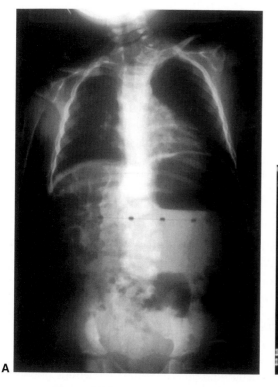

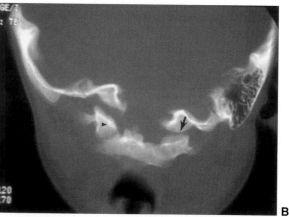

**A**   **B**

**Figure 22.9** This boy, 4 years and 10 months of age, presented with a torticollis. **A:** The antero-posterior radiograph of his entire spine, taken with him in the standing position, documents the head tilt to the left, along with left-sided hemivertebrae in the left lower cervical spine. Also note the multiple hemivertebrae in the thoracic and lumbar spine. **B:** A computed tomography scan with frontal reconstruction clearly demonstrates an absent lateral mass of C1 (*arrow*) with a normal right lateral mass (*arrowhead*). This represents a Doubousset type II, C1 unilateral absence.

developed spinal cord. The ideal age for posterior fusion is between 5 and 8 years, corresponding to the age at which the canal size reaches adult proportions.

*Familial Cervical Dysplasia.* The epidemiology of this recently described atlas deformity (81) is not known. Clinical presentation varies from an incidental finding to a passively correctable head tilt, suboccipital pain, decreased cervical motion, or a clunking of the upper cervical spine.

Plain radiographs are difficult to interpret. Various anomalies of C1, most commonly a partial absence of the posterior ring of C1, are typically seen. Various anomalies of C2 also commonly exist, for example, a shallow hypoplastic left facet. Other dysplasias of the lateral masses, facets, and posterior elements are seen, as are occasional spondylolistheses. Occiput–C1 instability is seen frequently, whereas C1-C2 instability rarely occurs. The delineation of this complex anatomy is often seen best with a CT scan and three-dimensional reconstruction (Fig. 22.10). When symptoms of instability are present, MRI in flexion and extension is recommended in order to assess the presence and magnitude of neural compression. Instability of the occipitocervical junction caused by the malformation may lead to neural compromise.

Nonsurgical treatment consists of observation every 6 to 12 months to ensure that instability does not develop, either clinically (e.g., progressive weakness and fatigue or objective signs of myelopathy) or radiographically on lateral flexion and extension radiographs. Surgical intervention is recommended for persistent pain, torticollis, and neurologic symptoms. A posterior fusion from the occiput to C2 is usually required, after gradual preoperative reduction using an adjustable halo cast (80).

*Atlantoaxial Rotary Displacement.* Atlantoaxial rotary displacement is one of the most common causes of childhood torticollis. Rotary displacements are characteristically

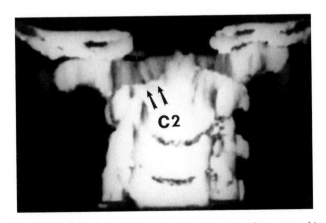

**Figure 22.10** A three-dimensional computerized tomographic scan of the upper cervical cord of a child with familial cervical dysplasia. The left superior facet of C2 is shallow and hypoplastic (*arrows*). (From Saltzman CL, Hensinger RN, Blane CE, et al. Familial cervical dysplasia. *J Bone Joint Surg Am* 1991;73-A:163–171, with permission.)

a pediatric problem, but they may occur in adults. There are several causes. Because the resultant radiographic findings and treatment regimens are the same for all pediatric causes, they are discussed as a unit and individual exceptions are noted where necessary.

The confusing terminology includes *rotary dislocation, rotary deformity, rotational subluxation, rotary fixation,* and *spontaneous hyperemic dislocation* (82,83). *Atlantoaxial rotary subluxation* is probably the most accepted term for describing the common childhood torticollis. *Subluxation* is misleading, however, because cases of "subluxation" usually present within the normal range of motion of the atlantoaxial joint. *Rotary displacement* is a more appropriate and descriptive term because it includes the entire range of pathology, from mild subluxation to complete dislocation. If the deformity persists, the children present with a resistant and unresolving torticollis that is best termed *atlantoaxial rotary fixation* or *fixed atlantoaxial displacement.* Gradations exist between very mild, easily correctable rotary displacement to rigid fixation. Complete atlantoaxial rotary dislocation has rarely been reported in surviving patients.

The radiographic findings of rotary displacement are difficult to demonstrate (84). In rotary torticollis, the lateral mass of C1 that has rotated to the anterior appears wider and closer to the midline (medial offset), whereas the opposite lateral mass is narrower and away from the midline (lateral offset). The facet joints may be obscured because of apparent overlapping. The lateral view shows the wedge-shaped lateral mass of the atlas lying anteriorly (where the oval arch of the atlas normally lies) and the posterior arches failing to superimpose because of the head tilt (Fig. 22.11). These findings may suggest occipitalization of C1 because the neck tilt may cause the skull to obscure C1 in the radiographic image. It is believed that the normal relation between the occiput and C1 is maintained in children with atlantoaxial rotary displacement. A lateral radiograph of the skull may demonstrate the relative positions of C1 and C2 more clearly than a lateral radiograph of the cervical spine. This is because tilting of the head also tilts C1, which creates overlapping shadows and makes interpretation of a lateral spinal radiograph difficult.

With plain radiographs, the position of C1 and C2 in a child with subluxation appears to be the same as that in a normal child whose head is rotated. Open-mouth views are difficult to obtain and interpret, and the lack of cooperation and diminished motion on the part of the child often make it impossible to obtain these special views. Cineradiography has been recommended, but the radiation dose is high, and it still may be difficult to obtain the patient's cooperation because of muscle spasms (84,85). CT scans are helpful in this situation if they are done properly (86). A CT scan, when taken with the head in the torticollic position, may be interpreted by the casual observer as showing rotation of C1 on C2. If the rotation of C1 on C2 is within the normal range, as it usually is early in this

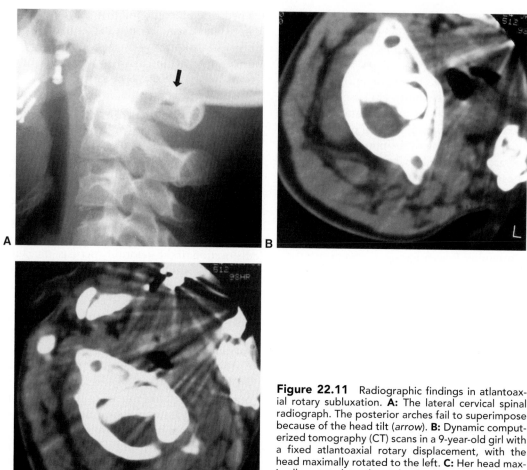

**Figure 22.11** Radiographic findings in atlantoaxial rotary subluxation. **A:** The lateral cervical spinal radiograph. The posterior arches fail to superimpose because of the head tilt (*arrow*). **B:** Dynamic computerized tomography (CT) scans in a 9-year-old girl with a fixed atlantoaxial rotary displacement, with the head maximally rotated to the left. **C:** Her head maximally rotated to the right, in this case, does not reach the midline. The ring of C1 is still in the exact relation to the odontoid as in **B**, indicating a fixed displacement.

condition, the observer may attribute this rotation to the positioning of the patient. A dynamic-rotation CT scan is helpful here. Views with the head maximally rotated to the right, then to the left, will demonstrate atlantoaxial rotary fixation when there is a loss of normal rotation (Fig. 22.11).

Rotary displacement can be classified into four types (Fig. 22.12) (82): type I is a simple rotary displacement without an anterior shift, type II is rotary displacement with an anterior shift of 5 mm or less, type III is rotary displacement with an anterior shift greater than 5 mm, and type IV is rotary displacement with a posterior shift. The amount of anterior displacement considered to be pathologic is greater than 3 mm in older children and adults and greater than 4 mm in younger children (29). Flexion and extension lateral-stress radiographs are suggested to rule out the possibility of anterior displacement.

Type I is the most common pediatric type. It is usually benign and frequently resolves by itself. Type II deformity is potentially more dangerous. Types III and IV are very rare, but because of the potential for neurologic involvement and even instant death, their management must be approached with great caution.

The etiology and pathoanatomy of the condition are not known completely (87). Several causative mechanisms are possible. Cervical spine fracture is rarely a cause. More commonly, atlantoaxial rotary displacement occurs following minor trauma [e.g., clavicle fractures (88)], after head and neck surgery including simple central line insertion (89), or after an upper respiratory tract infection. The children present with a "cock-robin" torticollis, and resist any attempt to move the head because of pain. The associated muscle spasm is noted on the side of the long sternocleidomastoid muscle. This is because the muscle is attempting to *correct* the deformity, unlike in congenital muscular torticollis in which the muscle *causes* the torticollis. If the deformity becomes fixed, the pain subsides but the torticollis persists, along with decreased neck motion. In longstanding cases, plagiocephaly and facial flattening may develop on the side of the tilt.

Spontaneous atlantoaxial subluxation with inflammation of adjacent neck tissues, also known as *Grisel syndrome*, is commonly seen in children after upper respiratory tract infections (Fig. 22.13). The children are frequently febrile (90). A direct connection exists between the

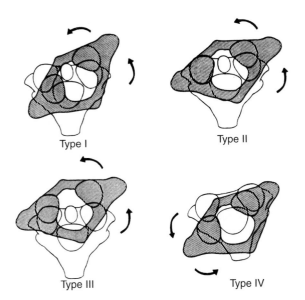

Type I      Type II

Type III      Type IV

**Figure 22.12** The four types of atlantoaxial rotary displacement. (From Fielding JW, Hawkins RJ. Atlanto-axial rotatory fixation. *J Bone Joint Surg Am* 1977;59-A:37–44, with permission.)

pharyngovertebral veins and the periodontal venous plexus and suboccipital epidural sinuses (91). This may provide a route for hematogenous transport of peripharyngeal septic exudates to the upper cervical spine, a possible anatomic explanation for the atlantoaxial hyperemia of Grisel syndrome. Regional lymphadenitis is known to cause spastic contracture of the cervical muscles. This muscular spasm, in the

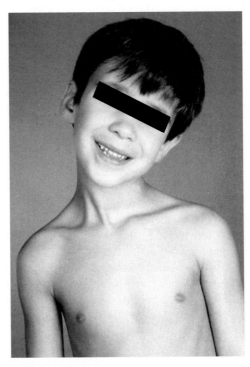

**Figure 22.13** A 5-year-old boy developed an atlantoaxial rotary subluxation after an upper respiratory viral infection (Grisel syndrome). It rapidly resolved after treatment with a soft collar and mild doses of diazepam.

presence of abnormally loose ligaments (hypothetically caused by the hyperemia of the pharyngovertebral vein drainage), could produce locking of the overlapping lateral joint edges of the articular facets. This situation prevents easy repositioning, resulting in atlantoaxial rotary displacement. The hyperemia after surgery of the oral pharynx, most frequently tonsillectomy and adenoidectomy, enhances the passage of the inflammatory products into the pharyngovertebral veins. It is known that patients may develop Grisel syndrome after otolaryngological procedures (92), especially with monopolar electrocautery (93). Kawabe et al. (94) have demonstrated meniscuslike synovial folds in the atlantooccipital and lateral atlantoaxial joints of children, but not in those of adults, and have found that the dens-facet angle of the axis is steeper in children than in adults. They postulate that excessive C1-C2 rotation, caused by the steeper angle and compounded by ligament laxity from an underlying hyperemia, allows the meniscuslike synovial folds to become impinged in the lateral atlantoaxial joint, leading to rotary fixation. The predominance of this syndrome in childhood correlates with the predilection for the adenoids to be maximally hypertrophied and inflamed at this same time, and located in the area drained by the pharyngovertebral veins.

Most atlantoaxial rotary displacements resolve spontaneously. Rarely, however, the pain subsides and the torticollis becomes fixed. The duration of symptoms and deformity dictates the treatment recommended (95).

Patients with rotary subluxation of less than 1 week's duration can be treated with immobilization in a soft cervical collar and rest for approximately 1 week. Close follow-up is mandatory. If spontaneous reduction does not occur with this initial treatment, hospitalization and the use of halter traction, muscle relaxants (e.g., diazepam), and analgesics are recommended next. Patients with rotary subluxation of more than 1 week but less than 1 month should be hospitalized immediately for cervical traction, relaxants, and analgesics. Gentle halo traction is occasionally needed in order to achieve reduction. The reduction is noted clinically and confirmed with a dynamic CT scan. If no anterior displacement is noted after reduction, cervical support should be continued only so long as symptoms persist. If there is anterior displacement, immobilization should be continued for 6 weeks to allow ligamentous healing to occur. In patients with rotary subluxation for more than 1 month, cervical traction (usually halo skeletal) can be tried for up to 3 weeks, but the prognosis is guarded. These children usually fall into two groups: those whose rotary subluxation can be reduced with halo traction but, despite a prolonged period of immobilization, resubluxate when the immobilization is stopped; and those whose subluxation cannot be reduced, and is fixed. It has been recently shown that patients with recurrence of deformity have a larger difference in the lateral mass–dens interval on the initial anteroposterior radiograph compared to those who do not have recurrence (96).

When the deformity is fixed, especially when anterior C1 displacement is present, the transverse atlantal ligament is compromised, presenting a potential for catastrophe. In this situation, posterior C1-C2 fusion should be performed. The indications for fusion are neurologic involvement, anterior displacement, failure to achieve and maintain correction, a deformity that has been present for more than 3 months, and recurrence of deformity following an adequate trial of conservative management (at least 6 weeks of immobilization after reduction). Before surgical fusion, halo traction is used for several days in order to obtain as much straightening of the head and neck as possible; a forceful or manipulative reduction should not be performed. Postoperatively, the child is simply positioned in a halo cast or vest in the straightened position obtained preoperatively; this usually achieves satisfactory alignment. A Gallie-type fusion with sublaminar wiring at the ring of C1 and through the spinous process of C2 is preferred to a Brooks-type fusion in which the wire is sublaminar at both C1 and C2. This is because of the decreased SAC at C2 and the consequent higher risk of neurologic injury. This wiring does not reduce the displacement but simply provides some internal stability for the arthrodesis. The overall results for a Gallie fusion are very good (Fig. 22.14) (97).

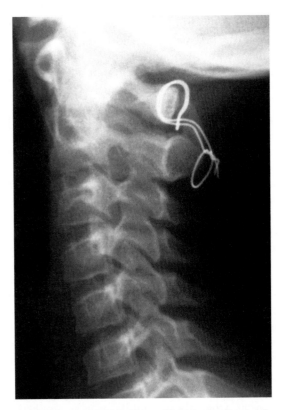

**Figure 22.14** The child in Figure 22.11 had a fixed deformity that occurred 6 months earlier, immediately after reconstructive maxillofacial surgery for Goldenhar syndrome. It did not respond to traction, including halo traction. She underwent a posterior C1-C2 (Gallie-type) fusion. A solid fusion was present 9 months later; clinically, the patient achieved 80 degrees of rotation to the left and 45 degrees of rotation to the right.

Long-term results do not indicate any significant abnormalities of the sagittal profile (98).

*Author's Preferred Treatment.* Patients with rotary subluxation of less than 1 week's duration are treated with immobilization in a soft cervical collar and rest for approximately 1 week. If spontaneous reduction does not occur, halter traction, muscle relaxants (e.g., diazepam), and analgesics are prescribed. Patients with rotary subluxation of more than 1 week but less than 1 month should be hospitalized immediately for cervical traction, relaxants, and analgesics. Gentle halo traction is occasionally needed to achieve reduction. All reductions are confirmed with a dynamic CT scan. In patients with rotary subluxation for more than 1 month, cervical traction (usually halo skeletal) can be tried for up to 3 weeks, but the prognosis is guarded. If reduction cannot be achieved or maintained, then posterior C1-C2 arthrodesis is recommended.

### Nonosseous Types
*Congenital Muscular Torticollis.* Congenital muscular torticollis, or congenital wry neck, is the most common cause of torticollis in the infant and young child, presenting at a median age of 2 months (99). The deformity is caused by contracture of the sternocleidomastoid muscle, with the head tilted toward the involved side and the chin rotated toward the opposite shoulder. A disproportionate number of these children have a history of a primiparous birth or a breech birth or other kind of difficult delivery. However, it has also been reported in children who were born normally and in those born by cesarean section (99–101).

The exact cause is not known and there are several theories. Because of the birth history, one theory is that a compartment syndrome occurs due to soft tissue compression of the neck at the time of delivery (102). Surgical histopathologic sections suggest venous occlusion of the sternocleidomastoid muscle (103). This occlusion may result in a compartment syndrome, as manifested by edema, degeneration of muscle fibers, and muscle fibrosis. This fibrosis is variable, ranging from small amounts to the entire muscle. It has been suggested that the clinical deformity is related to the ratio of fibrosis to remaining functional muscle. If ample muscle remains, the sternocleidomastoid will probably stretch with growth, and the child will not develop torticollis; if fibrosis predominates, there is little elastic potential, and torticollis will develop.

Another theory blames *in utero* crowding, since three in four of these children have the lesion on the right side (104), and up to 20% have developmental hip dysplasia (105). The fact that this condition can occur in children with normal birth histories or in children born by cesarean section challenges the perinatal compartment syndrome theory and supports the *in utero* crowding theory. The fact that it can occur in families (106–108) (supporting a genetic predisposition) also calls the compartment syndrome theory into question.

A third theory, supported by histopathologic evidence of denervation and reinnervation, cites a primarily neurogenic cause (109). The primary myopathy initially may result from trauma, ischemia, or both, and unequally involves the two heads of the sternocleidomastoid muscle. With continuing fibrosis of the sternal head, the branch of the spinal accessory nerve to the clavicular head of the muscle can be entrapped, leading to a later progressive deformity (109).

The final theory concerns mesenchymal cells remaining in the sternocleidomastoid from fetal embyrogenesis. Recent histopathologic studies have demonstrated the presence of both myoblasts and fibroblasts in sternocleidomastoid tumors in varying stages of differentiation and degeneration (110). The source of these myoblasts and fibroblasts is unknown. After birth, environmental changes stimulate these cells to differentiate, and the sternocleidomastoid tumor develops. Hemorrhagic and inflammatory reactions would be expected if the tumor were a result of perinatal birth trauma or intrauterine positioning, yet these cells were not seen in sternocleidomastoid histopathologic studies. The occurrence of torticollis depends on the fate of the myoblasts in the mass. If the myoblasts undergo normal development and differentiation, no persistent torticollis will occur and conservative treatment will likely succeed. If the myoblasts mainly undergo degeneration, then the remaining fibroblasts produce large amounts of collagen, with a scarlike contraction of the sternocleidomastoid muscle and the typical torticollis.

There are three clinical subgroups; those with sternocleidomastoid tumor (43% of cases), those with muscular torticollis (31%), and those with postural torticollis (22%) (111). The clinical features of congenital muscular torticollis depend on the age of the child. The condition is often discovered in the first 6 to 8 weeks of life. If the child is examined during the first 4 weeks of life, a mass or "tumor" may be palpable in the neck (100). Although it may be palpable, it is unrecognized up to 80% of the time (112). Characteristically, it is a nontender, soft enlargement beneath the skin, and is located within the sternocleidomastoid muscle belly. This so-called tumor reaches its maximum size within the first 4 weeks of life then gradually regresses. After 4 to 6 months of life the contracture and the torticollis are the only clinical findings. In some children the deformity is not noticed until after 1 year of age, which raises questions about both the congenital nature of this entity and the perinatal compartment syndrome theory. Recent studies (113) indicate that the rate of associated hip dysplasia in children with congenital muscular torticollis is 8%, lower than the previously cited 20% (105). The sternocleidomastoid tumor subgroup, the most severe group, presents at an earlier age and is associated with a higher incidence of breech presentation (19%), difficult labor (56%), and hip dysplasia (6.8%) (111).

If the deformity is progressive, skull and face deformities can develop (plagiocephaly), often within the first year of life. The facial flattening occurs on the side of the contracted muscle, and is probably caused by the sleeping position of the child (114). In the United States children usually sleep prone, and in this position it is more comfortable for them to lie with the affected side down. The face thus remodels to conform to the bed. If the child sleeps supine, reverse modeling of the contralateral skull occurs. In the child who is untreated for many years, the level of the eyes and ears becomes unequal and can result in considerable cosmetic deformity.

Radiographs of the cervical spine should be obtained in order to rule out associated congenital anomalies. Plain radiographs of the cervical spine in children with muscular torticollis are always normal, aside from the head tilt and rotation. If any suspicion exists about the status of the hips, appropriate imaging (e.g., ultrasonography or radiography) should be done, depending on the age of the child and expertise of the ultrasonographer.

Research MRI studies demonstrate abnormal signals in the sternocleidomastoid muscle, but no discrete masses within the muscle (102). The muscle diameter is two to four times greater than that of the contralateral muscle. In older patients the signals are consistent with atrophy and fibrosis, similar to those encountered in compartment syndromes of the leg and forearm.

As the deficit in cervical rotation increases, so does the incidence of a previous stenocleidomastoid tumor, hip dysplasia, and the likelihood of needing surgery increase (115,116). Treatment initially consists of conservative measures (100,101,112,117,118). Good results can be expected with stretching exercises alone, with one series reporting 90% success (117) and another 95% (116). Children with a sternocleidomastoid tumor respond less favorably to conservative stretching exercises than do those with a simple muscle torticollis; none of the children with postural torticollis need surgery (116). The extent of sternocleidomastoid fibrosis on ultrasound examination is also predictive of the need for surgery (119,120). In one series, conservative therapy was effective for all the patients in whom only the lower one-third of the muscle was involved with fibrosis; surgery was needed in 35% of the children in whom the entire length of the muscle was involved (121).

The exercises are administered by the caregivers and guided by the physiotherapist. The ear opposite the contracted muscle should be positioned to the shoulder, and the chin should be positioned to touch the shoulder on the same side as the contracted muscle. When adequate stretching has occurred in the neutral position, the exercises should be graduated up to the extended position, which achieves maximum stretching and prevents residual contractures. Treatment measures to be used along with stretching include room modifications; the child's toys and crib should be modified so that the neck is stretched when the infant is reaching for or looking at objects of interest. The exact extent of the efficacy of these stretching measures, compared against a natural history of spontaneous resolution, is not known (122); there are many anecdotal cases of spontaneous resolution. Occasionally, muscle stretching itself will result in partial or complete rupture of the sternocleidomastoid muscle (123).

If stretching measures are unsuccessful after 1 year of age (116,118,122,124), surgery is recommended. The child's neck and anatomic structures are larger by this age, making surgery easier. Established facial deformity or a limitation of more than 30 degrees of motion usually precludes a good result, and surgery is required to prevent further facial flattening and further cosmetic deterioration (118). Asymmetry of the face and skull can improve so long as adequate growth potential remains after the deforming pull of the sternocleidomastoid is removed; good but not perfect results can be obtained with surgery performed on children as old as 12 years (112,125).

The best time for surgical release is between the ages of 1 and 4 years (100,126); for those treated surgically before the age of 3 years excellent results can be expected in nearly all cases (125). Surgical treatments include a unipolar release (125) at the sternoclavicular or mastoid pole, bipolar release, middle third transection, and even complete resection. Although these surgical procedures are usually done open, endoscopic (127) and percutaneous (distal) approaches have been recently described (128). Bipolar release combined with a Z-plasty of the sternal attachment (Fig. 22.15) yielded 92% satisfactory results in one series, whereas only 15% satisfactory results were obtained with other procedures (124). Similar results, although not perfect, can be achieved even in older children by using a bipolar release technique (129). In a more recent series of surgical cases, excellent results were obtained with a unipolar release and aggressive postoperative stretching (125). Middle-third transection has also been reported to give 90% satisfactory results (130). Z-plasty lengthening maintains the V-contour of the neck and cosmesis, which the middle-third transection does not. Structures that can be

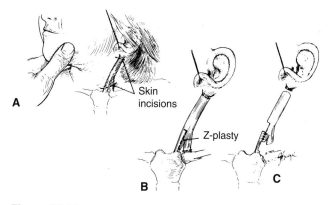

**Figure 22.15** The Z-plasty procedure for torticollis. **A:** The location of the skin incisions. **B:** The clavicular and mastoid attachments of the sternocleidomastoid muscle are cut, and a Z-plasty is performed. Note that the medial aspect of the sternal attachment is preserved. **C:** The completed procedure after release of the proximal muscle insertion. (From Ferkel RD, Westin GW, Dawson EG, et al. Muscular torticollis. A modified surgical approach. *J Bone Joint Surg Am* 1983;65-A:894–900, with permission.)

injured by surgery are the spinal accessory nerve, the anterior and external jugular veins, the carotid vessels and sheath, and the facial nerve. Skin incisions should never be located directly over the clavicle because of cosmetically unacceptable scar spreading; rather, they should be made one finger's breadth proximal to the medial end of the clavicle and sternal notch, and in line with the cervical skin creases. The postoperative protocol can vary from simple stretching exercises to cast immobilization. Some type of a bracing device to maintain alignment of the head and neck is probably a desirable part of the postoperative protocol.

*Author's Preferred Treatment.* In children diagnosed before 1 year of age, a regimen of stretching exercises and room modifications is tried first. If this approach fails, or if the child presents after 1 year of age, a bipolar sternocleidomastoid release is performed. Postoperative orthotic immobilization is used along with frequent physiotherapy for at least 3 months after surgery.

### Neurogenic Types

Although rare, these causes should be considered in the differential diagnosis of any atypical torticollis, especially when the condition is unresponsive or progressive in the face of therapy that is believed to be appropriate. The major neurogenic etiologies are central nervous system tumors (i.e., of the posterior fossa or spinal cord), syringomyelia with or without cord tumor, Arnold-Chiari malformation, ocular dysfunction, and paroxysmal torticollis of infancy.

Posterior fossa tumors can present with torticollis (131,132). The ophthalmologic literature (133) has described three children with torticollis, photophobia, and epiphora (tearing). In all three children, the diagnosis was delayed by an initial diagnosis of a local ocular inflammatory condition. The age at presentation ranged from 1 to 23 months. The delay in diagnosis ranged from 5 months to 4 years. The neoplastic diagnosis was not considered initially by the ophthalmologists because the primary signs of posterior fossa tumors are extraocular muscle paresis, nystagmus, and papilledema.

Cervical cord tumors can present with torticollis, often early in their course (134,135). Frequently the initial diagnosis is congenital torticollis, obstetric birth palsy, muscular dystrophy, or cerebral palsy (134). The peculiar, often overlooked signs of the tumor are spinal rigidity, early spinal deformity, and spontaneous or induced vertebral pain. In young children, pain may be expressed as irritability and restlessness (136).

Imaging of a child with a potential central nervous system tumor should consist of plain radiographs of the skull and cervical spine followed by CT scan and MRI. Vertebral angiography may also be needed, both diagnostically and in neurosurgical planning.

The Arnold-Chiari malformation (Fig. 22.8) is caudal displacement of the hindbrain, often with other congenital deformities of the brain stem and cerebellum (137,138). It may be associated with myelomeningocele (i.e., Chiari type II malformation). The Chiari type I malformation is a downward displacement of the medulla oblongata with extrusion of the cerebellar tonsils through the foramen magnum; it is encountered in older children. Dure et al. (137) described 11 children with Chiari type I malformations; torticollis was the presenting complaint of 1 of the 11 children, who was 5 years of age. It was associated with headaches and paracervical muscle spasm; the torticollis was left sided. As with tumors, the workup in a child with the potential diagnosis of Chiari malformation consists of plain radiographs of the skull and cervical spine followed by an MRI (137). The treatment is neurosurgical.

Ocular pathology accounts for up to one third of children with no obvious orthopaedic cause of torticollis (139). The torticollis is usually atypical (140). These children typically present at approximately 1 year of age. The face can be turned about a vertical axis, the head can be tilted to one shoulder with the frontal plane of the face remaining coronal, the chin can be elevated or depressed, or a combination of any of these positions can occur. These abnormal head positions optimize visual acuity and maintain binocularity. An ocular cause is likely if the head is tilted but not rotated or if the tilt changes when the child is lying versus sitting or standing up. Children with ocular torticollis have a full range of cervical motion without the fibrotic sternocleidomastoid muscle seen in congenital muscular torticollis. Ophthalmologic evaluation is usually positive for paralytic squint or nystagmus. Detailed tests conducted by an experienced ophthalmologist are diagnostic. Treatment for ocular torticollis is usually by ophthalmic surgery.

Paroxysmal torticollis of infancy is a rare, unusual, episodic torticollis lasting for minutes to days, with spontaneous recovery (141–143). The attacks usually occur in the morning and last from minutes to days, with a frequency ranging from less than one episode per month to three to four episodes per month. The attacks may be associated with lateral trunk curvature, eye movements or deviations, and alternating sides of torticollis. The children are usually girls (71%), the average age at onset is 3 months (range, 1 week to 30 months), and the average recovery period is 24 months (range, 6 months to 5 years). It has been suggested that paroxysmal torticollis of infancy is equivalent to a migraine headache (144,145) because family histories of migraines were reported for 29% of the patients in one study, or that it could be a forerunner of benign paroxysmal vertigo of childhood (142). Whatever the cause, it is usually self-limiting and does not require therapy. It may be linked to a mutation in the *CACNA1A* gene (145), which is associated with familial hemiplegic migraine.

### Sandifer Syndrome

This is a syndrome of gastroesophageal reflux, often from a hiatal hernia, and abnormal posturing of the neck and trunk, usually torticollis (146,147). The torticollis is likely an attempt of the child to decrease esophageal discomfort resulting from the reflux. The abnormal posturing may also present as opisthotonos or neural tics, and often mimics central nervous system disorders. Most patients present in infancy. The incidence of gastroesophageal reflux is high (up to 40% of infants) (148), with the principal symptoms being vomiting, failure to thrive, recurrent respiratory disease, dysphagia, various neural signs, torticollis, and respiratory arrest. The diagnosis of symptom-causing gastroesophageal reflux is frequently overlooked. On careful examination of these infants, it is found that the sternocleidomastoid muscle is not tight or short, and there is no tumor; this eliminates the possibility of congenital muscular torticollis. Further workup excludes dysplasias and congenital anomalies of the cervical spine as well as central nervous system disorders. In these situations the physician should consider Sandifer syndrome in the differential diagnosis.

Plain radiographs of the cervical spine eliminate congenital anomalies or dysplasias; contrast studies of the upper gastrointestinal tract usually demonstrate the hiatal hernia and gastroesophageal reflux (149). Esophageal pH studies may be necessary; many children, both asymptomatic and symptomatic, show evidence of gastroesophageal reflux (150). Treatment begins with medical therapy. If this fails, fundoplication can be considered, which is usually curative (151).

### Klippel-Feil Syndrome

Klippel-Feil syndrome consists of congenital fusions of the cervical vertebrae, clinically exhibited by the triad of a low posterior hairline, a short neck, and variably limited neck motion (Fig. 22.16A and B) (152). Its incidence is approximately 0.7% (153). Other associated anomalies are often present both in the musculoskeletal and other organ systems. The congenital fusions result from abnormal embryologic formation of the cervical vertebral mesenchymal anlages. This unknown embryologic insult is not limited to the cervical vertebrae and explains the other anomalies associated with the Klippel-Feil syndrome. In some instances the Klippel-Feil syndrome is familial, indicating a genetic transmission (154–156).

Approximately one-third of these children have an associated Sprengel deformity. Other anomalies associated with the syndrome are scoliosis (both congenital and idiopathic) (152), congenital limb deficiency (157), renal anomalies (158), deafness (159), synkinesis (mirror movements) (160), pulmonary dysfunction (161), and congenital heart disease (162). Radiographs demonstrate a wide range of deformities, ranging from simple block vertebrae to multiple and bizarre anomalies. Klippel-Feil syndrome can be divided into three types, depending upon the extent of vertebral involvement: type I involves the cervical and upper thoracic vertebrae, type II involves the cervical vertebrae alone, and type III involves the cervical vertebrae as

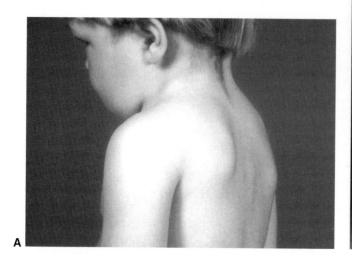
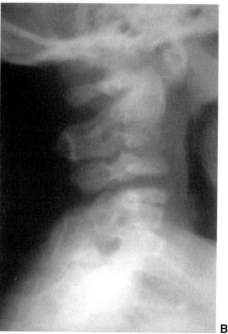

**Figure 22.16** This boy, 3 years and 6 months of age, presented with a short neck and reduced motion. **A:** Note the short neck and low posterior hair line. **B:** The lateral cervical spine radiograph demonstrates complete fusion of the posterior elements of C2 and C3, with reduced disc height anteriorly at C2-C3. Note the reduced space between C3 and C4, which most likely represents a cartilage fusion between C3 and C4 that will likely become an osseous fusion later.

well as lower thoracic or upper lumbar vertebrae (163). Associated scoliosis makes interpretation of the radiographs even more difficult. Flexion and extension lateral radiographs are used to assess for instability, and this should always be done prior to administering any general anesthetic. If instability is noted on the flexion and extension radiographs, the anesthesiologist should be informed accordingly. The anesthesiologist may elect to undertake intubation differently (e.g., awake nasotracheal, fiberoptic guided). Any segment adjacent to unfused segments may develop hypermobility and neurologic symptoms (164). A common pattern is fusion of C1 to C2 and of C3 to C4, leading to a high risk of instability at the unfused C2-C3 level (165). If the flexion and extension radiographs are difficult to interpret, a flexion and extension CT or MRI scan can be useful. A CT scan is especially helpful at the C1-C2 level in assessing the SAC; sagittal MRI is more helpful at other levels.

All children with Klippel-Feil syndrome should be further evaluated for other organ system problems. A general pediatric evaluation should be undertaken by a qualified pediatrician to ensure that no congenital cardiac or other neurologic abnormalities exist. Renal imaging should be done in all cases; simple renal ultrasonography is usually adequate for the initial evaluation (166). MRI should be performed whenever there is a clinical basis for any concern about neurologic involvement, in order to define the site and cause of neurologic pathology. Also, an MRI should be performed before any orthopaedic spinal procedure; this is to rule out any other intraspinal pathology that might not be seen clinically or radiographically (e.g., Arnold-Chiari malformation, tethered cord, nonosseous diastematomyelia) (167).

The natural history depends on whether renal or cardiac problems are present, since they have the potential to lead to organ system failure and death. Cervical spine instability (168) can develop with neurologic involvement, especially in the upper segments, or in patients with iniencephaly (168,169). The more numerous the occipitoatlantal anomalies, the higher the neurologic risk (170). Degenerative joint and disc disease develops in patients with lower segment instabilities. In adulthood, many patients with Klippel-Feil syndrome will complain of headaches, upper-extremity weakness, or numbness and tingling. On neurologic examination, subtle findings can be seen in up to half of these adults. Those with mirror-movement disorders are likely to have cervicomedullary neuroschisis (171). Degenerative disc disease, as seen on MRI scans, occurs in nearly 100% of these patients (172).

Because children with large fusion areas (Fig. 22.17) are at high risk for developing instabilities, strenuous activities should be avoided, especially contact sports. Other nonsurgical methods of treatment are cervical traction, collars, and analgesics when mechanical symptoms appear, usually in the adolescent or adult patient. Arthrodesis is needed for the management of neurologic symptoms caused by instability. Asymptomatic hypermobile segments pose a dilemma regarding stabilization.

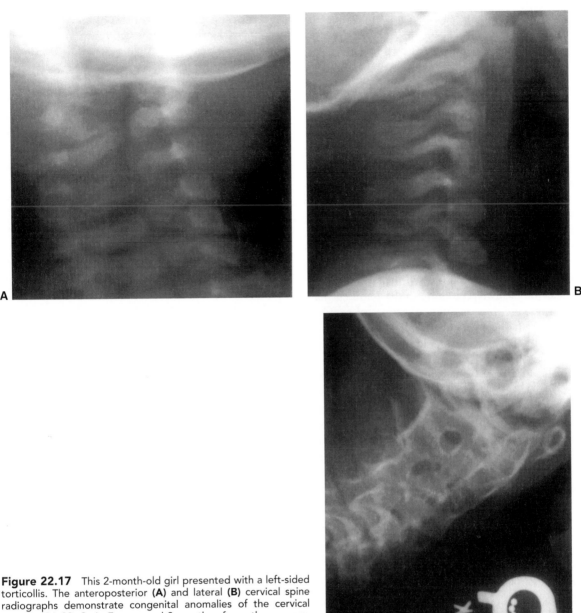

**Figure 22.17** This 2-month-old girl presented with a left-sided torticollis. The anteroposterior **(A)** and lateral **(B)** cervical spine radiographs demonstrate congenital anomalies of the cervical spine at C1-C2. **C:** At 7 years and 3 months of age these anomalies have further ossified and matured, demonstrating massive congenital fusions of the cervical spine.

Unfortunately, no guidelines exist for this problem. The need for decompression at the time of stabilization depends on the exact anatomic circumstance, as will the choice of combined anterior and posterior rather than simple posterior fusions. Surgery for cosmesis alone is usually unwarranted and risky.

### Author's Preferred Treatment

Once Klippel-Feil syndrome is diagnosed, it is mandatory that imaging of the genitourinary system be performed if it has not already been done. The patient is counseled against contact sports, especially collision sports (football, wrestling, ice hockey) and sports that may place the cervical spine under stress (e.g., gymnastics, diving, basketball,

soccer, volleyball). We typically ask the child what sports he/she likes to participate in, and then determine whether that sport is likely to place the cervical spine under stress. If so, that activity should be avoided. Arthrodesis is reserved for the very rare instances of symptomatic hypermobility.

### Os Odontoideum

Os odontoideum is a rare anomaly in which the tip of the odontoid process is divided by a wide transverse gap, leaving the apical segment without its basilar support (173). The exact rate of incidence is not known. It most likely represents an unrecognized fracture at the base of the odontoid or damage to the epiphyseal plate during the first few years of life (173,174). Either of these conditions can compromise the blood supply to the developing odontoid, resulting in the os odontoideum. MRI scans have further documented the presence of nuchal cord changes consistent with trauma (175). A congenital etiology has also been proposed (176), and may represent an embryological anomaly characterized by segmentation at the junction of the proximal $1\frac{1}{2}$ somites of the $2\frac{1}{2}$ somites from which the odontoid forms (177).

Localized neck pain is the usual symptom at presentation; transitory episodes of paresis, myelopathy, and cerebral brain stem ischemia due to vertebral artery compression from the upper cervical instability are less common. Sudden death rarely occurs.

Radiographs demonstrate an oval or round ossicle, with a smooth sclerotic border of variable size located in the position of the normal odontoid tip. It is occasionally located near the basioccipital bone in the foramen magnum area. There are three radiographic types of os odontoideum; round, cone, and blunt-tooth (178). The base of the dens is usually hypoplastic. The gap between the os and the hypoplastic dens is wider than in a fracture, usually well above the level of the facets. However, it may be difficult to differentiate an os odontoideum from nonunion following a fracture. Tomograms and CT scans are useful in further delineating the bony anatomy, and flexion and extension lateral radiographs help in assessing instability. The instability index and sagittal plane rotation angle can be measured (Fig. 22.18) (179). The presence of myelopathy is highly correlated with a sagittal plane rotation angle of 20 degrees or more and an instability index of 40% or higher; it is also most common in the round type of os odontoideum (178). Myelopathy is also associated with cystic or fibrocartilaginous masses behind the odontoid, within the transverse ligament, or at the level of the articulation between the os odontoideum and the remainder of the odontoid (176,180–182); these typically regress after successful stabilization and arthrodesis (183).

The neurologic symptoms are caused by cord compression from posterior translation of the os into the cord in extension or from the odontoid into the cord in flexion. Hypermobility at the C1 and C2 level may cause vertebral artery occlusion with ischemia of the brain stem and posterior fossa structures; this will result in seizures, syncope, vertigo, and visual disturbances.

Those with local pain or transient myelopathies often recover with immobilization. Subsequently, only nonstrenuous activities should be allowed, but curtailment of activities in the pediatric age group can be difficult. The risk of a small insult leading to catastrophic quadriplegia and death must be weighed. The long-term natural history is unknown.

Surgery is indicated when there is 10 mm or more of ADI, a SAC of 13 mm or less (33), neurologic involvement, progressive instability, or persistent neck pain. Surgery should also be strongly considered in patients who are asymptomatic but have an instability index greater than 40% and/or a sagittal plane rotation angle greater than 20 degrees. A Gallie fusion is recommended. The surgeon must be careful when tightening the wire so that the os is not pulled back posteriorly into the canal and cord, because the consequences would be disastrous. In small children, the wire may be eliminated. In all children, a Minerva or halo cast or vest is also used for at least 6 weeks, and often for 12 weeks. Recently, C1-C2 screw fixation has been reported to be helpful in treating pediatric atlantoaxial instability in children older than 4 years of age (184). In all children undergoing C1-C2 posterior arthrodesis, care should be taken to avoid fixation of the C1-C2 segment in hyperlordosis, as that will lead to subaxial cervical kyphosis postoperatively (185).

## Developmental and Acquired Stenoses and Instabilities

### Down Syndrome

Because of underlying collagen defects in children with this syndrome, cervical instabilities can develop at both the occiput-C1 and C1-C2 levels. The instability may occur at more than one level and in more than one plane (e.g., sagittal and rotary planes). With the advent of the Special Olympics, there has been much concern regarding the participation of children with Down syndrome, and much confusion regarding the appropriate approach to the

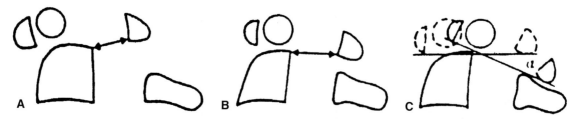

**Figure 22.18**  Radiographic parameters used for determining the instability index and sagittal plane rotation in os odontoideum. The minimum **(A)** and maximum **(B)** distance from the posterior border of the body of C2 to the posterior atlantal arch. The instability index = [(maximum distance − minimum distance)/maximum distance] × 100%. **C:** The change in the atlantoaxial angle between flexion and extension is the sagittal plane rotation. (From Watanabe M, Toyama Y, Fujimura Y. Atlantoaxial instability in os odontoideum with myelopathy. *Spine* 1996;21:1435–1439, with permission.)

problem of upper cervical instability in these children. Outlined in following text are the most recent recommendations regarding this problem.

The incidence of occiput-C1 instability has been reported to be as high as 60% in children with Down syndrome (37) and 69% in the adults (186). The vast majority are asymptomatic (187,188). Measurement reproducibility is poor (189), but a Powers ratio of less than 0.55 is more likely to be associated with neurologic symptoms (190) (Fig. 22.24A). No guidelines exist regarding the frequency of periodic screening or indications for surgery, with the exception of those for atlantooccipital fusion in the symptomatic child. Tredwell et al. (37) believe that treatment plans for these children should depend on the amount of room available for the cord rather than absolute values of displacement for both atlantoaxial and atlantooccipital instability.

Atlantoaxial instability in children with Down syndrome was first reported by Spitzer et al. (186) in 1961. Subsequently there have been many reports on this instability. However, there are none that document the true incidence of atlantoaxial dislocation (in contrast to instability), and there are no long-term studies of the natural history of this problem.

The incidence of atlantoaxial instability in children with Down syndrome has been estimated to range from 9% to 22% (37,191–193). The incidence of symptomatic atlantoaxial instability is much less; it was reported to be 2.6% (191) in a series of 236 patients with Down syndrome. Progressive instability and neurologic deficits are more likely to develop in boys older than 10 years (193). Children with Down syndrome have a significantly greater incidence of cervical skeletal anomalies, especially persistent synchondrosis and spina bifida occulta of C1, than do normal children (194). Also, children with both Down syndrome and atlantoaxial instability have an increased frequency of cervical spine anomalies compared with Down syndrome children without atlantoaxial instability (194). These spinal anomalies may be a contributing factor in the cause of atlantoaxial instability in these children.

Most children with atlantoaxial or occipitoatlantal hypermobility are asymptomatic. When symptoms occur, they are usually pyramidal tract symptoms, such as gait abnormalities, hyperreflexia, easy fatigability, and quadriparesis. Occasionally, local symptoms exist such as head tilt, torticollis, neck pain, and limited neck mobility. The neurologic deficits are not necessarily attributable to hypermobility of the atlantoaxial or occipitoatlantal joints. Neurologic symptoms in one series of adult patients with Down syndrome were equally common in those with an increased ADI as in those with a normal ADI (195). In this situation, further evaluation with flexion-extension CT or MRI scans is needed to assess for cord compression.

Rarely does sudden catastrophic death occur. In nearly all the patients, catastrophic injury to the spinal cord has been preceded by weeks to years of less severe neurologic abnormalities. In a review by the American Academy of Pediatrics, 41 cases of symptomatic atlantoaxial instability were compiled. In only 3 of these 41 children did the initiation or worsening of symptoms of atlantoaxial instability occur after trauma during organized sports activities (192).

In the past, screening of patients with Down syndrome by using lateral flexion-extension radiographs was recommended (196). However, symptomatic atlantoaxial instability is very rare, and the chances of a sports-related catastrophic injury even rarer. The reproducibility of radiographic screening for atlantoaxial and occipitoatlantal mobility is poor (188,189,197). Furthermore, the radiologic picture can change over time, most frequently from abnormal to normal (193). Because of all these factors, and in the absence of any evidence that a screening program is effective in preventing symptomatic atlantoaxial and occipitoatlantal mobility, lateral cervical radiographs are believed to be of unproven value, and the previous recommendations for screening radiographs by the American Academy of Pediatrics have been retired (192).

The identification of patients with symptoms or signs consistent with symptomatic spinal cord injury is thus more important than radiographs. Neurologic examination is often difficult to perform and interpret in these children (37). Parental education about the early signs of myelopathy is extremely important (e.g., increasing clumsiness, more episodes of falling, and worsening of upper-extremity function). A thorough history and neurologic examination of the patient are more important than screening radiographs before a decision is made about participation in sports. However, further research is needed in this confusing matter, and because of persistent concerns, the Special Olympics does not plan to remove its requirement that all Down syndrome athletes have radiographs of the cervical spine before participating in athletic events.

Because of this requirement, spinal radiographs are often obtained in the absence of neurologic symptoms. When such radiographs are available, they should be reviewed to determine whether there are any other associated anomalies, such as persistent synchondrosis of C2, spina bifida occulta of C1, ossiculum terminale, os odontoideum, and other less common anomalies. When the plain radiographs indicate atlantoaxial or atlantooccipital instability of 6 mm or more in an asymptomatic patient, CT and MRI scans in flexion and extension can determine the extent of neural encroachment and cord compression.

Once a patient with Down syndrome presents with radiographic instability, what treatment should be instituted? Those with asymptomatic atlantoaxial or occipitoatlantal hypermobility should probably be followed up with repeat neurologic examinations; the role of repeat radiographs, however, is unclear, as noted in the previous discussion. Because the risk of a catastrophic spinal cord injury is extremely low with organized sports in Down syndrome children in the absence of any neurologic findings, the avoidance of high risk activities must be individualized. For those children with sudden onset or recent progression of neurologic symptoms, immediate fusion should be undertaken if appropriate imaging confirms cord compromise. The most difficult question concerns the patient with upper cervical hypermobility with minimal or nonprogressive chronic symptoms. Before embarking upon arthrodesis, imaging with flexion-extension MRI (77) or CT scan should be undertaken to confirm cord compression from the hypermobility, and to eliminate other central nervous system causes of neurologic symptoms. A CT scan is faster, reducing the need for sedation, which can be potentially dangerous in these children. A CT scan also visualizes the C1-C2 relations that are necessary to measure the SAC. MRI is more useful for evaluating other central nervous system lesions. Even if successfully stabilized, patients with chronic symptoms often show little symptomatic improvement after arthrodesis (198).

Posterior cervical fusion at the levels involved is the recommended surgical treatment. The classic technique for posterior C1-C2 fusion uses autogenous iliac crest bone graft with wiring and postoperative halo cast immobilization. Internal fixation with wiring and/or transarticular screws (199) provides protection against displacement, shortens the time of postoperative immobilization, permits the possible use of less rigid forms of external immobilization, and is reported to aid in obtaining fusion (200). However, internal fixation with sublaminar wiring poses added risk. If the instability does not reduce as observed on routine films in the extension position, the patient would be at high risk for developing iatrogenic quadriplegia if sublaminar wiring and acute manipulative reduction were tried (201,202). For this reason it has been recommended that preoperative traction be used to effect the reduction. If reduction does not occur with traction, then only an onlay bone grafting should be performed, without sublaminar wiring (201). Sublaminar wiring at C2 is not recommended regardless of the success of reduction; sublaminar wiring at C2 was associated with the only death of a patient in one series (203). If wiring is to be performed, pliable, smaller caliber wires should be used. Satisfactory results can be obtained with onlay bone grafts and rigid external immobilization without internal fixation (204).

The patient with Down syndrome is at higher risk for postoperative complications (neurologic and other) after fusion (205–207). Neurologic complications can range from complete quadriplegia and death to Brown-Sequard syndrome (203). Another potential cause of neurologic impairment is overreduction if an unstable os odontoideum is present (203). A posterior translation of the ring of C1 and the os fragment into the SAC can result from this overreduction. In a study of the results of surgical fusion in 35 symptomatic Down syndrome children, 8 made a complete recovery, 14 showed improvement, 7 did not improve, 4 died, and the outcome for 2 is unknown (191). Patients with long-standing symptoms and marked neural damage showed little or no postoperative improvement, whereas patients with a more recent onset of symptoms usually

made an excellent recovery. Other complications are loss of reduction despite halo cast immobilization and resorption of the bone graft, with a stable fibrous union or an unstable nonunion (Fig. 22.19) (204,205).

The long-term results after cervical fusion are not yet known. Individuals with Down syndrome who undergo short cervical fusions are at risk for developing instability above the level of fusion, such as occiput-C1 after a C1-C2 fusion or C1-C2 after lower level fusions (208). This later instability occurred in four of five children between 6 months and 7 years after surgery.

***Author's Preferred Treatment.*** All children with Down syndrome, even those with normal flexion-extension lateral radiographs, should avoid collision sports (boxing, football, wrestling). This seems prudent in view of the known underlying ligamentous laxity and potential for development of cervical instability. Also, all children with Down syndrome should avoid any sports or activities that do or potentially may stress the cervical spine (e.g., boxing, football, wrestling, ice hockey, basketball, diving, and gymnastics). Certainly any child with progressive instability, although he or she is neurologically intact, should also not participate in any activities that have the potential to stress the cervical spine. These children should also be followed up closely from a clinical perspective to watch for the development of any neurologic signs or symptoms. Children with neurologic signs or symptoms and cervical instability should undergo arthrodesis, usually posterior. Most instabilities are corrected with simple positioning. Internal fixation is advised except for sublaminar wires at C2. If instability is present and does not reduce as seen on routine films taken in the extension position, the patient is at high risk for developing iatrogenic quadriplegia if sublaminar wiring and acute manipulative reduction were tried. Preoperative traction should be used in such a situation to effect reduction. If reduction does not occur, then only an onlay bone grafting should be performed without internal fixation. The high complication rate associated with these procedures should be remembered and parents should be counseled accordingly.

### Marfan Syndrome

Marfan syndrome affects ligamentous laxity and bone morphology. It is caused by a mutation in the glycoprotein fibrillin, which has been mapped to the long arm of chromosome 15. Abnormalities regarding the cervical spine in this syndrome have only recently been described (209,210). These are primarily abnormalities that are noted on radiographs. Focal cervical kyphosis involving at least three consecutive vertebrae occurs in 16% of patients with Marfan syndrome, with an average kyphosis of 22 degrees. The normal cervical lordosis is absent in 35% of patients. Atlantoaxial hypermobility is common, occurring in approximately 54% of patients. There is also an increased incidence of basilar impression (36%) seen on radiographs.

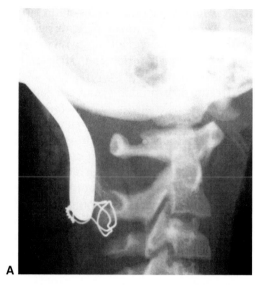

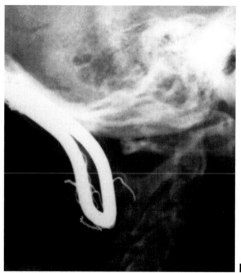

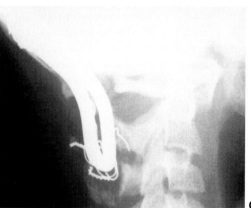

**Figure 22.19 A:** The child in Figure 22.3 underwent posterior cervical fusion from the occiput to C2 with internal fixation and autogenous iliac crest bone graft. **B,C:** Halo-vest immobilization was maintained for 4 months postoperatively and was followed by a Philadelphia collar. Despite this postoperative treatment, the boy progressed to a nonunion, evidenced by graft resorption, wire breakage, and subsidence of the Luque rectangle, although flexion and extension radiographs 1.5 years postoperatively showed a marked decrease in hypermobility. The atlantooccipital distance was 4 mm, with only a 1-mm change in the atlanto-dens interval; the space available for the cord measured 18 mm in flexion and 19 mm in extension. The child's neurologic symptoms also disappeared.

Unlike in Down syndrome, there is no increased incidence of cervical skeletal anomalies such as persistent synchondrosis and spina bifida occulta of C1. In spite of the abnormalities seen in patients with Marfan syndrome, symptoms and neurologic compromise are rare. The incidence of neck pain is not greater than that in the general population. Patients with Marfan syndrome should be advised to avoid sports with high-impact loading on the cervical spine; it does not appear necessary to routinely perform cervical spine radiographs for those undergoing general anesthesia. Atlantoaxial rotatory subluxation may be increased in those with Marfan syndrome, and this should be specially noted during surgical positioning.

### Nontraumatic Occipitoatlantal Instability

Nontraumatic occipitoatlantal instability is rare in the absence of any underlying syndrome (e.g., Down syndrome). Georgopoulos et al. (211) have described pediatric nontraumatic atlantooccipital instability. Congenital enlargement of the occipital condyles may have caused this instability by increasing motion at this joint. The presenting symptoms were severe vertigo in one 14-year-old boy and nausea with projectile vomiting in one 6-year-old girl.

These symptoms are postulated to be a result of vertebrobasilar arterial insufficiency resulting from the hypermobility at the occiput-C1 junction. The diagnosis of instability was suggested by plain radiographs initially and confirmed by cineradiography. Both children were treated with a posterior occiput-C1 fusion, and the symptoms resolved.

### Cerebral Palsy

Cervical radiculopathy and myelopathy in cerebral palsy (212–215) were first described in the athetoid types and subsequently in the spastic types. Patients with athetoid cerebral palsy develop cervical disc degeneration at a younger age than the general population. This degeneration progresses more rapidly and involves more levels than would normally be expected. Angular and listhetic instabilities also are more frequent and appear at a younger age (216). The combination of disc degeneration and listhetic instability predisposes these patients to a relatively rapid, progressive neurologic deficit.

The symptoms are brachialgia and weakness of the upper extremity with decreased functional use or increased paraparesis or tetraparesis (213–215). In ambulatory patients, a loss of ambulatory ability is often seen on presentation. Occasional loss of bowel and bladder control also occurs. Atlantoaxial instability has been recently described in patients with severe spastic quadriplegia; the symptoms are usually apnea, opisthotonos, torticollis, respiratory problems, muscle tone abnormalities and hyperreflexia, and bradycardia (217).

Radiographic findings (Fig. 22.20) include narrowing of the spinal canal and premature development of cervical spondylosis; malalignment of the cervical spine with localized kyphosis, increased lordosis, or both; and instability of the cervical spine manifested as spondylolisthesis. Flattening of the anterosuperior margins of the vertebral bodies and beaklike projections of the anteroinferior margins are radiographic findings relating to the spondylosis. Myelography demonstrates stenosis, disc protrusion, osteophyte projection, and blocks in dye flow, most commonly at the C3-C4 and C4-C5 levels.

The kyphosis, herniated discs, and osteophytes result in nerve root and cord compression. It is believed that the exaggerated flexion and extension of the neck in these young adults with cerebral palsy causes accelerated cervical degeneration and cervical stenosis earlier than in people who do not have cerebral palsy, who develop stenosis in

the late fourth and fifth decades of life. Exaggerated flexion and extension occur in patients with athetosis and writhing movements. Difficulty with head control also can cause exaggerated flexion and extension in patients with spastic cerebral palsy.

Treatment is primarily surgical. Anterior discectomy, resection of osteophytes, and interbody fusion have been the most effective methods. A halo cast is best and is well tolerated in some patients with athetosis (214). However, postoperative immobilization can be a problem for some other patients, thus some surgeons recommend a posterior wiring of the facets as well in order to minimize the duration of postoperative immobilization (213). Posterior laminectomy when performed alone (214) is contraindicated in patients with cerebral palsy with developmental cervical stenosis because this will increase the instability. Long-term follow-up of surgically treated patients demonstrates late disc degeneration and increased range of motion at adjacent segments in those who underwent anterior arthrodesis (219).

### Postlaminectomy Deformity

Cervical kyphosis is common after cervical laminectomy in children (220–226). This phenomenon is more likely in

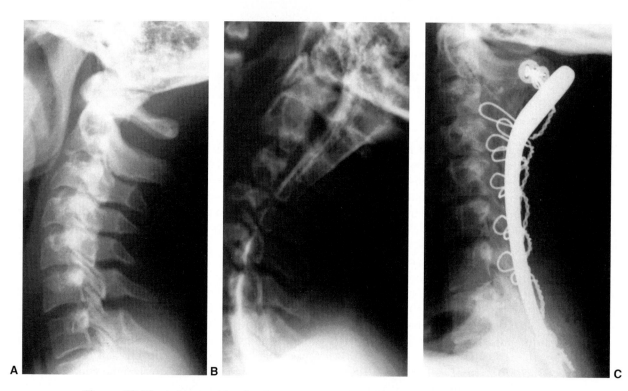

**A**    **B**    **C**

**Figure 22.20** A 14-year-old girl with spastic quadriparesis showed progressive loss of upper-extremity function with loss of ability to control her wheelchair and feed herself. She also complained of some mild neck pain. **A:** The lateral radiograph shows marked stenosis from C3 to C6, as evidenced by a spinal canal-to-vertebral body ratio (Torg ratio) of less than 0.8. **B:** The myelogram shows near complete block of the dye column from C3 to C5. This stenosis was treated with posterior laminectomy from C3 to C7 and posterior cervical fusion from C2 to T1 using Luque rectangle fixation with spinous process and facet wiring. **C:** Eight months postoperatively, there is stable fixation and solid facet joint fusion. The girl's upper-extremity strength is improved, and she is able to feed herself. [From Loder RT, Hensinger RN. Developmental abnormalities of the cervical spine. In: Weinstein SL, ed. *The pediatric spine: principles and practice* New York: Raven Press, 1994, with permission (218).]

immature, growing children. It has been duplicated in animal models; a C3-C6 laminectomy in growing cats uniformly resulted in kyphosis, whereas normal cervical curves were maintained in adult cats (227). The natural history of postlaminectomy kyphosis is unknown; however, the incidence of kyphosis when extensive cervical laminectomies are performed in childhood varies from 33% to 100%, with an overall average of 70% (225). Postlaminectomy kyphosis is weakly correlated with age (mean age at laminectomy, 10.5 years) and is not dependent upon the total number of levels decompressed or the location of these levels (225). Postlaminectomy lordosis is less common and is strongly correlated with a peak age at decompression of 4 years (225). In one study, 12 of 15 children who had undergone a cervical or cervicothoracic laminectomy prior to 15 years of age developed kyphosis (224). The normal posterior muscular attachments to the spinous processes and laminae, as well as facet capsules, the ligamentum nuchae, and the ligamentum flavum, are violated by the laminectomy. This loss of posterior supporting structures allows for a progressive deformity, which, if kyphotic in nature, can eventually result in neurologic symptoms and deficits. Early radiographic features show a simple kyphosis; later, vertebral body wedging and anterior translations of one vertebral body on another can develop. A late, severe deformity is the swan neck deformity (223). Neurologic problems result from cord stretch and compression from the anterior kyphotic vertebral bodies. MRI is useful in delineating the extent of cord attenuation and compression.

After a laminectomy, nonsurgical treatment starts with frequent radiographic follow-up studies; the role of prophylactic bracing is not yet known. When kyphotic deformities develop, anterior vertebral body fusion, followed by immobilization with a Minerva cast or halo cast or vest, is recommended (222) (Figs. 22.21 and 22.22). The role of a prophylactic posterior fusion at the time of laminectomy is not yet known (220), nor is the role of osteoplastic laminotomy instead of laminectomy (228), although this approach might not always be suitable in the context of the primary pathology.

## Other Syndromes

### Fetal Alcohol Syndrome

Central nervous system dysfunctions, growth deficiencies, facial anomalies, and variable major and minor malformations are the characteristics of fetal alcohol syndrome. The children present with developmental delay, especially in motor milestones, failure to thrive, mild to moderate retardation, mild microcephaly, distinct facies (hypoplasia of the facial bones and circumoral tissues), and congenital cardiovascular anomalies. The cervical findings are similar to those in Klippel-Feil syndrome. Radiography reveals congenital fusion of two or more cervical vertebrae, resembling Klippel-Feil syndrome, in approximately half of the children (229). The major visceral anomaly in fetal alcohol syndrome occurs in the cardiovascular system, whereas in Klippel-Feil syndrome the major anomaly is in the genitourinary system (229).

The natural history is not known. Radiographic imaging and treatment recommendations regarding the cervical spine are the same as those for Klippel-Feil syndrome.

### Craniofacial Syndromes

Cleft lip and/or palate is the most common craniofacial anomaly. It can be a solitary finding, but more often it is associated with other syndromes and anomalies. Children with cleft palate anomalies have a 13% to 18% incidence of cervical spinal anomalies compared with the 0.8% incidence in children undergoing orthodontia care for other reasons (230,231). This incidence is highest in patients with soft palate and submucous clefts (45%). These anomalies, usually spina bifida and vertebral body hypoplasia, are predominantly in the upper cervical spine. The potential for instability is unknown, as is the natural history. No documented information regarding treatment is available; however, the clinician should be aware of this association and make sound clinical judgments as needed. These patients also demonstrate a reduced cervical lordosis compared to those without cleft lip and/or palate (231).

### Craniosynostosis Syndromes

The craniosynostosis syndromes—Crouzon, Pfeiffer, Apert, Goldenhar, and Saethre-Chotzen—exhibit cervical spine fusions, atlantooccipital fusions, and butterfly vertebrae (232–237). Fusions are more common in Apert syndrome (71%) than in Crouzon syndrome (38%) (232). Upper cervical fusions are most common in Crouzon and Pfeiffer syndromes (234), whereas in Apert syndrome the fusions are more likely to be complex and involve C5 and C6 (232). However, this syndrome variation is not accurate enough for syndromic differentiation. Congenital cervicothoracic scoliosis with rib fusions is seen in Goldenhar syndrome, usually from hemivertebrae (234,238). C1-C2 instability in Goldenhar syndrome may be as high as 33%, and these children should be monitored carefully for this potential problem (239).

The cervical fusions are progressive with age; in younger children the vertebrae appear to be separated by intervertebral discs, but as the children grow older the vertebrae fuse. There are no specific, standard recommendations for treatment. The author recommends following the same principles as for Klippel-Feil syndrome. The main concern is the potential difficulty with intubation in these children. Odontoid anomalies are rare; however, if any question exists regarding the stability of the cervical spine, lateral flexion and extension radiographs should be obtained. Children with Goldenhar syndrome have a high incidence of C1-C2 instability (240). There a high incidence of diabetes among the mothers of children with Goldenhar syndrome; it has recently been suggested that children with

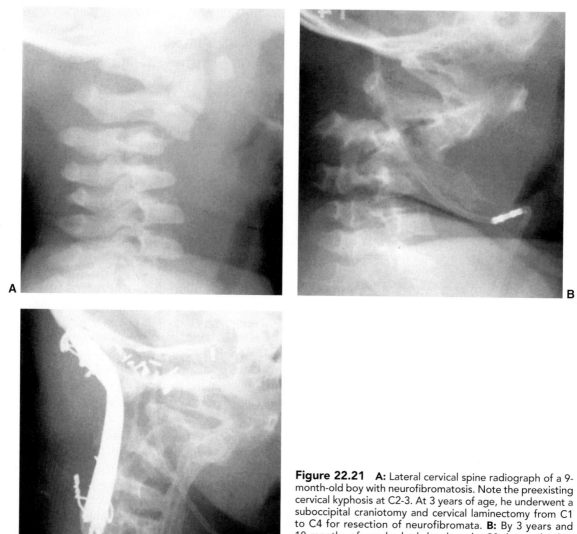

**Figure 22.21  A:** Lateral cervical spine radiograph of a 9-month-old boy with neurofibromatosis. Note the preexisting cervical kyphosis at C2-3. At 3 years of age, he underwent a suboccipital craniotomy and cervical laminectomy from C1 to C4 for resection of neurofibromata. **B:** By 3 years and 10 months of age he had developed a 90-degree kyphosis. **C:** He underwent combined anterior cervical fusion from C2 to C6 with a fibular strut graft and posterior cervical fusion from the occiput to C6 with internal fixation consisting of a Luque U-rod. Three years postoperatively, solid fusion with a residual 70-degree kyphosis is present.

Goldenhar syndrome should be assessed for maternal diabetes exposure, which should aid in counseling concerning cause and risk of recurrence (239).

### Skeletal Dysplasias

Skeletal dysplasias are discussed in detail in Chapter 8.

### Combined Soft Tissue and Skeletal Dysplasias

**Neurofibromatosis.** Neurofibromatosis is the most common single-gene disorder in humans. The proportion of patients with neurofibromatosis and cervical spine involvement is difficult to assess: 30% of neurofibromatosis patients in the series of Yong-Hing et al. (241) and 44% with neurofibromatosis and scoliosis or kyphosis had cervical spine lesions. The cervical lesions are often asymptomatic (241). Symptoms, when they do occur, include diminished or painful neck motion, torticollis, dysphagia, deformity,

and neurologic signs ranging from mild pain and weakness to paraparesis and quadriparesis (57,242). Neck masses constituted 20% of presenting symptoms in one study of patients with neurofibromatosis (243).

Radiographic features of neurofibromatosis in the cervical spine are vertebral body deficiencies and dysplasia or scalloping (241). This condition is often associated with kyphosis and foraminal enlargement (244). Lateral flexion and extension radiographs are recommended for all patients with neurofibromatosis before general anesthesia or surgery (241). MRI is helpful in assessing the involvement of neural structures and dural ectasia. CT scan is useful in evaluating the upper cervical spine complex and the bony definition of the neural foramen. The natural history regarding the cervical spine in patients with this condition is unknown, but those with severe kyphosis often develop neurologic deterioration.

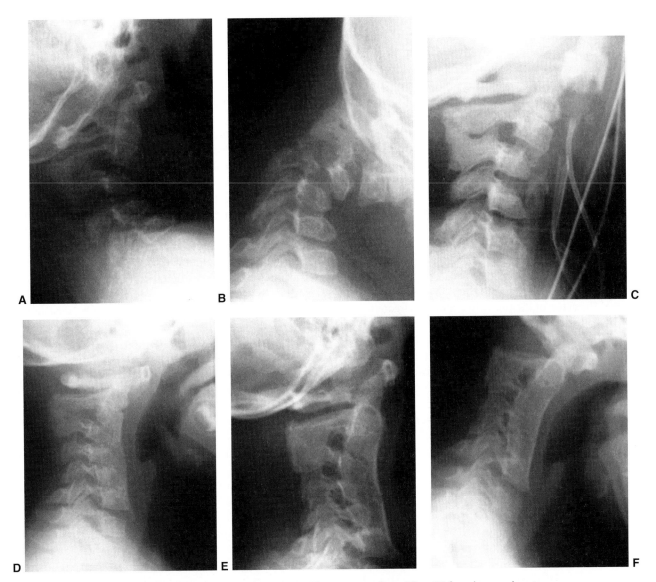

**Figure 22.22**  This girl underwent a cervical laminectomy from C2 to C6 for a low-grade astrocytoma of the cervical cord. At 1 year and 7 months of age, she had a postlaminectomy kyphosis that was 45 degrees in extension **(A)** and 82 degrees in flexion **(B)**. **C:** An anterior cervical discectomy and fusion from C2 to C6 was performed with autogenous iliac crest strut graft. Immediately after surgery, the kyphosis was corrected to 20 degrees. Halo-vest immobilization was used for 3 months. **D:** Solid incorporation of the fusion occurred by 6 months postoperatively. At 4 years and 7 months of age, flexion **(E)** and extension **(F)** lateral radiographs show maintenance of the correction, solid fusion, and no instability at the remaining levels.

Indications for surgery are cord or nerve root compression, C1–C2 rotary subluxation, pain, and neurofibroma removal (241,242). Laminectomy alone without accompanying arthrodesis is contraindicated (245). Fusion, with or without internal fixation, is usually achieved with simple interspinous wiring; a halo cast or vest is usually needed after surgery. Kyphosis requires both anterior and posterior fusion (Fig. 22.21). Pseudarthroses are frequent with isolated posterior fusions. Vascularized fibular grafts may be necessary to effect fusion in difficult cases (244,246). If there are no indications for surgical treatment, the patient should be followed up closely.

*Fibrodysplasia Ossificans Progressiva.*  Fibrodysplasia ossificans progressiva is an inheritable, autosomal dominant disorder (247) of connective tissue with progressive soft tissue ossification. The disorder itself is rare; most cases represent new spontaneous mutations. Eventually all patients with this disorder develop cervical spine changes (248), often starting in childhood. These patients usually present with neck stiffness (249) within the first 5 years of life. No cases of neurologic compromise have been reported. Other general clinical features are big toe malformations, reduction defects of all digits, deafness, baldness, and mental retardation. Early in the course of the disease small vertebral bodies and large pedicles are seen radiographically. Occasionally nuchal musculature ossification is also seen. Later, neural arch fusions are seen. This factor reflects the progressive ossification of the cervical spinal musculature, ligament ossification, and spontaneous fusion of the cervical discs and apophyseal joints. No effective medical treatment is known. Surgical treatment of the cervical spine is not necessary.

# TRAUMA

Injuries to the cervical spine are rare in children and occur more in boys than in girls. In one study, the age- and gender-adjusted incidence in the general population was 7.41 per 100,000 per year (250); this incidence was much less in children younger than 11 years, 1.19 per 100,000, than in adolescents (older than 11 years, 13.24 per 100,000). The cause of the injury in children is frequently a fall, whereas in adolescents it is frequently related to sports, recreational activities, or motor vehicle crashes. Children involved in side impact crashes are more likely to have cervical spine injuries than those involved in frontal crashes (251). Unrestrained children are more likely to sustain cervical spine injuries in motor vehicle crashes than restrained children (252,253). In general, children (younger than 11 years of age) are more likely to sustain ligamentous injuries and injuries to the upper cervical spine, whereas adolescents are more likely to sustain fractures and injuries to the lower cervical spine (250). In a large series of 1098 children with cervical spine injury, upper spine injuries occurred in 52%, lower cervical spine injuries in 28%, and both upper and lower injuries in 7% (254). Upper cervical spine injuries carry a significantly higher mortality than do lower cervical spine injuries (254). By the age of 10 years the bony cervical spine has reached adult configurations, and the injuries sustained are essentially those of the adult. Therefore, this chapter will concentrate on injuries sustained in the first decade of life.

Most children with potential cervical spine injuries have sustained polytrauma and frequently arrive immobilized on backboards and wearing cervical collars. If the child is comatose or semiconscious, if there are external signs of head injury, or if the child complains of neck pain, cervical spine radiographs are needed. All children involved in motor vehicle crashes who have head trauma and neck pain, or who have neurologic signs or symptoms, should have cervical spine radiographs (255,256). The views recommended for this initial screening are the cross-table lateral and anteroposterior views. The need for an open-mouth odontoid is controversial, especially in children less than 5 years of age (257,258). If the child is too critically ill to be positioned for all views, then the cross-table lateral view is adequate until a complete evaluation can be performed. Cervical spine precautions must be maintained until a complete evaluation has demonstrated no injury. Once a cervical injury has been identified, close scrutiny

must be undertaken to ensure that there are no other injuries in the remainder of the axial skeleton.

The child arriving in the emergency suite is often on a standard backboard. Young children have a disproportionately large head, and positioning them on a standard backboard leads to a flexed posture of the neck (Fig. 22.23A) (259). This flexion can lead to further anterior angulation or translation of an unstable cervical spine injury and can also cause pseudosubluxation, which in itself in an injured child can be difficult to interpret. To prevent this undesirable cervical flexion in young children during emergency transport and radiography, modifications must be made by either creating a recess for the occiput of the larger head or using a double mattress to raise the chest (Fig. 22.23B). A simple clinical guideline is to align the external auditory meatus with the shoulder.

Flexion and extension lateral radiographs may be necessary in order to determine the stability of the cervical spine; hyperflexion ligamentous injuries may not be seen immediately, and flexion and extension views a few weeks later, after the spasm has subsided, may document instability. In one series of children with ligamentous injuries of the cervical spine, 8 of 11 children with lower cervical instability were diagnosed between 2 weeks and 4 months after the trauma (260).

Secondary signs of spinal injury in children are often seen before the actual injury or fracture itself. Malalignment of the spinous processes on the anteroposterior radiograph should be regarded as highly indicative of a jumped facet joint. Widening of the posterior interspinous distances should be regarded as highly indicative of a posterior ligamentous injury. In adults, an increase in the retropharyngeal soft tissue space can indicate a hematoma in the setting of trauma, and raise the suspicion that an upper cervical fracture exists. In children, however, the pharyngeal wall is close to the spine in inspiration, whereas there may be a large increase in this space with forced expiration, as when the child cries (261). This should be remembered

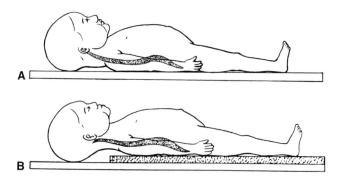

**Figure 22.23** **A:** Positioning a young child on a standard backboard forces the neck into a kyphotic position because of the relatively large head. **B:** Positioning a young child on a double mattress, which raises the chest and torso and allows the head to translate posteriorly, creates a normal alignment of the cervical spine. (From Herzenberg JE, Hensinger RN, Dedrick DK, et al. Emergency transport and positioning of young children who have an injury of the cervical spine. *J Bone Joint Surg Am* 1989;71-A:15–22, with permission.)

when considering the significance of prevertebral pharyngeal soft tissue in the cervical spine radiographs of a frightened, crying child.

CT scan is useful for further assessing the upper cervical spine, especially the ring of the atlas and, occasionally, the odontoid. As a rule, CT scan is not recommended for screening but only in order to further study suspicious areas on plain radiographs or in planning treatment. It should be used for studying all fractures of C1. MRIs are useful in assessing the spinal cord and discs. In an injured child, an MRI is the method of choice for assessing the cervical spine when (a) the child is obtunded and/or nonverbal, and a cervical spine injury is suspected; (b) the plain radiograph findings are equivocal; (c) neurologic symptoms are present without radiographic findings; or (d) there is inability to clear the cervical spine in a timely manner (262).

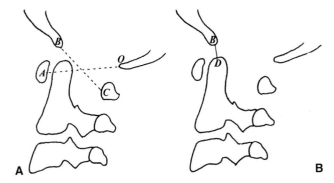

**Figure 22.24** The *BC:OA* ratio (Powers ratio) **(A)** and the *DB* distance **(B)** are used for assessing traumatic atlantooccipital dislocation. A ratio greater than 1.0 and a DB distance greater than 12.5 mm indicates the potential for atlantooccipital dislocation. (From Bulas DI, Fitz CR, Johnson DL. Traumatic atlanto-occipital dislocation in children. *Radiology* 1993;188:155–158, with permission.)

## Fractures and Ligamentous Injuries of the Occipital Complex to the C1-C2 Complex

### Atlantooccipital Dislocation

Atlantooccipital dislocation is rare (263), and most children do not survive it (264). Deployment of air bags has recently been associated with this injury in children (265–268). With the present rapid response to trauma victims and aggressive field care, more of these children now survive. These children are usually polytrauma victims with severe head injuries, and they present with a range of clinical neurologic pictures (263,264). In the past, those who survived had incomplete lesions, often demonstrating cranial nerve dysfunctions and varying degrees of quadriplegia. Many of the children who presently survive have complete loss of neurologic function below the brain stem and live only because of outpatient ventilatory support. Other presentations may range from a responsive child with hypotension or tachycardia to a patient in complete cardiac arrest. Occasionally, some patients present with normal findings on neurologic examination. As of 2001, there were 29 children with atlantooccipital dislocation who survived (269).

In severe cases the diagnosis is evident; however, some of the cases do not demonstrate marked radiographic displacement. In the past, a Powers ratio of greater than 1.0 (Fig. 22.24A) was used as an indication of the presence of atlantooccipital dislocation (270). This criterion can cause the practitioner to miss isolated distraction injuries, anterior atlantooccipital dislocations that have spontaneously reduced after injury, and posterior atlantooccipital injuries (263). For this reason, the distance between the tip of the dens and the basion (Fig. 22.24B) has been used as a sign, in which a distance of more than 12.5 mm indicates the potential for atlantooccipital dislocation. Recent studies have described the stabilizing nature of the tectorial membrane. When this membrane is disrupted, there is a high likelihood of atlantooccipital instability. If the C1-C2 to C2-C3 posterior interspinous ratio is greater than 2.5, there

is a high chance of tectorial membrane disruption, and MRI evaluation is warranted (271).

The first obstacle in the treatment of this injury is its diagnosis. If the suspicion of craniocervical trauma persists after inconclusive plain radiography, CT or MRI scans can be quite useful (Fig. 22.25). Subarachnoid hemorrhage at the craniocervical junction will be seen after atlantooccipital dislocation (272); a CT scan can also assist in assessing osseous alignment (273). Once diagnosed, standard respiratory and other supporting measures are given. Early definitive immobilization of the dislocation should be undertaken. The immobilization can be with a halo cast alone or with supplemental internal fixation and posterior fusion (272,274). Traction should be avoided because it can distract the joint and cause further neurologic injury (275). These children must be moved rapidly into an upright position in order to maximize pulmonary care. Late neurologic deterioration may indicate progressive hydrocephalus or retropharyngeal pseudomeningocele (276).

### Fractures of the Atlas

The Jefferson fracture is rare in children (277–279). It is caused by an axial load from the head into the lateral masses. Unlike in adults, a single fracture through the ring in children may be isolated, hinging on the synchondrosis (278,280) instead of a double break in the ring. Alternatively, a bifocal posterior arch fracture can occur—a Jefferson fracture variant (281). A transverse atlantal ligament rupture may occur as the lateral masses separate, resulting in C1-C2 instability.

CT scans are useful in both the diagnosis of this injury and the assessment of healing. This injury in children is not commonly seen on plain radiographs, which usually show only an asymmetry between the odontoid and the lateral masses. Even if it is clearly seen on plain radiographs, a CT scan should also be performed to confirm the diagnosis and to rule out a transverse alar ligament rupture. Treatment is usually simple immobilization with

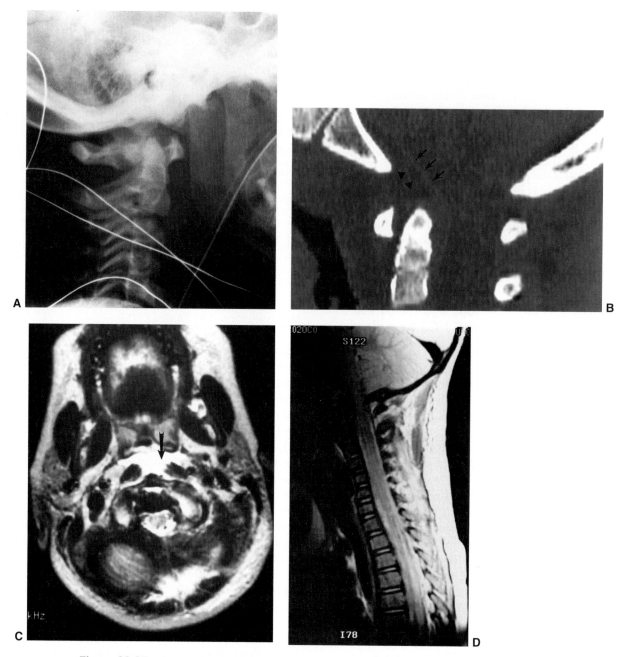

**Figure 22.25** This girl, 5 years and 6 months of age, was hit by a van from behind, and presented with bilateral palsies of the cranial nerve VI. **A:** The lateral radiograph of the upper cervical spine demonstrates a rotational malalignment: the basion hemi-shadows fail to overlap while the C1 arches nearly superimpose upon each other, raising the possibility of atlantooccipital dislocation. **B:** A computed tomography (CT) scan with sagittal reconstruction demonstrates elevation of the periosteum at the caudal level of the clivus (*arrows*) and hemorrhage (*arrowheads*). **C:** An axial image from the magnetic resonance imaging (MRI) scan demonstrates abnormal fluid accumulation immediately anterior to the atlantooccipital junction (*arrow*). **D:** The MRI scan sagittal view demonstrates subarachnoid space narrowing at the level of the foramen magnum and atlantooccipital joint.

a Minerva or halo cast. Rarely is surgery necessary unless rupture of the transverse alar ligament occurs, rendering the spine unstable. The timing of surgery needs to be individualized.

### Transverse Atlantoaxial Ligament Ruptures

Transverse atlantoaxial ligament ruptures may result from either severe or mild trauma (260). As seen on radiographs,

the ADI is increased, usually well beyond the normal 5 mm. Adequate ligamentous healing and stability are not achieved by simple immobilization. The recommended treatment is reduction in extension, posterior cervical C1-C2 fusion with autogenous bone graft, and immobilization with a halo or Minerva cast. A solid arthrodesis is documented on flexion and extension lateral radiographs after 2 to 3 months of immobilization. If the ligament is avulsed from the lateral masses of C1 and the bony avulsion attached to the ligament is close to the lateral mass, simple immobilization may be adequate (282).

### Odontoid Fractures

Odontoid fractures are a common pediatric cervical spine injury (283). They are usually physeal fractures of the dentocentral synchondrosis, usually Salter-Harris type I fractures. These may occur after major or minor trauma. Neurologic deficits are rare. These fractures usually displace anteriorly with the dens posteriorly angulated (Fig. 22.26). This fracture is usually seen only on the lateral view. If it is difficult to tell from the radiographs whether there is a fracture or merely a mild, normal, posterior angulation of the dens [which occurs in up to 4% of normal children (284)], dynamic flexion and extension CT scans with sagittal reconstructions can be performed to evaluate for any motion or instability.

Displaced odontoid fractures in children reduce easily with mild extension and posterior translation. In most circumstances the simple double mattress technique is all that is needed to obtain a reduction. After a few days of recumbence and early healing, the fracture can be immobilized easily with the use of a Minerva or halo cast. As with all physeal fractures, healing is rapid, and immobilization can usually be discontinued in 6 to 10 weeks. Flexion and extension lateral radiographs should be taken to confirm union with stability. These fractures, unlike those in adults, do not have a significant nonunion rate requiring subsequent C1-C2 fusion. The intact hinge of anterior periosteum most likely aids in the ease of reduction and accounts for the stability of reduction and rapid healing.

### Spondylolisthesis of C2

Spondylolisthesis of C2, also known as *hangman fracture* in adults, is rare in children. It most likely arises from hyperextension. Pizzutillo et al. (285) reported on a series of five cases in children. Care must be taken to not confuse this fracture with congenital anomalies that may mimic a hangman fracture and lead to overtreatment (286–289). Similarly, it may be caused by child abuse (290). These fractures readily heal with immobilization in either a Minerva or halo cast after gentle positioning to obtain a reduction. Traction by itself, as with most cervical injuries in children, should be avoided because it overdistracts the spine and is associated with an increased potential for nonunion and more serious neurologic injury. Posterior cervical fusion of C1-C3 is indicated for the rare case of nonunion or instability.

## Fractures and Ligamentous Injuries of C3-C7

These injuries are more common in older children and adolescents than in young children (250,291). The typical patterns of fracture are usually compression fractures of the vertebral body, or facet fractures and dislocations caused

by hyperflexion. These injuries are adult in pattern, and standard adult treatment should be used. Physeal fractures, usually of the inferior end plates, also can occur (292) because of hyperextension. In older children they are usually ring apophyseal fractures with minimal instability or neurologic damage. In younger children they usually involve the entire end plate. Physeal fractures are frequently not recognized in severely injured children, and they may be noted for the first time at autopsy (292). These fractures are associated with a high incidence of neurologic injury (Fig. 22.27). In these children, simple positioning (e.g., double mattresses or, rarely, traction) followed by immobilization is all that is needed for treatment. Because these are physeal injuries, healing is rapid.

Traumatic ligamentous instability may also occur in children (260). The pivot point for younger children is in the upper cervical spine because of the large size of the head, weak cervical musculature, incompletely ossified wedge-shaped vertebrae, physiologic ligamentous laxity, and horizontal facet joints in this region. The upper cervical spine offers little resistance to traumatic shear forces, which often result in ligamentous instability. The goal is to differentiate this traumatic ligamentous instability from pseudosubluxation using the posterior cervical line.

Traumatic subluxation of the axis is a recently described true ligamentous instability at C2-C3, and not pseudosubluxation. Most of the children with this condition sustained an injury with the head and neck in flexion, usually caused by falls or sports injuries (260,293). The patients complain of severe neck pain. Immediately after injury the instability may not be radiographically apparent, and becomes noticeable only after progressive kyphosis is noted. In younger children, avulsion of the cartilaginous tips of the C2 spinous process is not visible on plain radiographs or CT scan. Later on, the avulsion fragments become ossified. This late ossification, along with the development of C2-C3 kyphosis, leads to the diagnosis. In one study of ligamentous injuries of the cervical spine in children, 7 of 11 injuries occurred at the C2-C3 level. Treatment must be individualized; both simple immobilization and posterior cervical arthrodesis have been used with good results. When instability exists, treatment should consist of posterior cervical fusion with Minerva or halo immobilization (Fig. 22.28). However, children who have undergone arthrodesis for cervical spine injury do demonstrate decreased mobility and increased osteoarthritis at long-term follow-up (294). Treatment for a mild sprain is immobilization for comfort followed by flexion and extension radiographs several weeks to a few months later to ensure that late instability does not occur.

## Transient Quadriparesis

Transient quadriparesis is a neuropraxia of the cervical cord with transient quadriplegia. It is seen most often in collegiate and professional athletes (295,296), although there are several instances among younger athletes also

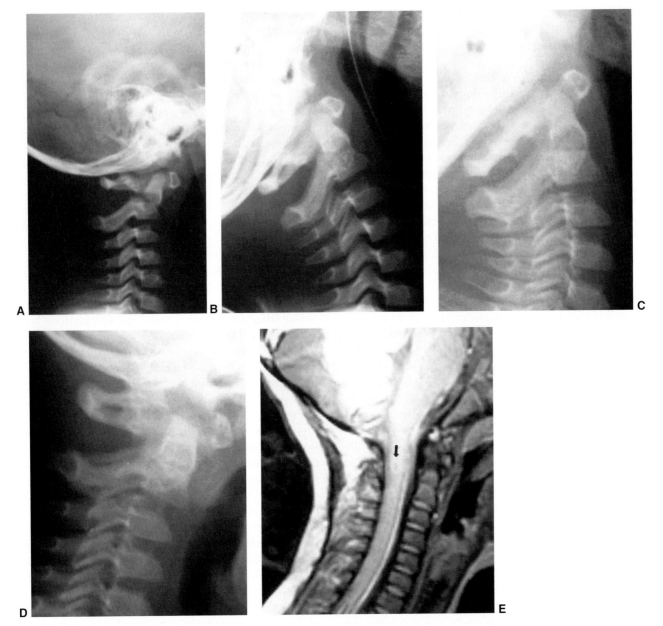

**Figure 22.26** This boy, 2 years and 9 months of age, was brought to the emergency department unable to move his upper extremities, and withdrew his lower extremities only in response to noxious stimuli. He had a reported history of falling off couches. On investigation, it became clear that the child had been battered. **A:** A lateral radiograph demonstrates the odontoid fracture through the dentocentral synchondrosis with anterior angulation and translation. A magnetic resonance imaging (MRI) scan did not reveal any abnormalities in the cord. **B:** Simple positioning with a double mattress allowed for reduction of the fracture; the child was maintained on a double mattress for several days to allow for subsidence of cord edema and early healing. He was then placed into a Minerva cast 10 days after the injury. The cast was removed 6 weeks after the injury, followed by immobilization with a soft collar. Flexion **(C)** and extension **(D)** radiographs demonstrated no instability with the healed fracture. **E:** The child improved remarkably. Two months after the injury he was running and walking without difficulty. There were some subtle upper-extremity changes, indicated by a change in hand dominance from right to left. MRIs showed signal changes in the cord (*arrow*), which were interpreted as development of an early posttraumatic syrinx.

(297). The incidence in the National Collegiate Athletic Association is 1.3 per 10,000 athletes per season (296).

The anteroposterior diameter of the spinal canal is decreased in the athletes with transient quadriparesis. The spinal cord is compressed on forced hyperextension or hyperflexion, causing the transient quadriparesis. Sensory changes such as burning pain, numbness, tingling, and loss of sensation and motor changes ranging from weakness to complete paralysis are seen. These episodes are transient, and recovery occurs in 10 to 15 minutes; neck pain is

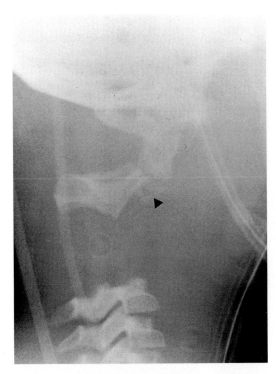

**Figure 22.27** This girl, 7 years and 2 months of age, sustained polytrauma and presented in an agonal state. A lateral radiograph demonstrates complete separation at the C2-C3 level along with an associated C2 hangman fracture. Also note the small fleck of bone (*arrowhead*) attached to the base of the C2 body; this likely represents an avulsion of the superior aspect of the body of C3 with the C2-C3 disc.

not present at the time of injury. Transient quadriparesis needs to be differentiated from a brachial plexus stretch, or "burner." Patients with the latter condition present with a monoparesis of the upper extremity and often with neck pain.

No fractures or dislocations are present. The ratio of the spinal canal to the vertebral body is decreased; a value of 0.8 for this ratio indicates significant developmental cervical stenosis. Congenital fusions, cervical instability, and intervertebral disc disease may also exist. In children, this spinal canal-to-vertebral body ratio is not as accurate, and is inconsistent in predicting spinal cord concussion (297). An MRI may be necessary in order to assess the presence or absence of a herniated nucleus pulposus.

The resolution of symptoms is universal. The only nonsurgical treatments that are needed are collars, analgesics, and antispasmodics. The efficacy of fusions for coexisting instability, discectomy for herniated nucleus pulposus, and decompression for congenital cervical stenosis is not known.

The major concern is whether the patient should continue to participate in athletic activities, and if he or she were to do so, what would be the risk of a permanent quadriplegia developing with a later episode. Torg et al. (298) believe that athletes with pure developmental spinal stenosis are not predisposed to more severe injuries

if they return to sports and that only those with instability or degenerative changes should be precluded from participation in contact sports. Odor et al. (299) found that one third of professional and rookie football players have a spinal canal ratio of less than 0.8 and that it is difficult to make decisions about continuing with the sport on the basis of this ratio alone. Eismont et al. (300), however, have shown that smaller cervical canals are correlated with significant neurologic injury in routine trauma. Considering this finding, and the fact that narrowing of the spinal canal correlates even more closely with spinal cord concussion in children (297), it is prudent to keep any child who has had a cervical cord concussion from playing contact sports until further epidemiologic data have been established.

## Spinal Cord Injury without Radiographic Abnormality

Spinal cord injury without radiographic abnormality (SCIWORA) occurs in 5% to 55% of all pediatric spinal cord injuries according to the neurosurgical literature (301); however, multicenter databases in a recent spinal cord injury study suggest that the incidence is much less (302). By definition, no disruption, malalignment, or other abnormalities are seen on plain radiographs. The immature and elastic pediatric spine is more easily deformed than that of an adult. Momentary displacement caused by external forces endangers the spinal cord without disrupting bone or ligaments. The four major factors involved in such injuries are hyperextension, flexion, distraction, and spinal cord ischemia. Ischemia may arise from cord contusion or direct vascular insult (303). Spinal stenosis is not a factor; in a recent study of 145 children with cervical SCIWORA (304), the average Torg ratio was greater than 1.0.

The neurologic deficit may range from complete loss of spinal cord function to partial cord deficits. The physiologic disruption of the spinal cord is not necessarily associated with anatomic disruption. Most deficits (78%) are cervical; patients with upper cervical SCIWORA are more likely to have severe neurologic lesions than patients with lower cervical SCIWORA. An MRI is most useful for studying the cord and disc-ligament complexes, and it correlates well with clinical outcome (305). Positive MRI findings are typically seen only in children with very severe neurologic involvement at presentation (306). The outcome usually is determined by the presenting neurologic status. Approximately one fourth of these children have a secondary deterioration in neurologic function.

There is some controversy regarding the best treatment approach. Pang and Pollack recommend immobilization in a Guilford brace for 3 months and complete avoidance of all sports (301). However, in the same series, no instability was noted in any of the children at initial evaluation, and only one child later developed instability as seen on flexion and extension radiographs. Without

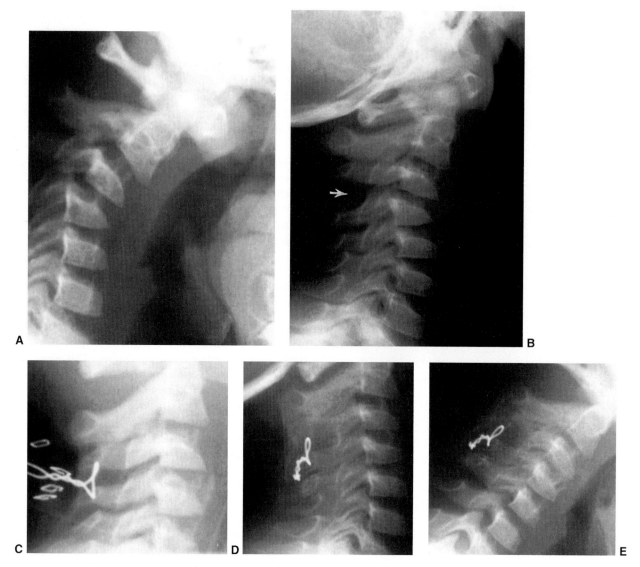

**Figure 22.28**   This boy, 4 years and 9 months of age, was run over by a snowmobile trailer 2 weeks before these radiographs were taken. He had complained of some neck pain and had been treated by chiropractic manipulation during these 2 weeks. The flexion **(A)** and extension **(B)** radiographs demonstrate marked instability at the C3-C4 interspace, which does not completely reduce, even with extension (*arrow*). **C:** He was treated by posterior fusion with iliac crest bone graft and interspinous wiring at C3-C4, as shown in this intraoperative radiograph. Halo-vest immobilization was used for 3 months. **D** and **E:** One year postoperatively, there was no instability at the C3-C4 level, but there was solid fusion, which had extended to C2 and C5, despite meticulous care not to expose the laminae of C2 and C5 or the interspinous ligaments of C2-C3 and C4-C5.

documented radiographic instability, the biomechanical usefulness of brace immobilization is questionable. Pang and Pollack, however, describe this as treatment for "incipient instability" (301). More recent studies question both the reality of the recurrence of a SCIWORA and the efficacy of bracing in the treatment of SCIWORA (304). Most ligamentous spine injuries, when allowed to heal with simple immobilization, do not return to the stability seen in the preinjury state; fusion is usually needed. It is atypical for SCIWORA to behave differently regarding instability, incipient or otherwise. Regardless of whether the child is braced, close follow-up of neurologic function is

needed. Flexion and extension radiographs should be taken after 3 months of bracing; any late development of instability requires surgical stabilization.

## Special Injury Mechanisms

### Birth Injuries and Battered Children
Birth trauma is a common cause of pediatric spinal cord injury and usually involves the cervical cord (307,308). Because of the increased incidence of cesarean section, the number of these cases is fortunately decreasing (309). As in SCIWORA, the vertebral column is more elastic than the

cord, and during delivery with prolonged distraction it may be tethered by nerve ends and blood vessels, injuring the cord but not the chondroosseous structures. Damage to the vertebral artery, with resultant ischemia of the cord, can also occur (310). In battered children, the large head, poorly supported by the cervical musculature, makes the upper cervical spine vulnerable to repeated shaking, leading to either SCIWORA or a fracture. In a recent Canadian study, the incidence of cervical spine injury is 4% of victims of shaken baby syndrome (311).

The diagnosis is difficult, especially with incomplete neurologic injury. Pure transection of the cord itself is rare (312). Temperature regulation dysfunction can cause fevers, reflex movements may be mistaken for voluntary movements, and respiratory distress can occur from paralyzed intercostal muscles. These patients may also present with symptoms that resemble a cerebral palsy–like picture (313) or sudden infant death syndrome (314). In one study, the diagnosis was delayed in three of four children, and the delay averaged 4.4 years from birth (315). Typically, no fractures are seen radiographically; MRI is often helpful in assessing cord damage. Anterior rupture of the lower cervical intervertebral discs is seen on pathologic examination in children who are victims of shaking (316).

Some children without complete transection can improve neurologically. Treatment is usually nonsurgical because these are very young infants. Bed rest, respiratory support, and physical therapy to prevent paralytic contractures should be instituted. Older children with bony injuries may need Minerva casts or halo immobilization. Surgical fusion with stabilization is rarely needed.

### Car Seat Injuries

Cervical fractures are being seen more often with the recent increase in the use of infant car seats (317–319). When these devices, which clearly make automobile travel safer for children, are not adequately tightened, serious and potentially fatal injuries can occur. The harness must be adjusted periodically to account for normal growth and seasonal changes in clothing thickness. Car seat styles that allow the main lock to be attached to the crotch strap (Fig. 22.29) prevent infants from sliding forward, which can apply hyperextension forces to the head, the neck, and the upper chest. Neurocentral synchondrosis separation between the body and the neural arches is a common pattern (318,320).

### Gunshot Wounds

Spinal injuries from gunshot wounds (321) have been on the increase; it has been reported that they account for one half of adolescent spinal cord injuries (322). One third of these injuries involve the cervical spine. Various degrees of neurologic loss are noted, with complete lesions in 75% of the patients in one series (321). Nonetheless, additional injuries to other body areas may cause more morbidity than the trauma to the neck.

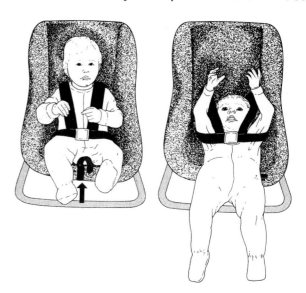

**Figure 22.29** A child in a car seat without locking the crotch strap (*arrow*) is in a dangerous situation that can allow serious injury in a collision. (From Conry BG, Hall CM. Cervical spine fractures and rear car seat restraints. *Arch Dis Child* 1987;62:1267–1268, with permission.)

In gunshot wounds to the neck, various degrees of fracture and intracanal bullets may be seen radiographically. Other imaging studies, such as arteriography and esophagography, are often needed in order to look for other injuries. Panendoscopy is useful for assessing injury to the trachea and esophagus. Spinal decompression is not indicated in either complete or incomplete lesions. For patients with complete injuries, removal of retained bullet fragments from the canal does not improve neurologic outcome. Patients who undergo decompression have a higher risk of meningitis and spinal instability, without any added benefit. Spinal instability is rare unless laminectomy is performed. Indications for neck exploration surgery are a positive arteriogram, impending airway obstruction, tracheal deviation, widened mediastinum, expanding hematoma, and appropriate pathology on panendoscopy. Routine exploration of the neck and wound is not advised.

## INFLAMMATORY AND SEPTIC CONDITIONS

### Juvenile Rheumatoid Arthritis

Juvenile rheumatoid arthritis is a chronic synovitis that can affect the joints of the cervical spine as well. The subtypes that usually involve the cervical spine are the polyarticular and systemic onset types; only rarely does the pauciarticular type affect the cervical spine (323).

Cervical spine involvement usually occurs in the first 1 to 2 years from disease onset and presents with stiffness. Pain and torticollis are rare, and when they occur in a patient with juvenile rheumatoid arthritis other causes should be explored, such as fracture, infection, and tumor.

Torticollis was present in only 4 of 92 children in the series of Fried et al. (324) and in 1 of 121 children in the series of Hensinger et al. (323). Abnormal neurologic findings are also infrequent in these children.

The radiographic features are classified into seven types (323):

1. Anterior erosion of the odontoid process
2. Anteroposterior erosion of the odontoid process (apple-core odontoid)
3. Subluxation of C1 on C2
4. Focal soft tissue calcification appearing adjacent to the ring of C1 anteriorly
5. Ankylosis of the apophyseal joints
6. Growth abnormalities
7. Subluxations between C2 and C7

The most common radiographic features in children with neck stiffness are soft tissue calcification at the leading edge of C1, anterior erosion of the odontoid process, and apophyseal joint ankylosis (Fig. 22.30). Although there may be mild hypermobility at C1-C2 with flexion

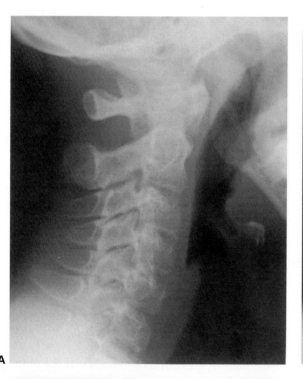

A

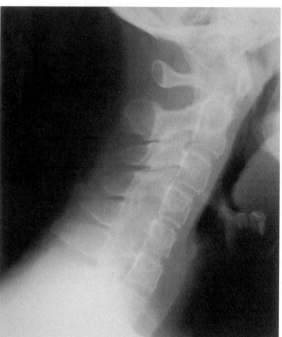

B

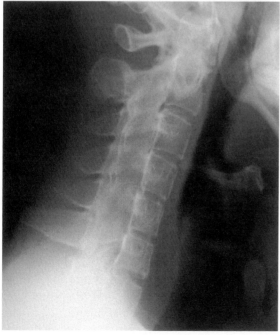

C

**Figure 22.30** Cervical spine radiographs of a boy with systemic onset juvenile rheumatoid arthritis. **A:** At 10 years of age, note the facet joint narrowing posteriorly from C2 to C6. **B:** At 17 years of age the facet joints from C3 to C6 have totally fused, with complete bony ankylosis. Also note the apple-core odontoid. **C:** By 21 years of age, there has been complete bony ankylosis between C2 and C3. The facet joint at C6-C7 is narrowed but not completely fused. Also note that the C4, C5, and C6 vertebral bodies are smaller in both height and depth.

and extension, true instability and myelopathy are rare. Basilar invagination, which often occurs in adult rheumatoid arthritis, also is rare in juvenile rheumatoid arthritis (324). The radiographic findings in juvenile rheumatoid arthritis that differ most from those in adult rheumatoid arthritis are late destruction of articular cartilage and bone, growth disturbances, spondylitis with associated vertebral subluxation and apophyseal joint ankylosis, and micrognathia (325,326). In five patients who had long-standing disease (average age, 19 years), Hallah et al. (327) described a nonreducible head tilt caused by collapse of an atlantoaxial lateral mass.

Other imaging studies are needed in the child with juvenile rheumatoid arthritis and neck pain. A bone scan is used for pinpointing the exact anatomic location of activity, and the anatomy is further studied with a CT scan. These studies can be helpful in looking for occult fractures, infections, and bony tumors.

Odontoid erosion results from the inflammatory synovitis and the pannus of the synovial ring surrounding the odontoid process. The pannus erodes the odontoid anteriorly and posteriorly, but leaves the apical and alar ligament attachments free, creating the apple-core lesion (Fig. 22.30B). This lesion is more susceptible to fracture, both from erosions and from vascular compromise to the odontoid, because the blood supply to the odontoid, which courses along its side (328), may be disturbed by the invading pannus. Ankylosis of the apophyseal joints is most common in the systemic onset subtype. In these young children, posterior ankylosis of the immature spine creates a tether, preventing further anterior growth. Decreased disc-space height and smaller vertebral bodies, both longitudinally and circumferentially, are the result (Fig. 22.30C) (325).

The treatment is generally nonsurgical, in conjunction with good rheumatologic care. Patients rarely develop flexion deformities; early in the course of the disease, a cervical collar may prevent this deformity (324). A cervical collar is recommended for patients who have involvement of the odontoid process or subaxial subluxation whenever they are in an automobile or other mode of travel. If these patients need surgery for any reason, intubation can be difficult because of the micrognathia, flexion deformity, and neck stiffness. Cervical fusion is rarely needed and should be reserved for children with documented instability or progressive neurologic deterioration.

## Intervertebral Disc Calcification

The first description of pediatric disc calcification was in 1924, and there are now more than 100 cases reported in the literature (329). It is slightly more common in boys than in girls (ratio of 7.5), with an average age at presentation of 8 years (range, 8 days to 13 years). It occurs most often in the cervical spine and is especially symptomatic when located there. The etiology is unclear. Theories

proposed are antecedent trauma (present in 30% of patients) and recent upper respiratory tract infections (present in 15% of patients, which may only reflect the normally high incidence of pediatric upper respiratory tract infections). There is no evidence to suggest metabolic disorders.

The most common clinical presentation is neck pain, which occurs in about one half of the children (329). The onset of symptoms is abrupt, between 12 and 48 hours. Twenty-three percent of the children are febrile on presentation. Torticollis occurs in one fourth of the children. Decreased cervical motion and spinal tenderness also can occur. Radicular signs and symptoms are rarely seen, and they are never without local symptoms. Myelopathy is rare (3 of 127 cases).

Calcified deposits are seen in the nucleus pulposus. The number of calcified discs averages 1.7 per child (Fig. 22.31). No protrusions have been seen in the asymptomatic group; 38% of the symptomatic children have detectable protrusions. Recent reports have also shown signal changes in the vertebrae on MRI scan (330).

Two thirds of the children are free of symptoms within 3 weeks and 95% are free of symptoms by 6 months. The radiographs show regression or disappearance of the calcific deposits in 90% of patients; approximately one half of the radiographic improvement occurs within 6 months. Children who are asymptomatic may not show regression on radiographic images, even when followed up for long periods. Children with multiple lesions show different rates of regression at the different disc levels. In some cases, persistent flattening of the vertebral bodies is noted into adulthood and may result in early degenerative changes (331).

Because of this natural history, treatment is symptomatic unless there is spinal cord compression. Analgesics, sedation, and cervical traction can all be used depending on the severity of symptoms. A short trial of a soft cervical collar also may be helpful. Contact sports should probably be avoided. Surgical intervention is rarely needed. Two cases have been reported in which anterior discectomy was performed (332,333).

## Pyogenic Osteomyelitis and Discitis

Pyogenic osteomyelitis and discitis is a spectrum of disease defined as a symptomatic narrowing of the disc space, often associated with fever and infection-like symptoms and signs. It affects all pediatric age ranges, and is more common in boys than in girls. The etiology is most likely infectious in nature; in about one third of the children an organism can be isolated, usually *Staphylococcus aureus* (334,335).

The children present with pain, difficulty in walking and standing, fever, and malaise. It usually involves the lumbar spine, with cervical involvement being rare. Early on there is a loss of disc-space height; later, end-plate irregularities

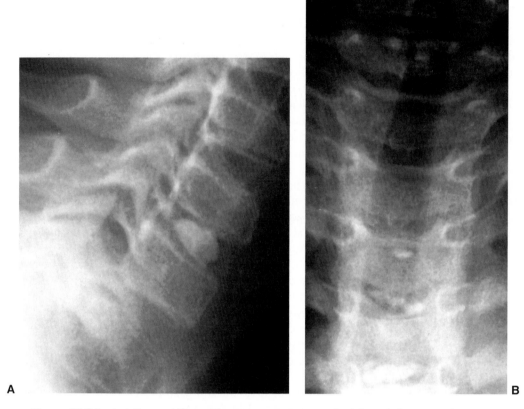

**Figure 22.31** **A:** A 7-year-old boy with symptomatic intervertebral disc calcification at the C6-C7 level, as seen on a lateral radiograph. **B:** He also showed asymptomatic involvement at the T3-T4, T4-T5, and T5-T6 levels, as seen on an anteroposterior radiograph.

on both sides of the disc appear. Bone scans are very useful in identifying the presence of discitis and osteomyelitis in a child with systemic symptoms when the anatomic location cannot be localized on clinical examination. The MRI findings are consistent with vertebral osteomyelitis (334,336). Other helpful diagnostic studies are the erythrocyte sedimentation rate and blood cultures. Disc and bone cultures are necessary only if the child does not respond to an initial course of rest and antibiotic treatment.

Many of these children spontaneously improve without treatment. The intervertebral disc space reconstitutes to varying degrees, but never to the normal height prior to illness. Sometimes spontaneous vertebral body fusion occurs. Initially, nonsurgical treatment is given. This includes rest, immobilization, and intravenous antistaphylococcal antibiotics. Surgery is necessary only if there is no response to nonsurgical management; usually, biopsy and culture to isolate the infectious agent is all that is needed.

## Tuberculosis

*Mycobacterium tuberculosis* infection in the cervical spine is rare compared with other levels of the spine. There will likely be an increase in North America because of the increasing number of immigrants from Third World countries, the rise of human immunodeficiency virus infection,

and the emergence of drug-resistant tuberculosis strains. There have been two very thorough reviews of this subject (337,338). Four of the 6 patients with upper cervical spine involvement and 24 of 40 with lower cervical spine involvement were children. Involvement at the cervicodorsal junction is also frequent in children (339).

In cases of upper cervical spine involvement the children present with neck pain and stiffness; torticollis, headaches, and constitutional symptoms may also be present. Neurologic symptoms vary from none to severe quadriparesis. In cases of lower cervical spine involvement the children present with the same symptoms, and in addition may have dysphagia, asphyxia, inspiratory stridor, and kyphosis. In children younger than 10 years, more diffuse and extensive involvement is seen, with large abscesses but with a decreased incidence of paraplegia and quadriplegia. The neurologic symptoms have a gradual onset over a period of 4 to 8 weeks. Sinus formation is not a prominent feature because of the thick cervical prevertebral fascia that contains the abscess. Cord compression occurs from the abscess and the kyphosis. Cultures and biopsies are not always positive. Because the infection is anterior, most cases will progress to spinal cord compression and paralysis if left untreated. Patients with involvement at the cervicodorsal junction have a very high incidence of neurologic loss (339).

Increased width of the retropharyngeal soft tissue space is seen radiographically, as are osteolytic erosions. Instability at the C1-C2 level can be seen in some children; rarely is there a fixed C1-C2 rotatory subluxation. A kyphosis is present in one fourth of patients with lower cervical spine involvement. Other useful imaging studies are chest radiography and renal studies.

Treatment involves antituberculous chemotherapy in all children. Surgery also is recommended for the cervical spine, because it gives rapid resolution of the pain, upper respiratory obstruction, and spinal cord compression. This is in contrast to the thoracic and lumbar spine, in which chemotherapy alone is an established method of treating tuberculosis (340). Debridement is performed with or without grafting. For children younger than 2 years, grafting is usually not needed. For children with upper cervical spine involvement, consideration should be given to anterior transoral drainage and fusion across the lateral facet joints. Most children need halo traction with reduction prior to drainage, if possible. Cervicodorsal involvement typically needs anterior decompression through an extended lower cervical approach (339).

## HEMATOLOGIC AND ONCOLOGIC CONDITIONS

The primary hematologic condition affecting the cervical spine is hemophilia (341). The involvement is usually asymptomatic, although mild neck discomfort may occur. Diminished lateral rotation may be noted on physical examination. Radiographic findings, which begin to occur in adolescence and early adulthood, consist of cystic changes in the vertebral bodies or end-plate irregularities. Rarely is C1-C2 instability present. These changes seen on radiographic examination can occur in patients with all degrees of severity of hemophilia. The pathoanatomy of these changes in the cervical spine is not known.

Many of these degenerative changes occur earlier in life than in the normal population; the natural history of these premature changes in the hemophiliac population is not known. There are no treatment recommendations at present, other than the standard precautions for patients with hemophilia.

### Benign Tumors

The common benign tumors that involve the pediatric cervical spine (342,343) are Langerhans cell histiocytosis, osteoid osteoma and osteoblastoma, osteochondroma, and aneurysmal bone cyst. All can be defined as neoplastic disorders without the propensity to metastasize. Although pathologically and physiologically benign, they can be clinically malignant if their surgical accessibility or risk of recurrence places the neural structures at high risk.

Most patients with benign cervical vertebral neoplasms are younger than 20 years of age and present with local neck pain (343). Radicular pain may occur in up to one-third of the patients (344); gross motor or sensory deficits are much less common. Neoplasms can cause torticollis. Probably the most common neoplasm causing childhood torticollis is osteoid osteoma. In one series, all four children with cervical osteoid osteomas presented with painful torticollis and decreased neck motion (345). In the literature, the incidence of torticollis is reported as ranging from 10% to 100% in children with cervical osteoid osteomas (346–348). The pain of an osteoid osteoma classically responds to aspirin or other nonsteroidal antiinflammatory medications. When basilar invagination is noted, Langerhans cell histiocytosis should be suspected (349).

With osteoid osteoma the typical radiographic feature is sclerosis (Fig. 22.32), although it is not always evident. Bone scans are very helpful in locating the lesion; CT scan is then used to further delineate the anatomy. The osteoid osteoma causes a sclerotic reaction in the surrounding bone but usually does not invade the epidural space. It is usually located in the laminae but can also be found in the pedicle and in the vertebral body. An osteoblastoma is usually a mixture of lytic and blastic elements (350). Bone scans are also positive but are usually not needed for determining the presence or absence of disease because most tumors are seen on plain radiographs. A CT scan is very helpful in further assessing the anatomy, especially the presence or absence of epidural invasion, which is common in osteoblastoma. Typically, osteoid osteomas and osteoblastomas are located in the posterior elements or pedicles (351) and, less commonly, in the vertebral body (352). Osteochondromas of the cervical spine (353–355) demonstrate the same typical radiographic appearance that they do in any other part of the body: expansile lesions with intact cortices and normal trabecular patterns, absence of calcification, and absence of soft tissue masses. One half of the patients have multiple osteochondromatosis. Most of these are in the laminae or spinous processes and can be mistaken for osteoblastomas. Aneurysmal bone cysts are typically expansile lytic lesions with a thin rim of cortical bone and may involve contiguous vertebral elements (e.g., the posterior elements, pedicle, and body). A CT scan is useful for determining the exact extent and the potential involvement and proximity of the vertebral artery and neural elements. Angiography may be needed. Aneurysmal bone cysts usually arise in the posterior elements (356). Eosinophilic granuloma usually exhibits vertebra plana as seen on radiographic images (357). The CT or MRI scan is useful in determining the potential encroachment on the neural structures. Eosinophilic granuloma usually arises in the vertebral body, with varying degrees of involvement and collapse.

In the cervical spine the main concern is the possible involvement of the vertebral artery and neural element because this can lead to neurologic dysfunction. The intense

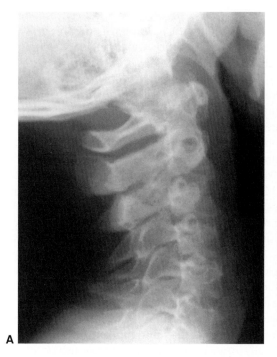
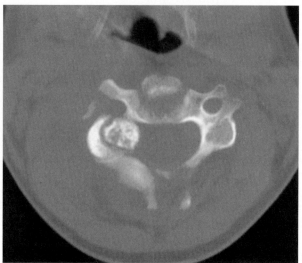

A

B

**Figure 22.32** A 13-year-old boy had a 2-year history of neck pain that did not resolve with long-term chiropractic treatment. **A:** Plain radiographs show a sclerotic nidus with a surrounding lucency at the level of the C3 pedicle and C2-C3 foramen. **B:** Computerized tomography (CT) scan confirms the typical appearance of an osteoid osteoma; note the proximity of the lesion to both the foramen and the nerve root as well as the vertebral artery.

inflammatory nature of the osteoid osteoma or osteoblastoma, which is so close to the neural elements, causes nerve root irritation. This irritation, pain, and muscle spasm may result in torticollis. Compressive myelopathy may also occur, especially in patients with epidural compression such as that seen with aneurysmal bone cysts (356,358,359).

The treatment of Langerhans cell histiocytosis of the cervical spine has traditionally consisted of immobilization (e.g., collars, Minerva casts) and low-dose irradiation. Immobilization is continued until early healing is seen radiographically. Low-dose irradiation should be reserved for lesions that are associated with neurologic deficits and are not surgically accessible. Multiple laminectomies should be avoided. Rarely has immobilization alone been used, and one of the children who underwent this treatment presented with total collapse of the vertebral body (357). Osteoid osteomas do not undergo malignant transformation. However, continued torticollis and pain may lead to fixed spinal deformities. For this reason the author advocates surgical resection. Pain relief with complete resection is dramatic. Significant complaints of postoperative pain resembling the preoperative pain indicate either incomplete resection or recurrence. For osteoblastoma and aneurysmal bone cysts, the primary treatment is surgical; nonsurgical treatment is used only as adjunctive therapy. The surgical goal is complete primary excision; however, this is often impossible because of the particular anatomic location of the cysts. In these situations,

adjunctive therapy is useful (e.g., radiotherapy for eosinophilic granuloma, or embolization for aneurysmal bone cysts if the nondominant vertebral artery is involved) (360). Intralesional injection using both steroids and calcitonin may be useful in the difficult case of an aneurysmal bone cyst (361).

Prophylactic fusion should be performed if the resection renders the spine unstable. The amount of resection necessary to render the spine unstable is not known in children; however, in adults resection of more than 50% of one facet likely leads to segmental instability (362). Because the development of postlaminectomy cervical instability is even more likely in children than in adults, the author recommends an arthrodesis along with any degree of facetectomy in children. Strong consideration should also be given to an arthrodesis after any degree of laminectomy. Multiple laminectomies should be avoided if at all possible; if it is necessary to perform laminectomies, then fusion and stabilization also should be performed. Anterior fusion is often necessary because of insufficient posterior elements after surgical excision; supplemental halo cast/vest or Minerva cast immobilization is usually needed if fusion is done. The overall surgical management is individualized and multidisciplinary (e.g., orthopaedics, neurosurgery, radiotherapy, interventional radiology). Surgical complications include recurrence, pseudarthrosis of the fusion, neurologic deterioration, and vertebral artery injury (363).

## Malignant Tumors

Most primary and metastatic malignant tumors involving the cervical spine occur in adults; rarely, the cervical spine in children can be involved by chordoma (364), leukemia, Ewing sarcoma (365), or metastatic neuroblastoma.

## REFERENCES

### Normal Embryology, Growth, and Development

1. O'Rahilly R, Meyer DB. The timing and sequence of events in the development of the human vertebral column during the embryonic period proper. *Anat Embryol* 1979;157:167–176.
2. Sensenig EC. The development of the occipital and cervical segments and their associated structures in human embryos. *Contrib Embryol Carnegie Inst* 1957;36:141–156.
3. O'Rahilly R, Muller F, Meyer DB. The human vertebral column at the end of the embryonic period proper. 1. The column as a whole. *J Anat* 1980;131:565–575.
4. Goodman FR. Limb malformations and the human *HOX* genes. *Am J Med Genet* 2002;112:256–265.
5. Connelly LE, Rogers JM. Methanol causes posteriorization of cervical vertebrae in mice. *Teratology* 1997;55:138–144.
6. Wéry N, Narotsky MG, Pacico N, et al. Defects in cervical vertebrae in boric acid-exposed rat embryos are associated with anterior shifts of *hox* gene expressed domains. *Birth Def Res (Part A)* 2003;67:59–67.
7. Kessel M, Gruss P. Homeotic transformations of murine vertebrae and concomitant alteration of Hox codes induced by retinoic acid. *Cell* 1991;67:89–104.
8. Li Z-L, Shiota K. Stage-specific homeotic vertebral transformations in mouse fetuses induced by maternal hyperthermia during somatogenesis. *Dev Dyn* 1999;216:336–348.
9. Ramirez-Solis R, Zheng H, Whiting J, et al. Hoxb-4 mutant mice show homeotic transformation of a cervical vertebra and defects in the closure of the sternal rudiments. *Cell* 1993;73:279–295.
10. Condie BG, Capecchi MR. Mice homozygous for a targeted disruption of *Hoxd-3* (*Hox-4.1*) exhibit anterior transformations of the first and second cervical vertebrae, the atlas and the axis. *Development* 1993;119:579–595.
11. Horan GSB, Wu K, Wolgemuth DJ, et al. Homeotic transformation of cervical vertebrae in *Hoxa-4* mutant mice. *Proc Natl Acad Sci U S A* 1994;91:12644–12648.
12. Tribioli C, Lufkin T. The murine *Bapx1* homeobox gene plays a critical role in embryonic development of the axial skeleton and spleen. *Development* 1999;126:5699–5711.
13. Leitges M, Neidhardt L, Haening B, et al. The paired homeobox gene Uncx4.1 specifies pedicles, transverse processes and proximal ribs of the vertebral column. *Development* 2000;127:2259–2267.
14. Subramanian V, Meyer BI, Gruss P. Disruption of the murine homeobox gene *Cdx1* affects skeletal identities by altering the mesodermal expression domains of *Hox* genes. *Cell* 1995;83:641–653.
15. van den Akker E, Forlani S, Chawengsaksophak K, et al. Cdx1 and Cdx2 have overlapping functions in anteroposterior patterning and posterior axis elongation. *Development* 2002;129:2181–2193.
16. McGaughran JM, Oates A, Donnai D, et al. Mutations in *PAX1* may be associated with Klippel-Feil syndrome. *Eur J Hum Genet* 2003;11:468–474.
17. Chi N, Epstein JA. Getting your Pax straight: Pax proteins in development and disease. *Trends Genet* 2002;18:41–47.
18. Wallin J, Wilting J, Koseki H, et al. The role of Pax-1 in axial skeletal development. *Development* 1994;120:1109–1121.
19. Rodrigo I, Hill RE, Balling R, et al. *Pax1* and *Pax9* activate *Bapx1* to induce chondrogenic differentiation in the sclerotome. *Development* 2003;130:473–482.
20. Smith CA, Tuan RS. Human PAX gene expression and development of the vertebral column. *Clin Orthop* 1994;302:241–250.
21. Peters H, Wilm B, Sakai N, et al. Pax1 and Pax9 synergistically regulate vertebral column development. *Development* 1999;126:5399–5408.
22. Villavicencio EH, Walterhouse DO, Iannaconne PM. The sonic hedgehog-patched-gli pathway in human development and disease. *Am J Hum Genet* 2000;67:1047–1054.
23. Weed M, Mundlos S, Olsen BR. The role of sonic hedgehog in vertebrate development. *Matrix Biol* 1997;16:53–58.
24. Kim JH, Kim PCW, Hui C-c. The VACTERL association: lessons from the sonic hedgehog pathway. *Clin Genet* 2001;59:306–315.
25. Ogden JA. Radiology of postnatal skeletal development. XI. The first cervical vertebrae. *Skeletal Radiol* 1984;12:12–20.
26. Ogden JA. Radiology of postnatal skeletal development. XII. The second cervical vertebra. *Skeletal Radiol* 1984;12:169–177.
27. Ogden JA, Murphy MJ, Southwick WO, et al. Radiology of postnatal skeletal development. XIII. C1-2 interrelationships. *Skeletal Radiol* 1986;15:433–438.
28. Remes VM, Heinänen MT, Kinnunen JS, et al. Reference values for radiological evaluation of cervical vertebral body shape and spinal canal. *Pediatr Radiol* 2000;30:190–195.
29. Locke GR, Gardner JI, van Epps EF. Atlas-dens interval (ADI) in children. A survey based on 200 normal cervical spines. *Am J Roentgenol* 1966;97:135–140.
30. Pennecot GF, Gouraud D, Hardy JR, et al. Roentgenographical study of the stability of the cervical spine in children. *J Pediatr Orthop* 1984;4:346–352.
31. Cattell HS, Filtzer DL. Pseudosubluxation and other normal variations in the cervical spine in children. *J Bone Joint Surg Am* 1965;47-A:1295–1309.
32. Fielding JW, Cochran GVB, Lawsing JF III, et al. Tears of the transverse ligament of the atlas. A clinical and biomechanical study. *J Bone Joint Surg Am* 1974;56-A:1683–1691.
33. Spierings ELH, Braakman R. The management of os odontoideum. *J Bone Joint Surg Br* 1982;64-B:422–428.
34. Steel HH. Anatomical and mechanical considerations of the atlanto-axial articulations. *J Bone Joint Surg Am* 1968;50-A:1481–1482.
35. Jauregui N, Lincoln T, Mubarak S, et al. Surgically related upper cervical spine canal anatomy in children. *Spine* 1993;18:1939–1944.
36. El-Khoury GY, Clark CR, Dietz FR, et al. Posterior atlantooccipital subluxation in Down syndrome. *Radiology* 1986;159:507–509.
37. Tredwell SJ, Newman DE, Lockitch G. Instability of the upper cervical spine in Down syndrome. *J Pediatr Orthop* 1990;10:602–606.
38. Wiesel SW, Rothman RH. Occipitoatlantal hypermobility. *Spine* 1979;4:187–191.
39. Gabriel KR, Mason DE, Carango P. Occipito-atlantal translation in Down's syndrome. *Spine* 1990;15:996–1002.
40. Shaw M, Burnett H, Wilson A, et al. Pseudosubluxation of C2 on C3 in polytraumatized children—prevalence and significance. *Clin Radiol* 1999;54:377–380.
41. Swischuk LE. Anterior displacement of C2 in children: physiologic or pathologic. A helpful differentiating line. *Radiology* 1977;122:759–763.
42. Dolan KD. Developmental abnormalities of the cervical spine below the axis. *Radiol Clin North Am* 1977;25:167–175.
43. Swischuk LE, Swischuk PN, John SD. Wedging of C-3 in infants and children: usually a normal finding and not a fracture. *Radiology* 1993;188:523–526.

### Congenital and Developmental Problems

44. Ballock RT, Song KM. The prevalence of nonmuscular causes of torticollis in children. *J Pediatr Orthop* 1996;16:500–504.
45. MacAlister A. Notes on the development and variations of the atlas. *J Anat Physiol* 1983;27:519–542.
46. Taylor AR, Chakravorty BC. Clinical syndromes associated with basilar impression. *Arch Neurol* 1964;10:475–484.
47. Burwood RJ, Watt I. Assimilation of the atlas and basilar impression. *Clin Radiol* 1974;25:327–333.
48. Epstein BS, Epstein JA. The association of cerebellar tonsillar herniation with basilar impression incident to Paget's disease. *Am J Roentgenol* 1969;107:535–542.
49. Hurwitz LJ, Shepherd WHT. Basilar impression and disordered metabolism of bone. *Brain* 1966;89:223–234.
50. Harkey HL, Crockard HA, Stevens JM, et al. The operative management of basilar impression in osteogenesis imperfecta. *Neurosurgery* 1990;27:782–786.
51. Pozo JL, Crockard HA, Ransford AO. Basilar impression in osteogenesis imperfecta. *J Bone Joint Surg Br* 1984;66-B:233–238.

52. Rush PJ, Berbrayer D, Reilly BJ. Basilar impression and osteogenesis imperfecta in a three-year-old girl: CT and MRI. *Pediatr Radiol* 1989;19:142–143.

53. Hayes M, Parker G, Ell J, et al. Basilar impression complicating osteogenesis imperfecta type IV: the clinical and neuroradiological findings in four cases. *J Neurol Neurosurg Psychiatry* 1999;66: 357–364.

54. Sawin PD, Menezes AH. Basilar invagination in osteogenesis imperfecta and related osteochondrodysplasias: medical and surgical management. *J Neurosurg* 1997;86:950–960.

55. Yamada H, Nakamura S, Tajima M, et al. Neurological manifestions of pediatric achondroplasia. *J Neurosurg* 1981;54:49–57.

56. Wong VCN, Fung CF. Basilar impression in a child with hypochondroplasia. *Pediatr Neurol* 1991;7:62–64.

57. Isu T, Miyasaka K, Abe H, et al. Atlantoaxial dislocation associated with neurofibromatosis. *J Neurosurg* 1983;58:451–453.

58. de Barros MC, Farias W, Ataide L, et al. Basilar impression and Arnold-Chiari malformation. *J Neurol Neurosurg Psychiatry* 1968;31:596–605.

59. Michie I, Clark M. Neurological syndromes associated with cervical and craniocervical anomalies. *Arch Neurol* 1968;18:241–247.

60. Teodori JB, Painter MJ. Basilar impression in children. *Pediatrics* 1984;74:1097–1099.

61. Chamberlain WE. Basilar impression (platybasia): bizarre developmental anomaly of occipital bone and upper cervical spine with striking and misleading neurologic manifestations. *Yale J Biol Med* 1939;11:487–496.

62. McRae DL. Bony abnormalities in the region of the foramen magnum: correlation of the anatomic and neurologic findings. *Acta Radiol* 1960;40:335–354.

63. McGregor M. Significance of certain measurements of skull in diagnosis of basilar impression. *Br J Radiol* 1948;21:171–181.

64. Pasztor E, Vajda J, Piffko P, et al. Transoral surgery for basilar impression. *Surg Neurol* 1980;14:473–476.

65. Menezes AH, van Gilder JC, Graf CJ, et al. Craniocervical abnormalities: a comprehensive surgical approach. *J Neurosurg* 1980; 53:444–454.

66. Wood DE, Good TL, Hahn J, et al. Decompression of the brain stem and superior cervical spine for congenital/acquired cranioverterbral invagination: an interdisciplinary approach. *Laryngoscope* 1990;100:926–931.

67. Hunt TE, Dekaban AS. Modified head-neck support for basilar impression with brain-stem compression. *Can Med Assoc J* 1982;126:947–948.

68. Menezes AH, VanGilder JC. Transoral-transpharyngeal approach to the anterior craniocervical junction. *J Neurosurg* 1988;69: 895–903.

69. Bharucha EP, Dastur HM. Craniovertebral anomalies (a report on 40 cases). *Brain* 1964;87:469–480.

70. Goel A, Bhatjiwale M, Desai K. Basilar invagination: a study based on 190 surgically treated patients. *J Neurosurg* 1998;88: 962–968.

71. McRae DL, Barnum AS. Occipitalization of the atlas. *AJR Am J Roentgenol* 1953;70:23–46.

72. Mesiwala AH, Shaffery CI, Gruss JS, et al. Atypical hemifacial microsomia associated with Chiari I malformation and syrinx: further evidence indicating that Chiari I malformation is a disorder of the paraxial mesoderm. *J Neurosurg* 2001;95:1034–1039.

73. Greenberg AD. Atlantoaxial dislocation. *Brain* 1968;91:655–684.

74. Wadia NH. Myelopathy complicating congenital atlantoaxial dislocation (a study of 28 cases). *Brain* 1967;90:449–472.

75. Kuhns LR, Loder RT, Rogers E, et al. Head-wag autotomography of the upper cervical spine in infantile torticollis. *Pediatr Radiol* 1998;28:464–467.

76. McRae DL. The significance of abnormalities of the cervical spine. *Am J Roentgenol* 1960;84:3–25.

77. Weng MS, Haynes RJ. Flexion and extension cervical MRI in a pediatric population. *J Pediatr Orthop* 1996;16:359–363.

78. Nicholson JT, Sherk HH. Anomalies of the occipitocervical articulation. *J Bone Joint Surg Am* 1968;50-A:295–304.

79. Doubousset J. Torticollis in children caused by congenital anomalies of the axis. *J Bone Joint Surg Am* 1986;68-A:178–188.

80. Graziano GP, Herzenberg JE, Hensinger RN. The halo-Ilizarov distraction cast for correction of cervical deformity. *J Bone Joint Surg Am* 1993;75-A:996–1003.

81. Saltzman CL, Hensinger RN, Blane CE, et al. Familial cervical dysplasia. *J Bone Joint Surg Am* 1991;73-A:163–171.

82. Fielding JW, Hawkins RJ. Atlanto-axial rotatory fixation. *J Bone Joint Surg Am* 1977;59-A:37–44.

83. Jackson G, Adler DC. Examination of the atlantoaxial joint following injury with particular emphasis on rotational subluxation. *Am J Roentgenol* 1956;76:1081–1094.

84. Fielding JW. Normal and selected abnormal motion of the cervical spine from the second cervical vertebra to the seventh cervical vertebra based on cineroentgenography. *J Bone Joint Surg Am* 1964;46-A:1779–1781.

85. Fielding JW. Cineroentgenography of the normal cervical spine. *J Bone Joint Surg Am* 1957;37:1280–1288.

86. Fielding JW, Stillwell WT, Chynn KY, et al. Use of computed tomography for the diagnosis of atlanto-axial rotatory fixation. *J Bone Joint Surg Am* 1978;60-A:1102–1104.

87. Mathern GW, Batzdorf U. Grisel's syndrome. Cervical spine clinical, pathologic, and neurologic manifestations. *Clin Orthop* 1989;244:131–146.

88. Bowen RE, Mah JY, Otsuka NY. Midshaft clavicle fractures associated with atlantoaxial rotatory displacement: a report of two cases. *J Orthop Trauma* 2003;17:444–447.

89. Brisson P, Patel H, Scorpio R, et al. Rotatory atlanto-axial subluxation with torticollis following central-venous catheter insertion. *Pediatr Surg Int* 2000;16:421–423.

90. Mezue WC, Taha ZM, Bashir EM. Fever and acquired torticollis in hospitalized children. *J Laryngol Otol* 2002;116:280–284.

91. Parke WW, Rothman RH, Brown MD. The pharyngovertebral veins: an anatomical rationale for Grisel's syndrome. *J Bone Joint Surg Am* 1984;66-A:568–574.

92. Yu KK, White DR, Weissler MC, et al. Nontraumatic atlantoaxial subluxation (Grisel syndrome): a rare complication of otolaryngological procedures. *Laryngoscope* 2003;113:1047–1049.

93. Tschopp K. Monopolar electrocautery in adenoidectomy as a possible risk factor for Grisel's syndrome. *Laryngoscope* 2002; 112:1445–1449.

94. Kawabe N, Hirotani H, Tanaka O. Pathomechanism of atlantoaxial rotatory fixation in children. *J Pediatr Orthop* 1989; 9:569–574.

95. Phillips WA, Hensinger RN. The management of rotatory atlanto-axial subluxation in children. *J Bone Joint Surg Am* 1989; 71-A:664–668.

96. Mihara H, Onari K, Hachiya M, et al. Follow-up study of conservative treatment for atlantoaxial rotatory displacement. *J Spinal Disord* 2001;14:494–499.

97. Fielding JW, Hawkins RJ, Ratzan SA. Spine fusion for atlantoaxial instability. *J Bone Joint Surg Am* 1976;58-A:400–407.

98. Parisine P, Di Silvestre M, Greggi T, et al. C1-C2 posterior fusion in growing patients. *Spine* 2003;28:566–572.

99. Ho BCS, Lee EH, Singh K. Epidemiology, presentation, and management of congenital muscular torticollis. *Singapore Med J* 1999;40:675–679.

100. Ling CM. The influence of age on the results of open sternomastoid tenotomy in muscular torticollis. *Clin Orthop* 1976;116: 142–148.

101. MacDonald D. Sternomastoid tumor and muscular torticollis. *J Bone Joint Surg Br* 1969;51-B:432–443.

102. Davids JR, Wenger DR, Mubarak SJ. Congenital muscular torticollis: sequela of intrauterine or perinatal compartment syndrome. *J Pediatr Orthop* 1993;13:141–147.

103. Whyte AM, Lufkin RB, Bredenkamp J, et al. Sternocleidomastoid fibrosis in congenital muscular torticollis: MR appearance. *J Comput Assist Tomogr* 1989;13:163–166.

104. Ling CM, Low YS. Sternomastoid tumor and muscular torticollis. *Clin Orthop* 1972;86:144–150.

105. Weiner DS. Congenital dislocation of the hip associated with congenital muscular torticollis. *Clin Orthop* 1976;121:163–165.

106. Thompson F, McManus S, Colville J. Familial congenital muscular torticollis. *Clin Orthop* 1986;202:193–196.

107. Hosalkar H, Gill IS, Gujar P, et al. Familial torticollis with polydactyly: manifestations in three generations. *Am J Orthop* 2001;30:656–658.

108. Engin C, Yavuz SS, Sahin FI. Congenital muscular torticollis: is heredity a possible factor in a family with five torticollis patients in three generations? *Plast Reconstr Surg* 1997;99:1147–1150.

109. Sarnat HB, Morrissy RT. Idiopathic torticollis: sternocleidomastoid myopathy and accessory neuropathy. *Muscle Nerve* 1981; 4:374–380.

110. Tang S, Liu Z, Quan X, et al. Sternocleidomastoid pseudotumor of infants and congenital muscular torticollis: fine structure research. *J Pediatr Orthop* 1998;18:214–218.

111. Cheng JCY, Tang SP, Chen TMK, et al. The clinical presentation and outcome of treatment of congenital muscular torticollis in infants—a study of 1086 cases. *J Pediatr Surg* 2000;35:1091–1096.

112. Coventry MB, Harris LE. Congenital muscular torticollis in infancy. *J Bone Joint Surg Am* 1959;41-A:815–822.

113. Walsh JJ, Morrissy RT. Torticollis and hip dislocation. *J Pediatr Orthop* 1998;18:219–221.

114. Brackbill Y, Douthitt TC, West H. Psychophysiologic effects in the neonate of prone versus supine placement. *J Pediatr* 1973; 81:82–84.

115. Cheng JCY, Au AWY. Infantile torticollis: a review of 624 cases. *J Pediatr Orthop* 1994;14:802–808.

116. Cheng JCY, Wong MWN, Tang SP, et al. Clinical determinants of the outcome of manual stretching in the treatment of congenital muscular torticollis in infants. *J Bone Joint Surg Am* 2001;83-A:679–687.

117. Binder H, Eng GD, Gaiser JF, et al. Congenital muscular torticollis: results of conservative management with long-term follow-up in 85 cases. *Arch Phys Med Rehabil* 1987;68:222–225.

118. Canale ST, Griffin DW, Hubbard CN. Congenital muscular torticollis. A long-term follow-up. *J Bone Joint Surg Am* 1982;64-A:810–816.

119. Cheng JC-Y, Metrewell C, Chen TM-K, et al. Correlation of ultrasonographic imaging of congenital muscular torticollis with clinical assessment in infants. *Ultrasound Med Biol* 2000;26:1237–1241.

120. Hsu T-C, Wang C-L, Wong M-K, et al. Correlation of clinical and ultrasonographic features in congenital muscular torticollis. *Arch Phys Med Rehabil* 1999;80:637–641.

121. Lin J-N, Chou M-L. Ultrasonographic study of the sternocleidomastoid muscle in the management of congenital muscular torticollis. *J Pediatr Surg* 1997;32:1648–1651.

122. Wei JL, Schwartz KM, Weaver AL, et al. Pseudotumor of infancy and congenital muscular torticollis: 170 cases. *Laryngoscope* 2001;111:688–695.

123. Cheng JCY, Chen TMK, Tang SP, et al. Snapping during manual stretching in congenital muscular torticollis. *Clin Orthop* 2001;384:237–244.

124. Ferkel RD, Westin GW, Dawson EG, et al. Muscular torticollis. A modified surgical approach. *J Bone Joint Surg Am* 1983;65-A:894–900.

125. Cheng JCY, Tang SP. Outcome of surgical treatment of congenital muscular torticollis. *Clin Orthop* 1999;362:190–200.

126. Tse P, Cheng J, Chow Y, et al. Surgery for neglected congenital torticollis. *Acta Orthop Scand* 1987;58:270–272.

127. Burstein FD, Cohen SR. Endoscopic surgical treatment for congenital muscular torticollis. *Plast Reconstr Surg* 1998;101:25–26.

128. Stassen LFA, Kerawal CJ. New surgical technique for the correction of congenital muscular torticollis (wry neck). *Br J Oral Maxillofac Surg* 2000;38:142–147.

129. Chen C-E, Ko J-Y. Surgical treatment of muscular torticollis for patients above 6 years of age. *Arch Orthop Trauma Surg* 2000; 120:149–151.

130. Gürpinar A, Kiristioglu I, Balkan E, et al. Surgical correction of muscular torticollis in older children with Jones technique. *J Pediatr Orthop* 1998;18:598–601.

131. Taboas-Perez RA, Rivera-Reyes L. Head tilt: a revisit to an old sign of posterior fossa tumors. *Bol Asoc Med P R* 1984;76:62–65.

132. O'Brien DF, Allcutt D, Caird J, et al. Posterior fossa tumours in childhood: evaluation of presenting clinical features. *Ir Med J* 2001;94:52–53.

133. Marmor MA, Beauchamp GR, Maddox SF. Photophobia, epiphora, and torticollis: a masquerade syndrome. *J Pediatr Ophthalmol Strab* 1990;27:202–204.

134. Giuffrè R, di Lorenzo N, Fortuna A. Cervical tumors of infancy and childhood. *J Neurosurg Sci* 1981;25:259–264.

135. Visudhiphan P, Chiemchanya S, Somburanasin R, et al. Torticollis as the presenting sign in cervical spine infection and tumor. *Clin Pediatr* 1982;21:71–76.

136. Rauch R, Jungert J, Rupprecht T, et al. Torticollis revealing as a symptom of acute lymphoblastic leukaemia in a fourteen-month-old girl. *Acta Paeditar* 2001;90:587–588.

137. Dure LS, Percy AK, Cheek WR, et al. Chiari type I malformation in children. *J Pediatr* 1989;115:573–576.

138. Wilkins RH, Brody IA. The Arnold-Chiari malformation. Neurological classics XXXVIII. *Arch Neurol* 1971;25:376–379.

139. Williams CRP, O'Flynn E, Clarke NMP, et al. Torticollis secondary to ocular pathology. *J Bone Joint Surg Br* 1996;78-B:620–624.

140. Rubin SE, Wagner RS. Ocular torticollis. *Surv Ophthalmol* 1986; 30:366–376.

141. Parker W. Migraine and the vestibular system in childhood and adolescence. *Am J Otol* 1989;10:364–371.

142. Snyder CH. Paroxysmal torticollis in infancy. A possible form of labyrinthitis. *Am J Dis Child* 1969;117:458–460.

143. Drigo P, Carli G, Laverda AM. Benign paroxysmal torticollis of infancy. *Brain Dev* 2000;22:169–172.

144. Al-Twaijri WA, Shevell MI. Pediatric migraine equivalents: occurrence and clinical features in practice. *Pediatr Neurol* 2002; 26:365–368.

145. Giffin NJ, Benton S, Goadsby PJ. Benign paroxysmal torticollis of infancy: four new cases and linkage to CACNA1A mutation. *Dev Med Child Neurol* 2002;44:490–493.

146. Murphy WJ Jr, Gellis SS. Torticollis with hiatus hernia in infancy. *Am J Dis Child* 1977;131:564–565.

147. Ramenofsky ML, Buyse M, Goldberg MJ, et al. Gastroesophageal reflux and torticollis. *J Bone Joint Surg Am* 1978;60-A:1140–1141.

148. Darling DB, Fisher JH, Gellis SS. Hiatal hernia and gastroesophageal reflux in infants and children: analysis of the incidence in North American children. *Pediatrics* 1974;54:450–455.

149. Darling DB. Hiatal hernia and gastroesophageal reflux in infancy and childhood. Analysis of the radiological findings. *Am J Roentgenol* 1975;123:724–736.

150. Jolley SG, Johnson DG, Herbst JJ, et al. An assessment of gastroesophageal reflux in children by extended pH monitoring of the distal esophagus. *Surgery* 1978;84:16–24.

151. Johnson DG, Herbst JJ, Oliveros MA, et al. Evaluation of gastroesophageal reflux surgery in children. *Pediatrics* 1977;59:62–68.

152. Hensinger RN, Lang JE, MacEwen GD. Klippel-Feil syndrome. A constellation of associated anomalies. *J Bone Joint Surg Am* 1974;56-A:1246–1253.

153. Brown MW, Templeton AW, Hodges FJ III. The incidence of acquired and congenital fusions in the cervical spine. *Am J Roentgenol* 1964;92:1255–1259.

154. Thompson E, Haan E, Sheffield L. Autosomal dominant Klippel-Feil anomaly with cleft palate. *Clin Dysmorphol* 1998;7:11–15.

155. Clarke RA, Kearsley JH, Walsh DA. Patterned expression in familial Klippel-Feil syndrome. *Teratology* 1996;53:152–157.

156. Clarke RA, Catalan G, Diwan AD, et al. Heterogeneity in Klippel-Feil syndrome: a new classification. *Pediatr Radiol* 1998;28:967–974.

157. Thomsen M, Krober M, Schneider U, et al. Congenital limb deficiencies associated with Klippel-Feil syndrome. A survey of 57 subjects. *Acta Orthop Scand* 2000;71:461–464.

158. Moore WB, Matthews TJ, Rabinowitz R. Genitourinary anomalies associated with Klippel-Feil syndrome. *J Bone Joint Surg Am* 1975;57-A:355–357.

159. Stark EW, Borton T. Klippel-Feil syndrome and associated hearing loss. *Arch Otolaryngol* 1973;97:415–419.

160. Gunderson CH, Solitare GB. Mirror movements in patients with the Klippel-Feil syndrome. *Arch Neurol* 1968;18:675–679.

161. Baga N, Chusid EL, Miller A. Pulmonary disability in the Klippel-Feil syndrome. *Clin Orthop* 1969;67:105–110.

162. Nora JJ, Cohen M, Maxwell GM. Klippel-Feil syndrome with congenital heart disease. *Am J Dis Child* 1961;102:110–116.

163. Thomsen MN, Schneider U, Weber M, et al. Scoliosis and congenital anomalies associated with Klippel-Feil syndrome types I-III. *Spine* 1997;21:396–401.

164. Hall JE, Simmons ED, Danylchuk K, et al. Instability of the cervical spine and neurological involvement in Klippel-Feil syndrome. *J Bone Joint Surg Am* 1990;72-A:460–462.

165. Epstein NE, Epstein JA, Zilkha A. Traumatic myelopathy in a seventeen-year-old child with cervical spinal stenosis (without fracture or dislocation) and a C2-3 Klippel-Feil fusion. *Spine* 1984;9:344–347.

166. Drvaric DM, Ruderman RJ, Conrad RW, et al. Congenital scoliosis and urinary tract abnormalities: are intravenous pyelograms necessary? *J Pediatr Orthop* 1987;7:441–443.

167. Ritterbusch JF, McGinty LD, Spar J, et al. Magnetic resonance imaging for stenosis and subluxation in Klippel-Feil syndrome. *Spine* 1991;16(Suppl. 10):539–541.

168. Pizzutillo PD, Woods M, Nicholson L, et al. Risk factors in Klippel-Feil syndrome. *Spine* 1994;19:2110–2116.

169. Sherk HH, Shut L, Chung S. Iniencephalic deformity of the cervical spine with Klippel-Feil anomalies and congenital evaluation of the scapula. *J Bone Joint Surg Am* 1974;56-A:1254–1259.

170. Rouvreau P, Glorion C, Langlais J, et al. Assessment and neurologic involvement of patients with cervical spine congenital synostosis as in Klippel-Feil syndrome: study of 19 cases. *J Pediatr Orthop B* 1998;7:179–185.

171. Royal SA, Tubbs S, D'Antonio MG, et al. Investigations into the association between cervicomedullary neuroschisis and mirror movements in patients with Klippel-Feil syndrome. *Am J Neuroradiol* 2002;23:724–729.

172. Guille JT, Miller A, Bowen JR, et al. The natural history of Klippel-Feil syndrome: clinical, roentgenographic, and magnetic resonance imaging findings at adulthood. *J Pediatr Orthop* 1995;15:617–626.

173. Fielding JW, Hesinger RN, Hawkins RJ. Os odontoideum. *J Bone Joint Surg Am* 1980;62-A:376–383.

174. Verska JM, Anderson PA. Os odontoideum. A case report of one identical twin. *Spine* 1997;22:706–709.

175. Kuhns LR, Loder RT, Farley FA, et al. Nuchal cord changes in children with os odontoideum: evidence for associated trauma. *J Pediatr Orthop* 1998;18:815–819.

176. Sakaida H, Waga S, Kojima T, et al. Os odontoideum associated with hypertrophic ossiculum terminale. *J Neurosurg* 2001;94:140–144.

177. Currarino G. Segmentation defect in the midodont process and its possible relationship to the congenital type of os odontoideum. *Pediatr Radiol* 2002;32:34–40.

178. Matsui H, Imada K, Tsuji H. Radiographic classification of os odontoideum and its clinical significance. *Spine* 1997;22:1706–1709.

179. Watanabe M, Toyama Y, Fujimura Y. Atlantoaxial instability in os odontoideum with myelopathy. *Spine* 1996;21:1435–1439.

180. Aksoy FG, Gomori JM. Symptomatic cervical synovial cyst associated with an os odontoideum diagnosed by magnetic resonance imaging. *Spine* 2000;25:1300–1302.

181. Chang H, Park J-B, Kim K-W. Synovial cyst of the transverse ligament of the atlas in a patient with os odontoideum and atlantoaxial instability. *Spine* 2000;25:741–744.

182. Chang H, Park J-B, Kim K-W, et al. Retro-dental reactive lesions related to development of myelopathy in patients with atlantoaxial instability secondary to os odontoideum. *Spine* 2000;25:2777–2783.

183. Jun B-Y. Complete reduction of retro-odontoid soft tissue mass in os odontoideum following the posterior C1-C2 transarticular screw fixation. *Spine* 1999;24:1961–1964.

184. Wang J, Vokshoor A, Kim S, et al. Pediatric atlantoaxial instability: management with screw fixation. *Pediatr Neurosurg* 1999;30:70–78.

185. Yoshimoto H, Ito M, Abumi K, et al. A retrospective radiographic analysis of subaxial sagittal alignment after posterior C1-C2 fusion. *Spine* 2004;29:175–181.

186. Spitzer R, Rabinowitch JY, Wybor KC. A study of the abnormalities of the skull, teeth, and lenses in mongolism. *Can Med Assoc J* 1961;84:567–568.

187. Matsuda Y, Sano N, Watanabe S, et al. Atlanto-occipital hypermobility in subjects with Down's syndrome. *Spine* 1995;20:2283–2286.

188. Selby KA, Newton RW, Gupta S, et al. Clinical predictors and radiological reliability in atlantoaxial subluxation in Down's syndrome. *Arch Dis Child* 1991;66:876–878.

189. Karol LA, Sheffield EG, Crawford K, et al. Reproducibility in the measurement of atlanto-occipital instability in children with Down syndrome. *Spine* 1996;21:2463–2468.

190. Parfenchuck TA, Bertrand SL, Powers MJ, et al. Posterior occipitoatlantal hypermobility in Down syndrome: an analysis of 199 patients. *J Pediatr Orthop* 1994;14:304–308.

191. Pueschel SM, Herndon JH, Gelch MM, et al. Symptomatic atlantoaxial subluxation in persons with Down syndrome. *J Pediatr Orthop* 1984;4:682–688.

192. Committee on Sports Medicine and Fitness of the American Academy of Pediatrics. Atlantoaxial instability in Down syndrome: subject review. *Pediatrics* 1995;96:151–154.

193. Burke SW, French HG, Roberts JM, et al. Chronic atlanto-axial instability in Down syndrome. *J Bone Joint Surg Am* 1985;67-A:1356–1360.

194. Pueschel SM, Scola FH, Tupper TB, et al. Skeletal anomalies of the upper cervical spine in children with Down syndrome. *J Pediatr Orthop* 1990;10:607–611.

195. Ferguson RL, Putney ME, Allen BL Jr. Comparison of neurologic deficits with atlanto-dens intervals in patients with Down syndrome. *J Spinal Disord* 1997;10:246–252.

196. Committee on Sports Medicine and Fitness of the American Academy of Pediatrics. Atlantoaxial instability in Down syndrome. *Pediatrics* 1984;74:152–154.

197. Wellborn CC, Sturm PF, Hatch RS, et al. Intraobserver reproducibility and interobserver reliability of cervical spine measurements. *J Pediatr Orthop* 2000;20:66–70.

198. Pueschel SM, Findley TW, Furia J, et al. Atlantoaxial instability in Down syndrome: roentgenographic, neurologic, and somatosensory evoked potential studies. *J Pediatr* 1987;110:515–521.

199. Brockmeyer DL, York JE, Appelbaum RI. Anatomical suitability of C1-2 transarticular screw placement in pediatric patients. *J Neurosurg (Spine 1)* 2000;92:7–11.

200. Taggard DA, Menezes AH, Ryken TC. Treatment of Down syndrome-associated craniovertebral junction abnormalities. *J Neurosurg (Spine 2)* 2000;93:205–213.

201. Nordt JC, Stauffer ES. Sequelae of atlantoaxial stabilization in two patients with Down's syndrome. *Spine* 1981;6:437–440.

202. Lundy DW, Murrary HH. Neurological deterioration after posterior wiring of the cervical spine. *J Bone Joint Surg Br* 1997;79-B:948–951.

203. Smith MD, Phillips WA, Hensinger RN. Fusion of the upper cervical spine in children and adolescents. An analysis of 17 patients. *Spine* 1990;16:695–701.

204. Rizzolo S, Lemos MJ, Mason DE. Posterior spinal arthrodesis for atlanto-axial instability in Down syndrome. *J Pediatr Orthop* 1995;15:543–548.

205. Segal LS, Drummond DS, Zanotti RM, et al. Complications of posterior arthrodesis of the cervical spine in patients with have Down syndrome. *J Bone Joint Surg Am* 1991;73-A:1547–1554.

206. Smith MD, Phillips WA, Hensinger RN. Complications of fusion to the upper cervical spine. *Spine* 1991;16:702–705.

207. Doyle JS, Lauerman WC, Wood KB, et al. Complications and long-term outcome of upper cervical spine arthrodesis in patients with Down syndrome. *Spine* 1996;21:1223–1231.

208. Msall M, Rogers B, DiGaudio K, et al. Long-term complications of segmental cervical fusion in Down syndrome. *Dev Med Child Neurol* 1991;33(Suppl. 64):5.

209. Hobbs WR, Sponseller PD, Weiss A-PC, et al. The cervical spine in Marfan syndrome. *Spine* 1997;22:983–989.

210. Herzka A, Sponseller PD, Pyeritz RE. Atlantoaxial rotatory subluxation in patients with Marfan syndrome. *Spine* 2000;25:524–526.

211. Georgopoulos G, Pizzutillo PD, Lee MS. Occipito-atlantal instability in children. *J Bone Joint Surg Am* 1987;69-A:429–436.

212. Ebara S, Harada T, Yamazaki Y, et al. Unstable cervical spine in athetoid cerebral palsy. *Spine* 1989;14:1154–1159.

213. Fuji T, Yonenobu K, Fujiwara K, et al. Cervical radiculopathy or myelopathy secondary to athetoid cerebral palsy. *J Bone Joint Surg Am* 1987;69-A:815–821.

214. Nishihara N, Tnabe G, Nakahara S, et al. Surgical treatment of cervical spondylotic myelopathy complicating athetoid cerebral palsy. *J Bone Joint Surg Br* 1984;66-B:504–508.

215. Reese ME, Msall ME, Owen S, et al. Acquired cervical impairment in young adults with cerebral palsy. *Dev Med Child Neurol* 1991;33:153–166.

216. Harada T, Ebara S, Anwar MM, et al. The cervical spine in athetoid cerebral palsy. *J Bone Joint Surg Br* 1996;78-B:613–619.

217. Tsirikos AI, Chang W-N, Shah SA, et al. Acquired atlantoaxial instability in children with spastic cerebral palsy. *J Pediatr Orthop* 2003;23:335–341.

218. Loder RT, Hensinger RN. Developmental abnormalities of the cervical spine. In: Weinstein SL, ed. *The pediatric spine: principles and practice.* New York: Raven Press, 1994.

219. Haro H, Komori H, Okawa A, et al. Surgical treatment of cervical spondylotic myelopathy associated with athetoid cerebral palsy. *J Orthop Sci* 2002;7:629–636.

220. Aronson DD, Kahn RH, Canady A, et al. Instability of the cervical spine after decompression in patients who have Arnold-Chiari malformation. *J Bone Joint Surg Am* 1991;73-A:898–906.

221. Cattell HS, Clark GL Jr. Cervical kyphosis and instability following multiple laminectomies in children. *J Bone Joint Surg Am* 1967;49-A:713–720.

222. Francis WR Jr, Noble DP. Treatment of cervical kyphosis in children. *Spine* 1988;13:883–887.

223. Sim FH, Svien HJ, Bickel WH, et al. Swan-neck deformity following extensive cervical laminectomy. *J Bone Joint Surg Am* 1974;56-A:564–580.

224. Yasuoka S, Peterson H, Laws ER Jr, et al. Pathogenesis and prophylaxis of postlaminectomy deformity of the spine after multiple level laminectomy: difference between children and adults. *Neurosurgery* 1981;9:145–152.

225. Bell DF, Walker JL, O'Connor B, et al. Spinal deformity after multiple-level cervical laminectomy in children. *Spine* 1994;19:406–411.

226. McLaughlin MR, Wahlig JB, Pollack IF. Incidence of post-laminectomy kyphosis after Chiari decompression. *Spine* 1997;22:613–617.

227. Lee K-S, Moon M-S. The effect of multilevel laminectomy on the cervical spine of growing cats. *Spine* 1993;18:359–363.

228. Hirabayashi K, Satomi K. Operative procedure and results of expansive open-door laminoplasty. *Spine* 1988;13:870–875.

229. Tredwell SJ, Smith DF, Macleod PJ, et al. Cervical spine anomalies in fetal alcohol syndrome. *Spine* 1982;7:331–334.

230. Sandham A. Cervical vertebral anomalies in cleft lip and palate. *Cleft Palate J* 1986;23:206–214.

231. Ugar DA, Semb G. The prevalence of anomalies of the upper cervical vertebrae in subjects with cleft lip, cleft palate, or both. *Cleft Palate Craniofac J* 2001;38:498–503.

232. Hemmer KM, McAlister WH, Marsh JL. Cervical spine anomalies in the craniosynostosis syndromes. *Cleft Palate J* 1987;24:328–333.

233. Louis DS, Argenta LC. The orthopaedic manifestations of Goldenhar's syndrome. *Surgical Rounds for Orthopaedics* 1987;43–46.

234. Sherk HH, Whitaker LA, Pasquariello PS. Facial malformations and spinal anomalies. A predictable relationship. *Spine* 1982;7:526–531.

235. Anderson PJ, Hall CM, Evans RD, et al. Cervical spine in Pfeiffer's syndrome. *J Craniofac Surg* 1996;7:275–279.

236. Moore MH, Lodge ML, Clark BE. Spinal anomalies in Pfeiffer syndrome. *Cleft Palate Craniofac J* 1995;32:251–254.

237. Anderson PJ, Hall CM, Evans RD, et al. The cervical spine in Saethre-Chotzen syndrome. *Cleft Palate Craniofac J* 1997;34:79–82.

238. Gibson JNA, Silence DO, Taylor TKF. Abnormalities of the spine in Goldenhar's syndrome. *J Pediatr Orthop* 1996;16:344–349.

239. Ewart-Toland A, Yankowitz J, Winder A, et al. Oculoauriculovertebral abnormalities in children of diabetic mothers. *Am J Med Genet* 2000;90:303–309.

240. Healey D, Letts M, Jarvis JG. Cervical spine instability in children with Goldenhar's syndrome. *Can J Surg* 2002;45:341–344.

241. Yong-Hing K, Kalamchi A, MacEwen GD. Cervical spine abnormalities in neurofibromatosis. *J Bone Joint Surg Am* 1979;61-A:695–699.

242. Craig JB, Govender S. Neurofibromatosis of the cervical spine. *J Bone Joint Surg Br* 1992;74-B:575–578.

243. Adkins JC, Ravitch MM. The operative management of von Recklinghausen's neurofibromatosis in children, with special reference to lesions of the head and neck. *Surgery* 1977;82:342–348.

244. Nijland EA, van den Berg MP, Wuisman PIJM, et al. Correction of a dystrophic cervicothoracic spine deformity in Recklinghausen's disease. *Clin Orthop* 1998;349:149–155.

245. Giaia G, Mandelli D, Capaccioni B, et al. Postlaminectomy cervical dislocation in von Recklinghausen's disease. *Spine* 1998;23:273–276.

246. Asazuma T, Yamagishi M, Nemoto K, et al. Spinal fusion using a vascularized fibular bone graft for a patient with cervical kyphosis due to neurofibromatosis. *J Spinal Disord* 1997;10:537–540.

247. Kaplan FS, McCluskey W, Hahn G, et al. Genetic transmission of fibrodysplasia ossificans progressiva. *J Bone Joint Surg Am* 1993;75-A:1214–1220.

248. Hall CM, Sutcliffe J. Fibrodysplasia ossificans progressiva. *Ann Radiol* 1978;22:119–123.

249. Connor JM, Smith R. The cervical spine in fibrodysplasia ossificans progressiva. *Br J Radiol* 1982;55:492–496.

## Trauma

250. McGrory BJ, Klassen RA, Chao EYS, et al. Acute fractures and dislocations of the cervical spine in children and adolescents. *J Bone Joint Surg Am* 1993;75-A:988–995.

251. Orzechowski KM, Edgerton EA, Bulas DI, et al. Patterns of injury to restrained children in side impact motor vehicle crashes: the side impact syndrome. *J Trauma Inj Infect Crit Care* 2003;54:1094–1101.

252. Kokoska ER, Keller MS, Rallo MC, et al. Characteristics of pediatric cervical spine injuries. *J Pediatr Surg* 2001;36:100–105.

253. Brown RL, Brunn MA, Garcia VF. Cervical spine injuries in children: a review of 103 patients treated consecutively at a level 1 pediatric trauma center. *J Pediatr Surg* 2001;36:1107–1114.

254. Patel JC, Tepas JJ III, Mollitt DL, et al. Pediatric cervical spine injuries: defining the disease. *J Pediatr Surg* 2001;36:373–376.

255. Lally KP, Senac M, Hardin WD Jr, et al. Utility of the cervical spine radiograph in pediatric trauma. *Am J Surg* 1989;158:540–542.

256. Rachesky I, Boyce WT, Duncan B, et al. Clinical prediction of cervical spine injuries in children. Radiographic abnormalities. *Am J Dis Child* 1987;141:199–201.

257. Buhs C, Cullen M, Klein M, et al. The pediatric trauma c-spine: is the 'odontoid' view necessary? *J Pediatr Surg* 2000;35:994–997.

258. Swischuk LE, John SD, Hendrick EP. Is the open-mouth odontoid view necessary in children under 5 years? *Pediatr Radiol* 2000;30:186–189.

259. Herzenberg JE, Hensinger RN, Dedrick DK, et al. Emergency transport and positioning of young children who have an injury of the cervical spine. *J Bone Joint Surg Am* 1989;71-A:15–22.

260. Pennecot GF, Leonard P, Gachons SPD, et al. Traumatic ligamentous instability of the cervical spine in children. *J Pediatr Orthop* 1984;4:339–345.

261. Ardraan GM, Kemp FH. The mechanism of changes in form of the cervical airway in infancy. *Med Radiogr Photogr* 1968;44:26–54.

262. Flynn JM, Closkey RF, Mahboubi S, et al. Role of magnetic resonance imaging in the assessment of pediatric cervical spine injuries. *J Pediatr Orthop* 2002;22:573–577.

263. Bulas DI, Fitz CR, Johnson DL. Traumatic atlanto-occipital dislocation in children. *Radiology* 1993;188:155–158.

264. Bucholz RW, Burkhead WZ. The pathological anatomy of fatal atlanto-occipital dislocations. *J Bone Joint Surg Am* 1979;61-A:248–250.

265. Giguere JF, St-Vil D, Turmel A, et al. Airbags and children: a spectrum of C-spine injuries. *J Pediatr Surg* 1998;33:811–816.

266. Angel CA, Ehlers RA. Atloido-occipital dislocation in a small child after air-bag deployment. *N Engl J Med* 2001;345:1256.

267. Bailey H, Perez N, Blank-Reid C, et al. Atlanto-occipital dislocation: an unusual lethal airbag injury. *J Emerg Med* 2000;18:215–219.

268. Okamoto K, Takemoto M, Okada Y. Airbag-mediated craniocervical injury in a child restrained with safety device. *J Trauma Inj Infect Crit Care* 2002;52:587–590.

269. Labbe J-L, Leclair O, Duparc B. Traumatic atlanto-occipital dislocation with survival in children. *J Pediatr Orthop B* 2001;10:319–327.

270. Powers B, Miller MD, Kramer RS, et al. Traumatic anterior atlanto-occipital dislocation. *Neurosurgery* 1979;4:12–17.

271. Sun PP, Poffenbarger GJ, Durham S, et al. Spectrum of occipitoatlantoaxial injury in young children. *J Neurosurg (Spine 1)* 2000;93:28–39.

272. Przybylski GJ, Clyde BL, Fitz CR. Craniocervical junction subarachnoid hemorrhage associated with atlanto-occipital dislocation. *Spine* 1996;21:1761–1768.

273. Matava MJ, Whitesides TE Jr, Davis PC. Traumatic atlanto-occipital dislocation with survival. *Spine* 1993;18:1897–1903.

274. Sponseller PD, Cass JR. Atlanto-occipital fusion for dislocation in children with neurologic preservation. *Spine* 1997;22:344–347.

275. Botelho RV, Palma AMS, Abgussen CMB, et al. Traumatic vertical atlantoaxial instability: the risk associated with skull traction. *Eur Spine J* 2000;9:430–433.

276. Naso WB, Cure J, Cuddy BG. Retropharyngeal pseudomeningocele after atlanto-occipital dislocation: report of two cases. *Neurosurgery* 1997;40:1288–1291.

277. Marlin AE, Williams GR, Lee JF. Jefferson fractures in children. *J Neurosurg* 1983;58:277–279.

278. Mikawa Y, Yamano Y, Ishii K. Fracture through a synchondrosis of the anterior arch of the atlas. *J Bone Joint Surg Br* 1987;69-B:483.

279. Judd DB, Liem LK, Petermann G. Pediatric atlas fracture: a case of fracture through a synchondrosis and review of the literature. *Neurosurgery* 2000;46:991–995.

280. Bayar MA, Erdem Y, Ozturk K, et al. Isolated anterior arch fracture of the atlas. Child case report. *Spine* 2002;27:E47–E49.

281. Abuamara S, Dacher J-N, Lechevallier J. Posterior arch bifocal fracture of the atlas vertebra: a variant of Jefferson fracture. *J Pediatr Orthop B* 2001;10:201–204.

282. Lo PA, Drake JM, Hedden D, et al. Avulsion transverse ligament injuries in children: successful treatment with nonoperative management. *J Neurosurg (Spine 3)* 2002;96:338–342.

283. Sherk HH, Nicholson JT, Chung SMK. Fractures of the odontoid process in young children. *J Bone Joint Surg Am* 1978;60-A:921–924.

284. Swischuk LE, Hayden CK Jr, Sarwar M. The posteriorly tilted dens. A normal variation mimicking a fractured dens. *Pediatr Radiol* 1979;8:27–28.

285. Pizzutillo PD, Rocha EF, D'Astous J, et al. Bilateral fracture of the pedicle of the second cervical vertebra in the young child. *J Bone Joint Surg Am* 1986;68-A:892–896.

286. Power DM, Cross JLL, Antoun NM, et al. Helical computed tomography and three-dimensional reconstruction of a bipedicular developmental anomaly of the C2 vertebra. *Spine* 1999;24:984–986.

287. Sheehan J, Kaptain G, Sheehan J, et al. Congenital absence of a cervical pedicle: report of two cases and review of the literature. *Neurosurgery* 2000;47:1439–1442.

288. Howard AW, Letts RM. Cervical spondylolysis in children: is it posttraumatic? *J Pediatr Orthop* 2000;20:677–681.

289. Grisoni NE, Ballock RT, Thompson GH. Second cervical vertebrae pedicle fractures versus synchondrosis in a child. *Clin Orthop* 2003;413:238–242.

290. Ranjith RK, Mullett JH, Burke TE. Hangman's fracture caused by suspected child abuse. *J Pediatr Orthop B* 2002;11:329–332.

291. Evans DL, Bethem D. Cervical spine injuries in children. *J Pediatr Orthop* 1989;9:563–568.

292. Lawson JP, Ogden JA, Bucholz RW, et al. Physeal injuries of the cervical spine. *J Pediatr Orthop* 1987;7:428–435.

293. Matsumoto M, Toyama Y, Chiba K, et al. Traumatic subluxation of the axis after hyperflexion injury of the cervical spine in children. *J Spinal Disord* 2001;14:172–179.

294. McGrory BJ, Klassen RA. Arthrodesis of the cervical spine for fractures and dislocations in children and adolescents. *J Bone Joint Surg Am* 1994;76-A:1606–1616.

295. Ladd AL, Scranton PE. Congenital cervical stenosis presenting as transient quadriplegia in athletes. *J Bone Joint Surg Am* 1986;68-A:1371–1374.

296. Torg JS, Pavlov H, Genuario SE, et al. Neurapraxia of the cervical spinal cord with transient quadriplegia. *J Bone Joint Surg Am* 1986;68-A:1354–1370.

297. Rathbone D, Johnson G, Letts M. Spinal cord concussion in pediatric athletes. *J Pediatr Orthop* 1992;12:616–620.

298. Torg JH, Naranja RJ, Pavlov H, et al. The relationship of developmental narrowing of the cervical spinal canal to reversible and irreversible injury of the cervical spinal cord in football players. An epidemiological study. *J Bone Joint Surg Am* 1996;78-A:1308–1314.

299. Odor JM, Watkins RG, Dillin WH, et al. Incidence of cervical spinal stenosis in professional and rookie football players. *Am J Sports Med* 1990;18:507–509.

300. Eismont FJ, Clifford S, Goldberg M, et al. Cervical sagittal spinal canal size in spine injury. *Spine* 1984;9:663–666.

301. Pang D, Pollack IF. Spinal cord injury without radiographic abnormality in children—the SCIWORA syndrome. *J Trauma* 1989;29:654–664.

302. Hendey GW, Wolfson AB, Mower WR, et al. Spinal cord injury without radiographic abnormality: results of the National Emergency X-radiography Utilization Study in Blunt Cervical Trauma. *J Trauma Inj Infect Crit Care* 2002;53:1–4.

303. Linssen WHJP, Praamstra P, Babreels FJM, et al. Vascular insufficiency of the cervical cord due to hyperextension of the spine. *Pediatr Neurol* 1990;6:123–125.

304. Bosch PP, Vogt MT, Ward WT. Pediatric spinal cord injury without radiographic abnormality (SCIWORA). The absence of occult instability and lack of indication for bracing. *Spine* 2002;27:2788–2800.

305. Grabb PA, Pang D. Magnetic resonance imaging in the evaluation of spinal cord injury without radiographic abnormality in children. *Neurosurgery* 1994;35:406–414.

306. Dare AO, Dias MS, Li V. Magnetic resonance imaging correlation in pediatric spinal cord injury without radiographic abnormality. *J Neurosurg (Spine 1)* 2002;93:33–39.

307. Abroms IF, Bresnan MJ, Zuckerman JE, et al. Cervical cord injuries secondary to hyperextension of the head in breech presentations. *Obstet Gynecol* 1973;41:369–378.

308. Byers RK. Spinal-cord injuries during birth. *Dev Med Child Neurol* 1975;17:103–110.

309. Morgan C, Newell SJ. Cervical spinal cord injury following cephalic presentation and delivery by caesarean section. *Dev Med Child Neurol* 2001;43:274–276.

310. Jones EL, Cameron AH, Smith WT. Birth trauma to the cervical spine and vertebral arteries. *J Pathol* 1970;100.

311. King WJ, MacKay M, Sirnick A. Shaken baby syndrome in Canada: clinical characteristics and outcomes of hospital cases. *Can Med Assoc J* 2003;168:155–159.

312. Shulman ST, Madden JD, Esterly JR, et al. Transection of spinal cord. A rare obstetrical complication of cephalic delivery. *Arch Dis Child* 1971;46:291–294.

313. Hillman JW, Sprofkin BE, Parrish TF. Birth injury of the cervical spine producing a "cerebral palsy" syndrome. *Am Surg* 1954;20:900–906.

## Inflammatory and Septic Conditions

314. Towbin A. Central nervous system damage in the human fetus and newborn infant. *Am J Dis Child* 1970;119:529–542.

315. Farley FA, Hensinger RN, Herzenberg JE. Cervical spinal cord injury in children. *J Spinal Disord* 1992;5:410–416.

316. Saternus K-S, Wighton-Kernbach G, Oehmichen M. The shaking trauma in infants—kinetic chains. *Forensic Sci Int* 2000;109:203–213.

317. Conry BG, Hall CM. Cervical spine fractures and rear car seat restraints. *Arch Dis Child* 1987;62:1267–1268.

318. Mousny M, Saint-Martin C, Danse E, et al. Unusual upper cervical fracture in a 1-year-old girl. *J Pediatr Orthop* 2001;21:590–593.

319. Winter SCA, Quaghebeur G, Richards PG. Unusual cervical spine injury in a 1 year old. *Injury* 2003;34:316–319.

320. Garton HJL, Park P, Papadopoulous SM. Fracture dislocation of the neurocentral synchondroses of the axis. *J Neurosurg (Spine 3)* 2002;96:350.

321. Kupcha PC, An HS, Cotler JM. Gunshot wounds to the cervical spine. *Spine* 1990;15:1058–1063.

322. Haffner DL, Hoffer MM, Wiedbusch R. Etiology of children's spinal injuries at Rancho Los Amigos. *Spine* 1993;18:679–684.

323. Hensinger RN, DeVito PD, Ragsdale CG. Changes in the cervical spine in juvenile rheumatoid arthritis. *J Bone Joint Surg Am* 1986;68-A:189–198.

324. Fried JA, Athreya B, Gregg JR, et al. The cervical spine in juvenile rheumatoid arthritis. *Clin Orthop* 1983;179:103.

325. Laiho K, Savolainen A, Kautiainen H, et al. The cervical spine in juvenile chronic arthritis. *Spine J* 2002;2:89–94.

326. Martel W, Holt JF, Cassidy JT. Roentgenologic manifestations of juvenile rheumatoid arthritis. *Am J Roentgenol* 1962;88:400–423.

327. Hallah JT, Fallahi S, Hardin JG. Nonreducible rotational head tilt and atlantoaxial lateral mass collapse. Clinical and roentgenographic features in patients with juvenile rheumatoid arthritis and ankylosing spondylitis. *Arch Intern Med* 1983;143:471–474.

328. Schiff DCM, Parke WW. The arterial supply of the odontoid process. *J Bone Joint Surg Am* 1973;55-A:1450–1456.

329. Sonnabend DH, Taylor TKF, Chapman GK. Intervertebral disc calcification syndromes in children. *J Bone Joint Surg Br* 1982; 64-B:25–31.

330. Herring JA, Hensinger RN. Cervical disc calcification. Instructional case. *J Pediatr Orthop* 1988;8:613–616.

331. Wong CC, Pereira B, Pho RWH. Cervical disc calcification in children. A long term review. *Spine* 1992;17:139–144.

332. Smith RA, Vohman MD, Dimon JH III, et al. Calcified cervical intervertebral discs in children. *J Neurosurg* 1977;46:233–238.

333. Oga M, Terada K, Kikuchi N, et al. Herniation of calcified cervical intervertebral disc causes dissociated motor loss in a child. *Spine* 1993;18:2347–2350.

334. Ring D, Johnston CE II, Wenger DR. Pyogenic infectious spondylitis in children: the convergence of discitis and vertebral osteomyelitis. *J Pediatr Orthop* 1995;15:652–660.

335. Wenger DR, Bobechko WP, Gilday DL. The spectrum of intervertebral disc-space infection in children. *J Bone Joint Surg Am* 1978;60-A:100–108.

336. Ring D, Wenger DR. Magnetic resonance-imaging scans in discitis. *J Bone Joint Surg Am* 1994;76-A:596–601.

337. Fang D, Leong JCY, Fang HSY. Tuberculosis of the upper cervical spine. *J Bone Joint Surg Br* 1983;65-B:47–50.

338. Hsu LCS, Leong JCY. Tuberculosis of the lower cervical spine (C2–C7). *J Bone Joint Surg Br* 1984;66-B:1–5.

339. Govender S, Parbhoo AH, Kumar KPS. Tuberculosis of the cervicodorsal junction. *J Pediatr Orthop* 2001;21:285–287.

340. Eighth Report of the Medical Research Council Working Party on Tuberculosis of the Spine. A 10-year assessment of a controlled trial comparing debridement and anterior spinal fusion in the management of tuberculosis of the spine in patients on standard chemotherapy in Hong Kong. *J Bone Joint Surg Br* 1982;64-B:393–398.

## Hematologic and Oncologic Conditions

341. Romeyn RL, Herkowitz HN. The cervical spine in hemophilia. *Clin Orthop* 1986;210:113–119.

342. Bohlman HH, Sachs BL, Carter JR, et al. Primary neoplasms of the cervical spine. *J Bone Joint Surg Am* 1986;68-A:483–494.

343. Levine AM, Boriani S, Donati D, et al. Benign tumors of the cervical spine. *Spine* 1992;17:S399–S406.

344. Sherk HH, Nolan JP Jr, Mooar PA. Treatment of tumors of the cervical spine. *Clin Orthop* 1988;233:163–167.

345. Raskas DS, Graziano GP, Herzenberg JE, et al. Osteoid osteoma and osteoblastoma of the spine. *J Spinal Disord* 1992;5:204–211.

346. Azouzi EM, Kozlowski K, Marton D, et al. Osteoid osteoma and osteoblastoma of the spine in children: report of 22 cases with brief literature review. *Pediatr Radiol* 1986;16:25–31.

347. Kirwan EOG, Hutton PAN, Pozo JL, et al. Osteoid osteoma and benign osteoblastoma of the spine: clinical presentation and treatment. *J Bone Joint Surg Br* 1984;66-B:159–167.

348. Nemoto O, Moser RP, van Dam BE, et al. Osteoblastoma of the spine: a review of 75 cases. *Spine* 1990;15:1272–1280.

349. Nanduri VR, Jarosz JM, Levitt G, et al. Basilar invagination as a sequela of multisystem Langerhan's cell histiocytosis. *J Pediatr* 2000;136:114–118.

350. Schwartz HS, Pinto M. Osteoblastomas of the cervical spine. *J Spinal Disord* 1990;3:179–182.

351. Ozaki T, Liljenqvist U, Hillmann A, et al. Osteoid osteoma and osteoblastoma of the spine: experiences with 22 patients. *Clin Orthop* 2002;397:394–402.

352. Suttner NJ, Chandy KJ, Kellerman AJ. Osteoid osteomas of the body of the cervical spine. Case report and review of the literature. *Br J Neurosurg* 2002;16:69–71.

353. Cohn RS, Fielding JW. Osteochondroma of the cervical spine. *J Pediatr Surg* 1986;21:997–999.

354. Novick GS, Pavlov H, Bullough PG. Osteochondroma of the cervical spine: report of two cases in pre-adolescent males. *Skeletal Radiol* 1982;3:13–15.

355. Oga M, Nakatani F, Ikuta K, et al. Treatment of cervical cord compression, caused by hereditary multiple exostosis, with laminoplasty. *Spine* 2000;25:1290–1292.

356. Capanna R, Albisinni U, Picci P, et al. Aneurysmal bone cyst of the spine. *J Bone Joint Surg Am* 1985;67-A:527–531.

357. Sherk HH, Nicholson JT, Nixon JE. Vertebra plana and eosinophilic granuloma of the cervical spine in children. *Spine* 1978;3:116–121.

358. Stillwell WT, Fielding JW. Aneurysmal bone cyst of the cervicodorsal spine. *Clin Orthop* 1984;187:144–146.

359. Garneti N, Dunn D, El Gamal E, et al. Cervical spondyloptosis caused by an aneurysmal bone cyst. *Spine* 2003;28:E68–E70.

360. Disch SP, Grubb RL Jr, Gado MH, et al. Aneurysmal bone cyst of the cervicothoracic spine: computed tomographic evaluation of the value of preoperative embolization. *Neurosurgery* 1986;19: 290–293.

361. Gladden ML Jr, Gillingham BL, Hennrikus W, et al. Aneursymal bone cyst of the first cervical vertebrae in a child with percutaneous intralesional injection of calcitonin and methylprednisolone. *Spine* 2000;25:527–530.

362. Zdeblick TA, Warden KE, McCabe R, et al. Cervical stability after foraminotomy. *J Bone Joint Surg Am* 1992;74-A:22–27.

363. Smith MD, Emery SE, Dudley A, et al. Vertebral artery injury during anterior decompression of the cervical spine. *J Bone Joint Surg Br* 1993;75-B:410–415.

364. Sibley RK, Day DL, Dehner LP, et al. Metastasizing chordoma in early childhood: a pathological and immunohistochemical study with review of the literature. *Pediatr Pathol* 1987;7:287–301.

365. Freiberg AA, Graziano GP, Loder RT, et al. Metastatic vertebral disease in children. *J Pediatr Orthop* 1993;13:148–153.

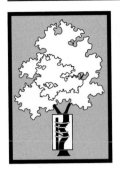

# 23

# The Upper Limb

*Peter M. Waters*

This chapter addresses the evaluation and treatment of the more common upper-limb and hand congenital anomalies, traumatic and posttraumatic conditions, neuropathic problems, and growth deformities. The sections of this chapter examine major diagnostic categories and anatomic regions. The reader will find more information regarding upper-extremity development (Chapter 2), fractures (Chapter 32), and limb deficiency (Chapter 30) in other chapters of this text.

Treatment of any upper limb or hand problem in a child should address the issues of function, growth, cosmetic deformity, and the emotional concerns of the child and family. All are important factors in determining a successful outcome. The orthopaedist's goals are to enhance the ability to place the hand in space; to improve deficiencies in grasp, release, or pinch function; and to improve skin mobility and sensibility (1). The treatment of physeal abnormalities improves growth-related loss of motion and function, and reduces pain and musculoskeletal deformity (2). Extensive time and counseling are important so as to address the concerns of the child and parents regarding the alteration in self-image that can occur with any hand deformity.

# CONGENITAL DEFORMITIES

## Pathogenesis

In utero, the arm bud appears 26 days after fertilization and 24 hours before the appearance of the leg bud. Growth is in a proximal-to-distal manner. Development is guided by the apical ectodermal ridge inducing the mesoderm to condense and differentiate (3). The upper limb anlage is initially continuous and extends to a hand paddle by day 31. The digital rays develop by day 36 with fissuring of the hand paddle, initially in the central rays, followed by the border digits. Mesenchymal differentiation also begins in a proximal-to-distal manner with chondrification, enchondral ossification, joint formation, and muscle and vascular development. Joint formation and digital separation require apoptosis, or programmed cell death. The entire process is complete by 8 weeks after fertilization (4). Other major organ system development is occurring simultaneously, which explains the associated cardiac, craniofacial, musculoskeletal, and renal anomalies that can occur with upper limb malformations.

Homeobox, or HOX genes regulate the development of the limb (5). Their genetic expression controls the timing and extent of growth by regulating mesenchymal cells. At present, the understanding of the genetic basis of limb development, and therefore of the occurrence of congenital anomalies, is expanding rapidly (6–12). For example, a mutation at the HOXD13 site has been identified as a cause of polysyndactyly (13). A further understanding of the role of genetics in limb development may revolutionize the treatment of congenital deficiencies.

Congenital anomalies occur in approximately 6% to 7% of live births, with 1% being multiple anomalies. It has been estimated that between 1 in 531 and 1 in 626 live births involve upper-extremity anomalies (14,15). Only 1% to 2% of these congenital differences are the result of chromosomal abnormalities. However, 75% of 233 missed abortions studied were noted to have an abnormal karyotype, with 18% having a morphologic defect and normal karyotype (16). At present, only a small percentage of these are known to be caused by defined genetic events. In most cases, the cause of the congenital malformation is still unknown, but expanding genetic information provides optimism for increased knowledge in the near future.

## Classification

There is no perfect classification system for congenital differences of the hand and upper limb. The present accepted classification system for congenital differences was proposed by Swanson (17) and revised by the Congenital Anomalies Committee of the International Federation of Societies for Surgery of the Hand (18). This classification is based on embryologic failure, and defines deficiencies as terminal or intercalary, with a subclassification into longitudinal and transverse deficiencies. The subcategories are as follows: (i) failure of formation of parts; (ii) failure of differentiation of parts; (iii) duplication; (iv) overgrowth; (v) undergrowth; (vi) constriction band syndrome; and (vii) generalized skeletal abnormalities. However, there have been reports of inconsistencies in classifying congenital anomalies of the upper limb by this system. A more descriptive method has been shown to be valid (19,20).

This chapter focuses on the major anomalies in each classification group, but presents them by anatomic region. Caring for the child with congenital differences involves more than surgical skill. From the moment of birth, these children may potentially be viewed by their parents, family, and society as being impaired; eventually, they will begin to view themselves the same way (21,22). It is critical that the treating surgeon helps provide the emotional support and caring that allow the parents and child to appropriately grieve the loss of a normal hand (23). It is helpful to provide them with in-depth knowledge of the cause and treatment options (24). This process starts with the initial newborn visit, and continues throughout the growth and development of the child into an independent, self-reliant adult (25). Support groups are useful for many of these children and their families.

The children who have normal central nervous systems will not be impaired. They will merely develop their skills in a "different" way from their peers. They may need the help of skilled and caring parents, siblings, therapists, teachers, coaches, prosthetists, and surgeons in order to achieve their goals and dreams. Being part of helping these children grow into unique and independent adults is exciting and rewarding for the surgeon.

# ENTIRE LIMB INVOLVEMENT

## Neuromuscular

### Cerebral Palsy

Cerebral palsy is a nonprogressive disorder of the central nervous system. It occurs in 5 in 1000 live births, and may be caused by perinatal anoxia, intraventricular hemorrhage, or congenital cerebral vascular accidents. It occurs most commonly in premature infants weighing less than 1500 g (26,27). The resultant hemiplegia or quadriplegia can lead to significant upper-extremity deformities and functional deficits. In hemiplegia, these individuals predominantly use the affected extremity as an assist for the unaffected extremity. In the quadriparetic, both upper limbs will have significant deformities and deficits. The quality of use of an affected extremity is dependent on many factors, including the presence of contractures, voluntary motor control, discriminatory sensibility, learning disabilities, and visual deficits (28–32). This section focuses on the deformities and deficits relating to elbow flexion, forearm pronation, wrist palmar flexion and ulnar deviation, finger flexion, and thumb-in-palm deformity in these patients.

***Upper-limb Contractures.*** Nearly three fourths of patients with hemiplegia develop a forearm pronation contracture (33). The presence of a significant pronation contracture limits the ability to perform bimanual tasks (31,34). Individuals with contractures greater than 60 degrees will either perform activities with one hand or use the dorsum of the affected hand or forearm to assist the unaffected hand. These individuals may benefit from surgical correction of their pronation deformity in order to improve the assistive function of that extremity. This can often be performed with simultaneous procedures to improve thumb-in-palm, wrist palmar flexion, or digital flexion deformities (35).

Elbow flexion contractures are often mild in patients with hemiplegia (33,36). Although approximately 50% of these patients will have a flexion contracture, most of these contractures are less than 30 degrees and do not limit function (37,38). There may be an associated radial head dislocation in a small number of patients, and this should be assessed radiographically before operative intervention (39). Patients with quadriparesis have greater degrees of elbow flexion contracture. However, these contractures rarely affect their ability to use their motorized wheelchairs, computers, or communication boards. In the caredependent, nonfunctional quadriparetic, contractures may become severe enough to affect hygiene and care. If skin breakdown develops or is imminent, then surgery may be necessary.

Wrist and hand involvement are common in cerebral palsy. Limited motor function occurs with: (i) poor release because of wrist and finger flexor spasticity and weak digital extension; (ii) inadequate grasp because of wrist palmar flexion spasticity and weak wrist extension; and (iii) minimal pinch because of thumb-in-palm deformity. Discriminatory sensibility is deficient in more than 50% of these children. Poor voluntary control of the upper extremity limits functional placement of the hand in space (31,33). In addition, many of these children have visual and cognitive abnormalities that further impair hand function. At best, most patients with spasticity have assistive hand function.

These children generally posture into elbow flexion, forearm pronation, wrist and palmar flexion, thumb-in-palm,

and interphalangeal swan-neck deformities. These deformities may be a combination of spasticity and contractures. Pronation deformity and thumb-in-palm contracture seem to affect function the most (33). The combination of neurologic impairment and disuse affects growth in length and girth of the affected arm and hand (33).

Upper-extremity classification systems have been used for assessing function in patients with cerebral palsy (39,40) (Fig. 23.1). The House classification of function has 9 levels, extending from 0 (does not use) to 8 (complete spontaneous use) (Table 23.1). In this useful scheme, there are four subgroups of patient function: 0 (no use), 1 to 3 (passive assist), 4 to 6 (active assist), and 7 and 8 (spontaneous use). Because spasticity changes with stress, growth, and central nervous system changes, it may be difficult on any one visit to accurately define a patient's level of function. This system is used with the input of the patient, family, and physical therapist in order to best define a patient's overall status. It is used for assessing the outcome of treatments (35). Both the Melbourne Assessment of Unilateral Upper Limb Function and the Pediatric Evaluation of Disablility Inventory (PEDI) have been validated for upper-limb function assessment in children with cerebral palsy. The Melbourne Assessment of Unilateral Upper Limb Function has very high internal consistency and high inter- and intraobserver reliability, making it a reliable tool in assessing function and outcome of interventions in patients with cerebral palsy (41,42).

*Treatment*

NONOPERATIVE CARE. In broad terms, the treatment options include: observation of the patient's growth and development; the use of therapy, including splints; injections, such as phenol or Botox; and performing surgical reconstruction.

Physical therapy, starting in infancy, is the standard treatment for children with cerebral palsy. The rationale is that, although the central nervous system deficit is static, the peripheral manifestations of spasticity and muscle imbalance are progressive with growth. By maintaining range of motion with passive therapy, it is hoped that contractures will be prevented (33,43). In addition, it is hoped that the affected child is capable of learned motor behavior leading to functional improvement over time, developmentally, and through formal therapy (44,45). At present, formal therapy is used during the period of infancy. This is most intense in the first year of life, and progresses to a home program with less formal supervision. In many states, early intervention programs end at 3 years of age. Monitoring of function and range of motion are performed less regularly thereafter, sometimes through the school system. During growth spurts that increase spasticity and lessen range of motion, or with specific activities that the patient finds difficult to do, brief periods of formal therapy are often reinitiated, but the therapeutic benefit has not been statistically established (33).

Besides passive range-of-motion and active-use programs, splints are often used. These may be daytime or

**CHILDREN'S HOSPITAL ORTHOPAEDIC HAND SURGERY HEMIPLEGIA EVALUATION**

Date _____ /___ /___

Evaluation Number _____

Involved Upper Extremity  (circle one)    L        R

☐ New Patient  ☐ Return Visit

MR No. _____

Date _____

Pt. Name _____

Date of Birth _____

Sex  (circle one)    M        F

**Parent History**

| | No | Yes | | dk |
|---|---|---|---|---|
| Hand splint ever | ☐ | ☐ | | ☐ |
| Hand splint now | ☐ | ☐ | | ☐ |
| night use | ☐ | ☐ | | ☐ |
| day use | ☐ | ☐ | | ☐ |
| Hx Upper Ext surgery | ☐ | ☐ | | ☐ |
| Green Procedure | ☐ | ☐ | | ☐ |
| Web release | ☐ | ☐ | | ☐ |
| Elbow release | ☐ | ☐ | | ☐ |
| Pronator release | ☐ | ☐ | | ☐ |
| Other UE Surg | ☐ | ☐ | | ☐ |

type: _____

(List date of surgeries. procedure, on back of page)

| | No | Yes | | dk |
|---|---|---|---|---|
| Hx seizures | ☐ | ☐ | | ☐ |

| | low | ave | high | |
|---|---|---|---|---|
| Intelligence | ☐ | ☐ | ☐ | ☐ |
| Motivation | ☐ | ☐ | ☐ | ☐ |

**Sensation Exam**

| | cos | ast | ind | | not test |
|---|---|---|---|---|---|
| Function | ☐ | ☐ | ☐ | | ☐ |

| | mm: | <6 | 6-10 | >10 | | nt |
|---|---|---|---|---|---|---|
| Two-Point Desc. | | ☐ | ☐ | ☐ | | ☐ |

| | # recog | 0 | 1 | 2 | 3 | nt |
|---|---|---|---|---|---|---|
| Obj. Rec. | | ☐ | ☐ | ☐ | ☐ | ☐ |

| | # recog | 0 | 1 | 2 | 3 | nt |
|---|---|---|---|---|---|---|
| Palm graphesthesia | | ☐ | ☐ | ☐ | ☐ | ☐ |

| | No | Yes | | nt |
|---|---|---|---|---|
| Rough | ☐ | ☐ | | ☐ |

| | No | Yes | |
|---|---|---|---|
| Proprioception | ☐ | ☐ | |

**Motor Exam**

| | unable | min | max | | nt |
|---|---|---|---|---|---|
| Grasp | ☐ | ☐ | ☐ | | ☐ |
| Release | ☐ | ☐ | ☐ | | ☐ |

| | No | Yes | | nt |
|---|---|---|---|---|
| Grasp reflex | ☐ | ☐ | | ☐ |
| Key pinch | ☐ | ☐ | | ☐ |
| Pulp pinch | ☐ | ☐ | | ☐ |
| Tip pinch | ☐ | ☐ | | ☐ |

| | I | IIA | IIB | III | nt |
|---|---|---|---|---|---|
| Zancolli | ☐ | ☐ | ☐ | ☐ | ☐ |

| | I | II | | III | nt |
|---|---|---|---|---|---|
| Bleck | ☐ | ☐ | | ☐ | ☐ |
| Mowery | ☐ | ☐ | | ☐ | ☐ |

**THUMB-IN-PALM**

- Type I    MC Adduction
- Type II   MC Ad + MCP flexion
- Type III  MC Ad + MCP ext/instability
- Type IV   MC Ad + MCP/IP flexion

**Deformities**

| | No | Yes | | nt |
|---|---|---|---|---|
| Thumb MCP hyperext. | ☐ | ☐ | | ☐ |
| Thumb MCP stability | ☐ | ☐ | | ☐ |
| First Web Contracture | ☐ | ☐ | | ☐ |
| Swan Deformity | ☐ | ☐ | | ☐ |
| DIP hyperextension | ☐ | ☐ | | ☐ |
| Pronator Deformity | ☐ | ☐ | | ☐ |
| Elbow Flex Deformity | ☐ | ☐ | | ☐ |
| Thumb in Palm | ☐ | ☐ | | ☐ |
| Active Supinator? | ☐ | ☐ | | ☐ |
| Web Angle (degrees) | ☐ | | | |

**Size**

| | | AFF | UNAFF |
|---|---|---|---|
| Circumference | arm | ☐ | ☐ |
| | forearm | ☐ | ☐ |
| Distance | O-MF | ☐ | ☐ |
| | O-UL | ☐ | ☐ |
| Hand width | | ☐ | ☐ |

**ADL**    (1=NU  2=AST  3=Ind)

| | | |
|---|---|---|
| ☐ Buttons | ☐ Hand | ☐ Screw |
| ☐ Pants/Shirt | ☐ Groom | ☐ Knob |
| ☐ Zipper | ☐ Teacup | ☐ Bottle |
| ☐ Utencils | ☐ Knots | ☐ Purse |

**Voluntary Control**

| Tendon | Good | Fair | Poor |
|---|---|---|---|
| EPL | | | |
| AbPL | | | |
| EPB | | | |
| FPL | | | |
| FCR | | | |
| FCU | | | |
| BR | | | |
| ECRB/L | | | |

**Functional Classification**

**Class**

| | | |
|---|---|---|
| 0 | Does not use | Does not use |
| 1 | Poor Passive Assist. | Uses as stabilizing weight only |
| 2 | Fair Passive Assist. | Can hold object placed in hand |
| 3 | Good Passive Assist. | Can hold onto object and stabilize for use in other hand |
| 4 | Poor Active Assist. | Can actively grasp object and hold it weakly |
| 5 | Fair Active Assist. | Can actively grasp object and stabilize it well |
| 6 | Good Active Assist. | Can actively grasp object and manipulate it against other hand |
| 7 | Spontaneous use-partial | Can perform bimanual activities easily and occasionally uses the hand spontaneously |
| 8 | Spontaneous use-complete | Uses the hand completely independently without reference to the other hand |

**Figure 23.1**  Data sheet for prospective analysis of hemiplegic function used at Children's Hospital, Boston.

nighttime splints. As Manske has observed, it is unclear whether they are cost-effective and alter long-term outcome (43). No objective study has been performed. However, most caretakers use splints in children with developing contractures. Daytime splints are recommended only if they improve function in patients with dynamic contractures. Recently, constraint therapy with casting of the unaffected limb has been advocated in order to improve the function of the affected limb in children with hemiplegia (46). A single randomized study has shown this to be effective. It has been shown that patients with hemiplegia do not maximally utilize their motor capabilities in the affected limb in functional tasks (47). Constraint therapy

may better enable these patients to maximize their motor function in the affected limb, but there are emotional issues that make this treatment difficult for some families and caregivers. In a small cohort of patients with cerebral palsy (48), it has been shown that functional electrical stimulation (FES) is effective in the short term (up to 3 months) in improving hand function, when applied to the extensor muscles of the wrist and hand. Its long-term effectiveness and applicability to all types, degrees, and ages of patients with cerebral palsy is still unclear.

Injection may provide useful information about the outcome of surgical procedures. At present, Botox is the

**TABLE 23.1**

**HOUSE CLASSIFICATION OF UPPER EXTREMITY AND HAND FUNCTION FOR PATIENTS WITH CEREBRAL PALSY**

| Level | Designation | Activity Level |
| --- | --- | --- |
| 0 | Does not use | Does not use |
| 1 | Poor passive assist | Uses as stabilizing weight only |
| 2 | Fair passive assist | Can hold on to object placed in hand |
| 3 | Good passive assist | Can hold on to object and stabilize it for use by other hand |
| 4 | Poor active assist | Can actively grasp object and hold it weakly |
| 5 | Fair active assist | Can actively grasp object and stabilize it well |
| 6 | Good active assist | Can actively grasp object and manipulate it against other hand |
| 7 | Spontaneous use, partial | Can perform bimanual activities easily and occasionally uses the hand spontaneously |
| 8 | Spontaneous use, complete | Uses hand completely independently without reference to the other hand |

most common form of neuromuscular injection (35,49), replacing xylocaine (50,51) and phenol (52,53). It is used at an initial dose of 1 to 2 U per kg of body weight, and should not exceed 6 U/kg/month. Injection into pronator, flexor carpi ulnaris (FCU), and thumb adductor are most often performed. Therapy should be performed aggressively to stretch agonistic musculotendinous units and strengthen antagonists. To date, Botox has been most effective in patients with high motivation to train, good motor learning capacity, and no fixed contracture or limiting spasticity (54). Its role in patients with contractures is limited and less effective, although these patients may show the greatest involvement. Its effectiveness in young children has not yet been studied critically. There are several ongoing prospective studies of Botox injections in the upper extremity and hand, so more definitive information should soon be available on the indications and effectiveness of its use in all age groups and at all levels of involvement. At this stage, in our institution, we use Botox injections in the upper limbs in (i) younger patients with marked spasticity or developing contractures; and (ii) older patients with limitations, for whom surgery is not indicated. Complications involve the formation of antibodies to Botox that limit further effective injections and leading to deterioration of upper limb function for the first 1 to 3 weeks postinjection in some patients.

OPERATIVE CARE. The broad indications for surgery in patients with cerebral palsy include: (i) contractures that cause hygiene and care problems not solved by therapy, splints, or casts; (ii) muscle imbalance or contractures that cause functional deficits that may be improved by tendon transfers, musculotendinous lengthening, and/or joint stabilization procedures; and (iii) cosmetic concerns (28–32,55). It may be difficult to identify the individual who will have

improved function through surgical reconstruction. As Smith so aptly pointed out, careful preoperative assessment is necessary in order to select the appropriate patients and operations (27). Video recordings of activities of daily living and validated multiple-task assessment scales, such as the Jebsen scale, can be helpful in defining functional limitations. Preoperative video assessments and House classifications are reliable and useful for surgical planning (56).

Surgery has been shown to effectively improve the level of function in all forms of cerebral palsy (35,57,58). The best candidates are patients with hemiplegia and good voluntary control, sensibility, and motivation. The principle of surgery is to restore muscle imbalance by lengthening or releasing tight, spastic muscles and by augmenting weak, stretched muscles by tendon transfers and tenodesis procedures. Unstable joints need to be stabilized by soft tissue or arthrodesis procedures in order to maximize the outcome of tendon reconstruction. Multiple upper-extremity rebalancing procedures performed under one anesthesia seem to be best. This can also be performed in conjunction with simultaneous lower-extremity procedures if the patient and surgeons can tolerate it. It cannot be stressed enough to the patient and family that surgery will not achieve a normal hand. Even the best outcome will result in deficiencies of function, cosmesis, and sensibility. Patients, families, and surgeons need to be realistic about the expected results. However, in properly selected patients, surgery will clearly improve function and patient satisfaction (35,57,58). This is evident in individuals using the dorsum of the hand or forearm for bimanual tasks. Thumb-in-palm deformity is usually markedly improved with surgery (57). The goal must be well defined and specific to the peripheral manifestation of the incurable, central disorder of cerebral palsy.

Mital cited excellent results with surgical release of elbow flexion contractures in patients with hemiplegia (36). He recommended release of the lacertus fibrosus, Z-lengthening of the biceps tendon, and musculotendinous lengthening of the brachialis fascia. In mild contractures, release of the lacertus fibrosus and musculotendinous lengthening of the brachialis alone may be sufficient.

More extensive elbow contractures are present in severe quadriparetics. The Z-lengthening of the biceps tendon and release of the brachialis fascia advocated by Mital (36) are not sufficient to obtain adequate release in these patients. In patients with contractures greater than 90 degrees and skin breakdown, extensive release of the muscle origins from the medial and lateral epicondyles, biceps and brachialis tendons, and anterior elbow capsule is necessary so as to solve the hygiene and care-related problems that accompany these conditions.

Forearm hyperpronation significantly limits hand function (33) in patients with hemiplegia. Patients are forced to use the dorsum of the forearm for two-handed tasks. Wrist and finger flexion deformities are commonplace in patients with hemiplegia. The FCU is usually the major deforming force at the wrist. Transfer of the FCU to the wrist extensors alleviates the deformity and improves the strength of the antagonist. On occasion, the extensor carpi ulnaris (ECU) is the primary deforming force, as noted by more ulnar deviation than palmar flexion at the wrist. In these situations, the ECU is transferred to the extensor carpi radialis brevis (35). Simultaneous musculotendinous lengthenings of the finger flexors are necessary if the extrinsic finger flexors are tight in the neutral wrist position (32). Otherwise, the patient will develop a disabling clenched fist postoperatively. Z-lengthenings, superficialis-to-profundus flexor tendon transfers, and bony procedures are reserved for patients with severe contractures and limited function. In the unusual patient with passive digital extension but no active digital extension, the FCU, ECU, or pronator teres (PT) can be transferred into the extensor digitorum communis. This will improve both wrist and digital extension.

Thumb-in-palm deformity will limit dynamic pinch and grasp function, and make hygiene difficult to maintain in severe contractures. Static contractures in the web space are corrected with web-space Z-plasties and adductor releases. Hoffer et al. (59) have shown by dynamic electromyography that release of the transverse adductor alone may lead to better pinch postoperatively in selected patients. At times, the static contractures include the flexor pollicis longus and brevis, and these muscles need to be appropriately lengthened or released. Dynamic rebalancing is performed with tendon transfers to the weak abductors and extensors of the thumb. The donor muscles used are numerous, and include the palmaris longus, flexor carpi radialis, and brachioradialis, among others. The recipient tendons include the extensor pollices brevis and longus and the abductor pollicis longus. The treatment for

each patient should be individualized in order to correct his or her deformity and imbalance. Finally, the metacarpophalangeal (MCP) joint should be stable postoperatively. In most patients, this is achieved by muscle rebalancing. On occasion, a capsulodesis or arthrodesis procedure should be performed. Selected patients with thumb-in-palm deformity respond very favorably to surgical intervention (57).

Finally, some patients with cerebral palsy have disabling swan-neck deformities of the interphalangeal joints. If the fingers extend at the proximal interphalangeal (PIP) joint beyond 40 degrees and lock, the position can limit grasp and cause pain. Multiple operations have been advised, including flexor digitorum superficialis tenodesis (32), intrinsic muscle slide (32), lateral band rerouting (60), spiral oblique ligament reconstruction, and resection of the motor branch of the ulnar nerve. The lateral band rerouting procedure provides both intrinsic and extrinsic rebalancing and is effective in correcting the problem.

In summary, patients with cerebral palsy who have disabling dynamic spasticity and fixed contractures of the wrist and hand benefit from surgical reconstruction. Over a 25-year experience, House reported that, for 718 procedures in 134 patients with cerebral palsy, the functional improvement was 2.6 functional levels on the House scale of 0 to 9 (34). Patients with fair and good voluntary control had significantly better improvement in functional use scores than those with poor voluntary control. Often, the more severely involved patients (House levels 0 to 2) respond best to musculotendinous lengthenings, tenodesis, and joint stabilization procedures. More functional patients (House levels 3 to 6) improve with dynamic tendon transfers and releases. Both groups of patients tolerate multiple simultaneous procedures (Fig. 23.2). However, surgery will not create a normal hand. The goals of surgery need to be realistic and attainable. In properly selected patients, surgery will improve assistive function and cosmesis. For many of these children, especially adolescents, and their families, the functional and cosmetic improvements are quite marked and satisfying.

**Complications.** Deformity may recur, or function may fail to improve. Proper preoperative selection so as to assess functional deficits and the patient's level of cooperation may lessen the risk of these problems postoperatively (28). Hematoma formation, wound breakdown, and infection can occur after extensive elbow releases (61). The institutionalized patients with quadriparesis may be most at risk. If wound dehiscence occurs and the joint is exposed, coverage with a rotation flap is the treatment of choice.

### Brachial Plexopathy

Brachial plexus birth palsy is rare, with an incidence between 0.1% and 0.4% of live births (62,63). Fortunately, many infants with minor birth palsies recover fully. These are the infants who initiate recovery of all muscle groups in the first 1 to 2 months of life. However, in other infants,

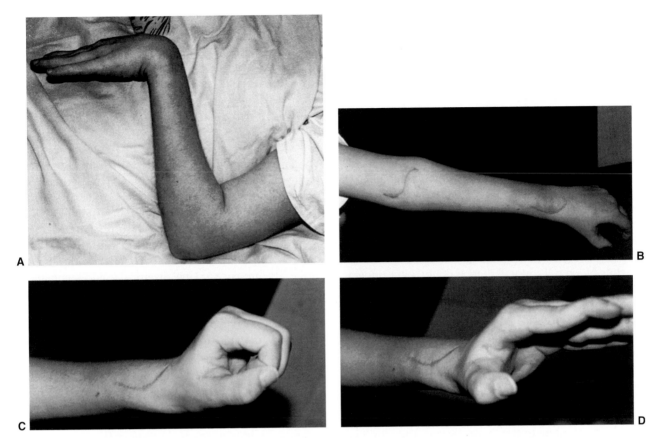

**Figure 23.2**  Clinical photographs of hemiplegic tendon transfers for improving hand and upper limb function. **A:** Preoperative view of dynamic elbow flexion, forearm pronation, wrist flexion, and ulnar deviation with poor assist function. **B:** Postoperative active elbow extension with maintenance of active elbow flexion. **C:** Postoperative active wrist extension with the thumb out of the palm for active pinch. **D:** Postoperative active grasp function with the thumb abducted and extended actively. (Courtesy of Ann Van Heest, MD)

permanent impairment does occur. It is most likely in infants who do not initiate antigravity motor recovery before 5 to 6 months of life (64–68). Horner syndrome is clearly a major risk factor for a poor outcome (67). Most infants have involvement of the upper trunk (C-5 to C-6, causing Erb palsy and, often, additional involvement of C-6 to C-7). Less often, the entire plexus (C-5 to T1) is affected. In rare instances, the lower trunk (C-7 to T1, causing Klumpke palsy) is most affected.

Perinatal risk factors include: infants who are large for gestational age; prolonged labor; previous births with brachial plexopathy; difficult delivery, including extraction techniques; and fetal distress. Shoulder dystocia is the mechanical factor that leads to an upper-trunk lesion in the difficult vertex delivery. Difficult arm extraction in a breech delivery can result in an avulsion injury of the upper trunk (69). The degree of impairment is related to the level and magnitude of injury to the plexus. Neural injury is defined by the type (stretch, rupture, avulsion) and severity (Sunderland grades I to V). Prognosis by natural history has been best defined by the spontaneous rate of recovery of muscle strength in the first 3 to 6 months of infancy. Gilbert and Tassin (68) described the recovery of antigravity biceps function in infancy as a predictor of the outcome of spontaneous recovery. This finding was confirmed in a similar study by Waters (67). Their results showed that infants who did not recover biceps function by 3 months of life were not normal after 2 years of age. Gilbert et al. recommend microsurgical reconstruction of the plexus in the first 3 to 6 months of life for infants who fail to recover biceps function (68,70,71). Michelow et al. (72) noted that return of biceps function alone had a 12% error rate in predicting outcome, as defined by long-term antigravity muscle strength. By using elbow flexion, elbow extension, wrist extension, finger extension, and thumb extension (the Toronto scale), their error rate for predicting outcome decreased to 5%. In this system, each muscle group is scored as 0 (no motion), 1 (motion present but limited), or 2 (normal motion), for a maximum score of 12. A score of less than 3.5 predicted a poor long-term outcome without microsurgery. In all studies, the presence of Horner syndrome, total plexus involvement, and failure of return of function by 3 to 6 months of life indicate a poor long-term outcome.

Clinical examination of an infant for motor-sensory function can be limited. It is important to distinguish true paralysis from the pseudoparalysis that comes with a neonatal clavicle fracture, humeral fracture, or septic shoulder. There can be clinical overlap because fractures also occur in infants with shoulder dystocia and infantile brachial plexopathy. Plain radiographs will identify the infant with clavicle and humeral fractures. In the neonate, these fractures heal within 10 to 21 days. If restriction in range of motion persists after 1 month, there will most likely be a concomitant brachial plexopathy. In the rare infant with a septic shoulder there will be evidence of systemic illness (altered vital signs, change in appetite, toxicity), marked irritability with glenohumeral range of motion, and abnormal white blood cell count. If there is doubt, ultrasonography will reveal the effusion, and arthrocentesis will be confirmatory.

The pupils should be assessed for Horner syndrome. Motor examination is limited to observation of spontaneous activity and stimulated movement by primitive reflexes in the infant. The Moro startle reflex and the asymmetric tonic neck reflex can elicit upper-trunk movement in infants in the first 6 months of life. Classification of nerve injury in the ambulatory child has included physical assessment according to the Mallet system. The modified Mallet system classifies upper-trunk function by grading hand-to-mouth, hand-to-neck, and hand-on-spine activity,

global abduction, and global external rotation from 0 (no function) to V (normal function). Grades II, III, and IV are illustrated (Fig. 23.3). The Toronto active motion scale is also utilized to define the degree of motor recovery, grades I through IV being gravity-assisted and grades V through VII being against gravity. These classification systems have been shown to be reliable in intra- and interobserver analysis (73).

Radiography can demonstrate an associated fracture of the clavicle or proximal humerus. Radiographic assessment of the severity of brachial plexus injury has used myelography, combined computed tomography (CT) scan and myelography, and magnetic resonance imaging (MRI). Kawai et al. (74) compared the results of all three techniques with operative findings. MRI and combined myelography and CT scan were more reliable than myelography alone. The presence of large diverticulae and meningoceles was indicative of root avulsion. Small diverticulae were diagnostic only 60% of the time. Electrodiagnostic studies, with electromyography and nerve conduction studies, are diagnostic of avulsion if there is no reinnervation after 3 months of age. However, the presence of reinnervation does not indicate the long-term quality of muscle recovery.

*Pathoanatomy.* Understanding the normal anatomy of the brachial plexus is critical to assessing and caring for an infant or child with brachial plexus palsy (Fig. 23.4). The brachial plexus supplies every muscle of the upper extremity except the trapezius. It is made up of spinal cord nerve

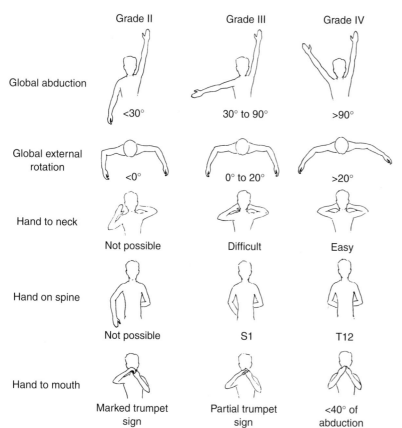

**Figure 23.3** Mallet classification for function about the shoulder in patients with brachial plexus birth palsy. Grade 0 is no function; grade V is normal function; and grades II through IV are depicted for hand-to-mouth, hand-to-neck, external rotation, and hand-to-sacrum activity.

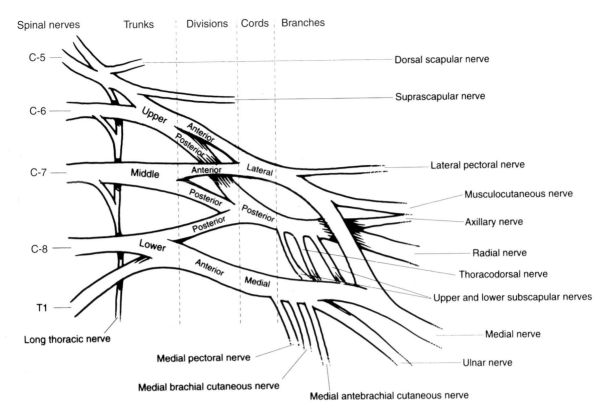

| Spinal nerves | Trunks | Divisions | Cords | Branches |

C-5 — ————————————— Dorsal scapular nerve

————————————— Suprascapular nerve

C-6 —

Upper

Anterior

Posterior

C-7 — Middle

Anterior

Lateral ————————————— Lateral pectoral nerve

Posterior

Posterior

————————————— Musculocutaneous nerve

————————————— Axillary nerve

C-8 — Lower

Posterior

Anterior

Medial

————————————— Radial nerve

————————————— Thoracodorsal nerve

————————————— Upper and lower subscapular nerves

T1 —

————————————— Medial nerve

Long thoracic nerve

————————————— Ulnar nerve

Medial pectoral nerve

Medial brachial cutaneous nerve

Medial antebrachial cutaneous nerve

**Figure 23.4** Brachialplexus anatomy.

root contributions from C-5 to T1. Prefixed cords (22% of the specimens) receive a contribution from C-4. Postfixed cords are rare (1%) and receive a contribution from T2. The C-5 and C-6 roots join to form the upper trunk. The C-7 root alone becomes the middle trunk. The C-8 and T1 roots become the lower trunk. Each trunk has an anterior and a posterior division. The anterior divisions of the upper and middle parts of the trunk form the lateral cord. The posterior divisions of all three parts of the trunk form the posterior cord. The anterior division of the lower trunk continues as the medial cord. The terminal branches of the cords form the major nerves of the upper extremity. The upper and lower subscapular and thoracodorsal nerves branch off from the posterior cord before it bifurcates into the radial and axillary nerves. The medial cord branches are the medial pectoral, medial brachial cutaneous, and medial antebrachial cutaneous nerves, terminating in the medial contribution to the median nerve and the ulnar nerve. The lateral cord supplies the lateral pectoral nerve and the lateral branch of the median nerve, and terminates as the musculocutaneous nerve. In infantile brachial plexopathy, any of these nerves can be affected. However, the most severe injuries are avulsions of the nerve roots. The most common injuries are postganglionic ruptures of the upper trunk.

### Treatment

*Nonsurgical.* As mentioned in the preceding text, all infants with brachial plexus birth palsies should be monitored for

spontaneous recovery in the first 3 to 6 months of life. During this time it is important to maintain glenohumeral range of motion, especially passive external rotation (75). This will lessen the risk of progressive glenohumeral dysplasia and dislocation (65–67,75–78). Many infants will initiate recovery in the first 6 to 8 weeks of life, and progress to a normal result. Infants who do not initiate recovery until after 3 months of life may be candidates for microsurgery or reconstructive surgery.

*Microsurgery*

The optimal timing for microsurgical intervention is still debated. The range used clinically is from 1 month to after 6 months of life (63,67–71). The indications include absence of biceps recovery, Toronto score less than 3.5, and total plexopathy with Horner syndrome. At present, most centers throughout the world agree that an infant with a flail extremity and Horner syndrome should have microsurgical reconstruction between 1 and 3 months of life. A child with complete absence of upper-trunk function (shoulder abduction, elbow flexion) should have surgery between 3 and 6 months of life. However, the controversy regarding the best timing for microsurgery, whether it should be done at 3, 4, 5, 6 or even 9 months, is still unresolved. This creates difficulties for parents who are trying to do what is best for their infants. There is an ongoing prospective study sponsored by the Pediatric Orthopedic Society of North America (POSNA) which hopes to resolve this issue. Microsurgery involves resection of the neuroma and bypass nerve grafting or nerve transfer procedures. On the basis of the information published in peer-reviewed journals, there seems to be no role for neurolysis alone in a patient at any age, especially in the infant older than 6 months of age. The recommended surgical technique involves exploration of the brachial plexus and reconstruction of avulsion and nonconducting rupture injuries. If the proximal trunk or nerve roots are intact, sural nerve grafting across the neuroma is preferred. In the presence of an avulsion, intercostal and spinal accessory nerve transfers are performed. The surgery will not restore normal function, but there is improvement when compared to natural history outcome alone (67,68). The controversy regarding the exact timing of intervention (e.g., whether to intervene at 3 months of age or at 6 months of age in an infant with no upper-trunk function) may not be resolved without a prospective, randomized study.

*Shoulder Surgery*

Children with chronic upper-trunk plexopathy may develop external rotation weakness and internal rotation contractures about the shoulder. This muscle imbalance will progressively alter the glenohumeral joint (65,66) (Table 23.2). Function, especially with the arm in above-horizontal activities, will be impaired (64,66). These children clearly benefit from surgical intervention (66,72). In the situation of dislocation in an infant (65,76,78,79), open reduction and capsulorrhaphy or arthroscopic release and reduction are indicated (Fig. 23.5). Such children have limited external rotation that affects function.

In young children with nearly normal glenohumeral joints (normal or mild increase in glenoid retroversion, grades I and II) or slight posterior subluxation (mild, grade III), anterior musculotendinous lengthening of the pectoralis major and/or subscapularis muscles and posterior latissimus dorsi and teres major transfer to the rotator cuff (77,80) will improve function (67). In addition, dynamic

### TABLE 23.2

**COMPUTED TOMOGRAPHY/MAGNETIC RESONANCE IMAGING (CT/MRI) CLASSIFICATION OF GLENOHUMERAL DEFORMITY IN CHRONIC BRACHIAL PLEXUS BIRTH PALSIES**

| Type | CT scan/MRI findings |
|------|----------------------|
| I | Normal glenohumeral joint |
| II | Minimal glenoid hypoplasia (>5 degrees increased retroversion) |
| III | Posterior subluxation of the humeral head |
| IV | Development of a false glenoid |
| V | Posterior flattening of the humeral head |
| VI | Infantile dislocation |
| VII | Proximal humeral growth arrest |

Findings are additive, with increasing severity from type I to type V. From Waters PM, Smith GR, Jaramillo D. Glenohumeral deformity secondary to brachial plexus birth palsy. *J Bone Joint Surg* 1998;80(5): 668–677, with permission.

rebalancing of the muscle forces about the shoulder at a young age has the potential advantages of restoring more normal anatomy and preventing progressive glenohumeral joint deformity. Glenohumeral joint remodeling appears to have limited utility with extraarticular musculotendinous rebalancing procedures alone. The benefit of arthroscopic release and reduction, as opposed to open reduction and stabilization, is still unclear in terms of long-term remodeling of a dysplastic joint, but both have been shown to be effective in reducing the humeral head, as verified by postoperative MRI. In the older child with more established and progressive deformity of the glenohumeral joint (more severe posterior glenoid flattening, advanced grade III), development of a false glenoid (grade IV) (Fig. 23.6), or humeral head dislocation and deformity (grade V), the deterioration of the joint is usually too advanced to tolerate a soft-tissue procedure. In these situations, humeral derotation osteotomy is indicated and will also improve function (67).

On rare occasions there are patients who need both osteotomy and tendon transfer. These patients are in the middle range of deformity (grade III). To date, it has been difficult to identify this small subset of patients preoperatively. Therefore, the transfer alone is performed initially, and only if the result is suboptimal more than 1 year later is the secondary-stage osteotomy performed. The role of glenoid osteotomy, its risks, and its benefits are still being defined as it relates to grade III and mild grade IV patients.

*Elbow and Forearm Reconstruction*

Elbow flexion and forearm supination deformities can occur with a permanent Klumpke (C-8 to T1) or mixed brachial plexus lesion. Contractures, bony deformity, and joint instability are the result of muscle imbalance in a growing child. In the rare case of a patient with residual C-8 to T1 neuropathy with recovery of C-5 to C-6 function, the elbow and forearm deformities are secondary to an intact biceps muscle in the presence of weak or absent triceps, pronator teres, and pronator quadratus muscles. Progressively, the biceps creates an elbow flexion and supination deformity from unopposed muscular activity. Soft-tissue contractures develop, followed by rotation deformities of the radius and ulna (81). Radial head dislocation may occur (82). The wrist and hand are often in extreme dorsiflexion because of unopposed wrist dorsiflexors. In the position of forearm supination, gravity further exacerbates the dorsiflexion deformity. The patient is left without use of the hand, and performs bimanual activities using the volar and ulnar forearm as an assist. Often, shoulder abduction and internal rotation are required in order to improve assistive function. Activities that require simultaneous elbow flexion and forearm pronation, such as dressing, eating, and writing (83), are significantly limited. In addition, the forearm and hand posture is a major cosmetic concern to both the patient and the family (84).

The biceps tendon can be treated by Z-lengthening and rerouting around the radius to convert it from a supinator

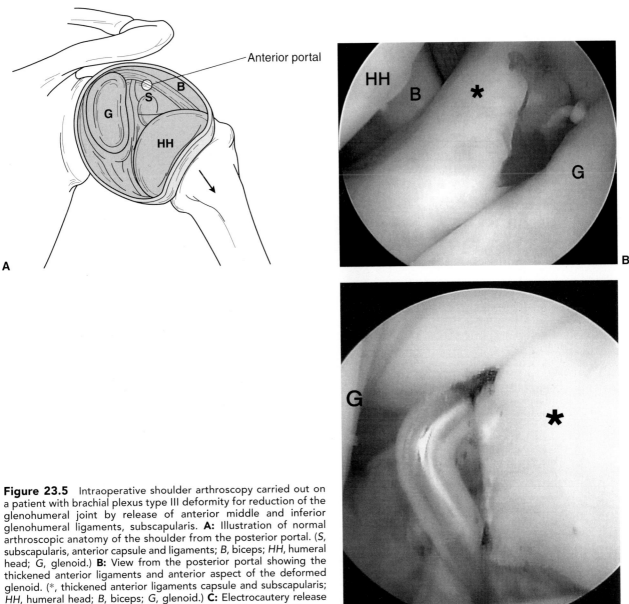

**Figure 23.5** Intraoperative shoulder arthroscopy carried out on a patient with brachial plexus type III deformity for reduction of the glenohumeral joint by release of anterior middle and inferior glenohumeral ligaments, subscapularis. **A:** Illustration of normal arthroscopic anatomy of the shoulder from the posterior portal. (*S*, subscapularis, anterior capsule and ligaments; *B*, biceps; *HH*, humeral head; *G*, glenoid.) **B:** View from the posterior portal showing the thickened anterior ligaments and anterior aspect of the deformed glenoid. (*, thickened anterior ligaments capsule and subscapularis; *HH*, humeral head; *B*, biceps; *G*, glenoid.) **C:** Electrocautery release of the anterior middle and inferior glenohumeral ligaments. A concomitant latissimus dorsi and teres major tendon transfer was perfomed along with posterior capsulorraphy.

to a pronator. This will improve elbow extension and forearm pronation. Surgically, the biceps tendon is identified as it inserts into the radial tuberosity. By dissecting lateral to the tendon, the brachial artery and median nerve are protected. A long Z-plasty of the tendon is performed from the musculotendinous junction to the insertion site. The distal attachment of the tendon is rerouted posteriorly around the radial neck, from medial to lateral. Care must be taken to stay adjacent to the radial neck so as to avoid injury or compression of the radial nerve. The distal tendon is reattached to its proximal counterpart in a lengthened position. This converts the biceps into a forearm pronator (83–85).

In the presence of a supination contracture, if the rerouting procedure alone is carried out, it will fail because of recurrence of the deformity. Zancolli (83) suggested performing simultaneous interosseous membrane release. However, active pronation was maintained in only 50% of patients who underwent this procedure. Bony correction of the forearm deformity can be performed more predictably. Manske et al. (85) proposed staged procedures of tendon rerouting and forearm osteoclasis. Waters and Simmons (84) described simultaneous tendon rerouting and osteotomy, using internal fixation to avoid multiple operations and loss of alignment. In both techniques, the forearm is positioned in approximately 20 to 30 degrees of pronation.

These patients clearly have significant improvement in their functional capabilities. Bimanual tasks, such as lifting, carrying, and transferring, are easier. The affected extremity

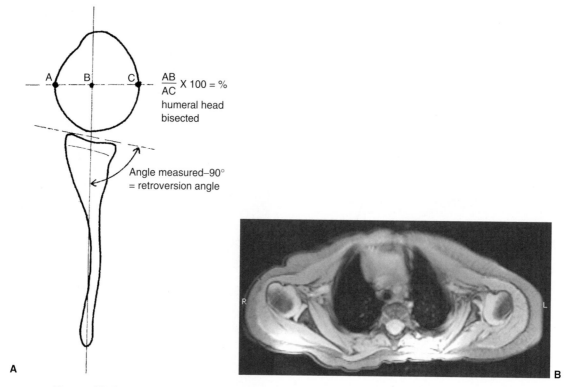

**A**

**B**

**Figure 23.6** **A:** Schematic showing the method of measuring the glenoscapular angle (glenoid vision) and the percentage of posterior subluxation of the humeral head. To measure the glenoscapular angle, a line is drawn parallel to the scapula and a second line is drawn tangential to the joint. The second line connects the anterior and posterior margins of the glenoid. The cartilaginous margins are used on magnetic resonance images. The osseous margins are used on computed tomographic scans. The intersecting line connects the center point of the first line (approximately the middle of the glenoid fossa) and the medial aspect of the scapula. The angle in the posterior medial quadrant is measured with a goniometer (*arrow*), and 90 degrees is then subtracted from this measurement to determine the glenoid version. The percentage of posterior subluxation is measured by defining the percentage of the humeral head that is anterior to the same scapular line. The greatest circumference of the head is measured as the distance from the scapular line to the anterior portion of the head. This ratio [the distance to the anterior aspect of the humeral head (*AB*) divided by the circumference of the humeral head (*AC*), multiplied by 100] is the percentage of subluxation. **B:** Magnetic resonance imaging of a type IV deformity with posterior humeral head subluxation and the development of a false glenoid. The glenoid is markedly retroverted. The contralateral glenohumeral joint is normal for age.

becomes a better assistive extremity to the unaffected side. The wrist and hand now have greater assisted palmar flexion and resolution of their dorsiflexion deformity. In addition, the patients are usually pleased with the cosmetic results.

### Arthrogryposis

Arthrogryposis multiplex congenita is a syndrome of unknown cause that presents at birth with contractures of the joints and muscle weakness (see Chapter 9). The incidence is approximately 1 in 3,000 live births (86). The clinical syndrome is variable and includes classic arthrogryposis (amyoplasia), distal arthrogryposis, and syndromic involvement (87). The classification of arthrogryposis makes the distinction between myopathic and neuogenic types; however, muscle biopsies and electromyography have not been shown to be helpful in determining the mode of therapy for these children (88). Intelligence is usually average or above average. Sensibility is normal.

Upper-extremity involvement is frequent, with 72% of the 114 patients in the Gibson and Urs study being affected (89). The wrist was most commonly involved, followed by the hand, elbow, and shoulder. In the classic presentation, the elbow is usually contracted in extension at birth. The shoulder is internally rotated with the forearm pronated. Often, there is wrist palmar flexion and ulnar deviation, and the fingers have flexion deformities. The thumb is usually adducted and flexed in the palm (89–91). These children often have incomplete syndactylies of all web spaces. The first web-space contracture is usually the most functionally significant. There is usually marked intrinsic muscle weakness. There may be camptodactyly or symphalangism of the PIP joints. All of this will limit hand function in these children (92).

Involvement is generally bilateral. The absence of both passive and active elbow flexion is a significant functional liability in these children. The goal of orthopaedic management of the arthrogrypotic elbow is to improve self-feeding and independent hygiene skills by achieving both passive and active elbow flexion. The goal of treatment of the hand is to improve pinch, grasp, and release functions.

### Treatment

*Nonoperative Care.* Initial care is with physical therapy to improve passive range of motion. Repetitive, gentle, passive manipulation of the involved joints may progressively lessen the contracture. This process is tedious and requires meticulous, gentle care by both the therapist and the family. Corrective splints and serial casts have been used with varying success. Caution is necessary because of the risk of fractures or dislocations that can occur as a complication of aggressive treatment of resistant contractures. At the elbow, the goal of therapy is to achieve at least 90 degrees of passive elbow flexion by 2 years of age. Most patients can achieve the desired passive elbow flexion through therapy (93). However, if this is not obtained, operative posterior elbow release and triceps V-Y lengthening are recommended (93–97). When passive elbow flexion is obtained, therapy should then emphasize the use of adaptive trunk sway, head tilt, and table-assisted passive elbow flexion to improve feeding and hygiene tasks. Finally, if subsequent active elbow flexion does not develop, active elbow flexion tendon transfer should be considered at approximately 5 years of age (93). Most of these children will have deficient biceps and brachialis musculature, and will fail to develop active elbow flexion.

Initial treatment of the wrist and hand should involve passive range of motion and nighttime splinting. The goal of therapy in the hand is to improve motion of the joints and digital strength. Fortunately, in many children the condition improves with growth and therapy during the first several years of life. Serial casting or splinting is often used for the wrist deformity, but this procedure is associated with a high rate of recurrence. If passive motion cannot be improved, surgical releases and tendon transfers may be necessary (98).

### Operative Care

POSTERIOR CAPSULOTOMY AND TRICEPS LENGTHENING. As mentioned in the preceding text, children who fail to achieve a functional arc of flexion at the elbow with manipulative therapy, splints, and casts, are candidates for operative elbow posterior capsulotomy and triceps lengthening. Surgery can be performed when the child is 2 years of age. If it is delayed well beyond this age, progressive bony deformity can occur. The goal of operative intervention is to achieve at least 90 degrees of passive elbow flexion. Initially, the dominant extremity should have surgery. The presence of passive elbow flexion will improve independence in feeding, hygiene, play, and school activities (84,93).

Surgical exposure is by a standard posterior approach to the elbow. The triceps tendon is incised in an inverted V. The angle of the V should be acute enough to allow for appropriate triceps lengthening. The ulnar nerve is protected during the medial incision of the tendon. The distal flap of the triceps is elevated from the elbow capsule, but often the triceps and the capsule are confluent distally. The triceps lengthening alone usually does not improve passive elbow flexion. A transverse incision in the elbow capsule is then made. Full passive elbow flexion is gained. The triceps tendon is lengthened in a V-Y manner at 90 degrees of flexion.

TENDON TRANSFERS FOR ELBOW FLEXION. Children with arthrogryposis who have passive elbow flexion of greater than 90 degrees and no active elbow flexion are candidates for tendon transfer. The transfers to be considered include: (i) triceps (93,94); (ii) pectoralis major using the sternocostal origin; (iii) pectoralis major using the entire musculature on a neurovascular pedicle (95); (iv) latissimus dorsi (93,96); (v) lateral and proximal reinsertion of the flexor-pronator origin; (vi) sternocleidomastoid with a free tendon graft; and (vii) pectoralis minor with a free tendon graft. Each of these transfers has been described in limited series in the arthrogrypotic elbow. Until recently, no objective criteria had been proposed for comparing the results of these various transfers (84,93). The muscle considered for transfer must be expendable and of sufficient strength to function actively against gravity after transfer. Each transfer has its inherent negative attributes: triceps transfer may weaken assistive ambulation in patients with lower-extremity involvement, and may result in a flexion contracture; pectoralis major transfer may create asymmetric breast appearance in women; Steindler flexorplasty may worsen wrist and finger flexion contractures. Information gained to date indicates that the triceps transfer is most effective in improving strength, active range of motion, and function (84,93).

The triceps muscle is strong in most children with arthrogryposis. With transfer, it is usually successful in providing active elbow flexion in a functional arc. However, the triceps is important for crutch ambulation, rising from a sitting position, and wheelchair transfers in patients with lower-extremity involvement and should be used cautiously for tendon transfer in these children. This operation involves the transfer of the antagonist to elbow flexion and leaves the patient without an active elbow extensor postoperatively. This can lead to progressive elbow flexion deformity with growth (93).

There are two options for transfer of the pectoralis major muscle for elbow flexion. The first choice is transfer of the sternocostal origin, as originally described by Clark (99). This transfer can be problematic because the partial transfer may be too weak to provide antigravity strength for feeding and facial hygiene. In addition, the pectoralis major muscle crosses the shoulder and may lose strength in trying to move both the shoulder and the elbow.

The second choice is transfer of the entire pectoralis major muscle on its neurovascular pedicles, as advocated by Carroll and Kleinman (95) and Doyle et al. (100). This operation has had favorable results in limited series of arthrogrypotic elbows. It involves transferring the insertion of the pectoralis major to the acromion. The origins of the clavicular and sternocostal heads, with attached anterior rectus abdominis fascia, are inserted distally into the proximal radius. The medial and lateral pectoral nerves and the lateral thoracic vessels are preserved. This transfer has the mechanical advantage of a linear contraction for elbow flexion and does not involve the loss of any strength in stabilizing or moving the shoulder. The proximal advancement of the insertion to the acromion or clavicle improves the lever arm and mechanical advantage of the transfer. In addition, the pectoralis minor can be transferred with the pectoralis major for further strength of transfer. However, it may create an asymmetric appearance of the breasts in women, and this has been raised as an argument against transfer (84).

In patients with significant lower-extremity involvement, with weak triceps or pectorals, or with failed pectoralis major or triceps transfers, a bipolar latissimus dorsi transfer, as described by Zancolli and Mitre (96), may be the optimal choice. Preoperative assessment of the strength of the latissimus is important before transfer, but at times this is difficult to assess. An experienced pediatric physical therapist with extensive muscle evaluation experience may be helpful. Biopsy of the muscle has been tried, but is not predictive of outcome with transfer.

In summary, physical therapy should be initiated in infancy to obtain and maintain passive range of motion of the elbow. This will frequently result in passive elbow flexion of greater than 90 degrees. If by 24 months of age nearly full passive elbow flexion has not been achieved, elbow capsulotomy and triceps lengthening are recommended. After 4 years of age, tendon transfer for elbow flexion in the dominant arm is recommended, with consideration given to intelligence, ipsilateral and contralateral upper-limb function, lower-extremity involvement, and available motors for transfer. All transfers have had success, but partial or complete triceps-to-biceps transfer gives the most predictably good results (84,93).

WRIST AND HAND RECONSTRUCTION. The wrist palmar flexion contracture is addressed with FCU lengthening or transfer to the wrist extensors. Unfortunately, in many of these children the transfer is more of a tenodesis procedure than a dynamic transfer. In addition, there is often bony deformity, even in the very young. Smith (27) had recommended a proximal row carpectomy to correct the wrist flexion contracture. However, there are frequently carpal coalitions present that preclude that procedure. A dorsal, carpal, closing-wedge osteotomy can correct the deformity in the presence of a carpal coalition. This is an excellent procedure to correct the bone and wrist joint deformity that does not respond to therapy (91). Simultaneous FCU transfer can be performed to rebalance the wrist. An alternative

to carpal osteotomy is a dorsal closing osteotomy of the radius and ulna dorsal osteotomies (87). However, these create an "S" deformity to the distal forearm, and physeal remodeling with growth tends to lead to recurrent wrist flexion deformity.

The thumb-in-palm contracture is addressed with a Z-plasty syndactyly release. Care must be taken not to over-release the adductor, because it may be providing the bulk of the pinch strength. Dynamic transfers for thumb abduction and extension are predominantly tenodesis procedures because of the limited strength of the donor muscles. Many of these children will have permanent limited motion and strength in their hands. Fortunately, their high level of intelligence allows them to be very adaptive in their functioning.

## ELBOW AND FOREARM REGION

### Congenital Dislocations

#### Congenital Radial Head Dislocations
Congenital dislocation of the radial head is a rare condition that may not be diagnosed until school age. It is usually an isolated condition, but it may be present in association with other congenital malformations and syndromes, including arthrogryposis and Cornelia de Lange, Larsen, and nail-patella syndromes (101–104). It may be associated with radioulnar synostosis (105,106) or other musculoskeletal anomalies, such as congenital hip dislocation, club feet, brachydactyly, clinodactyly, tibial fibular synostosis, congenital below-elbow amputation, and radial or ulnar club hand. Dislocations associated with Madelung deformity or familial osteochondromatosis (106) may be acquired, and will be considered elsewhere in this chapter.

Congenital radial head dislocation may be bilateral or unilateral (107). It is defined by the direction of subluxation or dislocation. Most congenital dislocations are posterior or posterolateral. It is important to distinguish the congenital dislocation from the posttraumatic dislocation. Because the condition frequently presents late, this distinction can be confusing (103,107). This is especially true for unilateral anterior dislocations in otherwise healthy children (108–110). Radiographic criteria have been established to distinguish this lesion from a chronic, traumatic dislocation. These include: a small, dome-shaped radial head; a hypoplastic capitellum; ulnar bowing with volar convexity in the anterior dislocation and dorsal convexity in the posterior dislocation; and a longitudinal axis of the radius that does not bisect the capitellum. The presence of these characteristics in the absence of any history of trauma to the affected elbow has been seen as evidence of a congenital radial head dislocation (84,103,111–116). In addition, bilateral involvement, the presence of other musculoskeletal or systemic malformations, and a positive family history make a congenital cause more likely.

*Clinical and Radiographic Features.*  Children with radial head dislocations often present after infancy. The most common reasons for presentation are (i) limited elbow extension; (ii) posterolateral elbow mass/prominence; and (iii) pain with activities, especially athletics (84,117). The elbow extension loss is frequently less than 30 degrees, and not of functional significance. This loss of motion is usually not noted early in life. The mass may be noted in infancy. Radiocapitellar incongruity can be a cause of pain and disability later in life (107,117). Unfortunately, many children present late with pain resulting from radiocapitellar articular changes. There is often chronic discomfort with school and sports activities. On occasion, these children may present with an acute loss of motion attributable to a loose osteochondral fragment. Some individuals remain asymptomatic, and the cosmesis of the deformity is their major concern.

On physical examination, the elbow may have cubitus valgus. A flexion contracture of up to 30 degrees often occurs with a posterior subluxation/dislocation. Hyperextension and/or loss of flexion may occur with an anterior dislocation. The radial head is palpable in its dislocated position. A congenital dislocation is not reducible by forceful manipulation, and should not be misinterpreted as a nursemaid's pulled elbow or a Monteggia lesion. There is usually limited forearm rotation, with supination being affected more than pronation. Clicking and crepitus may be present when there is intraarticular pathology (84).

Radiographs reveal the subluxation/dislocation (Fig. 23.7). The longitudinal axis of the radius does not bisect the capitellum, regardless of the angle of the radiograph. The radius and ulna are of different lengths. The ulna is bowed, with volar convexity in an anterior dislocation and dorsal convexity in the more common posterior dislocation. The capitellum is hypoplastic. The radial head will be dome-shaped, with a long, narrow radial neck.

*Natural History.*  The presence of a congenital dislocated radial head is not an indication for operative intervention. Many patients with this disorder have no functional limitation and no pain. Their mild limitation of motion may not restrict them in any significant way. The degree of cubitus valgus is usually mild, and does not seem to put them at risk for ulnar neuropathy. Therefore, in most cases a definitive diagnosis followed by observation is most appropriate. If the patient develops pain, functional or progressive limitation of motion, or restriction of elbow-related activities, then surgery needs to be considered (84).

### Treatment

*Operative Care.*  Ideally, the care of a congenital dislocated radial head would involve open reduction and restoration of normal anatomy. This has led many surgeons to consider open reduction of a congenital dislocation if the child presents in infancy (101,105,111,118). The logic is that if the radial head can be reduced early in infancy, the deformity of the capitellum and the forearm may not occur or remodel with growth. This may prevent the long-term complications of pain, loss of motion, and osteochondral loose bodies. However, there have been only a small number of published cases of open reduction of congenital radial head dislocations (105,118,119). Techniques have included ulnar osteotomy and lengthening, radial shortening and osteotomy, annular ligamentous reconstruction, and the use of limb-lengthening devices to reduce the radial head (115,118–120). Sachar and Mih's report of open reduction through an anconeus approach, followed by annular ligament reconstruction, is the most promising series to date. They described seven cases of open reduction of a congenitally dislocated radial head with good success (118). Their operative findings included an abnormality of the annular ligament that was surgically correctable. The indications for this procedure, and the age limit, are still being defined in this relatively rare condition. It is reasonable in specialized centers to consider open reduction of the congenitally dislocated radial head in the infant younger than 1 to 2 years of age, provided the family is well informed of the *limited* nature of the information regarding this procedure. Hopefully, clinical surgical research in this area will define the indications and techniques for open reduction and annular ligament reconstruction in congenital radial head dislocations.

Most children with congenital radial head dislocation present later than infancy. Therefore, the most common procedures for this problem are excision of loose bodies and excision of the radial head. The indications for excision of a loose osteochondral fragment are the presence of

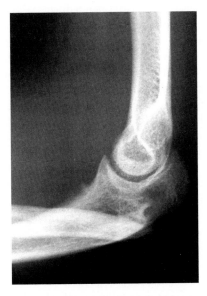

**Figure 23.7**  Lateral radiograph of congenital posterolateral dislocation of the radial head. There is evidence of tapering of the radial head and neck posteriorly, bowing of the ulna posteriorly, and a small dome-shaped radial head. These patients often have limited elbow extension and develop intraarticular pain at the abnormal radiocapitellar articulation in adolescence.

pain, clicking or locking, and loss of motion. Usually, degenerative changes are too advanced for repair of the osteochondral fragment. There is some controversy regarding the indications and timing for excision of the radial head. In the skeletally immature patient, the concern is the potential development of postoperative complications (see "Complications," below). These concerns have not been supported in the published literature on excision of the congenitally dislocated radial head. Most of these children do not present until adolescence with pain or progressive restriction of motion. In our series, the youngest patient with excision of a symptomatic congenital radial head without complication was 8 years of age (107). However, the presence of an asymptomatic dislocated radial head alone, without painful, progressive restricted range of motion, is not an indication for radial head excision. Indications for radial head excision must include progressive pain, progressive loss of motion, and progressive restriction of activities (84), regardless of age.

COMPLICATIONS. Throughout the 20th century, standard textbooks and journal articles have denounced the concept of radial head excision in the skeletally immature individual. Postoperative complications of progressive cubitus valgus and potential associated ulnar neuropathy, proximal migration of the radius with recurrent radiocapitellar impingement, radioulnar synostosis, and reformation of the radial head have been cited (111,112,121–123). However, most of these problems occurred after radial head excisions to treat trauma. The admonishment never to excise a radial head in a skeletally immature individual still holds true in the posttraumatic situation. These complications are rare after excision for congenital radial head dislocations (107).

Reformation of the radial head is the most common problem with excision of a congenital dislocation (122, 124,125). If it leads to recurrent radiocapitellar impingement, limitation of motion, and/or pain, then repeat radial head excision should be performed. Wrist pain does occur in the long term but seems to be mild and nonrestrictive (107). Fortunately, iatrogenic radial nerve injury is rare.

### Congenital Humeroulnar Dislocations

Dislocation of the ulnotrochlear joint is exceedingly rare. Mead and Martin described a family with aplasia of the trochlea and humeroulnar dislocations (126). Ulnotrochlear dislocations have also been seen in hyperelasticity syndromes. These situations are rarer than the unusual posttraumatic persistent or recurrent dislocation.

A congenital dislocation will result in limited range of elbow motion that can affect function. The dislocation is usually palpable on examination. There may be axial malalignment, such as cubitus valgus. If severe, the valgus deformity can result in ulnar neuropathy. In recurrent dislocations secondary to hyperelasticity or associated with syndromes such as Rubinstein-Taybi syndrome (127), the elbow instability is palpable and even audible on examination.

On occasion, the recurrent instability can lead to osteochondral injury that will cause pain, clicking, or even locking on examination.

Elbow dislocation can also be seen with ulnar dysplasia and ulnar dimelia (128–131). The dysplastic ulnotrochlear joint in ulnar club hand can lead to elbow problems that limit motion and function. Ulnar dimelia, or mirror hand, is exceedingly rare. The forearm and elbow in this condition consist of two ulnae and no radius. This means that there are two olecranon processes articulating with the distal humerus. There are usually two poorly defined trochleae and no capitellum present. The olecranon processes may face one another. There is significant limitation of elbow and forearm rotation (84,132,133).

If the child presents before ossification of the secondary centers, it may be difficult to define the dislocation anatomically by plain radiography. MRI will be diagnostic, but will require sedation or general anesthesia in infants. Ultrasonography may be diagnostic in skilled hands (84).

**Natural History.** Children with congenital dislocations will have limited elbow and forearm range of motion and strength, and this will affect function. They must compensate with shoulder, wrist, or trunk range of motion to perform recreational activities and activities of daily living. If left unreduced, chronic arthritic pain could develop. However, this is not well documented.

In children with recurrent instability, pain may develop secondary to osteochondral injury. This can lead to osteochondral loose bodies and arthrosis-like pain.

### Treatment

*Operative Care.* The isolated, congenital elbow dislocation has been rarely treated with open reduction (84,127). These cases and operations are rare enough that generalized comment is difficult. The more abnormal the anatomy, the less likely that operative intervention will be successful.

In recurrent instability, ligamentous reconstruction, transposition of the biceps tendon insertion to the coronoid process, and an anterior bone-block procedure have all been advocated (127,128). The choice or combination of procedures depends on the pathologic anatomy and the degree of instability.

It is the rare congenital elbow dislocation associated with ulnar dimelia and ulnar club hand that may warrant surgical reconstruction. Although ulnar dysplasia will be described in more detail in the section dealing with the wrist, it is worthwhile to discuss elbow reconstruction in this section. In type II ulnar club hand there is partial absence of the ulna distally (128,130). The proximal ulna articulates with the humerus but is usually unstable. With growth, the radius migrates proximally, leading to progressive loss of elbow flexion and extension. A supination deformity of the forearm may develop that limits forearm rotation (130). In these circumstances, creation of a single-bone forearm may improve cosmesis, stabilize the forearm, and improve elbow motion (132,128). As described by

Bayne (128), with this procedure the ulnar anlage is completely excised and the adjacent ulnar artery and nerve are protected. Radial osteotomy is then performed proximally. The radius is placed distal to the ulna in an end-to-end manner. Intramedullary fixation is performed to connect the proximal ulna to the distal radius. If there is significant bowing of the radius distal to the osteotomy site, a second osteotomy is performed with passage of the intramedullary wire. If it is difficult to attain end-to-end fixation, then side-to-side fusion is acceptable. Resection of the dislocated proximal radius can be performed simultaneously or up to 6 months later. If there is any question of neurovascular compromise, it is advisable to delay the proximal radius excision (128). At the time of proximal radius excision, the posterior interosseus radial nerve should be exposed and protected.

Wood recommends that reconstruction of the complex elbow deformity associated with ulnar dimelia should begin at the elbow with excision of the lateral olecranon process (132). Reconstruction of ligamentous structures may be necessary after excision in order to provide elbow stability. Excision of the lateral olecranon will reportedly provide improved passive elbow flexion and extension, but limitation in active elbow flexion may continue because of deficiencies in the biceps and brachialis musculature. Tendon transfers for active elbow flexion have reportedly had limited success (132). This condition (and reconstruction) is so rare that in-depth analysis of treatment options is not possible.

## Congenital Synostoses

These entities are classified as failure of differentiation of parts with skeletal involvement. In this section, congenital radioulnar and elbow synostoses will be discussed.

### Congenital Radioulnar Synostosis

Congenital synostosis of the proximal radius and ulna is a rare malformation of the upper limb. It is caused by a failure of the radius and ulna to separate, usually proximally.

During the embryonic period of fetal development, the humerus, radius, and ulna are conjoined. Longitudinal segmentation begins distally. For a time, the proximal ends are united and share a common perichondrium. Genetic or teratogenic factors that are as yet unknown may disrupt proximal radioulnar joint development, leading to a bony synostosis. This represents a type I deformity. If rudimentary joint development occurs before developmental arrest, a rudimentary radial head will develop with a less severe degree of coalition. This is a type II deformity (134).

During this period of intrauterine development, the forearm is anatomically in a position of varying degrees of pronation (135). Failure of formation of the proximal radioulnar joint at this stage of differentiation will leave the forearm in its fetal position of pronation. With rare exceptions (136), the forearm is fixed in pronation with congenital radioulnar synostosis (135).

Congenital radioulnar synostosis is usually an isolated event. There is a 3:2 ratio of boys to girls. Positive family histories have been reported (102,137,138). It is a bilateral occurrence 80% of the time (139). The condition is also seen in disorders such as acropolysyndactyly (Carpenter syndrome), acrocephalosyndactyly (Apert syndrome), arthrogryposis, acrofacial dysostoses of Najjar and mandibulofacial dystosis, and Klinefelter syndrome and its variants (140,141).

Although radioulnar synostosis is usually an isolated event, there may be associated anomalies of the musculoskeletal, cardiovascular, thoracic, gastrointestinal, renal, and central nervous systems. Cardiac anomalies include tetralogy of Fallot and ventricular septal defects. Thoracic anomalies include hypoplasia of the first and second ribs and the pectoral musculature. Renal anomalies involve anatomic malformations that can be screened by ultrasonography. In the central nervous system, associated problems include microcephaly, hydrocephalus, encephalocele, mental retardation, delay in attaining developmental milestones, and hemiplegia. Musculoskeletal problems include clubfeet, dislocated hips, polydactyly, syndactyly, and Madelung deformity (84,105,139,142).

**Clinical and Radiographic Features.** These children present for evaluation when they have a functional deficit. Generally, the degree of fixed forearm pronation determines the disability and the age of presentation. The presence of bilateral synostosis in marked pronation significantly limits function, and leads to an earlier presentation. Most children will present for evaluation by school age. Radioulnar synostosis is often first noted by a teacher or daycare worker when comparing the affected child with peers performing the same tasks (84).

Functional complaints are variable and include: (i) difficulty in holding or using small objects such as spoons or pencils; (ii) inability to dress owing to poor manipulation of belt buckles or buttons; (iii) backhanded positioning when holding objects such as bottles or toys; and (iv) difficulty competing in sports requiring upper-extremity dexterity. Feeding and accepting objects with an open palm are often difficult (84,139).

On physical examination, the elbow often has loss of its normal carrying angle and has a flexion deformity. The flexion contracture is usually minimal. Shortening of the forearm is more apparent in unilateral cases. Rotational hypermobility of the wrist compensates for the lack of forearm rotation (136,138). Despite this ligamentous laxity, patients do not appear to develop symptoms of carpal instability.

Almost all patients present in fixed pronation. In the series by Simmons et al. (139), approximately 40% of patients presented with pronation of less than 30 degrees, 20% had pronation fixed between 30 and 60 degrees, and 40% had more than 60 degrees of pronation. Pronation of greater than 60 degrees is most limiting.

Radiographs of patients with congenital radioulnar synostosis show anatomic variations from minor radial head deformities in patients with limited forearm rotation to full synostosis and absence of the radial head in patients with no rotation (105) (Fig. 23.8). The more extensive synostoses are usually fixed in more pronounced pronation. Plain radiographic classifications have distinguished partial and complete synostoses. In the partial synostosis there is often a rudimentary radial head present, but it is posteriorly or posterolaterally subluxated. In the complete synostosis the radial head is absent, and the proximal radius and ulna are a single bony mass. There is always an increased anterior bow of the radius. On occasion, the synostosis can extend into the middiaphysis of the forearm.

Occasionally, a patient will present with limited forearm rotation and normal radiographs. MRI of the proximal radius and ulna may reveal a cartilaginous synostosis that has yet to ossify or a fibrous tether that limits motion (84).

**Natural History.** In the absence of functional limitation, children with radioulnar synostosis should be observed. Children can often compensate for lack of forearm rotation if they have (i) synostosis in neutral-to-mild pronation (less than 60 degrees), (ii) significantly compensatory radiocarpal and intercarpal wrist rotation, and (iii) unilateral disease (84). These children present because they, their parents, and/or their teachers notice them performing home, school, or recreational tasks differently from their peers. However, when questioned extensively, it becomes apparent that they are without pain or functional disability (138). These children and their families are best served by counseling regarding the diagnosis and functional issues of their problem, and reassurance that operative intervention would be unlikely to improve their condition.

**Treatment.**

*Operative Care.* The ideal treatment would be to restore normal forearm rotation. Many surgical attempts to do so have been tried. Reported procedures have included division of the bony bridge (135); resection of the synostotic proximal radius to save the bicipital tuberosity, with (143–145) and without (146) muscle interposition; division of the interosseous membrane; and muscle, fat, fascia, or silastic interposition after synostosis excision (137,147). All had limited success at restoring motion. Artificial joint replacement, with a metallic swivel in the intramedullary canal of the radius between the supinator and pronator teres, also failed (145). Tagima et al. (147) reported improved forearm rotation with synostosis takedown, radial osteotomy, and interposition of either a silastic or a free fascial lateral arm flap. Intraoperatively, synostosis takedown procedures can dramatically improve motion, but there is a high incidence of loss of motion in 6 to 12 months after surgery. At present, the functional gain does not seem to warrant this surgical intervention.

The alternative to synostosis excision is derotation osteotomy. The goal is to place the hyperpronated hand in a more functional position. The dominant extremity is given priority in bilateral cases. It is easiest to perform the osteotomy through the synostosis distal to the coronoid process. Before the procedure, an intramedullary ulnar Kirschner wire is placed to maintain control of the osteotomy. After completion of the osteotomy, the forearm can be rotated into the desired position of correction and can be held in this position by either percutaneous pins or external fixation (148). Generally, patients undergoing derotation osteotomy have a fixed preoperative position of 60 to 100 degrees of pronation. The final corrected position is often 0 to 20 degrees of pronation (84). Ogino and Hikino advocated measuring the preoperative

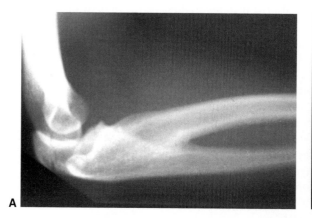
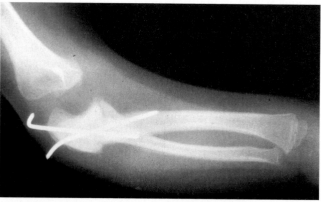

**Figure 23.8  A:** Preoperative radiograph of a congenital radioulnar synostosis. There is complete fusion of the proximal radius and ulna, and posterior dislocation of the radial head. The entire ulna is mildly hypoplastic. **B:** Postoperative radiograph of a derotation corrective osteotomy for this patient. A longitudinal wire is passed down the medullary canal of the ulna across the synostosis site. This Kirschner wire starts from the proximal ulnar apophysis. The osteotomy cut is performed through the synostosis. The transfixing wire is obliquely placed to secure the corrective derotation to a position of 0 to 20 degrees of pronation.

compensatory wrist supination to define the desired operative osteotomy correction (136). Once this position is achieved a second percutaneous Kirschner wire transfixes the osteotomy site obliquely, from the proximal ulna to the distal radius, across the derotated synostosis (Fig. 23.8). Because there is a high risk of compartment syndrome postoperatively (139,149), it is important to avoid internal fixation that would require a second operation for removal if neurovascular compromise occurs. Resection of bone at the synostosis site (136), or dorsal and volar fasciotomies through the operative incision, lessen the risk of compartment syndrome postoperatively (84) and should be performed routinely.

Patients undergoing derotation osteotomies have been noted to show significant improvement in function and cosmesis. Bimanual tasks are easier. Single-handed tasks, such as holding a fork, no longer require backhanding in extreme hyperpronation. Activities of daily living, such as dressing and feeding, are performed more independently and with less adaptive shoulder and trunk motion.

COMPLICATIONS. The most significant complication is postoperative compartment syndrome. It has been reported in one third of patients undergoing derotation osteotomy. This is attributable to changes in the vascularity and volume of the forearm compartments with derotation osteotomies in the range of 60 to 90 degrees. Compartment syndrome is more common in osteotomies with greater than 85 degrees of rotational correction. Prophylactic forearm fasciotomy, or resection of a segment of synostotic bone, reduces the incidence of this complication. If compartment syndrome is developing, the compressive dressings should be removed promptly, and the limb should be placed horizontally at the level of the heart. Compartment pressure measurements are routinely performed in the presence of tense compartments in a child with the clinical appearance of compartment syndrome. In pediatric patients an increasing analgesia requirement and a high level of anxiety are the most diagnostic clinical signs of compartment syndrome (150). Removal of the oblique transfixing Kirschner wire is performed if removal of dressings and proper elevation fail to improve the situation. Removal of the oblique Kirschner wire allows the forearm to rotate to its preoperative position, lessens the tension on the interosseous vessels, and may reduce the pressure of the forearm compartments. Finally, if these maneuvers do not resolve the problem, emergent skin and fascia decompression is mandatory (84,139).

With removal of the Kirschner wire in compartment syndrome there is a risk of loss of operative correction. The longitudinal ulnar Kirschner wire helps maintain control of the osteotomy site and allows for controlled, repeat derotation 5 to 10 days later. Although more rigid internal fixation may seem more desirable, it unnecessarily complicates the procedure, especially if compartment syndrome develops.

## Elbow Synostosis

Elbow synostosis is very rare. It occurs in isolation or in association with syndromic conditions. Humeroradial synostosis is more common than ulnotrochlear synostosis (151–153). The elbow flexion may range from 60 to 90 degrees. Often, there is also limited or no forearm motion. On examination, there will be no elbow motion.

Elbow synostosis is often associated with other upper limb malformations, such as ulnar clubhand (153). It has been described in siblings with humeroradial synostosis, indicating a potential genetic inheritance pattern. It frequently occurs with phocomelia variants (151). The limitation of elbow motion limits function, particularly if the affected extremity is dominant. The placement of a functional hand in space is limited by the lack of flexion-extension at the elbow. Compensatory trunk, head, and shoulder motion is difficult to adapt. Associated hand anomalies can further limit function (84).

*Treatment.* Attempts at synostosis excision and restoration of elbow motion have had minimal success. Techniques have included excision with muscle, fat, silastic interposition, or distraction arthroplasties. Although intraoperatively the motion can be improved, recurrence of the synostosis usually develops postoperatively. The use of continuous passive motion devices or distraction elbow hinge devices has not improved results (84). If the ankylosis leads to dysfunctional positioning of the hand in space, such as in the presence of an ulnar clubhand, corrective osteotomy is indicated. Most often, this is a derotation osteotomy at the level of the synostosis (151). Correction of a marked flexion deformity acutely increases the risk of neurovascular compromise. There is no role for total elbow arthroplasty, because of the possibility of early mechanical failure (84).

## Musculoskeletal

### Osteochondromatosis

Deformity of the forearm is common in multiple hereditary osteochondromatosis, with between 30% and 60% of patients affected in various series (154–156). The most frequent problem seems to be distal ulnar osteochondroma, which selectively slows the growth of the ulna in the presence of continued radial growth. The resultant relative shortening of the ulna can lead to progressive bowing of the radius and/or possible radial head dislocation. At the wrist there is increased radial angulation of the distal epiphysis, with ulnar deviation of the hand and ulnar translocation of the carpus (156–159). These deformities can lead to progressive loss of forearm rotation. If radial head dislocation occurs, loss of elbow motion can occur and pain may develop. This section focuses on the treatment of ulnar shortening, progressive radial bowing, and radial head subluxation. The principles outlined here for osteochondromatosis have also been used in congenital syndromes with forearm growth discrepancies, such as Conradi and Morquio syndromes (84).

***Natural History.*** There are very limited natural history data on patients with deformity secondary to osteochondromatosis of the upper extremity. There is ample information on the indications for, and the results of, surgical excision of osteochondromas and forearm reconstruction for these patients with deformities (160–162). The Shriners group in St. Louis (163) attempted to obtain natural history data by surveying their patients by telephone. Their data suggest that adults with forearm, wrist, and hand deformities from osteochondromatosis do reasonably well with activities of daily living and occupational tasks. Unfortunately, their data were limited because they could not reach many of their patients, and no patients were examined.

***Treatment Indications.*** The presence of an osteochondroma alone is not an indication for surgical excision. Excision of an osteochondroma will not predictably improve growth or prevent recurrence with growth. However, if the osteochondroma is a source of pain, limitation of motion, or neurovascular or muscular impingement, then excision is indicated. In addition, children with forearm osteochondromatosis may present with progressive deformity, loss of pronation and supination, and wrist or elbow pain related to joint subluxation. The limitations of forearm rotation may be caused by impingement of osteochondromas distally or proximally. When the loss of motion is secondary to impingement alone, rotation will improve with osteochondroma excision (156,157). In the presence of progressive forearm deformity, loss of rotation may also be related to bony malalignment, proximal radial head subluxation, or distal radioulnar joint dislocation. In these situations, rotation and radiocapitellar alignment can be improved by corrective radial osteotomy and ulnar lengthening (160). In the presence of radial head dislocation, reconstruction is very difficult. Attempts at reduction of the radial head by osteotomy or distraction lengthening techniques have had limited long-term success. Radial head excision has been advocated after skeletal maturity (161,162). The creation of a single-bone forearm may be the necessary salvage procedure in this complex deformity, and this can be performed at a very young age with successful results (156,162,164,165).

***Operative Management.*** Operative intervention is indicated in the presence of either progressive deformity that limits motion or radiocapitellar joint instability. The indications, specifically in terms of deformity, are ulnar shortening by more than 1.5 cm, increasing distal radial articular angle greater than 30 degrees, ulnar carpal translocation greater than 60%, progressive radial bowing, and radial head subluxation (160). The key to managing radiocapitellar instability is to treat it before frank dislocation occurs. Once the radial head is dislocated, obtaining and maintaining reduction is difficult.

Most patients with forearm deformities secondary to osteochondromatosis can be treated with a single-stage operative correction. The ulnar shortening is addressed by simultaneous excision of the osteochondroma and Z-lengthening of the ulna. After the Z-osteotomy, distraction lengthening is carried out intraoperatively with an external fixator. When the desired lengthening is achieved, a plate is applied to maintain the length until bony healing is complete (84) (Fig. 23.9). This lengthening technique is, in essence, a rebalancing of the forearm skeleton. It realigns the proximal and distal radioulnar joints. In one series, lengthenings of 1 to 2.3 cm, leading to a neutral ulnar variance at the wrist, were obtained in a single stage (160). In most patients forearm rotation was improved by an average of 40 degrees (84,160). Results indicate improved range of motion and function with minimal risk of complications.

There are rare situations in osteochondromatosis in which correction cannot be obtained in a single procedure (120,166–168). The option then is to perform serial lengthenings or gradual distraction osteoclasis. Up to 13 cm of length has been obtained by distraction techniques (166,167). However, the rate of complications with distraction osteoclasis in the forearm has been cited as between 60% and 100%. Therefore, forearm lengthenings by distraction techniques should be performed cautiously by those skilled in the technique. The techniques available for distraction lengthening include unilateral external fixation frames (169–171), classic Ilizarov technique (170), and hybrid fixation using transverse Ilizarov wires fixed at 90 degrees to half pins (168,172). Most surgeons performing distraction lengthening now use a hybrid technique so as to lessen the risk of neurovascular and muscle entrapment complications (166–168,172). The fixator is preassembled as part of preoperative planning, with a half ring proximally and a full ring distally. In situations requiring angular correction, appropriate hinges need to be applied in order to obtain correction. Because each case is unique, the specifics of application are difficult to address in a review such as this. However, certain principles need to be adhered to. The pins need to be placed in the safe zone so as to lessen the risk of complications. Passive digital flexion and extension need to be at the full range intraoperatively after pin placement to ensure postoperative maintenance of motion. The preferred site for corticotomy is the proximal ulna metaphysis to enhance regeneration of bone (168). Lengthening begins 3 to 5 days after surgery and progresses at a rate of 1 mm per day, usually with an advance of 0.25 mm four times per day. Maintenance of passive and active range of motion of the shoulder, elbow, and digits is critical. Clearly, the loss of hand function is not worth the advantage of increased forearm length. Prevention and treatment of expected pin-track infection require meticulous pin care and liberal use of oral antibiotics. After the desired lengthening is achieved, the external fixator is left in place until there is sufficient regenerate bone to allow removal without the risk of fracture. In general, the fixator

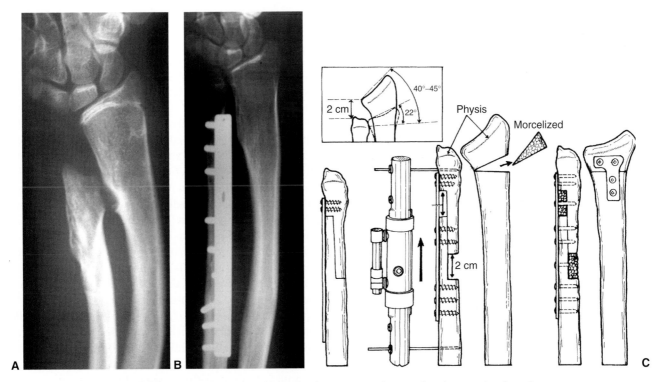

**Figure 23.9 A:** Preoperative radiograph of a patient with osteochondromatosis, ulnar shortening, and mild radial deformity, with recent progressive loss of forearm rotation. **B:** Postoperative radiograph of single-stage lengthening of the ulna and radial osteotomy. **C:** Illustration of the lengthening technique.

is left in place for at least twice the time necessary to obtain lengthening (84).

In the presence of radial head dislocation, the distraction technique has been used in an attempt to reduce the radial head before correcting the forearm deformity (120,168,172). A separate ring and olive wire are placed in the proximal radius. Progressive distal migration of the radial head has been used for radiocapitellar reduction. Once the radial head is reduced, the forearm correction is performed as described in the preceding text. However, recurrent subluxation, stiffness of the joint, and pain have occurred after radial head reduction (84). The limited success of this procedure in this situation does not seem to warrant its use.

The creation of a radioulnar synostosis is indicated for either painful radial head dislocation or radius and ulna instability that is not salvageable by other means. In these circumstances, it can result in a stable, pain-free extremity (161). Radial head excision is performed to decompress the radiocapitellar joint and improve the range of motion of the elbow. Correction of the deformities of the radius and ulna is performed at the same time as the radioulnar synostosis with internal fixation and bone grafting. Some increased length can be achieved with the single-stage procedure. The distal ulna and proximal radial resected bone are utilized as bone graft. Neutral rotation to 20 degrees of pronation is desired. Although this procedure is rarely indicated, these patients have excellent long-term results (161).

### Pseudarthrosis

Congenital pseudarthrosis of the forearm is rare and clearly associated with neurofibromatosis. Wood (173) summarized the cases of forearm pseudarthrosis in the medical literature, and noted that, according to the published papers, 5% of patients with neurofibromatosis have pseudarthrosis of the upper or lower limb, whereas more than 50% of patients with congenital pseudarthrosis of the forearm have definitive neurofibromatosis, multiple café-au-lait spots, or a positive family history of neurofibromatosis. Congenital pseudarthrosis is most often seen in the tibia, but it has been described in all the long bones.

The survey by Wood (173) found 46 cases of forearm pseudarthrosis. The ulna alone was involved in 20 cases (Fig. 23.10), the radius alone in 15 cases, and both ulna and radius were involved in 11 cases. Twenty-three of these patients had either neurofibromatosis (18 patients) or a positive family history of neurofibromatosis (5 patients). Reports of this disorder range from a single case to up to 6 patients (174).

As in tibial pseudarthrosis, all reports describing treatment options for this problem outline the difficulty of obtaining union with conventional cast immobilization or corticocancellous autografting or allografting, with and without internal fixation techniques. The role of distraction lengthening techniques for congenital pseudarthrosis of the forearm is unclear. There are several reports of the use of vascularized fibular grafts (174,175) to heal the

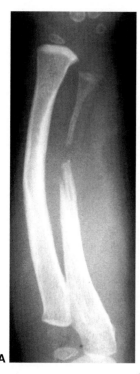 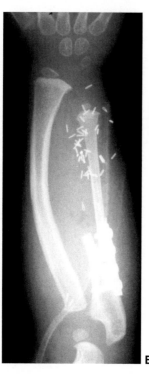

**Figure 23.10 A:** Preoperative radiograph of congenital pseudarthrosis of the ulna. Note the hypoplasia and tapering of the distal ulna. **B:** Postoperative radiograph of the vascularized fibular transfer, with proximal epiphyseal and physeal transfer, to establish distal ulnar growth. If the patient is very young, the microvascular transfer must include revascularization of both the diaphysis and epiphysis of the fibula so as to obtain physeal growth. The most distal metallic clip indicates the top of the fibular epiphysis in the reconstructed distal radioulnar joint.

pseudarthrosis. These reports indicate a high rate of union when vascularized fibular transfer is carried out. This is the preferred treatment for this disorder at present. In the forearm, the fibula is internally fixed to the proximal ulna. Distally, the fibula is secured either to the soft tissues of the distal radioulnar joint and the triangular fibrocartilage complex (TFCC) or to the residual distal ulna, provided it is not too dysplastic and dysvascular. The vascular anastomosis is end-to-side in relation to the ulnar artery. At the donor site of a skeletally immature patient, the distal fibula is fixed to the tibia so as to prevent valgus ankle instability after harvesting a vascularized fibular graft (173,176). The proximal fibular epiphysis can be transferred in the young patient to allow for growth. In this situation, the separate vascular supplies to the fibular diaphysis and epiphysis need to be preserved and maintained with the transfer and vascular anastomosis. The soft-tissue support of the lateral knee must be reconstructed.

Creation of a single-bone forearm has been performed successfully as a salvage procedure (117). In the presence of an associated radial head dislocation, this may be the only successful option (84).

## WRIST REGION

### Congenital

#### Radial Dysplasia

Radial dysplasia is classified as a failure of longitudinal formation. It occurs in 1 in 30,000 to 1 in 100,000 live births (177,178). The underdevelopment, or aplasia, of the radius is universally associated with hypoplasia or absence of the thumb and of the radial aspect of the carpus (179). The radial or preaxial deficiency has been classified by Bayne and Klug (177) into four types, ranging from a present but defective distal radial epiphysis (type I), to complete absence of the radius (type IV). James et al. modified this classification system to include type N, which has normal radial and carpal length thumb hypoplasia, and type O, which has normal radial length but carpal abnormalities (180). The severity of the radial deficiency determines the extent of the associated deficiencies of the thumb, digits, ulna, and elbow (Fig. 23.11). Therefore, the wide spectrum of anatomic deficiency includes mild radial deviation of the wrist and minimal thumb hypoplasia; complete absence of the thumb and radius; camptodactyly of the index, long, and ring fingers; foreshortening of the ulna; and a stiff elbow.

*Pathogenesis.* The pathogenesis of longitudinal deficiency of the radius is unknown. It has been postulated that injury to the apical ectodermal ridge during upper limb development is the cause (7,148). Factors such as intrauterine compression, an inflammatory process, vascular insult, maternal drug exposure (thalidomide, insulin), and irradiation have all been raised as possible etiologic causes (1). There is no known genetic cause except when radial deficiency is associated with other congenital abnormalities. The pattern of inheritance is autosomal dominant or autosomal recessive, depending on the syndrome. There are many associated congenital syndromes, including cardiac, craniofacial, hematopoietic, musculoskeletal, gastrointestinal, and renal organ syndromes. There are associated chromosomal abnormalities, including trisomy 13, 18, and 21. The occurrence is most often sporadic.

*Associated Anomalies.* Although radial longitudinal deficiency can occur in isolation, it is commonly associated with other congenital malformations. Forty percent of patients with unilateral radial club hand and 27% of patients with bilateral radial club hand have associated malformations (181). It is imperative that these problems be assessed by clinical, radiographic, and laboratory evaluations as appropriate. These organ system malformations may present in a nonsyndromic pattern. Congenital cardiac, genitourinary, respiratory, skeletal, and neurologic problems occur in children with radial dysplasia. Similarly, many syndromes have been described in association with longitudinal deficiency of the radius. The most common

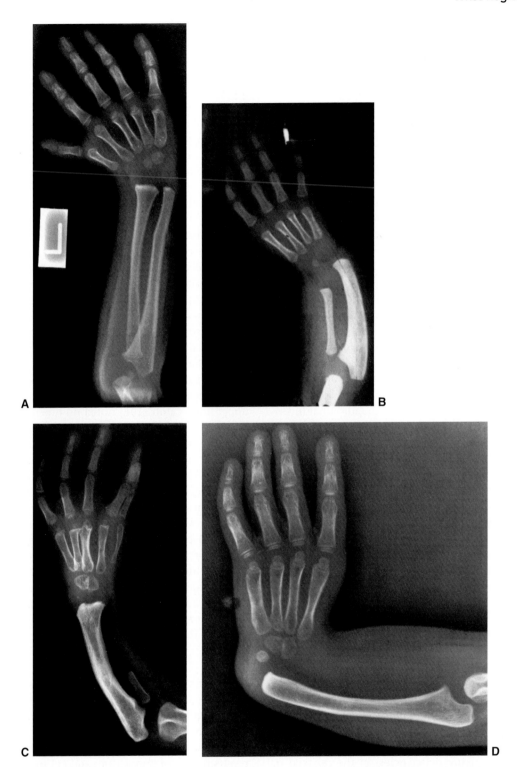

**Figure 23.11** Classification of radial dysplasia types I through IV as represented by radiographs. **A:** In type I, the ulnar variance is positive as a result of the foreshortened distal radius. **B:** In type II, both the proximal and distal radial physes have deficient growth, with more radial shortening and ulnar bowing. **C:** In type III, the radius is partially absent. **D:** In type IV, the radius is completely absent.

are Holt-Oram syndrome, Fanconi anemia, thrombocytopenia with absent radius, and the "VACTERLs" syndromes of abnormal vertebrae, anus, cardiovascular tree, trachea, renal system, and limb buds. (The classic "VATER" syndrome comprised vertebral anomalies, anal atresia, tracheoesophageal fistula, and renal anomalies.) (182–184). Holt-Oram syndrome is an autosomal dominant disease characterized by upper-limb malformations and major cardiac malformations (185). The gene for Holt-Oram syndrome has been identified. Fanconi anemia also has an autosomal dominant inheritance pattern. In infancy, there are usually characteristic facial features (microphthalmos, strabismus, hearing deficits) (186). Pancytopenia often does not present until later in childhood. Fanconi anemia can be identified by a mitomycin C test, but it is now advocated that all infants with radial-sided defects be assessed early for Fanconi anemia with the diepoxybutane (DEB) test, since a delay in diagnosis can have serious consequences (187). Thrombocytopenia with absent radius is also from autosomal recessive inheritance. The thrombocytopenia is present at birth. The platelet count usually improves with growth, and hand surgery should be delayed until it is safe (186,188).

*Clinical Features.* The clinical presentation of radial dysplasia depends on the severity of the malformation. Bayne et al. (189) have tried to clarify the spectrum of clinical deformity by classifying radial club hands from type I to type IV. Type IV deficiency is the most common. Type I deformity involves a defective distal radial physis. This leads to a minor foreshortening of the radius and a prominent distal ulna. Although there is mild radial deviation of the wrist throughout life, problems with radioulnar incongruity, such as triangular fibrocartilage tears, ulnocarpal impaction syndrome, and distal radioulnar joint pain or loss of motion, usually do not occur. The major clinical issue is the associated thumb hypoplasia with opposition weakness. Type II deficiency involves limited proximal and distal radial physeal growth. As a consequence, the wrist is more radially deviated, and the ulna bows. The thumb hypoplasia is usually more significant, with more deficiency of the radial carpus. Type III deficiency is the absence of the distal two thirds of the radius. The wrist is more severely deviated, and the hand has limited mechanical support. The ulna is thickened and bowed. The associated thumb and finger abnormalities of hypoplasia and camptodactyly are more common and severe. Type IV deficiency involves complete absence of the radius. The ulnar bowing is marked. The thumb is usually absent. The index, long, and even ring fingers are often involved. The elbow may have limited range of motion. There is marked limitation of hand, wrist, and forearm function.

*Pathoanatomy.* Radial dysplasia involves skeletal malformations and soft-tissue deficiencies on the preaxial or radial side of the hand, wrist, and forearm. The severity of the soft-tissue loss parallels the skeletal deficiency. The preaxial muscles arise from the lateral epicondyle, and are normally innervated by the radial nerve. Therefore, the radial wrist extensors and brachioradialis are either absent or deficient. The pronator-flexor muscle mass is affected when its skeletal insertion sites are absent or hypoplastic. These structures may consist of only fibrous tissue (radial anlage) that maintains or worsens the deformity of the

wrist and hand with growth. Similarly, the neurovascular structures will be affected. The posterior interosseous and sensory branches of the radial nerve will be absent in a severe deformity. The radial artery is usually absent. The ulnar nerve and artery are usually present and unaffected. The blood supply to the hand comes through the ulnar artery, and at times the interosseous vessels or a persistent median artery. The median nerve is usually present and serves as a neural supply to the hand along with the ulnar nerve. However, the more severe the deformity of the hand and wrist, the more limited the neural and vascular supply will be to the hand.

*Natural History.* Generally, children with longitudinal deficiency of the radius have an unaffected central nervous system. As with any congenital upper limb malformation, children's creative minds allow them to perform all activities of life. However, they may need to use adaptive mechanisms. These generally include a spherical grip and lateral pinch to compensate for the absence of opposition (190). Fifty to sixty-two percent of patients with radial dysplasia have unilateral involvement. Even with severe unilateral radial dysplasia, these children will adapt their skills by increasing their use of the contralateral, normal hand and upper limb. Lamb (191) noted no functional impairment in patients with unilateral involvement. Individuals with bilateral involvement have more difficulty. Activities of daily living, such as hygiene, eating, and dressing, are affected. Adaptive techniques and alteration of clothes are often necessary. However, as Bora et al. (192,193) reported, despite these adaptive modifications, patients without surgical correction were more limited than surgically treated patients. Finally, the issue of the cosmetic and psychological impact of radial dysplasia is difficult to quantify. The social setting is constantly changing, and peer perception plays a major role in an involved individual's self-perception. Parental and family perception and coping will surely have a profound effect on a developing child's self-image. There is limited objective psychologic information at present.

*Treatment.* Treatment should address the following problems with radial dysplasia: (i) unstable wrist with lack of support for the hand; (ii) digital weakness secondary to radially deviated wrist; (iii) intrinsic digital weakness and deformity; (iv) thumb hypoplasia or aplasia that results in lack of opposition; and (v) foreshortened ulna. All of these deformities affect function in the patient with radial dysplasia. In addition, there are significant cosmetic deformities in these children that can be improved by intervention.

*Nonsurgical Intervention.* The options for nonsurgical intervention in these children are corrective casting, bracing, and physical therapy. In infancy, the first goal is to achieve passive correction of the radial deviation deformity. In mild cases, this involves merely a home exercise program of wrist ulnar deviation, extension, and distraction stretching. In more severe cases, care involves corrective casting or splinting to gradually stretch the contracted soft tissues, and then maintain the correction. The splints are used in conjunction with a passive range-of-motion program. If attempts to correct the static radial deviation contracture are not successful within 6 to 12 weeks of vigorous therapy and skilled bracing or casting, the use of distraction external fixation to obtain soft-tissue and musculoskeletal alignment should be considered (194).

Once passive motion has been achieved, it is necessary to maintain the correction. Again, in mild forms of the condition, this can be done nonsurgically. A nighttime corrective splinting program during infancy and times of rapid growth is useful. This treatment is adequate for most type I and type II malformations. In severe cases, the lack of a stable wrist out of the splint impairs hand and limb function. These children are candidates for operative correction at 6 to 12 months of age.

*Surgical Intervention.* There are two indications for surgery: persistent wrist radial deviation contracture (Fig. 23.12), and functionally limiting thumb deficiency. The surgical options for the wrist contracture and lack of support for the hand have included bone graft procedures to the ulna, centralization, radialization, and wrist fusion (195). Surgical options for thumb aplasia are pollicization and microvascular toe-to-thumb transfer. Thumb hypoplasia can be surgically corrected with first web-space deepening, MCP joint stabilization, and opponensplasty tendon transfer. Less clear indications exist for the surgical treatment of digital camptodactyly, ulnar foreshortening, and radial hypoplasia in type II deformities.

Potential contraindications for surgery include: (i) lack of elbow flexion, such that the wrist deviation enables the patient to perform hand-to-mouth and hand-to-neck activities; (ii) severe index digital deformity and weakness that will result in failed pollicization; and (iii) severe medical problems that pose a risk to the patient's well-being.

The earliest forms of surgical correction for radial dysplasia involved improving the radial deviation deformity and lack of wrist support for the hand by grafting bone to the ulna. Albee (196), Starr (197), Entin (198), and Riordan (199) described the use of nonvascularized bone grafts from the proximal fibula to the ulna in Y-configuration to support the carpus and hand. These procedures resulted in significant short-term improvement. However, the transplant usually failed to grow, leading to recurrent deformity. Vascularized bone grafting has recently been advocated by Vilkki (200), in rare circumstances. Centralization of the carpus over the third metacarpal has been a standard treatment (191–193). Soft-tissue release of the radial contracture, contouring of the ulna to match the carpus, and capsular reefing are performed. Stabilization is performed with pin fixation until healing is achieved. The problem with centralization is a high incidence of recurrence. Lamb (191) advocated modifying the technique by notching the carpus to inset the distal ulna. This lessened recurrence, but also decreased wrist motion and increased early ulnar physeal closure postoperatively. Function is clearly impaired when there is less than 30 degrees of wrist motion postoperatively. Buck-Gramcko (201) introduced radialization during the thalidomide crisis. The centralization procedure is modified by aligning the ulna with the second metacarpal. Tendon transfers from the radial aspect of the wrist (extensor carpi radialis and flexor carpi radialis, if present) to the dorsal, ulnar wrist are performed in order to rebalance the wrist and hand. The quality of the radial muscles clearly affects the success of the radialization procedure. With both centralization and radialization, correction is performed at the wrist. If there is a concomitant ulnar bow of greater than 30 degrees, ulnar osteotomy should also be performed. This usually involves a multiple-level open osteotomy and intramedullary fixation.

In the rare situations in which passive correction of the wrist is not possible by splinting, casting, or therapy, distraction and correction with an external fixator is performed. As described by Kessler (194), this can be performed in infancy (Fig. 23.13). Often, after 3 to 6 weeks of external fixation an open centralization or radialization procedure is performed. Wrist fusion is not performed in young patients, because this leads to loss of wrist motion and potential loss of ulnar physeal growth. However,

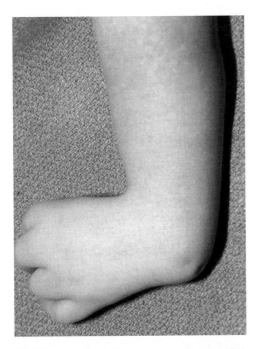

**Figure 23.12** A patient with complete absence of the radius and thumb aplasia. Note the foreshortening of the forearm, 90-degree radial deviation at the wrist, and dimpling of the skin over the distal ulna, with the proximal and radially subluxated carpus and hand.

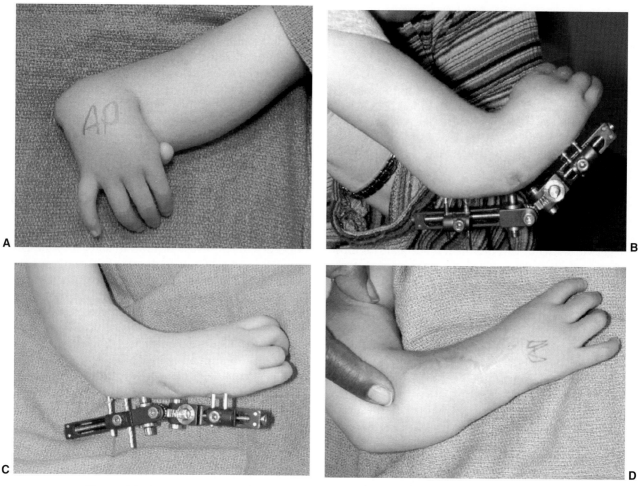

**Figure 23.13** Clinical photographs of a patient undergoing progressive distraction lengthening to stretch the soft tissues, bring the hand out to length, and reduce the wrist over the ulna. This patient has a markedly foreshortened forearm. Preoperatively, there was volar, radial, and proximal subluxation of the carpus and hand that was not correctable with exercises and splinting. **A–D:** Preoperative **(A)**, early postoperative after fixator application **(B)**, after correction just before fixator removal **(C)**, and final result after centralization **(D)**. (Case and illustrations courtesy of Dr Allan Peljovich.)

Catagni et al. (202) performed wrist fusion in conjunction with distraction lengthening in adolescent and young adult patients with recurrent deformity.

Generally, wrist reconstruction is performed before thumb reconstruction. Ideally, thumb reconstruction should be performed before the child is 18 months of age, because the learning ability for the pinch movement becomes limited once the central nervous system matures to this stage. In mild forms of radial dysplasia, the thumb hypoplasia causes functional problems involving decreased first web space, MCP joint instability, and weak thenar muscles. The first web space can be deepened with Z-plasties or rotation flaps (203,204). Release of adductor and first dorsal interosseous fascia is often necessary. The MCP joint can be stabilized with local fascia or use of extra flexor digitorum superficialis tendon length for ligament reconstruction. On occasion, MCP joint chondrodesis (fusion of the proximal phalanx epiphysis to the metacarpal head) or arthrodesis is appropriate. Opponensplasty is performed simultaneously with use of the abductor digiti quinti (205), ring-finger flexor digitorum superficialis (94), or accessory digital extensors. All have had reported success in providing opposition strength. Thumb aplasia is best addressed with pollicization (204,206). Toe-to-thumb microvascular transfers have been reported, but to date the results are less successful than those of index-finger pollicization. Overall, the quality of the index-finger donor determines the quality of the subsequent thumb. If there is significant camptodactyly, the thumb will be stiffer, weaker, and less often used in pinch activities than if the index has full passive mobility and intrinsic and extrinsic strength. In a well-performed pollicization, the results are functionally and cosmetically pleasing to the patient, family, and surgeon.

COMPLICATIONS. Recurrent deformity and premature closure of the distal ulnar physis are the two major complications of wrist reconstruction. The occurrence of these problems depends on the procedure performed (centralization versus radialization) and the quality of the preoperative musculoskeletal and soft-tissue anatomy. With radialization, the goal is to dynamically rebalance the wrist and maintain motion. If this fails to occur, radial deviation and flexion deformity will recur with growth. In addition, if there is limited elbow flexion, excessive flexion and radial deviation of the wrist will be used by the patient to compensate while carrying out activities of daily living such as oral hygiene and feeding. This contributes to the recurrence rate.

Physeal arrest is more common with centralization procedures. The forearm is already foreshortened, and this is further exacerbated by loss of distal growth. Because 70% to 80% of forearm growth comes from the distal physis, postoperative growth arrest is a major cosmetic and functional problem.

Finally, in patients with radial dysplasia, pollicization procedures can have poorer results in terms of opposition strength and active range of motion (207). The opposition weakness may be improved by opponensplasty transfer (208,209), but there should be a strong donor if the procedure is to succeed. Otherwise, the patient will continue to compensate with lateral digital pinch on the ulnar side of the hand.

### Ulnar Dysplasia/Ulnar Club Hand

Ulnar, or postaxial, longitudinal deficiency is less common than either radial or central longitudinal deficiency. It is classified as a failure of formation of parts. The incidence was found by Birch-Jensen to be 1 in 100,000 live births (178). Ogden et al. cited a boy-to-girl ratio of 3:2, with only 25% of the patients showing bilateral involvement (210).

Most cases are sporadic, but there are reports of familial occurrence, too (211–214). It also occurs as a part of rare, identified, inheritable syndromes, such as ulnar mammary (Schnitzel) syndrome, Klippel-Feil syndrome (215,216), and some nongenetic syndromes such as Cornelia de Lange syndrome. It is associated with musculoskeletal system malformations in up to 50% of cases. Contralateral upper-extremity deficiencies of phocomelia, transverse arrest, radial deficiency, and aphalangia occur commonly. Similarly, lower-extremity deficiencies, such as proximal femoral focal and fibular deficiencies, occur in almost one half of the cases. Unlike those with radial dysplasia, it is uncommon for patients with ulnar deficiency to have associated major organ system malformations. Ogino and Kato's experimental data may explain this finding (217). They produced major deficiencies in rat fetuses by injecting the mothers with the antimetabolite Myleran. The timing of injection during the gestational period determined the limb malformation produced. For example, ulnar deficiencies were produced by earlier injections than were radial deficiencies. Fetuses that had ulnar deficiencies had more lethal cardiac malformations. This may explain why there are fewer major organ system malformations and a lower incidence of ulnar deficiency among live births.

**Clinical Features.** Bayne classified ulnar deficiency into four groups based on the musculoskeletal abnormalities of the elbow and forearm (218). Most clinicians use this system to define and establish treatment plans for these patients. Type I deficiency is hypoplasia of the ulna. Both distal and proximal physes of the ulna are present, but decreased in growth. There is minimal, nonprogressive bowing of the radius, and a variable presentation of hand malformations. Type II deficiency is the most common type and involves partial absence of the radius. There is a fibrous anlage extending from the distal ulna to the carpus. The hand is ulnarly deviated, with bowing of the radius, and these deformities may be progressive with growth. The elbow is stable if there is sufficient proximal ulna present. Again, digital malformations or absences are variable. Type III deficiency involves complete absence of the ulna. There is no ulnar anlage. The radius, wrist, and hand are usually straight. The elbow is unstable as a result of the lack of an olecranon. Hand malformations and absences are common. Type IV deficiency involves synostosis of the distal humerus to the proximal radius. There is an ulnar anlage present from the distal humerus to the carpus, with marked bowing of the radius and ulnar deviation of the hand. Hand anomalies are common also in type IV deformities (Fig. 23.14).

Cole and Manske (219) further classified ulnar deficiency by the presenting hand malformations. They divided the disorder into four types according to the deficiency of the first web space and thumb. Type A is a normal thumb and first web space. Type B involves a mild web contracture and thumb hypoplasia. Type C involves marked hypoplasia of the thumb with rotation of the thumb into the plane of motion of the other digits. Type D is absence of the thumb. In their series, 73% of the 55 patients had thumb deficiencies. This was similar to Broudy and Smith's findings of 16 hypoplastic thumbs and 5 absent thumbs in 26 patients with ulnar club hand (220).

In addition, in these patients the limb is foreshortened and usually internally rotated. The glenoid may be dysplastic. The radial head is often dislocated, and range of motion of the elbow is limited in up to 40% of cases (221). These abnormalities make placement of the hand in space difficult. The hand malformations limit pinch, grasp, and release functions. Reconstructive surgery is indicated for improving hand and wrist orientation, thumb opposition, and digital motion and strength.

**Treatment.** There is a scarcity of data regarding the natural history of untreated ulnar dysplasia. In 1927, Southwood stated, "From the functional viewpoint, therefore, the deformed limb is much more useful than its anatomical condition would lead one to expect" (222). This malformation is not associated with central nervous system deficiencies. As with all congenital malformations in individuals with normal brains, the patients will perform activities well, but differently. Treatment has to improve function and cosmesis, if it is to be warranted.

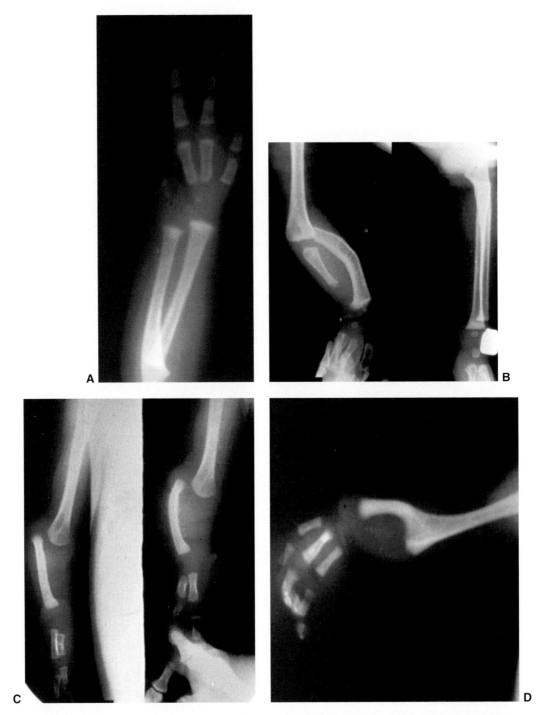

**Figure 23.14** Classification of ulnar dysplasia types I through IV as represented by radiographs. **A:** Type I dysplasia represents deficiency of both the proximal and distal ulnar physes, with foreshortening of the ulna and mild bowing of the radius. **B:** Type II is the most common type and represents partial absence of the radius. **C:** Type III involves complete absence of the radius with an unstable elbow joint. **D:** Type IV includes complete absence of the radius and humeroulnar synostosis.

Nonsurgical treatment has predominantly involved physical therapy and corrective casting or splinting. In types I and III deficiencies, the mild ulnar deviation of the wrist and hand may be improved with serial casting, splinting, and passive exercises starting in infancy. In types II and IV deficiencies, the ulnar anlage may make nonsurgical correction of the severe ulnar deviation of the hand and wrist impossible.

There is considerable debate regarding the treatment of the hand that is severely ulnarly deviated and that does not respond to casting/splinting. There is limited information to allow for critical evaluation of the options of (i) leaving the patient alone, (ii) performing excision of the ulnar anlage, and (iii) corrective radial osteotomy. Some of the confusion exists because not all of these deformities are progressive (223). As Flatt (1) makes clear, it is difficult to critically evaluate the literature because of limited objective measurements in previous studies. He correctly points to the low incidence of this disorder as hampering objective assessment of the therapeutic options. As with many rare conditions, only multicenter, prospective studies can definitively answer the questions.

The lack of this information allows for subjective interpretation of the treatment options, leading to reluctance to pursue aggressive surgical intervention. Within these limits, an attempt is made to outline treatment options and recommendations for wrist deformity, elbow instability, and digital and thumb deficiencies.

Resection of the ulnar anlage is indicated for progressive ulnar deviation of the wrist and hand of greater than 30 degrees. This can occur in types II and IV deficiencies (1,224). Through an ulna-based incision, the anlage is identified as it inserts into the carpus. The ulnar artery and nerve should be protected. Resection should be performed until neutral positioning of the wrist can occur intraoperatively. If there is associated marked ulnar deviation of the radius, concomitant radial osteotomy can be performed. However, it is imperative to assess the location of the radial head and the status of forearm rotation before proceeding with anlage excision and consideration of radial osteotomy.

If there is a dislocated radial head and limited forearm rotation preoperatively in the type II deformity, anlage excision, resection of the radial head, and creation of a single-bone forearm should be carried out simultaneously. If there is acceptable forearm rotation preoperatively, it is best to correct only the wrist deformity and to monitor the status of the forearm and elbow with growth. Resection of the radial head for cosmetic reasons should be performed cautiously, because even the dislocated head may be providing some elbow stability in these patients.

Similarly, creation of a single-bone forearm may result in improved cosmesis, but the loss of forearm rotation may cause an unacceptable loss of function. In patients with type IV deficiency, there may be associated internal rotation posture to the arm that limits placement of the hand in space. If this is present, simultaneous external rotation osteotomy of the limb and ulnar anlage excision should be performed. This is clearly the case with patients with bilateral deformity who are unable to reach their mouths preoperatively.

Repair of digital and thumb deficiencies is indicated. Syndactyly is common and should be corrected in infancy. Thumb hypoplasia or absence should also be repaired in infancy. Broudy and Smith (220) described a modified pollicization procedure for the malpositioned thumb in the plane of motion of the other fingers. Tendon transfers for intrinsic and extrinsic muscle deficiencies of the thumb and fingers are indicated if there are adequate donors available.

### Madelung Deformity

Madelung (225), in 1878, described a growth deformity of the distal radius. For reasons that are still unknown, the volar, ulnar aspect of the distal radial physis slows or stops growing prematurely. The continued normal growth of both the ulnar physis and the remaining dorsal, radial aspect of the radial physis results in ulnar overgrowth, carpal subluxation, and radial articular deformity (Fig. 23.15). Madelung deformity usually occurs in girls, and is most often bilateral (226). It may not become clinically apparent until the adolescent growth spurt, which is when most patients present. It is generally sporadic in presentation. It is also associated with Leri-Weill syndrome, a dyschondrosteosis form of mesomelic dwarfism that is inherited in an autosomal dominant manner (224,227). In addition, Madelung deformity has been associated with Hurler mucopolysaccharidosis, Turner syndrome, osteochondromatosis, achondroplasia, and Ollier disease (228). True Madelung deformity should be distinguished from a posttraumatic or postinfectious deformity.

*Clinical and Radiographic Features.* The clinical and radiographic picture is dependent on the age at presentation and the severity of the growth arrest. Generally, by the time the affected children are brought for treatment, there is marked deformity, limitation of motion, and activity-related pain. Because the condition is usually bilateral, the subtle growth deformity that occurs before the adolescent growth spurt is often ignored. However, with early presentation there is a slight positive ulnar variance and loss of the volar, ulnar aspect of the radial lunate fossa (Fig. 23.15). The carpus subluxates volarly and into the gap between the radius and the ulna. These patients may have mild symptoms of ulnocarpal impaction with power grip activities, and distal radioulnar joint incongruity with forearm rotation. More often, individuals with Madelung deformity present late with marked deformity. There is an increased tilt of the radial articular surface from the dorsal radial corner of the styloid to the volar, ulnar aspect of the depleted lunate fossa. The ulnar variance is more positive, with carpal overlap and dorsal subluxation. The carpus migrates more proximal into the increasing diastasis between the radius and the ulna on anteroposterior radiographs. These patients have more pain and limitation of motion, especially forearm rotation and wrist extension.

*Pathoanatomy.* The skeletal features are well described. As mentioned previously, the arrest of the volar, radial aspect of the distal radial physis causes subsequent deformity of the radiocarpal, radioulnar, and ulnocarpal joints. Vickers and Nielsen (229), Linscheid (230), and Ezaki (226) have described abnormal tethering of soft tissues from the distal radius to the carpus and ulna. These have included aberrant ligaments (228,229) and pronator quadratus muscle insertions (230). It is unclear whether these structures are responsible for the growth deformity of the radius. Vickers

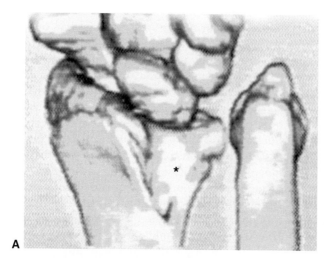

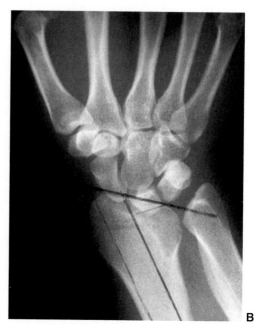

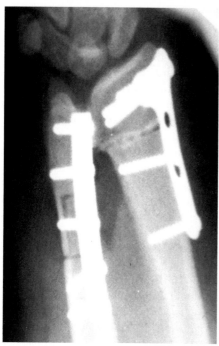

**Figure 23.15 A:** Magnetic resonance imaging (MRI) of severe Madelung deformity. Note that the lunate fossa (*) is markedly deficient and oriented ulnarly. **B:** Preoperative three-dimensional MRI of a patient with Madelung deformity and debilitating ulnocarpal and radioulnar pain. There is nearly complete deficiency of the lunate fossa and subluxation of the carpus ulnarly, volarly, and proximally. The ulna has a positive variance. **C:** Postoperative radiograph of a radiodorsal closing-wedge osteotomy of the radius and ulnar Z-shortening osteotomy in this patient. This procedure restored radial articular alignment, corrected the ulnocarpal impaction, and reduced the distal radioulnar joint.

and Nielsen's successful treatment of Madelung deformity by excision of the volar tethering soft tissues and prophylactic physiolysis of the volar radial physis indicates that there may be a causal relationship.

*Treatment.* The early descriptions of the treatment of Madelung deformity advocated treatment only for symptomatic patients at skeletal maturity (231). Originally, the mere presence of the deformity was not an indication for operative intervention in the asymptomatic patient, regardless of age. However, the growth discrepancy is easier to treat if it is dealt with early. Young patients become

symptomatic and the range of function of the limbs becomes restricted with increasing growth deformity. Vickers and Nielsen advocated early intervention with physiolysis (229). The treatment principle is similar to that for Blount disease, with resection of the abnormal volar, ulnar physeal region of the radius and fat interposition. At the same time, any aberrant, tethering anatomic structures are excised. Their case series indicates restoration of radial growth and prevention of progressive deformity. Some patients with Madelung deformity can present at a very young age with marked deformity and complete lack of a lunate fossa for carpal support. In these patients it is difficult to carry out successful reconstruction surgery, and there is a high rate of recurrent deformity with growth. Combined radial and ulnar osteotomies are necessary for initial correction. Repeat surgery is not uncommon. An alternative treatment for the patient presenting early is to perform ulnar and radial epiphysiodesis in order to prevent progressive or recurrent deformity and symptoms. In the patient with bilateral disease, this treatment leads to foreshortened upper limbs without side-to-side discrepancy.

The treatment for a patient presenting late with marked deformity and symptoms is more problematic. The radial deformity can be addressed by an osteotomy. Techniques described include a dome osteotomy, dorsal radial closing-wedge osteotomy, or volar opening-wedge radial osteotomy and bone grafting. The ulnar overgrowth is treated with an ulnar-shortening procedure (Fig. 23.16). Alternative methods of ulnar shortening include resection of the distal ulna and a Sauve-Kapandji procedure. However, there may already be significant deterioration of the articular cartilage, wrist ligaments, or triangular fibrocartilage, resulting in continued pain and limitation of motion postoperatively.

# HAND REGION

## Congenital

### Cleft Hand and Symbrachydactyly

Central defects of the hand have been described in the past as typical or atypical. Since 1992, the International Federation of Societies of Surgery of the Hand has classified typical cleft hands as *cleft hands* and atypical cleft hands as part of *symbrachydactyly*. Cleft hands represent a partial or complete longitudinal deficiency in the central portion of the hand. The elbow, forearm, and wrist are usually normal. There are often ulnar and radial-sided syndactylies and digital hypoplasia. Cleft hands often occur in conjunction with cleft feet. In that situation, there is an autosomal dominant inheritance pattern. However, the penetrance is variable, with approximately one third of the known carriers of the gene having no malformations (232,233). Genetic identification has been localized to the p63 gene on chromosome 3q27 (234–236). In addition, the phenotypic expression in affected individuals is variable. Cleft hands are also associated with other syndromes and malformations such as cleft lip/palate (ectrodactyly, ectodermal dysplasia, cleft syndrome), other craniofacial syndromes, Cornelia de Lange syndrome, congenital heart disease, ocular malformations, and imperforate anus (233,237). The incidence is estimated at between 1 in 90,000 and 1 in 100,000 live births (178,238,239). Various classification schemes have been used. Most have focused on the nature of the deformities (240,241). Manske and Halikis proposed a classification system of cleft hands based on the thumb and first web space (242). This scheme aids the surgeon in surgical reconstruction decisions and therefore may be the most useful classification.

Symbrachydactyly is defined by unilateral central digital deficiencies and simple syndactylies. It is a sporadic event without genetic inheritance. There are no associated anomalies. The feet are normal. It is a unilateral process, often with multiple absent digital rays. There are often finger nubbins present, which is a situation not seen in cleft hands. Symbrachydactyly is a transverse deficiency that may or may not be a separate entity from transverse absence of digits (233). These entities are distinct from the amputations associated with constriction band syndrome.

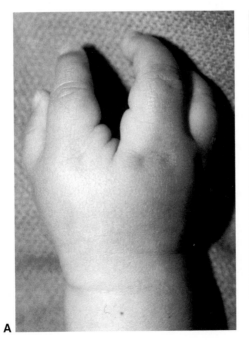 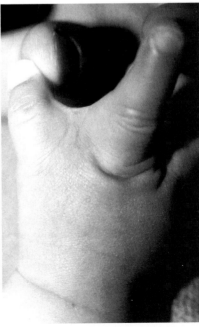

**Figure 23.16** **A:** Cleft hand with absent middle ray. **B:** Incomplete syndactyly of the first web space in the same patient. Closure of the cleft must include deepening of the first web space to maintain maximum hand function.

Symbrachydactyly should be viewed as a clinical entity distinct from cleft hand, with a very different treatment plan.

### Treatment

*Cleft Hands.* As Flatt (1) poignantly stated, "The cleft hand is a functional triumph and a social disaster." The wide central cleft allows for outstanding grasp, release, and pinch functions. Sensibility is normal. The cleft hand, therefore, functions usually without limits.

Treatment of the cleft hand centers on closure of the cleft. However, surgical closure of the cleft must be accompanied by appropriate treatment of the first web space and thumb to avoid limiting the patient. The skin flaps designed for cleft closure, however, must take into account the status of the first web space (Fig. 23.16). If the first web space is normal or mildly narrowed (Manske types I and IIA), simple cleft closure, such as with a Barsky flap (243), can be performed. If necessary, a simultaneous but separate Z-plasty widening of the first web space can be performed (Manske types IIA and IIB). If the first web space has a marked syndactyly (Manske type III), the flap designs use the redundant skin of the cleft closure to create a first web space. The adduction contracture of the thumb is released, and the index ray is transposed ulnarly at the same time. The Snow-Littler, Ueba, and Miura flaps (244–246) all involve transposition of the cleft skin to the first web space, with simultaneous transposition of the index ray ulnarly. If there is a transverse bone across the cleft, this must be removed in order to prevent progressive deformity. Often there is a conjoined flexor and extensor across the base of the cleft that has to be released. Sometimes carpal closing-wedge osteotomy is necessary to close the cleft. In addition, the stability of the index- and ring-finger MCP joints should be maintained or restored. Associated fourth web space syndactylies are separated with Z-plasties and skin grafts. There may be associated camptodactyly or clinodactyly of the adjacent digits requiring corrective splinting or surgery.

*Symbrachydactyly.* The treatment of symbrachydactyly in the United States is probably the most individualized of that of any of the congenital malformations. The range of options include (i) leaving the child alone; (ii) nonvascularized transfers to the soft-tissue nubbins of the phalanges (247,248); (iii) microvascular toe transfer(s) (249–253); (iv) web-space deepening; (v) digital distraction lengthening or bone grafting (254); and (vi) use of a prosthetic. In addition, families and patients are very interested in the possibilities of transplantation and laboratory cellular growth of digits. There is no definitive answer at present. The choice is greatly influenced by the family's desires and the surgeon's experience and biases. There are few peer-reviewed published studies regarding functional and cosmetic outcomes that would guide the decision more objectively. However, there are clear principles to help guide all parties as to the best choice for them.

The primary goal is to improve pinch. In the presence of a normal thumb and web space, all of the choices for treatment will work. In this situation, treatment options focus on the quality of the other digital rays. If the soft-tissue pockets of the digits are adequate, nonvascularized transfer of the proximal phalanx of the toes is a very good choice. Although it will not provide normal digital length, it will provide stability for lateral pinch. This must be performed before 18 months of age and include the periosteum and collateral ligaments (247,255). The proximal phalanx is harvested through an extensor-tendon-splitting dorsal approach. The proximal phalanx is harvested extraperiosteally, while protecting the neighboring tendons and neurovascular structures. At the metatarsophalangeal joint, the collateral ligaments, dorsal capsule, and volar plate are detached proximally from the metatarsal, while leaving intact their distal attachments to the phalanx. At the PIP joint, those soft tissues are left attached to the middle phalanx. With transfer to the hand, the proximal soft tissues of the toe phalanx are sutured to the corresponding soft tissues of the recipient site. The best results for phalangeal survival and growth are realized when this procedure is performed before 1 year of age. The quality of the soft-tissue pocket clearly affects the outcome. Multiple phalangeal transfers can be performed simultaneously. In the presence of a normal thumb and first web, digital lengthening can be performed. In addition, digital lengthening has been performed successfully after nonvascularized toe phalangeal transfer (254). Finally, prosthetic use has been tried. The major problems with prostheses are that children function as well or better without them because the prostheses are insensate. In the adolescent and adult, a cosmetic prosthesis may be used for social reasons (240). It should be noted that the finest cosmetic prostheses are very expensive.

If there is a deficient first web space, deepening of the web with release of the adduction contracture is appropriate. At times, this may require resection or transfer of the index metacarpal (Fig. 23.16) in order to achieve a useful web for pinch and grasp functions. If there is absence of the thumb, then digital transposition or microvascular transfer is indicated.

Microvascular toe transfer should be performed only if: the patient is a child older than 2 years; the family is well-informed about all aspects of the surgery and possible outcomes; there are proximal nerves, vessels, tendons, and muscles available for creating a viable and functional transfer; there is carpal or metacarpal support for the transfer; and there is an experienced surgical team (217). Unfortunately, although this procedure is being performed more commonly nowadays, objective data regarding functional, cosmetic, and psychologic outcomes are still minimal in relation to children.

### Constriction Band Syndrome

*Constriction band syndrome,* also known as *amnionic band syndrome,* or *amnion disruption sequence* is the result of disruption of the inner placental wall, the amnion. This early amnionic rupture often results in oligohydramnios and amnionic bands. The fibrous bands from the amnionic wall wrap around the digits, causing constricting digital bands, amputations, and syndactylies (256–258). Streeter (259) was the first to propose that this syndrome is a mechanical deformation rather than a malformation.

There is no inheritance pattern. This syndrome occurs in 1 in 15,000 live births (260). It is associated with other musculoskeletal deformations in 50% of cases, the most common being clubfeet. There may be devastating cleft lip and facial deformations as a result of deforming amnionic bands. There are no associated major organ system malformations.

In the hand, the ring finger is most frequently affected. This may be because in a clenched fist, the ring finger is the longest. The band may merely cause an indentation. However, if it is circumferential, the constriction ring may lead to distal edema or cyanosis (Fig. 23.17). Intrauterine amputations are the result of vascular insufficiency caused by the tourniquetlike bands. At times, this can be noted at birth with a necrotic or severely compromised phalanx distal to a constricting band. Syndactyly occurs when the bands attach adjacent digits (Fig. 23.18). There are often skin clefts proximal to the syndactyly, indicating the embryonic formation of a web space before the amnionic rupture and subsequent deformation. The extremity proximal to the band is normal. The development of the underlying tendons, nerves, vessels, and muscles is also normal.

***Clinical Treatment.*** Impending tissue necrosis is an indication for emergent removal of the band to relieve vascular compromise. This is a rare situation, usually seen only in the neonatal period. Removal of neonatal constricting bands

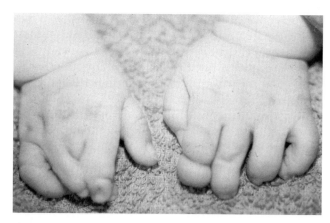

**Figure 23.18** Bilateral amnionic band syndrome with deep constriction rings on the left hand and partial acrosyndactyly and amputations on the right hand.

that are causing vascular compromise can generally be performed outside the operating room. The band will literally unravel or debride like an eschar. Improved venous drainage is almost immediate.

Multiple minor band indentations without vascular compromise or functional or cosmetic problems do not require treatment. Constricting rings that cause distal deformity are treated with excision of the constriction ring and staged Z-plasty reconstruction. Complete excision of the ring is necessary to recontour the digit or limb. The depth of excision can extend to the periosteum. Such digits usually have chronic impaired venous outflow with marked distal swelling. In these situations, it is imperative to preserve distal venous drainage and the deep neurovascular structures. Careful dissection of the veins, arteries, and nerves is performed on both sides of the deep constricting band. These structures are then delicately freed from the band to preserve their longitudinal integrity. It is recommended that complete circumferential excision not be performed in one procedure. Rather, excision up to 270 degrees at one time may be safest for preservation of vascular inflow and outflow. Z-plasties are performed after ring excision, so as to prevent recurrence.

Syndactyly release with Z-plasties and skin grafts follows the basic principles outlined in the section on syndactyly. The unique features of amnionic band syndrome are acrosyndactyly secondary to constricting bands and the presence of epithelialized incomplete web-space proximal to the syndactyly.

In the rare situation of constricting bands causing progressive deformity in digits of unequal length, early digital separation is necessary. More often, the acrosyndactyly separation can be performed after 6 months of life. There is usually limited skin for coverage, and creative flap design is needed to cover all the web spaces. Abundant skin graft is necessary. Distal release of complex syndactylies may require excision of osseous or cartilaginous synostoses. The embryologic remnant of the web is usually too distal and small to

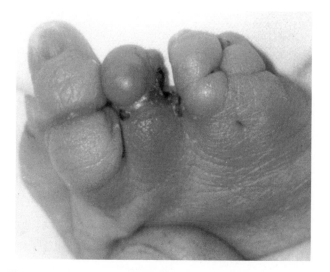

**Figure 23.17** An amnionic band causing digital ischemia in a neonate in the newborn nursery. This condition is rare, and requires immediate removal of the band in order to prevent further soft-tissue digital loss.

serve as an acceptable web reconstruction. Excision of that epithelial tract is usually performed. If that primitive web is used, it often must be deepened secondarily.

The most severe cases involve absence or deficiency of the thumb. The reconstruction can include metacarpal or phalangeal transposition from the index finger (261,262), nonvascularized toe phalangeal transfer, or vascularized toe transfer. It is imperative to reconstruct the thumb for pinch and proper grasp and release functions in these patients.

Because the underlying tissues are normal, as is the central nervous system, these patients have outstanding hand function after reconstruction. There are clear cosmetic differences, but minimal functional differences between them and their peers.

### Syndactyly

Syndactyly is one of the most common congenital deformities. It occurs because of a failure of separation of the digital rays *in utero*. Normal differentiation of digits occurs during the fifth to eighth weeks of gestation. Failure of normal programmed cell death results in *syn* (together) *dactylos* (digits). The incidence is between 1 in 2000 and 1 in 2500 live births (1). It can occur in isolation or as part of a syndromic condition. It is often an inheritable condition, whether in isolation or as part of a syndrome. It is bilateral and symmetric in up to 50% of patients. It is more common in boys than in girls.

Syndactyly is classified by the extent of, and the tissues involved in, the webbing. Digital separation *in utero* starts distally and proceeds proximally. Normally, the third web space is the most distal web, followed by the second, fourth, and first web spaces. The normal commissure of the web extends over 30% to 35% of the length of the proximal phalanx (263). The bones, joints, tendons, and neurovascular structures separate before the skin does. If separation fails to occur or ends prematurely, syndactyly

results. If it extends over the entire length of the phalanges, then it is complete. Complete syndactyly is when the web is more distal than is normal (Fig. 23.19); complex syndactyly is when there is osseous connection between the digits; and simple syndactyly is when the digits are joined by skin only (263). Acrosyndactyly involves webbing of the tips of all the digits. Syndactyly can also be a part of other major developmental problems in the hand that affect hand function, such as brachydactyly, camptodactyly, clinodactyly, symphalangism, and polydactyly. These are the most complicated syndactylies in terms of surgical decisions and care. As noted in the preceding section, syndactyly secondary to amnionic band syndrome is not a malformation, but an *in utero* disruption, and will be considered separately.

***Clinical and Radiographic Features.*** Syndactyly most often affects the third web space of the hand. It is sequentially less common in the fourth, second, and, finally, first web space (1). It may be associated with syndactyly of the toes. In isolated syndactyly, often one of the parents will have an incomplete syndactyly of the fingers and/or toes. As mentioned in the preceding text, there are many chromosomal, craniofacial syndromic, and generalized syndromic conditions associated with syndactyly. These all need to be evaluated before treating the syndactyly. The most important aspect of the hand evaluation for syndactyly is determination of the quality of the affected digits. In simple syndactyly, these digits are usually normal except for their skin union. In more complex situations, the digits may have malalignment, limited motion, and limited strength after surgical separation. Plain radiographs will reveal osseous union and marked joint and bony malalignment. However, in infancy, the areas of chondral abnormalities in the joints, physes, and between digits exhibiting syndactyly will not be visible on plain radiographs. MRI and arteriography are

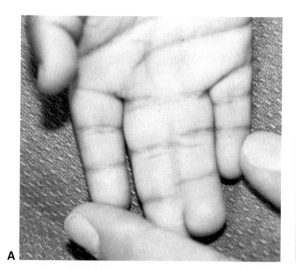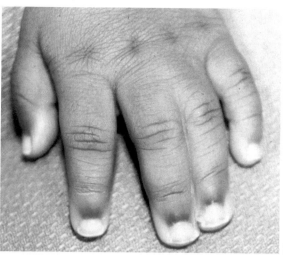

A                                                                                          B

**Figure 23.19   A,B:** A 1-year-old child with complete simple third web-space syndactyly. In this patient, the distal eponychial folds and nail plates are already separate. The underlying joints, tendons, nerves, and blood vessels should be separate and normal.

used only in very complex situations to define digital anatomy preoperatively.

*Treatment.* Patients with incomplete syndactyly may choose not to undergo surgical separation. If the syndactyly does not extend beyond the PIP joint, this will not limit function. However, it may affect wedding ring wear in the third web space, and for this reason, some patients request separation.

Most parents and children with complete syndactyly desire separation of the digits for functional and cosmetic reasons. There are rare situations in which a family declines surgery for complete syndactyly. Because of the discrepancy in the lengths of the adjacent digits, this usually results in some degree of bony malalignment and joint contracture. This is most marked in the border digit syndactylies (first and fourth web spaces), and least marked in the third web space. Leaving the digits joined also precludes independent function of the affected digits. There are also syndromic and chromosomal situations in which the overall health or mental capacity of the patient does not warrant the risks of surgical separation. Finally, there are situations of complex syndactyly in which the affected digits are too hypoplastic, malaligned, or stiff to warrant separation. Otherwise, the standard treatment is surgical separation of the affected digits.

Unfortunately, separation is not as simple as parents wish, that is, the simple division of the conjoined skin. The uncovered soft tissues result in linear scars with long-term joint contractures, digital malalignment, and loss of motion and function (223,264). Standard treatment now consists of: (i) local rotation flap coverage for the commissure; (ii) zig-zag incisions, avoiding the interdigital creases to prevent scar contractures; and (iii) full-thickness skin grafts to cover all areas of the digits not covered by local flaps (Fig. 23.20). In addition, special attention is given to the eponychial reconstruction with either local flaps or composite grafting (265).

Surgery is generally performed in infancy, when anesthesia and surgical handling of the tissues are safe. There is some controversy regarding the best age for surgery (1,266) but in most institutions it is performed at approximately 12 months of age (267). After 6 months of age, the anesthesia risk is equivalent throughout childhood. With magnification, surgery can be performed safely and skillfully during infancy. The only controversy concerns surgical healing and scarring. Neonatal releases result in more scarring. There is some evidence that surgical release performed at approximately 18 months of age may result in less scarring and recurrent web contractures than release during infancy (268). However, this is a very difficult developmental age for elective surgical intervention.

Complete separation of the digits in the neonatal period has had a higher rate of complications. Border digits of unequal length need to be separated earlier to lessen angular and rotatory deformity in the longer digit (Fig. 23.21).

In incomplete syndactyly that is proximal to the PIP joint, surgery usually involves the use of local flaps such as double-opposing Z-plasties and "stickman" or "dancing girl" flaps. Separation may not be to normal depth, but patients often prefer to avoid skin grafting (269). If the incomplete syndactyly extends to the middle phalangeal region, full-thickness skin grafting is necessary.

In simple, complete syndactyly, surgery involves the use of a dorsal rotation flap into the web, Z-plasty flaps the length of the digits, and full-thickness skin grafts to

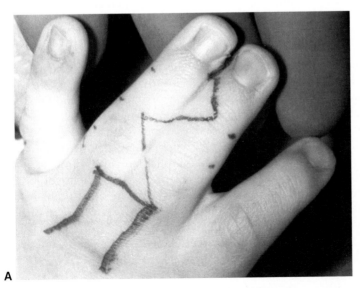
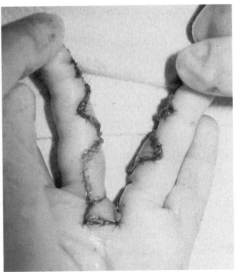

**Figure 23.20** **A:** Intraoperative photograph of a 1-year-old child with complete syndactyly treated with dorsal rotation flap coverage and Z-plasties, as outlined. Note the skin marks on the lateral borders of the ring and long fingers to outline the apex and base of each Z-plasty. This allows for precision placement of corresponding volar and dorsal Z-plasties. **B:** Intraoperative photograph after dorsal-to-volar rotation flap coverage for web space, Z-plasties, and full-thickness skin grafting.

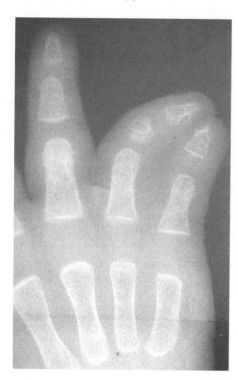

**Figure 23.21** Radiograph of complex syndactyly of the fourth web space with progressive deformity of the ring finger. This should be released early in infancy to prevent progressive deformity. The abnormal middle phalanx of the ring finger may still require corrective osteotomy.

cover the defects. It is important to have a vascularized flap for web skin reconstruction. This is usually done with a dorsal rectangular flap but may also involve a dorsal metacarpal island flap (270–272). The fascial connections between the digits extending from Grayson and Cleland ligaments need to be separated. Any synostosis or synchondrosis union of the distal phalanges should be divided. Conjoined nails are divided, and the exposed eponychial and paronychial regions are reconstructed with local flaps or composite grafts (273,274). If the common digital nerve extends beyond the desired web deepening, epineural separation is performed proximally. If the common digital artery bifurcates distally, ligation of one of the proper digital arteries may be necessary for obtaining the desired separation. This is one of the major reasons why surgery is not performed on both sides of a single digit in multiple syndactylies.

Complex syndactylies are more likely to have abnormal underlying joints, bones, neurovascular structures, muscles, or tendons. The separation of skin follows the same principles as in complete syndactyly. If there is significant digital malalignment, skin incisions may need to be modified so as to maximize coverage. After separation of the skin, all abnormal connections of fascia, tendons, bones, joints, nerves, and arteries need to be addressed individually. Phalangeal deformity may require osteotomy. Instability of the joints may require ligamentous reconstruction. Stiffness of the joints, camptodactyly, or symphalangism may need

to be dealt with subsequently. Neural, vascular, and nail problems are managed in a manner similar to those described for complete syndactyly. Tendon reconstruction is performed primarily if possible. Brachydactyly is usually addressed subsequently, if at all.

Acrosyndactyly separation begins early in life, especially if it is bilateral. Adjacent webs are not separated simultaneously. Generally, the first and third webs are separated together, as are the second and fourth webs. Abundant full-thickness skin graft is usually required. Sufficient time between procedures (3 to 6 months) lessens worries about flap necrosis and scar contracture. In syndromic conditions, such as Apert syndrome, the acrosyndactyly is more complex, and normalcy may never be achieved (275,276).

*Complications.* Fortunately, the most worrisome complication, an avascular digit, is almost never encountered and should be avoidable. Adhering to the axiom of never operating on both sides of a digit during the same procedure prevents the occurrence of this devastating complication. Careful dissection of the digital vessels in complex situations lessens the risk of avascularity at the initial or subsequent operations. Preoperative vascular studies in complicated situations prepare the surgeon and allow him or her to avoid intraoperative surprises and dangers. Flap necrosis and scar contracture are more common. The flaps should be secured without tension, and their vascularity should be checked with deflation of the tourniquet at the completion of the procedure. If in doubt, lessen the tension and use skin graft. Skin graft failure is usually caused by inadequate immobilization and excessive shear forces applied to the grafts. Secure immobilization with the compressive dressing, long-arm cast, and sling and swathe bandages is necessary for protecting the grafts. Infection is rare but will result in marked scar contractures that require reoperation. Long-term issues that have been reported regarding skin graft sites include contracture formation, graft breakdown (both incidences are seen more often with split thickness grafts), hyperpigmentation, and hair growth (both incidences are seen more often with full thickness grafts) (277). Nail deformity and poor eponychial coverage are common when there is an initial conjoined nail. The use of composite grafts seems to lessen the incidence of these complications. Web-space creep is common with growth, but often does not require reoperation unless digital contractures develop. The use of local rotation flaps and skin grafts will resolve this problem. Keloid formation is rare but has been shown to be associated with primary digital enlargement before syndactyly separation (278). Finally, angular deformity may require osteotomy or joint reconstruction.

### Polydactyly

Polydactyly is a common congenital malformation. It can occur on the radial (preaxial), central, or ulnar (postaxial) portion of the hand. Preaxial, or thumb, polydactyly usually occurs in isolation and will be addressed in the section dealing with the thumb. Central polydactyly is very rare and is usually associated with syndactyly; the underlying digits are rarely normal. It can be inherited in an autosomal dominant manner. It affects girls more than boys, and is often bilateral. Postaxial or small-finger polydactyly has a variable racial incidence, with the occurrence in African Americans estimated to be as high as 1 in 300 live births, and that in whites estimated to be 1 in 3000 live births (279–281). It is often bilateral. Polydactyly has been classified by Stelling (282) and Turek (283) into three types. Type I involves soft tissue alone and is very common in the African American population. Type II involves phalangeal duplication articulating with a single or bifid metacarpal head. Type III involves a complete ulnar ray duplication, including the metacarpal. There is also a universal classification of polydactyly proposed by Buck-Gramcko and Behrens (260) that denotes the digit involved by a Roman numeral (I to V) and the extent of bifurcation by abbreviation [DIST (distal), DIP (distal interphalangeal), MID (middle), PIP (proximal interphalangeal), PROX (proximal), MCP (metacarpophalangeal), MET (metacarpal), CMC (carpometacarpal), C (carpal), IC (intercarpal), and RUD (rudimentary polydactyly)]. The major issue for the surgeon is not the classification of the polydactyly, but whether excision with reconstruction, or reconstruction alone, is warranted. Only postaxial soft-tissue polydactyly (type I, or rudimentary) can be treated by excision alone. All other forms require reconstruction. Central polydactyly is usually an isolated malformation, and postaxial polydactyly in African Americans is almost always an isolated malformation. Postaxial polydactyly in whites without a positive family history may be associated with chromosomal abnormalities, other syndromes, or other malformations.

*Treatment.* Soft-tissue polydactyly on the ulnar side can be treated with excision during the newborn period (Fig. 23.22). Unfortunately, too often this has been performed with a suture ligature by inexperienced hands. The result is a persistent nubbin caused by incomplete excision of the base of the digit. If a suture ligature is used, it must bring about necrosis of the entire digit. Otherwise, it may be best to perform an elliptical excision under local anesthesia. Care is taken to ligate the digital vessels with this excision. Other than failure to completely excise the digit, complications are rare, and the hand is normal afterward. There have been reports of traumatic neuromas along with hypertrophic scars that have led to late problems and the need for repeat surgery (284, 285). The parents should be aware of the future genetic implications for them and their children.

More complex postaxial polydactylies require excision and reconstruction in the operating room (Fig. 23.22). In addition to excising the redundant parts, transfer of the hypothenar muscles (abductor digiti quinti, flexor digiti quinti) from the sixth to the fifth digit is necessary. In type II polydactyly, the MCP joint collateral ligaments are also transferred to the reconstructed fifth digit. If the metacarpal head is enlarged or bifid, intraarticular osteotomy is appropriate. In this procedure, the origins of the collateral ligament and the metacarpal physis should be preserved. In type III polydactyly, the entire ray is resected, and the basilar joint is stabilized. The outcome of surgery in both type II and type III malformations is usually cosmetic and functional normalcy.

Treatment of central synpolydactyly is much more complex (286,287). The major decision is whether it is feasible to achieve independently functioning digits. The choices are to leave the digits conjoined, to attempt reconstruction to a five-digit hand, or to perform ray resections of part or all of the synpolydactyly. Often the involved digits have bone and joint malalignment, hypoplasia, and poor motor, nerve, and vascular supplies. The reconstructed digit is usually smaller, stiffer, weaker, and malaligned. The family needs to be well aware of this, so that their expectations are realistic as far as surgical reconstruction and digital function are concerned. Treatment decisions in this condition are often personal, based on the family's desires and the surgeon's preferences.

### Camptodactyly

Camptodactyly translates from Greek to mean *bent finger*. It involves a flexion deformity of the PIP joint, most commonly in the small finger. It may present in infancy or in adolescence. It may involve a single digit or multiple digits (Fig. 23.23).

Camptodactyly may be associated with multiple systemic malformations. Its incidence is unknown but has been cited at less than 1% of the general population (288,289). Most cases appear in infancy, and there is equal gender distribution (290). Less commonly, it may first appear in adolescence, usually in girls (291). Some cases are familial, with an autosomal dominant inheritance etiology and variable penetrance patterns. Most cases are isolated, without a positive family history. Up to two thirds of the patients have bilateral small-finger involvement. It is important to distinguish camptodactyly from neurologic causes of clawing or from posttraumatic butonniere deformities (292).

There is debate about the cause. In simple terms, there is an anatomic imbalance between the flexor and extensor mechanisms (290). This may be secondary to an abnormal insertion of the lumbricals, flexor digitorum superficialis, or retinacular ligaments (293–298). The volar skin is usually tight. With growth, these anatomic abnormalities cause PIP joint contracture and phalangeal bony abnormalities. The distal proximal phalanx becomes narrowed volarly and flattened dorsally, with loss of the normal contour of the head. The articular surface can become incongruous, with notching of the base of the middle phalanx (299). Initially, the patient can compensate for the PIP

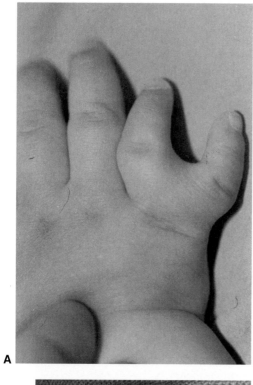

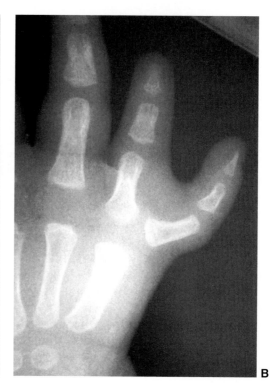

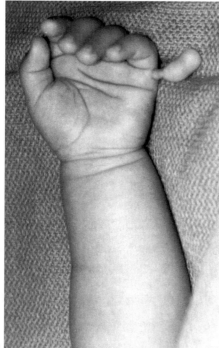

**Figure 23.22 A:** Complete postaxial polydactyly with phalangeal duplication with a conjoined metacarpal. **B:** Radiograph of the same patient. Reconstruction will consist of excision of the duplicate phalanges, contouring of the bifid metacarpal head, and transfer of the metacarpophalangeal joint ulnar collateral ligament and the hypothenar musculature to the reconstructed fifth digit. **C:** Simple polydactyly with only soft-tissue attachment. This can be excised in the newborn nursery under local anesthesia. Care must be exercised while performing suture ligature; the entire stalk should be excised so as to avoid leaving a residual nubbin.

joint flexion contracture by MCP and distal interphalangeal (DIP) joint hyperextension (Fig. 23.24). This keeps the digital pulp of the affected fingers in line with the other digital rays. Therefore, the mild contracture in the older child may not need treatment. However, as the contracture continues to progress beyond 30 degrees and toward 90 degrees, it becomes more difficult for the patient to compensate. Camptodactyly is usually progressive with growth.

*Treatment.* Treatment should attempt to restore normal flexor-extensor balance. The options for treatment are splinting and surgical reconstruction. Most clinicians recommend an initial treatment program of progressive passive extension and splinting with dynamic or progressive static splints. Parents are instructed to perform frequent home exercises for their infants; affected adolescents are similarly instructed to perform a home program for themselves. The

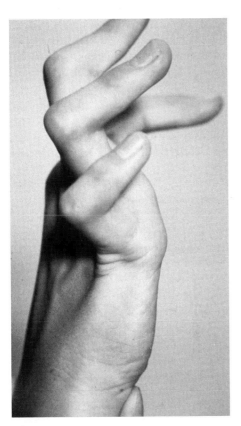

**Figure 23.23**   An adolescent patient with marked camptodactyly of the small, ring, and long fingers. There are proximal interphalangeal joint flexion contractures in each digit, and the patient is actively hyperextending the metacarpophalangeal joints to compensate for those contractures.

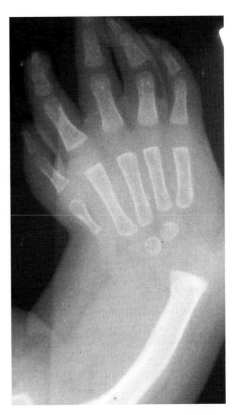

**Figure 23.24**   Radiograph of a thumb with type IIIB hypoplasia without a carpometacarpal joint and proximal thumb metacarpal. This is usually treated with pollicization. Less often, treatment is by reconstruction, potentially including a microvascular toe metatarsophalangeal transfer to form a thumb carpometacarpal joint. Note the radial dysplasia in this patient.

goal is to achieve full passive extension. It is hoped that active extension will follow. Many clinicians (291,300–302) report success with a splinting program in most cases. The best results are in mild cases in young patients. The patients are followed until the end of growth in order to treat recurrence if it occurs.

There is significant debate regarding the indications for surgery. McFarlane et al. strongly recommend surgical intervention to reconstruct the aberrant insertion of the lumbrical (297,298). However, the published surgical results are disappointing in terms of outcome (297,298, 301,303). Surgery is reserved for severe contractures that are not amenable to splinting treatment. Specifically, surgery shows best results in patients in whom the finger is flexed into the palm and obstructs use of the hand. The principle of surgical intervention is to correct the abnormal anatomy. This involves release of the aberrant lumbrical (288,297,298) or flexor digitorum superficialis (294) insertion in conjunction with volar Z-plasties and PIP joint release (303). Local flaps or full-thickness skin grafts are often necessary for volar skin coverage. Tendon transfer to the extensor mechanism is performed in patients with full passive extension of the PIP joint, but no active extension (304). The results of soft-tissue reconstruction often merely change the arc of motion rather than normalize it. Preoperatively,

patients have significant flexion contracture. Postoperatively, they generally have difficulty achieving full active and passive flexion.

There are frequently bony changes present at the PIP joint, and these preclude restoration of normal motion or alignment. Oldfield (305) and Flatt (1) have stated that, in the presence of marked radiographic evidence of bone and joint changes, corrective extension osteotomy may be most effective at improving alignment and function. The published data about this salvage operation are too limited to enable objective evaluation (288).

In summary, with treatment of camptodactyly it is unusual to achieve a perfectly aligned and mobile digit. Parents and patients should be aware of this from the outset. In addition, deformity can recur with growth and persistent muscle imbalance.

### Clinodactyly

Clinodactyly is abnormal angulation (>10 degrees) of the digit in the radioulnar plane. It is usually caused by a misshapen middle phalanx. The middle phalanx is trapezoidal, with less height on the radial side. This results in deviation at the DIP joint. Clinodactyly is most often seen in the small finger and is usually bilateral. This form of clinodactyly has an autosomal dominant inheritance (306–309). Clinodactyly is also frequently associated with syndromes (Holt-Oram, Turner, Silver, and Cornelia de Lange) and chromosomal abnormalities (trisomy 18 and 21), and should alert the primary neonatal examiner to look for associated malformations or problems. For example, clinodactyly of the thumb is seen in Rubinstein-Taybi syndrome (310,311) and diastrophic dwarfism (312,313). In addition, it is common with other congenital abnormalities of the hand. Mild clinodactyly, however, is commonplace in otherwise healthy individuals. In these situations the major issue is cosmesis. Function is affected only when the deformity is severe enough to impinge on the adjacent digit during flexion.

**Treatment.** Treatment is based on the degree of deformity. Most cases are mild and nonprogressive, and therefore do not warrant surgical intervention. Progressive, severe clinodactyly may interfere with flexion and grip. In these rare situations, the progressive deformity is secondary to altered physeal growth. The middle phalangeal physis may be a bracket delta phalanx. Treatment options are bracket resection and surgical realignment. Physeal bar resection and fat graft interposition have been reported by Vickers (314,315) to restore longitudinal growth and provide correction. Surgical realignment can be in the form of opening-wedge, closing-wedge, and reverse-wedge osteotomies. Osteotomy should be delayed until there is sufficient ossification of the middle phalanx to allow for precise cuts. Generally, this is around school age. The complications of osteotomy are persistent deformity and loss of interphalangeal motion. Loss of motion in a patient whose indication for surgery was purely cosmesis is unacceptable to most patients, their families, and surgeons.

# HAND: THUMB

Congenital deformities of the thumb occur in all categories of congenital hand anomalies described by the American Society and the International Federation of Societies for Surgery of the Hand. Failure of formation occurs with aplasia of the thumb, and this is often associated with other radial-sided longitudinal deficiencies. Failure of separation occurs with thumb-index syndactylies, which are common with other syndactyly syndromes. Duplication is seen in the form of thumb polydactyly, undergrowth as thumb hypoplasia, and overgrowth as macrodactyly and triphalangeal thumbs. Also, thumb abnormalities are common as part of constriction band syndrome or generalized musculoskeletal disorders. The list is exhaustive and this section will cover the more common congenital thumb malformations.

## Trigger Thumbs/Digits

Trigger thumb represents an abnormality of the flexor pollicis longus and its tendon sheath at the A1 pulley, where there is a palpable mass (Notta nodule), representing the flexor pollicis longus constriction at the A1 pulley. In the past, trigger thumbs were defined as congenital. However, this condition is *almost always* acquired in the first 2 years of life, as indicated by a prospective screening of neonates, which failed to record any trigger thumbs (316,317). The cause appears to be a size mismatch between the flexor pollicis longus and the A1 pulley, leading to progressive constriction. Unlike adult trigger digits, there does not appear to be an inflammatory component (318); 30% of the cases are bilateral. Isolated trigger thumbs have no associated syndromes. However, trigger digits are seen with neurologic syndromes (trisomy 18) and mucopolysaccharidoses (319). There is no familial inheritance pattern. Patients with trigger thumb present at ages ranging from infancy to school age. Often, the diagnosis is missed until local trauma brings attention to the thumb. In the emergency setting, the flexed interphalangeal joint can be mistaken for an interphalangeal joint dislocation. Radiographs are misleading because of limited phalangeal ossification. A palpable nodule at the A1 pulley is diagnostic. If the trigger is longstanding, compensatory hyperextension of the MCP joint develops to effectively bring the thumb out of the palm. In addition, mild radial deviation of the interphalangeal joint may develop, secondary to eccentric flexor pull.

### Treatment

In infants younger than 9 months of age, Dinham and Meggit (320) found that 30% of trigger thumbs may resolve spontaneously. In infants older than 1 year of age, less than 10% of trigger thumbs resolved spontaneously. Ger et al. (321) found lack of resolution in their patients after observation for 3 years. There is limited evidence that splinting is of benefit (322), and often it is not well tolerated. Surgical release of the constricting A1 pulley and flexor tendon sheath is the treatment of choice indicated in infants who show no spontaneous resolution by 1 year of age, and in any toddler or older child presenting with a locked trigger thumb. Incision is made transversely in the digital crease to lessen scarring. Care must be taken to avoid injury to the superficial digital neurovascular bundles. The oblique pulley has to be preserved so as to prevent flexor tendon bowstringing. Recurrence is extremely rare.

Trigger digits are more often multiple, and can be associated with central nervous system disorders and syndromes (trisomy 18, mucopolysaccharidoses). The pathology appears to predominate at the decussation of the flexor tendons under the A2 pulley, and not at the A1 pulley alone. The triggering appears to occur as the flexor digitorum profundus passes through the chiasm of the flexor digitorum superficialis. Surgical recurrence is high in pediatric trigger digits. This may be because A1 pulley release alone is not sufficient to solve the problem (323). Further opening of the chiasm or resection of a slip of the flexor digitorum superficialis is often necessary to prevent recurrence (319).

## Hypoplasia/Aplasia of the Thumb

Children with thumb hypoplasia or aplasia will have deficient prehension and grasp. Thumb hypoplasia or aplasia can occur in isolation, or be associated with other radial-sided deficiency syndromes (Holt-Oram and Fanconi syndromes). It is seen universally in radial dysplasia. It is also common in other congenital malformations (206,324), including those of the cardiac, craniofacial, musculoskeletal, renal, gastrointestinal, and hematopoietic systems. It may involve hypoplasia of the metacarpals (Cornelia de Lange syndrome and diastrophic dwarfism) or phalanges (Rubinstein-Taybi and Apert syndromes). The finding of a thumb deficiency in a neonate should prompt a thorough multiple-system examination for other malformations. In addition, a DEB screening for Fanconi anemia is recommended for all infants with radial-sided defects including thumb hypoplasia.

In general terms, thumb hypoplasia includes a contracted first web space, unstable MCP joint, thenar weakness, and interphalangeal joint stiffness or instability. Buck-Gramcko (325) and Manske et al. (326) have modified the Blauth (327) classification for thumb hypoplasia. This classification system is useful from the point of view of treatment considerations. There are five types of thumb hypoplasia in the Buck-Gramcko modification of the Blauth classification (Table 23.3). A type I thumb is essentially a normal thumb, except for diminished size. A type II thumb is even smaller and narrower, with a contracted first web space and thenar atrophy. Type III thumbs have marked atrophy or absence of both the intrinsic and extrinsic musculature. The thumb is globally unstable and underdeveloped. Manske et al. (326) further subdivided type III thumbs into A and B categories.

### TABLE 23.3

### MODIFIED BLAUTH CLASSIFICATION OF CONGENITAL THUMB HYPOPLASIA

| Type | Findings |
|---|---|
| I | Small thumb with hypoplasia of abductor pollicus brevis and opponens pollicus |
| II | Narrow first web space, laxity of the ulnar collateral ligament of the metacarpophalangeal joint, thenar muscle hypoplasia |
| III | Global thenar weakness and metacarpophalangeal joint collateral ligament instability, partial aplasia of the first metacarpal, extrinsic weakness |
| IIIA | As in the previous category, with proximal metacarpal and carpometacarpal joints present |
| IIIB | Absent proximal metacarpal, with deficient carpometacarpal joint |
| IV | *Pouce flottant* (floating thumb); no bony support |
| V | Thumb aplasia |

Findings are additive with increasing severity.
Adapted from Tada K, Kurisaki E, Yonenobu K, et al. Central polydactyly—a review of 12 cases and their surgical treatment. *J Hand Surg [Am]* 1982;7(5):460–465; Wood VE. Treatment of central polydactyly. *Clin Orthop Relat Res* 1971;74:196–205; Kay S. Camptodactyly. In: Green DP, Hotchkiss RN, Pederson WC. eds. *Green's operative hand surgery*, 4th ed. New York: Churchill-Livingstone, 1999:510, with permission.

Type IIIA thumbs have a stable carpometacarpal (CMC) joint, whereas type IIIB thumbs have absence of the proximal metacarpal and trapezium. Type IIIB thumbs have no basilar joint stability (Fig. 23.23). Type IV thumbs are the classic *pouce flottant* or "floating thumbs." A type V demonstrates complete aplasia of the thumb.

The pathoanatomy is dependent on the severity of the thumb hypoplasia. Universally, the thumb ray bones are smaller and narrower. The interphalangeal joint is usually underdeveloped and stiff. The first web space is contracted in all except the rare type I thumb. The MCP joint usually has ulnar collateral ligament insufficiency, but may be globally unstable. The thenar intrinsics are deficient, and they may be completely absent in the more severe forms of hypoplasia. The thumb's extrinsic musculature is progressively deficient in the classification scheme. The major anatomic determining factor for reconstruction is the status of the CMC joint. Type IIIB and type IV thumbs have no basilar joints. Plain radiographs are helpful in distinguishing the skeletal development, including the carpus and distal radius.

### Treatment

The choice in the treatment of children with thumb hypoplasia is whether to do surgery or not. If left alone, these children will adapt. They will use lateral pinch between the long and index fingers. However, the deficiencies in pinch, grasp, and fine motor activities will be significant. Surgical reconstruction can improve function and cosmesis, and should be advised (328).

Reconstruction of the hypoplastic thumb, therefore, includes first web space deepening; opponensplasty, with either the abductor digiti quinti or the ring-finger flexor digitorum superficialis tendon; and MCP joint stabilization, with either ligamentous reconstruction or arthrodesis. Blauth types I to IIIA should be reconstructed according to these principles (Fig. 23.25). The choice of first web-space deepening procedure includes two-part and four-part Z-plasties or the use of dorsal rotation flaps from the index finger, thumb, or hand. The degree of contracture determines the amount of skin necessary to provide a normal depth and breadth to the web for pinch and grasp activities. The abductor digiti quinti transfer for opposition can be used in the infant with a relatively stable MCP joint. Care must be taken to protect the proximal neurovascular pedicle to the abductor muscle, with dissection near the pisiform (193). In older children, or in patients with marked instability of the MCP joint, the ring-finger flexor digitorum superficialis is used for opposition. The additional tendon length can be used for ligamentous reconstruction. In addition to the flexor digitorum superficialis tendon, local fascia from the adductor can be mobilized for ligamentous augmentation at the MCP joint. If soft tissue procedures fail, or the instability at the MCP joint is too severe, fusion can be performed. The physis of the proximal phalanx should be preserved so as to maximize growth of the thumb ray. Chondrodesis of the metacarpal head to the epiphysis of the proximal phalanx is desirable.

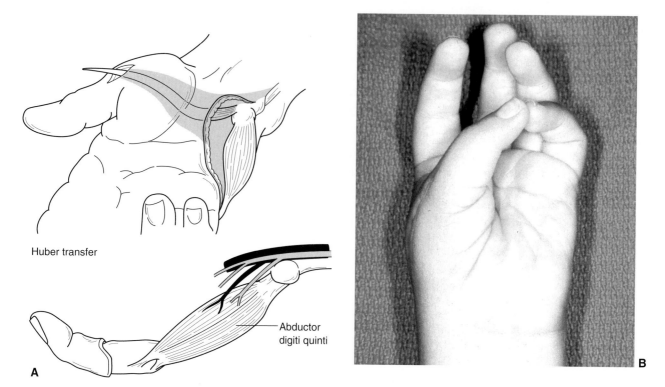

Huber transfer

Abductor
digiti quinti

**A**

**B**

**Figure 23.25**   **A:** Illustration of Huber opponensplasty transfer of abductor digiti quinti to the abductor pollicus brevis for a hypoplastic thumb reconstruction. It is imperative that the neurovascular bundle be preserved proximally during the transfer. **B:** Postoperative clinical photograph of opposition pinch in a patient with a Huber opponensplasty reconstruction.

Thumb hypoplasia with the absence of a basal joint (type IIIB), *pouce flottant* (type IV), or aplasia of the thumb (type V) are candidates for pollicization of the index finger. The major area of controversy is still the type IIIB thumb. In the absence of a CMC joint, the results of reconstruction have been disappointing (329). It is a difficult decision for the parents to accept pollicization in these children, because of the appearance of the thumb. However, reconstruction without a CMC joint leads to continued lateral pinch of the index and long fingers, rather than use of the reconstructed thumb. CMC joint reconstruction, with microvascular transfer of a toe metatarsophalangeal joint, has rarely been performed in children with type IIIB thumbs (329). This is an alternative to pollicization in these children. Surgery is performed later and is quite extensive. Pollicization involves the conversion of the triphalangeal index finger, without a basilar joint and a narrow web space, to a biphalangeal thumb with a CMC joint and a deep first web space. The removal of the index metacarpal and the use of the index metacarpal epiphysis as the trapezium enable the surgeon to properly position and cover the thumb. The technique described by Buck-Gramcko is used most commonly (203,204) (Fig. 23.26). In the congenital absence of the thumb, this is better than microvascular toe transfer. Thumb reconstruction or pollicization is generally performed between 6 and 18 months of age. The quality of the pollicized digit is dependent on the quality of the original index finger, in terms of tendon function and joint motion. Patients with thumb aplasia and radial dysplasia generally do more poorly, because the involved index finger has deficient musculature and camptodactyly. Manske and McCarroll performed secondary opposition transfers in children with poor pollicization (208). The best results are seen in children who have aplasia alone, and normal index fingers (Fig. 23.27).

## Thumb Duplication

### Preaxial Polydactyly

Thumb duplication may be a misnomer because it implies that there are two normal thumbs whereas, in fact, both thumbs are hypoplastic. In isolation, thumb duplication is usually a sporadic occurrence. It may be associated with genetic syndromes, such as acrocephalopolysyndactyly (Nocack and Carpenter types) and Holt-Oram or Robinow syndromes. If it is associated with a triphalangeal thumb or with duplication of the great toe, it may be autosomal dominant, with variable penetrance (330). The locus for preaxial polydactyly has been mapped to chromosome 7q36 (331) inheritance. Preaxial polydactyly is a rare occurrence, with an incidence estimated at 0.08 in 100,000 live births. There are many different classification systems, including the universal (332), Marks and Bayne (333), and Wassel (334) systems. Classification by the Wassel system

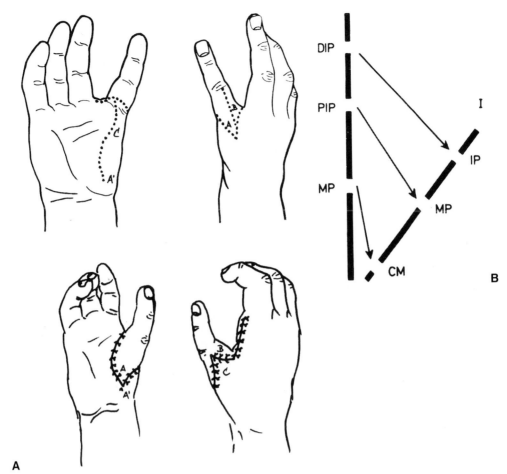

**Figure 23.26** Illustrations of the pollicization procedure as popularized by Buck-Gramcko. **A:** Outlines show the skin incisions that provide first web-space flap coverage as the pollex is positioned for opposition. The triphalangeal index finger is converted into a biphalangeal thumb. The index metacarpal is excised, except for the distal epiphysis. **B:** The changes in joints from the index finger to the thumb and the tendon transfers to provide opposition and pinch function are as follows: extensor indicis proprius → extensor pollicis longus; extensor digitorum II → abductor pollicis longus; interosseus palmaris I → adductor pollicis; interosseus dorsalis I → abductor pollicis brevis. *DIP*, distal interphalangeal; *PIP*, proximal interphalangeal; *MP*, metacarpophalangeal; *IP*, interphalangeal; *CM*, carpometacarpal; *I* number of finger.

is dependent on the number of bifid or duplicated phalanges or metacarpals, starting distally and progressing proximally (Fig. 23.28). A bifid distal phalanx is Wassel type I. A duplicated distal phalanx is type II (Fig. 23.28), constituting approximately 20% of all thumb duplications. A duplicated distal phalanx with a bifid proximal phalanx is type III. A thumb with duplicated proximal and distal phalanges is type IV, which is the most common type (approximately 40%) (Fig. 23.29). Duplicated proximal and distal phalanges with a bifid MTP is type V. Duplication of all phalanges and metacarpals is type VI. Any duplication with a triphalangeal thumb is type VII, which accounts for approximately 20% of thumb duplications.

The pathoanatomy is dependent on the type of polydactyly. The nails, bones, joints, ligaments, muscles, tendons, nerves, and blood vessels are split between the two digits. In addition, there can be hypoplasia or aplasia of any of the normal anatomic elements of a thumb. Plain radiographs will generally provide definitive information regarding skeletal pathoanatomy. Careful surgical exploration will define the soft-tissue anatomy.

***Treatment.*** Surgical reconstruction is the treatment of choice to improve function and cosmesis. Unlike postaxial polydactyly, ablation in the nursery is not recommended, even for the simplest preaxial polydactyly. Too often, the thenar musculature and collateral ligaments insert on the radius-based digit and can be lost with simple excision (335–337).

Treatment involves excision of the more hypoplastic thumb and reconstruction of the more developed thumb. Generally, the radius-based digit is excised. The soft-tissue elements usually bifurcate at the level of the skeletal split. Transfers of the shared or aberrant tendons, nerves, and ligaments to the reconstructed thumb are necessary in order to maximize outcome.

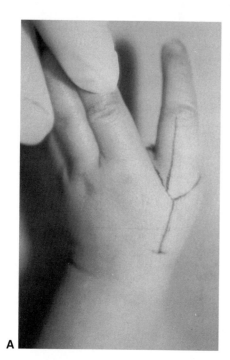 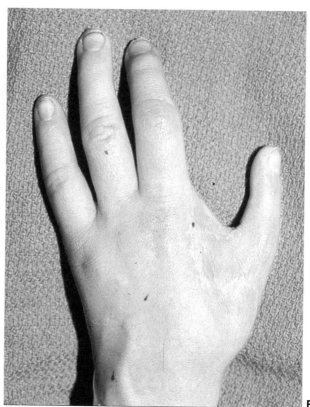

**Figure 23.27** **A:** A 1-year-old child with thumb aplasia. The surgical incisions for index pollicization are outlined. These flaps provide for deep first web space. **B:** Long-term follow-up clinical photograph of a pollicization.

The extensor pollicis longus tendon is usually bifid. The flexor pollicis longus usually inserts on the ulnar thumb, although it can be bifid or insert on the radial thumb. The thenar musculature and the radial collateral ligament to the MCP joint usually insert radially, especially in the common type IV polydactyly (Fig. 23.29). These should be transposed. The radial digital nerve may be present only in the radial thumb, and should be transposed to the radial aspect of the reconstructed thumb. The bifid proximal phalanx or metacarpal should be excised in types II and IV, respectively. Primary phalangeal or metacarpal osteotomy is indicated if there is axial malalignment. The more developed thumb often has a larger nail and distal phalanx. However, some Wassel type II malformations have almost equally sized distal phalanges and nails (Fig. 23.30). Surgical recombination of the distal phalanx and nail beds (Bilhaut-Cloquet procedure) in types I and II malformations has been disappointing because of poor nails, loss of joint motion, and physeal closure. It still appears best to accept the more hypoplastic distal phalanx than to consider recombination of the nail and phalanx (338). Adduction contracture of the first web space should be treated with Z-plasty to deepen the web space. The need for additional surgery with growth may be as high as 40% of cases.

Angular deformity of the proximal and distal phalanges into a zig-zag posture is the most common problem (339–342). Reconstruction with osteotomy, tendon transfers, ligament reconstruction, or arthrodesis may be necessary to improve both function and cosmesis.

## Triphalangeal Thumbs

Triphalangeal thumbs are usually inherited in an autosomal dominant manner. This is true whether they are associated with thumb polydactyly (343) or are seen in isolation. In inherited isolated triphalangeal thumbs, the genetic marker has been localized to chromosomal region 7q36 (344). The extra phalanx is the middle phalanx. It may be wedge-shaped or rectangular. The thumb may be in a position of opposition or in the plane of motion of the other fingers. The latter situation may indicate an index finger duplication with an absent thumb. This concept is supported not only by the clinical and radiographic appearance of the most radial digit, but also by the dermatoglyphics (345). The triphalangeal thumbs that were studied contained the radial loops normally seen in the index finger and not in the thumb.

Triphalangeal thumbs may be associated with musculoskeletal malformations, such as cleft feet and preaxial polydactyly (346); congenital heart disease, including Holt-Oram syndrome (347); hematopoietic abnormalities such as Fanconi and Blackfan-Diamond syndromes (348,349); and imperforate anus (350).

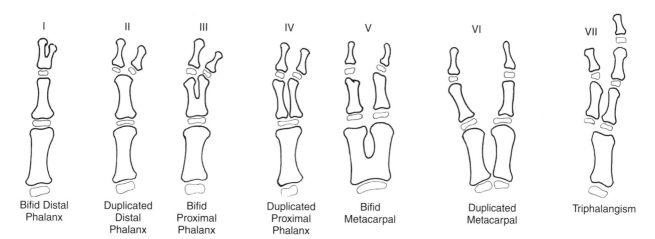

I — Bifid Distal Phalanx

II — Duplicated Distal Phalanx

III — Bifid Proximal Phalanx

IV — Duplicated Proximal Phalanx

V — Bifid Metacarpal

VI — Duplicated Metacarpal

VII — Triphalangism

**Figure 23.28** Wassel classification of thumb duplications. Type IV is the most common, with an incidence of 40%. Types II and VII have an incidence of approximately 20% each.

Classification and pathoanatomy are dependent on the type of triphalangism. Type I involves a delta middle phalanx with radial deviation deformity (Fig. 23.31). Type II involves a normal middle phalanx, but an opposable thumb. Type III is an index-finger duplication with all digits in the same plane. In types I and II triphalangism, the first web space is normal. In the five-fingered hand (type III), there is a contracted first web space that limits prehension. Similarly, usually the thenar musculature is normal in type I and type II triphalangeal thumbs, whereas it is absent in type III triphalangism. In addition, the triphalangeal thumb may be hypoplastic and have associated extrinsic musculature weakness.

### Treatment

Rarely, patients with triphalangeal thumbs prefer not to undergo surgical reconstruction. Patients with significant cosmetic abnormalities and limitation of pinch prefer

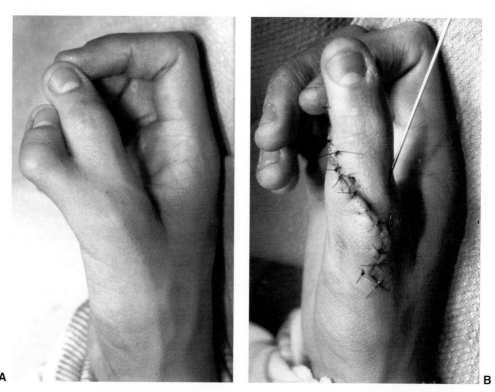

**Figure 23.29** **A:** An adolescent with the more common Wassel type IV thumb duplication. **B:** Results at the conclusion of the surgical reconstruction. Surgery included excision of the radial proximal and distal duplicated digits, transfer of the thenars and metacarpophalangeal joint radial collateral ligament to the reconstructed thumb, and contouring of the skin by excision of redundancy and Z-plasties.

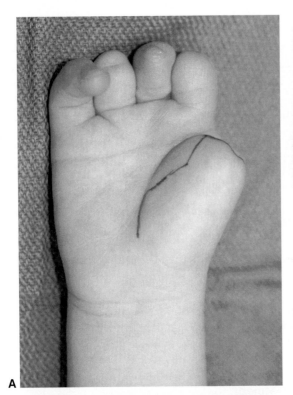

A

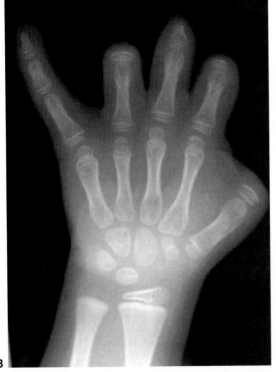

B

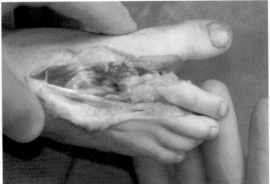

C

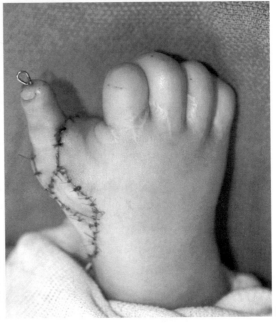

D

**Figure 23.30** **A:** Preoperative clinical photograph of a toddler with constriction band syndrome and congenital amputation of the thumb at the metacarpal–phalangeal joint level. **B:** Preoperative radiograph revealing the level of the congenital amputation through the proximal phalanx just beyond the epiphysis. **C:** Intraoperative anatomy of second toe donor harvest for microscopic transfer and thumb reconstruction. **D:** Immediate postoperative clinical photograph of toe transfer. This process led to normal thumb functioning and to a remarkable cosmetic result for the patient.

reconstruction for both functional and cosmetic reasons. A malaligned and elongated triphalangeal thumb in the same plane as the other digits is cosmetically anomalous and functionally limited for prehension activities.

Depending on the type of triphalangeal thumb, surgery may involve web-space deepening, excision of the extra phalanx (351), opposition transfer (352), or a modified pollicization procedure (352–354). The delta phalanx is usually excised to correct the length and angular deformity of the type I triphalangeal thumb (Fig. 23.31). If this procedure is performed in infancy, usually a stable interphalangeal joint can be reconstructed (355). In older children, or in children with abnormal phalanges and interphalangeal joints, a combination of shortening osteotomy and arthrodesis is preferred. In these situations, physeal growth of a biphalangeal digit should be preserved. In the five-fingered hand, a modified pollicization procedure is necessary so as to provide a deep first web space and an opposable thumb.

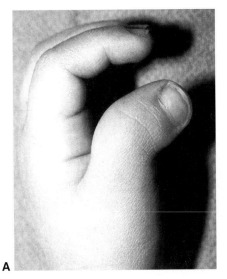
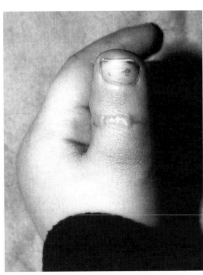

**Figure 23.31  A:** Triphalangeal thumb with a delta phalanx and a marked radial deviation deformity. **B:** Postoperative photograph after excision of the delta phalanx and rotation flap reconstruction of the soft tissues.

## TRAUMATIC INJURIES

Fractures to the pediatric hand are commonplace, accounting for approximately one fourth of all childhood fractures (356). The two peak ages for these fractures are adolescence (from sport-related activities) and infancy (from crush injuries). Most fractures are nondisplaced, nonphyseal injuries. Physeal injuries, however, can account for up to 40% of finger fractures (357,358), with a Salter-Harris II fracture of the small-finger proximal phalanx being the most common. Most pediatric hand fractures do well regardless of treatment (359). Malunion and growth disturbance are rare (357,360). However, there is a subset of pediatric hand injuries that will do poorly if not recognized and treated appropriately. The purpose of this section is to review fractures that are problematic.

### Overview

The bones of the digits have only one secondary center of ossification. These appear between birth and 3 to 4 years of age. The epiphyses of the phalanges are proximal. The epiphyses of the metacarpals are distal, except for the thumb, in which the physis is proximal. Distally in the thumb, there can be a second epiphysis or pseudoepiphysis. Ossification of the phalangeal condyles is progressive with growth, but in preschool children the condyles may be predominantly cartilaginous. Radiographic evaluation of injuries in young children may be difficult because of the chondral nature of the epiphysis and the intraarticular portions of the condyles. It is important to obtain true anteroposterior and lateral radiographs of the injured digits. In a diagnostically confusing situation, MRI scans of the fingers and hand should be performed.

To protect the anatomic healing of a traumatized digit in a young child, maximal protection is necessary. It is often necessary to protect the preschool-age child with a long-arm mitten cast. The older child often needs a short-arm mitten cast. Single-finger splinting is difficult to maintain, even in an adolescent. If the fracture is painful, or if it requires immobilization to maintain reduction, casting of the entire hand is appropriate. Fortunately, most pediatric fractures are nondisplaced and stable (361). The outcome will be successful regardless of immobilization technique. In these situations, the change is made to simple buddy taping as soon as it is comfortable. However, it is imperative not to mistake a problematic injury for a simple one and treat it with benign neglect. Such a mistake will lead to long-term loss of alignment, motion, and function, that may not be salvageable by secondary surgical reconstruction.

### Distal Phalanx Injuries

#### Nail-plate Injuries, Physeal Fractures, Mallet Fingers, and Tip Amputations

Most injuries to the distal phalangeal region are secondary to crush injury. These injuries are most common in the toddler and preschool age groups. The mechanism of injury is usually a digit caught in a door. Adults, often parents, are frequently involved in the accident, which makes the situation emotionally charged. The injuries can include partial or complete amputation, nail-bed laceration, and distal phalangeal fracture. All of these sites of trauma need to be addressed in the care of the child. In addition, time and energy need to be spent in helping the family cope with the emotional trauma.

***Tip Amputations.*** A distal phalangeal crush injury in a toddler usually includes a partial amputation with a nail-bed laceration and a distal phalangeal tuft fracture (Fig. 23.32). The fractures are generally minor avulsions that heal without problems. The partial amputation often extends dorsally through the nail bed, leaving some volar pulp intact. The volar soft-tissue attachments maintain the vascularity to the distal tip. Meticulous repair under conscious sedation and/or local anesthesia usually leads to normal long-term

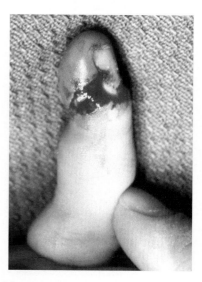

**Figure 23.32** Typical distal phalangeal crush injury with nail and pulp laceration. Repair requires nail-plate removal, absorbable suture repair of the lacerated nail bed, and anatomic closure of the eponychial skin.

outcome. The technique involves initial repair of the eponychial folds to properly align and stabilize the digit. It is imperative to then meticulously repair the nail-bed laceration with fine, absorbable suture (i.e., 6-0 chromic suture) and loupe magnification to prevent long-term nail deformity. The dorsal roof of the eponychium is preserved by placement of a spacer for several days after repair. Even when there is nearly complete amputation, with apparently nonviable distal tissue, soft-tissue repair almost always leads to survival of the tip. Uncomplicated repair of the partial amputation and nail-bed laceration will generally heal without permanent damage to the nail or phalanx. However, neglected nail-bed injuries are associated with a high rate of permanent deformity (354,362).

Care of the complete amputation at the level of the nail, or distally, is more controversial. First, this is a much more difficult situation emotionally for the child and family. The injury often occurs while the child is under adult supervision. There is usually significant stress and guilt associated with the amputation. The parents universally want the tissue replaced. However, this injury is beyond the trifurcation of the digital arteries near the level of the DIP joint, and so the tissue is not replantable. The debate concerns whether to suture the amputated part back on without vascular anastomoses (a composite graft), or to allow healing by secondary intention (363). Replacement of the amputated soft tissue initially makes the family feel better, but usually is not necessary. The amount of soft tissue amputated is small. The physis is proximal and not affected. Subsequent growth will be normal. The overall digital length, therefore, will be nearly normal. The cosmetics of composite grafting and healing by secondary intention are generally equal in the long term. Long-term sensibility and function seem to be equivalent. In addition,

in the short term, replacement of the amputated part may be more stressful for the family and child, with multiple dressing changes, superficial necrosis of the distal tip, and slow healing. Therefore, if the soft-tissue loss is minor, reassurance to the family of the long-term result, and treatment with serial dressing changes are best. This is true as well for the situation in which a minimal portion of exposed bone is debrided. However, if the piece includes the eponychium or the entire sterile and germinal matrix of the nail, composite grafting of the amputated part is preferred. There is a chance that this will heal and preclude secondary reconstructive surgery.

***Physeal Fractures and Nail-bed Entrapment.*** Some children will present with distal laceration and flexion posture of the distal phalanx, or mallet appearance. Radiographs will reveal a displaced physeal fracture with dorsal widening. Too often, these children are diagnosed as having mallet finger and treated with splinting. This is not an extensor tendon disruption. The extensor mechanism is intact because the terminal tendon inserts into the more proximal epiphysis. The deformity is caused by entrapment of the proximal nail bed (germinal matrix) in the physeal fracture site (364). If not recognized early, the open injury can become secondarily infected. The clinical appearance of the finger and the radiographic physeal changes may be interpreted as distal phalangeal osteomyelitis. However, antibiotic treatment alone or surgical debridement of the distal phalanx is not the proper treatment for this late-presenting fracture. Surgical repair of the nail bed is necessary in order to prevent long-term nail and distal phalanx growth problems. Under local, regional, or general anesthesia, the nail plate should be removed. By flexing the distal phalanx, the surgeon can gently extract the entrapped nail bed. The germinal matrix should be meticulously repaired so as to avoid long-term nail-plate problems. At times, this requires more proximal exposure by raising an eponychial flap. After repair of the nail bed, the nail plate can be replaced to preserve the dorsal roof of the eponychium and to provide an internal splint for repair of the fracture (364,365). Placement of a cautery hole in the nail plate will lessen the risk of subsequent hematoma and paronychial infection.

***Mallet Fingers.*** True mallet fingers are rare in the preadolescent child. In this age group, physeal fracture is more common. In the adolescent, mallet injuries with disruption of the extensor mechanism are more common and adultlike. As long as there is no entrapment of the germinal matrix, as noted in the preceding text, these injuries can be treated with immobilization. Rarely, the entire epiphysis can be displaced with the extensor mechanism (366,367). If recognized early, this injury should be treated with open reduction of the dislocated epiphysis. The rare, chronic mallet finger in the young child has been treated successfully with tenodermodesis (368).

## Phalanx Fractures

### Phalangeal Neck Fractures

Phalangeal neck fractures are problematic. They are usually caused by crush injury. As the child attempts to extract the affected digit, the condyles become entrapped and a fracture occurs in the subcondylar region (347,356,357,361, 369,370). The condylar fragment displaces into extension and often malrotates. The fragment is tethered by the collateral ligaments as it rotates dorsally up to 90 degrees. The condylar fragment is small, and has a precarious blood supply through the collateral ligaments. The subcondylar fossa is obliterated, blocking interphalangeal flexion (Fig. 23.33). If not properly recognized and treated, complications of malunion, loss of motion, and avascular necrosis can occur. Too often, the severity of the fracture is underappreciated in the urgent care setting. The patient presents late, with inappropriate immobilization and a significantly healed fracture. In addition, the fracture is unstable and will often displace after closed reduction (371). The treatment of choice is closed reduction and percutaneous pinning. In a young child, this can be accomplished with a single oblique pin. In an older child, crossed pins prevent malrotation. Placement of the pins in the distal fragment requires careful localization of the fragment and avoidance of the extensor mechanism. If open reduction is necessary, the collateral ligaments should not be dissected from the distal fragment. Careful dissection lessens the risk of avascular necrosis.

When there is marked callus, open reduction may cause avascular necrosis. The fracture has generally been healing too long for successful closed reduction and percutaneous pinning to be carried out. If there is still lucency along the fracture line, percutaneous osteoclasis can be performed (372). A pin is placed dorsally in the fracture site under fluoroscopic control, and used for reducing the fracture. The subcondylar fossa can be reconstituted, and the fracture can be pinned percutaneously.

If the fracture is completely healed upon referral, late subchondral fossa reconstruction can be performed if there is a bony block to flexion (370). An average of 90 degrees of PIP joint flexion has been obtained with subchondral fossa reconstruction (370). Remodeling of the fracture is rare because of the significant distance from the physis, but it has been described in case reports of both proximal and middle phalanx phalangeal neck fractures (373). Observation may be appropriate, but only if the patient is young, there is only malangulation and not malrotation, and the family is willing to wait for 1 or 2 years.

### Intercondylar Fractures

Intercondylar fractures in young children are often small osteochondral fractures. These carry a high risk of nonunion, malunion, and avascular necrosis (354,374). This is particularly true in the middle phalanx if the injury is a crush injury that alters the local blood supply. The fracture is intraarticular, generally displaced, and requires anatomic reduction for a successful outcome. Most often, the fracture has to be treated aggressively with open reduction. The collateral ligament attachments to the fragment are preserved so as to lessen the risk of avascular necrosis. On occasion, bone grafting is necessary for maintaining articular congruity and to prevent collapse. Even with well-performed open reduction, complications of this fracture can occur in the young patient (374). Avascular necrosis usually resolves by revascularization, but often not before collapse. Articular malunion can occur (Fig. 23.34). Loss of motion may not limit function.

In the adolescent, treatment of intercondylar fractures is similar to that in adults. Anatomic reduction and pin fixation are necessary to restore the joint surface and to prevent loss of reduction that can occur with this unstable fracture. Generally, the procedure can be performed closed, using distraction and a percutaneous towel clip to obtain reduction (375). Open reduction can be performed with a volar, midaxial, or dorsal approach. This is appropriate for fractures that cannot be reduced closed or for comminuted fractures. Restoration of an anatomic joint will lessen the risk of loss of motion, malalignment, or long-term arthritis (Fig. 23.34).

Diaphysis-level phalangeal fractures are rare in the young child, and more common in the teenager. The major issue in these fractures is malrotation (357) (Fig. 23.35).

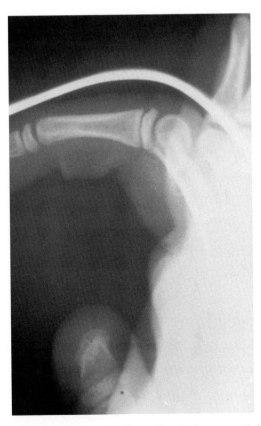

**Figure 23.33** Displaced phalangeal neck fracture with loss of the subchondral fossa. This leads to loss of digital flexion. This fracture requires prompt attention, anatomic reduction, and pin stabilization. If the fracture is left in the position shown here in the splint, there will be a problematic malunion.

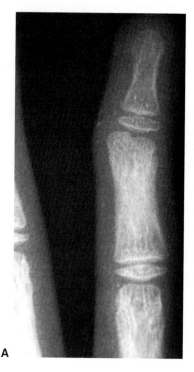

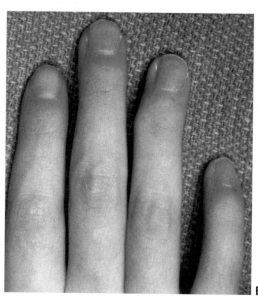

A

B

**Figure 23.34** **A:** Radiograph of a displaced intercondylar fracture with articular malunion. **B:** Clinical photograph of a similar patient. This injury requires acute anatomic reduction and pin stabilization to prevent long-term loss of motion, malalignment, and potential pain and arthritis.

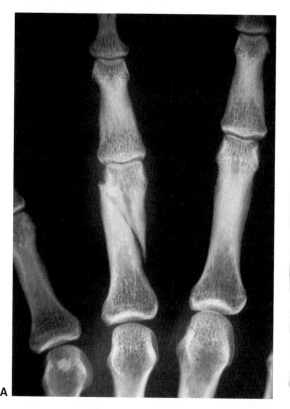

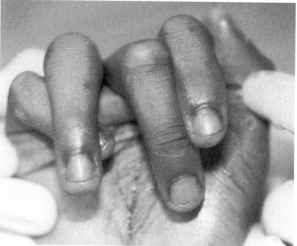

A

B

**Figure 23.35** **A:** Displaced proximal phalanx fracture with malrotation. **B:** Tenodesis testing reveals malrotation. By passively extending and flexing the wrist, the digits will passively flex and extend, respectively. Malalignment is evident.

Frequently, children will not actively move the finger in the acute setting to allow for accurate assessment of digital alignment. However, close inspection of the nail plates will reveal the digital malalignment. In addition, the examiner can test digital alignment by tenodesis of the wrist. With passive wrist extension, the fingers flex and point toward the volar scaphoid tubercle. Digital alignment is generally symmetric. Children will tolerate this test, even when they are in too much pain or are too frightened to actively move their digits. Tenodesis assessment should be performed on all phalangeal and metacarpal fractures, regardless of radiographic appearance. If closed treatment is chosen, a finger should never be immobilized by itself, but should be secured to the adjacent digits to prevent subsequent loss of reduction and malrotation.

If the fracture is malrotated and unstable, reduction with pin or screw stabilization is necessary (376,377). Although malrotation is uncommon, it is a major problem if missed until after healing. The malrotated digit impairs the function of the adjacent digits because the digits will overlap in flexion. At that stage, malrotation can be corrected only with osteotomy.

### Physeal Fractures

Physeal fractures constitute 30% to 70% of pediatric finger fractures (356–358,360). A Salter-Harris II fracture of the small finger is the most common of these fractures. Closed reduction of the abducted fracture is performed in MCP flexion so as to lessen the restraint of the more distal web space. The surgeon's thumb or a cylindrical object such as a pencil can be used. Postreduction stability is maintained by taping the digit loosely to the adjacent digit and applying a short-arm mitten cast. The less common type III physeal fracture requires open reduction if there is more than 2 mm of diastasis or articular step-off.

## Metacarpal Fractures

Distal metacarpal metaphyseal (boxer) fractures are common in adolescence. The mechanism is a closed fist injury, most often to the small-finger metacarpal. These fractures are usually juxtaphyseal and malaligned, with apex dorsal angulation. In the acute setting, closed reduction and cast immobilization with three-point fixation for 3 weeks is preferred for displaced fractures. This includes volar-to-dorsal pressure on the metacarpal head and dorsal-to-volar pressure on the more proximal shaft. Often, these patients will not seek medical attention until there is significant healing. Fortunately, the fracture is adjacent to the distal metacarpal physis, and the flexion malunion can remodel if there is sufficient growth remaining. This fact has led some clinicians to approach these fractures with neglect to allow for remodeling. Indeed, depending on the age of the patient, remodeling of the flexion deformity can occur. However, malrotation will not remodel. In addition, if remodeling is slow or fails to occur, the prominence of the metacarpal head in the palm can be limiting.

Unstable or multiple metacarpal fracture(s) are rare. They should be treated with closed reduction and percutaneous pinning. Two smooth pins are placed, under fluoroscopic control, from ulnar to radial, distal to the fracture site(s), from the 5th to the 4th or 3rd metacarpal, as necessary. Late open reduction of the juxtaphyseal fracture carries the risk of physeal injury and should be avoided. Diaphyseal fractures of the fifth metacarpal carry a higher risk of a malunion that will not remodel. Closed reduction and transverse percutaneous pinning to the adjacent metacarpals, or intramedullary pin fixation, is the treatment of choice. Corrective osteotomy may be necessary in the severe, malunited diaphyseal fracture that fails to remodel the flexion deformity with growth.

The major issue in other diaphyseal metacarpal fractures, especially if there are multiple metacarpal fractures, is malrotation. Active digital motion or passive tenodesis of the wrist will reveal malrotation. Anatomic reduction and pin, screw, or plate fixation will correct the malrotation.

## Thumb Fractures

The unique features of fractures of the thumb are seen in Salter-Harris III fractures of the proximal phalanx, and at the base of metacarpal fractures. The type III physeal fracture of the thumb proximal phalanx is the skeletally immature equivalent of an adult ulnar collateral ligament disruption (378) (Fig. 23.36). These fractures require open reduction and internal fixation in order to restore stability of the joint and anatomic alignment of the joint and physis. During surgical exposure, the surgeon should remember that the ligament is intact. Therefore, after adductor takedown, the MCP joint should be exposed through the fracture site rather than through inadvertent incision of the ligament. The long-term results of anatomic open reduction are excellent. Metaphyseal fractures at the base of the thumb metacarpal often displace (379). Immobilization and observation, even in displaced fractures, are appropriate as long as there are at least 2 years of growth remaining, because the malunited dorsoradial prominence will remodel during the ensuing 6 to 12 months (362) (Fig. 23.37). Most parents would prefer to wait for remodeling rather than have operative reduction and pinning. In the markedly displaced and unstable fracture, closed reduction and percutaneous pinning are appropriate. The presence of a Bennett fracture with articular malalignment requires anatomic alignment of the intraarticular component and pin fixation of the thumb metacarpal to the adjacent second metacarpal and carpus.

## Wrist Injuries

### Scaphoid Fractures

Scaphoid fractures occur from a fall on an outstretched wrist. The pain is often mild, rather than the severe pain a child or parent expects from an acute fracture. This leads some patients and families to ignore the acute injury and not present until late. When the child presents at the acute

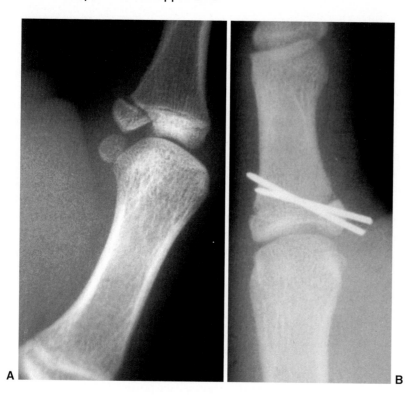

**Figure 23.36 A:** Salter-Harris III displaced proximal phalanx fracture of the thumb. This fracture requires open reduction and internal fixation in order to restore articular congruity and ligamentous stability. **B:** Postoperative radiograph of a similar patient with pins in place.

stage of the injury, there will be tenderness to palpation over the anatomic snuff-box (the region dorsoradially at the wrist between the extensor pollicis longus and the extensor pollicis brevis tendons), over the volar scaphoid

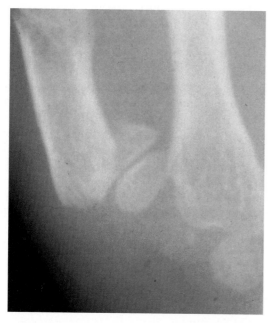

**Figure 23.37** Displaced base in a metacarpal thumb fracture. Because this fracture is juxtaphyseal, adjacent to the carpometacarpal joint with universal motion, its remodeling potential is almost unlimited if the patient is younger than 10 years. Treatment choices are closed reduction and pinning, or immobilization in a cast to allow for biologic remodeling for the ensuing 6 to 12 months of growth. This patient was treated in a cast.

tubercle, and upon axial compression of the thumb CMC joint. Radiographs may reveal the fracture. The best view is an anteroposterior view in 30 degrees of ulnar deviation (scaphoid view). If the radiographs are diagnostic for the fracture, long-arm immobilization in a thumb spica cast is best. If the radiographs are negative, but the child has tenderness at the site of the injury, as noted in the preceding text, protected immobilization for 2 weeks is advised. Repeat clinical and radiographic examination should be performed out of cast 2 weeks later if tenderness persists. If there is still doubt about the diagnosis, MRI or CT scan is advised. The CT scan shows the bony alignment better, but the MRI gives added information about the vascularity to the proximal pole, and better information about the cartilage surfaces in a young child. CT scans are used for assessing acute fractures in adolescents. MRI scans are used for assessing the acute injury in the child younger than 10 years of age. In the acute setting, MRI scans have been diagnostic for the exact site of injury, and can lead to appropriate treatment early (380,381).

Previously, it was reported that most scaphoid fractures in the skeletally immature patient were distal pole or avulsion fractures (374). Distal pole fractures heal readily with cast immobilization without risk of nonunion or avascular necrosis. However, scaphoid wrist fractures are becoming more common in the adolescent age group. These fractures can displace and carry the same risks of nonunion and avascular necrosis in the child as they do in the adult. Therefore, nonunions are becoming more commonplace (382,383). Treatment of an established nonunion in a child should be with open reduction, bone grafting, and,

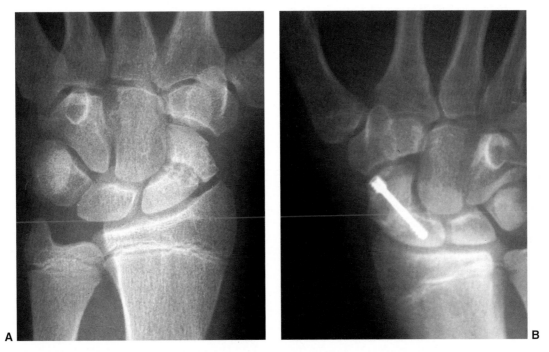

**Figure 23.38** **A:** Scaphoid nonunion in an adolescent. **B:** Postoperative iliac crest bone grafting and internal fixation for a similar scaphoid fracture nonunion.

potentially, internal fixation. Internal fixation screws have been used in children with both acute displaced wrist fractures and established nonunions (373,382,383) (Fig. 23.38). It is difficult to determine whether a bipartite scaphoid, even if bilateral, is congenital or posttraumatic. However, if it is symptomatic, it should be treated in the same way as a traumatic nonunion. The success of open reduction, bone grafting, and internal fixation for a scaphoid nonunion is high in children (382,383). Proximal pole fractures and nonunions have now been described in children and adolescents (384). These fracture nonunions have been treated successfully with vascularized bone graft from the distal radius to the scaphoid.

### Wrist Pain, Triangular Fibrocartilage Complex Tears, and Ligamentous Injuries.

*Atraumatic Ligamentous Instability.* Most adolescents with chronic wrist pain have overuse injuries. These patients often have generalized ligamentous laxity or a hyperelasticity syndrome. The wrist pain is similar to the patellofemoral knee pain and multidirectional shoulder instability pain seen in this age group. Overuse, growth, and resultant muscle weakness all contribute to instability of the joints. On physical examination, there is often systemic evidence of generalized laxity (elbow cubitus valgus, pes planus, knee hyperextension, passive hyperextension of the index finger parallel to the dorsal forearm, and thumb abduction to the volar forearm). At the wrist, there will be increased midcarpal translation to volar and dorsal applied stress. This passive midcarpal instability will be equivalent on both the

affected and the unaffected wrist. However, the affected side will often have painful clicking. Plain radiographs may reveal a volar tilt to the lunate on the lateral view. MRI scans and arthrograms appear normal. These children respond to alteration of activities and strengthening, as in other growth-related overuse injuries in the teenager. It is the author's experience that resistive strengthening with therapeutic putty is best.

*Traumatic Scapholunate Ligamentous Injuries.* Posttraumatic injuries to the scapholunate ligament rarely occur in children. Most descriptions of these injuries have been case reports (385). However, it is the author's experience that these traumatic ligamentous injuries are occurring more frequently with today's higher level of athletic competition in this age group. On physical examination, the tenderness is usually more focal than in atraumatic ligamentous laxity wrist pain. Asymmetric clicking with applied ligamentous stress testing is common. Static injuries are more common in adults, and will show an increased scapholunate distance and a flexed scaphoid on plain radiographs. Most scapholunate injuries in children are dynamic injuries, with normal plain radiographs. In addition, the scapholunate distance in children has been difficult to interpret because of eccentric ossification and the chondral nature of the carpus in the young. A recent study of pediatric wrist radiographs developed an age standard for scapholunate distances in both sexes (386). This will help in the evaluation of pediatric carpal injuries. MRI scans may reveal the ligamentous injury. Arthroscopic examination of the wrist is diagnostic and often therapeutic. Many of these injuries are partial tears of the ligament, with an associated chondral lesion of the radius. This leads to mechanical impingement that often responds favorably to arthroscopic debridement. It is rare that there will be a complete ligamentous disruption in this age group. However, symptomatic complete scapholunate disruptions need to be treated with ligamentous reconstruction.

### Triangular Fibrocartilage Complex Tears

Posttraumatic chronic wrist pain that does not respond to prolonged rest and therapy should be evaluated for intraarticular pathology. As in scaphoid fractures and intercarpal ligamentous injuries, the epidemiology of triangular fibrocartilage complex (TFCC) tears has changed to include the adolescent. Physical examination for TFCC tears includes ulnocarpal compressive testing, lunate-triquetral stress testing, and stress testing of the distal radioulnar joint. Painful clicking with these maneuvers, especially if asymmetric, may be indicative of a tear. However, many children with nondissociative laxity show similar findings on physical examination. Plain radiographs are normal. The MRI may be diagnostic, but there has been a high incidence of false-negative readings for adolescent TFCC tears.

In skilled hands arthroscopy is definitive for diagnosis, and often for treatment (Fig. 23.39).

TFCC tears occur in the skeletally immature patient. Most tears are associated with nonunion of ulnar styloid fractures, radial growth, ulnar overgrowth, and/or ulnocarpal impaction syndrome. Isolated tears also occur. In adolescents and children, these tears are usually peripheral tears that respond well to surgical repair (387). Isolated tears can be repaired arthroscopically. Tears associated with radial and ulnar bony deformities are repaired at the time of corrective osteotomy (Fig. 23.40). Treatment should also include appropriate excision of the ulnar styloid nonunion, shortening of the impacting ulna, osteotomy of the deformed radius, and stabilization of the distal radioulnar joint, if necessary (387).

## Dislocations

Most hyperextension injuries to the interphalangeal joints in children result in a tear of the volar plate. There may be associated minimal Salter-Harris III physeal avulsions of the adjacent phalanx (Fig. 23.41). These injuries are stable. Treatment should be brief immobilization for comfort, followed by buddy taping until the patient is asymptomatic.

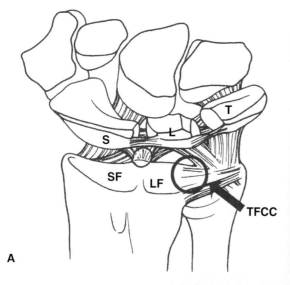

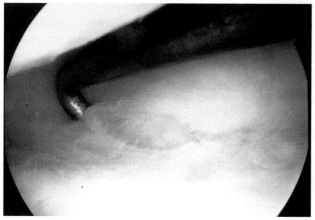

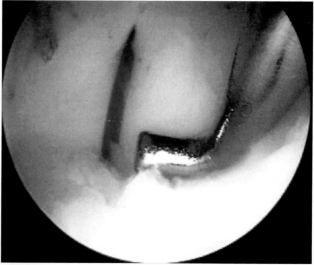

**Figure 23.39  A:** Illustration of intraarticular wrist anatomy, as seen from the dorsal 3/4 portal. (*S*, scaphoid; *L*, lunate; *SF*, scaphoid fossa; *LF*, lunate fossa; *T*, triquetrum; *TFCC*, triangular fibrocartilage complex). **B:** Arthroscopic photograph of a triangular fibrocartilage complex (TFCC) peripheral tear. The tear is along the peripheral edge of the TFCC, where the blood supply enters and aids in healing. In this situation, repair is by arthroscopic suture techniques. **C:** Intraoperative photograph of arthroscopic suture repair of peripheral TFCC tear.

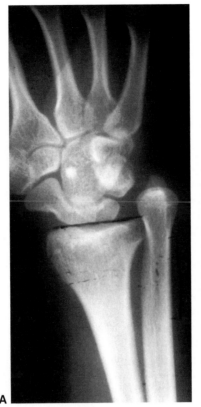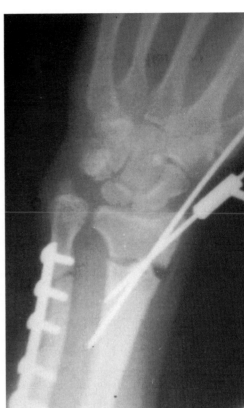

**Figure 23.40** **A:** Radiograph of ulnocarpal impaction associated with radial growth arrest, ulnar overgrowth, and a triangular fibrocartilage complex (TFCC) tear. **B:** Repair of the TFCC, ulnar shortening, and radial osteotomy with bone grafting were performed.

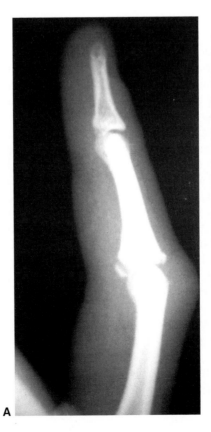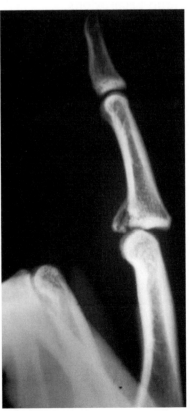

**Figure 23.41** Volar plate injuries. **A:** Nondisplaced minor volar and dorsal avulsion injuries. This injury requires minimal immobilization and prompt initiation of range-of-motion exercises to minimize the risk of permanent flexion contracture. **B:** This injury has a more significant fracture fragment and joint subluxation. It requires anatomic reduction of the proximal interphalangeal joint and an extension block splint to allow for motion within the range of joint stability.

Prolonged treatment with splints can lead to PIP joint stiffness. True interphalangeal dislocations occur less often. The dislocation is usually dorsal, and it occurs more commonly at the PIP joint than at the DIP joint. Closed reduction with distraction and dorsal-to-volar manipulation are generally successful.

Rarely, a displaced epiphysis, flexor tendon, or interposed volar plate can block reduction, demanding an open reduction procedure. MCP joint dislocation of the thumb or index finger can be simple or complex (371). Simple dislocations are reducible in the emergency setting. Complex dislocations are irreducible, and have an interposed volar plate blocking closed reduction. Plain radiographic evidence of widening and lateralization of the joint, as well as bayonet apposition of the proximal phalanx and metacarpal, indicate an irreducible situation.

Open reduction of a complex dislocation can be performed through a volar (388,389) or a dorsal (390,391) approach. In the volar approach, the radial neurovascular bundle is tented just beneath the skin by the metacarpal head. It is imperative to be cautious with the skin incision so as not to cause laceration. In either approach, the volar plate should be incised so as to allow reduction of the joint and anatomic realignment of the flexor tendons, sesamoids, and collateral ligaments. Postoperative treatment is by early protected motion with buddy taping and extension block splinting. Chronic instability is rare, but limitation of MCP motion is not. The digital neurapraxia secondary to the dislocation will resolve in this age group.

## Tendon Lacerations

The classification system, in terms of zones of injury for flexor tendon lacerations, is the same for the child as it is for the adult. The diagnosis of flexor tendon injury, operative care, and postoperative rehabilitation may be more difficult in the child. This is especially true in the toddler and preschool-aged child, whose ability for cooperation is limited. Often, the presenting digital cascade and digital excursion with wrist tenodesis serve as the basis for the diagnosis of flexor tendon laceration (Fig. 23.42). If in doubt, the clinician should explore the wound under anesthesia. Repair of the tendon lacerations in zones I and II requires meticulous technique with fine sutures. Repair can be performed electively in the first 1 to 2 weeks with equivalent results. However, if there is any concern regarding the vascular status of the digit, repair should be emergent, with exploration of the digital neurovascular bundles. In the infant, the core suture may be as fine as 6-0 and the epitenon suture may be 8-0. Postoperative immobilization in a cast for 4 weeks is effective protection. Subsequent rehabilitation is necessary in order to regain maximal passive and active motion.

There have been no differences in total active motion (TAM) between early mobilization protocols and cast immobilization for 4 weeks in children younger than 15

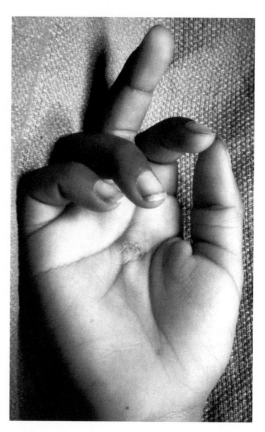

**Figure 23.42** Photograph of an altered digital flexion cascade with passive wrist extension tenodesis. This is diagnostic of a flexor tendon laceration in the long finger.

years (392). The results of isolated profundus tendon lacerations in zone I averaged 90% to 94% of normal TAM. Isolated profundus lacerations in zone I averaged 71% to 78% TAM. Combined superficialis and profundus lacerations in zone II averaged 72% TAM. However, if cast immobilization continued beyond 4 weeks there was a significant decrease in TAM, to 40% by 6 weeks. There was no difference in the results according to age groups from birth to 15 years.

Associated nerve or palmar plate injuries diminished the results slightly. Postoperative tendon rupture is rare. Two-stage reconstruction of unrecognized zone II lacerations in children younger than 6 years has had poorer results than in adults, with a higher rate of complications and a mean TAM of approximately 60% of normal. Results were better with supervised rehabilitation (393).

The principles of the treatment of extensor tendon lacerations in the adult apply to the child as well. Direct repair in the emergency room under sedation, or in the operating room under general anesthesia, is preferred. Cast immobilization in a protected position of wrist dorsiflexion and digital extension is continued for 4 weeks after repair. Results are excellent with primary repair. Associated fractures, dislocations, and flexor tendon injuries impair the results.

## Amputations

Complete or partial amputations of the distal fingertip are very common in children, and have been discussed in detail in the section on distal phalangeal injuries. Treatment of more proximal, complete digital amputations with replantation in children as young as 1 year of age is now standard. In children, the indications for replantation are more liberal than in adults, and include multiple-digit, thumb, midpalm, hand, and distal forearm amputations as well as single-digit amputations in zones I and II. Crush amputations from doors, heavy objects, or bicycle chains have a peak incidence at 5 years, whereas sharp amputations occur more commonly in adolescence. Digital survival rates from replantation range from 69% to 89% in pediatric series. More favorable digital survival was seen with sharp amputations, body weight greater than 11 kg, more than one vein repaired, bone shortening, interosseous wire fixation, and vein grafting of arteries and veins. Vessel size generally exceeds 0.8 mm in digital replants in children, and is not a technical problem for the skilled microvascular surgeon. Index- and long-finger replants have better survival than small-finger replants in children. A finger survival rate of 95% was seen in children if prompt reperfusion occurred after arterial repair with at least one successful venous anastomosis, compared with zero survival if one or both of these factors was absent (394). Neural recovery rates far exceed those cited in adults, with return of two-point discrimination of less than 5 mm often present (378). Tenolysis may rarely be necessary after tendon repair. Two-stage flexor tendon reconstruction in children has a higher rate of complications than in adults. Growth arrest or deformity is more common if there is a crush component to the amputation. These digits are rarely normal after replanting, although the results in children are better than in adults, in terms of sensibility and recovery of range of motion. Microvascular toe-to-thumb transfer is a very successful alternative to pollicization in the case of a failed thumb replant in a young child (395) (Fig. 23.43).

## Sprengel Deformity

Children with Sprengel deformity (396) often present with a decreased neck line, limited motion about the shoulder, or both. This is secondary to the embryonic failure of one, or sometimes both, scapulae to descend in utero. The abnormal elevation is in conjunction with hypoplasia and abnormal alignment of the scapula. Most often the scapula is small and shaped like an equilateral triangle rather than having a long medial border. The scapula in Sprengel deformity usually has abnormal anterior bending of the superior pole into the convexity of the upper thoracic region. There is often limited forward flexion and abduction of the shoulder because of lack of normal scapulothoracic motion and malpositioning of the glenoid. In up to 50% of cases there may be an associated omovertebral bar, which consists of a fibrous, cartilaginous, or bony connection between the superior medial angle of the scapula and the cervical spine (397). Frequently, there is associated abnormal regional anatomy

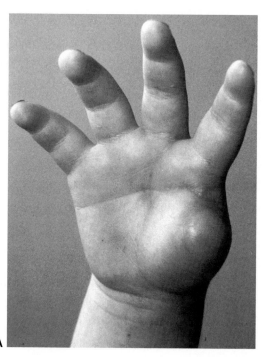
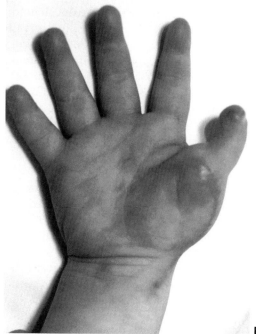

**Figure 23.43** **A:** Traumatic amputation of the thumb in a 2-year-old child. **B:** Postoperative photograph of the same patient after microvascular toe-to-thumb transfer for thumb reconstruction.

including scoliosis, spina bifida, clavicular abnormalities, rib anomalies, and Klippel-Feil syndrome, among others (398,399). Systemic abnormalities include renal and pulmonary disorders. In 10% to 30% of the cases, the condition is bilateral.

A classification by Cavendish (398) grades the severity of deformity in a rudimentary way: grade I is mild, with level glenohumeral joints and no deformity visible when the patient is dressed; grade 2 has level glenohumeral joints, with a lump in the neck region with the patient dressed; grade 3 is a moderate deformity with 2 to 5 cm of shoulder elevation; and grade 4 is severe, with elevation of the scapula to the vicinity of the occiput. The more severe the deformity, the more likely there are to be limitations of motion and function and associated regional anatomic anomalies. Surgery is indicated in children with severe cosmetic and functional limitations. Surgery does not correct the scapular hypoplasia, but is indicated for improving shoulder motion by restoring more normal positioning of the scapula and glenoid. This often consists of excising any omovertebral connections and surgically derotating and caudally relocating the scapula. Most of the procedures that are described include extraperiosteal resection of the superior pole of the scapula (398,400). Subperiosteal resection is associated with a high rate of recurrence (401,402). In addition to functional indications for surgery, most patients and families welcome the cosmetic improvement in the appearance of the neck line.

In the mild deformities, extraperiosteal excision of the superior pole of the scapula and any omovertebral connections alone may be satisfactory treatment. In the moderate and severe deformities, the scapula is also derotated and moved more distally in order to bring the glenoid into a more vertical orientation. The purpose of surgery is to improve the neck contour along with shoulder motion and function. Indications for functional improvement have been cited for preoperative abduction less than 110 to 120 degrees (397,403). Surgery is recommended most often in patients between 3 and 8 years of age (404–406). Surgery after 8 years of age is associated with the highest risk of nerve impairment; clavicular osteotomy is recommended in the older child in order to lessen the risk of brachial plexus impingement with scapular descent.

Surgical procedures for scapular descent have included the Woodward procedure (407), the Green procedure (408,409), and a vertical scapular osteotomy (410). The Woodward procedure moves the scapula distally by detachment and reattachment of the parascapular muscles at their origins on the spinal process. The Green procedure involves extraperiosteal detachment of the scapular insertion of the paraspinal muscles, and reattachment after the scapula has been moved distally with traction cables. Wilkinson and Campbell described a vertical scapular osteotomy in conjunction with a clavicular oseotomy in the older child for improving anterior release and scapular

relocation and for lessening the risk of neurologic injury. The modified Woodward procedure includes resection of the superior pole of the scapula in conjunction with surgical scapular descent and realignment. The results have been reported to have improved abduction in the range of 40 to 50 degrees (397,411) and achieved a satisfactory cosmetic result. Hypertrophic scar formation, however, has been cited often as a complication.

# REFERENCES

1. Flatt AE. *The care of congenital hand anomalies.* St. Louis, MO: Quality Medical Publishing, 1994.
2. McCarroll HR. Congenital anomalies: a 25-year overview. *J Hand Surg [Am]* 2000;25:1007.

## Congenital Deformities

3. Saunders JWJ, Cairns JM, Gasseling MT. The role of the apical ridge of ectoderm in the differentiation of the morphological structure and inductive specificity of limb parts in the chick. *J Morphol* 1957;101:57.
4. Ulthoff HK. *The embryology of the human locomotor system.* Berlin: Springer-Verlag New York, 1990.
5. Tabin C. The initiation of the limb bud: growth factors, Hox genes, and retinoids. *Cell* 1995;80:671.
6. Omi M, Ude H. Effects of digit tissue on cell death and ectopic cartilage formation in the interdigital zone in chick leg buds. *Dev Growth Differ* 1996;38:419.
7. Saunders JW Jr. The proximo-distal sequence of origin of the parts of the chick wing and the role of the ectoderm. 1948. *J Exp Zool* 1998;282(6):628–668.
8. Solursh M. Ectoderm as a determinant of early tissue pattern in the limb bud. *Cell Differ* 1984;15:17.
9. Summerbell D. A quantitative analysis of the effect of excision of the AER from the chick limb-bud. *J Embryol Exp Morphol* 1974;32:651.
10. Summerbell D. The zone of polarizing activity: evidence for a role in normal chick limb morphogenesis. *J Embryol Exp Morphol* 1979;50:217.
11. Tickle C. Experimental embryology as applied to the upper limb. *J Hand Surg [Br]* 1987;12:294.
12. Goodman FR. Limb malformations and the human HOX genes. *Am J Med Genet* 2002;112:256.
13. Muragaki Y, Mundlos S, Upton J, et al. Altered growth and branching patterns in synpolydactyly caused by mutations in HOXD13. *Science* 1996;272:548.
14. Lamb DW, Wynne-Davies R, Soto L. An estimate of the population frequency of congenital malformations of the upper limb. *J Hand Surg [Am]* 1982;7:557.
15. Conway H, Bowe J. Congenital deformities of hand. *Plast Reconstr Surg* 1956;18:286.
16. Philipp T, Philipp K, Reiner A, et al. Embryoscopic and cytogenetic analysis of 233 missed abortions: factors involved in the pathogenesis of developmental defects of early failed pregnancies. *Hum Reprod* 2003;18:1724.
17. Swanson AB. A classification for congenital limb malformations. *J Hand Surg [Am]* 1976;1:8.
18. Swanson AB, Swanson GD, Tada K. A classification for congenital limb malformation. *J Hand Surg [Am]* 1983;8:693.
19. Luijsterburg AJ, van Huizum MA, Impelmans BE, et al. Classification of congenital anomalies of the upper limb. *J Hand Surg [Br]* 2000;25:3.
20. Luijsterburg AJ, Sonneveld GJ, Vermeij-Keers C, et al. Recording congenital differences of the upper limb. *J Hand Surg [Br]* 2003;28:205.
21. Bradbury ET, Hewison J. Early parental adjustment to visible congenital disfigurement. *Child Care Health Dev* 1994;20:251.
22. Bradbury ET, Kay SP, Tighe C, et al. Decision-making by parents and children in paediatric hand surgery. *Br J Plast Surg* 1994;47:324.
23. Gath A. The impact of an abnormal child upon the parents. *Br J Psychiatry* 1977;130:405.

24. Netscher DT, Scheker LR. Timing and decision-making in the treatment of congenital upper extremity deformities. *Clin Plast Surg* 1990;17:113.

25. Varni JW, Setoguchi Y. Effects of parental adjustment on the adaptation of children with congenital or acquired limb deficiencies. *Journal of Dev Behav Pediatr* 1993;14(1):13–20.

## Entire Limb Involvement

26. Volpe JJ. *Neurology of the newborn.* Philadelphia, PA: WB Saunders, 1987.

27. Smith RJ. *Tendon transfers of the hand and forearm.* Boston, MA: Little, Brown and Company, 1987.

28. Zancolli EA, Goldner LJ, Swanson AB. Surgery of the spastic hand in cerebral palsy: report of the Committee on Spastic Hand Evaluation (International Federation of Societies for Surgery of the Hand). *J Hand Surg [Am]* 1983;8(5 Pt 2):766–772.

29. Skoff H, Woodbury DF. Management of the upper extremity in cerebral palsy. *J Bone Joint Surg Am* 1985;67(3):500–503.

30. Zancolli EA, Zachary EJ. Surgical rehabilitation of the spastic upper limb in the cerebral palsy. In: Lamb DW, ed. *The paralyzed hand.* Edinburgh: Churchill Livingstone, 1987:153.

31. Waters PM, Van Heest A. Spastic hemiplegia of the upper extremity in children. *Hand Clin* 1998;14(1):119–134.

32. Bleck EE. *Orthopaedic management of cerebral palsy.* Philadelphia, PA: WB Saunders, 1979.

33. Sakellarides HT, Mital MA, Lenzi WD. Treatment of pronation contractures of the forearm in cerebral palsy by changing the insertion of the pronator radii teres. *J Bone Joint Surg Am* 1981;63(4):645–652.

34. Van Heest AE, House JH, Cariello C. Upper extremity surgical treatment of cerebral palsy. *J Hand Surg [Am]* 1999;24(2): 323–330.

35. Koman LA, Gelberman RH, Toby EB, et al. Cerebral palsy. Management of the upper extremity. *Clin Orthop Relat Res* 1990;253:62–74.

36. Mital MA. Lengthening of the elbow flexors in cerebral palsy. *J Bone Joint Surg Am* 1979;61(4):515–522.

37. Pletcher DF, Hoffer MM, Koffman DM. Non-traumatic dislocation of the radial head in cerebral palsy. *J Bone Joint Surg Am* 1976;58(1):104–105.

38. House JH, Gwathmey FW, Fidler MO. A dynamic approach to the thumb-in palm deformity in cerebral palsy. *J Bone Joint Surg Am* 1981;63(2):216–225.

39. Phelps WM. Long-term results of orthopaedic surgery in cerebral palsy. *J Bone Joint Surg Am* 1957;39:53.

40. Mowery CA, Gelberman RH, Rhoades CE. Upper extremity tendon transfers in cerebral palsy: electromyographic and functional analysis. *J Pediatr Orthop* 1985;5(1):69–72.

41. Randall M, Carlin JB, Chondros P, et al. Reliability of the Melbourne assessment of unilateral upper limb function. *Dev Med Child Neurol* 2001;43(11):761–767.

42. Bourke-Taylor H. Melbourne Assessment of Unilateral Upper Limb Function: construct validity and correlation with the Pediatric Evaluation of Disability Inventory. *Dev Med Child Neurol* 2003;45(2):92–96.

43. Manske PR. Cerebral palsy of the upper extremity. *Hand Clin* 1990;6(4):697–709.

44. Pagliano E, Andreucci E, Bono R, et al. Evolution of upper limb function in children with congenital hemiplegia. *Neurol Sci* 2001;22(5):371–375.

45. Sterr A, Freivogel S, Voss A. Exploring a repetitive training regime for upper limb hemiparesis in an in-patient setting: a report on three case studies. *Brain Inj* 2002;16(12):1093–1107.

46. Willis JK, Morello A, Davie A, et al. Forced use treatment of childhood hemiparesis. *Pediatrics* 2002;110(1 Pt 1):94–96.

47. Sterr A, Freivogel S, Schmalohr D. Neurobehavioral aspects of recovery: assessment of the learned nonuse phenomenon in hemiparetic adolescents. *Arch Phys Med Rehabil* 2002;83(12): 1726–1731.

48. Wright PA, Granat MH. Therapeutic effects of functional electrical stimulation of the upper limb of eight children with cerebral palsy. *Dev Med Child Neurol* 2000;42(11):724–727.

49. Goldner JL, Koman LA, Gelberman R, et al. Arthrodesis of the metacarpophalangeal joint of the thumb in children and adults.

Adjunctive treatment of thumb-in-palm deformity in cerebral palsy. *Clin Orthop Relat Res* 1990;253:75–89.

50. Botte MJ, Keenan MA. Percutaneous phenol blocks of the pectoralis major muscle to treat spastic deformities. *J Hand Surg [Am]* 1988;13(1):147–149.

51. Gelberman RH. The upper extremity in cerebral palsy. In: Bora W, ed. *The pediatric upper extremity.* Philadelphia, PA: WB Saunders, 1986:323.

52. Keenan MA, Tomas ES, Stone L, et al. Percutaneous phenol block of the musculocutaneous nerve to control elbow flexor spasticity. *J Hand Surg [Am]* 1990;15(2):340–346.

53. Braun RM, Hoffer MM, Mooney V, et al. Phenol nerve block in the treatment of acquired spastic hemiplegia in the upper limb. *J Bone Joint Surg Am* 1973;55(3):580–585.

54. Autti-Ramo I, Larsen A, Taimo A, et al. Management of the upper limb with botulinum toxin type A in children with spastic type cerebral palsy and acquired brain injury: clinical implications. *Eur J Neurol* 2001;8(Suppl. 5):136–144.

55. Tonkin MA, Hughes J, Smith KL. Lateral band translocation for swan-neck deformity. *J Hand Surgery [Am]* 1992;17(2):260–267.

56. Waters PM, Zurakowski D, Patterson P, et al. Interobserver and intraobserver reliability of therapist-assisted videotaped evaluations of upper-limb hemiplegia. *J Hand Surg [Am]* 2004;29(2): 328–334.

57. Dahlin LB, Komoto-Tufvesson Y, Salgeback S. Surgery of the spastic hand in cerebral palsy. Improvement in stereognosis and hand function after surgery. *J Hand Surg [Br]* 1998;23(3):334–339.

58. Eliasson AC, Ekholm C, Carlstedt T. Hand function in children with cerebral palsy after upper-limb tendon transfer and muscle release.[see comment]. *Dev Med Child Neurol* 1998;40(9): 612–621.

59. Hoffer MM, Perry J, Garcia M, et al. Adduction contracture of the thumb in cerebral palsy. A preoperative electromyographic study. *J Bone Joint Surg Am* 1983;65(6):755–759.

60. Page CM. An operation for relief of flexion contracture in the forearm. *J Bone Joint Surg Am* 1923;5:233.

61. Manske PR, McCarroll HRJ, Hale R. Biceps tendon rerouting and percutaneous osteoclasis in the treatment of supination deformity in obstetrical palsy. *J Hand Surg [Am]* 1980;5:153.

62. Adler JB, Patterson RL Jr. Erb's palsy. Long-term results of treatment in eighty-eight cases. *J Bone Joint Surg Am* 1967;49(6): 1052–1064.

63. Hardy AE. Birth injuries of the brachial plexus: incidence and prognosis. *J Bone Joint Surg Br* 1981;63:98–101.

64. Wickstrom J. Birth injuries of the brachial plexus. Treatment of defects in the shoulder. *Clin Orthop Relat Res* 1962;23:187–196.

65. Pearl ML, Edgerton BW. Glenoid deformity secondary to brachial plexus birth palsy. *J Bone Joint Surg* 1998;5:659–667.

66. Waters PM, Smith GR, Jaramillo D. Glenohumeral deformity secondary to brachial plexus birth palsy. *J Bone Joint Surg* 1998;80(5):668–677.

67. Waters PM. Comparison of the natural history, the outcome of microsurgical repair, and the outcome of operative reconstruction in brachial plexus birth palsy. *J Bone Joint Surg* 1999;81(5): 649–659.

68. Gilbert A, Tassin JL. Reparation chirurgicale du plexus brachial dans la paralysie obstetricale. *Chirurgie* 1984;110:70–75.

69. Geutjens G, Gilbert A, Helsen K. Obstetric brachial plexus palsy associated with breech delivery. A different pattern of injury. *J Bone Joint Surg Br* 1996;78(2):303–306.

70. Gilbert A, Whitaker I. Obstetrical brachial plexus lesions. *J Hand Surg [Br]* 1991;16(5):489–491.

71. Meyer RD. Treatment of adult and obstetrical brachial plexus injuries. *Orthopedics* 1986;9(6):899–903.

72. Michelow BJ, Clarke HM, Curtis CG, et al. The natural history of obstetrical brachial plexus palsy. *Plast Reconstr Surg* 1994;93(4): 675–680; discussion 681.

73. Bae DS, Waters PM, Zurakowski D. Reliability of three classification systems measuring active motion in brachial plexus birth palsy. *J Bone Joint Surg Am* 2003;85-A(9):1733–1738.

74. Kawai H, Tsuyuguchi Y, Masada K. Identification of the lesion in brachial plexus injuries with root avulsion: a comprehensive assessment by means of preoperative findings, myelography, surgical exploration and intraoperative electrodiagnosis. Neuroorthopaedics 1989;7:15–23.

75. Kozin SH. Correlation between external rotation of the glenohumeral joint and deformity after brachial plexus birth palsy. *J Pediatr Orthop* 2004;2:189–193.

76. Pearl ML, Edgerton BW, Kon DS, et al. Comparison of arthroscopic findings with magnetic resonance imaging and arthrography in children with glenohumeral deformities secondary to brachial plexus birth palsy. *J Bone Joint Surg* 2003;85(5): 890–898.

77. Waters PM, Peljovich AE. Shoulder reconstruction in patients with chronic brachial plexus birth palsy. A case control study. *Clin Orthop Relat Res* 1999;364:144–152.

78. Moukoko D, Ezaki M, Wilkes D, et al. Posterior shoulder dislocation in infants with neonatal brachial plexus palsy. *J Bone Joint Surg Am* 2004;4:787–793.

79. Troum S, Floyd WE, Waters PM. Posterior dislocation of the humeral head in infancy associated with obstetrical paralysis. A case report. *J Bone Joint Surg* 1993;75:1370–1375.

80. Hoffer MM, Wickenden R, Roper B. Brachial plexus birth palsies, results of tendon transfers to the rotator cuff. *J Bone J Surg* 1978;60:691.

81. Leffert RD. Brachial plexus. In: DP G, ed. *Operative hand surgery*, 3rd ed. New York: Churchill Livingstone, 1993:1509.

82. Aitken J. Deformity of elbow joint as sequel to Erb's obstetrical paralysis. *J Bone J Surg Br* 1952;34:352.

83. Zancolli E. Paralytic supination contracture of the forearm. *J Bone J Surg* 1967;49:1275.

84. Waters PM, Simmons BP. Congenital abnormalities: elbow region. In: Peimer CA, ed. *Surgery of the hand and upper extremity*. New York: McGraw-Hill, 1996:2049.

85. Manske PR, McCarroll HRJ, Hale R. Biceps tendon rerouting and percutaneous osteoclasis in the treatment of supination deformity in obstetrical palsy. *J Hand Surg [Am]* 1980;5:233.

86. Fahy MJ, Hall JG. A retrospective study of pregnancy complications among 828 cases of arthrogryposis. *Genet Couns* 1990; 1(1):3–11.

87. Weeks PM. Surgical correction of upper extremity deformities in arthrogrypotics. *Plast Reconstr Surg* 1965;36(4):459–465.

88. Kang PB, Lidov HG, David WS, et al. Diagnostic value of electromyography and muscle biopsy in arthrogryposis multiplex congenita. *Ann Neurol* 2003;54:790.

89. Gibson DA, Urs ND. Arthrogryposis multiplex congenita. *J Bone Joint Surg* 1970;52(3):483–493.

90. Lloyd-Roberts GC, Lettin AWF. Arthrogryposis multiplex congenita. *J Bone Joint Surg Br* 1970;52:494.

91. Meyn M, Ruby L. Arthrogryposis of the upper extremity. *Orthop Clin North Am* 1976;7(2):501–509.

92. Ezaki M. Treatment of the upper limb in the child wtih arthrogryposis. *Hand Clin* 2000;16:703.

93. Van Heest A, Waters PM, Simmons BP. Surgical treatment of arthrogryposis of the elbow. *J Hand Surg [Am]* 1998;23(6): 1063–1070.

94. Bunnell S. Restoring flexion to paralytic elbow. *J Bone Joint Surg Am* 1951;33:566.

95. Carroll RE, Kleinman WB. Pectoralis major transplantation to restore elbow flexion to the paralytic limb. *J Hand Surg [Am]* 1979;4(6):501–507.

96. Zancolli E, Mitre H. Latissimus dorsi transfer to restore elbow flexion. An appraisal of eight cases. *J Bone Joint Surg Am* 1973; 55(6):1265–1275.

97. Williams PF. The elbow in arthrogryposis. *J Bone Joint Surg Br* 1973;55(4):834–840.

98. Smith DW, Drennan JC. Arthrogryposis wrist deformities: results of infantile serial casting. *J Pediatr Orthop* 2002;22:44.

99. Clark J. Reconstruction of biceps brachii by pectoralis major transplantation. *Br J Surg* 1946;34:180.

100. Doyle JR, James PM, Larsen LJ, et al. Restoration of elbow flexion in arthrogryposis multiplex congenita. *J Hand Surg [Am]* 1980;5(2):149–152.

## Elbow and Forearm Region

101. Williams PF. The elbow in arthrogryposis. *J Bone Joint Surg Br* 1973;55(4):834–840.

102. Bergsma D. *Birth defects compendium*, 2nd ed. New York: Alan R. Liss (The National Foundation, March of Dimes), 1979.

103. Dobyns JH. Congenital abnormalities of the elbow. In: Morrey BF, ed. *The elbow and its disorders*. Philadelphia, PA: WB Saunders, 1985:161.

104. Fidalgo Valdueza A. The nail-patella syndrome. A report of three families. *J Bone Joint Surg Br* 1973;55(1):145–162.

105. Mital MA. Congenital radioulnar synostosis and congenital dislocation of the radial head. *Orthop Clin North Am* 1976;7(2): 375–383.

106. Wynne-Davies R. *Heritable disorders in orthopedic practice*. Oxford: Blackwell Science, 1973.

107. Campbell CC, Waters PM, Emans JB. Excision of the radial head for congenital dislocation. *J Bone Joint Surg Am* 1992;74(5): 726–733.

108. Bucknill TM. Anterior dislocation of the radial head in children. *Proc R Soc Med* 1977;70(9):620–624.

109. Danielisz L. Congenital dislocation of the head of the radius and elbow injury. *Arch Chir Neerl* 1971;23(2):163–171.

110. Danielsson LG, Theander G. Traumatic dislocation of the radial head at birth. *Acta Radiol Diagn* 1981;22(3B):379–382.

111. Almquist EE, Gordon LH, Blue AI. Congenital dislocation of the head of the radius. *J Bone Joint Surg Am* 1969;51(6):1118–1127.

112. Lloyd-Roberts GC, Bucknill TM. Anterior dislocation of the radial head in children: aetiology, natural history and management. *J Bone Joint Surg Br* 1977;59-B(4):402–407.

113. Mardam-Bey T, Ger E. Congenital radial head dislocation. *J Hand Surg [Am]* 1979;4(4):316–320.

114. McFarland B. Congenital dislocation of the head of the radius. *Br J Surg* 1936;24:41.

115. Hirayama T, Takemitsu Y, Yagihara K, et al. Operation for chronic dislocation of the radial head in children. Reduction by osteotomy of the ulna. *J Bone Joint Surg Br* 1987;69(4):639–642.

116. Exarhou EI, Antoniou NK. Congenital dislocation of the head of the radius. *Acta Orthop Scand* 1970;41(5):551–556.

117. Bell SN, Morrey BF, Bianco AJ Jr. Chronic posterior subluxation and dislocation of the radial head. *J Bone Joint Surg Am* 1991; 73(3):392–396.

118. Sachar K, Mih AD. Congenital radial head dislocations. *Hand Clin* 1998;14(1):39–47.

119. Brennan JS, Krause ME, Harrey D. Annular ligament construction for congenital anterior dislocation of both radial heads. *Clin Orthop* 1963;29:205.

120. Villa A, Paley D, Catagni MA, et al. Lengthening of the forearm by the Ilizarov technique. *Clin Orthop Relat Res* 1990;250: 125–137.

121. Lewis RW, Thibodeau AA. Deformity of the wrist following resection of the radial head. *Surg Gynecol Obstet* 1937;64:1079.

122. King BB. Resection of the radial head and neck: an end-result study of thirteen cases. *J Bone Joint Surg Am* 1939;21:839.

123. Sojbjerg JO, Ovesen J, Gundorf CE. The stability of the elbow following excision of the radial head and transection of the annular ligament. An experimental study. *Arch Orthop Trauma Surg* 1987;106(4):248–250.

124. Kelly DW. Congenital dislocation of the radial head: spectrum and natural history. *J Pediatr Orthop* 1981;1(3):295–298.

125. Sutro CJ. Regrowth of bone at the proximal end of the radius following resection in this region. *J Bone Joint Surg Am* 1935;17:867.

126. Mead C, Martin M. Aplasia of the trochlea: an original mutation. *J Bone Joint Surg Am* 1963;45:379.

127. Wood V. Congenital elbow dislocations. In: Buck-Gramcko D, ed. *Congenital malformations of the hand and forearm*. London: Churchill Livingstone, 1998:487.

128. Bayne LG. Ulnar club hand. In: Green DP, ed. *Operative hand surgery*, 3rd ed. New York: Churchill Livingstone, 1993:298.

129. Ogden JA, Watson HK, Bohne W. Ulnar dysmelia. *J Bone Joint Surg Am* 1976;58(4):467–475.

130. Riordan CD. Congenital absence of the radius, 15 year follow up. *J Bone Joint Surg Am* 1955;37:1129.

131. Lloyd-Roberts GC. Treatment of defects of the ulna in children by establishing cross-union with the radius. *J Bone Joint Surg Br* 1973;55(2):327–330.

132. Wood VE. Ulnar dimelia. In: Green DP, ed. *Operative hand surgery*, 3rd ed. New York: Churchill Livingstone, 1993:490.

133. Tsuyuguchi Y, Tada K, Yonenobu K. Mirror hand anomaly: reconstruction of the thumb, wrist, forearm, and elbow. *Plast Reconstr Surg* 1982;70(3):384–387.

134. Wilkie DPD. Congenital radio-ulnar synostosis. *Br J Surg* 1914;1:366.

135. Green WT, Mital MA. Congenital radio-ulnar synostosis: surgical treatment. *J Bone Joint Surg Am* 1979;61(5):738–743.

136. Ogino T, Hikino K. Congenital radio-ulnar synostosis: compensatory rotation around the wrist and rotation osteotomy. [erratum appears in J Hand Surg [Br] 1987 Oct;12(3):402]. *J Hand Surg [Br]* 1987;12(2):173–178.

137. Hansen OH, Andersen NO. Congenital radio-ulnar synostosis. Report of 37 cases. *Acta Orthop Scand* 1970;41(3):225–230.

138. Cleary JE, Omer GE Jr. Congenital proximal radio-ulnar synostosis. Natural history and functional assessment. *J Bone Joint Surg Am* 1985;67(4):539–545.

139. Simmons BP, Southmayd WW, Riseborough EJ. Congenital radioulnar synostosis. *J Hand Surg [Am]* 1983;8(6):829–838.

140. Giuffre L, Corsello G, Giuffre M, et al. New syndrome: autosomal dominant microcephaly and radio-ulnar synostosis. *Am J Med Genet* 1994;51(3):266–269.

141. Robinson GC, Miller JR, Dill FJ. Klinefelter's syndrome with the XXYY sex chromosomes complex. *J Pediatr* 1964;65:266.

142. Sachar K, Akelman E, Ehrlich MG. Radioulnar synostosis. *Hand Clin* 1994;10(3):399–404.

143. Morrison J. Congenital radio-ulnar synostosis. *Br J Med* 1892; 2:1337.

144. Cross AR. Congenital bilateral radioulnar synostosis. *Am J Dis Child* 1939;58:1259.

145. Kelikian H. *Congenital deformities of the hand and forearm.* Philadelphia, PA: WB Saunders, 1974.

146. Stretton JL. Congenital synostosis of radio-ulnar articulations. *Br Med J* 1905;2:1519.

147. Tagima T, Ogisho N, Kanaya F. Follow-up study of joint mobilization of proximal radio-ulnar synostosis. Paper presented at: American Society of Surgery of the Hand meeting, Cincinnati, OH, 1994.

148. Boireau P, Laville JM. Rotational osteotomy technique for congenital radio-ulnar synostosis with central medullary nailing and external fixation. *Rev Chir Orthop Reparatrice Appar Mot* 2002;88:812.

149. Nieman KM, Gould JS, Simmons BP. Injuries to and developmental deformities of the elbow in children. In: Bora FW, ed. *The pediatric upper extremity: diagnosis and management*, Philadelphia, PA: WB Saunders, 1986:213.

150. Kadiyala K, Waters P. Upper extremity compartment syndromes. *Hand Clin* 1998;14:467.

151. Dobyns J, Wood V, Bayne L. Congenital hand deformities. In: Green DP, ed. *Operative hand surgery*, 3rd ed. New York: Churchill Livingstone, 1993:251.

152. Murphy HS, Hanson CG. Congenital humeroradial synostosis. *J Bone Joint Surg Am* 1945;27:712.

153. Leisti J, Lachman RS, Rimoin DL. Humeroradial ankylosis associated with other congenital defects (the "boomerang arm" sign). *Birth Defects Orig Artic Ser* 1975;11(5):306–307.

154. Solomon L. Hereditary multiple exostosis. *J Bone Joint Surg Br* 1963;45:292.

155. Jaffe HL. Hereditary multiple exostosis. *Arch Pathol* 1943;36:335.

156. Shapiro F, Simon S, Glimcher MJ. Hereditary multiple exostoses. Anthropometric, roentgenographic, and clinical aspects. *J Bone Joint Surg Am* 1979;61(6A):815–824.

157. Bock GW, Reed MH. Forearm deformities in multiple cartilaginous exostoses. *Skeletal Radiol* 1991;20(7):483–486.

158. Fogel GR, McElfresh EC, Peterson HA, et al. Management of deformities of the forearm in multiple hereditary osteochondromas. *J Bone Joint Surg Am* 1984;66(5):670–680.

159. Masada K, Tsuyuguchi Y, Kawai H, et al. Operations for forearm deformity caused by multiple osteochondromas. *J Bone Joint Surg Br* 1989;71(1):24–29.

160. Arms DM, Strecker WB, Manske PR, et al. Management of forearm deformity in multiple hereditary osteochondromatosis. *J Pediatr Orthop* 1997;17(4):450–454.

161. McCornack EB. The surgical management of hereditary multiple exostosis. *Orthop Rev* 1981;10:57.

162. Rodgers WB, Hall JE. One-bone forearm as a salvage procedure for recalcitrant forearm deformity in hereditary multiple exostoses. *J Pediatr Orthop* 1993;13(5):587–591.

163. Waters PM, Van Heest AE, Emans J. Acute forearm lengthenings. *J Pediatr Orthop* 1997;17(4):444–449.

164. Lowe HG. Radio-ulnar fusion for defects in the forearm bones. *J Bone Joint Surg Am* 1991;18:316.

165. Murray RA. The one-bone forearm: a reconstruction procedure. *J Bone Joint Surg Am* 1955;37:366.

166. Catagni MA, Szabo RM, Cattaneo R. Preliminary experience with Ilizarov method in late reconstruction of radial hemimelia. *J Hand Surg Am* 1993;18(2):316–321.

167. Tetsworth K, Krome J, Paley D. Lengthening and deformity correction of the upper extremity by the Ilizarov technique. *Orthop Clin North Am* 1991;22(4):689–713.

168. Dahl MT. The gradual correction of forearm deformities in multiple hereditary exostoses. *Hand Clin* 1993;9(4):707–718.

169. Pritchett JW. Lengthening the ulna in patients with hereditary multiple exostoses. *J Bone Joint Surg Br* 1986;68(4):561–565.

170. Cheng JC. Distraction lengthening of the forearm. *J Hand Surg Br* 1991;16(4):441–445.

171. Irani RN, Rushen NM, Petrucelli R. Ulnar lengthening for negative ulnar variance in hereditary multiple osteochondromas. *J Bone Joint Surg Br* 1992;1:143.

172. Paley D. Lengthening and deformity of the upper arm. Paper presented at: American Society of Surgery of the Hand Congenital Differences Workshop, Salt Lake City, UT, 1994.

173. Wood VE. Congenital pseudarthrosis of the forearm. In: Green DP, Hotchkiss RN, Pederson WC, eds. *Green's operative hand surgery*, 4th ed. New York: Churchill Livingstone, 1999:541.

174. Bell DF. Congenital forearm pseudarthrosis: report of six cases and review of the literature. *J Pediatr Orthop* 1989;9(4):438–443.

175. Allieu Y, Gomis R, Yoshimura M, et al. Congenital pseudarthrosis of the forearm-two cases treated by free vascularized fibular graft. *J Hand Surg Am* 1981;6(5):475–481.

176. Weiland AJ, Weiss AP, Moore JR, et al. Vascularized fibular grafts in the treatment of congenital pseudarthrosis of the tibia. *J Bone Joint Surg Am* 1990;72(5):654–662.

## Wrist Region

177. Bayne LG, Klug MS. Long-term review of the surgical treatment of radial deficiencies. *J Hand Surg [Am]* 1987;12(2):169–179.

178. Birch-Jensen A. *Congenital deformities of the upper extremities.* Copenhagen: Ejnar Munksgaard Forlag, 1950.

179. Manske PR, McCarroll HR Jr, Swanson K. Centralization of the radial club hand: an ulnar surgical approach. *J Hand Surg [Am]* 1981;6(5):423–433.

180. James MA, McCarroll HRJ, Manske PR. The spectrum of radial longitudinal deficiency: a modified classification. *J Hand Surg [Am]* 1999;24:1145.

181. Goldberg MJ, Bartoshesky LE. Congenital hand anomaly: etiology and associated malformations. *Hand Clin* 1985;1(3): 405–415.

182. Barry JE, Auldist AW. The Vater association: one end of a spectrum of anomalies. *Am J Dis Child* 1974;128(6):769–771.

183. Beals RK, Rolfe B. VATER association. A unifying concept of multiple anomalies. *J Bone Joint Surg Am* 1989;71(6):948–950.

184. Carroll RE, Louis DS. Anomalies associated with radial dysplasia. *J Pediatr* 1974;84(3):409–411.

185. Goldstein R. Hypoplastic anemia with multiple congenital anomalies (Franconi syndrome). *Am J Dis Child* 1955;89:618.

186. Hall JG. Thrombocytopenia and absent radius (TAR) syndrome. *J Med Genet* 1987;24(2):79–83.

187. Esmer C, Sanchez S, Ramos S, et al. DEB test for Fanconi anemia detection in patients with atypical phenotypes. *Am J Med Genet* 2004;124A:35.

188. Hedberg VA, Lipton JM. Thrombocytopenia with absent radii. A review of 100 cases. *Am J Pediatr Hematol Oncol* 1988;10(1):51–64.

189. Bayne LG, Costas BLL, Lourie GM. The upper limb. In: Morrissy RT, Weinstein SL, eds. *Lovell and Winter's pediatric orthopaedics*, 4th ed. Philadelphia, PA: Lippincott-Raven, 1996:781.

190. Skerik SK, Flatt AE. The anatomy of congenital radial dysplasia. Its surgical and functional implications. *Clin Orthop Relat Res* 1969;66:125–143.

191. Lamb DW. Radial club hand. A continuing study of sixty-eight patients with one hundred and seventeen club hands. *J Bone Joint Surg Am* 1977;59(1):1–13.

192. Bora FW Jr, Nicholson JT, Cheema HM. Radial meromelia. The deformity and its treatment. *J Bone Joint Surg Am* 1970;52(5): 966–979.

193. Bora FWJ, Carniol PJ, Martin E. Congenital anomalies of the upper limb: radial club hand. In: Bora FWJ, ed. *The pediatric upper extremity: diagnosis and management*. Philadelphia, PA: WB Saunders, 1986:28.

194. Kessler I. Centralisation of the radial club hand by gradual distraction. *J Hand Surg [Br]* 1989;14(1):37–42.

195. Tonkin MA. Radial longitudinal deficiency (radial dysplasia, radial clubhand). In: Green DP, Hotchkiss RN, Pederson WC, eds. *Green's operative hand surgery*, 4th ed. New York: Churchill Livingstone, 1999:344.

196. Albee FH. Formation of radius congenitally absent, condition seven years after implantation of bone graft. *Ann Surg* 1928; 87:105.

197. Starr DE. Congenital absence of the radius: a method of surgical correction. *J Bone Joint Surg Am* 1945;27:572.

198. Entin MA. Reconstruction of congenital aplasia of radial component. *Surg Clin North Am* 1964;44:1091.

199. Riordan CD. Congenital absence of the radius. *J Bone Joint Surg Am* 1955;37:1129.

200. Vilkki SK. Distraction lengthening and microvascular bone transplantation in the treatment of radial club hand. Paper presented at: American Society for Surgery of the Hand Congenital Differences Workshop, Salt Lake City, UT, 1994.

201. Buck-Gramcko D. Radialization as a new treatment for radial club hand. *J Hand Surg [Am]* 1985;10(6 Pt 2):964–968.

202. Catagni MA, Szabo RM, Cattaneo R. Preliminary experience with Ilizarov method in late reconstruction of radial hemimelia. *J Hand Surg [Am]* 1993;18(2):316–321.

203. Lister G. Reconstruction of the hypoplastic thumb. *Clin Orthop Relat Res* 1985;195:52–65.

204. Buck-Gramcko D. Pollicization of the index finger. Method and results in aplasia and hypoplasia of the thumb. *J Bone Joint Surg Am* 1971;53(8):1605–1617.

205. Huber E. Hilfsoperation bei Medianuslahmug. *Dtsch Z Chir* 1921;162:271.

206. Carroll RE. Pollicization. In: Green DP, ed. *Operative hand surgery*, 2rd ed. New York: Churchill Livingstone, 1988:2263.

207. Gilbert A. Pollicizations in radial club hand. Paper presented at: Second International Workshop on Congenital Differences of the Upper Limb, Salt Lake City, UT, 1994.

208. Manske PR, McCarroll HR. Abductor digiti minimi opponensplasty in congenital radial dysplasia. *J Hand Surg [Am]* 1978;3:552.

209. Manske PR, McCaroll HR Jr. Index finger pollicization for a congenitally absent or nonfunctioning thumb. *J Hand Surg [Am]* 1985;10(5):606–613.

210. Ogden JA, Watson HK, Bohne W. Ulnar dysmelia. *J Bone Joint Surg Am* 1976;58(4):467–475.

211. Bamshad M, Krakowiak PA, Watkins WS, et al. A gene for ulnar-mammary syndrome maps to 12q23-q24.1. *Hum Mol Genet* 1995;4(10):1973–1977.

212. Robert AS. A case of deformity of the forearm and hands with an unusual history of hereditary congenital deficiency. *Ann Surg* 1886;3:135.

213. Turnpenny PD, Dean JC, Duffty P, et al. Weyers' ulnar ray/oligodactyly syndrome and the association of midline malformations with ulnar ray defects. *J Med Genet* 1992;29(9):659–662.

214. Wulfsberg EA, Mirkinson LJ, Meister SJ. Autosomal dominant tetramelic postaxial oligodactyly. *Am J Med Genet* 1993;46(5): 579–583.

215. Chemke J, Nisani R, Fischel RE. Absent ulna in the Klippel-Feil syndrome: an unusual associated malformation. *Clin Genet* 1980;17(2):167–170.

216. Franceschini P, Vardeu MP, Dalforno L, et al. Possible relationship between ulnar-mammary syndrome and split hand with aplasia of the ulna syndrome. *Am J Med Genet* 1992;44(6):807–812.

217. Ogino T, Kato H. Clinical and experimental studies on ulnar ray deficiency. *Handchir Mikrochir Plast Chir* 1988;20(6):330–337.

218. Bayne LG. Ulnar club hand (ulnar deficiencies). In: Green DP, ed. *Operative hand surgery*, 3rd ed. New York: Churchill Livingstone, 1993:288.

219. Cole RJ, Manske PR. Classification of ulnar deficiency according to the thumb and first web. *J Hand Surg [Am]* 1997;22(3): 479–488.

220. Broudy AS, Smith RJ. Deformities of the hand and wrist with ulnar deficiency. *J Hand Surg [Am]* 1979;4(4):304–315.

221. Johnson J, Omer GE Jr. Congenital ulnar deficiency. Natural history and therapeutic implications. *Hand Clin* 1985;1(3):499–510.

222. Southwood AR. Partial absence of the ulna and associated structures. *J Anat* 1926-1927;61:346.

223. Raus EE. Repair of simple syndactylism in the healthy neo-newborn. *Orthop Rev* 1984;13:498.

224. Beals RK, Lovrien EW. Dyschondrosteosis and Madelung's deformity. Report of three kindreds and review of the literature. *Clin Orthop Relat Res* 1976;116:24–28.

225. Madelung V. Die Spontane Subluxaion der Hand nach vorne. *Verh Dtsch Ges Chir* 1878;7:259.

226. Ezaki M. Madelung's deformity. In: Green DP, Hotchkiss RN, Pederson WC, eds. *Green's operative hand surgery*. New York: Churchill Livingstone, 1999:528.

227. Felman AH. Dyschondrosteosis: mesomelic dwarfism of Leri and Weill. *Am J Dis Child* 1970;120:329.

228. Nielsen JB. Madelung's deformity. A follow-up study of 26 cases and a review of the literature. *Acta Orthop Scand* 1977;48(4): 379–384.

229. Vickers D, Nielsen G. Madelung's deformity: treatment by osteotomy of the radius and Lauenstein procedure. *J Hand Surg [Am]* 1987;12(2):202–204.

230. Linscheid RL. Madelung's Deformita. *Correspondence Newsletter no. 24. Correspondence Club American Society for Surgery of the Hand.* 1979.

231. Ranawat CS, DeFiore J, Straub LR. Madelung's deformity. An end-result study of surgical treatment. *J Bone Joint Surg Am* 1975;57(6):772–775.

## Hand Region

232. Scherer SW, Poorkaj P, Allen T, et al. Fine mapping of the autosomal dominant split hand/split foot locus on chromosome 7, band q21.3-q22.1. [see comment]. *Am J Hum Genet* 1994;55(1):12–20.

233. Kay SPJ. Congenital hand deformities: cleft hand. In: Green DP, Hotchkiss RN, Pederson WC. eds. *Green's operative hand surgery*. New York: Churchill Livingstone, 1999:402.

234. Ianakiev P, Kilpatrick MW, Toudjarska I, et al. Split-hand/split-foot malformation is caused by mutations in the p63 gene on 3q27. *Am J Hum Genet* 2000;67:59.

235. Barrow LL, van Bokhoven H, Daack-Hirsch S, et al. Analysis of the p63 gene in classical EEC syndrome, related syndromes, and non-syndromic orofacial clefts. *J Med Genet* 2002;39:559.

236. Witters I, Van Bokhoven H, Goossens A, et al. Split-hand/split-foot malformation with paternal mutation in the p63 gene. *Prenat Diagn* 2001;21:1119.

237. Buss PW. Cleft hand/foot: clinical and developmental aspects. *J Med Genet* 1994;31(9):726–730.

238. Calzolari E, Manservigi D, Garani GP, et al. Limb reduction defects in Emilia Romagna, Italy: epidemiological and genetic study in 173,109 consecutive births. *J Med Genet* 1990;27(6):353–357.

239. Froster-Iskenius UG, Baird PA. Limb reduction defects in over one million consecutive live births. *Teratology* 1989;39:127.

240. Ogino T. Cleft hand. *Hand Clin* 1990;6(4):661–671.

241. Watari S, Tsuge K. A classification of cleft hands, based on clinical findings: theory of developmental mechanism. *Plast Reconstr Surg* 1979;64(3):381–389.

242. Manske PR, Halikis MN. Surgical classification of central deficiency according to the thumb web. *J Hand Surg [Am]* 1995; 20(4):687–697.

243. Barsky AJ. Cleft hand: classification incidence and treatment. Review of the literature and report of nineteen cases. *J Bone Joint Surg Am* 1964;46:1707.

244. Snow JW, Littler JW. Surgical treatment of cleft hand. *Transactions of the society of plastic and reconstructive surgery, 4th congress in Rome*. Amsterdam: Excerpta Medica Foundation, 1967:888.

245. Ueba Y. Plastic surgery for the cleft hand. *J Hand Surg [Am]* 1981;6(6):557–560.

246. Miura T, Komada T. Simple method for reconstruction of the cleft hand with an adducted thumb. *Plast Reconstr Surg* 1979; 64(1):65–67.

247. Goldberg NH, Watson HK. Composite toe (phalanx and epiphysis) transfer in the reconstruction of the aphalangic hand. *J Hand Surg [Am]* 1982;7:454.

248. Buck-Gramcko D. The role of nonvascularized toe phalanx transplantation. *Hand Clin* 1990;6(4):643–659.
249. Buck-Gramcko D. Cleft hands: classification and treatment. *Hand Clin* 1985;1(3):467–473.
250. Ducloyer P, Saffar P *Les malformations congenitales du membre superieur*. Paris: Expansion Scientifique Francaise, 1991.
251. Buck-Gramcko D, Pereira JA. Proximal toe phalanx transplantation for bony stabilization and lengthening of partially aplastic digits. *Ann Chir Main Memb Super* 1990;9(2):107–118.
252. Cowen NJ, Loftus JM. Distraction augmentation manoplasty: technique of lengthening digits or entire hands. *Orthop Rev* 1978;7:45.
253. Entin MA. Reconstruction of congenital abnormalities of the upper extremities. *J Bone Joint Surg Am* 1975;57:727.
254. Vilkki SK. Advances in microsurgical reconstruction of the congenitally adactylous hand. *Clin Orthop Relat Res* 1995;(314):45–58.
255. Seitz WH Jr, Dobyns JH. Digital lengthening. With emphasis on distraction osteogenesis in the upper limb. *Hand Clin* 1993; 9(4):699–706.
256. Pillet J. Esthetic hand prosthesis. *J Hand Surg [Am]* 1983;8:778.
257. Kay S. Hypoplastic and absent digits. In: Green DP, Hotchkiss RN, Pederson WC, eds. *Green's operative hand surgery*, 4th ed. New York: Churchill Livingstone, 1999:368.
258. Kino Y. Clinical and experimental studies of the congenital constriction band syndrome, with an emphasis on its etiology. *J Bone Joint Surg Am* 1975;57(5):636–643.
259. Streeter GL. Focal deficiencies in fetal tissue and their relation to intrauterine amputation. *Contributions to embryology*, Vol. 22. Washington, DC: Carnegie Institution, 1930:126.
260. Patterson TJS. Congenital ring-constrictions. *Br J Plast Surg* 1961;14:1.
261. Dobyns JH. Segmental digital transposition in congenital hand deformities. *Hand Clin* 1985;1(3):475–482.
262. Soiland H. Lengthening a finger with the "on-the-top" method. *Acta Chir Scand* 1961;122:184.
263. Light TR. Congenital anomalies: syndactyly, polydactyly and cleft hands. In: Peimer CA, ed. *Surgery of the hand and upper extremity*, New York: McGraw-Hill, 1996:2111.
264. Jones NF, Upton J. Early release of syndactyly within six weeks of birth. *Orthop Trans* 1992;17:360.
265. Sommerkamp T, Ezaki M, Carter P. The pulp plasty: a composite graft for complete syndactyly fingertip separations. *J Hand Surg [Am]* 1992;17:15.
266. Toledo LC, Ger E. Evaluation of the operative treatment of syndactyly. *J Hand Surg [Am]* 1979;4(6):556–564.
267. Percival NJ, Sykes PJ. Syndactyly: a review of the factors which influence surgical treatment. *J Hand Surg [Br]* 1989;14(2): 196–200.
268. Keret D, Ger E. Evaluation of a uniform operative technique to treat syndactyly. *J Hand Surg [Am]* 1987;12(5 Pt 1):727–729.
269. Shinya K. Dancing girl flap: a new flap suitable for web release. *Ann Plast Surg* 1999;43:618.
270. Withey SJ, Kangesu T, Carver N, et al. The open finger technique for the release of syndactyly. *J Hand Surg [Br]* 2001;26:4.
271. Aydin A, Ozden BC. Dorsal metacarpal island flap in syndactyly treatment. *Ann Plast Surg* 2004;52:43.
272. Dao KD, Shin AY, Billings A, et al. Surgical treatment of congenital syndactyly of the hand. *J Am Acad Orthop Surg* 2004;12:39.
273. Tagaki S, Hosokawa K, Haramoto U, et al. A new technique for the treament of syndactyly with osseous fusion of the distal phalanges. *Ann Plastic Surg* 2000;44:660.
274. Golash A, Watson JS. Nail fold creation in complete syndactyly using Buck-Gramcko pulp flaps. *J Hand Surg [Br]* 2000;25:11.
275. Fearon JA. Treatment of the hands and feet in Apert syndrome: an evolution in management. *Plast Reconstr Surg* 2003;112:1.
276. Chang J, Danton TK, Ladd AL, et al. Reconstruction of the hand in Apert syndrome: a simplified approach. *Plast Reconstr Surg* 2002;109:465.
277. Deunk J, Nicolai JP, Hamburg SM. Long-term results of syndactyly correction: full-thickness versus split-thickness skin grafts. *J Hand Surg [Br]* 2003;28:125.
278. Muzaffar AR, Rafols F, Masson J, et al. Keloid formation after syndactyly reconstruction: associated conditions, prevalence, and preliminary report of a treatment method. *J Hand Surg [Am]* 2004;29:201.
279. Frazier TM. A note on race specific congenital malformation rates. *Am J Obstet Gynecol* 1960;80:184.
280. Nathan PA, Keniston RC. Crossed polydactyly. *J Hered* 1940; 31:25.
281. Woolf CM, Myrianthopoulos NC. Polydactyly in American negroes and whites. *Am J Hum Genet* 1973;25(4):397–404.
282. Stelling F. The upper extremity. In: Ferguson AB, ed. *Orthopaedic surgery infancy and childhood*, Baltimore, MD: JB Lippincott, 1963:304.
283. Turek SL. *Orthopaedic principles and their applications*. Philadelphia, PA: JB Lippincott Co, 1976.
284. Heras L, Barco J, Cohen A. Unusual complication of ligation of rudimentary ulnar digit. *J Hand Surg [Br]* 1999;24:750.
285. Leber GE, Gosain AK. Surgical excision of pedunculated supernumerary digits prevents traumatic amputation neuromas. *Pediatr Dermatol* 2003;20:108.
286. Tada K, Kurisaki E, Yonenobu K, et al. Central polydactyly—a review of 12 cases and their surgical treatment. *J Hand Surg [Am]* 1982;7(5):460–465.
287. Wood VE. Treatment of central polydactyly. *Clin Orthop Relat Res* 1971;74:196–205.
288. Kay S. Camptodactyly. In: Green DP, Hotchkiss RN, Pederson WC. eds. *Green's operative hand surgery*, 4th ed. New York: Churchill-Livingstone, 1999:510.
289. Jones KG, Marmor L, Lankford LL. An overview on new procedures in surgery of the hand. *Clin Orthop Relat Res* 1974;9(0): 154–167.
290. Engber WD, Flatt AE. Camptodactyly: an analysis of sixty-six patients and twenty-four operations. *J Hand Surg [Am]* 1977; 2(3):216–224.
291. Benson LS, Waters PM, Kamil NI, et al. Camptodactyly: classification and results of nonoperative treatment. *J Pediatr Orthop* 1994;14(6):814–819.
292. Larner AJ. Camptodactyly in a neurology outpatient clinic. *Int J Clin Pract* 2001;55:592.
293. Millesi H. Camptodactyly. In: Littler JW, Cramer LM, Smith JW. eds. *Symposium on reconstructive surgery*. St Louis, MO: Mosby, 1974:175.
294. Smith RJ, Kaplan EB. Camptodactyly in similar atraumatic flexion deformities of the proximal interphalangeal joints of the fingers. *J Bone Joint Surg Am* 1968;50:1187.
295. Koman LA, Toby EB, Poehling GG. Congenital flexion deformities of the proximal phalangeal joint in children: a subgroup of camptodactyly. *J Hand Surg [Am]* 1990;15:582.
296. Courtenmanche AD. Camptodactyly: etiology and management. *Plast Reconstr Surg* 1969;44:451.
297. McFarlane RM, Classen DA, Porte AM, et al. The anatomy and treatment of camptodactyly of the small finger. *J Hand Surg [Am]* 1992;17(1):35–44.
298. McFarlane RM, Curry GI, Evans HB. Anomalies of the intrinsic muscles in camptodactyly. *J Hand Surg [Am]* 1983;8(5 Pt 1): 531–544.
299. Buck-Gramcko D. Camptodactyly. In: Bowers WH, ed. *The interphalangeal joints*. Edinburgh: Churchill Livingstone, 1987:200.
300. Hori M, Nakamura R, Inoue G, et al. Nonoperative treatment of camptodactyly. *J Hand Surg [Am]* 1987;12(6):1061–1065.
301. Ogino T, Kato H. Operative findings in camptodactyly of the little finger. *J Hand Surg [Br]* 1992;17(6):661–664.
302. Miura T, Nakamura R, Tamura Y. Long-standing extended dynamic splintage and release of an abnormal restraining structure in camptodactyly. *J Hand Surg [Br]* 1992;17(6):665–672.
303. Siegert JJ, Cooney WP, Dobyns JH. Management of simple camptodactyly. *J Hand Surg [Br]* 1990;15(2):181–189.
304. Carneiro RS. Congenital attenuation of the extensor tendon central slip. *J Hand Surg [Am]* 1993;18(6):1004–1007.
305. Oldfield MC. Dupuytren's contracture. *Proc R Soc Med* 1954; 47:361.
306. Hersh AH, DeMarinis F, Stecher RM. On the inheritance and development of clinodactyly. *Am J Dis Child* 1940;60:1319.
307. McKusick VA. *Mendelian inheritance in man: catalogs of autosomal dominant, autosomal recessive, and X linked phenotypes*, 2nd ed. Baltimore, MD: The Johns Hopkins University Press, 1968.
308. Poznanski AK, Pratt GB, Manson G, et al. Clinodactyly, camptodactyly, Kirner's deformity, and other crooked fingers. *Radiology* 1969;93(3):573–582.

309. Poznanski AK. Anomalies of the hand - general considerations. *The hand in radiographic diagnosis*. Philadelphia, PA: WB Saunders, 1984;1:173–180.
310. Poznanski AK. Rubinstein-Taybi syndrome (broad thumbs syndrome). In: Poznanski AK, ed. *The hand in radiologic diagnosis*, Philadelphia, PA: WB Saunders, 1974:369.
311. Rubinstein JH. The broad thumbs syndrome: progress report 1968. *Birth Defects Orig Artic Ser* 1969;5:25.
312. Amuso SJ. Diastrophic dwarfism. *J Bone Joint Surg Am* 1968; 50:113.
313. Taybi H. Diastrophic dwarfism. *Radiology* 1963;80:1.
314. Vickers DW. Langenskiold's operation (physolysis) for congenital malformations of bone producing Madelung's deformity and clinodactyly. *J Bone Joint Surg Br* 1984;66:778.
315. Vickers D. Clinodactyly of the little finger: a simple operative technique for reversal of the growth abnormality. *J Hand Surg Br* 1987;12(3):335–342.

### Hand: Thumb

316. Rodgers WB, Waters PM. Incidence of trigger digits in newborns. *J Hand Surg [Am]* 1994;19(3):364–368.
317. Slakey JB, Hennrikus WL. Acquired thumb flexion contracture in children: congenital trigger thumb. *J Bone Joint Surg Br* 1996; 78(3):481–483.
318. Buchman M, Gibson T, McCallum D. Transmission electron microscopic pathoanatomy of congenital trigger thumbs. *J Pediatr Orthop* 1999;19:411.
319. Van Heest AE, House J, Krivit W, et al. Surgical treatment of carpal tunnel syndrome and trigger digits in children with mucopolysaccharide storage disorders. *J Hand Surg [Am]* 1998; 23(2):236–243.
320. Dinham JM, Meggitt BF. Trigger thumbs in children. A review of the natural history and indications for treatment in 105 patients. *J Bone Joint Surg Br* 1974;56(1):153–155.
321. Ger E, Kupcha P, Ger D. The management of trigger thumb in children. *J Hand Surg [Am]* 1991;16(5):944–947.
322. Tsuyuguchi Y, Toda K, Kawaii H. Splint therapy for trigger fingers in children. *Arch Phys Med Rehabil* 1983;64:75.
323. Cardon LJ, Ezaki M, Carter PR. Trigger finger in children. *J Hand Surg [Am]* 1999;24:1156.
324. Kleinman WB, Strickland JW. Thumb reconstruction. In: Green DP, Hotchkiss RN, Pederson WC. eds. *Green's operative hand surgery*, 4th ed. New York: Churchill Livingstone, 1999:2068.
325. Buck-Gramcko D. Congenital absence and hypoplasia of thumb. In: Strickland JW, ed. *The thumb, the hand, the upper limb*, Edinburgh: Churchill Livingstone, 1971:1605.
326. Manske P, McCarroll H, James M. Type IIIA hypoplastic thumb. *J Hand Surg [Am]* 1995;20:246.
327. Blauth W. Der hypoplastiche Daumen. *Arch Orthop Unfallchir* 1967;62:225.
328. Abdel-Ghani H, Amro S. Characterisitics of patients with hypoplastic thumb: a prospective study of 51 patients with the results of surgical treatment. *J Pediatr Orthop B* 2004;13:127.
329. Shibata M, Yoshizu T, Seki T. Reconstruction of a congenital hypoplastic thumb with use of a free vascularized metatarsophalangeal joint. *J Bone Joint Surg Am* 1998;80:1469.
330. Orioli IM, Castilla EE. Thumb/hallux duplication and preaxial polydactyly type I. *Am J Med Genet* 1999;82:219.
331. Heus HC, Hing A, van Baren MJ, et al. A physical and transcriptional map of the preaxial polydactyly locus on chromosome 7q36. *Genomics* 1999;57:342.
332. Light T, Buck-Gramcko D. Polydactyly: terminology and classification. In: Buck-Gramcko D, ed. *Congenital malformations of the hand and forearm*, London: Churchill Livingstone, 1998:217.
333. Marks TW, Bayne LG. Polydactyly of the thumb: abnormal anatomy and treatment. *J Hand Surg [Am]* 1978;3(2):107–116.
334. Wassel HD. The results of surgery for polydactyly of the thumb. *Clin Orthop Relat Res* 1969;64:175–193.
335. Benetar N. Thumb duplication: simple surgery for a common problem? *Handchir Mikrochir Plast Chir* 2004;36(2–3):137–140.
336. Mih AD. Complications of duplicate thumb reconstruction. *Hand Clin* 1998;14(1):143–149.
337. Seidman GD, Wenner SM. Surgical treatment of the duplicated thumb. *J Pediatr Orthop* 1993;13(5):660–662.
338. Masuda T, Sekiguchi J, Komuro Y, et al. "Face to face": a new method for the treatment of polydactyly of the thumb that maximises the use of available soft tissue. *Scand J Plast Reconstr Surg Hand Surg* 2000;34:79.
339. Kawabata H, Masatomi T, Shimada K, et al. Treatment of residual instability and extensor lag in polydactyly of the thumb. [see comment]. *J Hand Surg [Br]* 1993;18(1):5–8.
340. Lourie GM, Consts BL, Bayne LG. The zig-zag deformity in preaxial polydactyly. *J Hand Surg [Br]* 1995;20:561.
341. Miura T. An appropriate treatment for postoperative Z-formed deformity of the duplicated thumb. *J Hand Surg [Am]* 1977; 2(5):380–386.
342. Tada K, Yonenobu K, Tsuyuguchi Y. Duplication of the thumb: a retrospective view of two hundred and thirty-seven cases. *J Bone Joint Surg Am* 1983;65:584.
343. Jaeger M, Refior HJ. The congenital triangular deformity of the tubular bones of hand and foot. *Clin Orthop Relat Res* 1971;81: 139–150.
344. Dobbs MB, Dietz FR, Gurnett CA, et al. Localization of dominantly inherited isolated triphalangeal thumb to chromosomal region 7q36. *J Orthop Res* 2000;18:340.
345. Shiono H, Ogino T. Triphalangeal thumb and dermatoglyphics. *J Hand Surg [Br]* 1984;9(2):151–152.
346. Phillips RS. Congenital split foot (lobster claw) and triphalangeal thumbs. *J Bone Joint Surg Br* 1971;53:247.
347. Newbury-Ecob RA, Leanage R, Raeburn JA, et al. Holt-Oram syndrome: a clinical genetic study. *J Med Genet* 1996;33(4):300–307.
348. Aase JM, Smith DW. Congenital anemia and triphalangeal thumb. *J Pediatr* 1969;74:471.
349. Diamond LR, Allen DM, Magill FB. Congenital (erythroid) hypoplastic anemia: a 25 year study. *Am J Dis Child* 1961;102:403.
350. Townes PL, Brocks ER. Hereditary syndrome of imperforate anus with hand, foot, and ear anomalies. *J Pediatr* 1972;81(2):321–326.
351. Milch H. Triphalangeal thumb. *J Bone Joint Surg Am* 1951;33:692.
352. Buck-Gramcko D. Hand surgery in congenital malformations. In: Jackson IT, ed. *Recent advances in plastic surgery*, New York: Churchill Livingstone, 1981:115.
353. Barsky AJ. *Congenital anomalies of the hand and their surgical treatment*. Springfield, IL: Charles C Thomas Publisher, 1958.
354. Wood VE. Treatment of the triphalangeal thumb. *Clin Orthop Relat Res* 1976;00(120):188–200.
355. Horii E, Nakamura R, Makino H. Triphalangeal thumb without associated abnormalities: clinical characteristics and surgical outcomes. *Plast Reconstr Surg* 2001;108:902.

### Traumatic Injuries

356. Landin LA. Fracture patterns in children. Analysis of 8,682 fractures with special reference to incidence, etiology and secular changes in a Swedish urban population 1950-1979. *Acta Orthop Scand* 1983;202:1–109.
357. Hastings H II, Simmons BP. Hand fractures in children. A statistical analysis. *Clin Orthop Relat Res* 1984;188:120–130.
358. Barton NJ. Fractures of the phalanges of the hand in children. *Hand* 1979;11(2):134–143.
359. Rang M. *Children's fractures*, 2nd ed. Philadelphia, PA: JB Lippincott, 1983.
360. Fischer MD, McElfresh EC. Physeal and periphyseal injuries of the hand. Patterns of injury and results of treatment. *Hand Clin* 1994;10(2):287–301.
361. Leonard MH, Dubravcik P. Management of fractured fingers in the child. *Clin Orthop Relat Res* 1970;73:160–168.
362. DaCruz DJ, Slade RJ, Malone W. Fractures of the distal phalanges. *J Hand Surg [Br]* 1988;13(3):350–352.
363. Louis DS, Jebson PJ, Graham TJ. Amputations. In: Green DP, Hotchkiss RN, Pederson WC, eds. *Green's operative hand surgery*, 4th ed. New York: Churchill Livingstone, 1999:48.
364. Seymour N. Juxta-epiphyseal fracture of the terminal phalanx of the finger. *J Bone Joint Surg Br* 1966;48:347.
365. Wood VE. Fractures of the hand in children. *Orthop Clin North Am* 1976;7(3):527–542.
366. Waters PM, Benson LS. Dislocation of the distal phalanx epiphysis in toddlers. *J Hand Surg [Am]* 1993;18(4):581–585.
367. Michelinakis E, Vourexaki H. Displaced epiphyseal plate of the terminal phalanx in a child. *Hand* 1980;12(1):51–53.

368. DeBoeck H, Jaeken R. Treatment of chronic mallet finger in children by tenodermodesis. *J Pediatr Orthop* 1992;12:351.

369. Dixon GL Jr, Moon NF. Rotational supracondylar fractures of the proximal phalanx in children. *Clin Orthop Relat Res* 1972;83: 151–156.

370. Simmons BP, Peters TT. Subcondylar fossa reconstruction for malunion of fractures of the proximal phalanx in children. *J Hand Surg [Am]* 1987;12(6):1079–1082.

371. Green DP. Hand injury in children. *Pediatr Clin North Am* 1977; 24:903.

372. Waters PM, Taylor B. Percutaneous osteoclasis and reduction of malangulated phalangeal neck fractures in children. *J Hand Surg [Am]* 2004;29(4): 707–711.

373. Mintzer CM, Waters OM, Brown DJ. Remodeling of a displaced phalangeal neck fracture. *J Hand Surg [Br]* 1994;19:594.

374. Light TR. Injury to the immature carpus. *Hand Clin* 1988;4(3): 415–424.

375. Weiss AP, Hastings H II. Distal unicondylar fractures of the proximal phalanx. *J Hand Surg [Am]* 1993;18(4):594–599.

376. Campbell RM Jr. Operative treatment of fractures and dislocations of the hand and wrist region in children. *Orthop Clin North Am* 1990;21(2):217–243.

377. Green DP, Anderson JR. Closed reduction and percutaneous pin fixation of fractured phalanges. *J Bone Joint Surg Am* 1973;55(8): 1651–1654.

378. Gabuzda G, Mara J. Bony gamekeeper's thumb in a skeletally immature girl. *Orthopedics* 1991;14(7):792–793.

379. Jehanno P, Iselin F, Frajman JM, et al. Fractures of the base of the first metacarpal in children. Role of K-wire stabilisation. *Chir Main* 1999;18(3):184–190.

380. Bretlau T, Christensen OM, Edstrom P, et al. Diagnosis of scaphoid fracture and dedicated extremity MRI. *Acta Orthop Scand* 1999;70(5):504–508.

381. Brydie A, Raby N. Early MRI in the management of clinical scaphoid fracture. *Br J Radiol* 2003;76(905):296–300.

382. Mintzer CM, Waters PM, Simmons BP. Nonunion of the scaphoid in children treated by Herbert screw fixation and bone grafting. A report of five cases. *J Bone Joint Surg Br* 1995;77(1):98–100.

383. Mintzer CM, Waters PM. Surgical treatment of pediatric scaphoid fracture nonunions. *J Pediatr Orthop* 1999;19(2):236–239.

384. Waters PM, Stewart S. Surgical Treatment of Non-union and Avascular Necrosis of the Proximal Scaphoid in Adolescents. *J Bone Joint Surg Am* 2002;84(6):915–920.

385. Gerard FM. Post-traumatic carpal instability in a young child. A case report. *J Bone Joint Surg Am* 1980;62(1):131–133.

386. Kaawach W, Ecklund K, Di Canzio J, et al. Normal ranges of scapholunate distance in children 6 to 14 years old. *J Pediatr Orthop* 2001;21(4):464–467.

387. Terry CL, Waters PM. Triangular fibrocartilage injuries in pediatric and adolescent patients. *J Hand Surg [Am]* 1998;23(4): 626–634.

388. Becton JL, Christian JD Jr, Goodwin HN, et al. A simplified technique for treating the complex dislocation of the index metacarpophalangeal joint. *J Bone Joint Surg Am* 1975;57(5): 698–700.

389. Bohart PG, Gelberman RH, Vandell RF, et al. Complex dislocations of the metacarpophalangeal joint. *Clin Orthop Relat Res* 1982(164):208–210.

390. Green DP, Terry GC. Complex dislocations of the metacarpophalangeal joint. *J Bone Joint Surg Am* 1973;55:1480.

391. McLaughlin HL. Complex "locked" dislocation of the metacarpophalangeal joint. *J Trauma* 1965;5:683.

392. O'Connell SJ, Moore MM, Strickland JW, et al. Results of zone I and zone II flexor tendon repairs in children. *J Hand Surg [Am]* 1994;19(1):48–52.

393. Amadio PC. Staged flexor tendon reconstruction in children. *Ann Chir Main Memb Super* 1992;11(3):194–199.

394. Baker GL, Kleinert JM. Digit replantation in infants and young children: determinants of survival. *Plast Reconstr Surg* 1994; 94(1):139–145.

395. Devaraj VS, Kay SP, Batchelor AG, et al. Microvascular surgery in children. *Br J Plast Surg* 1991;44(4):276–280.

396. Sprengel O. Die angeborene Verschiebung des Schulterblattes nach oben. *Arch Klin Chir* 1891;42:545.

397. Carson WG, Lovell WW, Whitesides TE Jr. Congenital elevation of the scapula. Surgical correction by the woodward procedure. *J Bone Joint Surg Am* 1981;63:1199.

398. Cavendish ME. Congenital elevation of the scapula. *J Bone Joint Surg Br* 1972;54:395.

399. Hesinger RN. Orthopedic problems of the shoulder and neck. *Pediatr Clin North Am* 1986;33:1495.

400. Greitemann B, Rondhuis JJ, Karbowski A. Treatment of congenital elevation of the scapula. 10 (2–18) year follow-up of 37 cases of Sprengel's deformity. *Acta Orthop Scand* 1993;64:365.

401. Schrock RD. Congenital elevation of the scapula. *J Bone Joint Surg Am* 1926;8:207.

402. Jeannopoulos CL. Observations on congential elevation of the scapula. *Clin Ortop* 1961;20:132.

403. Neer CICI, ed. *Shoulder reconstruction*. Philadelphia, PA: WB Saunders, 1990.

404. Robinson RA, Braun RM, Mack P, et al. The surgical importance of the clavicular component of Sprengel's deformity. *J Bone Joint Surg Am* 1967;49A:1481.

405. Orrell KG, Bell DF. Structural abnormality of the clavicle associated with Sprengel's deformity. A case report. *Clin Orthop Relat Res* 1990;258:157–159.

406. Klisic P, Filipovic M, Uzelac O, et al. Relocation of congenitally elevated scapula. *J Pediatr Orthop* 1981;1:43.

407. Woodward JW. Congenital elevation of the scapula. Correction by release and transplantation of the muscle origins. A preliminary report. *J Bone Joint Surg Am* 1961;43A:219.

408. Green WT. The surgical correction of congenital elevation of the scapula (Sprengel's deformity). *J Bone Joint Surg Am* 1957;39A: 1439.

409. Leibovic SJ, Ehrlich MG, Zaleske DJ. Sprengel deformity. *J Bone Joint Surg Am* 1990;72:192.

410. Wilkinson JA, Campbell D. Scapular osteotomy for Sprengel's shoulder. *J Bone Joint Surg Br* 1980;62-B:486.

411. Grogan DP, Stanley EA, Bobechko WP. The congenital undescended scapula. Surgical correction by the woodward procedure. *J Bone Joint Surg Br* 1983;65:598.

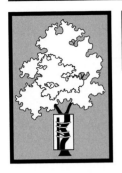

# 24 Developmental Hip Dysplasia and Dislocation

*Stuart L. Weinstein*

## GROWTH DISTURBANCE OF THE PROXIMAL FEMUR

In the pediatric orthopaedic literature, the longstanding terminology of *congenital dysplasia* or *congenital dislocation of the hip* (CDH) has been progressively replaced by the term *developmental dysplasia* or *developmental dislocation of the hip* (DDH). (The term *congenital dysplasia* is attributed to Hippocrates; *congenital* implies that a condition existed at birth.) The American Academy of Orthopaedic Surgeons

(1), the Pediatric Orthopaedic Society of North America, and the American Academy of Pediatrics have endorsed the name change of this entity from CDH to DDH, because the latter is more representative of the wide range of abnormalities seen in this condition (2).

The term *developmental* is more encompassing and is taken in the literal sense of organ growth and differentiation, including the embryonic, fetal, and infantile periods. This terminology includes all cases that are clearly congenital and those that are developmental, incorporating subluxation, dislocation, and dysplasia of the hip. Because this change in terminology has not yet been incorporated into the *International Classification of Diseases*, the term "CDH," which has existed in the literature for years, will continue to be used in many publications.

One of the most confusing areas in DDH is the terminology used in discussing the condition. What different investigators mean by "instability," "dysplasia," "subluxation," and "dislocation" varies considerably. In this chapter, the term "DDH" denotes developmental dysplasia of the hip and encompasses all the variations of the condition described. Within this spectrum are two entities: *dysplasia* and *dislocation*. In the newborn, the term *dysplasia* refers to any hip with a positive *Ortolani* sign. This sign is the sensation the examiner feels upon provoking the femoral head into subluxation (i.e., partial contact between the femoral head and acetabulum), dislocation (i.e., no contact between the femoral head and the acetabulum), or reduction from either of these positions. It is often difficult to make the distinction between these two entities, especially given the subtleties of arthrographic and ultrasonographic classifications. Because further subclassification in the newborn has no influence on treatment, the author prefers to use the term *dysplasia* to encompass these entities and other variations. The term *dislocation* refers here only to complete, irreducible dislocations.

# NORMAL GROWTH AND DEVELOPMENT OF THE HIP JOINT

For the hip joint to grow and develop in a normal way, there must be a genetically determined balance of growth of the acetabular and triradiate cartilages and a well-located and centered femoral head. Embryologically, the components of the hip joint, the acetabulum, and the femoral head develop from the same primitive mesenchymal cells (3–6) (Fig. 24.1). A cleft develops in the precartilaginous cells at about the 7th week of gestation. This cleft defines the acetabulum and the femoral head. By the 11th week of intrauterine life, the hip joint is fully formed (5–7). Theoretically, the 11th week is the earliest time at which a dislocation could develop, although this rarely happens (7). Acetabular development continues throughout intrauterine life, particularly by means of growth and development of the labrum (3,6). In the normal hip at birth, the femoral head is deeply seated in the acetabulum and held within

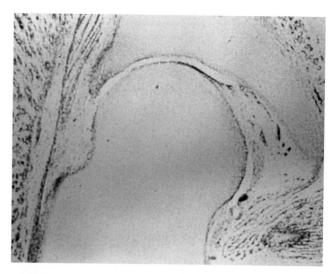

**Figure 24.1** Embryonic hip. The components of the hip joint, the acetabulum, and the femoral head develop from the same primitive mesenchymal cells. A cleft develops in the precartilaginous cells at about the 7th week of gestation, defining the acetabulum and the femoral head.

the confines of the acetabulum by the surface tension of the synovial fluid. It is extremely difficult to dislocate a normal infant's hip, even after incising the hip joint capsule (8,9). The retaining force is similar to that of a suction cup. Hips in newborns with DDH are not merely normal hips with capsular laxity; they are pathologic entities.

After birth, continued growth of the proximal femur and the acetabular cartilage complex is extremely important to the continuing development of the hip joint (3,7,10–12). The growth of these two members of the hip joint is interdependent.

## Acetabular Growth and Development

The *acetabular cartilage complex* (Fig. 24.2) is a three-dimensional structure that is triradiate medially and cup-shaped laterally. The acetabular cartilage complex is interposed between the ilium above, the ischium below, and the pubis anteriorly. Acetabular cartilage forms the outer two-thirds of the acetabular cavity, and the nonarticular medial wall of the acetabulum is formed by a portion of the ilium above, the ischium below, and portions of the triradiate cartilage.

Thick cartilage, from which a secondary ossification center, the *os acetabulum* (discussed later in this chapter), develops in early adolescence, separates the acetabular cavity from the pubic bone (11). The fibrocartilaginous labrum is at the margin of the acetabular cartilage, and the joint capsule inserts just above its rim (13) (Fig. 24.3).

The triradiate cartilage is a triphalangic structure. Each phalangis is composed of very cellular hyaline cartilage. This cartilage contains many canals. Each side of each limb of the triradiate cartilage has a growth plate. One phalangis

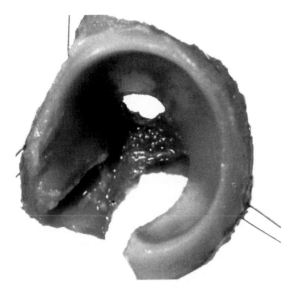

**Figure 24.2** Normal acetabular cartilage complex of a 1-day-old infant. The ilium, ischium, and pubis have been removed with a curet. The lateral view shows the cup-shaped acetabulum. (From Ponseti IV. Growth and development of the acetabulum in the normal child: anatomical, histological and roentgenographic studies. *J Bone Joint Surg Am* 1978;60:575.)

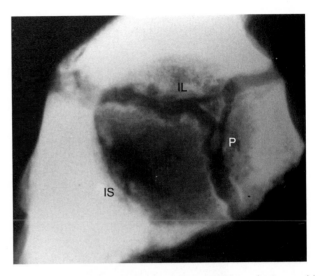

**Figure 24.4** Lateral radiograph of the acetabulum of a 9-year-old girl. Two centers of ossification are seen within the cartilage adjoining the pubis (*P*) and appear to be developing within the vertical phalange of the triradiate cartilage. The positions of the ischium (*IS*) and the ilium (*IL*) are indicated. (From Ponseti IV. Growth and development of the acetabulum in the normal child: anatomical, histological and roentgenographic studies. *J Bone Joint Surg Am* 1978;60:575.)

is oriented horizontally between the ilium and the ischium. One phalangis is oriented vertically and interposed between the pubis and the ischium. The third phalangis is located anteriorly and slanted superiorly between the ilium and the pubis (Fig. 24.4). The triradiate cartilage is the common physis of these three pelvic bones. Interstitial growth within the triradiate cartilage causes the hip joint to expand in diameter during growth (14).

The entire *acetabular cartilage complex* is composed of very cellular hyaline cartilage (Fig. 24.3). The lateral portion of the acetabular cartilage is homologous with other epiphyseal cartilages of the skeleton (15). This is important in understanding normal growth and development and the

shape of the acetabulum in skeletal dysplasias and injury. The labrum, or fibrocartilaginous edge of the acetabulum, is at the margin of the acetabular cartilage. The hip joint capsule inserts just above the labrum. The capsule insertion is continuous with the labrum below, and with the periosteum of the pelvic bones above.

Articular cartilage covers the acetabular cartilage on the side that articulates with the femoral head. On the opposite side is a growth plate, with its degenerating cells facing toward the pelvic bone that it opposes. New bone formation occurs in the metaphysis adjacent to the degenerating cartilage cells. Growth of the acetabular cartilage occurs by means of interstitial growth within the cartilage and appositional growth under the perichondrium. This fact is most important when considering various innominate bone osteotomies, because surgical injury (by aggressive periosteal stripping or osteotome placement) to this important area may jeopardize further acetabular growth.

## Growth of the Proximal Femur

In the infant the entire proximal end of the femur, including the greater trochanter, the intertrochanteric zone, and the proximal femur, is composed of cartilage. Between the 4th and 7th months of life, the proximal femoral ossification center appears. This bony centrum and its cartilaginous anlage continue to enlarge (although at a slowly decreasing rate) until adult life, at which stage only a thin layer of articular cartilage remains over it. The proximal femur and the trochanter enlarge by appositional cartilage cell proliferation (16).

The three main growth areas in the proximal femur are the physeal plate, the growth plate of the greater trochanter,

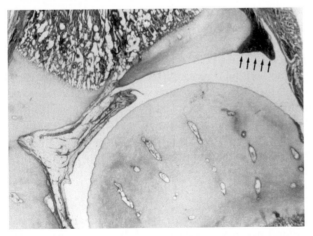

**Figure 24.3** Coronal section through the center of the acetabulum in a full-term infant. Note the fibrocartilaginous edge of the acetabulum, the labrum (*arrows*), at the peripheral edge of the acetabular cartilage. The hip capsule inserts just above the labrum.

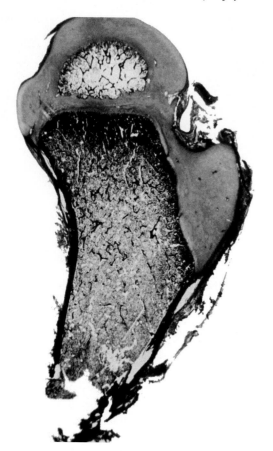

**Figure 24.5** The proximal femur in an infant has three physeal plates: the growth plate of the greater trochanter, the growth plate of the proximal femoral physeal plate, and the growth plate of the femoral neck isthmus connecting the other two plates.

and the femoral neck isthmus (16) (Fig. 24.5). A balance among the growth rates of these centers accounts for the normal configuration of the proximal femur, the relation between the proximal femur and the greater trochanter, and the overall width of the femoral neck. The growth of the proximal femur is affected by muscle pull, the forces transmitted across the hip joint by weightbearing, normal joint nutrition, circulation, and muscle tone (16–18). Any alterations in these factors may cause profound changes in the development of the proximal femur (19,20).

During infancy, a small cartilaginous isthmus connects the trochanteric and femoral growth plates along the lateral border of the femoral neck and is a reflection of their previous common origin. This growth cartilage contributes to the lateral width of the femoral neck and remains active until maturity.

It is the normal growth of these three physes that determines the femoral neck configuration in the adult. Disturbances in growth in any of these three growth plates, by whatever mechanism, alter the shape of the proximal femur. Hyperemia secondary to surgery or inflammatory conditions may stimulate growth in any or all of these growth plates (16).

The proximal femoral physeal plate contributes approximately 30% to the overall growth in length of the femur, and 13% to the growth of the limb. Any damage to or disruption of the blood supply to this plate disrupts the growth at this plate and results in a varus deformity because the trochanter and the growth plate along the femoral neck continue to grow (16,21). Partial physeal arrest patterns may be caused by damage to portions of the proximal femoral physeal plate. The relation between the growth of the trochanter and the physis of the proximal femur should remain constant; it is measured by the articular trochanteric distance, which is the distance between the tip of the greater trochanter and the superior articular surface of the femoral head. The greater trochanter is usually classified as a traction epiphysis, depending on normal abductor pull for growth stimulation. The trochanter, like the proximal femur, grows appositionally.

## Determinants of Shape and Depth of the Acetabulum

Experimental studies and clinical findings in humans with unreduced dislocations suggest that the main stimulus for the concave shape of the acetabulum is the presence of a spherical femoral head (10,15,22–24). Harrison determined that the acetabulum failed to develop in area and depth after femoral head excision in rats (15). He also demonstrated atrophy and degeneration of the acetabular cartilage, although the growth plates of the triradiate cartilage remained histologically normal, as did the length of the innominate bones. These experimental findings are characteristic of humans who have had untreated hip dislocations (Fig. 24.6).

For the normal depth of the acetabulum to increase during development, several factors must act in concert. There must be a reduced spherical femoral head. There must also be normal interstitial and appositional growth within the acetabular cartilage, and periosteal new bone formation must occur in the adjacent pelvic bones (10,11). The depth of the acetabulum is further enhanced at puberty by the development of three secondary centers of ossification (Fig. 24.7). These three centers are homologous with other epiphyses in the skeleton (11,15). The *os acetabulum* develops in the thick cartilage that separates the acetabular cavity from the pubis. The os acetabulum is the epiphysis of the pubis and forms the anterior wall of the acetabulum. The epiphysis of the ilium, the *acetabular epiphysis*, forms a major portion of the superior edge of the acetabulum. A third, small epiphysis also forms in the ischial region and contributes to its normal growth (11,15,25).

Normal acetabular growth and development occur through balanced growth of the proximal femur, the acetabular and triradiate cartilages, and the adjacent bones. This balance, which is probably genetically determined, may be faulty in DDH. There is ample evidence to suggest that an adverse intrauterine environment also plays an important role in the pathogenesis of hip dysplasia (11,26–30).

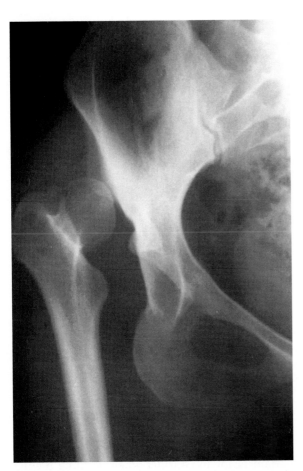

**Figure 24.6** Untreated dislocation of the hip. Note the lack of the concave shape and the shallowness of the acetabulum.

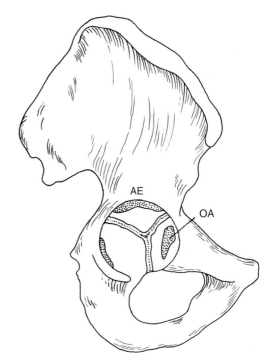

**Figure 24.7** Diagram of the right innominate bone of an adolescent. The os acetabulum (*OA*) is shown within the acetabular cartilage adjoining the pubic bone. The acetabular epiphysis (*AE*) is within the acetabular cartilage adjoining the iliac bone, and another small epiphysis is within the acetabular cartilage adjoining the ischium **(left)**. (Adapted from Ponseti IV. Growth and development of the acetabulum in the normal child: anatomical, histological and roentgenographic studies. *J Bone Joint Surg Am* 1978;60:575.)

## PATHOANATOMY

### Dislocations in Newborns

In the newborn with DDH, the tight fit between the femoral head and the acetabulum is lost. The femoral head can be made to glide in and out of the acetabulum, with a palpable sensation known clinically as the *Ortolani sign* (11,18,31,32). DDH in the newborn refers to a spectrum of anatomic abnormalities, from mild dysplastic changes to the severe pathoanatomic changes that are found in the rare idiopathic teratologic dislocation, and more commonly in teratologic dislocations associated with conditions such as myelomeningocele and arthrogryposis.

The most common pathologic change in the newborn with DDH is a hypertrophied ridge of acetabular cartilage in the superior, posterior, and inferior aspects of the acetabulum. This ridge was referred to by Ortolani as the *neolimbus* (18,32). The neolimbus is composed of hypertrophied acetabular cartilage (9,31) (Fig. 24.8). There often is a trough or groove in the acetabular cartilage caused by secondary pressure of the femoral head or neck. It is over this ridge of acetabular cartilage that the femoral head glides in and out of the acetabulum, with the palpable sensation referred to as the Ortolani sign (9,18,32).

There is empiric evidence that the pathologic changes are reversible in the typical newborn with DDH, because there is a 95% success rate of treatment using simple devices such as the Pavlik harness and the von Rosen splint (33). These pathologic changes are typical of 98% of DDH cases that occur at or around birth. However, approximately 2% of newborns have teratologic (antenatal) dislocations not associated with a syndrome or neuromuscular condition (25,28). In these rare cases, the pathologic and clinical findings are similar to those seen in late-diagnosed DDH, which is described later in this chapter.

### Acetabular Development in Developmental Hip Dysplasia

Acetabular development in treated DDH cases may be different from that described for the normal hip. This is particularly true for late-diagnosed cases. The primary stimulus for normal growth and development comes from the femoral head within the acetabulum (10,23,24). When there is a delay in diagnosis and treatment, some aspects of normal growth and development are lost. The femoral head must be reduced as soon as possible, and the reduction must be maintained to provide the stimulus for acetabular development. If concentric reduction is maintained, the acetabulum has the potential for recovery and resumption of normal growth and development for many years (34–36).

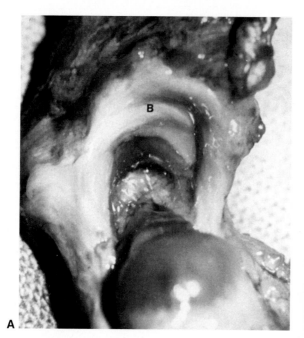
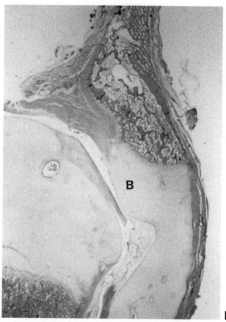

**Figure 24.8** **A:** Right acetabular cavity and femoral head of a newborn baby with bilateral congenital hip dysplasia. There is an acetabular bulge (*B*) or neolimbus along the upper acetabular cartilage, and the acetabular cavity is small. **B:** Frontal section of the same hip. The femoral head is very large in relation to the acetabular cavity. Note how the labrum is everted and adheres to the joint capsule above. The neolimbus (*B*) is composed of hypertrophied acetabular cartilage. (From Ishii Y, Weinstein SL, Ponseti IV. Correlation between arthrograms and operative findings in congenital dislocation of the hip. *Clin Orthop* 1980;153:138.)

The age at which a dysplastic hip can still return to "normal" after reduction remains controversial (33,35–43). The resumption and adequacy of acetabular development is a multifactorial problem that depends on the age at which the reduction is obtained and on whether the growth potential of the acetabular cartilage and the proximal femur is normal. The capacity of the acetabular cartilage to resume normal growth depends on its intrinsic growth potential, and whether it has been damaged by the subluxated or dislocated femoral head or by various attempts at reduction. In the patient with DDH who has been treated, especially in late-diagnosed cases, *accessory centers of ossification* contribute to acetabular development (Fig. 24.9). *Accessory centers of ossification* in the acetabulum are seen in only 2% to 3% of normal hips, and they rarely appear before 11 years of age. However, among patients treated for DDH, the centers may be present in as many as 60% of hips, usually appearing 6 months to 10 years after reduction (34–37,44) (Fig. 24.9). These *accessory centers* form in the peripheral acetabular cartilage, and may be a primary abnormality of dysplasia or, more likely, they are a secondary abnormality caused by pressure damage from the femoral head and/or neck in the subluxated or dislocated position or by damage secondary to closed or open treatment (see later discussion on obstacles to reduction). In treated DDH cases, these accessory centers of ossification should be sought on every sequential radiograph so as to determine whether acetabular development is progressing, as they may coalesce to form a normal acetabulum (Fig. 24.9). This is an

important factor to consider when deciding if surgical intervention is necessary to correct residual acetabular dysplasia. Although the presence of these centers indicates continued growth in the acetabular cartilage, they may be indicative of injury to the cartilage in this area. Their presence does not assure normal acetabular development.

## PATHOGENESIS, EPIDEMIOLOGY, AND DIAGNOSIS

### Causes of Developmental Dysplasia of the Hip

Many factors contribute to DDH. Genetic and ethnic factors play a key role, with the incidence of DDH as high as 25 to 50 in 1000 live births among Lapps and Native Americans and a very low rate among the southern Chinese population and persons of African descent (29,45–59).

A positive family history for DDH may be found in 12% to 33% of patients who have DDH (30,45,59). One study reported a tenfold increase in the incidence of DDH among the parents of index patients and a sevenfold increase among siblings compared with the incidence among the general population (45). There is some suggestion that anteversion of the femoral neck or acetabulum may be an etiologic factor (29,31,37,60–62).

The genetic effects on the hip joint in patients with DDH are revealed as primary acetabular dysplasia, various

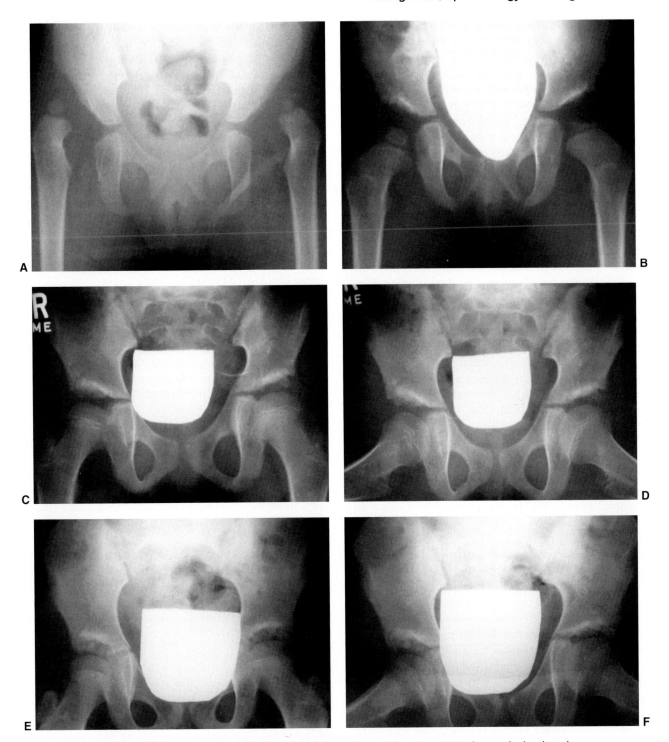

**Figure 24.9** **A:** An 18-month-old girl with bilateral high dislocations. Note the poorly developed acetabula with well-developed secondary acetabula. **B:** At 33 months of age, the irregular ossification centers in the left and right hip have coalesced, with a slight improvement in the acetabular index. **C:** When the girl is 7 years of age, an anteroposterior view shows the appearance of the accessory centers of ossification in the periphery of the acetabulum. **D:** The accessory centers of ossification are somewhat better appreciated in the abduction view at 7 years of age. **E:** An anteroposterior view at 8 years of age shows the coalescence of the accessory centers of ossification, increasing the depth of the acetabulum. Note the excellent sourcil formation. **F:** The accessory centers of ossification are well demonstrated in an abduction view at 8 years of age.

degrees of joint laxity, or a combination of both. Intrauterine mechanical factors, such as breech position or oligohydramnios, and neuromuscular mechanisms such as myelomeningocele, can profoundly influence genetically determined intrauterine growth (5,6,63,64). The first-born child is more likely to be affected than subsequent children. Any of the factors contributing to an "adverse" intrauterine environment may influence the development of the hip joint, and postnatal influences may also contribute to the development of DDH (5,30,65–67).

## Risk Factors and Incidence

Whites show an increased incidence of DDH among first-born children (8,26,27,68–71). The unstretched abdominal muscles and the primigravida uterus may subject the fetus to prolonged periods of abnormal positioning, forcing the fetus against the mother's spine. This restraint limits fetal mobility, especially hip abduction. The high rate of association of DDH with other intrauterine molding abnormalities, such as torticollis and metatarsus adductus, lends some support to the theory that the "crowding phenomenon" plays a role in the pathogenesis (8,71–73). Oligohydramnios, which is associated with limited fetal mobility, also is associated with DDH (8,71). The left hip is the most commonly affected hip; in the most common fetal position, this is the hip that is usually forced into adduction against the mother's sacrum (8,47,71).

DDH is more common among girls (80% of cases) and among children delivered in the breech presentation. In the general population, breech presentations occur in approximately 2% to 4% of vaginal deliveries. Carter and Wilkinson (26,27) reported that 17% of children with DDH had a breech presentation; Salter reported the incidence as 23% (74). Twice as many girls as boys are born breech (75). Fifty-nine percent of breech presentations are first-born children (26,27,75). Ramsey and MacEwen demonstrated that 1 of 15 girls born breech has evidence of hip instability. In animal studies, the prolonged maintenance of an abnormal position, such as the breech position, is associated with the production of DDH (23,24).

The postnatal environment may significantly influence the development of DDH. In societies that use swaddling (i.e., hips forced into adduction and extension) in the immediate postnatal period, the incidence of DDH is high, possibly as a result of the forceful positioning of the legs in extension and adduction, counter to normal newborn hip flexion and hamstring contractures (30,47,57,62,67,76–79).

The influence of hip capsular laxity on the development of DDH has been addressed by many investigators. Newborns with DDH may have capsular laxity. Hip capsular laxity has been implicated in the pathogenesis of DDH, because the diagnostic test for DDH, the Ortolani sign, depends on the head gliding in and out of the dysplastic acetabulum over a ridge of abnormal acetabular cartilage.

Proponents argue that because reversible dysplasia can be produced in animals by producing ligamentous laxity, the acetabular dysplasia seen in DDH is a secondary phenomenon (23,24,30,31,74,80). LeDamany demonstrated that the acetabulum is shallowest at birth (61). Ralis and McKibbin confirmed LeDamany's anatomic work in a small number of patients (80). They too demonstrated that the acetabulum was shallowest at birth and that this, combined with the normal laxity in the joint of the infant, makes the time around delivery a high-risk period for dislocation (80,81). These anatomic experiments were repeated by Skirving and Scadden in African neonates (29); in the African neonate, the acetabulum was deeper more frequently and in a narrower range, possibly explaining why DDH is almost nonexistent among persons of African descent. This finding also provides indirect evidence that acetabular dysplasia is a primary cause of DDH.

Laxity of the hip joint capsule is often seen in newborn infants and has been documented by ultrasonography (82). The laxity may allow some instability without a positive Ortolani sign. In postmortem examination of seven stillborn infants, the hips demonstrated instability with a negative Ortolani sign; arthrograms demonstrated slight pooling of the contrast media medially. On gross examination, the hip capsules were stretched, and the femoral heads could be pulled slightly away from the acetabula. However, the hips were anatomically and histologically normal, unlike the postmortem findings reported for all infants with positive Ortolani signs (9,11,32,55,83,84). In addition to the normal physiologic capsular laxity expected in the newborn, DDH is not a feature of conditions characterized by hyperlaxity, such as Down, Ehlers-Danlos, and Marfan syndromes (32).

Taking into account the epidemiologic and etiologic factors, a high-risk group of patients can be identified. This group includes any patient who has more than one of the factors listed in Table 24.1. If an infant manifests any combination of these factors, the physician should be alert to the possibility of DDH.

---

**TABLE 24.1**

**HIGH-RISK FACTORS FOR DEVELOPMENTAL DYSPLASIA OR DISLOCATION OF THE HIP**

Breech position
Female gender
Positive family history or ethnic background (e.g., Native American, Laplander)
Lower limb deformity
Torticollis
Metatarsus adductus
Oligohydramnios
Significant persistent hip asymmetry (e.g., abducted hip on one side, adducted hip on the other side)
Other significant musculoskeletal abnormalities

---

The incidence of DDH is influenced by geographic and ethnic factors and by the diagnostic criteria used by the examining physician. Another important factor is the diagnostic acumen of the examiner. The age of the patient at the time of diagnosis must be taken into account, because the physical findings and manifestations of the condition change with increasing delay in diagnosis (8,9,11,30,32,55, 71,82–88).

Most patients with DDH are detectable at birth (89,90). Despite screening programs for newborns, some cases are not detected, and some evidence suggests that a few cases may arise after birth (29,85,90–99). Moreover, whether acetabular dysplasia is primary or secondary to an unrecognized dislocation or subluxation that has reduced spontaneously remains uncertain.

## Diagnosis

The clinical diagnostic test for DDH was originally described by LeDamany in 1912 (61). LeDamany referred to the palpable sensation of the hip gliding in and out of the acetabulum as the *signe de ressaut*. In 1936, Ortolani, an Italian pediatrician, described the pathogenesis of this diagnostic sign (32,84). Ortolani called the palpable sensation the *segno dello scotto*. Fellander et al. likened this diagnostic sign to the femoral head gliding in and out of the acetabulum over a ridge and referred to this palpable sensation as the *ridge phenomenon* (100). This ridge, over which the femoral head glides in and out of the acetabulum, is composed of hypertrophied acetabular cartilage (9,31,32,84) (Fig. 24.8). Ortolani named the ridge the *neolimbus*.

Unfortunately, inadequate translation of LeDamany's and Ortolani's works into English resulted in the use of the term *click* to describe this diagnostic sign. High-pitched soft tissue clicks are often elicited in the hip examination of newborns. These clicks are usually transmitted from the trochanteric region or the knee and have no diagnostic significance (100). This poor understanding of the pathoanatomy of the primary diagnostic sign of DDH in the newborn has no doubt led to overdiagnosis and overtreatment of infants (101–104).

Another diagnostic test, the Barlow maneuver, is often referred to as the "click of exit." The Barlow maneuver is a provocative maneuver in which the hip is flexed and adducted and the femoral head is palpated to exit the acetabulum partially or completely over a ridge of the acetabulum (85). Many physicians refer to the Ortolani sign as the *click of entry*, which is caused when the hip is abducted, the trochanter is elevated, and the femoral head glides back into the acetabulum. Some physicians make treatment decisions on the basis of whether they feel that the hip is Ortolani-positive rather than Barlow-positive, the general opinion being that the Barlow-positive hip is more stable and hence may stabilize spontaneously. Because Ortolani and LeDamany described the palpable sensation as the femoral head exits or enters the acetabulum, the author prefers to use the Ortolani sign to refer to both the palpable sensation of subluxating or dislocating the hip and to reducing a subluxated or dislocated hip. The author also makes no distinction in treatment between patients exhibiting the Ortolani sign and those with the Barlow sign.

Newborn clinical screening programs estimate that 1 of every 100 newborns examined has evidence of some hip instability (i.e., positive Ortolani or Barlow sign), although the incidence of true dislocation is reported to be between 1 and 1.5 cases per 1000 live births (9,43,85,93–96, 101,105–110).

Complete irreducible dislocations are extremely rare in newborns and are usually associated with other generalized conditions, such as arthrogryposis, myelodysplasia, and other syndromes. These perinatal teratologic dislocations are at the extreme end of the DDH pathologic spectrum and account for only 2% of cases in newborn examination series (9,47,48,111,112). They are usually manifested because of the secondary adaptive changes more characteristic of the late-diagnosed case.

### Late Diagnosis

If the diagnosis of DDH is not made early, preferably in the newborn nursery, secondary adaptive changes develop (46). The most reliable physical finding in late-diagnosed DDH is limitation of abduction (Fig. 24.10). Limited abduction is a clinical manifestation of the various degrees of shortening of the adductor longus that are associated with hip subluxation or dislocation (48). Other manifestations of late-diagnosed DDH may include apparent femoral shortening, also called *the Galeazzi sign* (Fig. 24.11); asymmetry of the gluteal (113), thigh, or labial folds (114); and limb-length inequality (Fig. 24.12). In patients with bilateral dislocations, clinical findings include a waddling gait and hyperlordosis of the lumbar spine (Fig. 24.13).

If DDH goes undetected, normal hip joint growth and development are impaired. With increasing age at detection and reduction, and particularly in children older than 6 months, the obstacles (intraarticular and extraarticular)

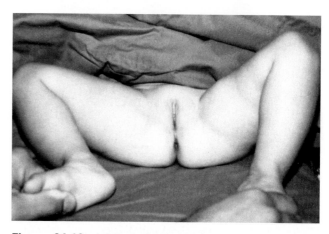

**Figure 24.10** A 15-month-old child with left hip dislocation. Note the limited abduction of the hip.

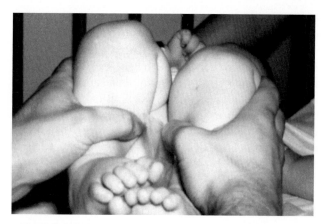

**Figure 24.11** A 15-month-old girl with developmental disloca-tion of the left hip. Note the apparent femoral shortening.

to concentric reduction become increasingly difficult to overcome by simple treatment methods such as use of the Pavlik harness, and closed or open reduction usually must be performed under general anesthesia. Restoration of nor-mal acetabular development is less likely as age at detec-tion increases (25,31,43,109,113–117).

In the late-diagnosed case, the extraarticular obstacles to reduction include the contracted adductor longus and the iliopsoas. These muscles are shortened because of the hip

being in the subluxated or dislocated position, allowing secondary muscle-shortening.

The intraarticular obstacles to reduction in late-diagnosed DDH include the ligamentum teres, the transverse acetabu-lar ligament, the constricted anteromedial joint capsule, and, rarely, an inverted and hypertrophied labrum (31,118). The most significant intraarticular obstacle to reduction, however, is some degree of anteromedial hip capsular constriction (31,119–123). The ligamentum teres may be thickened, and it may become the primary obstacle to reduction in some cases. In children of walking or crawling age, the ligamentum teres may be significantly elongated and enlarged. Its sheer bulk precludes concentric reduction without excision of the ligament. The transverse acetabular ligamentum may hypertrophy secondary to the constant pull of the ligamentum teres on its attachment at the base of the acetabulum (31,123). This effect decreases the diam-eter of the acetabulum.

A rare finding, other than in teratologic dislocations, is a true inverted labrum or *limbus* (i.e., hypertrophied labrum) (120) (Fig. 24.14). The acetabular labrum may be iatrogenically inverted, and may be an obstacle to reduc-tion in patients previously treated with unsuccessful closed reductions. Arthrograms are often misinterpreted as showing an inverted labrum (124); the shadow thought to be the inverted labrum or limbus is instead the neolim-bus (originally described by Ortolani) (9,31,125,126) (Fig. 24.15). This neolimbus is epiphyseal cartilage and is almost never an obstacle to reduction. It must not be removed, because removal impairs acetabular develop-ment (9,127). If the surgeon feels that this tissue is some-how impairing reduction, it should be radially incised but never excised. The cartilage of the neolimbus may be pri-marily abnormal or may be damaged by a traumatic open or closed reduction. A response to this damage may be responsible for the appearance of the previously discussed *accessory centers of ossification* seen in treated cases of DDH (9) (Fig. 24.9).

### Diagnostic Imaging and Radiography

Although the clinical examination remains the gold stan-dard (128), ultrasonography has gained popularity world-wide as a screening tool. Its cost-effectiveness has yet to be documented for screening for DDH on a wide scale.

The use of ultrasonography in the diagnosis and man-agement of children with DDH remains controversial (129–139). Many proponents strongly recommend that ultrasonography be used as a routine screening tool in the newborn nursery and that it be used extensively in the management of all DDH problems (140–142). The use of ultrasonography in orthopaedic practice was pioneered by Graf in Austria in the 1970s (143,144). Harcke et al. in the United States (145–148), Terjesen et al. in Norway (149–152), and Clarke in Great Britain (153–155) have been the prime evaluators of this tool for the diagnosis of DDH and other hip disorders.

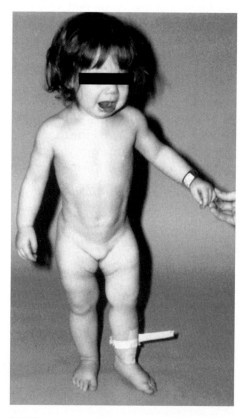

**Figure 24.12** A 1-year-old girl with developmental dislocation of the left hip was referred for toe walking. Note the apparent limb-length inequality and the asymmetry of the thigh and labial folds.

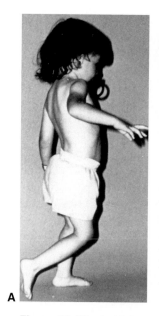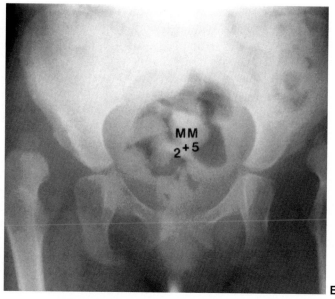

**Figure 24.13**  A girl, 2 years and 5 months of age, with bilateral hip dislocations. **A:** Note the waddling gait and hyperlordosis. **B:** Radiograph shows high bilateral dislocations and poorly developed acetabula with well-developed secondary acetabula where the femoral heads articulate with the ilia.

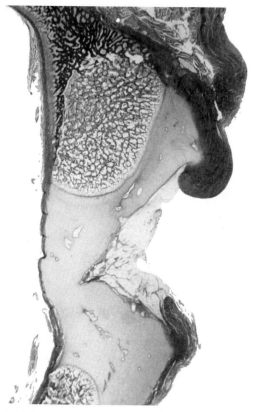

**Figure 24.14**  A coronal section of the acetabulum demonstrates the interned hypertrophic labrum (limbus) extending over the margin of a slightly thickened acetabular cartilage. The thick capsule extends upward above the inverted labrum, from which it is separated by a shallow groove. In this section through the ilium, the growth plate is slanted upward laterally, but endochondral ossification is normal. At the margin of the roof, periosteal bone growth is retarded. (From Ponseti IV. Morphology of the acetabulum in congenital dislocation of the hip: gross, histological and roentgenographic studies. *J Bone Joint Surg Am* 1978;60:586.)

Ultrasonography can be used in two basic ways to evaluate the child with DDH: morphologic assessment and dynamic assessment (156–161). The morphologic assessment, as pioneered by Graf, focuses primarily on critical evaluation of the anatomic characteristics of the hip joint (Fig. 24.16). This is accomplished by measuring two angles on the ultrasound image: the $\alpha$ angle, which is a measurement of the slope of the superior aspect of the bony acetabulum, and the $\beta$ angle, which evaluates the cartilaginous component of the acetabulum. The hip is classified into four types and several subtypes according to various factors (143,144) (Fig. 24.17). In the evaluation of Terjesen et al., the percentage of acetabular coverage of the femoral head (i.e., percent coverage) is a key measurement (149–152).

The morphologic approach to ultrasonography is widely practiced in Europe, but it has been criticized because of substantial interobserver and intraobserver variations in the measurement of angles, particularly the $\beta$ angle (146).

The availability of equipment with which motion can be observed in real time and in multiple planes provides a means of seeing what occurs during the Ortolani or Barlow maneuver. The use of dynamic ultrasonography, as popularized by Harcke et al. (145–147), has been criticized for being excessively operator-dependent and requiring a subjective assessment of the findings.

The indications for ultrasonography in the diagnosis and treatment of DDH are not universally established. Because there are many controversies yet to be resolved, ultrasonography cannot be advocated as a routine screening tool, even though (146) it is used as such in Europe. Prospective longitudinal studies documenting the outcomes of minor anatomic abnormalities found in ultrasonographic

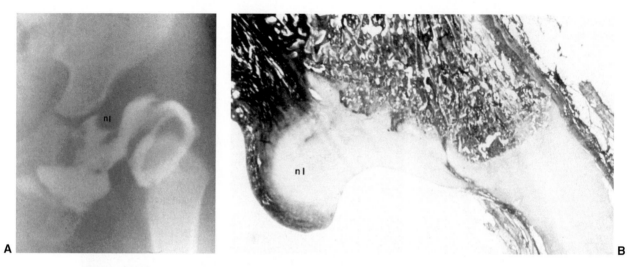

**Figure 24.15** **A:** Arthrogram of the left hip in a 15-month-old child with complete dislocation. Note the shadow of the neolimbus (*nl*). **B:** A histologic specimen demonstrates hypertrophied acetabular cartilage of the neolimbus (*nl*), consistent with the arthrographic appearance in **(A)**.

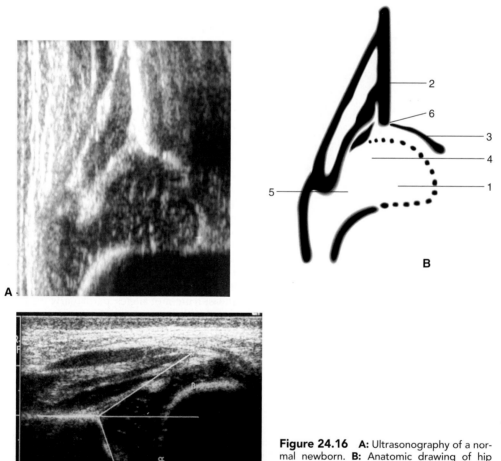

**Figure 24.16** **A:** Ultrasonography of a normal newborn. **B:** Anatomic drawing of hip landmarks (after Graf): *1*, femoral head; *2*, iliac limb; *3*, bony acetabular roof; *4*, acetabular labrum; *5*, joint capsule; *6*, osseous rim. **C:** The $\alpha$ and $\beta$ angles are identified on this ultrasonograph of a newborn.

| Type according to Graf | Bony roof/ bony roof angle $\alpha$ | Superior bony rim (bony promontory) | Cartilaginous roof / cartilage roof angle $\beta$ | Age | |
|---|---|---|---|---|---|
| TYPE I<br>mature hip | Good<br>$\alpha \geq 60$ | Angular / slightly rounded ("blunt") | Covers the femoral head<br>I a ⇨ $\beta$ <55 (extending far distance over the femoral head)<br>I b ⇨ $\beta$ >55 (extending short distance over the femoral head) | Any age | 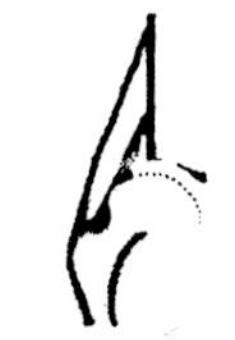 |
| TYPE II a (+)<br>physiological immature ⇨ appropriate for age | Adequate (satisfactory)<br>$\alpha = 50 - 59$<br>(minimal degree of maturity is attained-look at the "sonometer") | Rounded | Covers the femoral head | 0 to 12 weeks | 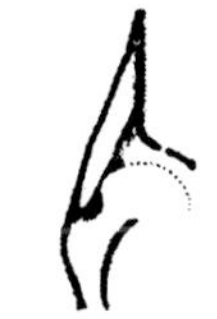 |
| TYPE II a (–)<br>physiological immature ⇨ maturational deficient | Deficient<br>$\alpha = 50 - 59$<br>(minimal degree of maturity is not attained-look at the "sonometer") | Rounded | Covers the femoral head | >6 to 12 weeks | |
| TYPE II b<br>delay of ossification | Deficient<br>$\alpha = 50 - 59$ | Rounded | Covers the femoral head | >12 weeks | |
| EXCEPTION: Type II<br>coming to maturity | Deficient | Angular (!) | Covers the femoral head, (echogenic because of ossification!) | Any age | |
| TYPE II c (critical range)<br>II c stable/II c unstable | Severely deficient<br>$\alpha = 43 - 49$ | Rounded to flattened | Still covers the femoral head<br>$\beta$ <77 | Any age | 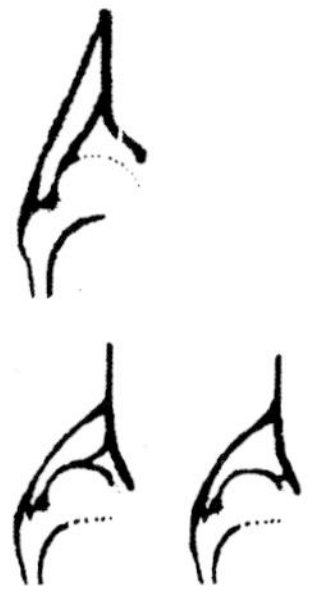 |
| TYPE D<br>decentering hip ⇨ $\beta$ >77 | Severely deficient<br>$\alpha = 43 - 49$ | Rounded to flattened | Displaced<br>$\beta$ >77 | | |
| TYPE III a<br>eccenteric hip ⇨ $\alpha$ >43 | Poor<br>$\alpha$ <43 | Flattened | Pressed upwards - without structural alteration<br>(devoid of echoes) proximal perichondrium goes up to the contour of the iliac wall | Any age | |
| TYPE III b<br>eccenteric hip ⇨ $\alpha$ <43 | Poor<br>$\alpha$ <43 | Flattened | Pressed upwards - with structural alteration<br>(they are echogenic) proximal perichondrium goes up to the contour of the iliac wall | | |
| TYPE IV<br>eccenteric hip ⇨ $\alpha$ <43 | Poor<br>$\alpha$ <43 | Flattened | Pressed downwards<br>horizontal or mulded proximal perichondrium | | |

**Figure 24.17**    Hip types based on ultrasonographic results. (Courtesy of Prof. R. Graf, Stolzalpe, Austria.)

examinations need to be completed (162,163). Its routine use in newborn nurseries has resulted in overdiagnosis (above the expected incidence) of DDH and cannot be considered cost-effective (164–167). Its use in only high-risk infants may eventually prove cost-effective (167,168). However, Clarke et al. showed that screening all high-risk infants and all infants who had any abnormality on physical examination did not reduce the prevalence of late-diagnosed cases (154,155,169).

Some centers advocate the use of ultrasonography in all Ortolani-positive infants to assess stability at the completion of treatment (146). An ideal use for ultrasonography is for "guided reduction" of a dislocated hip in an infant (170), in other words, for monitoring the progress of reduction of a subluxated or dislocated hip being treated in a Pavlik harness. Ultrasonography is used at 7- to 10-day intervals to check the progress of reduction of the hip and its stability during Pavlik harness treatment. This may temporarily obviate the need for radiographic evaluation. Other uses for ultrasonography in the treatment of DDH include monitoring of the hip position while the patient is in traction before attempting reduction and evaluating closed reductions in the operating room. The distinct advantage of ultrasonography is that it provides some anatomic evaluation of the hip joint without exposing the infant to radiation.

Debate continues regarding the appropriate planes for evaluation and whether an orthopaedic surgeon, the treating physician, or a radiologist with expertise in ultrasonography should perform the evaluation. In the newborn, DDH is not a radiographic diagnosis; the diagnosis should be made by clinical evaluation, which may be enhanced by ultrasonography if the examination results are questionable. Some investigators have used vibration arthrometry (171–173).

After the newborn period (4 to 6 weeks of age), the diagnosis of DDH should be confirmed by radiography. Many radiographic measurements can be made, but there are wide interobserver and intraobserver variations in these measurements (174,175). Because it is difficult to standardize the radiographic positioning of infants, many centers use positioning frames (176).

When monitoring the treatment of children with DDH, it is essential to notice changes in the radiographic measurements over time, and not to make significant decisions based on a single radiograph. The classic radiographic features of late-diagnosed DDH include: an increased acetabular index (28,177–182); disruption of the Shenton line; a widened pelvic floor (183); an absent teardrop figure (184–190); delayed appearance of the femoral ossific nucleus on the involved side or dissimilar sizes of the ossific nuclei; abnormality in Smith centering ratios (23,24,36); decreased femoral head coverage; and failure of the medial metaphyseal beak of the proximal femur, and, subsequently, the secondary ossification center, to be located in the lower inner quadrant defined by the Hilgenreiner and Perkins lines (87,191,192) (Fig. 24.18A). When the triradiate cartilage is closed, the acetabular angle of Sharp (i.e., from the inferior edge of the teardrop figure to the edge of the acetabulum) is a useful measurement of acetabular dysplasia (193).

In children younger than 8 years, the acetabular index is a reasonable measure of acetabular development (174). Measurement of the center-edge (CE) angle becomes useful only in the patient who is more than 5 years of age, and is most useful in the adult patient (44) (Fig. 24.18B). Radiographs show only the ossified portion of the pelvic bones and the proximal femur. Excellent acetabular coverage of the femoral head may be found, albeit by unossified cartilage (Fig. 24.19). If this cartilage does not ossify, the residual dysplasia may eventually lead to subluxation and degenerative joint disease.

The Shenton line provides only a qualitative estimate of dysplasia during the first few years of life. After 3 or 4 years of age, the Shenton line should be intact on all views of the hip; thereafter, any disruption of the Shenton line indicates an abnormality in the relation between the proximal femur and the acetabulum. As will be emphasized in the section on methods of treatment, this relation must be restored in order to prevent degenerative joint disease in later life (25,44,57,62,116).

Magnetic resonance imaging (MRI) has been used for DDH diagnosis and evaluation, as well as for documentation of femoral head–acetabular relationships after closed or open reduction (194,195). With advances in software, this modality will no doubt provide useful information in the future, but the need for anesthesia in infants and children limits its utility (196–199).

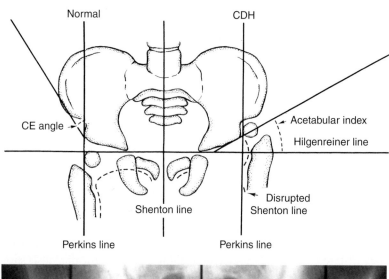

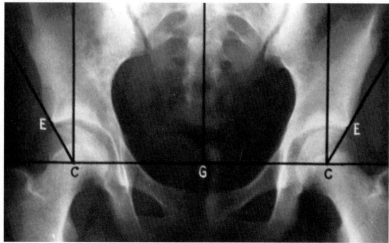

**Figure 24.18** **A:** Radiographic parameters. *CDH*, congenital dysplasia of the hip; *CE Angle*, center-edge angle. **B:** Center-edge angle of Wiberg. *C*, Center of the femoral head; *E*, bony edge of the acetabulum; *G*, gravity line.

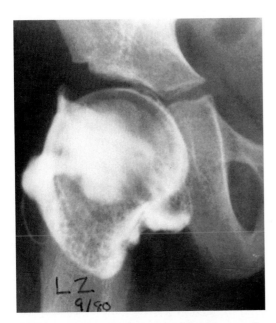

**Figure 24.19** Arthrogram of a 5-year-old girl 3 years after open reduction. Note the excellent coverage of the femoral head by unossified acetabular cartilage.

# NATURAL HISTORY

## Course in Newborns

The natural history of untreated DDH in the newborn is quite variable. Yamamuro and Doi followed up 52 patients whose hips had positive Ortolani signs for a 2-year period without treatment for the first 5 months. Of the 12 they called "dislocated" hips, 3 (25%) were radiographically normal at 5 months of age. Of the 42 which they called "subluxable" hips, 24 (57%) were normal at 5 months (79).

Barlow reported that 1 of every 60 infants born has instability (i.e., positive Barlow sign) of one or both hips (85). More than 60% of these stabilize during the first week of life, and 88% stabilize during the first 2 months, without treatment. The remaining 12% become true congenital dislocations and persist in the absence of treatment. Pratt et al. did a follow-up, for an average of 11.2 years, of 18 "dysplastic" hips in patients who had been diagnosed on the basis of clinical and radiographic parameters at an age younger than 3 months., They found that 15 of these hips were radiographically normal (78).

Coleman followed up 23 untreated patients who had been diagnosed as having DDH on the basis of clinical and radiographic criteria at younger than 3 months. He found that 26% of the femoral heads became completely dislocated, 13% had partial contact of the femoral head with the acetabulum, 39% remained located but retained dysplastic features, and 22% were normal (47).

Most unstable hips in newborns stabilize soon after birth, some may go on to subluxation (partial contact of femoral head with the acetabulum) or dislocation, and some may remain located (intact Shenton line) but retain anatomic dysplastic features. Because it is not possible to predict the outcome of unstable hips in newborns, all newborns with clinical hip instability, as manifested by a positive Ortolani or Barlow sign, should be treated.

## Course in Adults

In adults, the natural history of untreated complete dislocation varies, and is affected by societal considerations (56,65,194–197). Despite complete dislocation, there may be little or no functional disability.

The natural history of complete dislocation depends on the presence or absence of two factors: a well-developed false acetabulum and bilaterality (26,57,66,115,200,201). Wedge and Wasylenko demonstrated only a 24% chance of a good clinical outcome with a well-developed false acetabulum, but with a moderately developed or absent false acetabulum, the patients had a 52% chance of a good clinical outcome (57,66). Of 42 patients with complete dislocations, 13 had radiographically confirmed degenerative joint disease, such as loss of joint space, cyst formation, sclerosis, osteophyte formation, and flattening of the femoral head. Of these 13 patients, 10 (76%) had poor clinical outcomes.

Milgram reported the gross and histologic features of a case of bilateral DDH discovered at postmortem examination (202). This 74-year-old man had no hip or thigh pain and only mild backache for 5 years before his death. The femoral head had no articulation with any portion of the ilium, and was covered with a thickened, markedly elongated hip joint capsule. The only degenerative changes were where the lesser trochanter abutted the overhanging superior acetabular rim. In the absence of a false acetabulum, most patients with complete dislocations do well, maintaining good range of motion with little functional disability (Fig. 24.20). Completely dislocated hips with

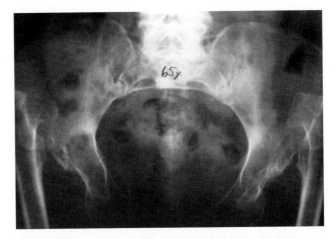

**Figure 24.20** A 65-year-old woman with bilateral, untreated developmental dislocations of the hips complained of some low back pain, but had no hip pain. She had a waddling gait and hyperlordosis.

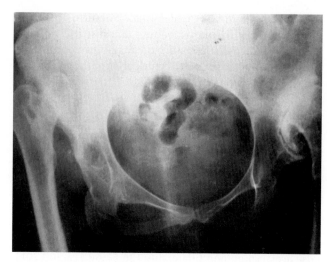

**Figure 24.21** Radiograph of a 43-year-old woman with complete dislocation of both hips. She is asymptomatic on the right side but has disabling symptoms from the left hip. She has no false acetabulum on the right, but has a well-developed false acetabulum on the left with secondary degenerative changes. [From Weinstein SL. Natural history of congenital hip dislocation (CDH) and hip dysplasia. *Clin Orthop* 1987;225:62, with permission.]

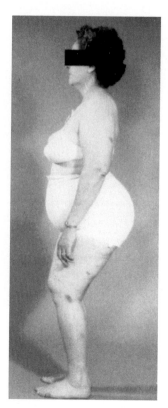

**Figure 24.22** A 45-year-old woman with bilateral complete dislocations, hip flexion deformity, and marked hyperlordosis. The patient's only reported symptoms concerned her back.

well-developed false acetabula are more likely to develop radiographically visible degenerative joint disease changes and poor clinical outcomes (Fig. 24.21). Factors that lead to the formation or lack of formation of a false acetabulum remain unknown (25).

Back pain may occur in patients with bilateral dislocations. It is thought that this pain is secondary to the hyperlordosis of the lumbar spine that is associated with bilateral dislocations (25,57,66,202–204) (P. Melvin, R. Johnston, I.V. Ponseti, *personal communication*) (Fig. 24.22).

In unilateral complete dislocations, secondary problems of limb-length inequality, ipsilateral knee deformity and pain, scoliosis, and gait disturbance are common. Limb-length inequalities of as much as 10 cm have been reported in patients with unilateral dislocations. These patients develop flexion–adduction deformities of the hip, which may lead to valgus deformities of the knee. The valgus knee deformity is often associated with attenuation of the medial collateral ligament and degenerative joint disease of the lateral compartment, although some medial compartment disease has also been described (25,57,66,116,201), (P. Melvin, R. Johnston, I.V. Ponseti, *personal communication*). The same factors that are involved in the development of secondary degenerative disease in the false acetabulum and in the associated clinical disability in bilateral cases affect unilateral dislocations also.

## Course of Dysplasia and Subluxation

The natural history of dysplasia and subluxation in untreated patients is important because of the likelihood that these findings can be extrapolated to residual dysplasia and subluxation after treatment (116,200,205–210).

After the neonatal period, the term *dysplasia* has an anatomic definition as well as a radiographic definition. *Anatomic dysplasia* refers to inadequate development of the acetabulum, the femoral head, or both (48). All subluxated hips (i.e., those in which there is some contact between the femoral head and the acetabulum) are by definition anatomically dysplastic. On film, the major difference between *radiographic dysplasia* and *radiographic subluxation* is determined by the integrity of the Shenton line. In *radiographic subluxation*, the Shenton line is disrupted and the femoral head is superiorly, laterally, or superolaterally displaced from the medial wall of the acetabulum. In *radiographic dysplasia*, the normal Shenton line relation is intact (57,66,211,212) (Fig. 24.23). In the literature describing the natural history of DDH, these two radiographic and clinical entities are often not separated. Moreover, secondary degenerative changes may convert a *radiographically dysplastic* hip into a *radiographically subluxated* hip (202,204,208,209, 212–214) (Figs. 24.24 and 24.25).

Anatomic abnormalities are seen roentgenographically in subluxation and dysplasia, but the natural histories of these two radiographic entities are different. Residual radiographic subluxation after treatment of DDH invariably leads to degenerative joint disease and clinical disability (25,65,67,116,202,207,209,212). The rate of deterioration is directly related to the severity of the subluxation and the age of the patient (209,212).

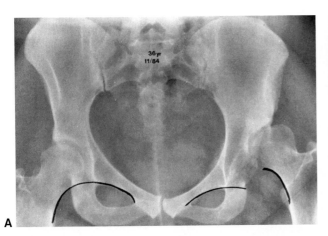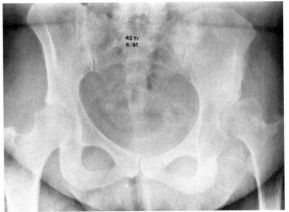

**Figure 24.23** Radiographic subluxation and dysplasia. **A:** A 36-year-old woman with bilateral anatomically abnormal (dysplastic) hips. The left hip is radiographically subluxated, with the Shenton line disrupted, and the right hip is radiographically dysplastic, with the Shenton line intact. **B:** Seven years later, note the marked loss of joint space in the secondary acetabulum of the left hip and very early disruption of the Shenton line on the right. The right hip is asymptomatic, and the left hip is about to undergo total hip arthroplasty.

There is considerable evidence that residual radiographic acetabular dysplasia leads to secondary degenerative joint disease, especially in women, although there are no predictive radiographic parameters (202,208,209,212,214,215). The reasons for degenerative changes in radiographically dysplastic hips are probably mechanical in nature and related to increased contact stress over time. A certain threshold of "overpressure" (product of time and pressure, involving years of exposure to pressure above a 2-megapascal (MPa) level, leading to damage) (216,217) may correlate with poor long-term outcome. Aspherical femoral heads (e.g., secondary to aseptic necrosis) tend to experience even more severe degrees of overpressure. It appears that radiographic degenerative joint disease correlates with the magnitude of the overpressure and the time of exposure (216). This overpressure may cause problems at a much younger age, with symptoms of "acetabular rim syndrome" (see Page 1021) (218).

Physical signs of radiographic hip dysplasia may not be visible. Cases of radiographic hip dysplasia are either diagnosed only incidentally on the basis of radiographs taken for other reasons, or after the patient develops symptoms (26,27,44,75,214). Stulberg and Harris found that 50% of their patients with radiographic dysplasia and degenerative joint disease had radiographic evidence of dysplasia in the other hip (214). Melvin et al., in their unpublished 30- to 50-year follow-up of DDH, demonstrated that 40% of the patients with DDH showed radiographic evidence of dysplasia in the opposite hip (P. Melvin, R. Johnston, I.V. Ponseti, *personal communication*). It has been estimated that 20% to 50% of degenerative joint disease of the hip is secondary to subluxation or residual radiographic acetabular dysplasia (44,57,212,214,215,219–221). Wiberg suggested that there was a direct correlation between the onset of radiographically determined degenerative joint disease and the amount of dysplasia as measured by the decrease in the CE angle (44) (Fig. 24.16).

Cooperman et al., in a radiographic study of degenerative joint disease and its relation to the severity of radiographic acetabular dysplasia, reviewed the 17 cases on which Wiberg based his conclusions (212). They concluded that 7 of 17 hips were actually subluxated. These subluxated hips were the most anatomically dysplastic; their CE angles averaged 2 degrees, and all 7 had radiographically seen degenerative changes by the time the patients were 42 years of age. The other 10 hips in Wiberg's series were radiographically dysplastic. They had intact Shenton lines and an average CE angle of 10 degrees. None of these patients developed radiographic degenerative joint disease before 39 years of age; however, degenerative changes became apparent radiographically by 57 years of age. In this review of Wiberg's series, the decrease in CE angle was associated with an increase in anatomic acetabular dysplasia and an increased likelihood that the hip would be subluxated. Subluxation was the primary factor in the development of degenerative joint disease in this group. Subluxation predictably leads to degenerative joint disease and clinical disability over time.

Cooperman et al. described 32 hips (28 patients) with radiographic evidence of acetabular dysplasia (i.e., CE angle less than 20 degrees, but without subluxation and with the Shenton line intact), at an average follow-up of 22 years (212). All the patients eventually developed radiographic evidence of degenerative joint disease. However, there was no linear correlation between the CE angle and the rate of development of degenerative joint disease, as had been suggested previously by Wiberg. A decreased CE angle was associated solely with increasing radiographic evidence of acetabular dysplasia and not with subluxation, because patients with subluxation had been excluded in this series. Cooperman et al. demonstrated that radiographic evidence of acetabular dysplasia leads to radiographically detectable degenerative joint disease, but the

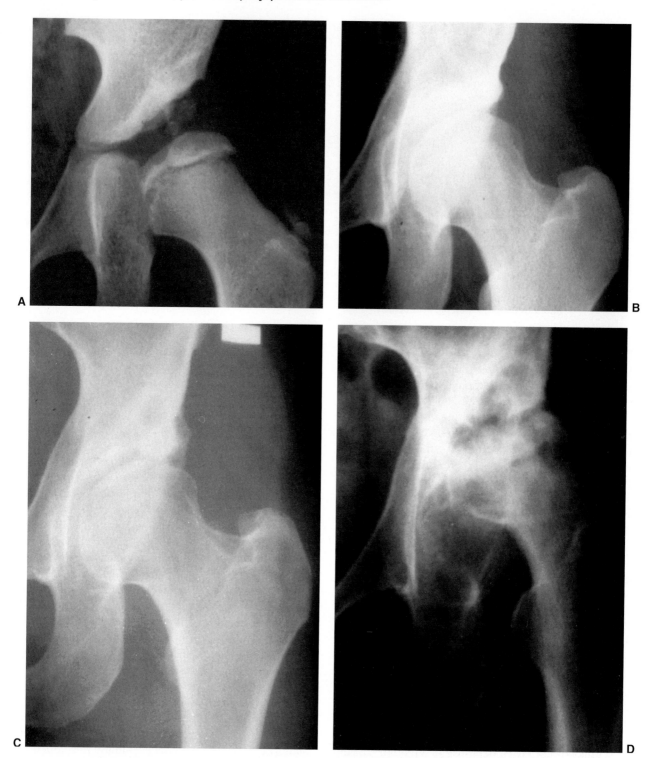

**Figure 24.24**    Anteroposterior radiographs made after closed reduction of developmental dislocation of the hip that had been performed when the patient was 2 years and 4 months of age.
**A:** Thirty-nine months after reduction, when the patient was 5 years and 7 months of age, the
accessory centers of ossification are visible in the acetabular cartilage. **B:** Fifteen years after
reduction, when the patient was 17 years of age, the Shenton line is intact and there is mild,
acetabular dysplasia. **C:** Forty-two years after reduction, when the patient was 44 years of age,
degenerative changes are present. **D:** Fifty-one years after reduction, when the patient was 53 years
of age, the hip is subluxed and shows severe degenerative changes (Iowa Hip Rating, 48 of 100
points). The patient subsequently underwent total hip replacement. (From Malvitz TA, Weinstein SL.
Closed reduction for congenital dysplasia of the hip: functional and radiographic results after an
average of thirty years. *J Bone Joint Surg Am* 1994;76:1777.)

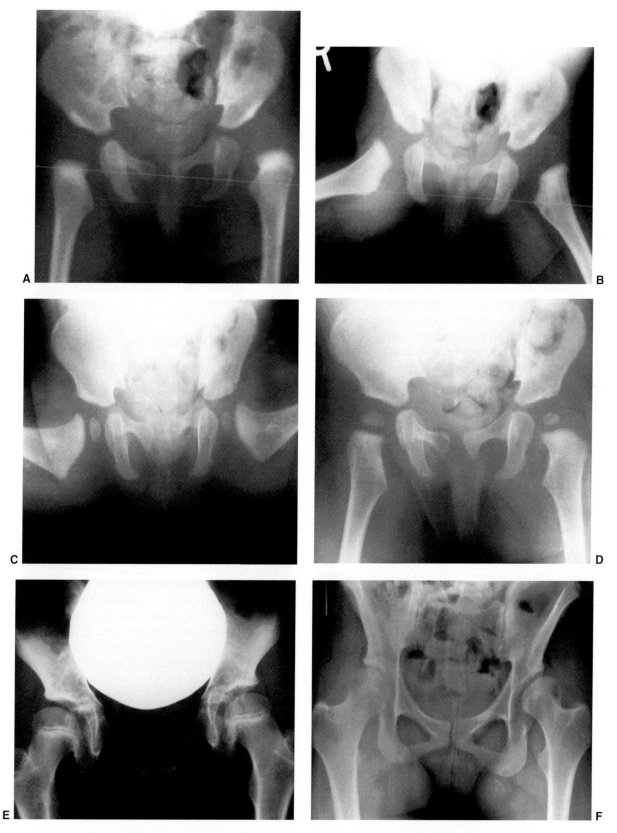

**Figure 24.25**  **A:** Anteroposterior view of a 4-month-old girl with left hip dislocation and right hip subluxation. **B:** Abduction view. **C:** Abduction view at 7 months of age, 3 months after closed treatment. **D:** Anteroposterior view at 7 months of age, 3 months after closed treatment. **E:** Anteroposterior view at 7 years of age. Note the mild anatomic dysplasia of both hips. **F:** Anteroposterior view at 15 years of age. Note the bilateral anatomic dysplasia. The right hip is radiographically dysplastic, and the left hip is radiographically subluxated.

process may take decades. This study also demonstrated that the conventional radiographic parameters used for describing dysplasia (e.g., CE angle, acetabular index of Sharp, percent coverage, depth, inclination) could not predict the rate at which a radiographically confirmed dysplastic hip joint would develop radiographic evidence of degenerative joint disease.

Stulberg and Harris demonstrated that there is no radiographic picture of degenerative joint disease that is uniquely associated with preexisting acetabular dysplasia (214). In 80% of patients with dysplasia, the CE angle is usually less than 20 degrees, but acetabular shallowness, as measured by acetabular depth, affects all of these patients. The investigators also demonstrated that the CE angle, the criterion most commonly used to quantitate dysplasia, could be affected by many factors, including positioning for the radiographs and the changes accompanying the normal development of degenerative joint disease. The secondary degenerative changes in a dysplastic acetabulum may give the hip a normal-appearing CE angle. In their series of 130 patients with primary or idiopathic degenerative joint disease, Stulberg and Harris were able to demonstrate that 48% showed evidence of primary acetabular dysplasia, and that acetabular dysplasia frequently occurred in women with degenerative joint disease.

Additional evidence for the association between radiographic evidence of acetabular dysplasia and degenerative joint disease comes from the southern Chinese population. In an epidemiologic study from Hong Kong, where the incidence of childhood hip disease is low, the incidence of adult osteoarthritis (nontraumatic) was also shown to be low (53,54).

Wedge and Wasylenko reported three peak periods of pain in subluxation, depending on the severity of the subluxation (57,66). Patients with the most severe subluxation usually had the onset of symptoms during the 2nd decade of life. Those with moderate subluxation presented during their 3rd and 4th decades, and those with minimal subluxation usually experienced the onset of symptoms around the 5th decade.

Patients who present soon after the onset of symptoms rarely have the classic signs of degenerative joint disease such as decreased joint space, cyst formation, double acetabular floor, and inferomedial femoral head osteophytes. The only radiographic feature present at the onset of symptoms may be increased sclerosis in the weight-bearing area. This increased sclerosis is secondary to increasing osteoblastic stimulation in response to the decreased weight-bearing surface area; the increase of the normal per-unit load strains the bone. The mechanism of pain in these instances is open to speculation.

In cases of subluxation, the mean age at onset of symptoms is 36.6 years in women and 54 years in men. Severe degenerative changes become evident radiographically approximately 10 years later, by 46.4 years of age in women and 69.6 years of age in men.

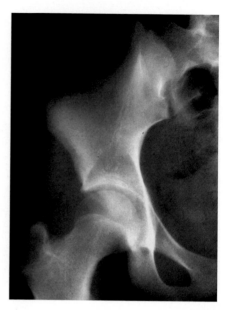

**Figure 24.26**  The "gold standard" normal hip at maturity: note intact Shenton line, well-developed and appropriately shaped teardrop, down-sloping sourcil, and normal gothic arch above the sourcil.

Patients with subluxated hips usually experience onset of symptoms at a younger age than patients with complete dislocations do. After pain and radiographically evident degenerative disease start, the disease progresses rapidly. Harris reported that symptoms of degenerative joint disease associated with radiographic evidence of acetabular dysplasia occurred early in life and that almost 50% of the patients in his series with acetabular dysplasia had their first reconstructive procedure before 60 years of age, with fewer than 5% having their first reconstruction after 60 years of age (215).

At maturity, the ideal radiograph should have a well-developed teardrop; a normal femoral neck-shaft angle; an intact Shenton line; a down-sloping sourcil and a well-developed gothic arch (Fig. 24.26). Any deviation from this radiographic appearance may lead to degenerative joint disease over the long term (57,116,184,208,209, 212–214).

## TREATMENT OF HIP DISLOCATION

### Newborns and Infants Younger Than 6 Months of Age

On the basis of the understanding of normal growth and development of the hip, the fundamental treatment goals in DDH are the same, regardless of the age of the patient. The first goal is to obtain reduction and maintain that reduction to provide an optimal environment for the development of the femoral head and acetabulum (115). As has been demonstrated by many follow-up studies of treated DDH, the acetabulum has the potential for development for many years after reduction as long as the reduction is maintained (34,36,37). The femoral head and femoral anteversion can remodel if the reduction is maintained (209,222). Further intervention is necessary only to alter an otherwise adverse natural history, as in the treatment of residual dysplasia and the prevention or treatment of subluxation. The later the diagnosis of DDH is made, the more difficult it is to achieve these goals, the less potential there is for acetabular and proximal femoral remodeling, and the more complex are the required treatments. With increasing age and complexity of treatment the risk of complications is greater, and the patient is more likely to develop degenerative joint disease.

The diagnosis of DDH should ideally be made in the newborn nursery (223). If the diagnosis is made in the nursery, treatment should be initiated immediately (224). Triple diapers or abduction diapers have no place in the treatment of DDH in the newborn. They give the family a false sense of security and are generally ineffective. Any success with the use of triple diapers or abduction diapers could be attributed to the natural resolution of the disorder.

The most commonly used device for the treatment of DDH in the newborn is the Pavlik harness (Fig. 24.27). Although other devices are available (e.g., von Rosen splint, Frejka pillow), the Pavlik harness remains the most commonly used device worldwide (35,81,225–236). When appropriately applied, the Pavlik harness prevents the hip extension and adduction that can lead to redislocation, but it allows further flexion and abduction, which lead to reduction and stabilization. By maintaining the Ortolani-positive hip in a Pavlik harness on a full-time basis for 6 weeks, hip instability resolves in 95% of cases (236).

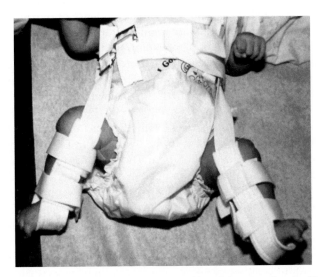

**Figure 24.27** Newborn with bilateral hip dislocations in a Pavlik harness. Appropriately applied, the harness prevents hip extension and adduction which can lead to redislocation, but allows further flexion and abduction, which lead to reduction and stabilization.

The Pavlik harness may be used effectively until 6 months of age for any child with residual dysplasia, subluxation, or complete dislocation. After 6 months of age the failure rate for the Pavlik harness is greater than 50%, because it is difficult to maintain the increasingly active and crawling child in the harness.

Mubarak et al. and others described the disadvantages associated with the use of the Pavlik harness for the treatment of DDH (33,237). They pointed out that failures of treatment most often result from problems related to the physician, the device, or the patient.

The physician-related errors fall into two categories: inappropriate application and persistence of inadequate treatment. The Pavlik harness is contraindicated in patients with significant muscle imbalance, such as those with myelodysplasia or cerebral palsy. It is also contraindicated in patients who have significant stiffness of the joints, such as children with arthrogryposis. The harness will fail if it is applied in a child with excessive ligamentous laxity, as seen in Ehlers-Danlos syndrome (33).

The persistence of inadequate treatment is the result of many factors. If treatment with the harness is to be successful, physicians should be well versed in its appropriate application and the adjustments that are necessary throughout the course of treatment. It is important that the physician recognize when a treatment failure has occurred, so as not to prolong treatment with the harness and cause secondary pathologic changes, called *Pavlik harness disease* (238). Persistence of treatment may damage the femoral head, injure the acetabular cartilage, and impair future bone growth. An inappropriately applied harness is a failure of the physician, not a failure of the orthotic (237,239).

Another major Pavlik harness problem is related to the specific orthotic device. Not all Pavlik harnesses are the same; the strap attachment sites vary. However, since the article by Mubarak et al. in 1981, most harnesses on the market meet the requisite standards that those authors outlined (33,237).

Some problems are related to the patient. Certain family, social, and educational situations make compliance impossible. In these situations, the Pavlik harness would be inappropriate, and closed reduction and casting may be the more judicious approach. The family must be educated about the importance of the harness, its care and maintenance, how the child should be bathed while wearing the harness, and the consequences of failure. Family noncompliance can lead to failure, and the use of a visiting nurse may be helpful in these situations.

The method of application of the harness (Fig. 24.27) should be demonstrated to the family members. The chest halter strap should be positioned at the nipple line, and the shoulder straps are to be set to hold the cross strap at this level. The leg and foot stirrups must have their anterior and posterior straps oriented anteriorly and posteriorly to the child's knees. Hip flexion should be set at 100 to 110 degrees. These straps should be in the anterior axillary line. The posterior abduction strap should be at the level of the child's scapula and adjusted to allow comfortable abduction within the *safe zone* (240), which is defined as the arc of abduction and adduction, that is, between redislocation and comfortable, unforced abduction. The posterior strap acts as a checkrein to prevent the hip from adducting to the point of redislocation. Ultrasonography is a useful means of documenting relocation of the Ortolani-positive hip.

There is great variability in treatment regimens with the Pavlik harness. If the Pavlik harness is used for stabilizing an unstable hip (i.e., an Ortolani- or Barlow-positive hip), the harness is used full time for 6 to 12 weeks after clinical stability is achieved. The author's preference is to use the harness full time for 6 weeks beyond the point when stability is reached. Most hips stabilize in days to weeks. The harness is checked at 7- to 10-day intervals to assess hip stability and to adjust the flexion and abduction straps to allow for growth of the infant. In the author's opinion, clinical examination is usually sufficient to check on the progress at each visit; but if uncertainty is present, ultrasonography may be used; radiographs are unnecessary.

In a child younger than 6 months who has a complete dislocation, the Pavlik harness may be used in a trial of ultrasound-monitored reduction. In this case, the harness must be applied with enough hyperflexion and abduction to point the femoral head toward the triradiate cartilage. This situation is the ideal indication for the use of ultrasonography to follow the reduction. When the harness is used in this situation, the infant should be checked at 7 to 10 days to determine whether the reduction is being accomplished. Clinical examination alone may be adequate, but initial radiographs or ultrasound should be obtained in order to document adequate flexion and redirection of the femoral neck toward the triradiate cartilage in the harness. After clinical stability is achieved, radiography is not indicated until approximately 3 months of age to assess acetabular development (Fig. 24.28). Ultrasonography is an excellent means of documenting progress toward and completion of successful reduction (241).

Although the Pavlik harness has provided a 95% overall success rate for the treatment of the Ortolani-positive hip, the success rate for using the harness to guide the reduction of a subluxated or dislocated hip in a child younger than 6 months of age is 85% (33,228,236,242).

The use of the Pavlik harness can be associated with complications; most of these complications are iatrogenic and can be avoided. Inferior dislocations may occur with prolonged excessive hip flexion (243–245). Hyperflexion may also induce femoral nerve compression neuropathy; this condition generally resolves after the harness is removed. It is important during each examination to make certain that the patient has active quadriceps function. Brachial plexus palsy may occur from compression by the shoulder straps, and knee subluxations may occur from improperly positioned straps.

Skin breakdown may occur in the groin creases and in the popliteal fossa if great care is not taken in keeping these areas clean and dry. Instruction with regard to bathing and skin care is essential.

The most disastrous consequence of Pavlik harness treatment is damage to the cartilaginous femoral head and the proximal femoral physeal plate (246,247). This is usually secondary to forced abduction in the harness or to persistent use of the harness, despite the failure of reduction, in a complete dislocation.

## Children 6 Months to 2 Years of Age

It is difficult to maintain a child older than 6 months of age in a Pavlik harness because of the child's activity levels. In this age group subluxated or dislocated hips should be treated by closed or open means as necessary, because success rates using the Pavlik harness are less than 50%.

In the late-diagnosed patient or the patient who fails treatment with the Pavlik harness, the obstacles to reduction are different, treatment has greater risks, and the results are far less predictable. The principal goals in the treatment of the late-diagnosed patient are similar to those for the newborn. The goal is to obtain reduction, to maintain that reduction so as to provide an adequate environment for femoral head and acetabular development, and to avoid proximal femoral growth disturbance (Fig. 24.29).

### Traction

For patients older than 6 months of age at diagnosis and those who have failed a trial of Pavlik harness reduction, closed reduction is indicated. In some centers, treatment by closed reduction and spica cast immobilization is preceded by a period of skin or skeletal traction (248–258) (Fig. 24.30). Traction theoretically stretches contracted muscles, allows reduction without excessive force, decreases the need for open reduction, and reduces the incidence of proximal femoral growth disturbance resulting from avascular necrosis (AVN). The use of prereduction traction, and its effectiveness at accomplishing what it is touted to do, are controversial topics (259,260). In 1991, Fish et al. sought the opinions of the members of the Pediatric Orthopaedic Society of North America on this topic (261). Most pediatric orthopaedic surgeons thought that traction did reduce the incidence of necrosis in the treatment of DDH. Only 5% of responders did not use traction in their practice. In the author's opinion, this practice pattern has changed considerably over the last 13 years, with far fewer pediatric orthopaedic surgeons employing prereduction traction.

The purpose of traction is to allow gradual relaxation of secondarily contracted muscles, such as the iliopsoas and adductor longus; theoretically, this allows reduction without creating excessive joint forces, thereby decreasing the incidence of AVN and reducing the need for open reduction. These ideas are lacking the support of scientifically valid studies (260).

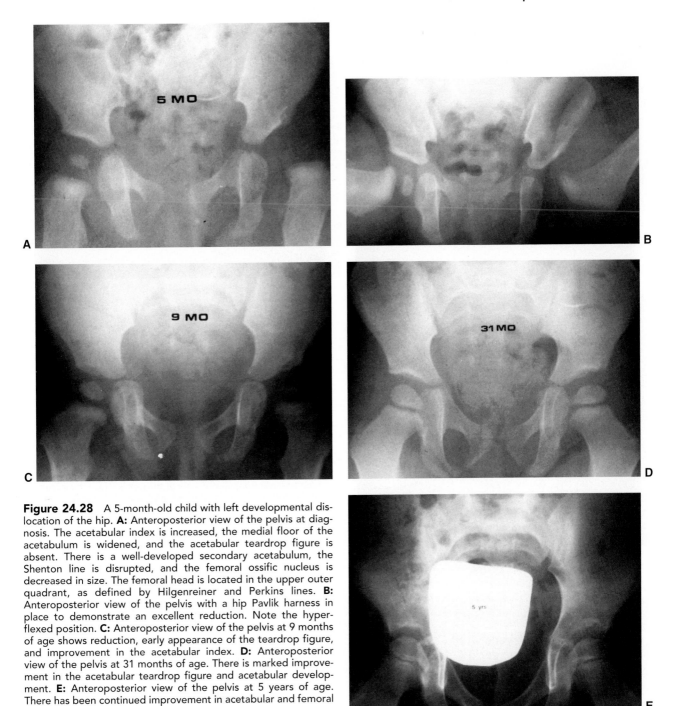

**Figure 24.28** A 5-month-old child with left developmental dislocation of the hip. **A:** Anteroposterior view of the pelvis at diagnosis. The acetabular index is increased, the medial floor of the acetabulum is widened, and the acetabular teardrop figure is absent. There is a well-developed secondary acetabulum, the Shenton line is disrupted, and the femoral ossific nucleus is decreased in size. The femoral head is located in the upper outer quadrant, as defined by Hilgenreiner and Perkins lines. **B:** Anteroposterior view of the pelvis with a hip Pavlik harness in place to demonstrate an excellent reduction. Note the hyperflexed position. **C:** Anteroposterior view of the pelvis at 9 months of age shows reduction, early appearance of the teardrop figure, and improvement in the acetabular index. **D:** Anteroposterior view of the pelvis at 31 months of age. There is marked improvement in the acetabular teardrop figure and acetabular development. **E:** Anteroposterior view of the pelvis at 5 years of age. There has been continued improvement in acetabular and femoral head development.

Gage and Winter studied a group of patients in order to quantify prereduction hip positions, and concluded that there was a direct correlation between inadequate traction and the incidence of growth disturbance (251). Weiner et al. found that in patients younger than 1 year traction for longer than 21 days substantially reduced the rate of growth disturbance (256). Buchanan et al. recommended a minimum of 2 weeks of traction until achievement of a 2+ traction station using the Gage and Winter scale (248). Skeletal traction was gradually increased over several weeks, and an average of 39% of body weight was usually required

for achieving this position. In contrast, Cooperman et al. studied 30 DDH hips with aseptic necrosis and 30 hips without necrosis and found, at an average 39-year follow-up, that the degree of initial displacement that had to be overcome in order to obtain reduction was comparable in both groups and that it was not a factor in the development of proximal femoral growth disturbance (262). Some of the worst outcomes were seen in patients with minimal superior dislocation. Schoenecker and Strecker demonstrated that the results of traction were not as good as the results of femoral shortening in older patients with DDH (263).

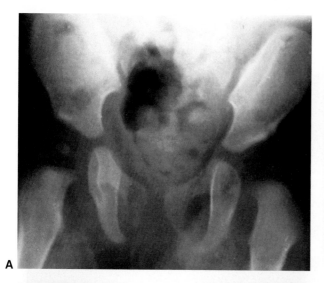

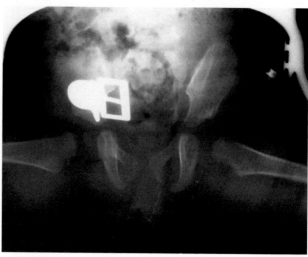

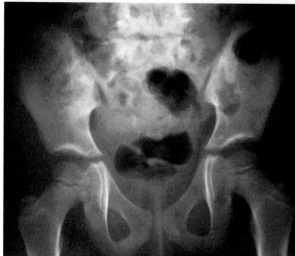

**Figure 24.29** A 6-month-old girl with apparent left hip subluxation and acetabular dysplasia secondary to excessive anteversion. **A:** Diagnostic anteroposterior view of the pelvis. Note the increased acetabular index, the poorly developed teardrop figure, and the small ossific nucleus. **B:** Anteroposterior view of the pelvis in the fixed abduction brace. Excellent reduction of the hip has been achieved. **C:** Anteroposterior view of the same patient at 5 years of age. The left hip appears normal.

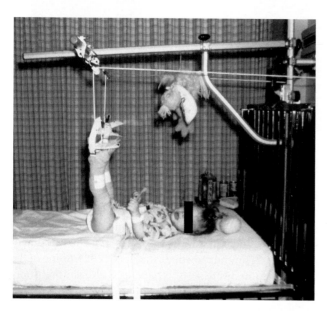

**Figure 24.30** A 1-year-old child with bilateral hip dislocations in traction.

Gibson and Benson (210) thought that although preliminary traction protects against growth disturbance, there was no relation between the original degree of displacement of the proximal femur and the final outcome (264). A recent study by Kutlu et al. (265), looking at traction as a single variable in a series of patients treated by closed reduction, showed that traction did not affect the rate of necrosis.

With respect to traction facilitating reduction, the assessment of the adequacy of closed reduction and the need for open reduction varies and is subjective. Several articles on open and closed reduction without the use of preliminary traction report incidences of proximal femoral damage comparable to those found in series in which prereduction traction was used (43,266–268). These researchers think that the main obstacles to reduction are intraarticular and therefore would not be affected by the use of traction. Controversy also exists about the amount of weight applied, the direction of application of the force, and the duration of applied traction. There are no clinical or experimental studies of the direct effects of traction, and there are no well-controlled studies that analyze the effect of traction as a single variable (260).

Surgeons who choose to use prereduction traction generally consider that 1 to 2 weeks of skin or skeletal traction are sufficient. However, a recent report on the successful use of traction to attain reduction in patients more than 6 months of age, reported a mean time in traction of 8 weeks (269). Skin traction is the most commonly used method, although some physicians recommend skeletal traction (239). Skin tapes should be applied above the knee to distribute the traction over a large area (Fig. 24.30). Elastoplast tape is applied loosely over tincture of benzoin from the ankle to the upper thigh. It is important not to stretch the Elastoplast tape at all; it should merely lie on the skin in a circumferential manner, with each edge directly opposing the preceding edge. Buck traction tapes are then applied from above the ankle to the thigh and to the foot plate; weights may be added to both legs, so that the buttocks "lightly" touch the bed. The author has used this method without adverse consequences. The direction of application of the traction forces (e.g., overhead, longitudinal, divaricated) and the duration of traction (days to months) vary worldwide.

The complications of traction include skin loss and ischemia of the lower extremities; these are attributable to inappropriate application. Neurocirculatory checks must be performed frequently, and traction must be applied in a carefully supervised manner.

In appropriate circumstances, traction may be used at home (270–272). This markedly decreases the costs associated with hospitalization. Patients are usually hospitalized for 24 hours to allow their parents to become familiar with the traction apparatus, to learn how to monitor neurocirculatory status, and to become totally familiar with the potential risks and danger signs. The patient and family must be cooperative; a visiting nurse is often helpful in instituting this program.

### Closed Reduction

Closed reductions are performed in the operating room. Gentle reduction must be done under general anesthesia. The hip is gently manipulated into the acetabulum by flexion, traction, and abduction. An open or percutaneous adductor tenotomy is usually necessary in these cases because of secondary adduction contracture, and for increasing the "safe zone" (arc of adduction–abduction in which the hip remains located), thereby lessening the incidence of proximal femoral growth disturbance.

The adequacy of closed reduction is somewhat subjective. In my opinion, anatomic reduction is the only acceptable reduction (Fig. 24.31). Because large portions of the femoral head and acetabulum are cartilaginous, arthrography is a useful tool in assessing the obstacles to and the adequacy of reduction (271,273–275). Dynamic arthrography using fluoroscopy helps to achieve both of these goals. Intraoperative ultrasonography may also be used. The use of the femoral head as a "dilating sound" to overcome the

intraarticular obstacles to reduction may cause damage to the femoral head and make open reduction more difficult (238,276,277).

The reduction is maintained in a well-molded plaster cast. Reduction, after casting, should be documented by radiography, computed tomography (CT) scan, MRI, or ultrasonography (31,164,278–283) (Fig. 24.32). The author prefers to use plaster of paris because of its "moldability," but some surgeons prefer to use synthetic materials. The plaster must be well-molded dorsal to the greater trochanters so as to prevent redislocation (Fig. 24.32). In the author's experience, most successful reductions are lost in the postoperative period by poorly applied and molded casts. The "human position" of hyperflexion and limited abduction is the preferred position (284,285) (Fig. 24.33). The amount of apparent hip flexion during cast application is often greater than the flexion seen on radiographs. Wide, forced abduction or forced abduction with internal rotation should be avoided because these approaches are associated with an increased incidence of proximal femoral growth disturbance (Fig. 24.34).

The duration of time required for maintenance of reduction in the plaster cast varies considerably. The author prefers to maintain the plaster below the knee on the involved side and above the knee on the uninvolved side for approximately 6 weeks, regardless of the patient's age. After that time, the plaster on the involved side (or sides) is cut to above the knee to allow some hip rotation and range of motion for the knee for an additional 6 weeks.

Most physicians use abduction orthotic devices for some period after cast removal. Some use them on a full-time basis (except for bathing) for several months, then part-time, usually during the night and napping hours, until acetabular development has caught up with that of the opposite, normal side (generally 18 to 24 months) or surgical intervention is planned. The use of abduction orthotic devices after reduction of DDH varies widely. The theory behind the use of the fixed abduction brace is that there may still remain mild instability that can be corrected by the fixed abduction brace that maintains the stable relation between the femoral head and the acetabulum, yet allows some hip mobility. Empirical evidence exists for its efficacy in cases of mild hip instability (Fig. 24.29). The complications associated with the use of a fixed abduction device include skin breakdown and proximal femoral growth disturbance. It is important to ensure, while positioning the device, that the hip is not placed in extreme positions of abduction that could interrupt the vascular supply to the proximal femur.

### Open Reduction

In patients 6 months to 2 years of age, open reduction is indicated if there is failure of closed treatment, persistent subluxation, soft tissue interposition, or reducible but unstable reductions other than in extreme positions of abduction. There had been a theory in recent years that the

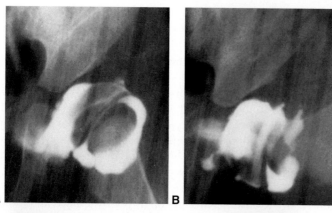

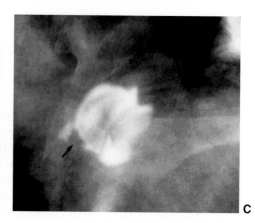

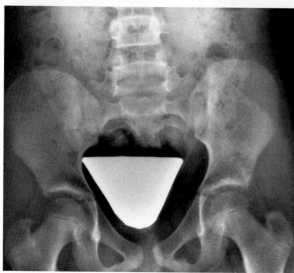

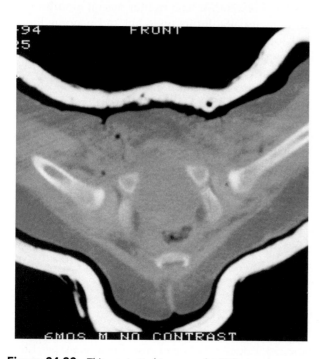

**Figure 24.31** Arthrograms demonstrate closed reduction of developmental dysplasia of the left hip in an 8-month-old infant. **A:** Untreated. **B:** Reduced. There is no pooling of dye medially. The acetabular cartilage completely covers the femoral head. **C:** Reduction in a plaster cast. Note the arthrographic shadow of the transverse acetabular ligament (*arrow*). **D:** Nine years after reduction. Note the symmetric acetabular and proximal femoral development.

**Figure 24.32** This computed tomography (CT) scan documents a successful closed reduction of a right hip dislocation. The plaster cast is molded dorsal to the greater trochanters in order to help prevent redislocation.

incidence of damage to the proximal femur is decreased if open reduction is delayed until the femoral ossific nucleus is present (286,287). This notion has recently been dispelled (288–290).

The goals of open treatment are to obtain reduction, maintain the reduction, avoid damage to the femoral head, and provide an optimal environment for acetabular and proximal femoral development. Open reduction of a DDH may be accomplished through a variety of surgical approaches (40,43,119,121–123,182,240,291–297).

The most commonly used surgical approach to open reduction is the anterolateral Smith-Petersen approach with a modified "bikini" incision, as described by Salter and Dubos (283). This is a standard approach to the hip joint and is familiar to most surgeons. In the late-diagnosed patient with DDH, any associated capsular laxity can be plicated through this approach. If the surgeon thinks that a secondary procedure, such as pelvic osteotomy, is necessary, it also can be accomplished through the same surgical approach (40,295–297).

One of the advantages of the anterior Smith-Petersen approach is that the hip is immobilized in a functional position, with minimal hip flexion and some degree of abduction. If this approach is used in conjunction with a

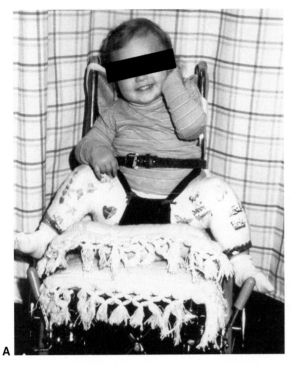

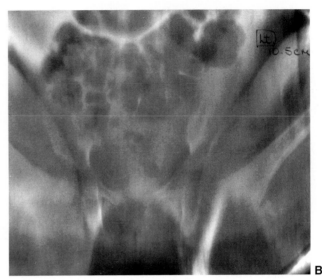

**Figure 24.33  A:** The "human position" of hyperflexion and limited abduction is the preferred position after closed reduction. This patient underwent bilateral reductions. **B:** Single-cut tomogram documents the hyperflexed, minimal abduction position.

capsular plication, the postoperative immobilization period is usually 6 to 8 weeks.

The disadvantages may include greater blood loss than with the various medial and anteromedial approaches, possible damage to the iliac crest apophysis and the hip abductors, and postoperative stiffness. If this approach is used in bilateral cases, the procedures are usually staged at 2- to 6-week intervals.

The various medial approaches have the advantage of approaching the hip joint directly over the site of the obstacles to reduction (43,121–123,293,298–303). The medial approach described by Ferguson is in the plane between the adductor brevis and the adductor magnus (119,304). Advocates of this approach claim that its advantages include minimal soft tissue dissection, direct access

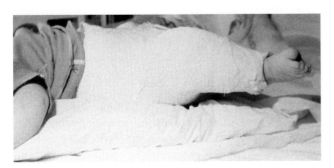

**Figure 24.34**  Wide abduction should be avoided. This position is associated with a high incidence of damage to the proximal femoral epiphysis and the physeal plate.

to the medial joint capsule and the iliopsoas tendon, avoidance of damage to the iliac apophysis and abductor muscles, minimal blood loss, and excellent cosmesis. However, it is a less familiar approach to most surgeons, and visualization is somewhat impaired. Capsular repair cannot be accomplished through this approach. The stability of the reduction is maintained only by the postoperative cast. This approach is somewhat difficult to use in older patients, and no concomitant surgical procedures can be performed through the same incision. Concern has also been expressed about a possible higher incidence of proximal femoral growth disturbance after use of this approach (305).

A third approach to open reduction in this age group is the anteromedial approach originally described by Ludloff and modified by Weinstein and Ponseti (43,109,115,121, 264,306–309). The approach is made in the interval between the femoral neurovascular bundle and the pectineus muscle. The advocates of this approach cite minimal blood loss (transfusion is never necessary) and the fact that it is the most direct approach to the obstacles to reduction. There is minimal muscle dissection in this approach; only the iliopsoas and the adductor longus are sectioned. Both hips can be reduced during the same operative procedure, the scar is extremely cosmetic, and there is no damage to the hip abductor muscles or the iliac apophysis. Postoperative stiffness is not a problem.

However, there are several disadvantages to the anteromedial approach. It is not a familiar approach to most

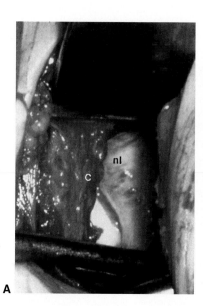
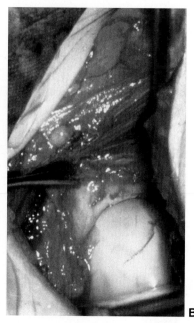

**Figure 24.35   A:** Open reduction through an anteromedial approach in a 14-month-old child. Note the anterior joint capsular edge (*c*) and the neolimbus (*nl*). **B:** The hip is reduced under direct view. The femoral head is well seated in the acetabulum, and the anterior edge of the hip capsule is everted by a hemostat.

surgeons. Only open reduction can be accomplished; no secondary procedures can be performed through this incision. It is difficult to use in older patients because of the depth of the hip joint and the difficulty with visualization. The surgeon who decides that capsular plication should be performed cannot do it through this approach. The medial femoral circumflex vessels (the primary blood supply to the proximal femur) are in the operative field. Moreover, visualization is claimed by some to be poor, and the approach is associated with a higher incidence of aseptic necrosis (305,310). In the author's experience of more than 200 cases, the visualization is excellent (Fig. 24.35) and the incidence of aseptic necrosis during a minimum 4-year follow-up is approximately 14%, which is well in line with the results of other series of open reductions (123,311). Capsular plication appears to be unnecessary in this age group, because in a successful closed reduction the capsule tightens and the scar induced by the surgical procedure helps to provide capsular stability. This approach, however, depends on the placement of a well-molded cast. The approach to casting after reduction is the same as that described earlier for closed reduction. A certain degree of capsular stability is gained through the prolonged postoperative immobilization that is necessary. No residual stiffness has been reported.

Following cast removal most physicians use some form of abduction orthosis for varying periods of time, as discussed in the preceding text. When using any of the approaches other than the anterior approach with capsular plication, the author uses a fixed abduction orthosis for 2 months on a full-time basis and then at night and nap time until acetabular development has normalized (generally 18 to 24 months) or further surgical intervention is planned for correcting residual dysplasia.

In assessing acetabular development after open or closed reduction, it is important to look for accessory ossification centers (Fig. 24.9). These give the treating physician an idea of whether the cartilage in the region of the neolimbus in the periphery of the acetabulum has the potential for ossification and normal acetabular development, or whether secondary acetabular procedures will be necessary.

In patients younger than 2 years, a secondary acetabular or femoral procedure is rarely required. The potential for acetabular development after closed or open reduction is excellent and continues for 4 to 8 years after the reduction (36,37,43,312–314). The most rapid improvement in acetabular development—as measured by parameters such as the acetabular index, development of the teardrop figure, and thinning of the medial floor—occurs in the first 18 months after surgery (34,36,37,43,312,315–317). Femoral anteversion and any coxa valga associated with the untreated condition have an excellent chance to resolve during this time. However, some surgeons think that every child with DDH older than 18 months should undergo pelvic osteotomy accompanying open reduction, because of the poor acetabular development potential (40,295, 296,318,319).

## Children Older Than 2 Years

In a child older than 2 years at the time of diagnosis of DDH, open reduction is usually necessary. In this age group, the treating surgeon must also consider whether to perform concomitant femoral shortening in conjunction with the open reduction. In children older than 3 years, femoral shortening to avoid excessive pressure on the proximal femur leads to far lower rates of proximal femoral growth disturbance than does preliminary traction followed by open reduction (263,320–323) (Fig. 24.36). Schoenecker and Strecker reported a 54% incidence of aseptic necrosis with a 32% incidence of redislocation, when skeletal traction was used in patients older than 3 years (263). A theoretical advantage of open reduction accompanied by femoral shortening is that it can be used for correcting any anatomic abnormality, such as excessive femoral anteversion. The disadvantages of femoral shortening include the need for a second incision and internal fixation for the osteotomy, and a further operation for hardware removal.

The age range of 2 to 3 years is considered a "gray zone;" some surgeons advocate preliminary traction before open reduction, but an increasing number of surgeons prefer to perform concomitant femoral shortening (324–326). In this age range, because the potential for acetabular development is markedly diminished, many surgeons recommend a concomitant acetabular procedure, either in conjunction with the open reduction or 6 to 8 weeks after it (327). The decision about whether to perform a secondary acetabular procedure is subjective. The author prefers to judge stability at the time of open reduction (328). If good stability is evident, the author prefers to observe acetabular development for the next few years, and if acetabular development is not improving by radiographic criteria (e.g., decreasing acetabular index, improvement in teardrop appearance

and shape) (183), the author considers secondary acetabular procedures (329,330). Most surgeons have been adopting earlier rather than later intervention for residual dysplasia, as the results are more predictable with fewer complications (317).

The most common accompanying acetabular procedure performed in this age group in conjunction with open reduction is innominate osteotomy as described by Salter (40,331) and by Pemberton (39,332–336). Anatomic deficiency of the acetabulum in this age group is usually anterior, and the Salter innominate osteotomy gives anterior coverage, although at the expense of posterior coverage. The Pemberton osteotomy provides anterior coverage, and also various degrees of lateral coverage, depending on the direction of the osteotomy cuts.

In this age group the standard anterolateral approach described by Smith-Petersen with the Salter modification is the ideal approach, because it enables capsular plication, immobilization of the hip joint in a more functional position, and innominate osteotomy, all at the same time and through the same incision.

After 3 years of age, open reduction of the hip should be accompanied by femoral shortening, and probably by a concomitant acetabular procedure, depending on hip stability at the time of surgery (317,323,326,337,338). The acetabular procedure may be performed at the time of

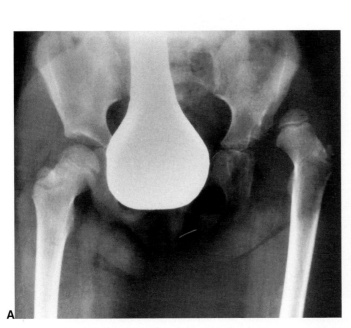
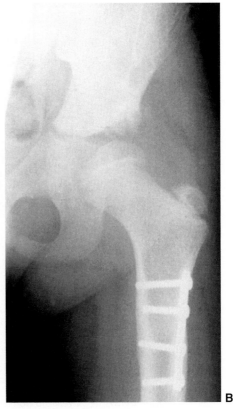

**Figure 24.36** **A:** Preoperative anteroposterior radiograph of a 4-year-old girl with developmental dislocation of the left hip. **B:** Eighteen months after reduction and femoral shortening, accessory centers of ossification are appearing in the lateral portion of the acetabular cartilage.

open reduction, 6 weeks later, or at a later date, depending upon acetabular development and the surgeon's judgment.

## SEQUELAE AND COMPLICATIONS

### Residual Femoral and Acetabular Dysplasia After Closed or Open Treatment

On the basis of studies of the natural history of DDH, it is the goal of treatment to have a radiographically confirmed normal hip at maturity in order to prevent degenerative joint disease in the future (Fig. 24.26). Hip subluxations must be corrected. The evidence demonstrates that residual acetabular dysplasia, even in the absence of subluxation, eventually leads to degenerative joint disease, so this also should be corrected (339,340). The goal of treatment of DDH is to have a hip as anatomically normal as possible by the end of skeletal growth.

#### Evaluation of Hip Dysplasia

When evaluating the patient with persistent dysplasia, the relation between the acetabulum and the femur should be assessed. Anatomic dysplasia can involve the acetabulum, the proximal femur, or both. In patients with DDH, the deficiency is most commonly on the acetabular side, or the dysplasia is significantly greater on the acetabular side. If there has been a disturbance of proximal femoral growth

secondary to previous treatment, the femoral side may be more dysplastic.

Dysplasias of the hip joint can be evaluated with radiographs taken with the patient in the standing position, when possible, and with the standard evaluations of acetabular development: the acetabular index, the acetabular angle of Sharp, and the CE angle. In most young children with DDH the acetabular deficiency is anterior, and in adolescents and adults with DDH, the acetabular deficiencies can be anterior, posterior, or global, (40,74, 295,341–345) and there also may be evidence of acetabular retroversion (346). Excessive femoral anteversion can be ascertained clinically, but is most accurately measured by CT scan (347). There has been an increased interest in evaluating dysplasia by means of three-dimensional CT scan (210,345,348,349). However, CT scan cannot show the cartilaginous component of the proximal femur or the acetabulum; therefore, it is most useful for mature patients or those close to maturity.

The best means of evaluating acetabular dysplasia in the mature patient includes three-dimensional CT scan (126,350–355), the false profile view, and plain radiography (356) (Fig. 24.37).

### The Role of Proximal Femoral Osteotomy

Deformities of the femoral neck assume significance only if they lead to subluxation of the joint: lateral subluxation with extreme coxa valga or anterior subluxation with

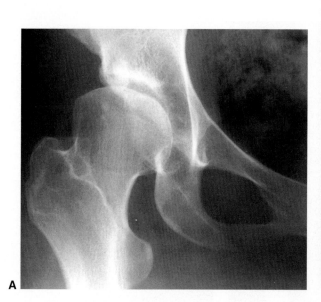
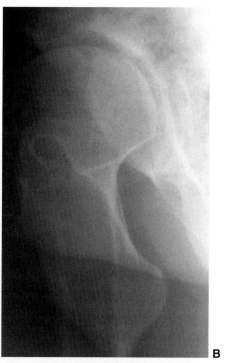

**Figure 24.37** A 34-year-old woman with residual dysplasia, who had undergone closed reduction for right developmental dysplasia of the hip at 16 months of age. She now has mild pain. **A:** Anteroposterior view of the hip. **B:** False profile lateral view demonstrating anterior deficiency of the acetabulum.

excessive anteversion (182). In general, patients with DDH have normal neck-shaft angles. They may have persistent anteversion that gives the radiologic appearance of subluxation (disrupted Shenton Line).

After reduction is obtained, the femoral neck anteversion corrects spontaneously in most patients with DDH (357). If acetabular dysplasia persists for 2 to 3 years after closed or open reduction and the patient has residual anteversion, proximal femoral rotational osteotomy may be considered. When the Shenton line is disrupted, the proper relation of the proximal femur can usually be restored by derotation osteotomy, with or without various degrees of varus. The varus derotation osteotomy is used alone in such cases by surgeons who think that redirection of the femoral head toward the center of the acetabulum stimulates normal acetabular development (154,181,204,358–367). If the proximal femoral varus derotation osteotomy is to be used for "stimulating" more normal acetabular development in patients with persistent femoral anteversion, it must be performed in children younger than 4 years (358). After 8 years of age, no improvement in acetabular dysplasia can result from this procedure alone.

Before performing varus derotation osteotomy, the surgeon must ensure that the femoral head can be concentrically reduced as seen on an anteroposterior pelvic radiograph with the patient's legs abducted 30 degrees and maximally internally rotated (Fig. 24.38). This position allows visualization of the actual angle of the femoral neck. If concentric reduction is not documented, this procedure should be accompanied by open reduction.

In small children, any leg-length discrepancy resulting from varus osteotomy should resolve by growth stimulation and restoration of the normal neck-shaft angle (368). In teenagers, however, more than a 15-degree lessening of the neck-shaft angle may result in limb shortening. If the varus osteotomy is excessive, it can cause lateralization of the shaft, shifting the mechanical axis medial to the knee joint and leading to mechanical abnormalities at the knee (369). Proximal femoral osteotomy may, in some cases, be indicated in order to correct residual deformity from a partial physeal arrest resulting from aseptic necrosis; however, minimal literature exists on this procedure.

If the osteotomy is transfixed with smooth wires, they can be removed after 6 to 8 weeks. Internal fixation devices are usually removed 12 to 18 months postoperatively; if they are not removed in young children, they become encased within the proximal femur, and this could pose problems if future operations become necessary.

In the adolescent or adult patient with residual acetabular dysplasia and a disrupted Shenton line in whom there is no potential for acetabular growth and remodeling, changing the orientation of the proximal femur does not increase the weight bearing area, but only shifts the weight-bearing area to another portion of the femoral head (370–372). Proximal femoral osteotomies in the adolescent or adult group are indicated only as adjuncts to pelvic operations and in extreme cases of coxa valga and subluxation (182,371) (Fig. 24.39).

### Role of Pelvic Osteotomies

Indications for the treatment of residual radiographic acetabular dysplasia after closed or open reduction (or discovered incidentally) depend on the age of the child and whether the patient has symptoms (373). The goal of treatment is to restore the anatomy to as near normal as possible by the time skeletal maturity is attained. As discussed previously, after concentric reduction is obtained and maintained, the potential for acetabular development continues for many years (34,36,37,43,209). However, after 4 years of age, this potential for restoration of normal anatomy is markedly decreased.

Correction of residual acetabular dysplasia theoretically provides for a better weight-bearing surface for the femoral head, restores the normal biomechanics of the hip and reduces contact pressures (345), and may increase the longevity of the hip by preventing degenerative joint disease. However, only prospective, long-term follow-up studies of these procedures can provide unambiguous answers.

In the young child, acetabular deficiencies are generally assessed by arthrography and by inspection at the time of open reduction. In reduced hips with residual dysplasia, the author has found that the problem is not one of deficiency of the acetabulum, but a failure of the peripheral acetabular cartilage to ossify (Fig. 24.40). In most cases, an arthrogram at the time of surgery shows excellent coverage of the femoral head by the unossified acetabular cartilage. This cartilage fails to undergo normal development because it is intrinsically abnormal or because it was damaged by the femoral head in the unreduced position, causing pressure necrosis. Given enough time, some of this acetabular cartilage may resume normal ossification and correct a large amount of the dysplasia. However, in the author's experience of a large number of patients treated with open and closed reduction, this does not happen in many cases, and intervention should be undertaken after the acetabulum has had a reasonable chance to develop on its own (123,209,374). Any osteotomy of the iliac bone and the neovascularity stimulated by it in healing may increase the ossification of the otherwise unossified acetabular cartilage. In any case, the redirection of the acetabulum restores more normal bony anatomy and normal biomechanics that may also be factors in stimulating ossification (239).

Shelf procedures were described before 1900 and were used widely until the mid-1950s, when Chiari described his medial displacement osteotomy (375). Later, Salter, Pemberton, and others described various pelvic osteotomies for redirecting the acetabulum and covering the femoral head with articular cartilage. Although intuitively it seems better to cover the femoral head with articular cartilage than to rely on fibrous metaplasia, it is impossible to be certain whether the long-term results of shelf arthroplasty will be

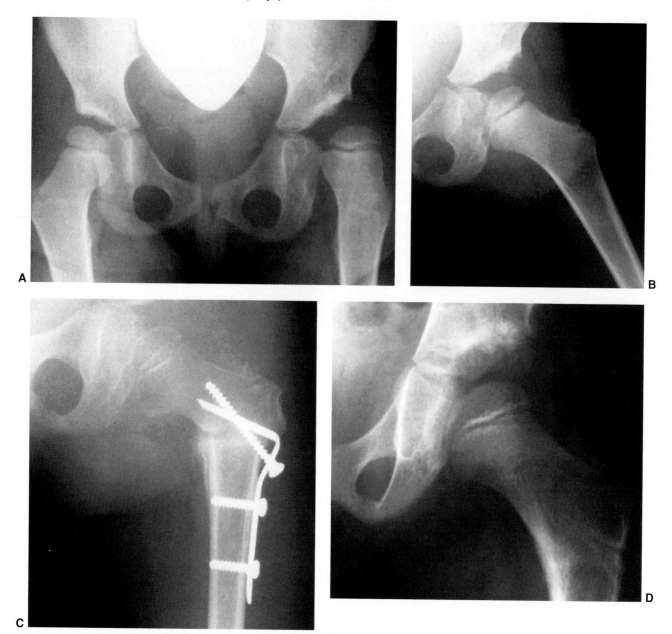

**Figure 24.38**  A 3-year-old girl 2 years after closed reduction. **A:** Anteroposterior view of the pelvis. Note the persistent acetabular dysplasia and apparent coxa valga. **B:** The radiograph shows the leg abducted approximately 30 degrees and maximally internally rotated. The femoral head is seated well within the acetabulum, and the Shenton line is restored. **C:** Anteroposterior view of the left hip 6 weeks after varus derotation osteotomy. **D:** Anteroposterior view of the left hip 18 months after varus derotation osteotomy, with hardware removed. The Shenton line has been restored; persistent acetabular dysplasia remains, but development of the teardrop figure improved, and accessory centers of ossification have appeared in the periphery of the acetabular cartilage.

less successful than those osteotomies that provide articular cartilage coverage (376,377).

Traditionally, the treatment options for residual acetabular dysplasia are divided into four groups. The first group consists of osteotomies of the pelvis that redirect the entire acetabulum. This redirection provides coverage of the femoral head by acetabular articular cartilage. These osteotomies include the Salter innominate osteotomy (40,74,295–297, 327,378–380) (Fig. 24.40), the Sutherland double-innominate osteotomy (381), the triple-innominate osteotomies of Tonnis (182,382–386), Steel (387–392), and Ganz (369,393–396), the spherical osteotomies of Wagner (397–399) and Eppright (372,400), and others (401–409). These procedures involve complete cuts through various pelvic bones and rotation of the acetabulum.

The general prerequisites for rotational osteotomy include complete concentric reduction and release of muscle contractures, including the iliopsoas and hip adductors;

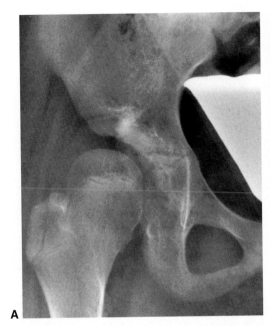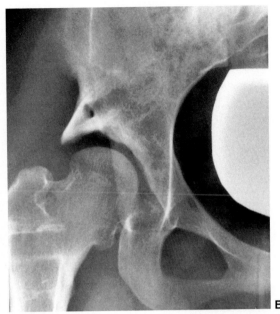

**Figure 24.39** A 10-year-old girl whose developmental dysplasia of the hip was diagnosed at 5 years of age. She had previously undergone open reduction, but had residual proximal femoral and acetabular deformities. **A:** Preoperative anteroposterior radiograph of the pelvis. **B:** Three years after varus derotation osteotomy and Staheli slotted acetabular augmentation.

a congruous joint; and good range of motion. Rotational pelvic osteotomies in the face of subluxation may lead to severe damage to the femoral head. These procedures are best performed before 6 years of age, but the age limits vary considerably, depending on the surgeon.

The Salter innominate osteotomy, which hinges on the symphysis pubis, is better performed in the infant, child, or adolescent, because of the flexibility of the symphysis pubis in young patients. However, this osteotomy can be performed in adults as well (297). The procedure is more likely to succeed when the CE angle is greater than 10 degrees.

The double-innominate osteotomy of Sutherland and Moore, although rarely performed today, aims to allow greater rotation of the pelvic fragment by cutting through the pubis, instead of merely hinging on it (381). Complications of this procedure can involve injury to the spermatic cords, bladder, and urethra. The triple-innominate osteotomy allows even greater coverage by means of cuts of all three hip bones.

An important factor to be considered when planning correction of acetabular dysplasia by one of the rotational procedures is the amount of dysplasia that needs to be corrected. The amount of coverage obtained by osteotomies such as the Salter procedure is limited, whereas osteotomies that cut all three pelvic bones provide the ability to obtain greater coverage (367,410–412). The closer the cuts are placed to the acetabulum, the greater the femoral head coverage. The triple-innominate osteotomies described by Tonnis and Ganz provide greater rotational possibilities than the one described by Steel (Fig. 24.41). The osteotomies that are

closest to the acetabulum (e.g., Eppright, Wagner, and Naito procedures) provide the greatest potential for redirection, but these require significant technical expertise and have higher rates of complications.

The second group among the treatment options includes acetabuloplasties that involve incomplete cuts and hinge on different aspects of the triradiate cartilage, such as the acetabular procedures described by Pemberton (39,314,316,332,334–336,413–415) and Dega (416–420). These procedures can theoretically decrease the volume of the acetabulum because they depend on the triradiate cartilage as the fulcrum.

Although seemingly obvious, it should be pointed out that osteotomies that depend on the triradiate cartilage as the fulcrum must be done in patients with open triradiate cartilage. Procedures which involve hinging on the triradiate cartilage, such as the Pemberton osteotomy, have the potential to injure the triradiate cartilage and cause premature closure, but these complications are not common (414,416). Procedures that must cross the triradiate cartilage and that would definitely induce closure, such as the Ganz osteotomy, cannot be done in patients with open triradiate cartilage.

A third group of acetabular reconstructive procedures involves placing bone over the hip joint capsule on the uncovered portion of the femoral head. These procedures provide coverage of the femoral head by capsular fibrous metaplasia (421,422). They include the various shelf procedures (423–429) and the medial displacement osteotomy described by Chiari (375–377,422,430–436). In 1981, Staheli and Chew introduced a modification of a previously

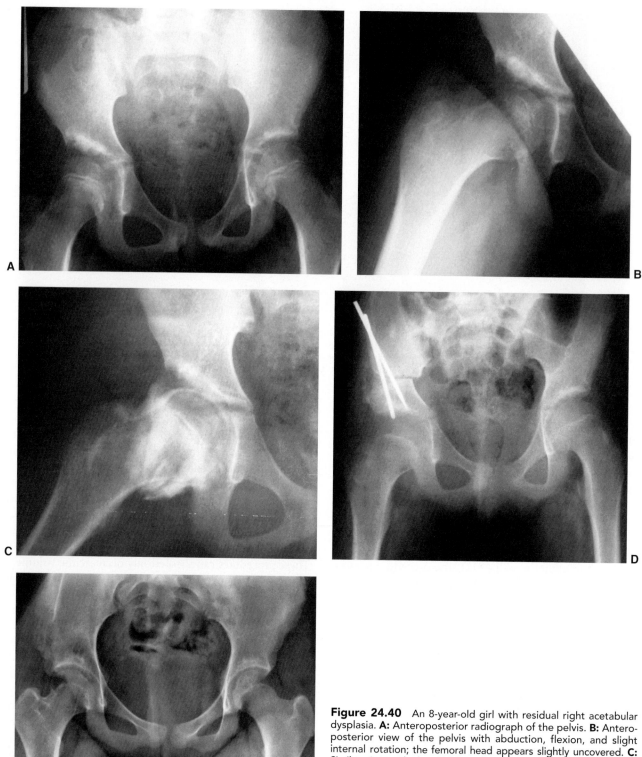

**Figure 24.40** An 8-year-old girl with residual right acetabular dysplasia. **A:** Anteroposterior radiograph of the pelvis. **B:** Anteroposterior view of the pelvis with abduction, flexion, and slight internal rotation; the femoral head appears slightly uncovered. **C:** Similar view with the addition of an arthrographic dye. Note the excellent coverage of the proximal femur by unossified acetabular cartilage. **D:** Immediately after the innominate osteotomy. **E:** Four years after the innominate osteotomy.

described shelf arthroplasty, and this gained widespread acceptance for use on its own in significant anatomic dysplasia, and also in conjunction with various rotational procedures as an augmentation to provide increased femoral head coverage (429) (Figs. 24.39, 24.42).

The shelf arthroplasty (Fig. 24.42) and the Chiari osteotomy (Figs. 24.43 and 24.44) may be performed in well-reduced hips, but they are usually reserved for hips that lack significant femoral head coverage because of inability to acquire such coverage with articular cartilage by

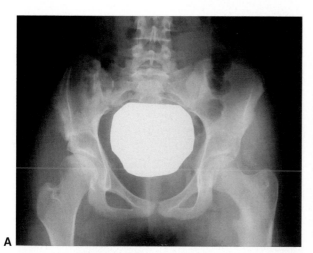
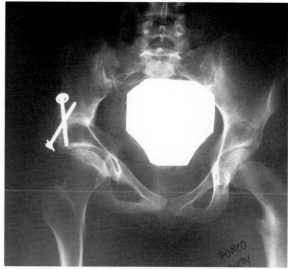

**Figure 24.41** A 16-year-old patient with residual dysplasia after treatment for developmental dislocation of the hip (DDH) and pain. **A:** Preoperative anteroposterior radiograph. **B:** Anteroposterior radiograph 2 years after a triple innominate osteotomy.

means of one of the other procedures mentioned in the preceding text (413,414). Many of these procedures can be performed in patients with early degenerative changes in the hope of delaying the necessity for arthroplasty or fusion. Further discussion of these issues is beyond the scope of this chapter.

The Chiari medial displacement osteotomy hinges on the symphysis pubica, with the distal fragment displacing medially and upward (Figs. 24.43 and 24.44). This medialization results in reduction of the lever arm in order to reduce joint loading. Abductor muscle function is theoretically improved. Patients may limp for as long as 1 year. There is some concern that bilateral Chiari osteotomies may interfere with a woman's ability to deliver children. This is one of the few procedures for which long-term results are available, and these show that, in the absence of subluxation and degenerative joint disease, good long-term outcomes may persist for many years (128,432,437–447).

The fourth group of procedures includes hybrids of the above groups, such as addition of a shelf to a Salter or Pemberton innominate osteotomy when the surgeon feels that inadequate coverage has been obtained by the primary procedure.

### Asymptomatic Mature Patient with Incidentally Discovered Hip Dysplasia

Decision-making is somewhat difficult and controversial in the case of the asymptomatic mature patient with hip dysplasia. For the asymptomatic adolescent with minimal radiographic dysplasia (because degenerative arthritis is a probability but not a certainty), the author prefers to inform the family about the potential for an adverse natural history and recommend surgery only at the onset of symptoms. There is usually a long interval between the

onset of symptoms and degenerative joint disease as evidenced on radiographic images (66). The patient can be reassured that if symptoms develop surgical treatment can help in avoiding long-term degenerative joint disease. However, faced with an adolescent with radiographic evidence of subluxation, regardless of the symptoms, the author recommends surgical correction, because without treatment an adverse natural history is certain.

### Acetabular Rim Syndrome

Over the last several years, as more has been learned about the natural history of hip dysplasia (25,66,209,212, 216,217,343) much attention has been focused also on acetabular rim syndrome (overload of the acetabular rim) (218) in young adults as a primary disease, or as a residual of childhood hip disease. These patients may present with sudden onset of sharp groin pain. They may describe symptoms such as sudden "locking" or a clicking sensation (412). These sensations are precipitated by movements that combine hip flexion, adduction, and internal rotation. Patients may also experience sudden "giving way" sensations. As the site of acetabular rim overload is usually anterior, symptoms are provoked on physical examination by the so-called impingement test. This test brings the anterior aspect of the femoral neck in contact with the anterior acetabulum by internally rotating the hip as it is gradually flexed to 90 degrees and adducted. In acetabular rim syndrome, the patient's original symptom of pain (usually in the groin) will be reproduced. Films taken in a weight-bearing situation and false profile lateral views will show evidence of dysplasia, as previously discussed. One may also see evidence of an acetabular rim fracture suggestive of the rim overload (218,412). A gadolinium-enhanced MRI arthrogram of the hip is the

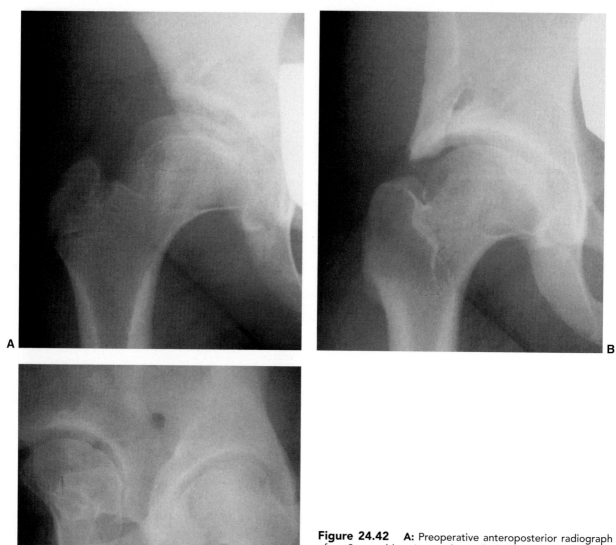

**Figure 24.42   A:** Preoperative anteroposterior radiograph of an 8-year-old patient with residual dysplasia and proximal femoral growth disturbance. **B:** Anteroposterior radiograph 2 years after shelf arthroplasty. **C:** False profile lateral radiograph 2 years after operative procedure.

best test for assessing labral disease (448,449), and a three-dimensional CT scan is the best diagnostic study for ascertaining the acetabular deficiencies.

In a symptomatic patient with hip dysplasia and no or very minimal evidence of arthritis, one of the joint-preserving operations (Ganz, Salter, Tonnis, Naito, Steel, etc., as described in the preceding text) is indicated in order to try to improve an otherwise poor long-term prognosis. A radiograph with the leg in maximal abduction must demonstrate that the femoral head is reduced, covered, and congruent and that good joint space is maintained. These are absolute prerequisites for considering a periacetabular osteotomy (PAO) (Fig 24.41). Labral pathology may have to be dealt with in conjunction with the PAO procedure.

In extreme cases of degenerative joint disease in the late teens or early adult years, hip fusion or total joint arthroplasty may be the only treatment alternatives available.

These circumstances are rare among patients younger than 30 years and are beyond the scope of this text.

### Disturbance of Growth of the Proximal Femur

The most disastrous complication associated with the treatment of DDH involves various degrees of growth disturbance of the proximal femur, including the epiphysis and the physeal plate. This is commonly referred to by the term *aseptic necrosis*. Because there has never been a study of a pathologic specimen from a patient with what is called *aseptic necrosis*, the author prefers to use the term *proximal femoral growth disturbance* (209). These growth disturbances can be precipitated experimentally by creating vascular injuries in animals; the results resemble the growth disturbances seen in humans with treated DDH. The disturbance to growth may be caused by vascular insults to the epiphysis or the physeal plate, or by pressure injury to the epiphyseal cartilage or the physeal plate

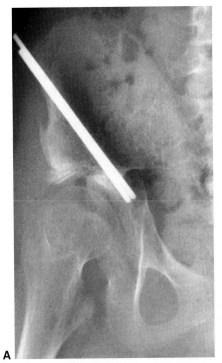
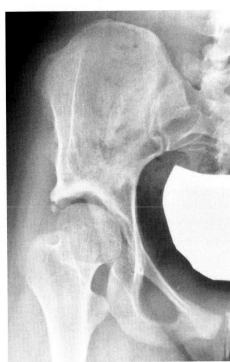

**Figure 24.43** An 11-year-old girl with pain and residual right hip subluxation with severe acetabular dysplasia. **A:** Immediately after the right Chiari osteotomy. Note the additional graft placed anteriorly. **B:** Eight years after the operation, there is excellent remodeling of the acetabulum with sourcil development.

(262,276,277,450–452,453–464). The blood supply to the proximal femur is described in Chapter 25.

Growth disturbance of the proximal femur in DDH occurs only in patients who have been treated. This may also occur in the other normal hip in a patient who has been treated for the involved hip (465,466). The reported incidence of proximal femoral growth disturbance varies from 0% to 73% (209,211,410,411,467–469). Different

opinions exist about the reasons for this variation (470–472). The use of prereduction traction (201,209,211,248,251, 265,455,467,473), adductor tenotomy (279,457, 474), open or closed reduction (43,119,124,305,455,475–477), the force applied during reduction (467,474,478,479), the position in which the patient is immobilized postoperatively (242,248,251,285,276,444,458,460–462,480), and the age at reduction (248,251,256,458) have all been implicated

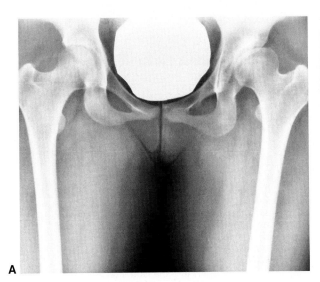
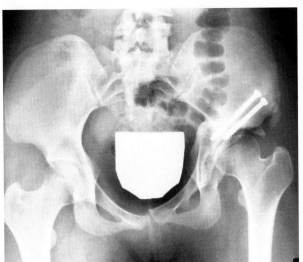

**Figure 24.44** This girl underwent open reduction of the left dysplastic hip at 18 months of age. She presented at 17 years of age with subluxation, as seen on the radiograph. **A:** Preoperative anteroposterior view of the pelvis. **B:** Eight weeks after Chiari osteotomy. Note the additional graft placed anteriorly.

as etiologic factors. Others think that the incidence may be much less variable than the means by which it is assessed (209,471).

In an extensive study of the development of ischemic necrosis published by the German Society for Orthopaedics and Traumatology (3,318), conservatively treated hips and operatively treated hips were evaluated in order to determine the factors associated with the development of ischemic necrosis (182). The factors associated with necrosis included: high dislocations and dislocations with inversion of the labrum; narrowing of the introitus between the superior labrum and the transverse ligament in the position of reduction; inadequate depth of reduction of the femoral head (greater than 3 mm from the acetabular floor); the age of the patient (older than 12 months); immobilization in

60 or more degrees of abduction for joint instability; and adductor tenotomy.

Westin et al. believed that the marked variation in the reported incidence indicated a lack of definition of terms (473). Thomas et al. concluded that there was some association between the reported incidence in a given series and the rigor with which the diagnosis had been sought (471). Buchanan et al. concluded that if signs of growth disturbance were not present within 12 months of reduction they were highly unlikely to appear (248).

Bucholz and Ogden (451) and Kalamchi and MacEwen (455) identified a lateral physeal arrest pattern that may not be evident until a patient is older than 12.5 years (mean, 9 years) (Fig. 24.45). This is the most common pattern of growth disturbance reported. Kalamchi and MacEwen

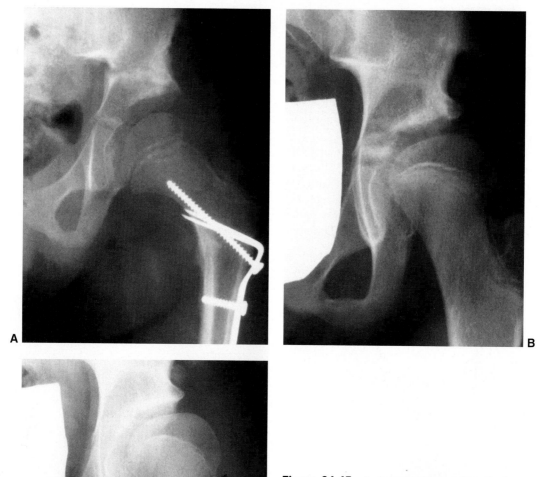

**Figure 24.45  A:** Anteroposterior view of a 5-year-old girl, 3 months after varus derotation osteotomy, an innominate osteotomy for residual dysplasia. She had undergone an open reduction procedure 3 years previously. **B:** Anteroposterior view at 9 years of age. Note the valgus tilt to the proximal femur. **C:** Anteroposterior view at 11 years of age. Note the lateral tether, a typical type II physeal plate tether, and how the tether produces hip subluxation. A physeal growth arrest pattern may not be evident until a patient is 9 years of age or older.

stressed that it may be difficult to identify this group early, and studies reporting growth disturbances with follow-up periods of less than 12 years must be regarded as preliminary and may not reflect the actual incidence of proximal growth disturbance (455).

The incidence of proximal femoral growth disturbance increases with delay in reduction (251,256). Younger patients have a lower rate of growth disturbance. Kalamchi and MacEwen, however, documented an increase in the incidence of the severe form (type IV) in younger patients (455). Salter et al. (285) and Ogden (460,461) proposed that the femoral head in DDH is most vulnerable to ischemic changes during the first 12 to 18 months of life, when it is composed mostly of cartilage. According to some orthopaedic specialists the risk of total head involvement becomes somewhat less after the appearance of the femoral ossific nucleus, although, as mentioned in the preceding text, this concept has recently been challenged (256,288).

Several factors associated with an increased incidence of proximal femoral growth disturbance have been documented in the clinical setting and in experimental studies. These include extremes in positioning of the proximal femur in abduction and abduction with extreme medial rotation. Extremes in position can cause compression of the medial femoral circumflex vessel as it passes the iliopsoas tendon and compression of the terminal branch between the lateral femoral neck and the acetabular margin (285,460,461). Anatomic and experimental investigations have persistently shown that strong medial rotation with concomitant abduction, and extreme abduction alone (i.e., the Lorenz position), can compromise the blood flow to the capital femoral epiphysis. If the hip is maximally abducted against firm resistance, the blood flow can be completely or almost completely arrested. The same is true in forced medial rotation. The blood vessels, and consequently the blood supply to the proximal femur, can be occluded by compression, either outside the femoral head or as the vessels cross through the epiphyseal cartilage (285,277,464). Schoenecker et al. showed a diminution of epiphyseal profusion with increasing pressure, which was relieved after the external fixation device was removed (276,463).

The extreme positions of abduction, frequently called the *frog-leg position* (Fig. 24.34) used in cases of unrelieved adduction contracture, as seen in dislocations, uniformly result in severe growth disturbances of the epiphysis (284,285,463).

Extreme positions can also cause pressure necrosis of the vulnerable epiphyseal cartilage and the physeal plate. This has been experimentally shown by Law et al. (457) and by Schoenecker et al. (463). These studies and others demonstrated the severe effects of cartilage necrosis (182,285,277). These effects can also be precipitated by circumscribed pressure, such as using the vulnerable femoral head as a "dilating sound" to overcome the intraarticular obstacles to reduction.

Severin advocated placing the femoral head in close apposition to the acetabulum in order to induce regression of the

obstacles to reduction (124). The idea is that sustained pressure from the femoral head causes the labrum to adapt itself to the spherical contour of the head. This maneuver can be used for obtaining reduction, but the price may be an increased incidence of necrosis (182,474); and hence the author's unwillingness to use the femoral head as a "dilating sound" to obtain closed reduction. Although the use of pre-reduction traction has been implicated as a factor in reducing the incidence of necrosis, the German Orthopaedic Study Group did not find this to be the case (182).

The continued use of closed techniques in an attempt to make the femoral head overcome the intraarticular obstacles to reduction can lead to severe necrosis (182). If closed reduction is attempted, in the author's opinion the only acceptable result is an anatomically perfect reduction; otherwise, the hip must be reduced openly so as to prevent damage to the vulnerable femoral head (182,481,482).

The most widely used classification of proximal femoral growth disturbance is that of Salter et al. (285) (Table 24.2). The author disagrees with the inclusion of coxa magna, because coxa magna is often seen after open reduction as a result of the stimulation of blood flow to the proximal femur (483–485). It is also often difficult to ascertain whether some of the residual deformities seen after treatment for DDH are alterations in the proximal femur secondary to disturbances that occurred before the reduction, or whether they are the result of complications associated with the reduction. One of the most common deformities seen is the flattening of the medial aspect of the proximal femur, which occurs because of pressure of the femoral head lying against the ilium before reduction.

Another area of uncertainty relates to temporary irregular ossification of the femoral epiphysis, and whether this

### TABLE 24.2

**SALTER'S CLASSIFICATION OF GROWTH DISTURBANCE OF THE FEMORAL HEAD**

| Class | Features |
|---|---|
| 1 | Failure of the appearance of the ossific nucleus of the femoral head within 1 year after reduction |
| 2 | Failure of growth of an existing ossific nucleus within 1 year after reduction |
| 3 | Broadening of the femoral neck within 1 year after reduction |
| 4 | Increased radiographic bone density, followed by fragmentation of the femoral head |
| 5 | Residual deformity of the femoral head and neck when reossification is complete; these deformities include coxa magna, coxa plana, coxa vara, and a short, broad femoral neck. |

From Salter RB, Kostiuk J, Dallas S. Avascular necrosis of the femoral head as a complication of treatment for congenital dislocation of the hip in young children: a clinical and experimental investigation. *Can J Surg* 1969;12:44.

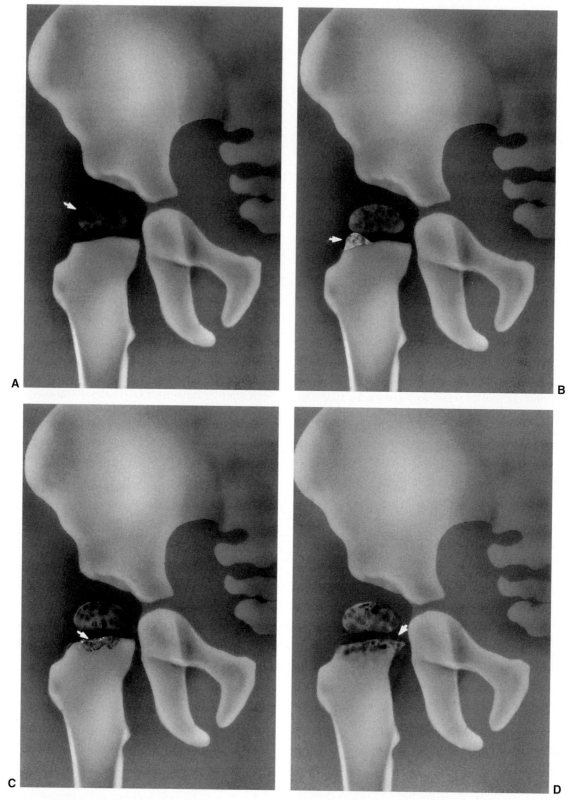

**Figure 24.46** Classification of proximal femoral growth disturbances. **A:** Group I. **B:** Group II. **C:** Group III. **D:** Group IV. (Adapted from Kalamchi A, MacEwen GD. Avascular necrosis following treatment of congenital dislocation of the hip. *J Bone Joint Surg Am* 1980;62:876.)

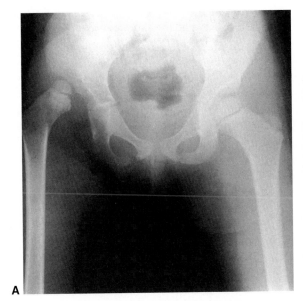
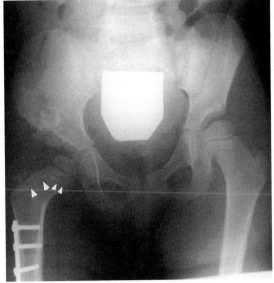

**Figure 24.47** A 3-year-old girl with right developmental dysplasia of the hip. **A:** Preoperative radiograph. **B:** Ten months after operative open reduction, femoral shortening, and Pemberton osteotomy. Note the presence of growth arrest line at the proximal femur (O'Brien lines; *arrows*); also note similar lines on the opposite, normal hip.

represents damage to the epiphyseal cartilage or merely multiple ossification centers that eventually coalesce. These areas may be analogous to the accessory centers of ossification seen in the periphery of the acetabulum. This pattern usually does not result in growth disturbance of the proximal femur. Only long-term follow-up studies of this entity can resolve this issue.

Kalamchi and MacEwen developed a classification of necrosis, emphasizing the growth disturbances associated with various degrees of physeal arrest (455). This classification (Fig. 24.46) puts all the growth disturbances seen in the ossific nucleus into one category if they are not associated with physeal involvement. Bucholz and Ogden provided an additional classification based on patterns of vascular supply resulting in partial or total ischemia (451). There are few studies documenting the interobserver or intraobserver reliability of these classifications of growth disturbance. As many as 25% of hips may not fit into any particular classification.

O'Brien et al. discussed the importance of identification of growth disturbance lines in predicting future deformity of the proximal femur (486,487) (Fig. 24.47). These growth arrest lines may provide the physician with early evidence of a future problem. However, the utility of this approach must await long-term follow-up studies.

There are long-term follow-up studies of patients having proximal femoral growth disturbance (182,262,488). The results indicate that any alteration or disturbance of proximal femoral growth decreases the longevity of the hip. As previously discussed, recent attention has focused on femoral acetabular impingement syndrome in patients with residual deformities of the proximal end of the femur, and their effect on the induction of labral tears and early osteoarthritis. (489–491)

In the treatment of the residual effects of necrosis, reduction must be maintained by corrective femoral and/or acetabular procedures (492,493). With arrest of the proximal femoral physeal plate, trochanteric overgrowth ensues, producing an abductor lurch (Fig. 24.48). If the problem is identified, greater trochanteric physeal plate arrest may be carried out, and this may maintain articular

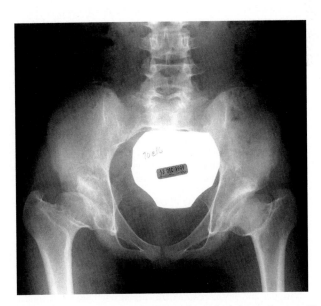

**Figure 24.48** A 14-year-old girl with residual dysplasia, type III growth arrest, and trochanteric overgrowth. The patient had bilateral open reductions at 14 months of age. She had a type III growth arrest of the proximal femur with resultant disturbance of growth and corresponding acetabular deformity and trochanteric overgrowth. Her Trendelenburg test was negative. Some patients with this deformity have an abductor lurch, necessitating distal transfer of the greater trochanter.

trochanteric distance if performed in children younger than 8 years (21,454,455,494,495,); otherwise, distal transfer of the greater trochanter may be necessary (417, 456–458,496–498).

The key to the diagnosis and management of DDH is early detection. This results in a 95% success rate of treatment with a low risk of complications. It is the initial treating physician who has the greatest chance of successfully achieving a normal hip. Orthopaedic surgeons must educate primary care colleagues in making the diagnosis early and initiating prompt referral.

## REFERENCES

### Growth Disturbance of the Proximal Femur

1. Surgeons Advisory Statement, American Academy of Orthopaedic Surgeons. "CDH" should be "DDH". Park Ridge, IL: American Academy of Orthopaedic Surgeons, 1991.
2. Klisic P, Jankovic L, Basara V. Long-term results of combined operative reduction of the hip in older children. J Pediatr Orthop 1988;8:532.

### Normal Growth and Development of the Hip Joint

3. Gardiner HM, Dunn PM. Controlled trial of immediate splinting versus ultrasonographic surveillance in congenitally dislocatable hips. Lancet 1990;336:1553.
4. Lee J, Jarvis J, Uhthoff HK, et al. The fetal acetabulum: a histomorphometric study of acetabular anteversion and femoral head coverage. Clin Orthop 1992;281:48.
5. Strayer LM. Embryology of the human hip joint. Yale J Biol Med 1943;16:13.
6. Strayer LM Jr. Embryology of the human hip joint. Clin Orthop 1971;74:221.
7. Watanabe RS. Embryology of the human hip. Clin Orthop 1974;98:8.
8. Dunn PM. The anatomy and pathology of congenital dislocation of the hip. Clin Orthop 1976;119:23.
9. Ponseti IV. Morphology of the acetabulum in congenital dislocation of the hip: gross, histological and roentgenographic studies. J Bone Joint Surg Am 1978;60:586.
10. Harrison TJ. The influence of the femoral head on pelvic growth and acetabular form in the rat. J Anat 1961;95:127.
11. Ponseti IV. Growth and development of the acetabulum in the normal child: anatomical, histological and roentgenographic studies. J Bone Joint Surg Am 1978;60:575.
12. Gardner E, Gray D. Prenatal development of the human hip joint. Am J Anat 1950;87:163.
13. Walker JM. Histological study of the fetal development of the human acetabulum and labrum: significance in congenital hip disease. Yale J Biol Med 1981;54:255.
14. Portinaro NM, Murray DW, Benson MKD. Microanatomy of the acetabular cavity and its relation to growth. J Bone Joint Surg Br 2001;83-B:377–383.
15. Harrison TJ. The growth of the pelvis in the rat: a mensoral and morphological study. J Anat 1958;92:236.
16. Siffert RS. Patterns of deformity of the developing hip. Clin Orthop Relat Res 1981;160:14.
17. Gage JR, Canny JM. The effects of trochanteric epiphysiodesis on growth of the proximal end of the femur following necrosis of the capital femoral epiphysis. J Bone Joint Surg Am 1980;62:785.
18. Osborne D, Effmann E, Broda K, et al. The development of the upper end of the femur with special reference to its internal architecture. Radiology 1980;137:71.
19. Schofield CB, Smibert JG. Trochanteric growth disturbance after upper femoral osteotomy for congenital dislocation of the hip. J Bone Joint Surg Br 1990;72:32.
20. Sugano NN, Noble PC, Kamaric E, et al. The morphology of the femur in developmental dysplasia of the hip. J Bone Joint Surg Br 1998;80:711.
21. Iverson LJ, Kalea V, Eberle C. Relative trochanteric overgrowth after ischemic necrosis in congenital dislocation of the hip. J Pediatr Orthop 1989;9:391.
22. Coleman CR, Slager RF, Smith WS. The effect of environmental influence on acetabular development. Surg Forum 1958;9:775.
23. Smith WS, Ireton RJ, Coleman CR. Sequelae of experimental dislocation of a weight-bearing ball-and-socket joint in a young growing animal. J Bone Joint Surg Am 1958;40:1121.
24. Smith WS, Coleman CR, Olix ML, et al. Etiology of congenital dislocation of the hip. J Bone Joint Surg Am 1963;45:491.
25. Weinstein SL. Natural history of congenital hip dislocation [CDH] and hip dysplasia. Clin Orthop 1987;225:62.
26. Carter CO, Wilkinson J. Congenital dislocation of the hip. J Bone Joint Surg Br 1960;42:669.
27. Carter CO, Wilkinson JA. Genetic and environmental factors in the etiology of congenital dislocation of the hip. Clin Orthop 1964;33:119.
28. Coleman SS. Diagnosis of congenital dysplasia of the hip in the newborn infant. J Bone Joint Surg Am 1956;162:548.
29. Skirving AP, Scadden WJ. The African neonatal hip and its immunity from congenital dislocation. J Bone Joint Surg Br 1979;61:339.
30. Wynne-Davies R. Acetabular dysplasia and familial joint laxity: two etiological factors in congenital dislocations of the hip. J Med Genet 1970;7:315.

### Pathoanatomy

31. Ishii Y, Weinstein SL, Ponseti IV. Correlation between arthrograms and operative findings in congenital dislocation of the hip. Clin Orthop 1980;153:138.
32. Ortolani M. Congenital hip dysplasia in the light of early and very early diagnosis. Clin Orthop 1976;119:6.
33. Mubarak S, Garfin S, Vance R, et al. Pitfalls in the use of the pavlik harness for treatment of congenital dysplasia, subluxation and dislocation of the hip. J Bone Joint Surg Am 1981;63:1239.
34. Harris NH, Lloyd-Roberts GC, Gallien R. Acetabular development in congenital dislocation of the hip with special reference to the indications for acetabuloplasty and pelvic or femoral realignment osteotomy. J Bone Joint Surg Br 1975;57:46.
35. Harris IE, Dickens R, Menelaus MB. Use of the pavlik harness for hip displacements. Clin Orthop 1992;281:29.
36. Lindstrom JR, Ponseti IV, Wenger DR. Acetabular development after reduction in congenital dislocation of the hip. J Bone Joint Surg Am 1979;61:112.
37. Harris NH. Acetabular growth potential in congenital dislocation of the hip and some factors upon which it may depend. Clin Orthop 1976;119:99.
38. Mardam-Bey TH, MacEwen GD. Congenital hip dislocation after walking age. J Pediatr Orthop 1982;2:478.
39. Pemberton PA. Pericapsular osteotomy of the ilium for treatment of congenital subluxation and dislocation of the hip. J Bone Joint Surg Am 1965;87:65.
40. Salter RB. Innominate osteotomy in treatment of congenital dislocation of the hip. J Bone Joint Surg Br 1961;43:72.
41. Schwartz D. Acetabular development after reduction of congenital dislocation of the hip: a follow-up study of fifty hips. J Bone Joint Surg Am 1965;47:705.
42. Somerville EW. A long-term follow-up of congenital dislocation of the hip. J Bone Joint Surg Br 1978;60:25.
43. Weinstein SL, Ponseti IV. Congenital dislocation of the hip. J Bone Joint Surg Am 1979;61:119.
44. Wiberg G. Studies on dysplastic acetabula and congenital subluxation of the hip joint. Acta Chir Scand 1939;83(Suppl. 58):1.

### Pathogenesis, Epidemiology, and Diagnosis

45. Bjerkreim I, Arseth PH. Congenital dislocation of the hip in Norway: late diagnosis CDH in the years 1970 to 1974. Acta Paediatr Scand 1978;67:329.
46. Bjerkreim I, Johansen J. Late diagnosed congenital dislocation of the hip. Acta Orthop Scand 1987;58:504.
47. Coleman SS. Congenital dysplasia of the hip in the Navajo infant. Clin Orthop 1968;56:179.
48. Coleman SS. Congenital dysplasia and dislocation of the hip. Louis, MO: Mosby, 1978.

49. Czeizel A, Szentpetery J, Kellermann M. Incidence of congenital dislocation of the hip in hungary. *Br J Prev Soc Med* 1974;28:265.

50. Edlestein J. Congenital dislocation of the hip in the Bantu. *J Bone Joint Surg Br* 1966;48:397.

51. Getz B. The hip in Lapps and its bearing on the problem of congenital dislocation. *Acta Orthop Scand Suppl* 1955;22.

52. Heikkila E. Congenital dislocation of the hip in Finland: an epidemiologic analysis of 1035 cases. *Acta Orthop Scand* 1984;55:125.

53. Hoagland FT, Yau AC, Wong WL. Osteoarthritis of the hip and other joints in Southern Chinese in Hong Kong. *J Bone Joint Surg Am* 1973;55:545.

54. Hoaglund FT, Healey JH. Osteoarthrosis and congenital dysplasia of the hip in family members of children who have congenital dysplasia of the hip. *J Bone Joint Surg Am* 1990;72:1510; erratum 1991;73:293.

55. Pompe Van Meerdervoort HF. Congenital musculoskeletal disorders in the South African Negro. *J Bone Joint Surg Br* 1977;59:257.

56. Rabin DL, Barnett CR, Arnold WD, et al. Untreated congenital hip disease: a study of the epidemiology, natural history and social aspects of the disease in a Navajo population. *Am J Public Health* 1965;55:1.

57. Wedge JH, Wasylenko MJ. The natural history of congenital dislocation of the hip: a critical review. *Clin Orthop* 1978; 137:154.

58. Albinana JM, Morcuende JA, Delgado E, et al. Radiologic pelvic asymmetry in unilateral late diagnosed developmental dysplasia of the hip. *J Pediatr Orthop* 1995;15:753.

59. Haasbeek JF, Wright JG, Hedden DM. Is there a difference between the epidemiologic characteristics of hip dislocation diagnosed early and late? *Can J Surg* 1995;38:437.

60. Fabry G, MacEwen GD, Shands AR Jr. Torsion of the femur: a follow-up study in normal and abnormal conditions. *J Bone Joint Surg Am* 1973;55:1726.

61. LeDamany P. La luxation congenitale de la hanche. *Etudes d'anatomie comparee d'anthropogenie normale et pathologique, deductions therapeutique.* Paris: Feliz Alcan, 1912.

62. Wedge JH, Munkacsi I, Loback D. Anteversion of the femur and idiopathic osteoarthrosis of the hip. *J Bone Joint Surg Am* 1989;71:1040.

63. Walker JM. Morphological variants in the human fetal hip joint: their significance in congenital hip disease. *J Bone Joint Surg Am* 1980;62:1073.

64. Walker JM, Goldsmith CH. Morphometric study of the fetal development of the human hip joint: significance for congenital hip disease. *Yale J Biol Med* 1981;54:411.

65. Palmen K. Prevention of congenital dislocation of the hip: the Swedish experience of neonatal treatment of hip joint instability. *Acta Orthop Scand Suppl* 1984;208:1.

66. Wedge JH, Wasylenko MJ. The natural history of congenital disease of the hip. *J Bone Joint Surg Br* 1979;61:334.

67. Yamamuro T, Ishida K. Recent advances in the prevention, early diagnosis, and treatment of congenital dislocation of the hip in Japan. *Clin Orthop* 1984;184:34.

68. Albinana J, Quesada JA, Certucha JA. Children at high risk for congenital dislocation of the hip: late presentation. *J Pediatr Orthop* 1993;13:268.

69. Asher MA. Orthopedic screening: especially congenital dislocation of the hip and spinal deformity. *Pediatr Clin North Am* 1977;24:713.

70. Asher MA. Screening for congenital dislocation of the hip, scoliosis, and other abnormalities affecting the musculoskeletal system. *Pediatr Clin North Am* 1986;33:1335.

71. Dunn PM. Prenatal observation on the etiology of congenital dislocation of the hip. *Clin Orthop* 1976;119:11.

72. Kumar SJ, MacEwen GD. The incidence of hip dysplasia with metatarsus adductus. *Clin Orthop* 1982;164:234.

73. Weiner DS. Congenital dislocation of the hip associated with congenital muscular torticollis. *Clin Orthop* 1976;121:163.

74. Salter R. Etiology, pathogenesis, and possible prevention of congenital dislocation of the hip. *Can Med Assoc J* 1968;98:933.

75. Wilkinson JA. A postnatal survey for the congenital displacement of the hip. *J Bone Joint Surg Br* 1972;54:40.

76. Abd-el-Kader-Shaheen M. Mehad: the Saudi tradition of infant wrapping as a possible aetiological factor in congenital dislocation of the hip. *J R Coll Surg Edinb* 1989;34:85.

77. Kutlu A, Memik R, Mutlu M, et al. Congenital dislocation of the hip and its relation to swaddling used in turkey. *J Pediatr Orthop* 1992;12:598.

78. Pratt WB, Freiberger RH, Arnold WD. Untreated congenital hip dysplasia in the Navajo. *Clin Orthop* 1982;162:69.

79. Yamamuro T, Doi H. Diagnosis and treatment of congenital dislocation of the hip in newborns. *J Jpn Orthop Assoc* 1965;39:492.

80. Ralis A, McKibbin B. Changes in shape of the human hip joint during its development and their relation to its stability. *J Bone Joint Surg Br* 1973;55:780.

81. McKibbin B. Anatomical factors in the stability of the hip joint in the newborn. *J Bone Joint Surg Br* 1970;63:148.

82. Dunn PM. Congenital dislocation of the hip (CDH): necropsy studies at birth. *J R Soc Med* 1969;62:1035.

83. Palmen K. Preluxation of the hip joint: diagnosis and treatment in the newborn and the diagnosis of congenital dislocation of the hip joint in Sweden during the years 1948-1960. *Acta Paediatr Scand Suppl* 1961;129:1.

84. Ortolani M. *Nuovi criteri diagnostici profilattico correttvi.* Bologna: Cappelli, 1948.

85. Barlow TG. Early diagnosis and treatment of congenital dislocation of the hip. *J Bone Joint Surg Br* 1962;44:292.

86. Danielsson LG, Nilsson BE. Attitudes to CDH [guest editorial]. *Acta Orthop Scand* 1984;55:244.

87. Hilgenreiner H. Aur Fruhdiagnose und Fruhbehandlung der angeborenen Huftgelenkuerrenkung. *Med Klin* 1925;21:1385.

88. MacNicol MF. Results of a 25-year screening programme for neonatal hip instability. *J Bone Joint Surg Br* 1990;72:1057.

89. Hadlow V. Neonatal screening for congenital dislocation of the hip: a prospective 21-year survey. *J Bone Joint Surg Br* 1988;70:740.

90. Hansson G, Nachemson A, Palmen K. Screening of children with congenital dislocation of the hip joint on the maternity wards in Sweden. *J Pediatr Orthop* 1983;3:271.

91. Ilfeld FW, Westin GW. "Missed" or late-diagnosed congenital dislocation of the hip: a clinical entity. *Isr J Med Sci* 1980; 16:260.

92. Ilfeld FW, Westin GW, Makin M. Missed or developmental dislocation of the hip. *Clin Orthop* 1986;203:276.

93. Jones D. An assessment of the value of examination of the hip in the newborn. *J Bone Joint Surg Br* 1977;59:318.

94. MacKenzie IG, Wilson JG. Problems encountered in the early diagnosis and management of congenital dislocation of the hip. *J Bone Joint Surg Br* 1981;63:38.

95. Noble TC, Pullan CR, Craft AW, et al. Difficulties in diagnosing and managing congenital dislocation of the hip. *Br Med J* 1978;2:620.

96. Walker G. Problems in the early recognition of congenital hip dislocation. *Br Med J* 1971;3:147.

97. Chan AC, Cundy P, Foster BK, et al. Late diagnosis of congenital dislocation of the hip and presence of a screening programme: South Australia population-based study. *Lancet* 1999;54:1514.

98. Darmonov A. Clinical screening for congenital dislocation of the hip. *J Bone Joint Surg Am* 1996;78:383.

99. Godward SDC. Surgery for congenital dislocation of the hip in the UK as a measure of outcome of screening. *Lancet* 1998; 351:1149.

100. Fellander M, Gladnikoff H, Jacobsson E. Instability of the hip in the newborn. *Acta Orthop Scand Suppl* 1970;130:36.

101. Fredensborg N, Nilsson BE. Overdiagnosis of congenital dislocation of the hip. *Clin Orthop* 1976;119:89.

102. Czeizel A, Tusnady G, Vaczo G, et al. The mechanism of genetic predisposition in congenital dislocation of the hip. *J Med Genet* 1975;12:121.

103. Czeizel AE, Intody Z, Modell B. What proportion of congenital abnormalities can be prevented? *Br Med J* 1993;306:499.

104. Jones DA. Neonatal hip stability and the Barlow test: a study in stillborn babies. *J Bone Joint Surg Br* 1991;73:216.

105. Robinson R. Effective screening in child health. *Br Med J* 1998; 316:1.

106. Churgay CA, Caruthers BS. Diagnosis and treatment of congenital dislocation of the hip. *Am Fam Physician* 1992;45:1217.

107. Frankenburg WK. To screen or not to screen: congenital dislocation of the hip [Editorial]. *Am J Public Health* 1981;71:1311.

108. von Rosen S. Diagnosis and treatment of congenital dislocation of the hip in the newborn. *J Bone Joint Surg Br* 1962;44:284.

109. Weinstein SL. The medial approach in congenital dislocation of the hip. *Isr J Med Sci* 1980;16:272.

110. Duppe H, Danielsson LG. Screening of neonatal instability and of developmental dislocation of the hip. A survey of 132,601 living newborn infants between 1956 and 1999. *J Bone Joint Surg Br* 2002;84(6):878–885.

111. Hass J. *Congenital dislocation of the hip.* Springfield, IL: Charles C Thomas Publisher, 1951.

112. Stanisavljevic S. *Diagnosis and treatment of congenital hip pathology in the newborn.* Baltimore, MD: Williams & Wilkins, 1964.

113. D'Souza LH, Hynes K, McManus F. Radiological screening for congenital dislocation in the infant at risk. *J Bone Joint Surg Br* 1996;78:319.

114. Ando M, Gotoh E. Significance of inguinal folds for diagnosis of congenital dislocation of the hip in infants aged three to four months. *J Pediatr Orthop* 1990;10:331.

115. Weinstein SL. Closed versus open reduction of congenital hip dislocation in patients under 2 years of age. *Orthopedics* 1990;13:221.

116. Weinstein SL. Congenital hip dislocation: long-range problems, residual signs, and symptoms after successful treatment. *Clin Orthop* 1992;281:69.

117. Danielsson L, Late-diagnosed DDH. A prospective 11 year follow up of 71 consecutive patients (75 hips). *Acta Orthop Scand* 2000;71(3):232–242.

118. Hattori T, Ono Y, Kitakoji T, et al. Soft tissue interposition after closed reduction in developmental dysplasia of the hip: the long term effect on acetabular development and aseptic necrosis. *J Bone Joint Surg Br* 1999;81:385.

119. Ferguson AB Jr. Treatment of congenital dislocation of the hip in infancy using the medial approach. In: Tachdjian MO, ed. *Congenital dislocation of the hip.* New York: Churchill Livingstone, 1982:283.

120. Leveuf J. Results of open reduction of "true" congenital luxation of the hip. *J Bone Joint Surg Am* 1948;30:875.

121. Ludloff K. The open reduction of the congenital hip dislocation by an anterior incision. *Am J Orthop Surg* 1913;10:438.

122. Mau H, Dorr WM, Henkel L, et al. Open reduction of congenital dislocation of the hip by Ludloffs method. *J Bone Joint Surg Br* 1971;53:1281.

123. Morcuende JA, Weinstein SL, Dolan L, et al. DDH: results of treatment after reduction by an anteromedial surgical approach at a minimum four year follow-up. *J Bone Joint Surg* 1997;79A:810.

124. Severin E. Contribution to the knowledge of congenital dislocation of the hip. *Acta Chir Scand Suppl* 1941;63:84.

125. Weintroub S, Green I, Terdiman R, et al. Growth and development of congenitally dislocated hips reduced in early infancy. *J Bone Joint Surg Am* 1979;61:125.

126. Lee DY, Choi IH, Lee CK, et al. Assessment of complex hip deformity using three-dimensional CT image. *J Pediatr Orthop* 1991;11:13.

127. O'Hara JN. Congenital dislocation of the hip: acetabular deficiency in adolescence (absence of the lateral acetabular epiphysis) after limbectomy in infancy. *J Pediatr Orthop* 1989;9:640.

128. Benson MKD, Evans JDC. The pelvic osteotomy of chiari: an anatomical study of the hazards and misleading radiographic appearance. *J Bone Joint Surg Br* 1976;58:163.

129. Bialik V, Reuveni A, Pery M, et al. Ultrasonography in developmental displacement of the hip: a critical analysis of our results. *J Pediatr Orthop* 1989;9:154.

130. Czubak J, Kotwicki T, Ponitek T, et al. Ultrasound measurements of the newborn hip. Comparison of two methods in 657 newborns [comment]. *Acta Orthop Scand* 1998;69(1):21–24.

131. Omeroglu H, Bicimoglu A, Koparal S, et al. Assessment of variations in the measurement of hip ultrasonography by the Graf method in developmental dysplasia of the hip. *J Pediatr Orthop B* 2001;10(2):89–95.

132. Marks DS, Clegg J, Al-Chalabi AN. Routine ultrasound screening for neonatal hip instability: can it abolish late-presenting congenital dislocation of the hip? *J Bone Joint Surg Br* 1994;76:534.

133. Morin C, Harcke HT, MacEwen GD. The infant hip: real-time US assessment of acetabular development. *Radiology* 1985;157:673.

134. Polanuer PA, Harcke HT, Bowen JR. Effective use of ultrasound in the management of congenital dislocation and/or dysplasia of the hip. *Clin Orthop* 1990;252:176.

135. Stone MH, Clarke NM, Campbell MJ, et al. Comparison of audible sound transmission with ultrasound in screening for congenital dislocation of the hip. *Lancet* 1990;336:421.

136. Uden A, Lindberg H, Josefsson PO, et al. Sonography in the diagnosis of neonatal hip instability. *Acta Orthop Scand* 1988;59(Suppl. 227):94.

137. Feldman DS. How to avoid missing congenital dislocation of the hip. *Lancet* 1999;354:1490.

138. Frank P, Jones D. Neonatal detection of developmental dysplasia of the hip (DDH). *J Bone Joint Surg Br* 1999;81:560.

139. Jones D. Neonatal detection of developmental dysplasia of the hip (DDH). *J Bone Joint Surg Br* 1998;80:943.

140. Bialik VB, Bialik GM, Blazer S, et al. Developmental dysplasia of the hip: a new approach to incidence. *Pediatrics* 1999;103:93.

141. Falliner AH, Hahne HJ, Hassenpflug J. Sonographic hip screening and early management of developmental dysplasia of the hip. *J Pediatr Orthop B* 1999;8:112.

142. Paton RS, Srinivasan MS, Shah B, et al. Ultrasound screening for hips at risk in developmental dysplasia: is it worth it? *J Bone Joint Surg Br* 1999;81:255.

143. Graf R. The diagnosis of congenital hip-joint dislocation by the ultrasonic compound treatment. *Arch Orthop Trauma Surg* 1980; 97:117.

144. Graf R. Hip sonography in infancy: procedure and clinical significance. *Fortschr Med* 1985;103:62.

145. Harcke HT, Lee MS, Sinning L, et al. Ossification center of the infant hip: sonographic and radiographic correlation. *AJR Am J Roentgenol* 1986;147:317.

146. Harcke HT, Kumar SJ. The role of ultrasound in the diagnosis and management of congenital dislocation and dysplasia of the hip. *J Bone Joint Surg Am* 1991;73:622.

147. Harcke HT. Imaging in congenital dislocation and dysplasia of the hip. *Clin Orthop* 1992;281:22.

148. Harcke H. The role of ultrasound in diagnosis and management of developmental dysplasia of the hip. *Pediatr Radiol* 1995;25:225.

149. Terjesen T, Bredland T, Berg V. Ultrasound screening of the hip joints. *Acta Orthop Scand* 1988;59(Suppl. 227):93.

150. Terjesen T, Runden T, Tangerud A. Ultrasonography and radiography of the hip in infants. *Acta Orthop Scand* 1989;60:651.

151. Terjesen T, Bredland T, Berg V. Ultrasound for hip assessment in the newborn. *J Bone Joint Surg Br* 1989;71:767.

152. Terjesen T. Femoral head coverage evaluated by ultrasonography in infants and children. *Mapfre Med* 1992;3(Suppl. 1):41.

153. Clarke NM, Harcke HT, McHugh P, et al. Real-time ultrasound in the diagnosis of congenital dislocation and dysplasia of the hip. *J Bone Joint Surg Br* 1985;67:406.

154. Clarke NMP, Clegg J, Al-Chalabi AN. Ultrasound screening of hips at risk for CDH: failure to reduce the incidence of late cases. *J Bone Joint Surg Br* 1989;71:9.

155. Clarke NM. Diagnosing congenital dislocation of the hip [editorial]. *Br Med J* 1992;305:435.

156. Bialik V, Wiener F. Sonography in suspected developmental dysplasia of the hip. *J Pediatr Orthop B* 1993;2:152.

157. Catterall A. The early diagnosis of congenital dislocation of the hip [Editorial]. *J Bone Joint Surg Br* 1994;76:515.

158. Dahlstrom H, Oberg L, Friberg S. Sonography in congenital dislocation of the hip. *Acta Orthop Scand* 1986;57:402.

159. Dahlstrom H, Friberg S, Oberg L. Current role of sonography in late CDH. *Acta Orthop Scand* 1988;59(Suppl. 227):94.

160. Engesaeter LB, Wilson DJ, Nag D, et al. Ultrasound and congenital dislocation of the hip: the importance of dynamic assessment. *J Bone Joint Surg Br* 1990;72:197.

161. Gardiner HM, Clarke NM, Dunn PM. A sonographic study of the morphology of the preterm neonatal hip. *J Pediatr Orthop* 1990;10:633.

162. Rosendahl K, Markestad T, Lie RT. Congenital dislocation of the hip: a prospective study comparing ultrasound and clinical examination. *Acta Paediatr* 1992;81:177.

163. Terjesen TH, Holen KJ, Tegnander A. Hip abnormalities detected by ultrasound in clinically normal newborn infants. *J Bone Joint Surg Br* 1996;78:636.

164. Hernandez RJ, Cornell RG, Hensinger RN. Ultrasound diagnosis of neonatal congenital dislocation of the hip. *J Bone Joint Surg Br* 1994;76:539.

165. Rosendahl KM, Markestad T, Lie RT, et al. Cost effectiveness of alternative screening strategies for developmental dysplasia of the hip. *Arch Pediatr Adolesc Med* 1995;149:643.

166. Rosendahl K, Markestad T, Lie RT. Developmental dysplasia of the hip: a population based comparison of ultrasound and clinical findings. *Acta Pediatr* 1996;85:64.

167. Terjesen T. Ultrasound as the primary imaging method in the diagnosis of hip dysplasia in children aged < 2 years. *J Pediatr Orthop B* 1996;5:123.

168. Holen KJ, Tegnander A, Bredland T, et al. Universal or selective screening of the neonatal hip using ultrasound? A prospective, randomized trial of 15, 529 newborn infants. *J Bone Joint Surg Br* 2002;84(6):886–890.

169. Boeree NR, Clarke NMP. Ultrasound imaging and secondary screening for congenital dislocation of the hip. *J Bone Joint Surg Br* 1994;76:525.

170. Taylor G, Clarke NMP. Monitoring treatment of developmental dysplasia of the hip with the pavlik harness: the role of ultrasound. *J Bone Joint Surg Br* 1997;79:719.

171. Kernohan WG, Beverland DE, McCoy GF, et al. Vibration arthrometry: a preview. *Acta Orthop Scand* 1990;61:70.

172. Kernohan WG, Cowie GH, Mollan RA. Vibration arthrometry in congenital dislocation of the hip. *Clin Orthop* 1991;272:167.

173. Kernohan WG, Trainor B, Nugent G, et al. Low-frequency vibration emitted from unstable hip in human neonate. *Clin Orthop* 1993;288:214.

174. Broughton NS, Brougham DI, Cole WG, et al. Reliability of radiological measurements in the assessment of the child's hip. *J Bone Joint Surg Br* 1989;71:6.

175. Weinstein S. Traction in developmental dislocation of the hip: is its use justified? *Clin Orthop* 1997;338:79.

176. O'Brien T, Barry C. The importance of standardized radiographs when assessing hip dysplasia. *Jr Med J* 1990;83:159.

177. Almby B, Lonnerholm T. Hip joint instability after the neonatal period. I. Value of measuring the acetabular angle. *Acta Radio Diagn* 1979;20:200.

178. Anda S, Terjesen T, Kvistad KA, et al. Acetabular angles and femoral anteversion in dysplastic hips in adults: CT investigation. *J Comput Assist Tomogr* 1991;15:115.

179. Anda S, Terjesen T, Kvistad KA. Computed tomography measurements of the acetabulum in adult dysplastic hips: which level is appropriate? *Skeletal Radiol* 1991;20:267.

180. Garvey M, Donoghue VB, Gorman WA, et al. Radiographic screening at four months of infants at risk for congenital hip dislocation. *J Bone Joint Surg Br* 1992;74:704.

181. Tonnis D. Normal values of the hip joint for the evaluation of x-rays in children and adults. *Clin Orthop* 1976;119:39.

182. Tonnis D, ed. *Congenital dysplasia and dislocation of the hip in children and adults.* New York: Springer-Verlag, 1987.

183. Papavasiliou VA, Piggott H. Acetabular floor thickening and femoral head enlargement in congenital dislocation of the hip: lateral displacement of femoral head. *J Pediatr Orthop* 1983;3:22.

184. Albinana J, Morcuende JA, Weinstein SL. Predictive value of the teardrop figure in congenital dislocation of the hip: a quantitative study, Annual Meeting 1994.

185. Kohler A. *Roentgenology.* London: Bailliere, Tindall & Cox, 1935.

186. Samani DJ, Weinstein SL. The pelvic tear-figure: a three-dimensional analysis of the anatomy and effects of rotation. *J Pediatr Orthop* 1994;14:650.

187. Smith JT, Matan S, Coleman SS, et al. The predictive value of the development of the acetabular teardrop figure in developmental dysplasia of the hip. Presented at the American Academy of Orthopaedic Surgeons Annual Meeting, San Francisco, CA, 1993.

188. Vare VB. The anatomy of the pelvic tear figure. *J Bone Joint Surg Am* 1952;34:167.

189. Albinana JM, Morevende JA, Weinstein SL. The teardrop in congenital dislocation of the hip diagnosed late: a quantitative study. *J Bone Joint Surg Am* 1996;78:1048.

190. Smith JM, Matan A, Coleman SS, et al. The predictive value of the development of acetabular teardrop figure in developmental dysplasia of the hip. *J Pediatr Orthop* 1997;17:165.

191. Bertol P, MacNicol MF, Mitchell GP. Radiographic features of neonatal congenital dislocation of the hip. *J Bone Joint Surg Br* 1982;64:176.

192. Perkins G. Signs by which to diagnose congenital dislocation of the hip, 1928 [Classical article]. *Clin Orthop* 1992;274:3.

193. Sharp IK. Acetabular dysplasia: the acetabular angle. *J Bone Joint Surg Br* 1961;43:269.

194. Bos CF, Bloem JL, Verbout AJ. Magnetic resonance imaging in acetabular residual dysplasia. *Clin Orthop* 1991;265:207.

195. Kashiwagi NS, Suzuki S, Kasahara Y, et al. Prediction of reduction in developmental dysplasia of the hip by magnetic resonance imaging. *J Pediatr Orthop* 1996;16:254.

196. Fisher R, O'Brien TS, Davis KM. Magnetic resonance imaging in congenital dysplasia of the hip. *J Pediatr Orthop* 1991;11:617.

197. Greenhill BJ, Hugosson C, Jacobsson B, et al. Magnetic resonance imaging study of acetabular morphology in developmental dysplasia of the hip. *J Pediatr Orthop* 1993;13:314.

198. Guidera KJ, Einbecker ME, Berman CG, et al. Magnetic resonance imaging evaluation of congenital dislocation of the hips. *Clin Orthop* 1990;261:96.

199. Johnson ND, Wood BP, Jackman KV. Complex infantile and congenital hip dislocation: assessment with MR imaging. *Radiology* 1988;168:151.

## Natural History

200. Henderson RS. Osteotomy for unreduced congenital dislocation of the hip in adults. *J Bone Joint Surg Br* 1970;52:468.

201. Visser JD. Functional treatment of congenital dislocation of the hip. *Acta Orthop Scand Suppl* 1984;206:1.

202. Milgram JW. Morphology of untreated bilateral congenital dislocation of the hips in a seventy-four-year-old man. *Clin Orthop* 1976;119:112.

203. Crawford AW, Slovek RW. Fate of the untreated congenitally dislocated hip. *Orthop Trans* 1978;2:73.

204. Chaptlchal GJ. The intertrochanteric osteotomy in the treatment of congenital dysplasia. *Clin Orthop* 1976;119:54.

205. Kerry R, Simonds GW. Long term results of late non operative reduction of developmental dysplasia of the hip. *J Bone Joint Surg Br* 1998;80:78.

206. Walker JM. Congenital hip disease in Cree-Ojibwa population: a retrospective study. *Can Med Assoc J* 1977;116:501.

207. Schwend RP, Pratt WB, Fultz J. Untreated acetabular dysplasia of the hip in the Navajo: a 34 year case series follow up. *Clin Orthop* 1999;36:108.

208. Fairbank JC, Howell P, Nockler I, et al. Relationship of pain to the radiological anatomy of the hip joint in adults treated for congenital dislocation of the hip as infants: a long-term follow-up of patients treated by three methods. *J Pediatr Orthop* 1986;6:539.

209. Malvitz TA, Weinstein SL. Closed reduction for congenital dysplasia of the hip: functional and radiographic results after an average of thirty years. *J Bone Joint Surg Am* 1994;76:1777.

210. Sherlock DA, Gibson PH, Benson MK. Congenital subluxation of the hip: a long-term review. *J Bone Joint Surg Br* 1985;67:390.

211. Berkeley ME, Dickson JH, Cain TE, et al. Surgical therapy for congenital dislocation of the hip in patients who are twelve to thirty-six months old. *J Bone Joint Surg Am* 1984;66:412.

212. Cooperman DR, Wallensten R, Stulberg SD. Acetabular dysplasia in the adult. *Clin Orthop* 1983;175:79.

213. Bombelli R. *Osteoarthritis of the hip.* Heidelberg: Springer-Verlag, 1983.

214. Stulberg SD, Harris WH. Acetabular dysplasia and development of osteoarthritis of the hip. *The hip: proceedings of the second open meeting of the hip society.* St. Louis, MO: Mosby, 1974:82.

215. Harris WH. Etiology of osteoarthritis of the hip. *Clin Orthop* 1986;213:20.

216. Hadley NA, Brown TD, Weinstein SL. The effect of contact pressure elevations and aseptic necrosis on the long-term outcome of congenital hip dislocation. *J Orthop Res* 1990;8:504.

217. Michaeli DM, Murphy SB, Hipp JA. Comparison of predicted and measured contact pressures in normal and dysplastic hips. *Med Eng Phys* 1997;19:180.

218. Klaue K, Durnin CW, Ganz R. The acetabular rim syndrome. *J Bone Joint Surg Br* 1991;73-B:423–429.

219. Lloyd-Roberts GC. Osteoarthritis of the hip: a study of the clinical pathology. *J Bone Joint Surg Br* 1955;37:8.

220. Murray RO. The aetiology of primary osteoarthritis of the hip. *Br J Radiol* 1965;38:810.
221. Solomon L. Patterns of osteoarthritis of the hip. *J Bone Joint Surg Br* 1976;58:176.

## Treatment of Hip Dislocation

222. Dimitriou JK, Cavadias AX. One-stage surgical procedure for congenital dislocation of the hip in older children: long-term results. *Clin Orthop* 1989;246:30.
223. Tredwell SJ. Neonatal screening for hip joint instability: its clinical and economic relevance. *Clin Orthop* 1992;281:63.
224. Dyson PH, Lynskey TG, Catterall A. Congenital hip dysplasia: problems in the diagnosis and management in the first year of life. *J Pediatr Orthop* 1987;7:568.
225. Atar D, Lehman WB, Tenenbaum Y, et al. Pavlik harness versus Frejka splint in treatment of developmental dysplasia of the hip: bicenter study. *J Pediatr Orthop* 1993;13:311.
226. Burger BJ, Burger JD, Bos CF, et al. Frejka pillow and Becker device for congenital dislocation of the hip: prospective 6-year study of 104 late-diagnosed cases. *Acta Orthop Scand* 1993;64:305.
227. Filipe G, Carlioz H. Use of the Pavlik harness in treating congenital dislocation of the hip. *J Pediatr Orthop* 1982;2:357.
228. Grill F, Bensahel H, Canadell J, et al. The Pavlik harness in the treatment of congenital dislocating hip: report on a multicenter study of the European Paediatric Orthopaedic Society. *J Pediatr Orthop* 1988;8:1.
229. Heikkila E. Comparison of the Frejka pillow and the von Rosen splint in treatment of congenital dislocation of the hip. *J Pediatr Orthop* 1988;8:20.
230. Hinderaker T, Rygh M, Uden A. The von Rosen splint compared with Frejka pillow: a study of 408 neonatally unstable hips. *Acta Orthop Scand* 1992;63:389.
231. Ilfeld FW, Makin M. Damage to the capital femoral epiphysis due to Frejka pillow treatment. *J Bone Joint Surg Am* 1977;59:654.
232. Iwasaki K. Treatment of congenital dislocation of the hip by the Pavlik harness: mechanism of reduction and usage. *J Bone Joint Surg Am* 1983;65:760.
233. Lempicki A, Wierusz-Kozlowska M, Kruczynski J. Abduction treatment in late diagnosed congenital dislocation of the hip: follow-up of 1,010 hips treated with the Frejka pillow 1967-76. *Acta Orthop Scand Suppl* 1990;236:1.
234. Pavlik A. Stirrups as an aid in the treatment of congenital dysplasias of the hip in children. *J Pediatr Orthop* 1989;9:157.
235. Pavlik A. The functional method of treatment using a harness with stirrups as the primary method of conservative therapy for infants with congenital dislocation of the hip, 1957 [classical article]. *Clin Orthop* 1992;281:4.
236. Cashman JP, Round J, Taylor G, et al. The natural history of developmental dysplasia of the hip after early supervised treatment in the Pavlik harness. A prospective, longitudinal follow up. *J Bone Joint Surg Br* 2002;84(3):418–425.
237. Viere RG, Birch JG, Herring JA, et al. Use of the Pavlik harness in congenital dislocation of the hip: an analysis of failures of treatment. *J Bone Joint Surg Am* 1990;72:238.
238. Jones GT, Schoenecker PL, Dias LS. Developmental hip dysplasia potentiated by inappropriate use of the Pavlik harness. *J Pediatr Orthop* 1992;12:722.
239. Moseley CF. The biomechanics of the pediatric hip. *Orthop Clin North Am* 1980;11:3.
240. Ramsey PS, Lasser S, MacEwen GD. Congenital dislocation of the hip: use of the Pavlik harness in the child during the first 6 months of life. *J Bone Joint Surg Am* 1976;58:1000.
241. Suzuki S. Ultrasound and the Pavlik harness in CDH. *J Bone Joint Surg Br* 1993;75:483.
242. Almby B, Hjelmstedt A, Lonnerholm T. Neonatal hip instability: reason for failure of early abduction treatment. *Acta Orthop Scand* 1979;50:315.
243. Bradley J, Wetherill M, Benson MK. Splintage for congenital dislocation of the hip: is it safe and reliable? *J Bone Joint Surg Br* 1987;69:257.
244. Rombouts JJ, Kaelin A. Inferior (obturator) dislocation of the hip in neonates: a complication of treatment by the Pavlik harness. *J Bone Joint Surg Br* 1992;74:708.
245. Fernandez Gonzalez J, Albinana J. Obturator dislocation in developmental dislocation of the hip: a complication during treatment. *J Pediatr Orthop B* 1996;5:129.

246. Suzuki S, Yamamuro T. Avascular necrosis in patients treated with the Pavlik harness for congenital dislocation of the hip. *J Bone Joint Surg Am* 1990;72:1048.
247. Suzuki S, Kashiwagi N, Kasahara Y, et al. Avascular necrosis and the Pavlik harness: the incidence of avascular necrosis in three types of congenital dislocation of the hip as classified by ultrasound. *J Bone Joint Surg Br* 1996;78:631.
248. Buchanan JR, Greer RBIII, Cotler JM. Management strategy for prevention of avascular necrosis during treatment of congenital dislocation of the hip. *J Bone Joint Surg Am* 1981;63:140.
249. Danzhou S, Hongzhi I, Weinmin Y, et al. Preoperative intermittent manual traction in congenital dislocation of the hip. *J Pediatr Orthop* 1989;9:205.
250. DeRosa GP, Feller N. Treatment of congenital dislocation of the hip: management before walking age. *Clin Orthop* 1987;225:77.
251. Gage JR, Winter RB. Avascular necrosis of the capital femoral epiphysis as a complication of closed reduction of congenital dislocation of the hip. *J Bone Joint Surg Am* 1972;54:373.
252. Kramer J, Schleberger R, Steffen R. Closed reduction by two-phase skin traction and functional splinting in mitigated abduction for treatment of congenital dislocation of the hip. *Clin Orthop* 1990;258:27.
253. Langenskjold A, Paavilainen T. The effect of traction treatment on the results of closed or open reduction for congenital dislocation of the hip: a preliminary report. In: Tachdjian MO, ed. *Congenital dislocation of the hip*, New York: Churchill Livingstone, 1982:365.
254. Lehman WB, Grant AD, Nelson J, et al. Hospital for Joint Diseases' traction system for preliminary treatment of congenital dislocation of the hip. *J Pediatr Orthop* 1983;3:104.
255. Morel G. The treatment of congenital dislocation and subluxation of the hip in the older child. *Acta Orthop Scand* 1975;46:364.
256. Weiner DS, Hoyt WA, Odell HW Jr. Congenital dislocation of the hip: the relationship of premanipulation traction and age to avascular necrosis of the femoral head. *J Bone Joint Surg Am* 1977;59:306.
257. Zionts LE, MacEwen GD. Treatment of congenital dislocation of the hip in children between the ages of one and three years. *J Bone Joint Surg Am* 1986;68:829.
258. Stucker RH, Huter T, Haberstroh J. The effect of traction treatment on blood flow in the immature hip: an animal study. *Z Orthop Ihre Grenzgeb* 1996;134:332.
259. Wenger DL, Lee CS, Kolman B. Derotational femoral shortening for developmental dislocation of the hip: special indications and results in the child younger than 2 years. *J Pediatr Orthop* 1995;15:768.
260. Weinstein SL. Traction in developmental dislocation of the hip. Is its use justified? *Clin Orthop* 1997;338:79–85.
261. Fish DN, Herzenberg JE, Hensinger RN. Current practice in use of prereduction traction for congenital dislocation of the hip. *J Pediatr Orthop* 1991;11:149.
262. Cooperman DR, Wallensten R, Stulberg SD. Post-reduction avascular necrosis in congenital dislocation of the hip. *J Bone Joint Surg Am* 1980;62:247.
263. Schoenecker PL, Strecker WB. Congenital dislocation of the hip in children: comparison of the effects of femoral shortening and of skeletal traction in treatment. *J Bone Joint Surg Am* 1984;66:21.
264. Fabry G. Open reduction by the Ludloff approach to congenital dislocation of the hip under the age of two. *Acta Orthop Belg* 1990;56:233.
265. Kutlu A, Ayata C, Cevat Ogun T, et al. Preliminary traction as a single determinant of avascular necrosis in developmental dislocation of the hip. *J Pediatr Orthop* 2000;20:579–584.
266. Coleman S. A critical analysis of the value of preliminary traction in the treatment of CDH. *Orthop Trans* 1987;13:180.
267. Kahle WK, Anderson MB, Alpert J, et al. The value of preliminary traction in the treatment of congenital dislocation of the hip. *J Bone Joint Surg Am* 1990;72:1043.
268. Quinn RH, Renshaw TS, DeLuca PA. Preliminary traction in the treatment of developmental dislocation of the hip. *J Pediatr Orthop* 1994;14:636.
269. Yamada N, Maeda S, Fujii G, et al. Closed reduction of developmental dislocation of the hip by prolonged traction. *J Bone Joint Surg Br* 2003;85-B(8):1173–1177.

270. Joseph K, MacEwen GD, Boos ML. Home traction in the management of congenital dislocation of the hip. *Clin Orthop* 1982;165:83.

271. Mubarak SJ, Beck LR, Sutherland D. Home traction in the management of congenital dislocation of the hips. *J Pediatr Orthop* 1986;6:721.

272. Voutsinas SA, MacEwen GD, Boos ML. Home traction in the management of congenital dislocation of the hip. *Arch Orthop Trauma Surg* 1984;102:135.

273. Ando M, Gotoh E, Matsuura J. Tangential view arthrogram at closed reduction in congenital dislocation of the hip. *J Pediatr Orthop* 1992;12:390.

274. Forlin E, Choi IH, Guille JT, et al. Prognostic factors in congenital dislocation of the hip treated with closed reduction: the importance of arthrographic evaluation. *J Bone Joint Surg Am* 1992;74:1140.

275. Renshaw TS. Inadequate reduction of congenital dislocation of the hip. *J Bone Joint Surg Am* 1981;63:1114.

276. Schoenecker PL, Lesker PA, Ogata K. A dynamic canine model of experimental hip dysplasia: gross and histological pathology, and the effect of position of immobilization on capital femoral epiphyseal blood flow. *J Bone Joint Surg Am* 1984;66:1281.

277. Salter RB, Field P. The effects of continuous compression on living articular cartilage. *J Bone Joint Surg Am* 1960;42:31.

278. Drummond DS, O'Donnell J, Breed A, et al. Arthrography in the evaluation of congenital dislocation of the hip. *Clin Orthop* 1989;243:148.

279. Gabuzda GM, Renshaw TS. Reduction of congenital dislocation of the hip. *J Bone Joint Surg Am* 1992;74:624.

280. Herring JA. Inadequate reduction of congenital dislocation of the hip [letter]. *J Bone Joint Surg Am* 1982;64:153.

281. McNally ET, Tasker A, Benson MK. MRI after operative reduction for developmental dysplasia of the hip. *J Bone Joint Surg Br* 1997;79:724.

282. Smith BG, Kasser JR, Hey LA, et al. Post reduction computed tomography in developmental dislocation of the hip. Part I. Analysis of measurement reliability. *J Pediatr Orthop* 1997;7:626.

283. Hernandez RJ. Concentric reduction of the dislocated hip: computed-tomographic evaluation. *Radiology* 1984;150:266.

284. Fogarty EE, Accardo NY. Incidence of avascular necrosis of the femoral head in congenital hip dislocation related of the degree of abduction during preliminary traction. *J Pediatr Orthop* 1981;1:307.

285. Salter RB, Kostiuk J, Dallas S. Avascular necrosis of the femoral head as a complication of treatment for congenital dislocation of the hip in young children: a clinical and experimental investigation. *Can J Surg* 1969;12:44.

286. Segal LS, Schneider DJ, Berlin JM, et al. The contribution of the ossific nucleus to the structural stiffness of the capital femoral epiphysis: a porcine model of DDH. *J Pediatr Orthop* 1999;19(4):433–437.

287. Segal LS, Berlin JM, Schneider DJ, et al. Chrondronecrosis of the hip. The protective role of the ossific nucleus in an animal model. *Clin Orthop* 2000;377:265–271.

288. Luhmann SS, Schoenecker PL, Anderson AM, et al. The prognostic importance of the ossific nucleus in the treatment of congenital dysplasia of the hip. *J Bone Joint Surg Am* 1998;80:1719.

289. Luhman SJ, Schoenecker PL, Anderson AM, et al. The prognostic importance of the ossific nucleus in the treatment of congenital dysplasia of the hip. *J Bone Joint Surg Am* 1998;80(12):1719–1727.

290. Luhman SJ, Bassett GS, Gordon JE, et al. Reduction of a dislocation of the hip due to developmental dysplasia. Implications for the need for further surgery. *J Bone Joint Surg Am* 2003;85-A(2):239–243.

291. Akazawa H, Tanabe G, Miyake Y. A new open reduction treatment for congenital hip dislocation: long-term follow-up of the extensive anterolateral approach. *Acta Med Okayama* 1990;44:223.

292. Dhar S, Taylor JF, Jones WA, et al. Early open reduction for congenital dislocation of the hip. *J Bone Joint Surg Br* 1990;72:175.

293. Mankey MG, Arntz CT, Staheli LT. Open reduction through a medial approach for congenital dislocation of the hip: a critical review of the Ludloff approach in sixty-six hips. *J Bone Joint Surg Am* 1993;75:1334.

294. McCluskey WP, Bassett GS, Mora-Garcia G, et al. Treatment of failed open reduction for congenital dislocation of the hip. *J Pediatr Orthop* 1989;9:633.

295. Salter RB. Role of innominate osteotomy in the treatment of congenital dislocation and subluxation of the hip in the older child. *J Bone Joint Surg Am* 1966;48:1413.

296. Salter RB, Dubos J-P. The first fifteen years' personal experience with innominate osteotomy in the treatment of congenital dislocation and subluxation of the hip. *Clin Orthop* 1974;98:72.

297. Salter RB, Hansson G, Thompson GA. Innominate osteotomy in the management of residual congenital subluxation of the hip in young adults. *Clin Orthop* 1984;182:53.

298. Katz K, Yosipovitch Z. Medial approach open reduction without preliminary traction for congenital dislocation of the hip. *J Pediatr Orthop B* 1994;3:82.

299. Mergen E, Adyaman S, Omeroglu H, et al. Medial approach open reduction for congenital dislocation of the hip using the Ferguson procedure: a review of 31 hips. *Arch Orthop Trauma Surg* 1991;110:169.

300. Monticelli G, Milella PP. Indications for treatment of congenital dislocation of the hip by the surgical medial approach. In: Tachdjian MO, ed. *Congenital dislocation of the hip*, New York: Churchill Livingstone, 1982:385.

301. O'Hara JN, Bernard AA, Dwyer NS. Early results of medial approach open reduction in congenital dislocation of the hip: use before walking age. *J Pediatr Orthop* 1988;8:288.

302. Roose PE, Chingren GL, Klaaren HE, et al. Open reduction for congenital dislocation of the hip using the Ferguson procedure: a review of twenty-six cases. *J Bone Joint Surg Am* 1979;61:915.

303. Konigsberg DE, Karol LA, Colby S, et al. Results of medial open reduction of the hip in infants with developmental dislocation of the hip. *J Pediatr Orthop* 2003;23(1):1–9.

304. Vedantam RC, Capelli AM, Schoenecker PL. Pemberton osteotomy for the treatment of developmental dysplasia of the hip in older children. *J Pediatr Orthop* 1998;18:254.

305. Simons GW. A comparative evaluation of the current methods for open reduction of the congenitally displaced hip. *Orthop Clin North Am* 1980;11:161.

306. Castillo R, Sherman FC. Medial adductor open reduction for congenital dislocation of the hip. *J Pediatr Orthop* 1990;10:335.

307. Cech O, Sosna A, Vavra J. Indications and surgical technique for open reposition of congenital dislocation of the hip after Ludloff [author's translation]. *Acta Chir Orthop Traumatol Cech* 1976;43:233.

308. Scapinelli R, Ortolani M Jr. Open reduction (Ludloff approach) of congenital dislocation of the hip before the age of two years. *Isr J Med Sci* 1980;16:276.

309. Sosna A, Rejholec M, Rybka V, et al. Long-term results of Ludloffs repositioning method. *Acta Chir Orthop Traumatol Cech* 1990;57:213.

310. Fisher EHI, Beck PA, Hoffer MM. Necrosis of the capital femoral epiphysis and medial approaches to the hip in piglets. *J Orthop Res* 1991;9:203.

311. Morcuende JM, Dolan LA, Weinstein SL, et al. Long term outcome after open reduction through an anteromedial approach for congenital dislocation of the hip. *J Bone Joint Surg Am* 1997;79:810.

312. Cherney DL, Westin GW. Acetabular development in the infant's dislocated hips. *Clin Orthop* 1989;242:98.

313. Noritake K, Yoshihashi Y, Hattori TTM. Acetabular development after closed reduction of congenital dislocation of the hip. *J Bone Joint Surg Br* 1993;75:737.

314. Akagi ST, Tanabe T, Ogawa R. Acetabular development after open reduction for developmental dislocation of the hip: 15 year follow up of 22 hips without additional surgery. *Acta Orthop Scand* 1998;69:17.

315. Brougham DI, Broughton NS, Cole WG, et al. The predictability of acetabular development after closed reduction for congenital dislocation of the hip. *J Bone Joint Surg Br* 1988;70:733.

316. Molina-Guerrero JA, Munuera-Martinez L, Esteban-Mugica B. Acetabular development in congenital dislocation on the hip. *Acta Orthop Belg* 1990;56:293.

317. Lalonde FD, Frick SL, Wenger DR. Surgical correction of residual hip dysplasia in two pediatric age groups. *J Bone Joint Surg Am* 2002;84-A(7):1148–1156.

318. Gallien R, Bertin D, Lirette R. Salter procedure in congenital dislocation of the hip. *J Pediatr Orthop* 1984;4:427.

319. Haidar RK, Jones RS, Vergroessen DA, et al. Simultaneous open reduction and salter innominate osteotomy for developmental dysplasia of the hip. *J Bone Joint Surg Br* 1996;78:471.

320. Klisic P, Jankovic L. Combined procedure of open reduction and shortening of the femur in treatment of congenital dislocation of the hips in older children. *Clin Orthop* 1976;119:60.

321. Daoud A, Saighi-Bououina A. Congenital dislocation of the hip in the older child: the effectiveness of overhead traction. *J Bone Joint Surg Am* 1996;78:30.

322. Fixen J, Li P. The treatment of subluxation of the hip in children over the age of four years. *J Bone Joint Surg Br* 1996;80:757.

323. Ryan MJ, Johnson LO, Quanbeck DS, et al. One stage treatment of congenital dislocation of the hip in children three to ten years old: functional and radiographic results. *J Bone Joint Surg Am* 1998;80:336.

324. Galpin RD, Roach JW, Wenger DR, et al. One-stage treatment of congenital dislocation of the hip in older children, including femoral shortening. *J Bone Joint Surg Am* 1989;71:734.

325. Heinrich SD, Missinne LH, MacEwen GD. The conservative management of congenital dislocation of the hip after walking age. *Clin Orthop* 1992;281:34.

326. Klisic PJ. Congenital dislocation of the hip: a misleading term [Brief Report]. *J Bone Joint Surg Br* 1989;71:136.

327. Bohm P, Brzuske A. Salter innominate osteotomy for the treatment of developmental dysplasia of the hip in children: results of seventy-three consecutive osteotomies after twenty-six to thirty-five years of follow up. *J Bone Joint Surg Am* 2002;84-A(2):178–186.

328. Zadeh HG, Catterall A, Hashemi-Nejad A, et al. Test of stability as an aid to decide the need for osteotomy in association with open reduction in developmental dysplasia of the hip. A long-term review. *J Bone Joint Surg Br* 2000;82-B(1):17–27.

329. Akagi S, Tanabe T, Ogawa R. Acetabular development after open reduction for developmental dislocation of the hip. 15 year follow up of 22 hips without additional surgery. *Acta Orthop Scand* 1998;69(1):17–20.

330. Albinana J, Dolan L, Spratt K, et al. Acetabular dysplasia after treatment for developmental dysplasia of the hip. Implications for secondary procedures. *J Bone Joint Surg* 2004;86B:876–886.

331. Waters P, Kurica K, Hall J, et al. Salter innominate osteotomies in congenital dislocation of the hip. *J Pediatr Orthop* 1988;8:650.

332. Coleman SS. The pericapsular (Pemberton) pelvic osteotomy and the redirectional (Salter) pelvic osteotomy. *Mapfre Med* 1992;3(Suppl. 1):124.

333. Coleman S. Prevention of developmental dislocation of the hip: practices and problems in the United States. *J Pediatr Orthop B* 1993;2:127.

334. Faciszewski T, Kiefer GN, Coleman SS. Pemberton osteotomy for residual acetabular dysplasia in children who have congenital dislocation of the hip. *J Bone Joint Surg Am* 1993;75:643.

335. Coleman S. The subluxating or wandering femoral head in developmental dislocation of the hip. *J Pediatr Orthop* 1995;15:785.

336. Ward WV, Vogt M, Grudziak J, et al. Severin classification system for evaluation of the results of operative treatment of congenital dislocation of the hip: a study of intraobserver and interobserver reliability. *J Bone Joint Surg Am* 1997;79:656.

337. Browne RS. The management of late diagnosed congenital dislocation and subluxation of the hip: with special reference to femoral shortening. *J Bone Joint Surg Br* 1979;61:7.

338. Wenger DR. Congenital hip dislocation: techniques for primary open reduction including femoral shortening. *Instr Course Lect* 1989;38:343.

## Sequelae and Complications

339. Weinstein SL, Mubarek SJ, Wenger DR. Developmental hip dysplasia and dislocation: Part I. *J Bone Joint Surg* 2003;85-A:1824–1832.

340. Weinstein SL, Mubarek SJ, Wenger DR. Developmental hip dysplasia and dislocation: part II. *J Bone Joint Surg* 2003;85A:2024–2035.

341. Barrett WP, Staheli LT, Chew DE. The effectiveness of the Salter innominate osteotomy in the treatment of congenital dislocation of the hip. *J Bone Joint Surg Am* 1986;68:79.

342. Lloyd-Roberts GC, Harris NH, Chrispin AR. Anteversion of the acetabulum in congenital dislocation of the hip: a preliminary report. *Orthop Clin North Am* 1978;9:89.

343. Murphy SB, Kijewski PK, Millis MB, et al. Acetabular dysplasia in the adolescent and young adult. *Clin Orthop* 1990;261:214.

344. Wientroub S, Boyde A, Chrispin AR, et al. The use of stereophotogrammetry to measure acetabular and femoral anteversion. *J Bone Joint Surg Br* 1981;63:209.

345. Hipp JA, Sugano N, Millis MB, et al. Planning acetabular redirection osteotomies based on joint contact pressures. *Clin Orthop* 1999;364:134–143.

346. Mast JW, Brunner RL, Zebrack J. Recognizing acetabular version in the radiographic presentation of hip dysplasia. *Clin Orthop* 2004;418:48–53.

347. Ruwi PA, Gage JR, Ozonoff MB, et al. Clinical determination of femoral anteversion. *J Bone Joint Surg Am* 1992;74:820.

348. Millis MB, Murphy SB. Use of computed tomographic reconstruction in planning osteotomies of the hip. *Clin Orthop* 1992;274:154.

349. Kim HW, Wenger DR. The morphology of residual acetabular deficiency in childhood hip dysplasia: a three dimensional computed tomographic analysis. *J Pediatr Orthop* 1997;17:637.

350. Atar D, Lehman WB, Grant AD. 2-D and 3-D computed tomography and magnetic resonance imaging in developmental dysplasia of the hip. *Orthop Rev* 1992;21:1189.

351. Azuma H, Taneda H, Igarashi H. Evaluation of acetabular coverage: three-dimensional CT imaging and modified pelvic inlet view. *J Pediatr Orthop* 1991;11:765.

352. Lang P, Genant H, Steiger P, et al. Three-dimensional digital displays in congenital dislocation of the hip: preliminary experience. *J Pediatr Orthop* 1989;9:532.

353. Lafferty CM, Sartoris DJ, Tyson R, et al. Acetabular alterations in untreated congenital dysplasia of the hip: computed tomography with multiplanar reformation and three-dimensional analysis. *J Comput Assist Tomogr* 1986;10:84.

354. Mendes DG. The role of computerized tomography scan in preoperative evaluation of the adult dislocated hip. *Clin Orthop* 1981;161:198.

355. O'Sullivan GS, Goodman SB, Jones HH. Computerized tomographic evaluation of acetabular anatomy. *Clin Orthop Relat Res* 1992;277:175.

356. Konishi N, Nagoya MD, Mieno T. Determination of acetabular coverage of the femoral head with use of a single anteroposterior radiograph: a new computerized technique. *J Bone Joint Surg Am* 1993;75:1318.

357. Doudoulakis JK, Cavadias A. Open reduction of CDH before one year of age: 69 hips followed for 13 (10-19) years. *Acta Orthop Scand* 1993;64:188.

358. Kasser JR, Bowen JR, MacEwen GD. Varus derotation osteotomy in the treatment of persistent dysplasia in congenital dislocation of the hip. *J Bone Joint Surg Am* 1985;67:195.

359. Monticelli G. Intertrochanteric femoral osteotomy with concentric reduction of the femoral head in treatment of residual congenital acetabular dysplasia. *Clin Orthop* 1976;119:48.

360. Niethard FU, Carstens C. Results of intertrochanteric osteotomy in infant and adolescent hip dysplasia. *J Pediatr Orthop B* 1994;3:9.

361. Williamson DM, Glover SD, Benson MK. Congenital dislocation of the hip presenting after the age of three years: a long-term review. *J Bone Joint Surg Br* 1989;71:745.

362. Blockey NJ. Derotation osteotomy in the management of congenital dislocation of the hip. *J Bone Joint Surg Br* 1984;66:485.

363. Chuinard EG. Femoral osteotomy in the treatment of congenital dysplasia of the hip. *Orthop Clin North Am* 1972;3:157.

364. Conforty B. Femoral osteotomy for correction of sequelae of conservative treatment of congenital dislocation of the hip. *Isr J Med Sci* 1980;16:284.

365. Lloyd-Roberts GC. The role of femoral osteotomy in the treatment of congenital dislocation of the hip. In: Tachdjian MO, ed. *Congenital dislocation of the hip*, New York: Churchill Livingstone, 1982:427.

366. Rejholec M, Stryhal F. Behavior of the proximal femur during the treatment of congenital dysplasia of the hip: a clinical long-term study. *J Pediatr Orthop* 1991;11:506.

367. Swenningsen S, Apalset K, Terjesen T. Osteotomy for femoral anteversion: complications in 95 children. *Acta Orthop Scand* 1989;60:401.

368. Karadimas JE, Holloway GM, Waugh W. Growth of the proximal femur after varus-derotation osteotomy in the treatment of congenital dislocation of the hip. *Clin Orthop* 1982;162:61.

369. Sangavi SS, Szoke G, Murray G, et al. Femoral remodeling after subtrochanteric osteotomy for developmental dysplasia of the hip. *J Bone Joint Surg Br* 1996;78:917.

370. Pellicci PM, Hu S, Garvin KL, et al. Varus rotational femoral osteotomies in adults with hip dysplasia. *Clin Orthop* 1991; 272:162.

371. Perlau RW, Wilson MG, Poss R. Isolated proximal femoral osteotomy for treatment of residua of congenital dysplasia or idiopathic osteoarthritis of the hip. *J Bone Joint Surg Am* 1996; 78:1462.

372. Robertson DE, Essinger JR, Imura S, et al. Femoral deformity in adults with developmental hip dyplasia. *Clin Orthop* 1996; 327:196.

373. Marafioti RL, Westin GW. Factors influencing the results of acetabuloplasty in children. *J Bone Joint Surg Am* 1980;62:765.

374. Albinana J, Weinstein SL, Morcuende JA, et al. DDH acetabular remodeling after open or closed reduction: timing for secondary procedures. *Orthop Trans* 1996;20:298.

375. Chiari K. Medial displacement osteotomy of the pelvis. *Clin Orthop* 1974;98:55.

376. Migaud H, Chantelot MC, Giraud F, et al. Long-term survivorship of hip shelf arthroplasty and Chiari osteotomy in adults. *Clin Orthop* 2004;418:81–86.

377. Ito I, Matsuno T, Minami A. A Chiari pelvic osteotomy for advanced osteoarthritis in patients with hip dysplasia. *J Bone Joint Surg Am* 2004;86-A:1439–1445.

378. Kalamchi A. Modified Salter osteotomy. *J Bone Joint Surg Am* 1982;64:183.

379. Millis MB, Hall JE. Transiliac lengthening of the lower extremity: a modified innominate osteotomy for the treatment of postural imbalance. *J Bone Joint Surg Am* 1979;61:1182.

380. McCarthy JJ, Fox JS, Curd AR. Innominate osteotomy in adolescents and adults who have acetabular dysplasia. *J Bone Joint Surg Am* 1996;78:1455.

381. Sutherland DH, Moore M. Clinical and radiographic outcome of patients treated with double innominate osteotomy for congenital hip dysplasia. *J Pediatr Orthop* 1991;11:143.

382. Tonnis D. A new technique of triple osteotomy for acetabular dysplasia in older children and adults. Abstracts of the 14th World Congress of the Society of International Chirurgiae Orthopaedicae et Traumatologiae, Kyoto, 1978.

383. Tonnis D, Behrens K, Tscharani F. A modified technique of the triple pelvic osteotomy: early results. *J Pediatr Orthop* 1981;1:241.

384. Tonnis D. Triple osteotomy close to the hip joint. In: Tachdjian MO, ed. *Congenital dislocation of the hip*, New York: Churchill Livingstone, 1982:555.

385. Tonnis D, Kasperczyk WJ. Acetabuloplasty and acetabular rotation. In: Freeman M, Reynolds D, eds. *Osteoarthritis in the young adult hip*, Edinburgh: Churchill Livingstone, 1988.

386. Tonnis D, Arning A, Bloch M, et al. Triple pelvic osteotomy. *J Pediatr Orthop* 1994;3:54.

387. Faciszewski T, Coleman S. Triple innominate osteotomy in the treatment of acetabular dysplasia. *J Pediatr Orthop* 1993; 13:426.

388. Guille JT, Forlin E, Kumar SJ, et al. Triple osteotomy of the innominate bone in treatment of developmental dysplasia of the hip. *J Pediatr Orthop* 1992;12:718.

389. Kumar SJ, MacEwen GD, Jaykumar AS. Triple osteotomy of the innominate bone for the treatment of congenital hip dysplasia. *J Pediatr Orthop* 1986;6:393.

390. Steel HH. Triple osteotomy of the innominate bone. *J Bone Joint Surg Am* 1973;55:343.

391. Steel HH. Triple osteotomy of the innominate bone. *Clin Orthop* 1977;122:116.

392. Hsin JS, Saluja R, Eilert RE, et al. Evaluation of the biomechanics of the hip following triple osteotomy of the innominate bone. *J Bone Joint Surg Am* 1996;78:855.

393. Ganz R, Vinh TS, Mast JW. A new periacetabular osteotomy for the treatment of hip dysplasias: technique and preliminary results. *Clin Orthop Relat Res* 1988;232:26.

394. Klaue K, Sherman M, Perren SM, et al. Extraarticular augmentation for residual hip dysplasia. *J Bone Joint Surg Br* 1993;75:750.

395. Trousdale RT, Cabanela ME. Lessons learned after more than 250 periacetabular osteotomies [comment]. *Acta Orthop Scand* 2003;74(2):119–126.

396. Hsieh PH, Shih CH, Lee PC, et al. A modified periacetabular osteotomy with use of the transtrochanteric exposure. *J Bone Joint Surg Am* 2003;85-A(2):244–250.

397. Wagner H. *The hip: proceedings of the fourth open scientific meeting of the Hip Society*. St. Louis, MO: Mosby, 1976.

398. Wagner H. Spherical acetabular osteotomy: long-term results. In: *Fourth harvard medical school course on osteotomy of the hip and knee*. Boston, MA: Harvard University Press, 1992.

399. Millis MB, Kaelin AJ, Schluntz K, et al. Spherical acetabular osteotomy for treatment of acetabular dysplasia in adolescents and young adults. *J Pediatr Orthop B* 1994;3:47.

400. Eppright RH. Dial osteotomy of the acetabulum in the treatment of dysplasia of the hip. *J Bone Joint Surg Am* 1976;58:726.

401. Nakamura T, Yamaura M, Nakamitu S, et al. The displacement of the femoral head by rotational acetabular osteotomy: a radiographic study of 97 subluxated hips. *Acta Orthop Scand* 1992;63:33.

402. Ninomiya S, Tagawa H. Rotational acetabular osteotomy for the dysplastic hip. *Clin Orthop* 1984;247:127.

403. Ninomiya S. Rotational acetabular osteotomy for the severely dysplastic hip in the adolescent and adult. *Clin Orthop* 1989;247:127.

404. Matsui MM, Masuhara K, Nishii T, et al. Early deterioration after modified rotational acetabular osteotomy for the dysplastic hip. *J Bone Joint Surg Br* 1997;79:220.

405. de Kleuver M, Huiskes R, Kauer JM, et al. Three dimensional displacement of the hip joint after triple pelvic osteotomy. A postmortem radiosterometric study. *Acta Orthop Scand* 1998; 69(6):585–589.

406. de Kleuver M, Kooijman MA, Kauer JM, et al. Pelvic osteotomies: anatomic pitfalls at the ischium. A Cadaver Study. *Arch Orthop Trauma Surg* 1998;117(6-7):376–378.

407. de Kleuver M, Kooijman MA, Kauer JM, et al. Anatomic basis of Tonnis' triple pelvic osteotomy for acetabular dysplasia. *Surg Radiol Anat* 1998;20(2):79–82.

408. de Kleuver M, Kooijman MA, Kauer JM, et al. Pelvic osteotomies: anatomic pitfalls at the pubic bone. A Cadaver Study. *Arch Orthop Trauma Surg* 1998;117(4-5):270–272.

409. de Kleuver M, Kapitein PJ, Kooijman MA, et al. Acetabular coverage of the femoral head after triple pelvic osteotomy: no relation to outcome in 51 hips followed for 8-15 years. *Acta Orthop Scand* 1999;70(6):583–588.

410. Rab GT. Preoperative roentgenographic evaluation for osteotomies about the hip in children. *J Bone Joint Surg Am* 1981;63:306.

411. Hansson LI, Olsson TH, Selvik G, et al. A roentgen stereophotogrammetric investigation of innominate osteotomy (Salter). *Acta Orthop Scand* 1978;49:68.

412. Garbuz DS, Masri BA, Haddad F, et al. Clinical and radiographic assessment of the young adult with symptomatic hip dysplasia. *Clin Orthop* 2004;418:18–22.

413. Eyre-Brook AL, Jones DA, Harris FC. Pemberton's acetabuloplasty for congenital dislocation or subluxation of the hip. *J Bone Joint Surg Br* 1978;60:18.

414. Leet AI, Mackenzie WG, Szoke G, et al. Injury to the growth plate after Pemberton osteotomy. *J Bone Joint Surg Am* 1999;81-A(2):169–176.

415. Nishiyama K, Sakamaki T, Okinaga A. Complications of Pemberton's pericapsular osteotomy: a report of two cases. *Clin Orthop Relat Res* 1990;254:205.

416. Labaziewicz L, Grudziak JS, Kruczynski J, et al. Combined one stage open reduction femoral osteotomy and Dega pelvic osteotomy for DDH. Presented at the American Academy of Orthopaedic Surgeons Annual Meeting, San Francisco, CA, 1993.

417. Lloyd-Roberts GC, Wetherill MH, Fraser M. Trochanteric advancement for premature arrest of the femoral capital growth plate. *J Bone Joint Surg Br* 1985;67:21.

418. Synder M, Zwierzchowski H. One-stage hip reconstruction with Dega's transiliac osteotomy in the treatment of congenital hip dislocation in children. *Beitr Orthop Traumatol* 1990;37:571.

419. Reichel H, Hoin W. Dega acetabuloplasty combined with intertrochanteric osteotomies. *Clin Orthop* 1996;323:234.

420. Grudziak JS, Ward WT. Dega osteotomy for the treatment of congenital dysplasia of the hip. *J Bone Joint Surg Am* 2001;83-A(6):845–854.

421. Albee FH. The bone graft wedge. *NY Med J* 1915;52:433.

422. Hiranuma S, Higuchi F, Inoue A, et al. Changes in the interposed capsule after Chiari osteotomy: an experimental study on rabbits with acetabular dysplasia. *J Bone Joint Surg Br* 1992;74:463.

423. Hamanishi C, Tanaka S, Yamamuro T. The Spitzy shelf operation for the dysplastic hip: retrospective 10 (5-25) year study of 124 cases. *Acta Orthop Scand* 1992;63:273.

424. Le-Saout J, Kerboul B, Lefevre C, et al. Results of 56 acetabular shelf operations: with a long follow-up. *Acta Orthop Belg* 1985;51:955.

425. Love BR, Stevens PM, Williams PF. A long-term review of shelf arthroplasty. *J Bone Joint Surg Br* 1980;62:321.

426. White RE Jr, Sherman FC. The hip-shelf procedure: a long-term evaluation. *J Bone Joint Surg Am* 1980;62:928.

427. Wiberg G. Shelf operation in congenital dysplasia of the acetabulum and in subluxation and dislocation of the hip. *J Bone Joint Surg Am* 1953;35:65.

428. Staheli LT. Surgical management of acetabular dysplasia. *Clin Orthop Relat Res* 1991;264:111.

429. Staheli LT, Chew DE. Slotted acetabular augmentation in childhood and adolescence. *J Pediatr Orthop* 1992;12:569.

430. Bailey TE Jr, Hall JE. Chiari medial displacement osteotomy. *J Pediatr Orthop* 1985;5:635.

431. Colton CL. Chiari osteotomy for acetabular dysplasia in young subjects. *J Bone Joint Surg Br* 1972;54:578.

432. Windhager R, Pongracz N, Schoenecker W, et al. Chiari osteotomy for congenital dislocation and subluxation of the hip: results after 20 to 34 years follow-up. *J Bone Joint Surg Br* 1991;73:890.

433. Winkler W, Weber A. Osteotomy of the pelvis (Chiari) [author's translation]. *Z Orthop Ihre Grenzgeb* 1977;115:167.

434. Mellerowicz HM, Matussek J, Baum C. Long term results of Salter and Chiari hip osteotomies in developmental hip dysplasia: a survey of over 10 years follow up with a new hip evaluation score. *Arch Orthop Trauma Surg* 1998;117:222.

435. Gangloff S, Onimus M. Chiari pelvic osteotomy: technique and indications. *J Pediatr Orthop* 1994;3:68.

436. Moll FK Jr. Capsular change following Chiari innominate osteotomy. *J Pediatr Orthop* 1982;2:573.

437. Betz RR, Kumar SJ, Palmer CT, et al. Chiari pelvic osteotomy in children and young adults. *J Bone Joint Surg Am* 1988;70:182.

438. Calvert PT, August AC, Albert JS, et al. The Chiari pelvic osteotomy: a review of the long-term results. *J Bone Joint Surg Br* 1987;69:551.

439. Dewaal Malefijt MC, Hodgland T, Nielsen HKL. Chiari osteotomy in the treatment of the congenital dislocation and subluxation of the hip. *J Bone Joint Surg Am* 1982;64:996.

440. Graham S, Westin GW, Dawson E, et al. The Chiari osteotomy: a review of 58 cases. *Clin Orthop* 1986;208:249.

441. Hogh J, MacNicol MF. The Chiari pelvic osteotomy: a long term review of clinical and radiographic results. *J Bone Joint Surg Br* 1987;69:365.

442. Lack W, Windhager R, Kutschera H, et al. Chiari pelvic osteotomy for osteoarthritis secondary to hip dysplasia. *J Bone Joint Surg Br* 1991;73:229.

443. Mitchell GP. Chiari medial displacement osteotomy. *Clin Orthop* 1974;98:146.

444. Rejholec M, Stryhal F, Rybka V, et al. Chiari osteotomy of the pelvis: a long-term study. *J Pediatr Orthop* 1990;10:21.

445. Reynolds DA. Chiari innominate osteotomy in adults: technique, indications and contraindications. *J Bone Joint Surg Br* 1986;68:45.

446. Rush J. Chiari osteotomy in the adult: a long-term follow-up study. *Aust N Z J Surg* 1991;61:761.

447. Zlati M, Radojevi B, Lazovi D, et al. Late results of Chiari's pelvic osteotomy: a follow-up of 171 adult hips. *Int Orthop* 1988;12:149.

448. Harris WH, Bourne RB, Oh I. Intra-articular acetabular labrum: a possible etiological factor in certain cases of osteoarthritis of the hip. *J Bone Joint Surg Am* 1979;61:510.

449. Nishina T, Saito S, Ohzono K, et al. Chiari pelvic osteotomy for osteoarthritis: the influence of the torn and detached acetabular labrum. *J Bone Joint Surg Br* 1990;72:765.

450. Brougham DI, Broughton NS, Cole WG, et al. Avascular necrosis following closed reduction of congenital dislocation of the hip: review of influencing factors and long-term follow-up. *J Bone Joint Surg Br* 1990;72:557.

451. Bucholz R, Ogden J. Patterns of ischemic necrosis of the proximal femur in nonoperatively treated congenital hip disease. In: *The hip: proceedings of the sixth open scientific meeting of the hip society.* St. Louis, MO: Mosby, 1978:43.

452. Campbell P, Tarlow SD. Lateral tethering of the proximal femoral physis complicating the treatment of congenital hip dysplasia. *J Pediatr Orthop* 1990;10:6.

453. Gotoh E, Ando M. The pathogenesis of femoral head deformity in congenital dislocation of the hip: experimental study of the effects of articular interpositions in pigs. *Clin Orthop* 1993;288:303.

454. Gregosiewicz A, Wosko I. Risk factors of avascular necrosis in the treatment of congenital dislocation of the hip. *J Pediatr Orthop* 1988;8:17.

455. Kalamchi A, MacEwen GD. Avascular necrosis following treatment of congenital dislocation of the hip. *J Bone Joint Surg Am* 1980;62:876.

456. Keret D, MacEwen GD. Growth disturbance of the proximal part of the femur after treatment for congenital dislocation of the hip. *J Bone Joint Surg Am* 1991;73:410.

457. Law EG, Heistad DD, Marcus ML, et al. Effect of hip position on blood flow to the femur in puppies. *J Pediatr Orthop* 1982;2:133.

458. Nicholson JT, Kopell HP, Mattei FA. Regional stress angiography of the hip: a preliminary report. *J Bone Joint Surg Am* 1954;36:503.

459. Ogden JA, Southwick WO. A possible cause of avascular necrosis complicating the treatment of congenital dislocation of the hip. *J Bone Joint Surg Am* 1973;55:1770.

460. Ogden JA. Anatomic and histologic study of factors affecting development and evolution of avascular necrosis in congenital hip dislocation. In: *The hip: proceedings of the second annual meeting of the hip society.* St. Louis, MO: Mosby, 1974:125.

461. Ogden JA. Changing patterns of proximal femoral vascularity. *J Bone Joint Surg Am* 1974;56:941.

462. Ogden JA. Normal and abnormal circulation. In: Tachdjian MO, ed. *Congenital dislocation of the hip,* New York: Churchill Livingstone, 1982:59.

463. Schoenecker PL, Bitz DM, Whiteside LA. The acute effect of position of immobilization on capital femoral epiphyseal blood flow: a quantitative study using the hydrogen washout technique. *J Bone Joint Surg Am* 1978;60:899.

464. Trueta RJ, ed. *Studies of the development and decay of the human frame.* Philadelphia, PA: WB Saunders, 1988.

465. Herold HZ. Avascular necrosis of the femoral head in children under the age of three. *Clin Orthop* 1977;126:193.

466. Herold HZ. Unilateral congenital hip dislocation with contralateral avascular necrosis. *Clin Orthop* 1980;148:196.

467. Crego CH Jr, Schwartzmann JR. Medial adductor open reduction for congenital dislocation of the hip. *J Bone Joint Surg Am* 1948;30:428.

468. Kalamchi A, Schmidt TL, MacEwen GD. Congenital dislocation of the hip: open reduction by the medial approach. *Clin Orthop* 1982;169:127.

469. Kruczynski J. Avascular necrosis of the proximal femur in developmental dislocation of the hip: incidence, risk factors, sequelae, and MR imaging for diagnosis and prognosis. *Acta Orthop Scand Suppl* 1996;268:1.

470. Pous JG, Camous JY, el-Blidi S. Cause and prevention of osteochondritis in congenital dislocation of the hip. *Clin Orthop* 1992;281:56.

471. Thomas IH, Dunin AJ, Cole WG, et al. Avascular necrosis after open reduction for congenital dislocation of the hip: analysis of causative factors and natural history. *J Pediatr Orthop* 1989;9:525.

472. Kruczynski J. Avascular necrosis after non operative treatment of developmental hip dislocation: prognosis in 36 patients followed 17-26 years. *Acta Orthop Scand* 1995;66:239.

473. Westin GW, Ilfeld FW, Provost J. Total avascular necrosis of the capital femoral epiphysis in congenital dislocated hips. *Clin Orthop* 1976;119:93.

474. Race C, Herring JA. Congenital dislocation of the hip: an evaluation of closed reduction. *J Pediatr Orthop* 1983;3:166.

475. Massie WK. Vascular epiphyseal changes in congenital dislocation of the hip: results in adults compared with results in coxa plana and in congenital dislocation without vascular changes. *J Bone Joint Surg Am* 1951;33:284.

476. Powell EN, Gerratana FJ, Gage JR. Open reduction for congenital hip dislocation: the risk of avascular necrosis with three different approaches. *J Bone Joint Surg Am* 1986;58:1000.

477. Scaglietti O, Calandriello B. Open reduction of congenital dislocation of the hip. *J Bone Joint Surg Br* 1962;44:257.

478. Esteve R. Congenital dislocation of the hip: a review and assessment of results of treatment with special reference to frame reduction as compared with manipulative reduction. *J Bone Joint Surg Br* 1960;42:253.

479. MacKenzie IG, Seddon HJ, Trevor D. Congenital dislocation of the hip. *J Bone Joint Surg Br* 1960;42:689.

480. Ponseti IV, Frigerio ER. Results of treatment of congenital dislocation of the hip. *J Bone Joint Surg Am* 1959;41:823.

481. Tonnis D. Surgical treatment of congenital dislocation of the hip. *Clin Orthop* 1990;258:33.

482. Tonnis D. An evaluation of conservative and operative methods in the treatment of congenital hip dislocation. *Clin Orthop* 1976;119:76.

483. Gamble JG, Mochizuki C, Bieck EE, et al. Coxa magna following surgical treatment of congenital hip dislocation. *J Pediatr Orthop* 1985;5:528.

484. O'Brien T, Salter RB. Femoral head size in congenital dislocation of the hip. *J Pediatr Orthop* 1985;5:299.

485. Imatani JM, Miyake Y, Nakatsuka Y, et al. Coxa magna after open reduction for developmental dislocation of the hip. *J Pediatr Orthop* 1995;15:337.

486. O'Brien T. Growth-disturbance lines in congenital dislocation of the hip. *J Bone Joint Surg Am* 1985;67:626.

487. O'Brien T, Millis MB, Griffin PP. The early identification and classification of growth disturbances of the proximal end of the femur. *J Bone Joint Sung Am* 1986;68:970.

488. Kim HW, Morcuende JA, Dolan LA, et al. Acetabular development in developmental dysplasia of the hip complicated by lateral growth disturbance of the capital femoral epiphysis. *J Bone Joint Surg Am* 2000;82-A(12):1692–1700.

489. Beck M, Leunig M, Parvizi J, et al. Anterior femoroacetabular impingement. Part II. Midterm results of surgical treatment. *Clin Orthop* 2004;418:67–73.

490. Lavigne M, Parvizi J, Beck M, et al. Anterior femoroacetabular impingment. Part I. Techniques of joint preserving surgery. *Clin Orthop* 2004;418:61–66.

491. Siebenrock KA, Wahab KHA, Werlen S, et al. Abnormal extension of the femoral head epiphysis as a cause of cam impingement. *Clin Orthop* 2004;418:54–60.

492. Bar-On EH, Huo MH, DeLuca PA. Early innominate osteotomy as a treatment for avascular necrosis complicating developmental hip dysplasia. *J Pediatr Orthop B* 1997;6:138.

493. Givon U, Schindler A, Ganel A, et al. Distal transfer of the greater trochanter revisited: long term follow up of nine hips. *J Pediatr Orthop* 1995;15:346.

494. Andrisano A, Marchiodi L, Preitano M. Epiphysiodesis of the great trochanter. *Ital J Orthop Traumatol* 1986;12:217.

495. Langenskjold A, Salenius P. Epiphysiodesis of the greater trochanter. *Acta Orthop Scand* 1967;38:199.

496. Bialik V, Rosenberg N. Transfer of greater trochanter. *J Pediatr Orthop B* 1994;3:30.

497. Fernbach SK, Poznanski AKK, Kelikian AS, et al. Greater trochanteric overgrowth: development and surgical correction. *Radiology* 1954;3:661.

498. MacNicol MF, Makris D. Distal transfer of the greater trochanter. *J Bone Joint Surg Br* 1991;73:838.

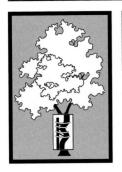

# 25

# Legg-Calvé-Perthes Syndrome

*Stuart L. Weinstein*

Legg-Calvé-Perthes disease remains one of the most controversial topics in all of pediatric orthopaedic surgery. The debate about its etiology and pathogenesis continues, and there is no unanimity regarding treatment. This chapter will review what is known about the condition, point out where controversies exist, and highlight the problems in decision making regarding treatment.

## EARLY HISTORY

Legg-Calvé-Perthes syndrome is a disorder of the hip in young children. The condition was described independently in 1910 by Legg (1), Calvé (2), Perthes (3), and Waldenstrom (4,5). In the late 19th century, however, Hugh Owen Thomas (6), Baker (7), and Wright (8) described patients with supposed hip joint infections that resolved without surgery, whose histories were consistent with Legg-Calvé-Perthes disease. Maydl (9), in 1897, reported this condition and thought it was related to congenital dislocation of the hip (10). Recent findings, discussed in this chapter's section on pathogenesis, suggest that Legg-Calvé-Perthes "disease" may more appropriately be called a syndrome.

In 1909, Arthur Legg presented a paper on five children who were limping after injury. This paper was published in 1910. He called this condition an "obscure affectation of the hip" and postulated that pressure secondary to injury caused flattening of the femoral head (1). In that same year, Calvé reported ten cases of a noninflammatory self-limiting condition that healed with flattening of the weight-bearing surface. He postulated that the cause of this condition was an abnormal or delayed osteogenesis. He reported coxa vara and increased femoral head size in these patients; on physical examination, all of the patients had decreased abduction (2). Perthes simultaneously reported six cases of what he termed "arthritis deformans juveniles." He postulated that this was an inflammatory condition (3). In his description of the condition, Waldenstrom postulated that the disease was a form of tuberculosis (4,5).

Perthes was the first investigator to describe the pathologic and histologic features of the disorder (11). He reported on a 9-year-old boy who had experienced symptoms for 2 years. Examination of a portion of the excised head revealed numerous cartilage islands throughout and "strings" connecting the cartilage of the joint and the physeal plate. Perthes noted that the marrow spaces were widened, with fatty infiltration; he saw no evidence of inflammation. He believed that the cartilage islands were new, and that this was an osteochondritis and not a tubercular process (11). Schwartz (12), an associate of Perthes, described the pathologic changes in a 7-year-old boy with a 2-year history of symptoms and reported similar findings. Waldenstrom (13) suggested the use of the term *coxa plana* to make the description of the disease consistent with that of other hip deformities, such as coxa vara and coxa valga. Sundt (14,15) published the first monograph on Legg-Calvé-Perthes syndrome, reporting on 66 cases and the pathology of the condition. The essential feature in all of his cases was the cartilaginous islands in the epiphysis. Sundt attributed the disease to an "osteodystrophy due to dysendocrinia of a hereditary disposition." He believed that individuals so predisposed would get Legg-Perthes disease after they sustained an injury (i.e., infection or trauma) to the hip. Sundt was the first to introduce the modern concept of the "susceptible child."

Phemister (16), reporting on the curettage findings in a 10-year-old child with an 8-month history of symptoms, described areas of bone necrosis, granulation tissue, old bone with new bone formation, and osteoclasts. He interpreted these findings as an inflammatory and infectious process. In 1922, Riedel (17) reported on two cases and presented the histology. He described the thickening of the articular cartilage and noted that the junction between the bone and the articular cartilage was filled with blood. He also noted that the physeal plate was destroyed and that there were many cartilage rests. Dead bone was surrounded by a rich granulation tissue, and many giant cells were present. He also noted that farther away from the main disease process, the marrow was fibrotic with inflammatory infiltrates. Riedel was the first investigator to notice that there were blastic and clastic changes working at the same time on the same bone trabeculae. In his second

specimen, he found regeneration of the cartilage in the subchondral area, cell atrophy, and some inflammatory cells. That same year, Waldenstrom (18) proposed the first radiographic classification of the disease process on the basis of the data from 22 patients who were followed up until the completion of their growth. Since then, most of the orthopaedic literature has centered on the etiologic, epidemiologic, and prognostic factors in Legg-Calvé-Perthes disease and follow-up of various treatment modalities (19–23).

## EPIDEMIOLOGY AND ETIOLOGY

Legg-Calvé-Perthes syndrome occurs most commonly in the age range of 4 to 8 years (24), but cases have been reported in children from 2 years of age to the late teenage years. It is more common in boys than in girls by a ratio of 4 or 5 to 1 (25). The incidence of bilaterality has been reported as 10% to 12% (24,26). Although the incidence of a positive family history in patients with Legg-Calvé-Perthes syndrome ranges from 1.6% to 20% (10,24,27–33), there is currently no evidence that this syndrome is an inherited condition (34).

Wynne-Davies and Gormley (24) reported on a series of 310 index patients with Legg-Calvé-Perthes syndrome. They noted that, of the children of index patients with the syndrome, only 2% had Legg-Calvé-Perthes syndrome. All twins in this series were discordant, including one monozygotic pair. Eleven percent had abnormal birth presentations, including breech and transverse, compared with the 2% to 4% incidence that would be expected in the general population. There is a higher incidence of Legg-Calvé-Perthes syndrome in later-born children, particularly the third to the sixth child, and a higher percentage in lower socioeconomic groups (35,36). Parents of the children with the syndrome also tend to be older than those in the general population (24,33,37).

Legg-Calvé-Perthes syndrome is more common in certain geographic areas, particularly in urban rather than rural communities, giving rise to the suspicion of a nutritional cause, possibly a trace element deficiency (35–43). There is also a recently reported strong association (33% of patients with the syndrome) of Legg-Calvé-Perthes disease with the psychological profile associated with attention deficit hyperactivity disorder (44). Malloy and Macmahon as well as Lappin et al. (45–47) noted that birth weight was lower in children with the syndrome. Harrison et al. (48) reported that children with Legg-Calvé-Perthes syndrome lagged behind their chronological age, and 89% of the involved individuals had delayed bone age. Ralston (49) and others demonstrated that this delay in skeletal maturation averages 21 months, but that during the healing stages of the disease there was recovery of height and weight through increased growth velocity (49–51). Race may also be a factor in the frequency of incidence of this condition. There is a higher frequency of occurrence of Legg-Calvé-Perthes syndrome among the Japanese, other Asians, Eskimos, and Central Europeans, and a lower frequency of occurrence among native Australians, Americans, Indians, Polynesians, and persons of African origin (10,40,52,53).

There is considerable evidence of anthropometric abnormalities in children with Legg-Calvé-Perthes syndrome. Cameron and Izatt (54) reported that boys with the syndrome were 1 inch shorter and girls with the syndrome were 3 inches shorter compared with healthy children. Burwell et al. (55–57) and others (35,58,59) demonstrated that children with the syndrome are smaller in all dimensions, except for head circumference, and shorter in the distal portions of the extremities as opposed to the proximal portions. Loder et al. (60), in a more recent study, demonstrated that bone age of the pelvis in boys was less delayed than that of the hand and wrist. In patients who have the disorder at a young age, the shortness in stature tends to correct during adolescence, whereas patients who have the disorder at an older age tend to be small throughout life (33). Eckerwall et al. (61) followed up 110 children with the disorder in a longitudinal study and showed that these children were shorter at birth, remained short during the entire growth period, and their growth velocity never changed. Burwell et al. (57) demonstrated an abnormality of growth hormone–dependent somatomedin in boys with Legg-Calvé-Perthes syndrome, whereas Tanaka et al. (62), Fisher (27), and Kitsugi et al. (63) reported contrary results.

Growth hormone regulates postnatal skeletal development. The effects of growth hormone on postnatal skeletal development are mediated, in part, by the somatomedins (insulinlike growth factors) (64). Somatomedin C insulinlike growth factor-1 (IGF1) is the principal somatomedin responsible for postnatal skeletal bone maturation (64). Plasma IGF1 levels have been reported to be significantly reduced in children with the disorder during the first 2 years after the diagnosis of Perthes disease. These alterations were accompanied by a tendency toward growth arrest and impaired weight gain. An acceleration in growth and weight gain is believed to accompany the healing stages of the disease, although a recent report by Kealey et al. disputes this growth acceleration following the active stages of the disease (65).

In plasma, nearly all IGF1 is bound to specific binding proteins. However, levels of the major binding protein, insulinlike growth factor binding protein 3 (IGFBP3), are normal during the first 2 years after the diagnosis of Perthes disease (66,67). Low levels of circulating IGF1 and failure of IGF1 to increase normally during the prepubertal years in patients with Perthes disease, in conjunction with reportedly normal growth hormone levels, raise the possibility of decreased responsiveness of growth-plate chondrocytes and hepatocytes (64). The combination of moderately reduced IGF1 levels with normal IGFBP3 has been reported in normal-variant short-statured children. The skeletal maturation delay and retarded bone age reported in patients with

Perthes disease, in conjunction with the findings described in the preceding text, could be considered to be a retention of the infantile hormone pattern (65).

Malnutrition is one factor that leads to low IGF levels, and this could be related to the reportedly higher incidence of Perthes disease in low-income families (42). The disproportionate skeletal development affecting the distal portions of the body reflects a tendency toward infantile body proportions. This correlates with the reduced IGF1 levels in the presence of normal levels of binding proteins (68). Controversy still exists in that a recent study by another group of investigators reported results opposite to those reported by Neidel et al. (67), with serum levels of IGF1 being normal and those of IGFBP3 being lower in children with Perthes disease, compared with controls (69). Another recent study, although confirming the skeletal maturation delay in children with Perthes disease, demonstrated no difference in IGF1 (measured with IGF2-blocked binding sites) and IGFBP3 serum concentrations with respect to bone age (70). This group disputed the claims of disturbance of the hypothalamic-pituitary-somatomedin axis in patients with Perthes disease. The reported differences in the various studies, in some cases, may be partly attributable to the methods used for measuring IGF1. There is an increased incidence of hernia in patients with Legg-Calvé-Perthes syndrome and their first-degree relatives. There is also an increased incidence of minor congenital abnormalities in patients with the syndrome (28,71–73).

The cause of Legg-Calvé-Perthes syndrome remains unknown. Many etiologic theories have been proposed. In the early part of the 20th century, most investigators thought that it was a disease of an inflammatory or infectious nature (3–5,74–76). Phemister (16,77) believed that the disease was an infectious process, although tissue cultures were negative. Axhausen (74) believed that it was caused by bacillary embolism in which the infection either was not manifested, or was too weak and healed quickly. As late as 1975, Matsoukas (78) demonstrated an association between Legg-Calvé-Perthes syndrome and prenatal rubella.

Until the 1950s, trauma was considered by many investigators to be the cause, or a significant contributing factor, of Perthes disease (1,79–85). As with most childhood orthopaedic conditions, a significant number of patients may relate an episode of trauma to the onset of symptoms.

Many investigators, particularly those from Eastern Europe, thought that Legg-Calvé-Perthes syndrome was of congenital origin, and that there was a relationship between this disease and congenitally dislocated hips (83–90). Glimcher (91) proposed that cytotoxic agents of external or endogenous origin may be responsible for bone cell death. A recent report showed the association of Perthes with delayed ossification of the proximal femoral epiphysis (92). At one time, Perthes disease was believed to be related to hypothyroidism (93–95); this has since been disproved (89,90). Recent reports demonstrate moderately increased plasma concentrations of free thyroxin and free triiodothyronine in patients with Perthes disease, compared with controls (68). It has yet to be conclusively determined whether the aforementioned factors contribute to causing Perthes disease, and whether IGF1 is at reduced levels in the early disease stages as reported. These findings do, however, provide additional evidence that growth-related systemic abnormalities exist in patients with Legg-Calvé-Perthes syndrome (68).

Transient synovitis has been thought, by many investigators, to be a precursor to the condition. Gershuni (96) reported that 25% of children with benign transient synovitis developed Legg-Calvé-Perthes disease, whereas Jacobs (97) reported three cases of Legg-Calvé-Perthes disease among 25 patients with acute transient synovitis. Although all hips with Perthes disease have synovitis, especially early in the course of the disease, and many have persistent synovitis for years (98–102), a review of the literature reveals that an average of 1% to 3% of patients with a history of transient synovitis later develop Legg-Calvé-Perthes syndrome (103–108). Chuinard (109) and Craig et al. (81,82) have proposed that excessive femoral neck anteversion is a causative factor in the development of Legg-Calvé-Perthes syndrome.

Most current etiologic theories involve vascular embarrassment. An insufficient blood supply to the proximal femur has been elucidated by many authors. The terminology used in the literature varies. However, there are three main sources of blood to the proximal femur: an extracapsular arterial ring, the ascending cervical (retinacular branches) vessels, and the artery of the ligamentum teres (110) (Fig. 25.1). The extracapsular ring is formed mostly by the medial and lateral femoral circumflex vessels. This ring gives rise to the ascending cervical branches, which are extracapsular, and these in turn give rise to the metaphyseal and epiphyseal branches. The anterior portion of the extracapsular ring is formed primarily by the lateral femoral circumflex artery. The posterior, lateral, and medial aspects of the ring are formed by the medial femoral circumflex artery. Chung (110) found that the greatest volume of blood flow to the femoral head comes through the lateral ascending cervical vessel (the termination of the medial femoral circumflex artery), which crosses the capsule in the posterior trochanteric fossa. Trueta and Pinto de Lima (111,112), and Chung (110) demonstrated that the anterior vascular anastomotic network (Fig. 25.1) is much less extensive than the posterior anastomotic network, particularly in specimens taken from patients 3 to 10 years of age, which correlates with the age range of Legg-Calvé-Perthes syndrome. Chung also demonstrated that the anterior anastomotic network was incomplete more often in boys, which correlates with the male predominance found in Legg-Calvé-Perthes syndrome. Ogden (113) reported the presence of vessels crossing the physeal plate in some of his specimens, but Chung disagreed, suggesting instead that the vessels do not actually cross the plate, but pass through the peripheral perichondral fibrocartilaginous complex.

Interruption of the blood supply to the femoral head in Perthes disease was first demonstrated in 1926, when Konjetzny (76) showed obliterative vascular thickening in a pathologic specimen. Theron (114) used selective angiograms to demonstrate obstruction of the superior retinacular artery in patients with Legg-Calvé-Perthes syndrome. In a recent angiographic study, Atsumi et al. showed that 68% of subjects with Perthes disease had interruption of the lateral epiphyseal arteries at their origin (115). In 1973, Sanchis et al. (116) proposed the second infarction theory. They experimentally infarcted the femoral head of animals

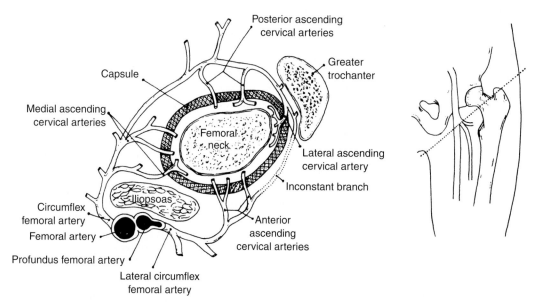

**Figure 25.1**  The blood supply to the normal proximal femur in a child. (From Chung SMK. The arterial supply of the developing proximal end of the human femur. *J Bone Joint Surg Am* 1976;58:961.)

labeled with tetracycline. They were unable to produce a typical histologic picture of Legg-Calvé-Perthes syndrome with only a single infarction. With a second infarction, however, they were able to show a more characteristic histologic picture of Legg-Calvé-Perthes syndrome. Inoue et al. (117) later correlated this double-infarction theory with human histologic material. Clinical correlation for this theory is provided by reports of recurrent Perthes disease (118,119) (Fig. 25.2). Salter and Thompson (120,121) proposed that Legg-Calvé-Perthes syndrome is a complication of aseptic necrosis, and that a fracture manifested radiographically by a subchondral radiolucent zone initiates the resorptive phase. Kleinman and Bleck (122) demonstrated increased blood viscosity in a group of patients with Legg-Calvé-Perthes syndrome, possibly leading to decreased blood flow to the femoral epiphysis. Vascular embarrassment, caused by intraosseous venous hypertension and venous obstruction, has been demonstrated by several authors (34,123,124).

Recently, attention has been centered on reports of protein C and S deficiencies in patients with Perthes syndrome (125–129). Thrombophilia induced by low levels of protein C or protein S, or by resistance to activated protein C, has been associated with the development of osteonecrosis and with arterial thrombosis (127–130). These investigators have suggested routine screening of: the levels of protein C, protein S, and lipoprotein(s); plasminogen activator inhibitor activity; and stimulated tissue-plasminogen activator activity in patients with Perthes syndrome (127). They believe that routine coagulation screening of children with Legg-Perthes disease has an additional advantage because of the familial nature of the autosomal dominant coagulopathies. These disorders are associated with thrombotic events in 60% of adult family members. The authors believe that the diagnosis of a coagulation disorder in a child with Legg-Perthes disease can and should lead to studies in first-degree relatives, with the goal of preventing thrombotic events in families. More recent literature has refuted the role of thrombophilia in causing Perthes disease (131–135).

## PATHOGENESIS

The histologic changes seen in Legg-Calvé-Perthes syndrome should be put in perspective. Few human specimens have been studied, and each such specimen represents only one stage in the disease process. Most specimens are from curettage or core biopsies, which show only one portion of the involved head at a time.

In the developing normal human femoral head, the secondary center of ossification is covered by cartilage comprising three zones (Fig. 25.3). The superficial zone has the morphologic properties of adult articular cartilage. Beneath this zone is the zone of epiphyseal cartilage, which is histochemically different. The zone becomes thinner as the skeleton matures and the epiphyseal bone enlarges in size. Underneath the epiphyseal cartilage is a thin zone formed by small clusters of cartilage cells that hypertrophy and

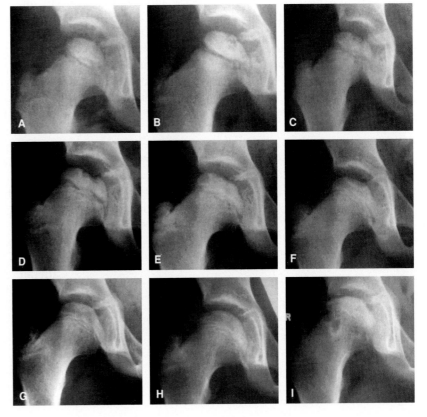

**Figure 25.2** A girl, 4 years and 8 months of age, was treated for left hip Perthes disease (late fragmentation phase) beginning in January 1983. Anteroposterior (**right, A–I**) and Lauenstein (**see pg. 1044, A–I**) views of the right hip at different stages, January 1983 to December 1987. **A:** View of the right hip at the time of initial presentation with no signs of involvement (January 1983). **B:** Early involvement, patient still asymptomatic (September 1983). **C–F:** Progressive healing of the right femoral epiphysis at May 1984 (**C**), August 1984 (**D**), May 1985 (**E**), and November 1985 (**F**). **G:** Femoral head was completely healed by December 1986. **H:** Recurrent changes in the density of the femoral head and a subchondral fracture that involves less than 50% of the head (Catterall group 2) was seen in June 1987. **I:** Complete involvement of the ossific nucleus (Catterall group 4) with diffuse metaphyseal reaction and cysts in December 1987. (From Martinez AG, Weinstein SL. Recurrent Legg-Calvé-Perthes' disease: case report and review of the literature. *J Bone Joint Surg Am* 1991;73:1081.)

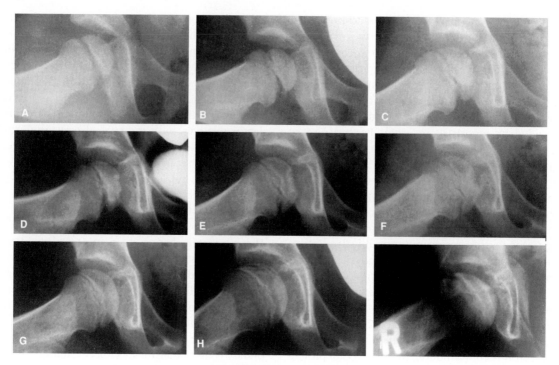

**Figure 25.2** (continued)

degenerate. Capillaries penetrate this zone from below, and bone forms at a much slower rate than in the metaphysis (136).

Histologic changes of the epiphyseal and physeal cartilage of patients with Legg-Calvé-Perthes syndrome (Figs. 25.4 and 25.5) were described as early as 1913. These and current studies demonstrate that the superficial zone of the epiphyseal cartilage covering the affected femoral head is normal but thickened. In the middle layer of the epiphyseal cartilage, however, two types of abnormalities are seen: areas of extreme hypercellularity, with the cells varying in size and shape and often arranged in clusters, and areas containing a

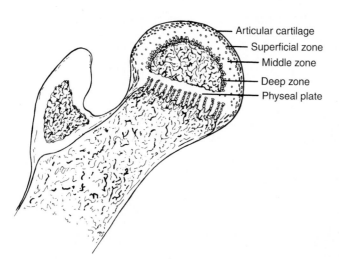

**Figure 25.3**   Proximal femur in a child.

loose fibrocartilage-like matrix. These abnormal areas in the epiphyseal cartilage have histochemical and ultrastructural properties that are different from normal cartilage and fibrocartilage. Areas of small secondary ossification centers are evident, with bony trabeculae of uneven thickness forming directly on the abnormal cartilage matrix (136–141). The superficial and middle layers of epiphyseal cartilage are nourished by synovial fluid and continue to proliferate, whereas only the deepest layer of the epiphyseal cartilage is dependent on the epiphyseal blood supply and is affected by the ischemic process (136,139,142–150).

The physeal plate also is abnormal in Legg-Calvé-Perthes syndrome. It shows evidence of cleft formation with amorphous debris and extravasation of blood. In the metaphyseal region, endochondral ossification is normal in some areas, but in others the proliferating cells are separated by a fibrillated cartilaginous matrix that does not calcify (Fig. 25.5). The cells in these areas do not degenerate but continue to proliferate without endochondral ossification, leading to tongues of cartilage extending into the metaphysis as bone growth proceeds in adjoining areas (136,137,141,151–153).

Catterall et al. (151) have demonstrated thickening, abnormal staining, sporadic calcification, and diminished evidence of ossification in the deep zone of the articular cartilage of the unaffected hip. They also demonstrated that the physeal plate in these unaffected hips is thinner than normal, with irregular cell columns and cartilage masses remaining unossified in the primary spongiosa.

Some of these cartilage changes have been seen in other epiphyseal plates, such as the greater trochanter and the

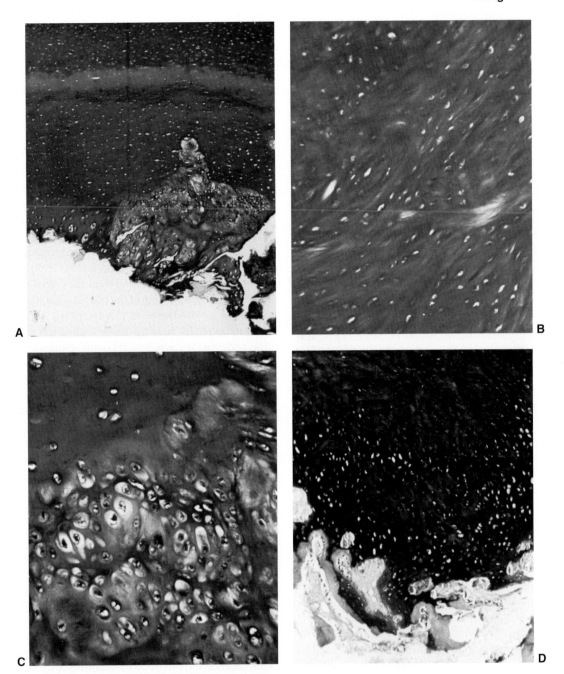

**Figure 25.4**  **A:** Superficial zone cartilage and epiphyseal cartilage of the femoral head. The superficial zone cartilage is normal and is Alcian blue-positive. The epiphyseal cartilage stains with periodic acid-Schiff, but only the perilacunar rims stain with Alcian blue. In the epiphyseal cartilage, there is an area of disorganized abnormal Alcian blue-positive cartilage. (Alcian blue with 0.6 mol per L magnesium chloride; original magnification, × 25.) **B:** Abnormal area of epiphyseal cartilage. The matrix has a fibrillated appearance and is strongly Alcian blue-positive. (Alcian blue with 0.6 mol per L magnesium chloride; original magnification, × 100.) **C:** Junction between the normal and abnormal epiphyseal cartilage. Normal cartilage is periodic acid-Schiff positive, whereas the abnormal cartilage is very cellular and retains Alcian blue positivity at high concentrations of magnesium chloride. (Alcian blue with 0.7 mol per L magnesium chloride; original magnification, × 165.) **D:** Extensive area of abnormal epiphyseal cartilage in the femoral head. Bone seems to form directly on the abnormal cartilage. Abnormal cartilage retains intense Alcian blue positivity at a high concentration of magnesium chloride, but loses that positivity and becomes strongly positive to periodic acid-Schiff at the bone-cartilage junction. (Alcian blue with 0.7 mol per L magnesium chloride, periodic acid-Schiff, and Weigert hematoxylin stains; original magnification, × 40.) (From Hresko MT, McDougall PA, Gorlin JB, et al. Prospective reevaluation of the association between thrombotic diathesis and Legg-Perthes disease. *J Bone Joint Surg Am* 2002;84(9):1613–1618.)

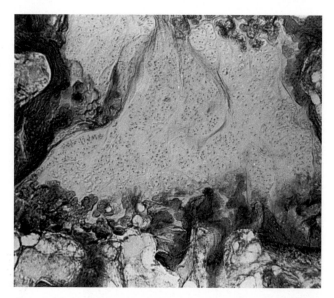

**Figure 25.5** Photomicrograph showing a large area of cartilage between the bone trabeculae of the femoral neck. (Original magnification, × 80.) (From Kealey WD, Mayne EE, McDonald W, et al. The role of coagulation abnormalities in the development of Perthes' disease. *J Bone Joint Surg Br* 2000;82(5):744–746.)

acetabulum (154). In the human specimens described by Ponseti (137), the physeal plate lesions were longstanding, as shown by the fact that there was only necrotic bone in the femoral head and no evidence of repair. Catterall et al. reported similar cartilaginous lesions in a patient with Catterall group 1 disease, in which there is no sequestrum formation (139,141) (Fig. 25.6). The various reported physeal plate and epiphyseal plate lesions resemble the lesions that Ponseti and Shepard produced in rats by administering aminonitrils (155). These epiphyseal and physeal plate changes, in conjunction with the unusual and precarious blood supply to the proximal femur, make the femoral head vulnerable to the effects of physeal plate disruption.

Surveys of patients with Legg-Calvé-Perthes syndrome confirm that the histologic abnormalities are accompanied by irregularities of ossification in other epiphyses, especially Kohler disease of the navicular (71,137,156). Harrison and Blakemore (157), studying 153 consecutive patients with unilateral Legg-Calvé-Perthes disease, found that 48% had contour irregularities in the contralateral normal capital epiphysis compared with 10% of the matched controls. Kandzierski et al. reported that 35% of patients with Perthes disease showed changes in the unaffected proximal femur in the first radiograph (145). Aire et al. (158) demonstrated that the unaffected hip showed anterior and lateral flattening at the time of diagnosis of the affected hip. These data suggest that Legg-Calvé-Perthes disease is a generalized process affecting other epiphyses, and therefore should not be referred to as a disease but should be called *Legg-Calvé-Perthes syndrome*.

Disorganization of the physeal plate, together with minimal trauma, may interrupt the continuity of retinacular

vessels, causing necrosis (136,137). This finding, in conjunction with the aforementioned epidemiologic, histologic, and radiologic data, supports the belief that Legg-Calvé-Perthes syndrome may be a localized manifestation of a generalized disorder of epiphyseal cartilage in the susceptible child (10,34,50,58,72,136,148,159,160).

## Radiographic Stages

Radiographically, Legg-Calvé-Perthes syndrome can be classified into four stages: initial, fragmentation, reossification, and healed. These stages are important in the formulation of treatment decisions that will be discussed later in this chapter. In the initial stage (18,161), one of the first signs of this condition is failure of the femoral ossific nucleus to increase in size because of a lack of blood supply (Fig. 25.7). The affected femoral head appears smaller than the opposite, unaffected ossific nucleus. Widening of the medial joint space, as initially described by Waldenstrom (18,162) (Fig. 25.7), is another early radiographic finding. Some researchers have theorized that widening is caused by synovitis. Others have proposed that this finding is secondary to decreased head volume caused by necrosis and collapse and a secondary increase in blood flow to the soft tissue parts, such as the ligamentum teres and pulvinar, causing the head to displace laterally (161,163). Synovitis is indeed present in patients with Perthes disease to varying degrees (98,99,101,102,164,165), but the medial joint space widening is probably most often an apparent radiographic phenomenon secondary to epiphyseal cartilage hypertrophy (Fig. 25.8).

In the initial stage, the physeal plate is irregular and the metaphysis is blurry and radiolucent (86) (Fig. 25.9A). The femoral ossific nucleus appears radiodense (166). This relative increase in radiodensity may be caused by osteopenia of the surrounding bone (167,168), or an increase in the mass of bone per unit area.

The second radiographic stage is called the *fragmentation phase* (18,161). Radiographically, the repair aspects of the disease become more prominent (Fig. 25.9B). The bony epiphysis begins to fragment, and there are areas of increased radiolucency and increased radiodensity. Increased radiodensity at this stage may be caused by new bone forming on old bone (169–173) and thickening of existing trabeculae (171). The subchondral radiolucent zone (i.e., crescent sign) first described by Waldenstrom (162,174), and later brought to wider attention by Caffey (175), is one of the very early signs of Legg-Calvé-Perthes syndrome in the fragmentation stage (Figs. 25.2 and 25.10). According to Salter and Thompson (121) and Salter and Bell (176), this radiographic finding results from a subchondral stress fracture, and the extent of this zone determines the extent of the necrotic fragment.

The third radiographic stage is the reparative or reossification phase (18,161). Radiographically normal bone density returns, with radiodensities appearing in areas that were formerly radiolucent. Alterations in the shape of the femoral head and neck become apparent (Fig. 25.9).

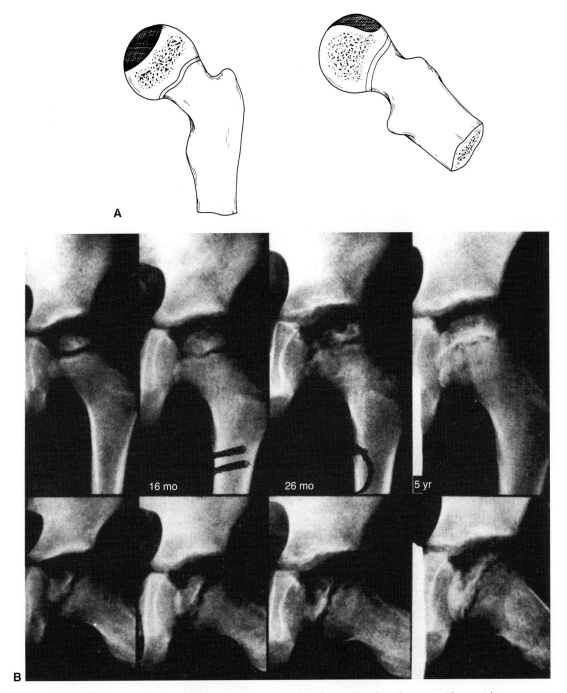

**Figure 25.6   A:** Catterall group 1 disease shows anterior femoral head involvement with no evidence of sequestrum, subchondral fracture line, or metaphyseal abnormalities. **B:** Catterall group 1 disease 1 week to 5 years after onset of symptoms.

The final stage is the healed phase. In this stage, the proximal femur may have residual deformity from the disease and the repair process (Fig. 25.9).

In the young child, Legg-Calvé-Perthes syndrome cannot be compared with aseptic necrosis after fracture of the neck of the femur or traumatic dislocations of the hip. In these situations, the vascular insult to the femoral head usually heals rapidly without going through the prolonged stages of fragmentation and repair that are seen in children with Legg-Calvé-Perthes syndrome (136,177,178).

## Pathogenesis of Deformity

The deformities of the femoral head that occur in Legg-Calvé-Perthes syndrome come about in many ways. First, there is growth disturbance in the epiphyseal and physeal

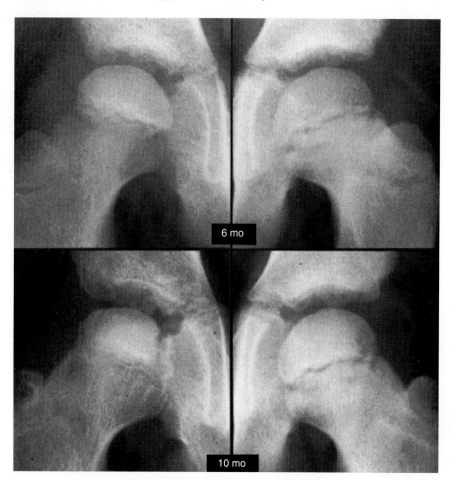

**Figure 25.7** Anteroposterior radiogram of a hip in a patient who developed Legg-Calvé-Perthes disease. On the initial film, taken 6 months after the onset of symptoms, the right ossific nucleus is smaller than the left, and the medial joint space is widened. Note also the retained density of the ossific nucleus compared with the normal hip and the relative osteopenia of the viable bone of the proximal femur and pelvis. Ten months after the onset of symptoms, the evolution of the radiographic changes is seen. (From McKibbin B, ed. *Recent advances in Perthes' disease.* Edinburgh: Churchill Livingstone, 1975.)

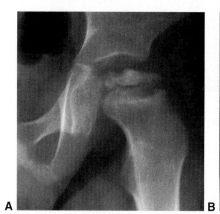
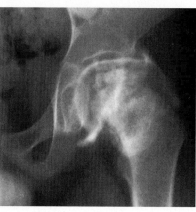
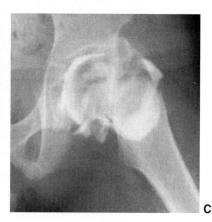

**Figure 25.8** A boy, 4 years and 9 months of age, with Catterall group 4 disease and at-risk status. **A:** Plain radiograph. **B:** Arthrogram in neutral abduction, adduction, and rotation. There is enlargement and flattening of the cartilaginous femoral head, and the lateral margin of the acetabulum is deformed by the femoral head. **C:** Arthrogram in abduction and slight external rotation. The femoral head hinges on the lateral edge of the acetabulum, further deforming the lateral acetabulum. Slight pooling of dye is seen medially. Note that the widened joint space is an apparent widening, not a real widening, and that it is secondary to continued growth of the superficial zone of cartilage in the absence of growth of the ossific nucleus.

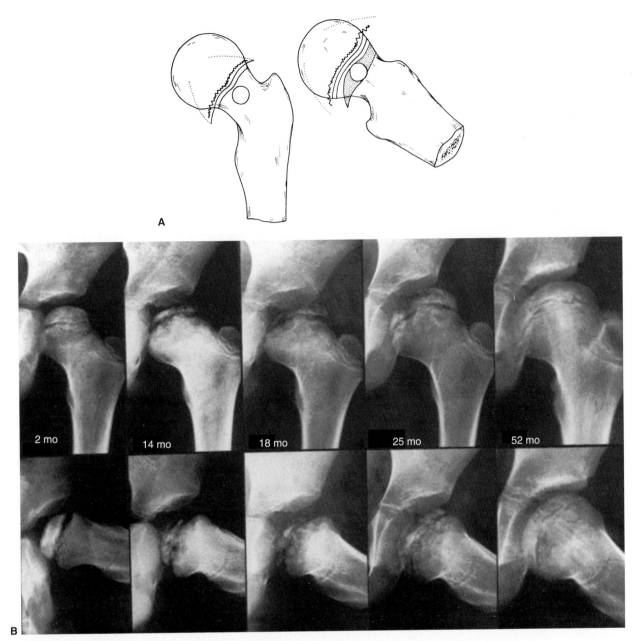

**Figure 25.9   A:** Catterall group 4 disease shows involvement of the whole head of the femur, with either diffuse or central metaphyseal lesions and with posterior remodeling of the epiphysis. **B:** Catterall group 4 disease, 2 months to 52 months after onset of symptoms. Note the stages: 14 months, fragmentation; 18 months, early reossification; 25 months, late reossification; 52 months, healed. Note also the growth-arrest line and evidence of reactivation of the growth plate along the femoral neck.

plates. In the physeal plate, this may result in premature closure with resultant deformity, such as central physeal arrest, causing shortening of the neck of the femur and trochanteric overgrowth (179,180) (Fig. 25.11). The repair process itself may cause physical compaction resulting from structural failure and displacement of tissue elements (91). During the healing process, the femoral head will deform according to the asymmetric repair process and the applied stresses. The molding action of the acetabulum during new bone formation may also play a role in this

process (181,182). With deformity of the femoral head, the acetabulum, particularly its lateral aspect, is deformed secondarily.

The articular cartilage of the femoral head shows changes in shape secondary to the disease process itself. The deepest layer of the articular cartilage is nourished by the subchondral blood supply. This layer is often devitalized in Legg-Calvé-Perthes syndrome (139,142–146,149). The superficial layers that are nourished by synovial fluid continue to proliferate, causing an increase in the thickness of

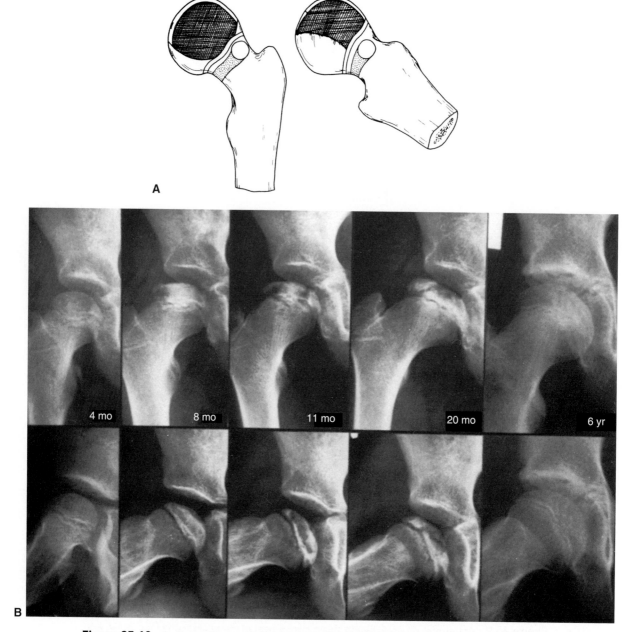

**Figure 25.10**   **A:** Catterall group 3 disease shows large sequestrum involving three-fourths of the femoral head. The junction between the involved and the uninvolved portions is sclerotic. Metaphyseal lesions are diffuse, particularly anterolaterally, and the subchondral fracture line extends to the posterior half of the epiphysis. The lateral column is involved. **B:** Catterall group 3 disease, 4 months to 6 years after symptom onset. Note the involvement of the lateral pillar, as well as the subchondral radiolucent zone on the radiograph taken 8 months after onset of symptoms.

the articular cartilage. With trabecular collapse and fracture and articular cartilage overgrowth, significant femoral head deformities develop that are manifested clinically as loss of abduction and rotation (Fig. 25.8).

The source of vessel ingrowth is under debate. Many investigators (142,143,183) have demonstrated that the new blood vessels arise from the metaphysis and the metaphyseal periosteum, and penetrate between the epiphysis and the joint cartilage into the epiphysis. Other investigators have shown metaphyseal vessels penetrating the physeal plate

into the epiphysis (113,184). When the blood supply of the subchondral area is restored, it generally comes from the periphery and moves to the center, first restoring endochondral ossification at the periphery and causing asymmetric growth (98,149) (Fig. 25.12). In addition, there is abnormal ossification of the disorganized matrix of the epiphyseal cartilage. Finally, there is periosteal bone growth and reactivation of the physeal plate along the femoral neck, with abnormally long cartilage columns leading to coxa magna and a widened femoral neck (136,137).

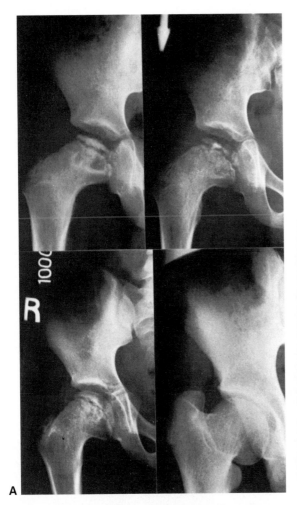
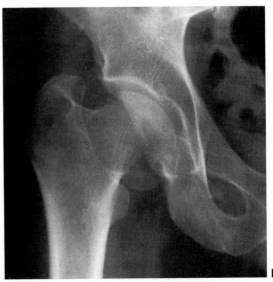

**Figure 25.11** **A:** A 6-year-old boy with Catterall group 4 disease. At 6 years and 2 months of age, fragmentation stage **(upper left)**. At 6 years and 9 months of age, early reossification stage **(upper right)**. At 8 years and 9 months of age, healed **(lower left)**. At 16 years and 2 months of age, skeletally mature **(lower right)**. The patient's hip healed with a central physeal arrest pattern. **B:** A 51-year-old patient at 45-year follow-up. He was asymptomatic and had a full range of motion (Iowa Hip Rating, 95 of 100 points). At maximal fragmentation the hip is classified as showing Catterall group 4, Salter-Thompson type B, and lateral pillar type C disease.

The actual deformity that develops is profoundly influenced by the duration of the disease. This, in turn, is proportional to the extent of the epiphyseal involvement, the age of the patient at the time of onset of the disease, the remodeling potential of the patient, and the stage of disease when treatment is initiated. An additional factor is the type of treatment chosen (185–188).

## Patterns of Deformity

Four basic patterns of residual deformity result from Legg-Calvé-Perthes syndrome: coxa magna, premature physeal arrest patterns, irregular femoral head formation, and osteochondritis dissecans (180,189). Coxa magna (Fig. 25.9) develops with ossification of the hypertrophied articular cartilage, and also from reactivation of the physeal plate along the femoral neck. This also occurs in conjunction with periosteal new bone formation along the femoral neck.

Premature physeal plate closure generally leads to one of two patterns of arrest: central or lateral. In the central arrest pattern, the femoral neck is short and the epiphysis is relatively round (Fig. 25.11). There is trochanteric overgrowth and mild acetabular deformity. In the lateral arrest pattern, the femoral head is tilted externally (Fig. 25.13). There is also trochanteric overgrowth. The epiphysis is oval, with a corresponding acetabular deformity (180,189).

The irregular femoral head may occur as a consequence of certain patterns of physeal arrest, or it may be an iatrogenic deformity from attempts at "containment" of a noncontainable head (Fig. 25.14). After the femoral head becomes deformed and is no longer containable within the acetabulum, the only motion that is allowed is in the flexion and extension plane, with abduction leading to hinging on the lateral edge of the acetabulum. This hinge abduction causes acetabular deformity, leading to femoral head deformity (190–192).

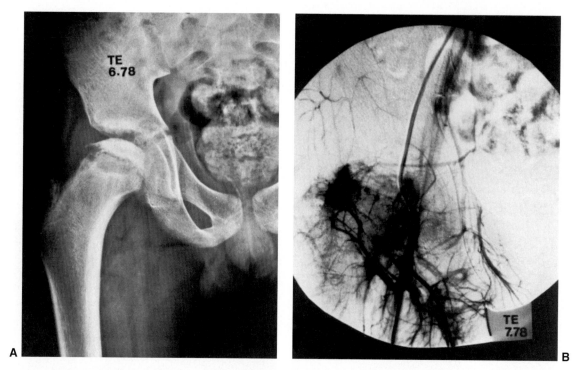

**Figure 25.12**  **A:** A 12-year-old boy with total femoral head involvement in the early fragmentation stage of the disease. **B:** Subtraction arteriogram demonstrating the avascularity of the central portion of the femoral head, with increased vascularity at the periphery. (Courtesy of J. G. Pous, MD, Montpellier, France.)

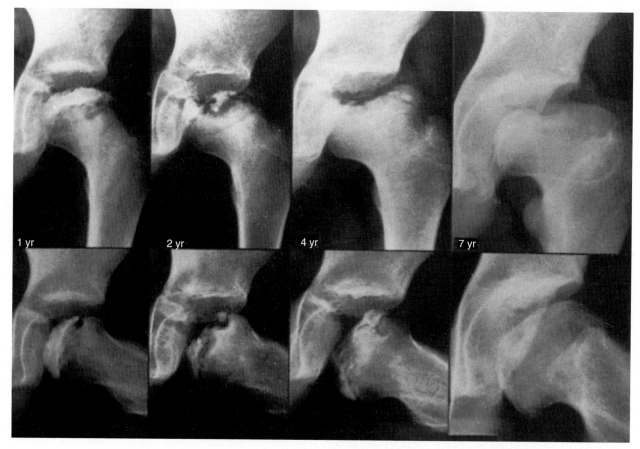

**Figure 25.13**  A 7-year follow-up from presentation in a patient with Catterall group 4 disease, who had a lateral growth-arrest pattern. At maximal fragmentation, the radiographic classification would be Salter-Thompson type B and lateral pillar type C disease. (From Weinstein SL. Perthes' disease: an overview. *Curr Orthop* 1988;2:181.)

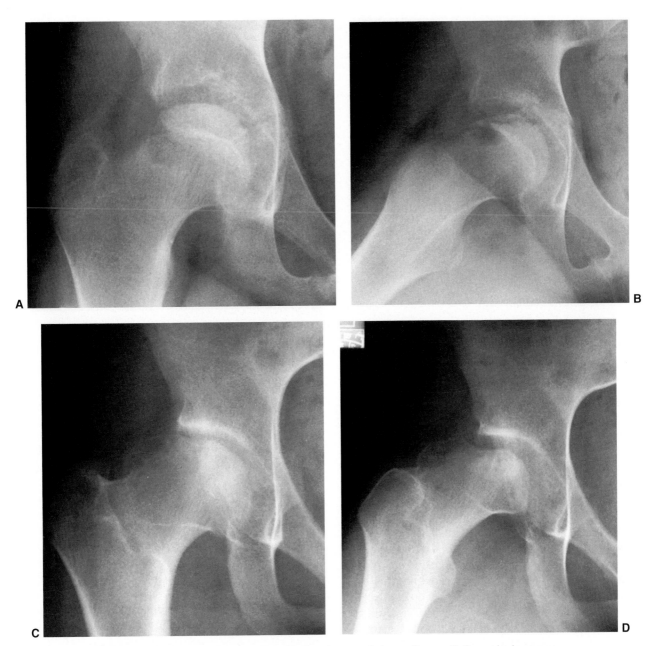

**Figure 25.14** A girl, 11 years and 3 months of age, with Catterall group 3 disease had a noncontainable femoral head, yet was treated for a long time in an abduction brace. **A,B:** Anteroposterior radiograph in the early fragmentation stage **(A)** and Lauenstein radiograph in the early fragmentation stage **(B)**. **C,D:** At age 14 years, the patient was skeletally mature, and had an irregular femoral head. Anteroposterior radiograph **(C)** and Lauenstein radiograph **(D)**. (From Weinstein SL. Perthes' disease: an overview. *Curr Orthop* 1988;2:181.)

The fourth and least common (3% incidence) residual deformity that occurs in Legg-Calvé-Perthes syndrome is osteochondritis dissecans (Fig. 25.15). This usually occurs when there is late onset of disease, and with prolonged, ineffectual repair (180,189,193–195).

## NATURAL HISTORY

The formulation of disease treatment requires that the treating physician knows what would happen to the patient in the absence of treatment (natural history), and what factors prognosticate an adverse outcome. The treating physician must determine which of these adverse prognostic factors can be affected by treatment. A treatment plan is then initiated, and long-term follow-up determines whether treatment favorably alters the course of the disease over the long term. The fundamental problem in developing treatment plans for patients with Legg-Calvé-Perthes syndrome is the paucity of natural history data (72,196–199).

Catterall (196) compared 46 untreated hips of Murley and Lloyd-Roberts with a matched control group of 51 hips treated with a weight-relieving caliper. The average age at diagnosis was 4 years and 6 months, and the average

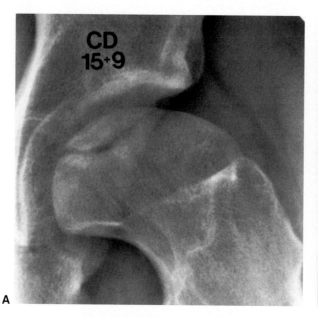
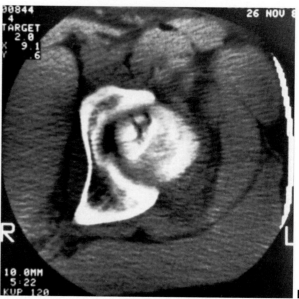

**Figure 25.15 A:** A 15-year-old boy, whose disease started at 8 years and 6 months of age, returned to the physician with pain and synovitis. Anteroposterior radiograph demonstrates osteochondritis of the femoral head. **B:** Computed tomographic (CT) scan shows multiple fragments that appear as one on the radiograph.

follow-up was 10 years and 5 months, with a range of 4 to 18 years. The patients were evaluated according to the grading system of Sundt, which requires some subjective assessments (200). The 10-year average follow-up in this series was too short to determine the outcomes for patients and thus the natural history of the disease, because most patients with childhood hip disease do well regardless of the radiographic appearance in their early years (201–204). In addition, no data are presented on the interobserver or intraobserver reliability of the outcome criteria.

Catterall also reported on 97 untreated patients from around the British Isles. The average follow-up in this series was only 6 years, and the results were graded according to the aforementioned system of Sundt (200). The outcomes in this group of patients (Table 25.1) are widely quoted in the literature as a comparison for outcomes of various treatment modalities. Unfortunately, very few articles in the literature use the same grading system for outcomes, and the follow-up of this group is too short to be defined as natural history.

The only other article labeled "natural history" in the literature (199) is not a natural history study but a study of patients from three centers, treated by different methods. This study attempted both to establish a relation between residual deformity and degenerative joint disease and to identify clinical and radiographic factors in the active phase of disease that would be predictive of hip deformity and degenerative joint disease. Therefore, as will be further discussed later in the chapter, decision making with reference to treatment is difficult because of the lack of true long-term natural history data.

## Long-term Follow-up Results

Although there is little information available on natural history, there are many long-term follow-up studies of patients with Legg-Calvé-Perthes syndrome. The long-term studies that are available suffer from the faults of retrospective long-term reviews in that most series contain only small numbers of patients, with many of the original patients not traced; original radiographs often are not available. Many of the longer series contain patients diagnosed in the years 1910 to 1940, when little was known about the disease, prognostic factors, and radiographic classifications. In most series, patients are combined regardless of what are now known to be prognostic factors: the extent of epiphyseal involvement, age at onset of the disease, age at

**TABLE 25.1**

**RESULTS FOR 97 UNTREATED HIPS**

**Catterall**

| Group | Good | Fair | Poor |
|---|---|---|---|
| Group 1 | 27 ⎤ | 1 | 0 |
| Group 2 | 25 ⎦ —92% | 6 | 2 |
| Group 3 | 4 | 7 | 11 ⎤ |
| Group 4 | 0 | 4 | 10 ⎦ —91% |
| Total | 56 (57%) | 18 (19%) | 23 (24%) |

Results graded by the system of Sundt (200).
From Catterall A. *Legg-Calvé-Perthes' disease.* Edinburgh: Churchill Livingstone, 1982.

the beginning of treatment, and stage of the disease at treatment initiation. Various treatment modalities are combined in many series, and control groups are generally absent. Because of these inherent problems, and the fact that different grading systems are used in judging clinical and radiographic end results, all of which lack interobserver and intraobserver reliability data, it is difficult to compare and contrast the various reported series. Despite these shortcomings, a great deal has been learned about the prognosis in Legg-Calvé-Perthes syndrome.

In reviewing long-term follow-up studies, it is apparent that results can improve with time, because remodeling potential continues until the end of growth (72,205) (Figs. 25.9 and 25.10). Mose wrote that, "for a precise prognosis, conclusions from any measurements ought not be made before the patient reaches the age of 16, when growth stops" (204). Reviews of the outcomes of treatment modalities before skeletal maturity must be viewed as preliminary reports.

Twenty to 40 years after the onset of symptoms, most (70% to 90%) patients with Legg-Calvé-Perthes syndrome are active and free of pain. Most patients maintain a good range of motion, despite the fact that few have normal-appearing radiographs. Clinical deterioration and symptoms of increasing pain, decreasing range of motion, and loss of function are observed only in patients with flattened irregular heads at the time of primary healing, and in patients with premature physeal closure, as indicated by femoral neck shortening, femoral head deformity, and trochanteric overgrowth (186) (Fig. 25.13).

Danielsson and Hernborg (206) reported a 33-year follow-up of 35 patients. Twenty-eight of the 35 patients were free of pain, with 34 of 35 functioning without restrictions. In a 34-year follow-up, Hall (207) reported satisfactory results in 71% of 209 cases. Perpich et al. (208) reported a 30-year follow-up of 37 patients. The average Iowa Hip Rating was 93 of a possible 100 points. Eighty-five percent of the patients had good clinical results, despite the fact that only 33% had spherical femoral heads, as rated by the Mose Sphericity Scale (204) (Fig. 25.16). Forty-three percent of the patients had poor Mose ratings; however, of these patients, 76% had good clinical results.

Ratliff (209) followed 34 patients for an average of 30 years and noted that 80% were fully active and free of pain, whereas only 40% were radiographically normal. He followed 16 of these patients for an additional 11 years (210) and noted that, despite the fact that only one-third of them had good anatomic results, "deterioration rarely occurred and many patients had no pain and [maintained] normal activity."

Yrjonen (201) followed 96 patients (106 hips), all of whom had noncontainment treatment, for an average of 35 years. At maturity, 61% had poor results by the Mose criteria. In a final follow-up, 48% had evidence of degenerative joint disease. However, at an average 35-year follow-up, only 4% had undergone total hip arthroplasty, with an additional

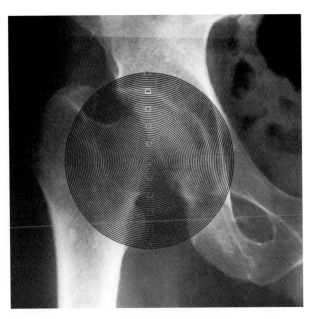

**Figure 25.16** Mose Sphericity Scale.

13% having clinical symptoms significant enough to warrant arthroplasty. Ippolito et al. (202) reported on 61 patients with an average follow-up of 25 years. Only 19% of their patients had poor results, as measured by the Iowa Hip Rating, at final follow-up. W.J. Cumming (personal communication, 1997) reported on 82 patients with 95 involved hips treated by prolonged frame recumbency, with an average follow-up of 38 years. Only 10% of the patients had required arthroplasty at follow-up, with an additional 10% having symptoms significant enough to warrant arthroplasty.

Gower and Johnston (211) reported on 30 nonoperated hips with an average 36-year follow-up. This series is representative of other 20- to 40-year long-term series reported in the literature. The average Iowa Hip Rating for these 30 patients was 91 points. The typical patient had minimal shortening, absent or mild hip pain, and minimal or no functional impairment with respect to their jobs and activities of daily living. Ninety-two percent of the patients had Iowa Hip Ratings higher than 80 points, and only 8% of them had undergone arthroplasty.

In follow-up studies beyond 40 years, hip function begins to deteriorate. In another study of the Iowa group of patients at 48-year follow-up, McAndrew and Weinstein (203) reported that only 40% of patients maintained an Iowa Hip Rating of better than 80 points. Forty percent of the patients had undergone arthroplasty, and an additional 10% had disabling osteoarthritis symptoms but had not yet undergone arthroplasty (Fig. 25.17). Further, at 48-year follow-up, 50% of the patients had disabling osteoarthritis and pain, and an additional 10% had Iowa Hip Ratings of less than 80 points. The prevalence of osteoarthritis in this group of patients was ten times that found in the general population in the same age range (186). Mose followed a group of patients into the 7th decade of life. All of the

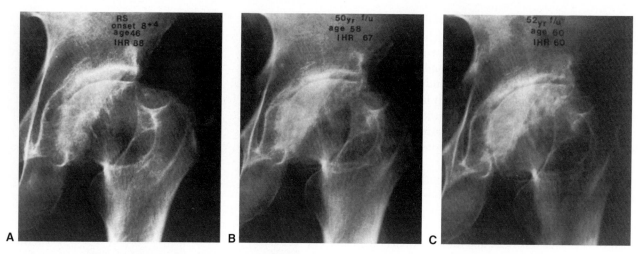

**Figure 25.17**   This patient had disease onset at 8 years and 3 months of age. At 46 years of age (38-year follow-up), the Iowa Hip Rating was 88 points **(A)**. At 58 years of age (50-year follow-up), there was a loss of 21 points on the Iowa Hip Rating, to 67 **(B)**. At 60 years of age, just before arthroplasty, the Iowa Hip Rating was 60 points **(C)**. (From Weinstein SL. Legg-Calvé-Perthes' disease: results of long-term follow-up. In: Fitzgerald RH Jr, ed. *The Hip: Proceedings of the Thirteenth Open Scientific Meeting of the Hip Society*. St. Louis, MO: Mosby, 1985:28.)

patients with irregular femoral heads had degenerative arthritis. Of those patients with femoral heads that Mose classified as "normal, ball shaped," no patient had degenerative joint disease by the middle of the 4th decade, but 67% had severe degenerative arthritis by the middle of the 7th decade (204). Therefore, the follow-up studies beyond 40 years demonstrate marked reduction of function, with most of the patients developing degenerative joint disease by the 6th and 7th decades (180,199,202–204).

## Prognostic Factors

In reviews of long-term series of patients with Legg-Calvé-Perthes syndrome, certain clinical and radiographic features have been identified that have prognostic value (186,190,201,212–216) (Table 25.2). The most important prognostic factor in determining the outcome is the residual deformity of the femoral head, coupled with hip joint incongruity (217–219). Femoral head deformity and joint incongruity are multifactorial problems. They are interrelated with all of the other prognostic factors. It must be kept in mind that Legg-Calvé-Perthes syndrome represents a

growth disturbance of the proximal femur; the epiphyseal and physeal cartilage is abnormal. Other key factors involved in the development of deformity include the extent of epiphyseal involvement and the varying degrees and patterns of premature physeal closure associated with this condition (220).

Stulberg et al. (199) established a relation between residual deformity and degenerative joint disease. This was accomplished by retrospectively examining the long-term outcomes of patients from three different centers treated by various methods (e.g., bed rest, spica cast, ischial weight bearing, brace, crutches, cork shoe lift on the normal side, combination of methods). They attempted to identify clinical and radiographic factors in the active phase of the disease that were predictive of the development of hip deformity. They proposed a radiographic classification of deformity relating to long-term outcome (Table 25.3). The more deformity there was at maturity (i.e., the higher the Stulberg classification), the worse the long-term outcome. However, as noted from long-term follow-up studies, it is the class 5 hips that deteriorate the earliest; they usually have significant symptoms by the end of the 4th decade (201–204). Patients with aspherical congruency (Stulberg class 3 and 4 disease) may have satisfactory outcomes for many years, with most patients undergoing significant functional deterioration in the 5th and 6th decades of life (201–204). This classification scheme, which attempts to classify a three-dimensional deformity using two-dimensional parameters, has been shown to have poor interobserver and intraobserver reliability (221). The general principles expressed by Stulberg et al. (199), however, have been shown to have validity with reference to long-term outcome studies. That is, the more out of round the femoral head is, and the greater the discrepancy between the shape of the femoral head and the shape of

## TABLE 25.2

### PROGNOSTIC FACTORS

Deformity of the femoral head
Hip joint incongruity
Age at onset of disease
Extent of epiphyseal involvement
Growth disturbance secondary to premature physeal closure
Protracted disease course
Remodeling potential
Type of treatment (?)
Stage at treatment initiation

## TABLE 25.3

### STULBERG CLASSIFICATION

| Class | Radiographic Features | Congruency |
|---|---|---|
| 1 | Normal hip | Spherical |
| 2 (Figs. 25.9 and 25.18) | Spherical femoral head, same concentric circle on anteroposterior and frog-leg lateral views, but with one or more of the following: coxa magna, shorter-than-normal neck, abnormally steep acetabulum | Spherical |
| 3 (Figs. 25.11 and 25.17) | Ovoid, mushroom-shaped (but not flat) head, coxa magna, shorter-than-normal neck, abnormally steep acetabulum | Aspherical |
| 4 (Fig. 25.13) | Flat femoral head and abnormalities of the head, neck, and acetabulum | Aspherical |
| 5 (Fig. 25.14) | Flat head, normal neck and acetabulum | Aspherical incongruency |

From Stulberg SD, Cooperman DR, Wallensten R. The natural history of Legg-Calvé-Perthes' disease. *J Bone Joint Surg Am* 1981;63:1095.

the acetabulum, the greater the chance of development of early degenerative joint disease.

O'Garra (222), Salter and Thompson (120,121), and others (72,137,190,196,223,224) have confirmed Waldenstrom's original finding that partial or anterior femoral head involvement leads to a more favorable prognosis than whole-head involvement. Catterall (72,138,196) demonstrated the importance of the extent of epiphyseal involvement with regard to prognosis, and he proposed four groups on the basis of the presence or absence of seven radiographic signs observed in 97 untreated hips (Figs. 25.6, 25.9, 25.10, and 25.18). He compared the final radiograph with the initial radiograph, using the clinical grading of Sundt (200); 90% of the patients who had good results were in group 1 or 2, whereas 90% of those who had poor results were in group 3 or 4. This commonly used classification has been criticized as being difficult to use in that there may be a great deal of interobserver error (213,225–227). It also has been criticized as being insufficiently prospective, because it may take up to 8 months for the hip to be far enough into the fragmentation phase to show the extent of epiphyseal involvement (228,229). Furthermore, it also has been noted that the classification may change when radiographs taken during the initial phase are compared with those taken at maximal fragmentation (229,230).

Salter and Thompson (121) described a simplified two-group classification based on prognosis and determined by the extent of the subchondral fracture line, which appears early in the course of the disease: in group A less than half of the head is involved (Catterall groups 1 and 2), and in group B more than half of the head is involved (Catterall groups 3 and 4). The major distinguishing factor between groups A and B is the presence or absence of a viable lateral column of the epiphysis. This intact lateral column (i.e., Catterall group 2, Salter-Thompson type A)

may shield the epiphysis from collapse and subsequent deformity (Fig. 25.18).

Maintenance of the integrity of the lateral column and the height of the femoral head has been described as important by several investigators (72,207,213,231,232). Hall (207) reported on the long-term follow-up (34 years) of 209 hips. He considered loss of femoral head height, as seen on the initial radiograph, to be an important prognostic sign. All of his patients in whom there had been a loss of 2 mm or more of height of the femoral head in the affected hip, compared with the unaffected hip, had unsatisfactory results in adult life. Patients in whom the height of the femoral head was within 2 mm of that of the unaffected hip on the initial radiograph had good results in all but six cases.

Herring et al. (213) proposed a radiographic classification based on the radiolucency of the lateral pillar of the femoral head on anteroposterior (AP) films during the

## TABLE 25.4

### LATERAL PILLAR CLASSIFICATION

| | |
|---|---|
| Type A | No involvement of the lateral pillar; lateral pillar is radiographically normal; possible lucency and collapse in the central and medial pillars, but full height of the lateral pillar is maintained |
| Type B | Greater than 50% of the lateral pillar height is maintained; lateral pillar has some radiolucency, with maintenance of bone density at a height between 50% and 100% of the original height of the lateral head |
| Type C | Less than 50% of lateral pillar height is maintained; lateral pillar becomes more radiolucent than in type B, and any preserved bone is at a height of <50% of the original height of the lateral pillar |

From Herring JA, Neustadt JB, Williams JJ, et al. The lateral pillar classification of Legg-Calvé-Perthes' disease. *J Pediatr Orthop* 1992;12:143.

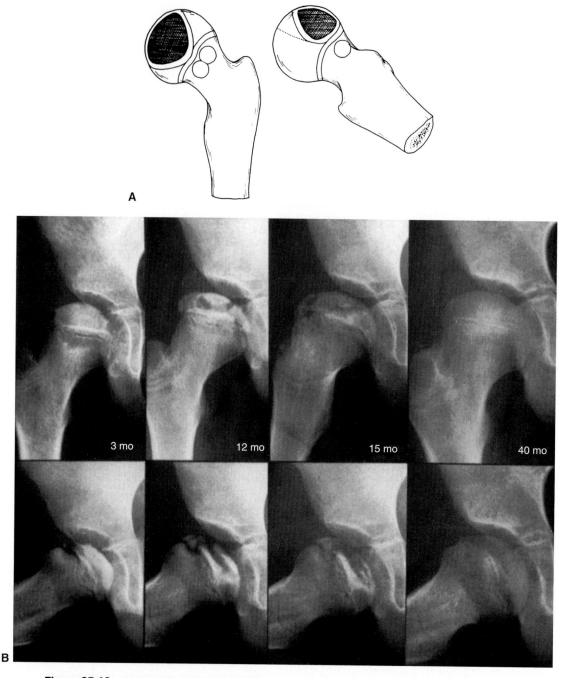

**Figure 25.18   A:** Catterall group 2 disease showing anterolateral involvement, sequestrum formation, and a clear junction between the involved and uninvolved areas. There are anterolateral metaphyseal lesions, and the subchondral fracture line is in the anterior half of the head. The lateral column is intact. **B:** Catterall group 2 disease. Three to 40 months after onset of symptoms, the lateral pillar is still intact.

fragmentation phase of the disease (Table 25.4) (Figs. 25.11, 25.13, and 25.19). The lateral pillar occupies the lateral 15% to 30% of the femoral head width on an AP radiograph. The central pillar occupies approximately 50% of the head width, and the medial pillar occupies 20% to 35% of the medial aspect of the head width on an AP radiograph.

Herring et al. reported on the outcomes of 93 hips in 86 patients with radiographic follow-up to maturity (213). Intraobserver reliability was reported to be 0.78, with a good correlation of outcome, as measured by the classification of Stulberg et al. (199). The importance of the integrity of the lateral column is seen in other classifications, with patients in Salter-Thompson type A and Catterall groups 1 and 2 having intact lateral columns. The results of treatment in long-term outcome studies show this to be an important prognostic factor (202,213,230,233,234) (Fig. 25.20). The reliability of this classification and its utility in Perthes disease will require further study (226,235).

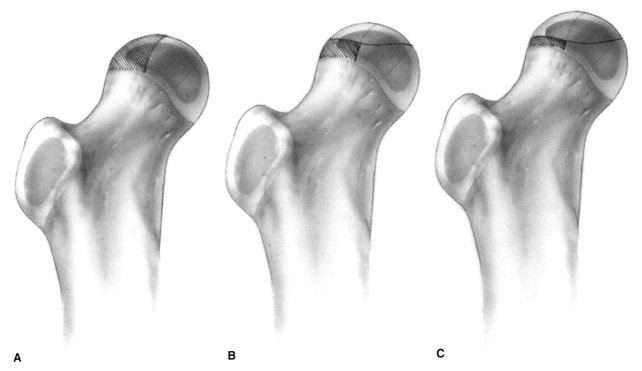

**Figure 25.19** Lateral pillar classification (see Table 25.4 for a description of **A**, **B**, and **C**).

In analyzing the unexpectedly poor results in each category, Catterall (72,190,196,236,237) identified certain radiographic signs, known as *at-risk signs*, that were associated with poor results (Fig. 25.21). Results in untreated patients show that there were no poor results in patients who did not have two or more of the radiographic at-risk signs during the active stage of the disease. Radiographic at-risk signs include the Gage sign (a radiolucency in the lateral epiphysis and metaphysis) and calcification lateral to the epiphysis. These two signs are indicative of early ossification in the enlarged epiphysis. They are present only when the head is deformed. These signs are present when the changes are reversible with treatment (72,238). A third at-risk sign is metaphyseal lesions. These metaphyseal radiolucencies may herald the potential for a growth disturbance of the physeal plate (153,239,240). The final two at-risk signs are lateral subluxation and a horizontal growth plate (241). Lateral subluxation is indicative of a widened head. A horizontal growth plate (adducted hip) is indicative of a developing femoral head deformity that, if left untreated, will lead to fixed deformity, hinge abduction, and subsequent further deformity. These radiographic at-risk signs are manifested clinically as loss of motion and adduction contracture. Catterall reported no poor results in patients who did not manifest at-risk signs. The validity of the Catterall classification and the at-risk signs has been confirmed by several series (229,242–249), but questioned by others (202,213,230,250).

Stulberg et al. (199) identified lateral and superior subluxation, which are indicative of significant growth disturbance and flattening of the femoral head, as the key factors associated with the development of class 3 and class 4 hips and poor long-term outcome (i.e., after 40 years). Disease onset after the age of 9 years and partial femoral head involvement, particularly anterosuperior quadrant involvement, were associated with the development of a class 5 hip and the early onset of degenerative joint disease (i.e., 3rd to 5th decade of life).

The duration of the disease is related to the extent of epiphyseal involvement. In general, the greater the extent of epiphyseal involvement, the longer the duration and course of the disease. End results are worse with prolonged disease duration (205,213,251,252). The extent of epiphyseal involvement is also related to the sex of the patient in that girls affected by Legg-Calvé-Perthes syndrome have a poorer prognosis than boys (253,254). This may be explained by the fact that there are more girls (who tend to be more skeletally mature than comparably aged boys, and hence have less remodeling potential) with Catterall group 3 or group 4 disease, which are the groups associated with a less favorable prognosis (159).

Age at onset of the disease is the second most significant factor related to outcome; only deformity is more significant. Eight years seems to be the watershed age in most long-term series (186,203,255–258); however, some authors believe that the prognosis is markedly worse for long-term outcome in patients older than 6 years at the onset of the disease (202). W.J. Cumming (personal communication, 1997) estimated that 45% of patients with onset of Perthes disease after the age of 6 years have undergone arthroplasty by age 60 years. Patients older than 11 or 12 years, even with Catterall group 2 or Salter-Thompson

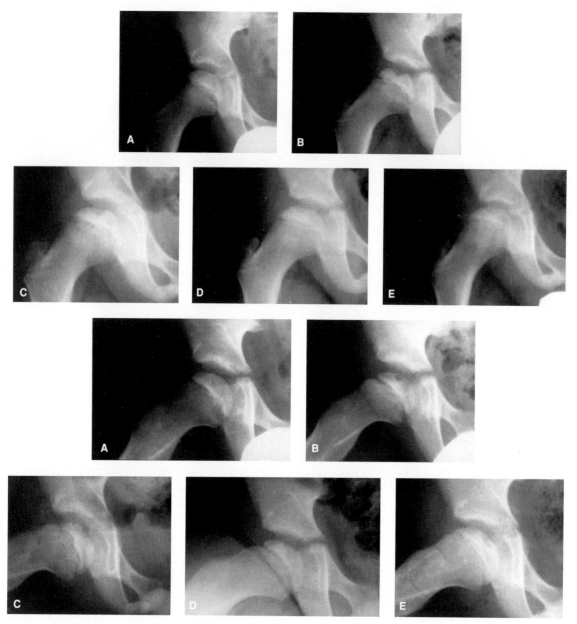

**Figure 25.20** Anteroposterior **(top, A–E)** and lateral **(bottom, A–E)** views of a 7-year-old boy who presented with hip pain and a limp. **A:** At presentation, the patient was in the initial radiographic stage of the disease; his prognosis was indeterminate. **B:** Six months after presentation, he had minimal loss of height of the lateral pillar and some radiolucency in that region, as well as significant bone resorption centrally. Note how the lateral pillar maintains its height throughout the course of the disease. **C–E:** One year **(C)**, 18 months **(D)**, and 3 years **(E)** after onset of disease. The patient had only mild symptoms on occasion, and maintained good range of motion throughout the course of the disease. Only symptomatic treatment was provided.

type A disease, may have poor anatomic and clinical results, even with treatment (259). Age at healing, however, is probably a more important factor (Fig. 25.11). The overall skeletal maturation delay (49) in patients with Legg-Calvé-Perthes syndrome, and the usual compensation for this delay during the pubertal growth spurt (50), contribute to the favorable prognosis in the young patient. The more immature the patient at the time of entering the reossification stage, the greater the potential for remodeling.

At-risk signs are also less likely to occur in younger patients, particularly those younger than 5 years.

The key factor relating to outcomes, and therefore to the prognosis, is the shape of the femoral head and its relationships to acetabular shape (congruency) and joint motion. The shape of the acetabulum depends on the geometric pattern within it during growth (181,260,261). In addition, the acetabulum continues to have significant potential for development until the patient is 8 or 9 years

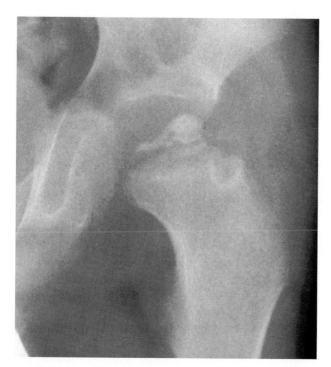

**Figure 25.21** A boy, 6 years and 5 months of age, with Catterall group 4 disease demonstrates all of the at-risk signs: Gage sign, calcification lateral to the epiphysis, metaphyseal lesions, lateral subluxation, and horizontal growth plate.

of age (85,87,262). If a young patient develops a deformity of the proximal femur because of Perthes disease, the immature acetabulum conforms to the altered shape of the femoral head. This may lead to the development of an aspherical congruency (Stulberg classes 3 and 4) that may be compatible with normal function for many years. In older patients (whether "older" means older than 6 years or older than 8 years is subject to debate), the acetabulum cannot conform to the shape of a deformed femoral head; there is thus a greater chance of the development of an incongruous relation between the two, leading to early degenerative joint disease (199,201–204,261,263).

The importance of premature physeal arrest secondary to the disease process cannot be overemphasized. Keret et al. (182), in a study of 80 patients with Legg-Calvé-Perthes syndrome, showed interference with physeal growth in 90% of them, with 25% having premature physeal closure. They demonstrated a direct correlation between the severity of physeal involvement and deformity of the femoral head. Clarke and Harrison (264) reported that 47% of 31 patients who presented with painful hips after Legg-Calvé-Perthes syndrome, at an average age of 27 years, showed evidence of premature physeal closure.

Various methods have been used to measure the sphericity of the femoral head and congruency at healing. Goff (10,52,265) used a transparent protractor with concentric circles drawn at 2 mm of radial difference to evaluate the shape of the femoral head. Mose further developed Goff's method and applied it clinically. This is the most commonly used

method of measuring sphericity (104,266–268) (Fig. 25.16). It is not clear from the criteria of Mose whether the measurement under consideration is the difference between the outline of the femoral head on the AP and lateral radiographs, or the deviation from a given circle, measured in millimeters, on either the AP or the lateral radiograph, or a combination of these two parameters. This variability in the application of the method of Mose et al. is evident in the literature on Legg-Calvé-Perthes syndrome (244,245,269–274).

In general, the template with concentric circles is superimposed on the AP and lateral radiograms. In the author's practice, if the outline of the femoral head is a perfect circle in both projections, it is rated good; less than 2 mm of deviation is rated fair; and more than 2 mm of deviation from a circle, in the AP or lateral projection, is rated poor. Regardless of the measurements used, it is important to realize that, with growth and remodeling of the femoral head and acetabulum, the various parameters used for measuring head deformity and congruency may change.

The shape of the femoral head and its congruency, as measured at skeletal maturity, are probably the most reliable indicators of prognosis and the development of degenerative joint disease. Catterall (72) showed, in a follow-up of untreated patients, that 33% of the patients improved in anatomic grade. Twenty percent of these patients improved two anatomic grades; all of these patients were younger than 5 years at the time of onset of the disease. However, it must also be remembered that the various deformities of the femoral head and anomalies in acetabular congruency are three-dimensional parameters that cannot be measured adequately on two-dimensional radiographs. Thus far, the only existing radiographic parameter that correlates with good clinical outcome is a perfectly spherical femoral head. Loss of sphericity by itself, however, does not necessarily lead to a poor long-term result (186,188,217).

Thompson and Westin (275) confirmed the work of Ferguson and Howorth (75), which demonstrated that after the femoral head is in the reossification stage of the disease, it will not deform further. If a treatment for femoral head deformity is to be successful, it must be instituted early in the course of the disease, that is, in the initial or fragmentation stage, hence the importance of radiographic staging of patients.

## CLINICAL PRESENTATION

Patients with Legg-Calvé-Perthes syndrome most commonly present with a history of an insidious onset of a limp. Most patients do not complain of much discomfort, unless specifically questioned about this aspect. Pain, when present, is usually activity-related and relieved by rest. Because of the mild nature of the symptoms, most patients do not present for medical attention until weeks or months after the clinical onset of disease. The pain is generally localized to the groin, or referred to the anteromedial thigh or knee region. Failure to recognize that the thigh or knee pain in the child may be secondary to hip pathology may cause further delay in the diagnosis. Some children present with more acute onset of symptoms. Seventeen percent of patients with Legg-Calvé-Perthes syndrome may have a history of related trauma (24,27,276).

## PHYSICAL EXAMINATION

The child with Legg-Calvé-Perthes syndrome usually presents with limited hip motion, particularly abduction and medial rotation. Early in the course of the disease, the limited abduction is secondary to synovitis and muscle spasm in the adductor group; however, with time and the subsequent emergence of deformities, the limitation of abduction may become permanent. Longstanding adductor spasm occasionally leads to adductor contracture. The Trendelenburg test in patients with Legg-Calvé-Perthes syndrome is often positive. These children most commonly have evidence of thigh, calf, and buttock atrophy from disuse secondary to pain. This is additional evidence of the longstanding nature of the condition before detection (1–5,185,265). Limb length should be measured; inequality is indicative of significant collapse of the femoral head and a poor prognosis. Evaluation of the patient's overall height, weight, and bone age may be helpful in ruling out skeletal dysplasias or growth disorders in the differential diagnosis, and may provide confirmatory evidence of the disorder. Laboratory studies are generally not helpful in Legg-Calvé-Perthes syndrome, although they may be necessary for ruling out other conditions (see section on differential diagnosis).

## IMAGING

In Legg-Calvé-Perthes syndrome, plain radiographs taken in the AP and frog-leg lateral positions are used in making the initial diagnosis, and also for assessing the subsequent clinical course. These radiographs are generally sufficient for the assessment of the patient and subsequent follow-up evaluations. From the plain radiographs, the extent of epiphyseal involvement (e.g., Catterall groups 1 to 4; Salter-Thompson type A or B; lateral pillar type A, B, or C) and the stage of the disease (initial, fragmentation, or reossification) can be determined. According to Salter and Thompson, if appropriate radiographs are taken within 4 months of the clinical onset of the disease, the subchondral radiolucent zone will be detectable (121). Catterall, however, states that this sign is helpful in only 25% of the cases, because it is present only transiently in the early phases of the disease (72). It is most important, while following the course of the disease, to view all radiographs sequentially and compare them with previous radiographs, so as to assess the stage of the reparative process and determine the constancy of the extent of epiphyseal involvement. Additional radiographic or imaging studies are rarely necessary but may be helpful in the initial assessment and also in the follow-up of the condition (277–279).

Radionuclide bone scanning with technetium and pinhole columnation (Fig. 25.22) may be helpful in the early stages of the disease, when the diagnosis is in question, particularly if the differential diagnosis is between transient synovitis and Perthes disease. Some investigators consider scintigraphy to be helpful in determining the extent of epiphyseal involvement and the prognosis (271,280–289).

Magnetic resonance imaging is widely available in medical centers. It appears to be sensitive in detecting infarction, but cannot yet accurately portray the stages of healing. Its role in the management of Perthes syndrome has yet to be defined. In the future, magnetic resonance imaging not only may help the clinician in the diagnosis, but may shed additional light on the underlying pathology of the condition (98,287,290–293) (Fig. 25.23).

Arthrography is useful primarily in demonstrating any flattening of the femoral head that may not be seen on plain

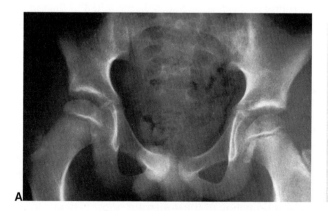
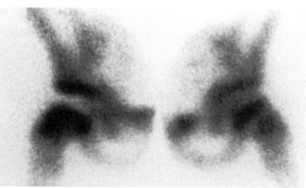

A          B

**Figure 25.22**    An 8-year-old boy with right hip pain. **A:** Anteroposterior radiograph demonstrates a slight increase in width and medial joint space; the femoral ossific nucleus is slightly smaller than the one on the opposite side. **B:** Technetium 99 radionuclide scan demonstrates decreased uptake in the entire right femoral head, with increased vascularity in the neck.

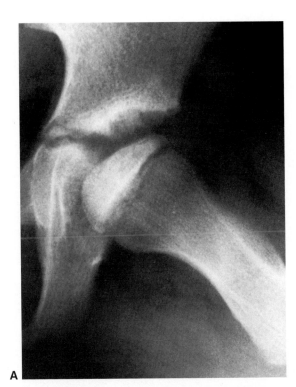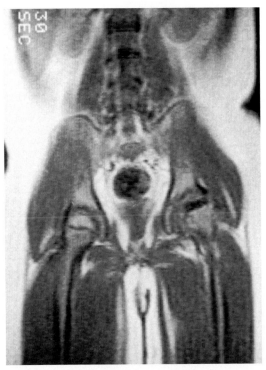

**Figure 25.23** A 6-year-old boy with Catterall group 3 disease in the early fragmentation stage. **A:** Plain radiograph shows apparent sparing of the posterior head. **B:** Magnetic resonance image demonstrates a complete absence of signal on the affected side. (Courtesy of Peter Scoles, MD, Case Western Reserve Medical School, Cleveland, Ohio.)

radiographs (Fig. 25.24). It can be used to demonstrate the hinge abduction (Fig. 25.8, 25.25, and 25.26) phenomenon with abduction of the leg (163,190,191,217,294). Arthrography, in conjunction with plain radiography or computed tomography, also may be useful in the diagnosis of osteochondritis dissecans secondary to Perthes disease. Arthrography is most useful for assessing the shape of the femoral head and its relation to the acetabulum, both of which are necessary for treatment decisions (Figs. 25.25 to 25.27). Where there is severe flattening of the femoral head, arthrography is helpful in determining containability before any treatment is started, whether it is Petrie casts or surgery. It is also useful in determining the best position of containment (e.g., internal or external rotation, and abduction or adduction) if surgical management is considered.

## DIFFERENTIAL DIAGNOSIS

The history of the patient, physical examination, and plain radiographs are usually sufficient for making a diagnosis of Legg-Calvé-Perthes syndrome (Table 25.5). Diagnosis early in the initial phase of the disease requires that it be differentiated from conditions such as septic arthritis, whether primary or secondary to proximal femoral osteomyelitis, and toxic synovitis (295–297). A complete blood count including white cell differential, erythrocyte sedimentation rate, C-reactive protein, and hip joint aspiration and analysis

of the fluid may be necessary in order to rule out infection. In patients with Legg-Calvé-Perthes syndrome all laboratory results are usually normal except the erythrocyte sedimentation rate, which may be slightly elevated. In early cases, if all of the laboratory and plain radiographic studies are normal, but doubt regarding the diagnosis persists, radionuclide scanning or magnetic resonance imaging may be helpful.

**TABLE 25.5**
**DIFFERENTIAL DIAGNOSIS**

Chondrolysis
Gaucher disease
Hemophilia
Hypothyroidism
Juvenile rheumatoid arthritis
Lymphoma
Mucopolysaccharidosis
Multiple epiphyseal dysplasia
Meyer dysplasia
Neoplasm
Old congenital dysplasia of the hip residuals
Osteomyelitis of the proximal femur
Septic arthritis
Sickle-cell disease
Spondyloepiphyseal dysplasia
Toxic synovitis
Traumatic aseptic necrosis

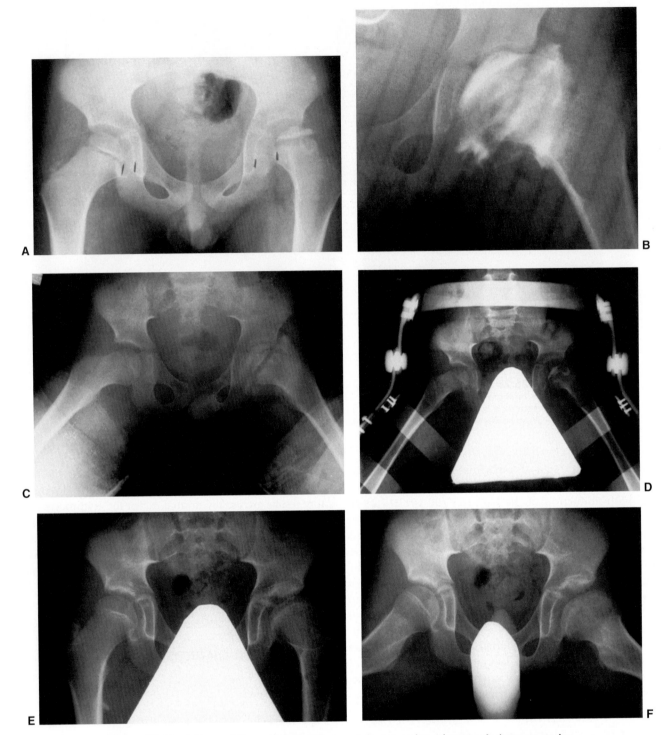

**Figure 25.24** A 5-year-old boy with Catterall group 4 disease and at-risk status. **A:** Anteroposterior radiograph on presentation. **B:** Anteroposterior arthrogram, in the same position as in **C**, after 10 days of traction. Note the relation between the lateral acetabular margin and the lateral margin of the cartilaginous femoral head, as well as the severe flattening of the femoral head. **C:** Anteroposterior radiogram in Petrie broomstick abduction plasters. The patient was maintained in casts for 6 weeks. **D:** Anteroposterior radiograph with pelvis abduction orthosis (weight bearing). **E:** Anteroposterior radiograph at age 13 years. Note residual deformity. **F:** Lauenstein radiograph at age 13 years.

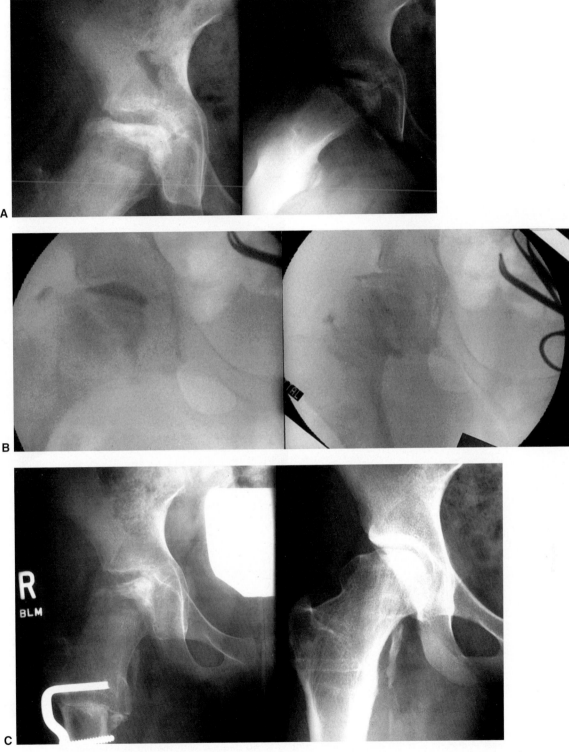

**Figure 25.25**  An 11-year-old girl with Catterall group 4 Perthes disease. The range of motion of the hip showed marked restriction of abduction (20 degrees) and rotation (10 degrees internal and external). All movement was painful. **A:** Preoperative anteroposterior **(left)** and Lauenstein **(right)** views. **B:** Intraoperative arthrograms demonstrating hinging on the lateral aspect of the acetabulum in abduction **(left)** with good congruity in adduction **(right). C:** Six-month **(left)** and 7-year **(right)** follow-ups after abduction osteotomy. At 7-year follow-up, the patient was free of pain, with 40 degrees of abduction, 20 degrees of adduction, flexion to 130 degrees, and 20 degrees of internal and external rotation. She has been pain-free since her surgery.

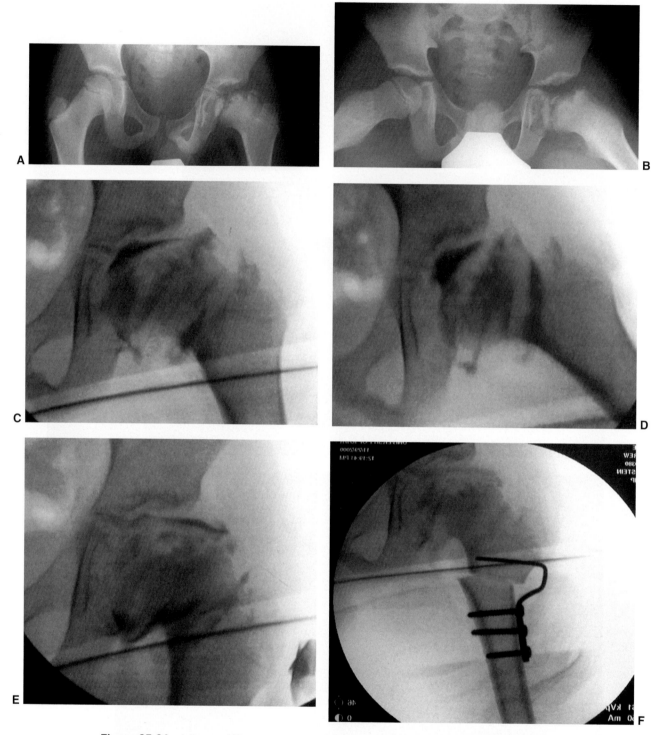

**Figure 25.26**   A 9-year-old boy presenting with hip pain, nonresponsive to nonsurgical measures. Clinical abduction is to 10 degrees; adduction is to 40 degrees with the hip in extension. **A:** Antero-posterior view of pelvis showing total femoral head involvement in reossification stage of disease. **B:** Lauenstein view. **C:** Arthrogram in neutral position showing considerable flattening of femoral head and slight impingement on lateral edge of the acetabulum. **D:** Arthrogram in abduction demonstrating hinge abduction. **E:** Arthrogram in adduction demonstrating reasonable congruity between femoral head and acetabulum; note normal contour of lateral acetabular edge. **F:** Abduction osteotomy allowing 45 degrees of abduction and 0 degrees of adduction. **G:** Three years postoperatively. Patient is pain-free with 45 degrees of abduction, 10 degrees of adduction, and good rotation. **H:** Lauenstein view 3 years postoperatively.

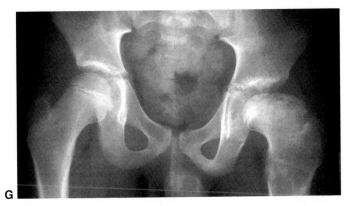
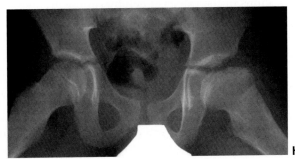

G

H

**Figure 25.26** (*continued*)

In patients with bilateral hip involvement, generalized disorders such as hypothyroidism and multiple epiphyseal dysplasia must be considered (298–300). In patients with bilateral involvement, particularly those with atypical radiographic features, care should be taken to obtain a detailed family history, measurements of height and weight should be recorded, and a bone survey should be done in order to rule out a metabolic or genetic condition (see Chapters 6 and 7). The possibility of Meyer dysplasia, a benign self-resolving condition, must be considered in children younger than 4 years of age (301).

## TREATMENT

For the past 75 years, many investigators (14,15,177,199, 200,302) have expressed a nihilistic attitude toward the role of therapy in this disease. Sundt (200) believed that treatment could not prevent degenerative joint disease. Because there is a paucity of long-term natural history data available, the question must be raised whether the outcome of Legg-Calvé-Perthes syndrome can be altered by any particular treatment. Although surgical management has become very popular today, long-term series of patients with uniform treatment, and matched for age, gender, stage, and extent of epiphyseal involvement, are necessary in order to determine the most effective treatment of Perthes syndrome.

Most patients (60%) with Legg-Calvé-Perthes syndrome do not need treatment (72,121,196,228,238,303). Treatment must be considered only for those patients who have an otherwise known poor prognosis based on prognostic factors gleaned from long-term follow-up. It is difficult to formulate specific treatments for patients because the natural history of the condition is not well known.

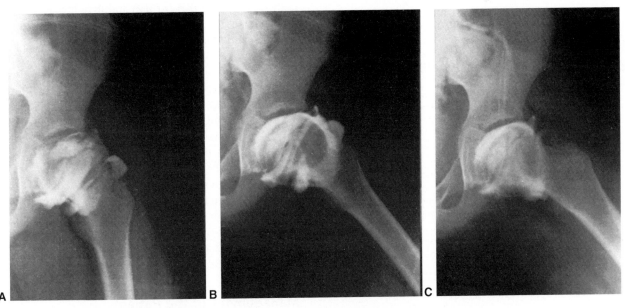

A

B

C

**Figure 25.27**  Arthrogram of a 6-year-old boy with Catterall group 4 disease. **A:** Neutral position. **B:** Abduction, external rotation, and slight flexion (the position that would be maintained by an abduction Scottish Rite-type orthosis). **C:** Abduction and internal rotation (the position that would be maintained by a varus derotation osteotomy or innominate osteotomy).

Also, most studies of current treatment methods lack interobserver and intraobserver reliability as regards classifications of the extent of epiphyseal involvement and outcome measures, and all the studies lack control groups. These factors, and other variables that exist in most series, make it difficult to support a "best" method of treatment.

Standard treatment algorithms are based on radiographic features of the various disease classification schemes. Under these protocols, no treatment is warranted in patients with a good prognosis (i.e., those with Catterall group 1, Salter-Thompson type A, or lateral pillar type A disease) (Table 25.6). Patients with a poor prognosis should be considered for treatment. These would include patients with Catterall groups 3 and 4 disease, Salter-Thompson type B disease, and lateral pillar type C disease. There is another large group of patients whose prognosis is indeterminate; these patients require careful follow-up, because they may need treatment at a later date. This group includes patients with Catterall group 2 disease (good prognosis in 90% of cases) and patients with lateral pillar type B disease. Because we have learned that the two major prognostic factors in outcome are deformity of the femoral head and age of the patient, these two factors must be taken into account in the decision-making process. Patients with deformity (arthrographically and/or clinically documented by persistent loss of motion, particularly abduction) younger than 8 years should be considered for treatment. Patients older than 8 years, especially girls, should be considered for treatment even in the absence of deformity. In the absence of treatment, such patients have a poor prognosis (257,258,304) because their growth potential is insufficient for any deformity of the proximal femur to be compensated for by a corresponding change in the shape of the acetabulum.

### TABLE 25.6

### TREATMENT OF LEGG-CALVÉ-PERTHES DISEASE

Poor prognosis group: treatment indicated
    Catterall 3 and 4
    Salter-Thompson B
    Lateral pillar C
    At risk clinically
    At risk radiographically, regardless of the disease extent
    Age <8 yr with deformity
    Age >8 yr (Catterall group 2, 3, and 4, with or without at-risk signs; lateral pillar B and C; Salter-Thompson B), with or without head deformity
Good prognosis group: no treatment necessary
    Catterall 1 and 2 (generally good prognosis in 90% of cases)
    Salter-Thompson A
    Lateral pillar A
Indeterminate prognosis group: may require treatment
    Catterall 2
    Lateral pillar B
In reossification stage: may require treatment

All patients should be treated if they manifest clinical at-risk signs (i.e., if they lose range of motion and have pain), or if they demonstrate several of the radiographic at-risk signs regardless of the extent of epiphyseal involvement. If the patient is already in the reossification or healing stage of the disease, little further deformity ensues, and no treatment is indicated unless the patient has symptoms (see the section "Treatment Options in the Noncontainable Hip and the Late-presenting Patient with Deformity" later in this chapter).

The earliest treatment methods used weight relief until the femoral head was reossified. These methods were based on the premise that weight relief would prevent the mechanical deformation of the head and early degenerative joint disease (89,305–307). These modalities included prolonged, strict bed rest, often in the hospital, and bed rest with or without various periods of traction on special frames or in spica casts. These methods of treatment were associated with disuse atrophy of muscles, osteopenia, shortening of the involved extremity, loss of thoracic kyphosis, urinary calculi, social and emotional problems, and high hospital costs (160,209,210,270,308–315).

The concept of weight relief as a treatment for Legg-Calvé-Perthes syndrome was challenged as early as 1927, when Legg stated that, "while the process suggesting weakness of bone structure is going on it is theoretically sound to allow no weight bearing but in practice relief from weight bearing in no way affects the end results" (316). In addition, prolonged immobilization and bed rest do not influence the radiographic course of the disease (228,248,249,317–319). Harrison and Menon (312) pointed out, as had Pauwels and others (160,320,321), that even at rest or during minimal activity significant forces act on the femoral head.

The cornerstone of treatment for Legg-Calvé-Perthes syndrome is referred to as *containment*. This concept was originally described by Parker (312) and Eyre-Brook (306). The rationale for this concept has been defined further by Harrison and Menon (312), Petrie and Bitenc (273), Salter (120,322), and others (323–328). The essence of containment is that, in order to prevent deformities of the diseased epiphysis, the femoral head must be contained within the depths of the acetabulum, thereby equalizing the pressure on the head and subjecting it to the molding action of the acetabulum. Containment is an attempt to reduce the forces through the hip joint by actual or relative varus positioning (329). Containment may be achieved by nonoperative or operative methods (330). The femoral head represents more than three-fourths of the sphere and the acetabulum only half of the sphere. Therefore, no method of containment can provide for a totally contained femoral head within the acetabulum during all portions of the gait cycle (149,327,328,331).

### Management of the Patient

The primary goals in the treatment of Legg-Calvé-Perthes syndrome are to prevent deformity (Stulberg classes 3, 4, and 5), stop growth disturbance, and thereby prevent degenerative joint disease. Attainment of these goals requires that each patient be assessed clinically and radiographically. Clinically, the patient is evaluated for clinical at-risk signs such as loss of motion, contracture of the joint, and pain. AP and frog-leg lateral radiographs are evaluated so as to determine the radiographic stage of the disease, the extent of epiphyseal involvement (Catterall group, Salter-Thompson type, or lateral pillar classifications), and the presence of radiographic at-risk signs. If treatment is to succeed in controlling subsequent deformity, it should be initiated in the initial or fragmentation phase of the disease (75,275).

Treatment is not indicated if the child demonstrates none of the clinical or radiographic at-risk signs; if he or she has Catterall group 1 or 2, Salter-Thompson type A, or lateral pillar type A disease; or if the disease is already in the reossification stage. A child who demonstrates clinical or radiographic at-risk signs regardless of the extent of epiphyseal involvement should receive treatment (185). Even patients with Catterall group 2 disease (or lateral pillar type B disease) who are at risk may have poor results without treatment (72) (W.J. Cumming, personal communication, 1997).

The first principle of treatment regardless of the definitive method of treatment chosen is restoration of motion. Motion of the joint enhances synovial nutrition and cartilage nutrition (332,333). This tenet of treatment cannot be overemphasized. The series that recorded the greatest success in treating patients for extensively involved femoral heads is that of Brotherton and McKibbin (323). These patients were treated with bed rest and containment. The end results in these patients were superior to those in another long-term study of patients treated with bed rest and containment on a frame (209,210). The only difference between the two treatment regimens was that in the former series motion was always maintained. Restoration of motion can be accomplished by bed rest alone, or with skin traction and progressive abduction to relieve the muscle spasms. The author recommends bed rest at home with nonsteroidal anti-inflammatory drugs (NSAIDs) on a round-the-clock basis and then reassessment in 1 week to assure that range of motion has considerably improved (to at least 45 degrees of abduction). Occasionally, surgical release of the contracted adductors may be necessary. Restoration of motion allows abduction of the hip, which reduces the forces on the hip joint and allows positioning of the uncovered anterolateral aspect of the femoral head in the acetabulum. Mobilization of the hip joint can also be achieved by rest followed by the use of progressive abduction plasters to stretch the hip adductor muscles while allowing hip flexion and extension. A full or almost full range of motion is usually obtainable within 7 to 10 days of treatment. Because of early deformity, complete abduction and internal rotation may not always be obtainable. Persistence of an adduction contracture is always associated with a serious femoral head deformity and will not respond to bed rest or to bed rest with traction (334).

Arthrography is a useful adjunct in determining whether the femoral head actually can be contained and, if so, in what position this is best accomplished (335) (Fig. 25.27). Arthrography can reveal any flattening of the femoral head that may not be seen on plain radiographs. More importantly, it can demonstrate the hinge abduction phenomenon (190,191,217) (Fig. 25.8, 25.25, and 25.26). Demonstration of the hinge abduction phenomenon, or the inability to contain the hip, is a contraindication to any type of containment treatment. Serious damage to the femoral head and acetabulum may result from trying to contain a noncontainable head (Fig. 25.14). Arthrography should be performed under general anesthesia. This also provides an opportunity to examine whether muscle spasm, contracture, or mechanical deformity is responsible for any apparent fixed deformities.

The treatment for Legg-Calvé-Perthes syndrome remains controversial, and there is disagreement regarding whether operative or nonoperative treatment is more beneficial. Although operative treatment is becoming increasingly popular, there is considerable debate about the benefits of each operative procedure. The shortage of natural history studies for comparison of the results of different modalities of treatment is another reason for the difficulty in resolving this controversy. In addition, the variability of criteria for inclusion of patients in studies, the use of different measurements to assess outcomes of treatment, the lack of interobserver and intraobserver reliability data, and the lack of untreated control groups make comparisons difficult.

In the earlier editions of this book, considerable space was devoted to describing the use of abduction bracing in the treatment of Perthes disease. Over the years, this modality has been replaced by more promising surgical interventions and is now rarely used by pediatric orthopaedic surgeons. It is mentioned in this edition for the historical perspective of the evolution of methods of treatment. Today the most widely used methods to maintain containment are femoral osteotomy, innominate osteotomy, and the use of a procedure earlier regarded as a salvage procedure, namely, lateral shelf acetabuloplasty. There is also growing interest in combined femoral and innominate surgical procedures.

## Nonoperative Treatment

In 1971, Petrie and Bitenc (273) reported excellent results from applying the principles of containment, using broomstick abduction with long-leg plasters (Fig. 25.24C). This series proved that weight bearing, with the femoral head contained, was not harmful. This method of treatment allows for weight bearing and maintenance of range of motion of the hip in the contained position. Successful results of this technique have been reported (336). Petrie casts are currently used by some surgeons after muscle-release procedures and capsulotomies for reducing femoral heads that are deformed and subluxated (337), or for maintaining containment after surgical treatment.

To avoid the repeated hospitalizations necessary for regaining knee and ankle motion, and to avoid the occasional flattening of the femoral condyles seen in patients treated with broomstick plasters, orthopaedists turned to the use of removal abduction orthoses, as typified by the Newington abduction brace (270), the Roberts orthosis (338), the Houston A-frame brace (339), and the Toronto Legg-Calvé-Perthes orthosis (169,340). These devices provide containment in the abducted internal rotation position.

The most widely used abduction orthosis was the Atlanta Scottish Rite orthosis or a modification thereof (Fig. 25.28). These devices were thought to provide for containment solely by abduction without fixed internal rotation (272, 274,341,342). They allowed free motion of the knee and ankle. Containment was provided by the abduction of the brace and the hip flexion required for walking with the legs in abduction. These devices are less cumbersome than other braces and are well tolerated by patients. On arthrography, the position of containment that would be maintained by an abduction orthosis of this variety would be demonstrated by abduction, slight flexion, and external rotation (Fig. 25.27). Containment had to be demonstrated on a radiograph with the patient in the weight-bearing position and in the brace (Fig. 25.24). The brace was worn on a full-time basis until the femoral head was in the reossification stage, when there was no further risk of collapse. Full-time bracing ranged from 6 to 18 months. The negative aspects of bracing included prolonged treatment times and the

need for compliance on the part of the patient. Some patients did not tolerate the brace for psychological reasons (343). This type of treatment was also difficult for girls and older patients to accept (344).

Although early radiographic anatomic results were comparable with those of previously used containment weight-bearing methods (274,342), follow-up reports of patients treated with these orthotic devices questioned the efficacy of this method of management (230,345,346). Martinez et al. (230) reported on 31 patients (34 hips) with severe Perthes disease (Catterall groups 3 and 4) that had been treated with weight-bearing abduction orthoses. The mean age of the patients when first seen was 6 years, and the mean duration of follow-up was 7 years. At follow-up, applying the Mose criteria, no hip had a good result, 35% had fair results, and 65% had poor results. On the basis of the classification of Stulberg et al., there were 41% class 2 results, 53% class 3 and 4 results, and 6% class 5 results. With respect to the lateral column, of the 20 hips in which collapse occurred, only 10% had Stulberg class 2 results, 35% had class 3 results, 45% had class 4 results, and 10% had class 5 results. By comparison, in the 14 hips in which collapse of the lateral column did not occur, 86% had Stulberg class 2 results and only 14% had class 3 results. Class 4 or 5 results were not found in hips in which a collapse did not occur. The authors concluded that although containment is the most widely accepted principle of treatment of Legg-Calvé-Perthes disease, little clinical

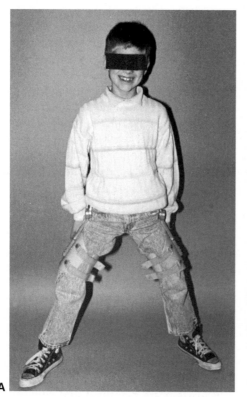
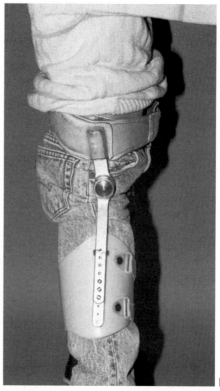

A                                                                    B

**Figure 25.28**  An abduction orthosis.

information supports the contention that bracing in abduction and external rotation, as provided by the Atlanta Scottish Rite orthosis and its modifications, is effective.

Meehan et al. (345) reported on 34 patients with Catterall group 3 or 4 disease, with an average age at diagnosis of 8 years. The average follow-up duration in this series was 6 years and 9 months. At follow-up, there were no Stulberg class 1 results, 3 class 2 results, 24 class 3 results, 6 class 4 results, and 1 class 5 result. The same investigators also arrived at a similar conclusion concerning the use of this orthotic device in the treatment of Perthes disease. In both of these studies the issue of compliance is not documented, and as with all studies of Perthes disease in the literature, control groups other than historic controls are absent. Because the radiographic outcomes in both of these studies were poor, it is questionable whether the orthosis itself adds anything to the treatment other than maintenance of range of motion. As expected, most patients with Perthes disease in both series were doing well clinically, as do most patients over the short term regardless of the extent of the deformity. The long-term prognosis for all but the Stulberg class 1 and 2 hips is guarded.

In the light of these results, bracing is rarely used today by pediatric orthopaedic surgeons in the treatment of Perthes disease. Because of the nihilistic attitude that many physicians share with regard to treatment for Perthes disease, they have begun treating patients with only maintenance of range-of-motion programs, including stretching exercises, nighttime abduction splinting, home traction, and other combinations. Long-term follow-up studies of these nonoperative range-of-motion regimens are needed in order to determine their efficacy.

## Surgical Treatment

Surgical methods of providing or maintaining containment are advocated by many investigators. Surgical containment methods offer the advantage of early mobilization and the avoidance of prolonged bracing or cast treatment. In addition, no end point for discontinuing treatment is required (337). Surgical containment may be approached from the femoral side, the acetabular side, or both sides of the hip joint. Procedures used for obtaining or maintaining containment in Legg-Calvé-Perthes syndrome are those that were originally used in the treatment of problems associated with developmental hip dysplasia and dislocation. The discussion that follows relates only to hips that are "containable" (relatively full range of motion, congruency between the femoral head and the acetabulum) and in the initial or fragmentation phase of the disease.

### Varus Osteotomy

Varus osteotomy, with or without associated derotation, offers the theoretical advantage of deep seating of the femoral head and positioning of the vulnerable anterolateral portion of the head away from the deforming influences of the acetabular edge (238,334,347–350). The varus position reduces the forces exerted by the joint on the femoral head (329,347). This procedure is thought to relieve the intraosseous venous hypertension and improve the disturbed intraosseous venous drainage reported in Legg-Calvé-Perthes syndrome, thereby speeding the healing process (123,124,144,347,348,351). A number of investigators disagree with these perceived benefits (352–354).

Prerequisites for varus derotation osteotomy include a full range of motion, congruency between the femoral head and the acetabulum, and the ability to contain the femoral head in the acetabulum in abduction and internal rotation (337,355) (Fig. 25.27). This assessment usually requires arthrography if the femoral head is well into the fragmentation phase. The procedure must be performed early, in the initial or fragmentation stage of the disease, in order to have any effect on later femoral head deformity (179,224,347).

The negative aspects of this treatment modality must be considered. Varus osteotomy, with or without derotation, usually requires the use of internal fixation and external mobilization in plaster for 6 weeks. The patient must incur the inherent risks and costs associated with at least one surgical procedure and most likely a second surgical procedure for hardware removal. The limb is temporarily shortened by the procedure. The varus angle must not exceed a neck-shaft angle of less than 110 degrees. The varus angle generally decreases with growth (190,356,357); however, if there has been physeal plate damage secondary to the disease, this remodeling potential may be lost, and the patient may have permanent shortening and temporary or permanent weakness of the hip abductors (144,357–361). The proponents of varus osteotomy, with or without derotation, report 70% to 90% satisfactory anatomic results using this method (144,224,347,348,358,360,362–372).

### Innominate Osteotomy

Innominate osteotomy provides for containment by redirection of the acetabulum, providing better coverage for the anterolateral portion of the femoral head. The femoral head is placed in relative flexion, abduction, and internal rotation with respect to the acetabulum in the weight-bearing position. Any shortening caused by the disease can be corrected (120,337,355,360,373–377). Prerequisites for innominate osteotomy include restoration of a full range of motion, a round or almost round femoral head, and congruency of the joint, demonstrated arthrographically. Treatment must be performed early in the course of the disease, and the head must be well seated in flexion, abduction, and internal rotation.

Innominate osteotomy is performed in a fashion similar to that for residual hip subluxation. The tendinous portion of the iliopsoas muscle is always released at the musculo-tendinous junction, and any residual contractures of the adductor muscles are released by subcutaneous adductor tenotomy (120,337). The osteotomy is fixed by two or three threaded pins for internal fixation. Partial weight bearing may be resumed in a cooperative child several days after surgery; however, in an uncooperative patient, immobilization in a spica cast for 6 weeks is required.

The disadvantages of innominate osteotomy are the associated risks and cost factors of the surgical procedure and the procedure for pin removal. Additionally, the operation is performed on the normal side of the joint. This procedure may increase the forces on the femoral head by lateralizing the acetabulum and increasing the lever arm of the abductors (347), although this supposition has so far not been substantiated. Innominate osteotomy may also cause a persistent acetabular configuration change where there was a previously normal acetabulum, leading to loss of motion, particularly flexion (378). Satisfactory anatomic results from this procedure range from 69% to 94% (337, 360,373–375,379–383).

There is significant biomechanical evidence to show that neither method of surgical containment, innominate or femoral osteotomy, may effectively shield an extensively necrotic segment of the femoral head from stress (327,328,384,385). Wenger (188) reported a high incidence of complications in surgically treated patients, even when the accepted methods were used and prerequisites were met.

### Varus Osteotomy Plus Innominate Osteotomy

Several short-term results of combined varus osteotomy plus innominate osteotomy have been reported in patients with severely involved Catterall group 3 or 4 disease. This combined procedure has the theoretical advantage of maximizing femoral head containment while avoiding the complications of either procedure alone. The femoral osteotomy directs the femoral head into the acetabulum, while theoretically reducing any increasing pressure or stiffness of the joint that would result from the pelvic osteotomy. The coverage provided by the innominate osteotomy reduces the degree of correction needed from the femoral osteotomy, thereby minimizing the complications of excessive neck-shaft varus, associated abductor weakness, and limb shortening. Advocates of this procedure also believe that permanent correction of the deformity, early weight bearing, and shortened treatment time are obtained. The disadvantages of the procedure include those mentioned for varus osteotomy and innominate osteotomy alone. Surgical time is increased, potential blood loss is magnified, and the combined procedures are technically more difficult. Satisfactory anatomic results from this combined procedure are reported in up to 78% of patients. As would be expected in short-term follow-up, the clinical results are excellent (386–390). The prerequisites for this operation include those for both varus and innominate osteotomies,

in a patient who probably would not achieve satisfactory coverage from either procedure alone.

### Shelf Arthroplasty

Recently, shelf arthroplasty has been proposed as a primary method of management in children older than 8 years with Catterall group 2, 3, or 4 disease with or without at-risk signs, lateral pillar type B or C disease, and Salter-Thompson type B disease; if subluxation is present, it must be reducible on a dynamic arthrogram (304,391) (Fig. 25.29). Contraindications include hips that do not meet the aforementioned criteria and the presence of hinge abduction. Only one intermediate-term follow-up study exists, but proponents of this method of treatment believe that containment of the femoral head by shelf arthroplasty, before significant deformity can develop, improves remodeling of the femoral head (304,392). The shelf procedure may cover the anterolateral portion of the head, preventing subluxation and lateral overgrowth of the epiphysis. Risk factors for poor results with this technique are age older than 11 years, female gender, and Catterall group 4 disease.

### Triple Innominate Osteotomy

Reports of the use of triple innominate osteotomy to treat Perthes disease have begun to surface in the literature (393,394). This procedure, originally introduced for the treatment of developmental hip dysplasia, is theoretically better able to cover the deforming femoral head. Only longer follow-ups will let physicians know if this will offer better long-term results compared with more commonly applied osteotomies.

### Arthrodiastasis

Recently reports have been published advocating the use of hip distraction (arthrodiastasis) for periods of 4 to 5 months, with or without soft tissue release, in older children with Perthes disease (395,396). A judgment about the usefulness of these procedures will have to await further follow-up.

Regardless of the method of containment chosen, any episode indicative of loss of containment, such as recurrent pain or loss of range of motion, must be treated aggressively with rest, traction, and reassessment of containment clinically and possibly radiographically.

## Treatment Options in the Noncontainable Hip and the Late-presenting Patient with Deformity

Patients presenting with deformity in the later stages (reossification) of the disease, those with noncontainable deformities, and those who have lost containment after undergoing either surgical or nonsurgical containment procedures present a management challenge. These patients

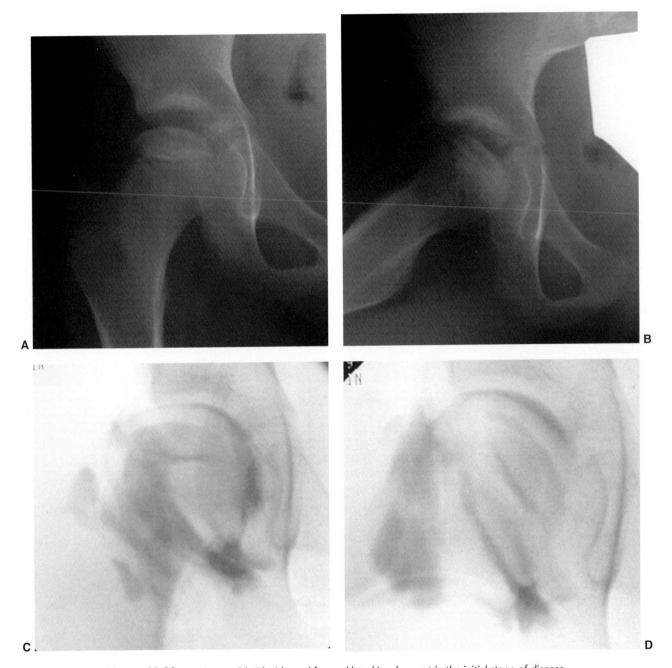

**Figure 25.29** An 8-year-old girl with total femoral head involvement in the initial stage of disease. **A:** Anteroposterior view. **B:** Lateral view. **C:** Intraoperative arthrogram in neutral position showing very mild flattening of the femoral head. **D:** Arthrogram in abduction showing no evidence of impingement. **E:** One year after shelf arthroplasty. **F:** Five years after shelf arthroplasty.

usually demonstrate hinge abduction on arthrography and have an extremely poor prognosis without additional treatment (186,203,237,337,397,398). They generally present with persistent pain, shortening of the involved extremity, and a fixed deformity, generally 10 to 15 degrees of fixed flexion and 15 to 20 degrees of fixed adduction (237,398). The salvage procedures to be considered at this point include abduction extension osteotomy (237,337,363,366,367, 398–401), lateral shelf arthroplasty, Chiari osteotomy, and cheilectomy. These procedures must be viewed as salvage procedures, with each having specific limited aims,

which may include pain relief, correction of limb-length inequality, increasing femoral head coverage, improvement in movement of the joint, and strengthening of a weak abductor (398).

### Abduction Extension Osteotomy

In patients in the active stage of the disease regardless of their age with a noncontainable hip or patients with a painful hip after healing who demonstrate hinge abduction, abduction extension osteotomy should be considered. Abduction extension osteotomy of the femur is indicated

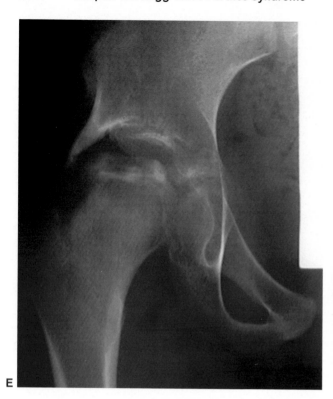

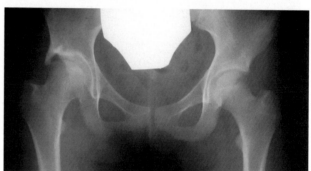

**Figure 25.29** *(continued)*

when arthrography demonstrates that the congruency of the joint is improved by the extended adducted position (Figs. 25.27 and 25.28). The preliminary results with this modality of treatment indicate improvement in limb length, decrease in limp, and improvement in function and range of motion (398). This procedure may be applied in either the active or the late stage of the disease, when arthrography demonstrates that the congruency of the joint is improved by the extended adducted position. This modality of treatment allows for realignment of the congruent position of the hip in the neutral weight-bearing position. Short-term results are promising (337,366,367,398).

### Shelf Arthroplasty

Lateral shelf acetabuloplasty may also be used in "salvage" situations, including lateral subluxation of the femoral head, inadequate coverage of the femoral head, and hinge abduction associated with severe Legg-Calvé-Perthes disease (402–407). In this scenario, the shelf would cover the enlarged femoral head in hopes of improving the outcome, much as shelves are used as salvage procedures in residual hip dysplasia cases (Fig. 25.30). One recent report does demonstrate resolution of hinge abduction (408). Using this method in the presence of hinge abduction would not be the author's preference as it does not reduce the lateral impingement of the head in abduction.

### Chiari Osteotomy

Chiari osteotomy improves the lateral coverage of the deformed femoral head, but does not reduce the lateral impingement in abduction and may exacerbate any existing abductor weakness (237,398). Chiari osteotomy may be useful in the enlarged, poorly covered femoral head that is beginning to develop symptoms of early degenerative joint disease. Although good preliminary results have been reported (400–406), the role of Chiari osteotomy in the treatment of Legg-Calvé-Perthes syndrome has yet to be defined.

### Femoral Acetabular Impingement

Cheilectomy removes the anterolateral portion of the femoral head that is impinging on the acetabulum in abduction (Fig. 25.31). It is indicated only in patients with functionally limiting and restricted range of motion. The procedure must be performed only after the physis is closed; otherwise, a slipped capital femoral epiphysis may ensue (399,409). Although cheilectomy may produce gratifying results with regard to improved range of motion, in some cases increasing stiffness may occur secondary to capsular adhesions at the osteotomy site (337). In addition, shortening associated with the femoral head deformity is not corrected. The entity of femoral acetabular impingement is discussed more fully in Chapter 24. Little long-term information, other than for cheilectomy, exists for impingement syndromes in Perthes disease.

### Osteochondritis Dissecans

Osteochondritis dissecans after Perthes syndrome may or may not be symptomatic (Fig. 25.15). If it is symptomatic, the pain may be intermittent. In patients with

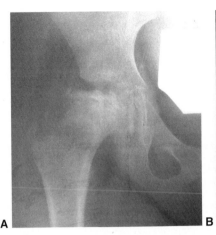 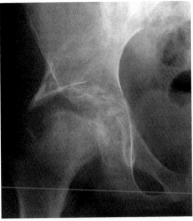 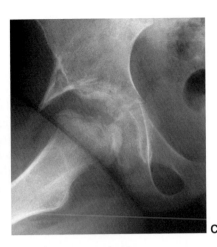

**Figure 25.30** A 9-year-old girl with Catterall group 4 and lateral pillar type C disease treated with lateral shelf arthroplasty. **A:** Note the marked loss of epiphyseal height. **B–C:** Anteroposterior **(B)** and Lauenstein **(C)** radiographs 1 year after operation. Note that the femoral head is in the reossification phase. The involved side is 1 cm shorter than the other. Abduction and internal rotation are to 15 degrees, external rotation is to 25 degrees, and flexion is to 100 degrees. (Courtesy of Fred Dietz, MD, University of Iowa, Iowa City, Iowa.)

pain, several treatment options are available. Symptomatic treatment with antiinflammatory agents and protective weight bearing may be used to promote healing. Persistent pain may warrant attempts at revascularization. This may include drilling of the fragment through the femoral neck and internal fixation, either percutaneously with pins or open with devices such as the Herbert screw. If the fragment becomes detached and cannot be reattached and causes mechanical catching symptoms, it may require removal

(191,410). There is a paucity of information on the natural history of the condition and the results of treatment.

In patients with Legg-Calvé-Perthes syndrome who have premature physeal arrest, trochanteric overgrowth may ensue (180,189). Such patients may develop a Trendelenburg gait and pain secondary to muscle fatigue. This has rarely been a significant problem in long-term reviews (186). However, distal and lateral advancement of the greater trochanter may be necessary (411,412).

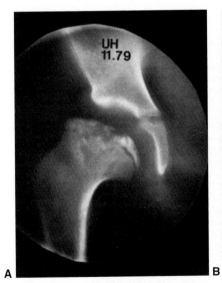 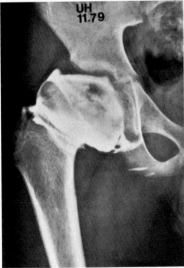 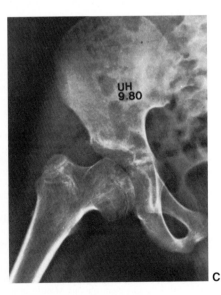

**Figure 25.31** A boy, 8 years and 6 months of age, with Catterall group 4 disease. The range of motion of the hip included flexion of 140 degrees, extension of 0 degree, abduction of 20 degrees, adduction of 30 degrees, internal rotation of 10 degrees, and external rotation of 30 degrees. **A:** Polytome indicating superolateral growth arrest. **B:** Arthrogram demonstrating femoral head flattening and enlargement, and deformation of the peripheral acetabulum. **C:** Abduction radiograph 7 months after cheilectomy. Range of motion at this time was 130 degrees of flexion, 20 degrees of extension, 50 degrees of abduction, 50 degrees of adduction, 45 degrees of internal rotation, and 40 degrees of external rotation. (Courtesy of J.G. Pous, MD, Montpellier, France.)

## FUTURE DEVELOPMENTS

Long-term series of patients with uniform treatment who are matched for age, gender, degree of epiphyseal involvement, and other diagnostic factors, compared with an untreated control group, will no doubt be required in order to determine the most effective treatment for Legg-Calvé-Perthes syndrome. As fundamental understanding of Legg-Calvé-Perthes syndrome increases, so does understanding of how various treatment modalities influence this complex growth disturbance.

## REFERENCES

### Early History

1. Legg AT. An obscure affection of the hip joint. *Boston Med Surg J* 1910;162:202.
2. Calvé J. Sur une forme particuliere de coxalgie greffe sur des deformations caracteristiques de l'extremite superieure de femur. *Rev Chir* 1910;42:54.
3. Perthes G. Uber arthritis deformans juvenilis. *Dtsch Z Chir* 1910;10:111.
4. Waldenstrom H. Der obere Tuberkulose collumnerd. *Z Orthop Chir* 1909;24:487.
5. Waldenstrom H. *Die tuberkulose des collum femoris im kindersalte ihre beziehungen zur huftgelenkentzundung.* Stockholm: 1910.
6. Thomas HO. *Contributions to surgery and medicine. Part II. Principles of the treatment of diseased joints.* London: HK Lewis, 1883.
7. Baker WM. Epiphyseal necrosis and its consequences. *Br Med J* 1883;2:416.
8. Wright GA. The value of determining the primary lesion in joint disease as an indication for treatment. *Br Med J* 1883;2:419.
9. Maydl K. Coxa vara arthritis deformans coxae. *Wien Klin Rudsch* 1897;10:153.
10. Goff CW. Legg-Calvé-Perthes syndrome (L.C.P.S.). *Clin Orthop* 1962;22:93.
11. Perthes G. Osteochondritis deformans juvenilis. *Arch Klin Chir* 1913;101:779.
12. Schwartz E. Eine typische erkrankung der oberen femurepiphyse. *Beitr Klin Chir* 1914;93:127.
13. Waldenstrom H. Coxa plana, osteochondritis deformans coxae, Calvé-Perthes schen krankheit, Legg's disease. *Zentralbl Chir* 1920;17:539.
14. Sundt H. Malum coxae: Calvé-Legg-Perthes. *Zentralbl Chir* 1920; 22:538.
15. Sundt H. *Malum coxae Calvé-Legg-Perthes.* Kristiania: Monographic, 1920.
16. Phemister DB. Perthes' disease. *Surg Gynecol Obstet* 1921;33:87.
17. Riedel G. Pathologic anatomy of osteochondritis deformans coxae juvenilis. *Zentralbl Chir* 1922;49:1447.
18. Waldenstrom H. The definitive forms of coxa plana. *Acta Radiol* 1922;1:384.
19. Wenger DR, Ward WT, Herring JA. Legg-Calvé-Perthes' disease. *J Bone Joint Surg Am* 1991;73:778.
20. Hilgenreiner H. Beitrag zur atiologie der osteochondritis coxae juvenilis. *Med Klin* 1933;29:234.
21. Jansen M. Platte huftpfanne und ihre folgen coxa plana: valga, vara und malum coxae. *Z Orthop Chir* 1925;46:234.
22. Slavik J. *Coxa plana: morbus Maydl-Calvé-Legg-Perthes.* Prague: Albertova Sbirka, 1956.
23. Weinstein SL. Legg-Calvé-Perthes' disease. *Instr Course Lect* 1983;32:272.

### Epidemiology and Etiology

24. Wynne-Davies R, Gormley J. The aetiology of Perthes' disease. *J Bone Joint Surg Br* 1978;60:6.
25. Barker DJP, Hall AJ. The epidemiology of Perthes' disease. *Clin Orthop* 1986;209:89.
26. Van den Bogaert G, De Rosa E, Moens P. Bilateral Legg Calvé Perthes disease: different from unilateral. *J Pediatr Orthop B* 1999;8:165.
27. Fisher RI. An epidemiological study of Legg-Perthes' disease. *J Bone Joint Surg Am* 1972;54:769.
28. Hall D, Harrison MHM. An association between congenital abnormalities and Perthes' disease of the hip. *J Bone Joint Surg Br* 1978;60:138.
29. Hall DJ. Genetic aspects of Perthes' disease: a critical review. *Clin Orthop* 1986;209:100.
30. O'Sullivan M, O'Rourke SK, MacAuley P. Legg-Calvé-Perthes' disease in a family: genetic or environmental. *Clin Orthop* 1985;199:179.
31. Vasseur PB, Foley P, Stevenson S, et al. Mode of inheritance of Perthes' disease in Manchester terriers. *Clin Orthop* 1989;244:281.
32. Wansborough RM, Carrie AW, Walker NF, et al. Coxa plana: its genetic aspects and results of treatment with long Taylor walking caliper. *J Bone Joint Surg Am* 1959;41:1959.
33. Wynne-Davies R. Some etiologic factors in Perthes' disease. *Clin Orthop* 1980;150:12.
34. Harper PS, Brotherton BJ, Cochlin D. Genetic risks in Perthes' disease. *Clin Genet* 1976;10:178.
35. Hall AJ, Barker DJ, Dangerfield PH, et al. Small feet and Perthes' disease: a survey in Liverpool. *J Bone Joint Surg Br* 1988;70:611.
36. Hall AJ, Barker DJ. Perthes disease in Yorkshire. *J Bone Joint Surg Br* 1989;71:229.
37. Hall AJ, Barker DJ, Dangerfield PH, et al. Perthes' disease of the hip in Liverpool. *Br Med J* 1983;287:1757.
38. Barker DJP, Dixon E, Taylor JF. Perthes' disease of the hip in three regions of England. *J Bone Joint Surg Br* 1978;60:478.
39. Catterall A. Legg-Calvé-Perthes' disease. *Instr Course Lect* 1989;38:297.
40. Chacko V, Joseph B, Seetharam B. Perthes' disease in South India. *Clin Orthop* 1986;209:95.
41. Hall AJ, Margetts BM, Barker DJ, et al. Low blood manganese levels in Liverpool children with Perthes' disease. *Paediatr Perinat Epidemiol* 1989;3:131.
42. Kealey WD, Moore AJ, Cook S, et al. Deprivation, urbanisation and Perthes' disease in Northern Ireland. *J Bone Joint Surg Br* 2000;82(2):167–171.
43. Peic S. Contribution to Perthes' disease. *Z Orthop* 1962;96:276.
44. Loder RT, Schwartz EM, Hensinger RN. Behavioral characteristics of children with Legg-Calvé-Perthes' disease. *J Pediatr Orthop* 1993;13:598.
45. Malloy MK, MacMahon B. Incidence of Legg-Calvé-Perthes' disease (osteochondritis deformans). *N Engl J Med* 1966; 275:998.
46. Malloy MK, MacMahon B. Birth weight and Legg-Perthes' disease. *J Bone Joint Surg Am* 1967;49:498.
47. Lappin K, Kealey D, Cosgrove A, et al. Does low birthweight predispose to Perthes' disease? Perthes' disease in twins. *J Pediatr Orthop B* 2003;12(5):307–310.
48. Harrison MHM, Turner MH, Jacobs P. Skeletal immaturity in Perthes' disease. *J Bone Joint Surg Br* 1976;58:37.
49. Ralston EL. Legg-Perthes' disease and physical development. *J Bone Joint Surg Am* 1955;37:647.
50. Cannon SR, Pozo JL, Catterall A. Elevated growth velocity in children with Perthes' disease. *J Pediatr Orthop* 1989;9:285.
51. Exner GU. Elevated growth velocity in children with Perthes' disease [Letter]. *J Pediatr Orthop* 1989;9:732.
52. Goff CW. Recumbency versus nonrecumbency treatment of Legg-Perthes' disease. *Clin Orthop* 1959;14:50.
53. Puny NA. The incidence of Perthes' disease in the population groups in the Eastern Cape region of South Africa. *J Bone Joint Surg Br* 1982;64:286.
54. Cameron J, Izatt MM. Legg-Calvé-Perthes' disease. *Scott Med J* 1960;5:148.
55. Burwell RG, Coates CL, Vernon CL, et al. Anthropometry and Perthes' disease: a preliminary report. *J Bone Joint Surg Br* 1976; 58:254.
56. Burwell RG, Dangerfield PH, Hall DJ, et al. Perthes' disease: an anthropometric study revealing impaired and disproportionate growth. *J Bone Joint Surg Br* 1978;60:461.
57. Burwell RG. Perthes' disease: growth and aetiology. *Arch Dis Child* 1988;63:1408.

58. Kristmundsdottir F, Burwell RG, Harrison MHM. Delayed skeletal maturation in Perthes' disease. *Acta Orthop Scand* 1987; 58:277.

59. Rao B, Joseph B, Chacko V, et al. Altered skeletal growth in Perthes' disease: an anthropomorphic study of children from rural India. *J Pediatr Orthop B* 1995;4:91.

60. Loder R, Farley FA, Herring JA, et al. Bone age determination in children with Legg-Calvé-Perthes disease: a comparison of two methods. *J Pediatr Orthop* 1995;15:90.

61. Eckerwall G, Wingstrand H, Haaglund G, et al. Growth in 110 children with Legg-Calvé-Perthes' disease: a longitudinal infancy childhood puberty growth model study. *J Pediatr Orthop B* 1996;5:181.

62. Tanaka H, Tamura K, Takano K, et al. Serum somatomedin A in Perthes' disease. *Acta Orthop Scand* 1984;55:135.

63. Kitsugi T, Kasahara Y, Seto Y, et al. Normal somatomedin-C activity measured by radioimmunoassay in Perthes' disease. *Clin Orthop* 1989;244:217.

64. Neidel J, Zander D, Hackenbroch MH. Low plasma levels of insulin-like growth factor I in Perthes' disease: a controlled study of 59 consecutive children. *Acta Orthop Scand* 1992;63:393.

65. Kealey WD, Lappin KJ, Leslie H, et al. Endocrine profile and physical stature of children with Perthes disease. *J Pediatr Orthop* 2004;24(2):161–166.

66. Neidel J, Zander D, Hackenbroch MH. No physiologic age-related increase of circulating somatomedin-C during early stage of Perthes' disease: a longitudinal study in 21 boys. *Arch Orthop Trauma Surg* 1992;111:171.

67. Neidel JSE, Zander D, Rutt J, et al. Normal plasma levels of IGF binding protein in Perthes' disease: follow up of a previous report. *Acta Orthop Scand* 1993;64:540.

68. Neidel J, Boddenberg B, Zander D, et al. Thyroid function in Legg-Calvé-Perthes' disease: cross-sectional and longitudinal study. *J Pediatr Orthop* 1993;13:592.

69. Matsumoto T, Enomoto H, Takahashi K, et al. Decreased levels of IGF binding protein 3 in serum from children with Legg Calvé Perthes' disease. *Acta Orthop Scand* 1998;69:125.

70. Grasemann H, Nicolai RD, Hauffa BP, et al. Skeletal immaturity, IGF-I and IGFBP-3 serum concentrations in Legg-Calvé-Perthes' disease. *Klin Padiatr* 1996;208:339.

71. Catterall A, Lloyd-Roberts GC, Wynne-Davies R. Association of Perthes' disease with congenital anomalies of genitourinary tract and inguinal region. *Lancet* 1971;1:996.

72. Catterall A. *Legg-Calvé-Perthes' disease.* Edinburgh: Churchill Livingstone, 1982.

73. Hall DJ, Harrison MHM, Burwell RG. Congenital abnormalities and Perthes' disease: clinical evidence that children with Perthes' disease may have a major congenital defect. *J Bone Joint Surg Br* 1979;61:18.

74. Axhausen G. Kohler's disease and Perthes' disease. *Zentralbl Chir* 1923;50:553.

75. Ferguson AB, Howorth MB. Coxa plana and related conditions at the hip. *J Bone Joint Surg Br* 1934;16:781.

76. Konjetzny GE. Zur pathologie und pathologischen anatomie der Perthes-Calvé schen krankheit. *Acta Chir Scand* 1943;74:361.

77. Phemister DB. Operation for epiphysitis of the head of the femur (Perthes' disease). *Arch Surg* 1921;2:221.

78. Matsoukas J. Viral antibody titers to rubella in coxa plana or Perthes' disease. *Acta Orthop Scand* 1975;46:957.

79. Bentzon PGK. Experimental studies on the pathogenesis of coxa plana and other manifestations of "local dyschondroplasia." *Acta Radiol* 1926;6:155.

80. Broder H. The late results in Legg-Perthes' disease and factors influencing them: a study of one hundred and two cases. *Bull Hosp Jt Dis* 1953;14:194.

81. Craig WA, Kramer WG, Watanabe R. Etiology and treatment of Legg-Calvé-Perthes syndrome. *J Bone Joint Surg Am* 1963; 45:1325.

82. Craig WA. Course of Legg-Calvé-Perthes: natural history, pathomechanics. *Orthop Rev* 1979;8:29.

83. Helbo S. *Morbus Calvé Perthes.* Odense: FynaTidendes Bogtrykkeri, 1954.

84. Leriche R. Recherches experimentales sur le me canisme de formation de l'osteochondrite de la hanche. *Lyon Chir* 1934; 31:610.

85. Lindstrom JR, Ponseti IV, Wenger DR. Acetabular development after reduction in congenital dislocation of the hip. *J Bone Joint Surg Am* 1979;61:112.

86. Bunger C, Solund K, Joyce F, et al. Carrageenan-induced coxitis in puppies. *Acta Orthop Scand* 1988;59:249.

87. Calot F. Uber neuere anschauungen in der pathologie der hufte auf grund der arbeiten der letzen jahre. *Z Orthop Chir* 1929;51:134.

88. Canestri G, Monzali GL. Osteocondrite postridut Lattante iva nella L.C.A.: l'osteochondrite apre reduction de la luxation congenitale de la hanche. *Lattante* 1957;28:537.

89. Gill AB. Legg-Perthes' disease of the hip: its early roentgenographic manifestations and its clinical course. *J Bone Joint Surg Br* 1940;22:1043.

90. Theodorou SD, Vlachos E, et al. Late Perthes disease after satisfactory treatment of congenital dislocation of the hip. *Clin Orthop Relat Res* 2004;420:220–224.

91. Glimcher MJ. Legg-Calvé-Perthes syndrome: biological and mechanical considerations in the genesis of clinical abnormalities. *Orthop Rev* 1979;8:33.

92. Kitoh H, Kitakoji T, Katoh M, et al. Delayed ossification of the proximal capital femoral epiphysis in Legg-Calve-Perthes' disease. *J Bone Joint Surg Br* 2003;85(1):121–124.

93. Cavanaugh LA, Shelton EK, Sutherland R. Metabolic studies in osteochondritis of the capital femoral epiphysis. *J Bone Joint Surg Br* 1936;18:957.

94. Emerick RW, Corrigan KF, Joistad AH Jr, et al. Thyroid function in Legg-Calvé-Perthes' disease: a new approach to an old problem. *Clin Orthop* 1954;4:160.

95. Gill AB. Relationship of Legg-Perthes' disease to the function of the thyroid gland. *J Bone Joint Surg Br* 1943;25:892.

96. Gershuni DH. Etiology of Legg-Calvé-Perthes syndrome. *Orthop Rev* 1979;8:49.

97. Jacobs BW. Early recognition of osteochondrosis of capital epiphysis of femur. *JAMA* 1960;172:527.

98. Hochbergs P. Magnetic resonance imaging in Legg-Calvé-Perthes' disease. Thesis, Lund University, Lund, Sweden, 1998.

99. Eckerwall G, Lohmander LS, Wingstrand H. Increased levels of proteoglycan fragments and stromelysin in hip joint fluid in Legg-Calvé-Perthes' disease. *J Pediatr Orthop* 1997;17:266.

100. Eckerwall G, Hochbergs P, Wingstrand H, et al. Sonography and intracapsular pressure in Perthes disease: 39 children examined 2–36 months after onset. *Acta Orthop Scand* 1994;65:575.

101. Suzuki S, Kasahara Y, Seto Y, et al. Arthroscopy in 19 children with Perthes' disease. *Acta Orthop Scand* 1994;65:581.

102. Vanpaemel L, Helders PJM, Kuis W, et al. Destructive synovitis in contralateral Perthes' disease: a report of 2 cases. *Acta Orthop Scand* 1994;65:585.

103. Haueisen DC, Weiner DS, Weiner SD. The characterization of transient synovitis of the hip in children. *J Pediatr Orthop* 1986;6:11.

104. Kallio P, Ryoppy S. Hyperpressure in juvenile hip disease. *Acta Orthop Scand* 1985;56:211.

105. Kallio P, Ryoppy S, Kunnamo I. Transient synovitis and Perthes: is there an etiologic connection? *J Bone Joint Surg Br* 1986;68:608.

106. Mukamel M, Litmanovitch M, Yosipovitch Z, et al. Legg Calvé Perthes' disease following transient synovitis: how often? *Clin Pediatr* 1985;24:629.

107. Wingstrand H, Bauer G, Brimar J, et al. Transient ischemia of the proximal femoral epiphysis in the child: interpretation of bone scintimetry for diagnosis in hip pain. *Acta Orthop Scand* 1985;56:197.

108. Wingstrand H, Egund N, Carlin NO, et al. Intracapsular pressure in transient synovitis of the hip. *Acta Orthop Scand* 1985;56:204.

109. Chuinard EG. Femoral osteotomy in treatment of Legg-Calvé-Perthes syndrome. *Orthop Rev* 1979;8:113.

110. Chung SMK. The arterial supply of the developing proximal end of the human femur. *J Bone Joint Surg Am* 1976;58:961.

111. Trueta J. The normal vascular anatomy of the human femoral head during growth. *J Bone Joint Surg Br* 1957;39:358.

112. Trueta J, Pinto de Lima CS. Studies of osteochondritis of the femoral head or Legg-Calvé-Perthes' disease. *Rev Ortop Traumatol Ed Lat Am* 1959;4:115.

113. Ogden JA. Changing patterns of proximal femoral vascularity. *J Bone Joint Surg Am* 1974;56:941.

114. Theron J. Angiography in Legg-Calvé-Perthes' disease. *Radiology* 1980;135:81.

115. Atsumi T, Yoshihara S, Hiranuma Y. Revascularization of the artery of the ligamentum teres in Perthes disease. *Clin Orthop Relat Res* 2001;386:210–217.

116. Sanchis M, Freeman MAR, Zahir A. Experimental stimulation of the blood supply to the capital epiphysis in the puppy. *J Bone Joint Surg Am* 1973;55:335.

117. Inoue A, Freeman MAR, Vernon-Roberts B, et al. The pathogenesis of Perthes' disease. *J Bone Joint Surg Br* 1976;58:483.

118. Katz JF. Recurrent Legg-Calvé-Perthes' disease. *J Bone Joint Surg Am* 1973;55:833.

119. Martinez AG, Weinstein SL. Recurrent Legg-Calvé-Perthes' disease: case report and review of the literature. *J Bone Joint Surg Am* 1991;73:1081.

120. Salter RB. Legg-Perthes' disease: the scientific basis for the methods of treatment and their indications. *Clin Orthop* 1980;150:8.

121. Salter RB, Thompson GH. Legg-Calvé-Perthes' disease: the prognostic significance of the subchondral fracture and a two group classification of the femoral head involvement. *J Bone Joint Surg Am* 1984;66:479.

122. Kleinman RG, Bleck EE. Increased blood viscosity in patients with Legg-Perthes' disease: a preliminary report. *J Pediatr Orthop* 1981;1:131.

123. Heildcinen E, Lanning P, Suramo I, et al. The venous drainage of the femoral neck as a prognostic sign of Perthes' disease. *Acta Orthop Scand* 1980;51:501.

124. Sutherland AD, Savage JP, Patterson DC, et al. The nuclide bone scan in the diagnosis and management of Perthes' disease. *J Bone Joint Surg Br* 1980;63:300.

125. Szepesi K, Posan E, Harsflavi J, et al. The most severe forms of Perthes' disease associated with the homozygous Factor V Leiden mutation. *J Bone Joint Surg Br* 2004;86(3):426–429.

126. Glueck CJ, Freiberg RA, Crawford A, et al. Secondhand smoke, hypofibrinolysis, and Legg-Perthes disease. *Clin Orthop* 1998; 352:159.

127. Glueck CJ, Crawford A, Roy D, et al. Association of antithrombotic factor deficiencies and hypofibrinolysis with Legg-Perthes disease. *J Bone Joint Surg Am* 1996;78:3.

128. Glueck C, Glueck HI, Greenfield D, et al. Protein C and S deficiency, thrombophilia, and hypofibrinolysis: pathophysiologic causes of Legg-Perthes disease. *Pediatr Res* 1994;35:383.

129. Glueck C, Freiberg R, Tracy T, et al. Thrombophilia and hypofibrinolysis: pathophysiologies of osteonecrosis. *Clin Orthop Relat Res* 1997;334:43.

130. Glueck C, Brandt G, Gruppo R, et al. Resistance to activated protein C and Legg-Perthes disease. *Clin Orthop Relat Res* 1997;338:39.

131. Hresko MT, McDougall PA, Gorlin JB, et al. Prospective reevaluation of the association between thrombotic diathesis and Legg-Perthes disease. *J Bone Joint Surg Am* 2002;84(9):1613–1618.

132. Kealey WD, Mayne EE, McDonald W, et al. The role of coagulation abnormalities in the development of Perthes' disease. *J Bone Joint Surg Br* 2000;82(5):744–746.

133. Koo KH, Song HR, Ha YC, et al. Role of thrombotic and fibrinolytic disorders in the etiology of Perthes' disease. *Clin Orthop Relat Res* 2002;399:162–167.

134. Hayek S, Kenet G, Lubetsky A, et al. Does thrombophilia play an aetiological role in Legg-Calvé-Perthes' disease? *J Bone Joint Surg Br* 1999;81:686.

135. Thomas D, Morgan G, Tayton K. Perthes' disease and the relevance of thrombophilia. *J Bone Joint Surg Br* 1999;81:691.

## Pathogenesis

136. Ponseti IV, Maynard JA, Weinstein SL, et al. Legg-Calvé-Perthes' disease: histochemical and ultrastructural observations of the epiphyseal cartilage and the physis. *J Bone Joint Surg Am* 1983; 65:797.

137. Ponseti IV. Legg-Perthes' disease. *J Bone Joint Surg Am* 1956; 38:739.

138. Catterall A. Legg-Calvé-Perthes' disease: classification and pathology. In: Fitzgerald RH Jr, ed. *The hip: Proceedings of the Thirteenth Open Scientific Meeting of the Hip Society*. St. Louis, MO: Mosby, 1985:24.

139. Catterall A, Pringle J, Byers PD, et al. A review of the morphology of Perthes' disease. *J Bone Joint Surg Br* 1982;64:269.

140. Dolman CL, Bell HM. The pathology of Legg-Calvé-Perthes' disease. *J Bone Joint Surg Am* 1973;55:184.

141. Jensen OM, Lauritzen J. Legg-Calvé-Perthes' disease. *J Bone Joint Surg Br* 1976;58:332.

142. Bernbeck R. Kritischenzum Perthes: problem der hufte. *Arch Orthop Unfallchir* 1950;44:445.

143. Bernbeck R. Zur pathogenese der jugendlichen huftokopfnekrose. *Arch Orthop Unfallchir* 1950;44:164.

144. Bohr H, Baadsgaard K, Sager P. The vascular supply to the femoral head following dislocation of the hip joint: an experimental study in newborn rabbits. *Acta Orthop Scand* 1965;35:264.

145. Kandzierski G, Karski T, Kozlowski K. Capital femoral epiphysis and growth plate of the asymptomatic hip joint in unilateral Perthes disease. *J Pediatr Orthop B* 2003;12(6):380–386.

146. Larsen FH, Reiman I. Calvé-Perthes' disease. *Acta Orthop Scand* 1973;44:426.

147. McKibbin B, Holdsworth FW. The nutrition of immature joint cartilage in the lamb. *J Bone Joint Surg Br* 1966;48:793.

148. Guerado E, Garces G. Perthes' disease. A study of constitutional aspects in adulthood. *J Bone Joint Surg Br* 2001;83(4):569–571.

149. McKibbin B, ed. *Recent advances in Perthes' disease*. Edinburgh: Churchill Livingstone, 1975.

150. Schiller MG, Axer A. Hypertrophy of the femoral head in Legg-Calvé-Perthes' syndrome (LCPS). *Acta Orthop Scand* 1972;43:45.

151. Catterall A, Pringle J, Byers PD, et al. Perthes' disease: is the epiphyseal infarction complete? A study of 2 cases. *J Bone Joint Surg Br* 1982;64:276.

152. Hoffinger SA, Henderson RC, Renner JB, et al. Magnetic resonance evaluation of "metaphyseal" changes in Legg-Calvé-Perthes' disease. *J Pediatr Orthop* 1993;13:602.

153. Smith RB, Ions GK, Gregg PJ. The radiological features of the metaphysis in Perthes' disease. *J Pediatr Orthop* 1982;2:401.

154. Gall EA, Bennett GA. Osteochondritis deformans of the hip (Legg-Perthes' disease) and renal osteitis fibrosa cystica: report of a case with anatomic studies. *Arch Pathol* 1942;33:866.

155. Ponseti IV, Shepard RS. Lesions of the skeleton and of other mesodermal tissues in rats fed sweet-pea (*Lathyrus odoratus*) seeds. *J Bone Joint Surg Am* 1954;36:1031.

156. Smith RB, Nevelos AB. Osteochondritis occurring at multiple sites. *Acta Orthop Scand* 1980;51:449.

157. Harrison MHM, Blakemore ME. A study of the "normal" hip in children with unilateral Perthes' disease. *J Bone Joint Surg Br* 1980;62:36.

158. Aire E, Johnson F, Harrison MHM, et al. Femoral head shape in Perthes' disease: is the contralateral hip abnormal? *Clin Orthop* 1986;209:77.

159. Catterall A. Thoughts on the etiology of Perthes' disease. *Iowa Orthop J* 1984;4:34.

160. Harrison MHM, Turner MH, Smith DN. Perthes' disease treatment with the Birmingham splint. *J Bone Joint Surg Br* 1982;64:3.

161. Jonsater A. Coxa plana, a histopathologic and arthrographic study. *Acta Orthop Scand Suppl* 1953;12:1.

162. Waldenstrom H. The first stages of coxa plana. *Acta Orthop Scand* 1934;5:1.

163. Kamegaya M, Moriya H, Tsuchiya K, et al. Arthrography of early Perthes' disease: swelling of the ligamentum teres as a cause of subluxation. *J Bone Joint Surg Br* 1989;71:413.

164. Wingstrand H. Legg-Calvé-Perthes' disease. *Acta Orthop Scand* 1994;65:573.

165. Wingstrand H. Significance of synovitis in Legg-Calvé-Perthes' disease. *J Pediatr Orthop B* 1999;8:156.

166. Bobechko WP, Harris WR. The radiographic density of avascular bone. *J Bone Joint Surg Br* 1960;42:626.

167. Ray RD, LaViolette D, Buckley HD, et al. Studies of bone metabolism. I. A comparison of the metabolism of strontium in living and dead bone. *J Bone Joint Surg Am* 1955;37:143.

168. Watson-Jones R, Roberts RE. Calcifications, decalcification and ossification. *Br J Surg* 1934;21:461.

169. Bobechko WP, McLaurin CA, Motloch WM. Toronto orthosis for Legg-Perthes' disease. *Artif Limbs* 1968;12:36.

170. Kemp HBS, Boldero JL. Radiological changes in Perthes' disease. *Br J Radiol* 1966;39:744.

171. Kenzora JE, Steele RE, Yosipovitch ZH, et al. Experimental osteonecrosis of the femoral head in adult rabbits. *Clin Orthop* 1978;130:8.

172. McKibbin B, Rails Z. Pathological changes in a case of Perthes' disease. *J Bone Joint Surg Br* 1974;56:438.

173. Phemister DB. Bone growth and repair. *Ann Surg* 1935;102:261.

174. Waldenstrom H. The first stages of coxa plana. *J Bone Joint Surg Br* 1938;20:559.

175. Caffey J. The early roentgenographic changes in essential coxa plana: their significance in pathogenesis. *Am J Roentgenol* 1968;103:620.

176. Salter RB, Bell M. The pathogenesis of deformity in Legg-Perthes' disease: an experimental investigation. *J Bone Joint Surg Br* 1968;50:436.

177. Brailsford JF. Avascular necrosis of bone. *J Bone Joint Surg Br* 1943;25:249.

178. Haliburton RA, Brockenshire FA, Barber JR. Avascular necrosis of the femoral capital epiphysis after traumatic dislocation of the hip in children. *J Bone Joint Surg Br* 1961;43:43.

179. Barnes JM. Premature epiphyseal closure in Perthes' disease. *J Bone Joint Surg Br* 1980;62:432.

180. Bowen JR, Foster BK, Hartzell CR. Legg-Calvé-Perthes' disease. *Clin Orthop* 1985;185:97.

181. Coleman RC, Slager RF, Smith WS. The effect of environmental influences on acetabular development. *Surg Forum* 1958;9:775.

182. Keret D, Harrison MHM, Clarke NMP, et al. Coxa plana: the fate of the physis. *J Bone Joint Surg Am* 1984;66:870.

183. Heitzman O. Epiphysenerkrankungen im wachstumsalter. *Klin Wochenschr* 1923;327.

184. Bohr HH. On the development and course of Legg-Calvé-Perthes' disease (LCPD). *Clin Orthop* 1980;150:30.

185. Weinstein SL. *Legg-Calvé-Perthes' disease.* St. Louis, MO: Mosby, 1983.

186. Weinstein SL. Legg-Calvé-Perthes' disease: results of long-term follow-up. In: Fitzgerald RH Jr, ed. *The hip: Proceedings of the Thirteenth Open Scientific Meeting of the Hip Society.* St. Louis, MO: Mosby, 1985:28.

187. Weinstein SL. The pathogenesis of deformity in Legg-Calvé-Perthes' disease. In: Uhthoff H, Wiley J, eds. *Behavior of the growth plate,* New York: Raven Press, 1988:79.

188. Wenger DR. Selective surgical containment for Legg-Perthes' disease: recognition and management of complications. *J Pediatr Orthop* 1981;1:153.

189. Bowen JR, Schreiber FC, Foster BK, et al. Premature femoral neck physeal closure in Perthes' disease. *Clin Orthop* 1982;171:24.

190. Catterall A. Legg-Calvé-Perthes syndrome. *Clin Orthop* 1981;158:41.

191. Grossbard GD. Hip pain in adolescence after Perthes' disease. *J Bone Joint Surg Br* 1981;63:572.

192. Reinker K. Early diagnosis and treatment of hinge abduction in Legg Perthes' disease. *J Pediatr Orthop* 1996;16:3.

193. Lecuire F, Rebouillat J. Long-term development of primary osteochondritis of the hip (Legg-Perthes-Calvé): apropos of 60 hips with a follow-up of more than 30 years. *Rev Chir Orthop* 1987;73:561.

194. Levine B, Kanat IO. Subchondral bone cysts, osteochondritis dissecans, and Legg-Calvé-Perthes' disease: a correlation and proposal of their possible common etiology and pathogenesis. *J Foot Surg* 1988;27:75.

195. Rowe SM, Kim HS, Yoon TR. Osteochondritis dissecans in Perthes' disease: report of 7 cases. *Acta Orthop Scand* 1989;60:545.

## Natural History

196. Catterall A. The natural history of Perthes' disease. *J Bone Joint Surg Br* 1971;53:37.

197. Chigwanda PC. Early natural history of untreated Perthes' disease. *Cent Afr J Med* 1992;38:334.

198. Norlin R, Hammerby S, Tkaczuk H. The natural history of Perthes' disease. *Int Orthop* 1991;15:13.

199. Stulberg SD, Cooperman DR, Wallensten R. The natural history of Legg-Calvé-Perthes' disease. *J Bone Joint Surg Am* 1981;63:1095.

200. Sundt H. Malum coxae Calvé-Legg Perthes. *Acta Chir Scand Suppl* 1949;148:1.

201. Yrjonen T. Prognosis in Perthes' disease after noncontainment treatment: 106 hips followed for 28–47 years. *Acta Orthop Scand* 1992;63:523.

202. Ippolito D, Tudisco C, Farsetti P. The long-term prognosis of unilateral Perthes' disease. *J Bone Joint Surg Br* 1987;69:243.

203. McAndrew MP, Weinstein SL. A long term follow-up of Legg-Calvé-Perthes' disease. *J Bone Joint Surg Am* 1984;66:860.

204. Mose K. Methods of measuring in Legg-Calvé-Perthes' disease with special regard to the prognosis. *Clin Orthop* 1980;150:103.

205. Herring JA, Williams JJ, Neustadt JN, et al. Evolution of femoral head deformity during the healing phase of Legg-Calvé-Perthes' disease. *J Pediatr Orthop* 1993;13:41.

206. Danielsson LG, Hernborg J. Late results in Perthes' disease. *Acta Orthop Scand* 1965;36:70.

207. Hall G. Some long-term observations of Perthes' disease. *J Bone Joint Surg Br* 1981;63:631.

208. Perpich M, McBeath A, Kruse D. Long term follow-up of Perthes' disease treated with spica casts. *J Pediatr Orthop* 1983;3:160.

209. Ratliff AHC. Perthes' disease: a study of 34 hips observed for 30 years. *J Bone Joint Surg Br* 1967;49:108.

210. Ratliff AHC. Perthes' disease: a study of 16 patients followed up for 40 years. *J Bone Joint Surg Br* 1977;59:248.

211. Gower WE, Johnston RC. Legg-Calvé-Perthes' disease, long-term follow-up of thirty-six patients. *J Bone Joint Surg Am* 1971;53:759.

212. Weinstein SL. Perthes' disease: an overview. *Curr Orthop* 1988;2:181.

213. Herring JA, Neustadt JB, Williams JJ, et al. The lateral pillar classification of Legg-Calvé-Perthes' disease. *J Pediatr Orthop* 1992;12:143.

214. Mukherjee A, Fabry G. Evaluation of the prognostic indices in Legg-Calvé-Perthes' disease. *J Pediatr Orthop* 1990;10:153.

215. Weinstein SL. Improving the prognosis in Legg-Calvé-Perthes' disease. *J Musculoskeletal Med* 1984;11:22.

216. Moberg A. *Legg-Calvé-Perthes' disease: an epidemiologic, clinical and radiological study.* Uppsala: Uppsala University, 1996.

217. Ismail A, Macnicol JF. Prognosis in Perthes' disease. *J Bone Joint Surg Br* 1998;80:310.

218. Yrjonen T. Long term prognosis in Legg-Calvé-Perthes disease: a meta analysis. *J Pediatr Orthop B* 1999;8:169.

219. Sponseller PD, Desai SS, Millis MB. Abnormalities of proximal femoral disease. *J Bone Joint Surg Br* 1989;71:610.

220. Moller PF. The clinical observations after healing of Calvé-Perthes' disease compared with final deformities left by that disease and the bearing of those final deformities on ultimate prognosis. *Acta Radiol* 1926;5:1.

221. Neyt J, Weinstein SL, Spratt K, et al. Stulberg classification system for evaluation of Legg-Calvé-Perthes' disease: intrarater and interrater reliability. *J Bone Joint Surg Am* 1999;81:1209.

222. O'Garra JA. The radiographic changes in Perthes' disease. *J Bone Joint Surg Br* 1959;41:465.

223. Ponseti IV, Cotton RL. Legg-Calvé-Perthes' disease: pathogenesis and evaluation. *J Bone Joint Surg Am* 1961;43:261.

224. Lloyd-Roberts GC, Catterall A, Salamon PB. A controlled study of the indications for the results of femoral osteotomy in Perthes' disease. *J Bone Joint Surg Br* 1976;58:31.

225. Agus H, Kalenderer O, Eryanilmaz G, et al. Intraobserver and interobserver reliability of Catterall, Herring, Salter-Thompson and Stulberg classification systems in Perthes disease. *J Pediatr Orthop B* 2004;13(3):166–169.

226. Gigante C, Frizziero P, Turra S. Prognostic value of Catterall and Herring classification in Legg-Calve-Perthes disease: follow-up to skeletal maturity of 32 patients. *J Pediatr Orthop* 2002;22(3):345–349.

227. Hardcastle PH, Ross R, Hamalainen M, et al. Catterall grouping of Perthes' disease: an assessment of observer error and prognosis using the Catterall classification. *J Bone Joint Surg Br* 1980;62:428.

228. Kelly FP, Canale ST, Jones RR. Legg-Calvé-Perthes' disease: long-term evaluation of noncontainment treatment. *J Bone Joint Surg Am* 1980;62:400.

229. Van Dam BE, Crider RJ, Noyes JD, et al. Determination of the Catterall classification in Legg-Calvé-Perthes' disease. *J Bone Joint Surg Am* 1981;63:906.

230. Martinez AG, Weinstein SL, Dietz FR. The weight-bearing abduction brace for the treatment of Legg-Perthes' disease. *J Bone Joint Surg Am* 1992;74:12.

231. Klisic P, Seferovic O, Blazevic U. Perthes' syndrome, classification and indications for treatment. *Orthop Rev* 1979;8:81.

232. Klisic P, Blazevic U, Seferovic O. Approach to treatment of Legg-Perthes' disease. *Clin Orthop* 1980;150:54.
233. Farsetti P, Tudisco C, Caterini R, et al. The Herring lateral pillar classification for prognosis in Perthes' disease: late results in 49 patients treated conservatively. *J Bone Joint Surg Br* 1995;77:739.
234. Ritterbusch JF, Shantharam SS, Gelinas C. Comparison of lateral pillar classification and Catterall classification of Legg-Calvé-Perthes' disease. *J Pediatr Orthop* 1993;13:200.
235. Lappin K, Kealey D, Cosgrove A. Herring classification: how useful is the initial radiograph? *J Pediatr Orthop* 2002;22(4):479–482.
236. Catterall A. Coxa plana. In: Apley AP, ed. *Modern trends in orthopaedics*. London: Butterworths, 1972.
237. Catterall A. Adolescent hip pain after Perthes' disease. *Clin Orthop* 1986;209:65.
238. Muirhead-Allwood W, Catterall A. The treatment of Perthes' disease: the results of a trial of management. *J Bone Joint Surg Br* 1982;64:282.
239. Aguirre M, Pellise F, Castellote A. Metaphyseal cysts in Legg-Calvé-Perthes' disease [Letter]. *J Pediatr Orthop* 1992;12:404.
240. Carroll NC, Donaldson J. Metaphyseal cysts in Legg-Calvé-Perthes' disease [Letter]. *J Pediatr Orthop* 1992;12:405.
241. Gershuni DH. Subluxation of the femoral head in coxa plana [Letter]. *J Bone Joint Surg Am* 1988;70:950.
242. Christensen FKS, Ejsted R, Luxiji T. The Catterall classification of Perthes: an assessment of reliability. *J Bone Joint Surg Br* 1978;60:166.
243. Clarke TE, Finnegan TL, Fisher RL, et al. Legg-Perthes' disease in children less than four years old. *J Bone Joint Surg Am* 1978;60:166.
244. Dickens DRV, Menelaus MB. The assessment of the prognosis of Perthes' disease. *J Bone Joint Surg Br* 1978;60:189.
245. Green NE, Beauchamp RD, Griffen PP. Epiphyseal extrusion as a prognostic index in Legg-Calvé-Perthes' disease. *J Bone Joint Surg Am* 1981;63:900.
246. Kamhi E, MacEwen D. Treatment of Legg-Calvé-Perthes' disease. *J Bone Joint Surg Am* 1975;57:651.
247. Mintowt-Czyz WJ, Tayton KJ. The role of weight relief in Catterall group IV Perthes' disease. *J Bone Joint Surg Br* 1982;64:247.
248. Mintowt-Czyz WJ, Tayton KJ. Indication for weight relief and containment in the treatment of Perthes' disease. *Acta Orthop Scand* 1983;54:439.
249. Simmons ED, Graham HK, Szalai JP. Interobserver variability in grading Perthes' disease. *J Bone Joint Surg Br* 1990;72:202.
250. Loder R, Farley FA, Hennsinger RN. Physeal slope in Perthes' disease. *J Bone Joint Surg Br* 1995;77:736.
251. Herring JA. Legg-Calvé-Perthes' disease: a review of current knowledge. *Instr Course Lect* 1989;38:309.
252. Lloyd-Roberts GC. The management of Perthes' disease. *J Bone Joint Surg Br* 1982;64:1.
253. Lovell WW, MacEwen GD, Stewart WR, et al. Legg-Perthes' disease in girls. *J Bone Joint Surg Br* 1982;64:637.
254. Guille J, Lipton GE, Szoke G, et al. Legg Calvé Perthes disease in girls: a comparison of the results with those seen in boys. *J Bone Joint Surg Am* 1998;80:1256.
255. Fabry K, Fabry G, Moens P. Legg-Calve-Perthes disease in patients under 5 years of age does not always result in a good outcome. Personal experience and meta-analysis of the literature. *J Pediatr Orthop B* 2003;12(3):222–227.
256. Joseph B, Mulpuri K, Varghese G. Perthes' disease in the adolescent. *J Bone Joint Surg Br* 2001;83(5):715–720.
257. Grasemann H, Nicolai RD, Patsalis T, et al. The treatment of Legg-Calvé-Perthes disease: to contain or not to contain. *Arch Orthop Trauma Surg* 1997;116:50.
258. Yasuda T, Tamura K. Prognostication of proximal femoral growth disturbance after Perthes' disease. *Clin Orthop Relat Res* 1996;329:244.
259. Cooperman DR, Stulberg SD. Ambulatory containment treatment in Legg-Calvé-Perthes' disease. In: Fitzgerald RH Jr, ed. *The hip: Proceedings of the Thirteenth Open Scientific Meeting of the Hip Society*. St. Louis, MO: Mosby, 1985:38.
260. Bellyei A, Mike G. Acetabular development in Legg-Calvé-Perthes' disease. *Orthopedics* 1988;11:407.
261. Kamegaya M, Shinada Y, Moriya H, et al. Acetabular remodelling in Perthes' disease after primary healing. *J Pediatr Orthop* 1992;12:308.
262. Weinstein SL, Ponseti IV. Congenital dislocation of the hip: open reduction through a medial approach. *J Bone Joint Surg Am* 1979;61:119.
263. Mazda K, Pennecot GF, Zeller R, et al. Perthes' after the age of twelve years: role of the remaining growth. *J Bone Joint Surg Br* 1999;81:696.
264. Clarke NMP, Harrison MHM. Painful sequelae of coxa plana. *J Bone Joint Surg Am* 1983;65:13.
265. Goff CW. *Legg-Calvé-Perthes' syndrome and related osteochondroses of youth*. Springfield, IL: Charles C Thomas Publisher, 1954.
266. Joseph B, Chacko V, Rao BS, et al. The epidemiology of Perthes' disease in south India. *Int J Epidemiol* 1988;173:603.
267. Joseph B. Morphological changes in the acetabulum in Perthes' disease. *J Bone Joint Surg Br* 1989;71:756.
268. Kahle WK, Coleman SS. The value of the acetabular teardrop figure in assessing pediatric hip disorders. *J Pediatr Orthop* 1992;12:586.
269. Katz JF. Protein-bound iodine in Legg-Calvé-Perthes' disease. *J Bone Joint Surg Am* 1955;37:842.
270. Curtis BH, Gunther SF, Gossling HR, et al. Treatment for Legg-Perthes' disease with the Newington ambulation-abduction brace. *J Bone Joint Surg Am* 1974;56:1135.
271. Comte F, De Rosa V, Zekri H, et al. Confirmation of the early prognostic value of bone scanning and pinhole imaging of the hip in Legg-Calvé-Perthes disease. *J Nucl Med* 2003;44(11):1761–1766.
272. King EW, Fisher RL, Gage JR, et al. Ambulation-abduction treatment in Legg-Calvé-Perthes' disease (LCPD). *Clin Orthop* 1980;150:43.
273. Petrie JG, Bitenc I. The abduction weightbearing treatment in Legg-Perthes' disease. *J Bone Joint Surg Br* 1971;53:54.
274. Purvis JM, Dimon JH III, Meehan PL, et al. Preliminary experience with the Scottish Rite Hospital abduction orthosis for Legg-Perthes' disease. *Clin Orthop* 1980;150:49.
275. Thompson G, Westin GW. Legg-Calvé-Perthes' disease: results of discontinuing treatment in the early reossification stage. *Clin Orthop* 1979;139:70.

## Clinical Presentation

276. Bunnell WP. Legg-Calvé-Perthes' disease. *Pediatr Rev* 1986;7:299.

## Imaging

277. Lee DY, Choi IH, Lee CK, et al. Assessment of complex hip deformity using three-dimensional CT image. *J Pediatr Orthop* 1991;11:13.
278. Naumann T, Kollmannsberger A, Fischer M, et al. Ultrasonographic evaluation of Legg-Calvé-Perthes' disease based on sonoanatomic criteria and the application of new measuring techniques. *Eur J Radiol* 1992;15:101.
279. Wirth T, LeQuesne GW, Paterson DC. Ultrasonography in Legg-Calvé-Perthes' disease. *Pediatr Radiol* 1992;22:498.
280. Calvér R, Venugopal V, Dorgan J, et al. Radionuclide scanning in the early diagnosis of Perthes' disease. *J Bone Joint Surg Br* 1981;63:379.
281. Danigelis JA, Fisher RL, Ozonoff MB, et al. 99m Tc-polyphosphate bone imaging in Legg-Perthes' disease. *Radiology* 1975;115:407.
282. Danigelis JA. Pinhole imaging in Legg-Perthes' disease: further observations. *Semin Nucl Med* 1976;6:69.
283. Deutsch SD, Gandsman E, Spraragen SC. Quantitative radioscintigraphy in the evaluation of hip pain in children. *Trans Orthop Res Soc* 1979;4:187.
284. Fisher RL, Roderique JW, Brown DC, et al. The relationship of isotopic bone imaging findings to prognosis in Legg-Perthes' disease. *Clin Orthop* 1980;150:23.
285. Kohler R, Seringe R, Borgi R. *Osteochondrite de la hanche*. Paris: Expansion Scientific Francais, 1981.
286. Suramo I, Puranen J, Heikkinen E, et al. Disturbed patterns of venous drainage of the femoral neck in Perthes' disease. *J Bone Joint Surg Br* 1974;56:448.
287. Kanildides C. Diagnostic radiology in Legg-Calvé-Perthes disease. *Acta Radiol Suppl* 1996;406:1.
288. Kaniklides C, Sahlstedt B, Lonnerholm T, et al. Conventional radiography and bone scintigraphy in the prognostic evaluation of Legg Calvé Perthes disease. *Acta Radiol* 1996;37:561.

289. Kaniklides C, Lonnerholm T, Moberg A, et al. Legg-Calvé-Perthes' disease: comparison of conventional radiography, MR imaging, bone scintigraphy and arthrography. *Acta Radiol* 1995;36:434.

290. Hosokawa M, Wook-Cheol K, Kubo T. Preliminary report on usefulness of magnetic resonance imaging for outcome prediction in early stage Legg Calvé Perthes disease. *J Pediatr Orthop B* 1999;8:161.

291. Jaramillo D, Kasser JR, Villegas-Medina OL, et al. Cartilaginous and growth disturbances in Legg-Calvé-Perthes disease: evaluation with MR imaging. *Radiology* 1995;197:767.

292. Uno A, Hattori T, Noritake K, et al. Legg-Calvé-Perthes disease in the evolutionary period: comparison of magnetic resonance imaging with bone scintigraphy. *J Pediatr Orthop* 1995;15:362.

293. Landes-Vasama T, Lamminen A, Merikanto J, et al. The value of MRI in early Perthes' disease: an MRI study with a 2 year follow-up. *Pediatr Radiol* 1997;27:517.

294. Roberts JM, Zink WP. Arthrographic classification of Legg-Perthes' disease. Presented at the Annual Meeting of the American Academy of Orthopaedic Surgeons, Las Vegas, NV, 1981.

## Differential Diagnosis

295. Bickerstaff D, Neill L, Booth A, et al. Ultrasound examination of the irritable hip. *J Bone Joint Surg Br* 1990;7:549.

296. Futami T, Kasahara Y, Suzuki S, et al. Ultrasonography in transient synovitis and early Perthes' disease. *J Bone Joint Surg Br* 1991;73:635.

297. Lucht U, Bunger C, Krebs B, et al. Blood flow in the juvenile hip in relation to changes of the intraarticular pressure: an experimental investigation in dogs. *Acta Orthop Scand* 1983;54:182.

298. Guille JT, Lipton GE, Tsirikos AI, et al. Bilateral Legg-Calve-Perthes disease: presentation and outcome. *J Pediatr Orthop* 2002;22(4):458–463.

299. Andersen PE Jr, Schantz K, Bollerslev J, et al. Bilateral femoral head dysplasia and osteochondritis: multiple epiphyseal dysplasia tarda, spondyloepiphyseal dysplasia tarda, and bilateral Legg-Perthes' disease. *Acta Radiol* 1988;29:705.

300. Ikegawa S, Nagano A, Nakamura K. A case of multiple epiphyseal dysplasia complicated by unilateral Perthes' disease. *Acta Orthop Scand* 1991;62:606.

301. Iwasaki K. The role of blood vessels within the ligamentum teres in Perthes' disease. *Clin Orthop* 1981;159:248.

## Treatment

302. Allen B. Graphic analysis of femoral growth in young children with Perthes' disease. *J Pediatr Orthop* 1997;17:255.

303. Blakemore ME, Harrison MHM. A prospective study of children with untreated Catterall group I Perthes' disease. *J Bone Joint Surg Br* 1979;61:329.

304. Daly K, Bruce C, Catterall A. Lateral shelf acetabuloplasty in Perthes' disease. *J Bone Joint Surg Br* 1999;81:380.

305. Danforth MS. The treatment of Legg-Calvé-Perthes' disease without weightbearing. *J Bone Joint Surg Br* 1934;16:516.

306. Eyre-Brook Al. Osteochondritis deformans coxae juvenilis, or Perthes' disease: the results of treatment by traction in recumbency. *Br J Surg* 1936;24:166.

307. Howarth B. Coxa plana. *Arch Pediatr* 1959;76:1.

308. Barranco SD, Traver RC, Friedman FM, et al. A comparative study of Legg-Perthes' disease. *Clin Orthop* 1973;96:304.

309. Eaton GO. Long-term results of treatment in coxa plana: a follow-up study of eighty-eight patients. *J Bone Joint Surg Am* 1967;49:1031.

310. Evans DL. Legg-Calvé-Perthes' disease: a study of late results. *J Bone Joint Surg Br* 1958;40:168.

311. Evans DL, Lloyd-Roberts GC. Treatment in Legg-Calvé-Perthes' disease. *J Bone Joint Surg Br* 1958;40:182.

312. Harrison MHM, Menon MPA. Legg-Calvé-Perthes' disease: the value of x-ray measurement in clinical practice with special reference to the broomstick plaster method. *J Bone Joint Surg Am* 1966;48:1301.

313. Heyman CH, Herndon CH. Legg-Perthes' disease: method for measurement of roentgenographic results. *J Bone Joint Surg Am* 1950;32:767.

314. Remvig Q, Mose K. Perthes' disease. *J Bone Joint Sung Br* 1961;43:855.

315. Siffert RS. Osteochondritis of the proximal femoral epiphysis. *Instr Course Lect* 1973;22:270.

316. Legg AT. The end results of coxa plana. *J Bone Joint Surg Br* 1927;25:26.

317. Bellyei A, Mike G. Weight bearing in Perthes' disease. *Orthopedics* 1991;14:19.

318. Mindell ER, Sherman MS. Late results in Legg-Perthes' disease. *J Bone Joint Surg Am* 1951;33:1.

319. Snyder CF. A sling for use in Legg-Perthes' disease. *J Bone Joint Surg Br* 1947;29:524.

320. Harrison MHM, Turner MH, Nicholson FJ. Coxa plana: results of a new form of splinting. *J Bone Joint Surg Am* 1969;51:1057.

321. Pauwels F. Des affections de la hanche d'origine mecanique et de lair traitement par l'osteotomie d'adduction. *Rev Chir Orthop* 1951;37:22.

322. Salter RB. Experimental and clinical aspects of Perthes' disease. *J Bone Joint Surg Br* 1966;48:393.

323. Brotherton BJ, McKibbin B. Perthes' disease treated by prolonged recumbency and femoral head containment: a long-term appraisal. *J Bone Joint Surg Br* 1977;59:8.

324. Denton J. Experience with Legg-Calvé-Perthes' disease (LCPD), 1968-1974, at the New York Orthopaedic Hospital. *Clin Orthop* 1980;150:36.

325. Katz JF. Conservative treatment of Legg-Calvé-Perthes' disease. *J Bone Joint Surg Am* 1967;49:1043.

326. Katz JF. Nonoperative therapy in Legg-Calvé-Perthes' disease. *Orthop Rev* 1979;8:69.

327. Rab GT, DeNatale JS, Herrmann LR. Three dimensional finite element analysis of Legg-Calvé-Perthes' disease. *J Pediatr Orthop* 1982;2:39.

328. Rab GT. Determination of femoral head containment during gait. *Biomater Med Devices Artif Organs* 1983;11:31.

329. Bombelli R. *Osteoarthritis of the hip.* Berlin: Springer-Verlag, 1983.

330. Grzegorzewski A, Bowen JR, Guille JT, et al. Treatment of the collapsed femoral head by containment in Legg-Calve-Perthes disease. *J Pediatr Orthop* 2003;23(1):15–19.

331. Rails Z, McKibbin B. Changes in shape of the human hip joint during its development and their relation to its stability. *J Bone Joint Surg Br* 1973;55:780.

332. Ekholm R. Nutrition of articular cartilage. *Acta Anat* 1955;24:329.

333. Maroudas A, Bullough P, Swanson SAV, et al. The permeability of articular cartilage. *J Bone Joint Surg Br* 1968;50:166.

334. Catterall A. The place of femoral osteotomy in the management of Legg-Calvé-Perthes' disease. In: Fitzgerald RH Jr, ed. *The hip: Proceedings of the Thirteenth Open Scientific Meeting of The Hip Society.* St. Louis, MO: Mosby, 1985:28.

335. Gershuni DH, Axer A, Handel D. Arthrography as an aid to the diagnosis and therapy in Legg-Calvé-Perthes' disease. *Acta Orthop Scand* 1980;51:505.

336. Richards BS, Coleman SS. Subluxation of the femoral head in coxa plana. *J Bone Joint Surg Am* 1987;69:1312.

337. Salter RB. The present status of surgical treatment of Legg-Perthes' disease: current concept review. *J Bone Joint Surg Am* 1984;66:961.

338. Roberts JM, Meehan P, Counts G, et al. Ambulatory abduction brace for Legg-Perthes' disease. Presented at the Annual Meeting of the American Academy of Orthopaedic Surgeons, Dallas, TX, 1974.

339. Donovan MM, Urquhart BA. Treatment with ambulatory abduction brace. *Orthop Rev* 1979;8:147.

340. Bobechko WP. The Toronto brace for Legg-Perthes' disease. *Clin Orthop* 1974;102:115.

341. Fackler CD. Nonsurgical treatment of Legg-Calvé-Perthes' disease. *Instr Course Lect* 1989;38:305.

342. Lovell WW, Hopper WC, Purvis JM. The Scottish rite orthosis for Legg-Perthes' disease. Presented at the Annual Meeting of the American Academy of Orthopaedic Surgeons, Dallas, TX, 1978.

343. Price CT, Day DD, Flynn JC. Behavioral sequelae of bracing versus surgery for Legg-Calvé-Perthes' disease. *J Pediatr Orthop* 1988;8:285.

344. MacEwen GD. Conservative treatment of Legg-Calvé-Perthes condition. In: Fitzgerald RH Jr, ed. *The hip: Proceedings of the Thirteenth Open Scientific Meeting of the Hip Society.* St. Louis, MO: Mosby, 1985:17.

345. Meehan PL, Angel D, Nelson JM. The Scottish Rite abduction orthosis for the treatment of Legg-Perthes' disease: a radiographic analysis. *J Bone Joint Surg Am* 1992;74:2.

346. Wang L, Bowen JR, Puniak MA, et al. An evaluation of various methods of treatment for Perthes' disease. *Clin Orthop Relat Res* 1995;314:225.

347. Axer A, Gershuni DH, Hendel D, et al. Indications for femoral osteotomy in Legg-Calvé-Perthes' disease. *Clin Orthop* 1980; 150:78.

348. Heikkinen E, Puranen J. Evaluation of femoral osteotomy in the treatment of Legg-Calvé-Perthes' disease. *Clin Orthop* 1980; 150:60.

349. Hoikka V, Poussa M, Yrjonen T, et al. Intertrochanteric varus osteotomy for Perthes' disease: radiographic changes after 2–16 year follow-up of 126 hips. *Acta Orthop Scand* 1991;62:549.

350. Lee DY, Seong SC, Choi IH, et al. Changes of blood flow of the femoral head after subtrochanteric osteotomy in Legg-Perthes' disease: a serial scintigraphic study. *J Pediatr Orthop* 1992;12:731.

351. Green NE, Griffen PP. Intra osseous venous hypertension in Legg-Perthes' disease. *J Bone Joint Surg Am* 1982;64:666.

352. Clancy M, Steel HH. The effect of an incomplete intertrochanteric osteotomy on Legg-Calvé-Perthes' disease. *J Bone Joint Surg Am* 1985;67:213.

353. Kendig RJ, Evans GA. Biologic osteotomy in Perthes' disease. *J Pediatr Orthop* 1986;6:278.

354. Marklund T, Tillberg G. Coxa plana: a radiological comparison of the rate of healing with conservative measures and after osteotomy. *J Bone Joint Surg Br* 1976;58:25.

355. Coleman SS. Observations on proximal femoral osteotomy and pelvic osteotomy. *Orthop Rev* 1979;8:139.

356. Mirovski Y, Axer A, Hendel D. Residual shortening after osteotomy for Perthes' disease. *J Bone Joint Surg Br* 1984;66:184.

357. Somerville EW. Osteotomy in treatment of Perthes' disease of the hip. *Orthop Rev* 1979;8:61.

358. Canario AT, Williams L, Weintraub S, et al. A controlled study of the results of femoral osteotomy in severe Perthes' disease. *J Bone Joint Surg Br* 1980;62:348.

359. Evans IK, Deluca PA, Gage JR. A comparative study of ambulation-abduction bracing and varus derotation osteotomy in the treatment of severe Legg-Calvé-Perthes' disease in children over 6 years of age. *J Pediatr Orthop* 1988;8:676.

360. Sponseller PD, Desai SS, Millis MB. Comparison of femoral and innominate osteotomies for the treatment of Legg-Calvé-Perthes' disease. *J Bone Joint Surg Am* 1988;70:1131.

361. Weiner SD, Weiner DS, Riley PM. Pitfalls in treatment of Legg-Calvé-Perthes' disease using proximal femoral varus osteotomy. *J Pediatr Orthop* 1991;11:20.

362. Noonan KJ, Price CT, Kupiszewski SJ, et al. Results of femoral varus osteotomy in children older than 9 years of age with Perthes disease. *J Pediatr Orthop* 2001;21(2):198–204.

363. Pecasse GA, Eijer H, Haverkamp D, et al. Intertrochanteric osteotomy in young adults for sequelae of Legg-Calvé-Perthes' disease—a long term follow-up. *Int Orthop* 2004;28(1):44–47.

364. Schmid OA, Hemmer S, Wunsche P, et al. The adult hip after femoral varus osteotomy in patients with unilateral Legg-Calvé-Perthes disease. *J Pediatr Orthop B* 2003;12(1):33–37.

365. Than P, Halmai V, Shaikh S, et al. Long-term results of derotational femoral varus osteotomy in Legg-Calvé-Perthes disease: 26-year follow-up. *Orthopedics* 2003;26(5):487–491.

366. Raney EM, Grogan DP, Hurley ME, et al. The role of proximal femoral valgus osteotomy in Legg-Calvé-Perthes disease. *Orthopedics* 2002;25(5):513–517.

367. Bankes MJ, Catterall A, Hashemi-Nejad A. Valgus extension osteotomy for 'hinge abduction' in Perthes' disease. Results at maturity and factors influencing the radiological outcome. *J Bone Joint Surg Br* 2000;82(4):548–554.

368. Coates CJ, Paterson JM, Woods KR, et al. Femoral osteotomy in Perthes' disease: results at maturity. *J Bone Joint Surg Br* 1990; 72:581.

369. Cordeiro EN. Femoral osteotomy in Legg-Calvé-Perthes disease. *Clin Orthop* 1980;150:69.

370. Landes-Vasama T, Marttinen EJ, Merikanto JE. Outcome of Perthes disease in unselected patients after femoral varus osteotomy and splintage. *J Pediatr Orthop B* 1997;6:229.

371. Hansson G, Wallin J. External rotational positioning of the leg after intertrochanteric combined varus derotational osteotomy in Perthes' disease. *Arch Orthop Traumatol Surg* 1997;116:108.

372. Joseph B, Srinivas G, Thomas R. Management of Perthes disease of late onset in southern India: the evaluation of a surgical method. *J Bone Joint Surg Br* 1996;78:625.

373. Yoon TR, Rowe SM, Chung JY, et al. A new innominate osteotomy in Perthes' disease. *J Pediatr Orthop* 2003;23(3):363–367.

374. Canale ST, D'Anca AF, Cotler JM, et al. Innominate osteotomy in Legg-Calvé-Perthes' disease. *J Bone Joint Surg Am* 1972;54:25.

375. Dekker M, VanRens TJG, Sloff TJJH. Salter's pelvic osteotomy in the treatment of Perthes' disease. *J Bone Joint Surg Br* 1981;68:282.

376. Salter RB. Perthes' disease: treatment by innominate osteotomy. *Instr Course Lect* 1973;22:309.

377. Salter RB. The scientific basis for innominate osteotomy for Legg-Calvé-Perthes' disease and the results in children with a bad prognosis. *Orthop Trans* 1985;9:203.

378. Coleman S, Kehl D. An evaluation of Perthes' disease: comparison of nonsurgical and surgical means. Presented at the Annual Meeting of the American Academy of Orthopaedic Surgeons, Las Vegas, NV, 1981.

379. Ingman AM, Paterson DC, Sutherland AD. A comparison between innominate osteotomy and hip spica in the treatment of Legg-Perthes' disease. *Clin Orthop* 1982;163:141.

380. Paterson DC, Leitch JM, Foster BK. Results of innominate osteotomy in the treatment of Legg-Calvé-Perthes' disease. *Clin Orthop* 1991;266:96.

381. Robinson HJ Jr, Putter H, Sigmond MB, et al. Innominate osteotomy in Perthes' disease. *J Pediatr Orthop* 1988;8:426.

382. Stevens P, Williams P, Menelaus M. Innominate osteotomy for Perthes' disease. *J Pediatr Orthop* 1981;1:47.

383. Moberg A, Hansson G, Kaniklides C. Results after femoral and innominate osteotomy in Legg-Calvé-Perthes' disease. *Clin Orthop Relat Res* 1997;334:257.

384. Ghaida HI, Hull ML, Rab GT. An instrumented brace for study of Legg-Calvé-Perthes' disease. *Biomater Med Devices Artif Organs* 1987;15:719.

385. Rab GT. Containment of the hip: a theoretical comparison of osteotomies. *Clin Orthop* 1981;154:191.

386. Craig WA, Kramer WG. Combined iliac and femoral osteotomies in Legg-Calvé-Perthes syndrome. *J Bone Joint Surg Am* 1974; 56:1314.

387. Crutcher JP, Staheli LT. Combined osteotomy as a salvage procedure for severe Legg-Calvé-Perthes' disease. *J Pediatr Orthop* 1992;12:151.

388. Olney BW, Asher MA. Combined innominate and femoral osteotomy for the treatment of severe Legg-Calvé-Perthes' disease. *J Pediatr Orthop* 1985;5:645.

389. Kim H, Wenger DR. Surgical correction of "functional retroversion" and "functional coxa vara" in Legg-Calvé-Perthes disease and epiphyseal dysplasia: correction of deformity defined by new imaging modalities. *J Pediatr Orthop* 1997;17:247.

390. Kim H, Wenger DR. "Functional retroversion" of the femoral head in Legg-Calvé-Perthes disease and epiphyseal dysplasia: analysis of head-neck deformity and its effect on limb position using three-dimensional computed tomography. *J Pediatr Orthop* 1997;17:240.

391. Willett K, Hudson I, Catterall A. Lateral shelf acetabuloplasty: an operation for older children with Perthes' disease. *J Pediatr Orthop* 1992;12:563.

392. Dimitriou JK, Leonidou O, Pettas N. Acetabulum augmentation for Legg-Calvé-Perthes disease: 12 children (14 hips) followed for 4 years. *Acta Orthop Scand Suppl* 1997;275:103.

393. Kumar D, Bache CE, O'Hara JN. Interlocking triple pelvic osteotomy in severe Legg-Calve-Perthes disease. *J Pediatr Orthop* 2002;22(4):464–470.

394. O'Connor PA, Mullhall KJ, Kearns SR, et al. Triple pelvic osteotomy in Legg-Calve-Perthes disease using a single antero-lateral incision. *J Pediatr Orthop B* 2003;12(6):387–389.

395. Maxwell SL, Lappin KJ, Kealey WD, et al. Arthrodiastasis in Perthes' disease. Preliminary results. *J Bone Joint Surg Br* 2004; 86(2):244–250.

396. Segev E, Ezra E, Wientroub S, et al. Treatment of severe late onset Perthes' disease with soft tissue release and articulated hip distraction: early results. *J Pediatr Orthop B* 2004;13(3):158–165.

397. Mose K, Hjorth J, Ulfeldt M, et al. Legg-Calvé-Perthes' disease: the late occurrence of coxarthrosis. *Acta Orthop Scand Suppl* 1977;169:1.

398. Quain S, Catterall A. Hinge abduction of the hip: diagnosis and treatment. *J Bone Joint Surg Br* 1986;68:61.

399. McKay DW. Cheilectomy of the hip. *Orthop Clin North Am* 1980;11:141.

400. Schepers A, Von Bormann PFB, Craig JJG. Coxa magna in Perthes' disease: treatment by Chiari pelvic osteotomy. *J Bone Joint Surg Br* 1978;60:297.

401. Van der Hayden AM, Van Tongerloo RB. Shelf operations in Perthes' disease. *J Bone Joint Surg Br* 1981;63:282.

402. Bennett JT, Mazurek RT, Cash JD. Chiari's osteotomy in the treatment of Perthes' disease. *J Bone Joint Surg Br* 1991;73:225.

403. Cahuzac JP, Onimus M, Trottmann F, et al. Chiari pelvic osteotomy in Perthes' disease. *J Pediatr Orthop* 1990;10:163.

404. Handlesmann JE. The Chiari pelvic shelving osteotomy. *Orthop Clin North Am* 1980;11:105.

405. Schepers A. The Chiari osteotomy in Perthes' disease. *S Afr Bone Joint Surg* 1996;6:3.

406. Koyama K, Higuchi F, Inoue A. Modified Chiari osteotomy for arthrosis after Perthes' disease. *Acta Orthop Scand* 1998;69:129.

407. Kruse RW, Guille JT, Bowen JR. Shelf arthroplasty in patients who have Legg-Calvé-Perthes' disease: a study of long-term results. *J Bone Joint Surg Am* 1991;73:1338.

408. Muratli HH, Can M, Yagmurlu MF, et al. The results of acetabular shelf procedures in Legg-Calvé-Perthes disease. *Acta Orthop Traumatol Turc* 2003;37(2):138–143.

409. Garceau GJ. Surgical treatment of coxa plana. Presented at the Joint Meeting of the Orthopaedic Associations of the English Speaking World. *J Bone Joint Surg Br* 1964;46:779.

410. Rowe SM, Moon ES, Yoon TR, et al. Fate of the osteochondral fragments in osteochondritis dissecans after Legg-Calvé-Perthes' disease. *J Bone Joint Surg Br* 2002;84(7):1025–1029.

411. Macnicol MF, Makris D. Distal transfer of the greater trochanter. *J Bone Joint Surg Br* 1991;73:838.

412. Matan A, Stevens P, Smith JT, et al. Combination trochanteric arrest and intertrochanteric osteotomy for Perthes' disease. *J Pediatr Orthop* 1996;16:10.

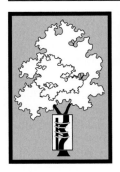

# 26

# Slipped Capital Femoral Epiphysis

*Robert M. Kay*

Slipped capital femoral epiphysis (SCFE) is defined as the displacement of the femoral head relative to the femoral neck and shaft. The term *slipped capital femoral epiphysis* is actually a misnomer. The femoral head is stabilized in the acetabulum, whereas the femoral neck and shaft move relative to the femoral head and acetabulum. In almost all cases of SCFE, the proximal femoral neck and shaft move anteriorly and rotate externally relative to the femoral head (1). If progression occurs to the point at which the femoral neck is completely anterior to the femoral head, then proximal migration of the femoral neck occurs as well.

## EPIDEMIOLOGY

The epidemiology of SCFE has been reported frequently in the last century. The male population with SCFE outnumbers the female population by 1.4 to 2.0 in most studies (2–11). The annual incidence is 2 to 13 per 100,000 and the cumulative risk is between 1 per 1000 and 1 per 2000 for the male population and is between 1 per 2000 and 1 per 3000 for the female population (8,12–14). Incidence of SCFE varies significantly among different populations, with higher incidences in those groups with higher mean body weights (15). Loder has noted more than a 40-fold difference in the incidence among differing races, with the highest rate being found in Polynesian children and the lowest rate being found in children from the Indo-Mediterranean region (15).

Most children with SCFE are peripubertal. Loder reported an average age of $12 \pm 1.5$ years for girls and $13.5 \pm 1.7$ years for boys in an international study carried out with more than 1600 patients (15). At the time of presentation, approximately 80% of the boys are reported to be between 12 and 15 years, and 80% of the girls between 10 and 13 years (8). Onset of SCFE is unusual for children of either sex less than 10 years old and for girls older than 14 and boys older than 16. Diagnosis of SCFE in such patients should raise the orthopaedist's suspicion that an underlying metabolic or systemic condition may have played a causative role.

The range of skeletal ages of children with SCFE has been reported to be significantly narrower than the range of their chronologic age (11,16,17). Most of the children with SCFE have open triradiate cartilage and are Risser 1 (18).

Obesity has been reported in 51% to 77% of patients with SCFE (6,15,19–21). Approximately 50% of the patients are at or above the 90th percentile for weight (22,23), and approximately 70% are above the 80th percentile (24). Obese children with slow maturation appear to be at especially high risk for SCFE (23).

Unilateral involvement is noted in 80% of children with SCFE at the time of presentation, with left hip involvement in most unilateral cases (12,13,15,25,26). In addition to the 20% who initially present with bilateral SCFE, 10% to 20% develop a symptomatic contralateral slip in adolescence (6,13,27–29). Long-term studies have reported radiographic evidence of a long-term bilateral involvement in as many as 80% of the patients (30), although most series report bilateral involvement at long-term follow-up in the 60% range in adulthood (13,28).

Some authors have noted significant seasonal variation in the incidence of SCFE at latitudes above 40 degrees, but not in lower latitudes (31–33). Others have not noted any seasonal variation (13). Such data appear to have little impact on the diagnosis and treatment of children with SCFE.

In summary, SCFE is most commonly seen in overweight, peripubertal children. Although any child presenting with hip, groin, thigh, or knee pain must be evaluated for possible hip pathology, the orthopaedist should be particularly suspicious of the possibility of SCFE in overweight, peripubertal children.

## ETIOLOGY

In most children with SCFE, the precise etiology is unknown. Regardless of the underlying etiology, the final common pathway appears to be a mechanical insufficiency of the proximal femoral physis to resist the load across it (34). SCFE may be thought of as occurring because of physiologic loads across an abnormally weak physis or abnormally high loads across a normal physis.

Conditions that weaken the physis include endocrine abnormalities, systemic diseases (such as renal osteodystrophy), and previous radiation therapy in the region of the proximal femur (35–40). Multiple mechanical factors have been postulated to account for abnormally high loads across the proximal femoral physis in children with SCFE, including obesity and anatomic variations in the proximal femoral and acetabular morphology.

### Endocrine Factors

The endocrinologic basis of SCFE has been studied both *in vivo* and *in vitro*. For more than 50 years, laboratory studies have demonstrated that estrogen strengthens and testosterone weakens the physis (41–43). These effects appear to be secondary to the impact that these hormones have on physeal width since mechanical strength of the physis varies inversely with physeal width (41,43,44).

Endocrinopathies appear to account for 5% to 8% of the SCFE cases, and SCFE has been estimated to be six times more common in patients who have an endocrinopathy than in those who do not (35–40,45–52). Although one recent study showed frequent endocrine abnormalities, most investigators have been unable to demonstrate consistent abnormalities in most children with SCFE (22,24,53,54).

The most common endocrinopathies in children with SCFE are hypothyroidism, panhypopituitarism, growth hormone (GH) abnormalities, and hypogonadism (35–40, 45–52). Other endocrine causes of SCFE include hyperparathyroidism or hypoparathyroidism (35,38,55). The increased prevalence of hypothyroidism in children with Down syndrome is a likely explanation for the increased risk of SCFE in these children (56–58).

The relative risk of SCFE is increased in children with GH deficiency, both prior to and during GH treatment (59–61). Other children with short stature and normal GH levels do not appear to share the same increased risk of SCFE (59,60). The initial diagnosis of hypothyroidism is often made after the diagnosis of SCFE; in most children with SCFE and GH deficiency, the endocrine abnormality is known prior to the diagnosis of SCFE (35).

SCFE has been noted to be most common in children around the time of puberty. It may be that the abnormalities in the complex interplay of hormones at puberty puts their hips at risk for SCFE (24,62). Laboratory studies in rats have also shown a decreased physeal strength at puberty (63).

Because the rate of endocrinopathy in children with SCFE is relatively low, previous authors have recommended against the routine screening of patients with SCFE without clinical evidence of an endocrinopathy (53). Burrow et al. reported that a person's height below the 10th percentile was the only useful screening characteristic for endocrine abnormalities; the sensitivity and the negative predictive value of using height below the 10th percentile as a cutoff were each reported to be at least 90% (46).

On the basis of the aforementioned data, routine screening of all patients with SCFE for any potential endocrine disease is not warranted. For children with suspected endocrine disease (including those who are younger than 10 years or older than 15 years and those who are of short stature), thyroid function tests should be carried out. GH levels should be checked for children of short stature. It is important to remember that most children with SCFE and thyroid dysfunction have no known history of any thyroid dysfunction at the time of presentation with SCFE. Among other children with both endocrinopathies and SCFE, the underlying endocrine disorder is often known prior to the diagnosis of SCFE.

## Other Systemic Diseases

Previous radiation therapy to the region of the femoral head also increases the risk of SCFE (64,65). The absolute risk of SCFE in patients with previous radiation therapy is unknown, although a risk as high as 10% has been cited (64). Unlike the typical patient with SCFE, children with SCFE following previous radiation therapy have been reported to have a median weight at the 10th percentile (65).

Renal osteodystrophy is associated with a sixfold to eightfold increased risk of SCFE (60). The incidence of SCFE has been reported as 0.03 to 0.64 per 1000 person-years among patients with end-stage renal disease receiving GH, with the highest rates in those patients who were on dialysis and receiving GH (66). Patients with renal osteodystrophy and SCFE are noted to be small in both weight and height (67).

The increased rate of SCFE associated with renal osteodystrophy is due to secondary hyperparathyroidism in these children, and medical management of the secondary hyperparathyroidism is of primary importance (67). If the hyperparathyroidism is controlled, slip progression will become rare, and surgical stabilization may not be necessary (67). Unlike the situation in other causes of SCFE, the displacement in patients with renal osteodystrophy is often through the metaphysis (35% of reported SCFE in one series), and other epiphyses have also been known to displace (67–69). Bilateral involvement has been reported in 82% to 95% of the patients with SCFE and renal osteodystrophy in large series studies (67,69). That many of these so-called SCFE cases do not occur through the physis may partly be the reason for the poorer results in the treatment of SCFE in children with renal osteodystrophy.

## Immunology

Elevated levels of serum immunoglobulins and the C3 component of complement have previously been reported in patients with SCFE (70). In patients with chondrolysis, serum immunoglobulin M (IgM) level was elevated as well (70). More recent studies have failed to show such abnormalities in serum levels, although synovial fluid abnormalities were noted in patients with SCFE (71,72). One study reported that plasma cells were a significant component of the synovitis in SCFE (71). In the same study, two of three patients with IgG and C3 present on synovial immunofluorescence developed chondrolysis (71). A later study revealed the presence of immune complexes in the synovial fluid in 10 of the 11 hips with SCFE (91%), but not in 2 of the 21 joints without SCFE (10%) (71,72). The role of these immune complexes in SCFE has not been defined.

## Genetics

A genetic basis for SCFE has not been definitively established. Among the patients with SCFE, a second member of their family has been reported to be affected in 3% to 7% of the cases in most series of studies carried out (11,21, 29,73–80). SCFE has been reported in identical twins (73,75,81), and has been found to have autosomal dominant inheritance with variable penetrance in familial cases (79,80). Whether this is due simply to a genetic predisposition for SCFE or due also to a tendency toward other risk features (such as obesity) remains unclear (79,82).

Some authors have reported an association of human leucocyte antigen (HLA) B12 with SCFE (73,75), whereas others have reported an association of HLA DR4 with SCFE (83). Other authors have noted that neither of these HLA phenotypes is a reliable marker of SCFE (84).

## Mechanical Factors

A variety of mechanical factors appear to play a role in the etiology of SCFE. Anatomic risk factors in the proximal femoral and acetabular morphology have been described. The high incidence of obesity in this patient population also suggests a mechanical role in the etiology of SCFE.

An association of SCFE with a decreased femoral anteversion has been reported, and this has been attributed to increased shear force across the proximal femoral physis in such patients (85,86). Anteversion values of the unaffected hips in the same patients were closer to normal (85).

Finally, reduced femoral anteversion has been noted in obese adolescents compared to adolescents of normal weight (87). This relative retroversion in obese adolescents may help explain the increased incidence of SCFE in this population group.

Decreased femoral neck–shaft angle in the hips of patients with SCFE compared to the hips of unaffected persons has also been reported (86). Such a decrease in the neck–shaft angle results in a more vertical physis, which may increase the shear force across the physis. Proximal femoral physeal inclination has previously been shown to change significantly between the ages of 9 and 12 years in humans, which is a potential contributing factor for SCFE (88). In the laboratory, the shear strength has also been shown to vary with physeal inclination (44).

Children with deeper acetabuli appear to be at greater risk for SCFE (89). The supposition is that with the capital femoral epiphysis anchored more deeply in the acetabulum, forces across the physis may be exaggerated, especially at the extremes of the range of motion. Variability in acetabular depth has been suggested as a potential cause for differences in the incidence of SCFE among different races. A recent study of acetabular morphology in patients with trauma calls this finding into question (90). It is possible that this study did not find such a correlation either because of limited sample size and/or because SCFE may simply be occurring in a small subset of the population who are outliers regarding such measures as acetabular depth.

Kordelle et al. have not found any difference in acetabular morphology in the affected and unaffected hips of children with SCFE (91). The lack of such acetabular differences is likely because SCFE generally occurs at an age at which little potential remains for acetabular remodeling, and this may help explain the high incidence of bilateral SCFE. Such bilateral acetabular symmetry in those with unilateral SCFE suggests that even if increased acetabular depth is a risk factor, there must be other etiologic factors involved as well.

Chung et al. reported that the mechanical forces across the femoral head during gait can be 6.5 times body weight and that such forces may be enough to cause a SCFE in an obese patient with a normal physis (92). Other authors have confirmed that mechanical forces across the hip during normal activities such as running are great enough to potentially cause SCFE (93).

In summary, the etiology of SCFE appears to be complex and is likely to be multifactorial. Endocrinopathies, other systemic diseases and local abnormalities (such as those caused by previous radiation exposure) have been noted to result in an increased risk of SCFE. Studies carried out on humans and animals indicate that such an increased risk of SCFE appears related to the impact that these maladies have on the strength of the growth plate. The association of hypothyroidism in children with Down syndrome and of secondary hyperparathyroidism in those with renal osteodystrophy explains the sometimes unclear risk profile of SCFE in certain groups of patients. Subtle abnormalities of hormonal balance at the time of puberty may also be partially responsible for SCFE in children without any definite systemic or hormonal abnormalities.

Mechanical factors also appear to play an etiologic role in the development of SCFE. Clearly, systemic and local factors alone cannot explain all the cases of SCFE because many patients with the aforementioned abnormalities do not develop a SCFE. In addition, most patients with SCFE provide evidence of increased forces across the proximal femoral physis due to one or more potential causes, including obesity and variations in the proximal femoral and/or acetabular morphology.

## CLINICAL FEATURES

Traditionally, classification of SCFE has been made on a temporal basis. Chronic slips are those causing symptoms for a period of at least 3 weeks, whereas acute slips are those that are symptomatic for less than 3 weeks. Acute-on-chronic slips are those with an acute exacerbation of the symptoms following a prodrome of symptoms of at least 3 weeks' duration. Chronic slips appear to account for 80% to 90% of all SCFE (2,15,94–96). Although not part of the preceding scheme, a "pre-slip" has been defined as a symptomatic hip with evidence of physiolysis prior to true movement of the femoral neck relative to the femoral head.

In 1993, Loder et al. suggested a new classification of SCFE based on physeal stability (97). An unstable SCFE was defined as occurring in an extremity upon which the patient could not bear weight either with or without crutches. With a stable slip, the child is able to bear weight on the involved extremity. Unstable SCFE account for 50% to 60% of acute SCFE and for 5% to 10% of all SCFE (95,97–99). This classification of SCFE based on stability has largely supplanted the aforementioned temporal classification scheme because of its improved ability to predict both osteonecrosis (ON) and poorer outcomes. Whereas ON is usually reported in 10% to 15% of acute SCFE, Loder et al. reported ON in 47% of unstable SCFE and 0% stable SCFE in their landmark paper (97). Even in cases of acute SCFE, only the unstable subset appear to be at significant risk for ON and a poor outcome (97,100).

The most common findings at presentation of SCFE include pain, limp, and decreased range of motion of the hip. Hip or groin pain in an obese, peripubertal child is highly suggestive of SCFE. However, hip pain is absent in as many as 50% of the children with SCFE, including up to 8% with a painless limp (101). Pain is localized to the knee and/or distal thigh in 23% to 46% of cases (4,6,101,102). Previous studies have noted that distal thigh and/or knee pain often result in significant misdiagnosis of SCFE, delay in diagnosis, unnecessary radiographs, increased slip severity, and sometimes in unnecessary knee arthroscopy (4,6, 20,76,101–103). These findings indicate the importance of examining the hip in all children presenting with distal thigh and/or knee pain.

Symptoms of SCFE are generally present for weeks to several months prior to presentation to the orthopaedist (15,104). Although patients report a specific inciting event as the cause of pain in approximately 50% of cases, severe trauma is rarely reported (101). Even when trauma is reported, further questioning often reveals a history of pain for weeks or months preceding the inciting event.

A significant proportion of the 5% to 10% of children with unstable SCFE present with an acute onset of severe hip pain in the absence of prodromal symptoms (15,96,105). Such SCFE often follow mild trauma.

As has been noted, most children with SCFE are obese. Short stature (height less than the 10th percentile) has been reported to be an indicator of increased risk for underlying systemic disease in children with SCFE (46). Loder and Greenfield noted that SCFE due to an underlying cause (such as underlying systemic disease or previous radiation exposure) was much greater in children older than 16 years and/or those who were below the 50th percentile for weight at the time of presentation (106).

When a child presents with hip, groin, thigh, or knee pain, care must be taken to evaluate both hips. The physician needs to be persistent when asking about symptoms in both hips, because a child often initially complains of only the more symptomatic hip in cases of bilateral SCFE.

One of the most helpful tip-offs in these patients is the observational gait analysis when the child walks into the examining room. The limp in children with SCFE is due to several gait deviations. Hip abductor weakness commonly manifests as a trunk lean to the affected limb in stance (Trendelenburg gait). If there is marked pain, an antalgic gait (decreased stance phase on the affected limb) will be present as well. Finally, because of the external rotation of the femoral neck and shaft (relative to the femoral head), the foot and knee progression angles on the affected side are often markedly external. Children with unilateral involvement have significant asymmetry of foot and knee progression angles with a unilateral Trendelenburg gait, whereas children with bilateral SCFE present with a more "waddling" gait bilaterally, and bilateral external foot and knee progression.

On physical examination, range of motion of the hips—including the rotational profile of the hips—should be measured and compared. Hip flexion to 90 degrees is unusual, and hip flexion contractures are common. Because hip flexion and extension are both lost, there is significant diminution of the sagittal arc. Hip abduction is significantly limited both actively and passively, and the hip abductors are weak.

Hip rotation is abnormal because of both the abnormal anatomy and the synovitis that accompany SCFE. Loss of the hip internal rotation is combined with preservation of (or even an increase in) external rotation. With a SCFE, the hip will automatically fall into external rotation (so-called obligate external rotation) as it is progressively flexed. Obligate external rotation of the hip(s) is essentially pathognomonic for SCFE. In cases of unilateral SCFE, comparison with the rotation of the contralateral hip clearly demonstrates this change in the arc of motion. In bilateral SCFE, both hips will demonstrate this shift toward external rotation.

In summary, any patient between the ages of 10 and 16 years who presents with a limp and pain in the groin, hip, thigh, or knee should be considered to have a SCFE until proven otherwise. Diagnoses such as pulled groin muscles are rarely correct in children, although such misdiagnoses are still commonly made in children with SCFE. The index of suspicion for the diagnosis of SCFE is markedly increased in obese, peripubertal children with a limp, external foot progression, and pain in the groin, hip, thigh, or knee. The index of suspicion is also very high in patients with a known history of endocrine abnormalities and in those with underlying diseases associated with endocrine abnormalities, such as Down syndrome and renal osteodystrophy.

# RADIOGRAPHIC FEATURES

## Radiographs

High-quality anteroposterior and lateral radiographs of each hip should be obtained to confirm the diagnosis of SCFE. Because of the high frequency of bilateral SCFE, bilateral imaging has been recommended for decades (20,107,108). In an unstable, acute SCFE, a lateral view is not obtained preoperatively in order to avoid causing pain and because of the potential for displacement of the SCFE.

On the anteroposterior view, widening and irregularity of the physis may be the only radiographic findings prior to, or with minimal, displacement of the femoral neck and shaft relative to the femoral head. Cowell noted that the displacement may not be evident in 14% of the anteroposterior views (101). Another common finding on the anteroposterior view is a decreased height of the capital femoral epiphysis when the epiphysis lies posterior to the femoral neck. As slipping progresses, the metaphysis appears progressively more lateral relative to the acetabular teardrop, and an increased radiodensity of the proximal metaphysis (the so-called "metaphyseal blanch") may be noted (109). Osteopenia of the affected hip is common as well.

Lateral views are more sensitive for detecting mild degrees of slip. With increased magnitude of slipping, the SCFE becomes evident on the anteroposterior view as well. Normally, a portion of the femoral head lies lateral to Klein's line (a line drawn along the lateral border of the femoral neck) (108) (Fig. 26.1A,B). A SCFE is present if the Klein's line lies cephalad to the femoral head, or if the amount of femoral head cephalad to the Klein's line is less than is seen for the contralateral hip.

Cross-table lateral views are often cited as more reliable than frog lateral views in the assessment of SCFE, which may be due to difficulties with the positioning of these children (110,111). However, using a femoral model, Loder reported that an accurate representation of the SCFE was obtained with either cross-table or frog lateral views when the femur is rotated externally by 30 degrees or less (112). The value of other specialized views, such as the Billing lateral, is still being debated (112,113).

The degree of slip is commonly quantified as the amount of femoral head displacement as a percentage of the femoral neck diameter, and was first described by Wilson in 1938 (20). Slips have been categorized as mild (less than 33%), moderate (33% to 50%), and severe (more than 50%) (6,21). Although frequently used, this measurement can be inconsistent because of variations in patient positioning and can change over the passage of time because of proximal femoral remodeling. This measurement should therefore be used only in the evaluation of SCFE prior to remodeling (114).

Southwick recommended measuring the angles between the proximal femoral physis and the femoral shaft, the so-called "head–shaft" angles, on both anteroposterior and

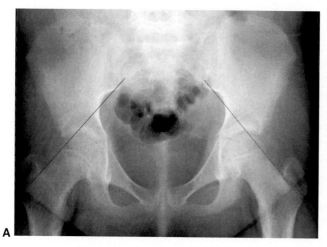
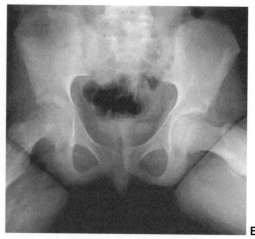

**Figure 26.1**   Radiographs of a 12-year-old boy with 3 months of hip pain show typical findings of a slipped capital femoral epiphysis (SCFE). **A:** Anteroposterior view demonstrates physeal widening, osteopenia, decreased epiphyseal height, increased metaphyseal-teardrop distance, and asymmetry of Klein's line. **B:** Although many of these features are seen on the anteroposterior view, the most striking feature is how much more easily the displacement is seen on the frog lateral view. The importance of obtaining lateral views when evaluating for SCFE cannot be overemphasized.

lateral radiographs (115). The difference between these two angles obtained at the affected and unaffected sides determines the degree of abnormal alignment, and are often referred to as *Southwick angles*. The lateral view gives an indication of posterior angulation. A difference of less than 30 degrees has been deemed mild, a difference of 30 degrees to 50 degrees moderate, and more than 50 degrees is deemed as severe (116).

The angle between the proximal femoral physis and femoral neck, the so-called "head–neck" angle, may be measured but is less reliable because remodeling adjacent to the SCFE may artificially decrease this number in the absence of clinically significant changes in femoral version.

## Other Imaging Studies

Radiographs are sufficient for the evaluation of most children with SCFE. However, additional imaging may be warranted in special circumstances, such as in the evaluation of a presumed "pre-slip" in a child with normal radiographs, or in the early evaluation of a patient with SCFE at risk for ON.

Computed tomography (CT) scans are rarely needed as a part of the initial assessment of children with SCFE (111). Some authors report that CT scan is more accurate than radiographs in evaluating the anatomy of SCFE (111), whereas others report comparable reliability between the two modalities (117,118). If a child presents very late in the course of SCFE, a CT scan may be useful in determining whether sufficient physeal closure has already occurred, thereby potentially precluding the need for an *in situ* fixation. A CT scan may also be helpful postoperatively in

determining whether any hardware used during surgery has accidentally penetrated the joint surface. This is particularly true in the case of femoral head collapse in association with ON of the femoral head.

Ultrasound has been championed by some authors, but currently appears to have little use in the routine evaluation of patients with SCFE (119–122). Previous studies using ultrasound images have indicated the presence of effusion in 42% to 60% of patients with SCFE (121,122). In experienced hands, ultrasound may have a role in confirming a suspected case of SCFE in the absence of any radiographic findings, but magnetic resonance imaging (MRI) is more commonly used in such situations.

MRI often plays an important role in the evaluation of hips of patients who are presumed to have SCFE but have normal radiographs, and MRI may also be used for the early detection of ON. The MRI findings in SCFE have been well described (118,123–125). Physeal widening, osseous edema adjacent to the physis, and the anatomic deformity associated with SCFE are typically seen, with the findings of physeal widening and irregularity as well as osseous edema adjacent to the physis seen in cases of "pre-slips" (125). In a child with suspected SCFE and normal radiographs, MRI is useful in determining whether a pre-slip is present (Fig. 26.2). Currently, MRI scanning is rarely used in evaluating patients with evident SCFE.

MRI may be used to assess femoral head circulation in order to evaluate for the presence of ON, as well as its extent and distribution if present. Unfortunately, metal artifact may significantly interfere with MRI signals. The findings of ON seen on MRI scans have not been correlated with subsequent radiographic findings and the clinical course of the affected hips.

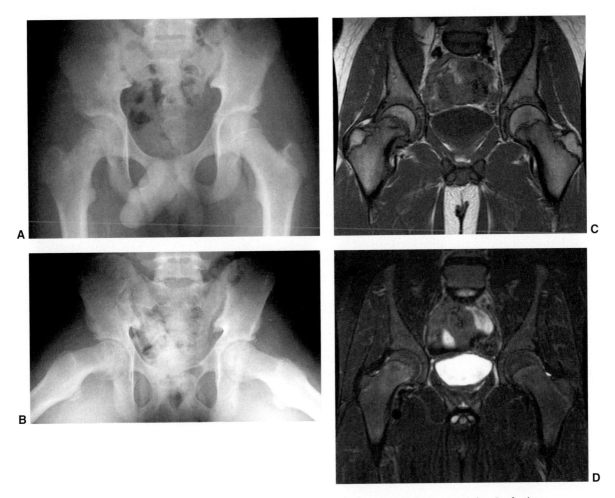

**Figure 26.2** A 12-year-old boy presented with pain in the right hip for two months. On further questioning, he reported some vague, intermittent symptoms in the left hip. Physical examination revealed pain in the right hip and obligate external rotation, but no such findings on the left. **A,B:** Anteroposterior and frog pelvis views at the time of presentation. A right slipped capital femoral epiphysis (SCFE) is evident, without definite plain radiographic changes on the left. **C,D:** Because of the vague left hip symptoms, magnetic resonance imaging (MRI) was done to rule out a left SCFE. MRI demonstrated physeal widening and irregularity (T1: flip angle 90, TR 700, TE 18) (seen best in **C**) and signal change on the right, mostly in the metaphysis in this case (fat saturation: flip angle 90, TR 4500, TE 75.37) (best seen in **D**), without any definite abnormalities on the left. Only the right hip underwent *in situ* fixation because of the normal physical examination and the lack of considerable MRI findings in the left hip. The patient denied ongoing pain in the left hip until nine months following *in situ* pinning of the right hip. He then had progressive pain in the left hip and re-presented to the orthopaedist one month later, at which time a mild left SCFE was noted and *in situ* fixation of the left hip was performed.

Bone scans may be used to assess femoral head viability in potential cases of ON of the femoral head, with decreased uptake being evident in cases of ON. Multiple studies have reported the utility of bone scanning in the detection of ON in SCFE (121,126,127). Sensitivity in detecting ON has been 100% in several series, although a false negative bone scan has been reported in a child who went on to develop mild ON (121,126–128).

Although pretreatment bone scans are quite sensitive, they are also associated with false positive results (i.e., an abnormal bone scan in a hip that does not develop ON). In two series, false-positive bone scans have been reported in one of the six (17%)(127) and two of three (67%) hips that were imaged (121).

## PATHOANATOMY

Because the femoral head is relatively fixed inside the acetabulum, the slip is best thought of as a slip of the proximal femoral neck and shaft relative to the femoral head. In children younger than 3 years, the perichondral ring imparts significant physeal stability, whereas the mammillary processes of the physis are primarily responsible for increasing physeal shear strength thereafter (92).

In laboratory rats, physeal cracks are evident in the planes of shear stress used to create SCFE (63). The mechanical patterns of physeal fracture and the zone through which physeal shear causes fractures has been shown in rabbits to vary with increasing age and with the direction of loading (129,130).

In humans, the direction of slip has been known for decades (1). In most cases, the proximal femoral neck and shaft migrate anteriorly and rotate externally, although slips have been noted to occur in other directions (131,132). Previous authors have confirmed this anatomy and suggested a torsional force as the cause of acute SCFE (133). With progression of the slip, the femoral neck may come to lie completely anterior to the femoral head. When this occurs, proximal migration of the proximal femur is possible (Fig. 26.3). However, most SCFE do not appear to progress to this point, and the apparent varus seen radiographically has been attributed to parallax (134,135). Degenerative changes, including cyst formation, may be seen in the anterior femoral neck and/or acetabulum because of impingement of the anterior femoral neck against the acetabulum during hip flexion, and such changes may be evident within years of the diagnosis of SCFE.

On the basis of computer modeling, Rab has noted that metaphyseal impingement limits the motion in severe SCFE (136). He reported that as the slip angle increases, progressively greater external hip rotation is necessary to avoid anterior impingement of the proximal femoral

metaphysis against the acetabulum during gait. Such levering can damage the anterosuperior acetabular cartilage and/or cause posterolateral labral injuries (136–139). Intraoperative evaluation by other authors has confirmed the mechanical impingement of the metaphysis against the superomedial acetabulum, with resulting cartilage and labral damage (140). Femoracetabular impingement has been suggested as a cause of idiopathic arthritis as well (141). As noted by Rab, as the proximal femur remodels and motion returns toward normal, an increasing portion of the remodeled metaphysis becomes an intraarticular weight-bearing surface, potentially contributing to late osteoarthritis (OA) (136).

Multiple studies have investigated the pathologic changes in SCFE (129,130,142–150). Multiple authors have noted the replacement of normal physis with abnormal cartilage, fibrocartilage, and fibrous tissue (147,150). The physis is often hypocellular, with increased amounts of ground substance in lieu of the normal columnar architecture (142,148). Others have noted a widening of the physis, with a loss of normal organization and the presence of clefts within the physis (149). Subsequent authors have confirmed the columnar disorganization with cartilage cell clumping in the physis, metaphysis, and epiphysis (148,150). Groups of cartilage cells have been noted between metaphyseal trabeculae (146,148,150). Collagen fibrils are markedly diminished in the hypertrophic zone (148). The resting zone is essentially normal (146,148). The proliferative zone has less densely packed collagen and increased disorganization, with ground substance replacing the normal chondrocytes. The hypertrophic zone is much larger than usual (up to 80% of the physeal width in comparison to 15% to 30% in normal physes) with marked disorganization, increased ground substance, and significant staining for glycoproteins (146,148). Cell degeneration and death have been noted in the proliferative and hypertrophic zones (142–144). The slip occurs through the proliferative and hypertrophic zones of the physis in an irregular pattern (62,146,148). Histologic sections of the physis in SCFE before and after *in situ* fixation demonstrate a return to a more normal architecture following fixation; such findings have been postulated to indicate that mechanical stabilization of the physis, with removal of the abnormal shear forces across the physis, allows at least a partial reversal of the pathology seen with SCFE (145).

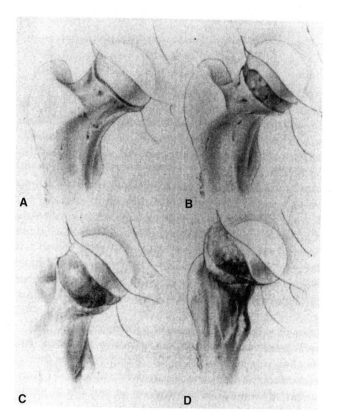

**Figure 26.3**  Pathoanatomy of SCFE is demonstrated. **A:** No displacement is seen. **B:** Rotation of the proximal femoral neck, with the femoral head (which is anchored in the acetabulum) posterior relative to the femoral neck. **C:** Progressive external rotation, with progressive posterior relation of the femoral head to the femoral neck. **D:** Proximal migration of the femoral neck due to the markedly posterior relation of the femoral head to the femoral neck. (From Morrissy RT. Principles of in situ fixation in chronic slipped capital femoral epiphysis. *Instr Course Lect* 1989;38:257–262, with permission.)

## BLOOD SUPPLY

ON is one of the few potentially devastating complications associated with SCFE, and understanding the proximal femoral blood supply is important in attempting to minimize the frequency of this complication. The blood supply of the proximal femur can be divided into the intraosseous and extraosseous components, as has been well documented by Crock and subsequently by Chung (151,152) (Fig. 26.4).

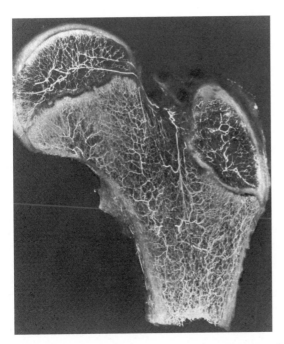

**Figure 26.4** A coronal section demonstrating vascularity of the proximal femur in a 13-year-old boy. Part of the vascular ring is visible at the base of the femoral neck, giving rise to the ascending cervical arteries which then enter the femoral head and supply blood to the superior head. (From Crock HV. A revision of the anatomy of the arteries supplying the upper end of the human femur. *J Anat* 1965;99:77–88, with permission.)

Chung noted that these components are present in an individual at birth and persist without significant change into adulthood (151). In cases of SCFE, the blood supply can be disrupted because of the SCFE itself (especially in cases with unstable SCFE), and it may also be compromised at the time of surgery.

It appears that the cause of ON is likely to be the disruption of the blood supply, which may occur because of displacement at the time of injury or at any time prior to operative fixation. Angiography performed in 12 patients with SCFE preoperatively showed filling of the superior retinacular artery in all seven stable slips and in only two of the five unstable slips (153). In one of the three unstable SCFE without preoperative filling of the superior retinacular artery, postoperative angiography demonstrated appropriate filling (153).

### Extraosseous Blood Supply

The extraosseous blood supply to the proximal femur may be disrupted in acute SCFE and has been well described. An arterial ring at the base of the femoral neck gives rise to ascending cervical arteries which penetrate the hip capsule and provide circulation to the femoral head, neck, and greater trochanter (151,152). The arterial ring at the base of the femoral neck consists of the lateral femoral circumflex artery, which runs anteriorly and constitutes the anterior portion of the arterial ring, and the medial femoral circumflex artery, which travels posteriorly and constitutes the medial, lateral, and posterior portions of the ring. The

ring is most commonly incomplete, without communication between the branches from the medial and lateral circumflex arteries.

Ascending cervical arteries (also known as retinacular vessels) arise from each portion of this extracapsular arterial ring and penetrate the hip capsule to enter the hip joint. The numerous branches from the lateral ascending cervical artery (which branch from the medial femoral circumflex artery) provide circulation to the greatest portion of the femoral head and neck. After penetrating the hip capsule, the ascending cervical arteries form a second arterial ring which is also usually incomplete. This intraarticular, subsynovial ring is smaller than the extracapsular ring and is located at the border between the articular surface of the femoral head and the femoral neck. These subsynovial vessels are consistently present medially and laterally and less commonly present anteriorly and posteriorly. The epiphyseal branches of these vessels cross the physis on the surface of the femoral head, enter the perichondral ring, and then cross into the epiphysis.

### Intraosseous Blood Supply

The intraosseous blood supply may be compromised by proximal femoral osteotomies or the internal fixation of SCFE. The ascending cervical arteries penetrate the intracapsular femoral neck, with different vessels supplying the metaphysis and epiphysis (151,152,154). The intraosseous blood supply of the femoral head is mainly located in its posterior and superior portions, with potential implications for the positioning of hardware (151). The extent of anastomoses between these vessels and the arterial branches of the ligamentum teres (which supply the medial third of the femoral head) appears to be quite limited (151,152,154).

## NATURAL HISTORY

In the short term, the natural history of the affected hip is one of progressive displacement, followed ultimately by stabilization of the slip and physeal closure. Although all slips must eventually cease progressing, the timing of cessation and the degree of the slip prior to cessation and physeal closure are unpredictable. Most slips progress slowly, although some may have significant, acute progression. The hips with such acute progression are the ones at the highest risk for significant complications.

Bilateral SCFE at the time of initial presentation accounted for approximately 20% of the children with SCFE in recent series (15,25,26). It is probable that this frequency will further increase with the increased awareness of the frequency of bilateral involvement and with the ongoing improvements in the imaging of SCFE.

An additional 10% to 20% of patients with SCFE are diagnosed with a contralateral SCFE in adolescence (6,13, 27–29). About 80% to 90% of symptomatic, contralateral

SCFE cases are diagnosed within 18 months of the diagnosis of the first slip, with 66% to 81% being diagnosed in the first year (15,25,116,155). The average duration between the diagnosis of the first and second slips in metachronous bilateral SCFE has been reported as 1.0 ± 0.8 years (15). Contralateral slips have been reported as late as 4 to 5 years following the initial SCFE (6,15,21).

The true frequency of bilateral SCFE at long-term follow-up appears to be approximately 60% (13,28), although rates of up to 80% have been reported (30). Many of the late contralateral SCFE cases reported in long-term radiographic follow-up are mild, asymptomatic slips (13,28,30). These data suggest that if 20% of the patients present with bilateral SCFE, then half of the 80% who present with unilateral SCFE will ultimately have a contralateral SCFE.

In the short term, 61% to 100% of children with endocrinopathies and SCFE have bilateral slips, although metachronous involvement is common (35,52). Because of this significant short-term risk, prophylactic pinning of the contralateral hip is recommended in patients with SCFE and endocrine disease (35,52).

In the long term, SCFE puts the hip at significant risk of OA, poorer results being associated with an increasing degree of SCFE (9,116,156–159). Hagglund et al. reported radiographic evidence of OA in 27% (28 of 104) of hips with SCFE at long-term follow-up (mean follow-up: 33 years) compared with 9% of control hips (9 of 101) (28). Carney and Weinstein reported a long-term follow-up (mean follow-up, 41 years) of 28 patients with 31 untreated SCFEs (between 1915 and 1952) and correlated the degree of the slips with radiographic and clinical scores (157). Patients with mild slips fared better than did those with moderate and severe slips with regard to radiographic changes and Iowa hip scores. At long-term follow-up, Iowa hip scores were at least 80 in all 17 hips with mild slips and in 9 of the 14 hips (64%) with moderate or severe slips. There was radiographic evidence of OA in 64% (9 of 14) of the mild slips and in 100% (13 of 13) of the moderate and severe slips.

Ordeberg et al. reported a 20- to 60-year follow-up (mean follow-up, 37 years) of 49 cases of SCFE that did not undergo primary treatment (159). They reported that only "a few" patients had restrictions regarding their work or social lives and that only 2 of 49 (4%) had required surgery for arthritis. Limb length discrepancy (LLD) of at least 2 cm was noted in 31% of the cases. The authors also noted that these results were far superior to a comparable group of patients treated with closed reduction and casting. Jerre noted superior results in untreated patients in Sweden as well (29).

Previous authors have noted that known cases of SCFE account for 2% to 9% of end-stage hip arthritis (160–164). A cadaveric study noted "post-slip" morphology in 8% of the skeletons and showed that OA was associated with such morphology (165).

A significant proportion of adults with "idiopathic" OA have been reported as having a stigma of pediatric hip disease, such as a "pistol grip" deformity. Murray reported an apparent association with SCFE in 40% of the adult hips thought to have degenerative arthritis as evidenced by the so-called "tilt deformity" of the femoral head (166). Stulberg et al. reported such deformity in 40% of patients with hip OA and no previously diagnosed hip disease (167). Stulberg et al., however, noted that the "tilt deformity" did not appear to be unique to SCFE (167). Resnick has suggested that the "tilt deformity" is not due to SCFE, but is due to the remodeling of the osteoarthritic hip (168).

In summary, 20% of patients with SCFE present with unilateral disease, an additional 10% to 20% develop a contralateral slip during adolescence, and 60% of the patients have bilateral SCFE which is evident at long-term follow-up. In all the cases of SCFE, OA appears to result, with worse slips being associated with increased rates and severity of the OA. Although SCFE leads to late degenerative changes, most hips function well into their 5th decade or later.

## TREATMENT

Once the diagnosis of SCFE is made, the child is admitted to the hospital and is confined to bed until surgery is performed, as has been recommended for decades (20). Under no circumstances should the child be allowed to bear weight once the diagnosis of an acute/unstable SCFE is made, as it may result in ON.

The goals of treatment in SCFE are early detection, prevention of further slipping, and avoidance of complications. Although attention is often focused on the affected hip, care of the unaffected hip (either through careful observation or through prophylactic treatment) cannot be forsaken.

Care of children with SCFE continues to advance along with our understanding of this disease. Increased vigilance and enhanced imaging allow the early detection of SCFE, and percutaneous fixation techniques allow for short hospital stays (or even outpatient surgery). With these enhancements in care, one recent study comparing treatment of children with SCFE at a pediatric hospital to the treatment given at a general hospital reported shorter hospital stays and lower hospital charges at the children's hospital (169).

As has been noted, SCFE puts the patient at long-term risk of OA, with the risk increasing along with the increase in the degree of slip. In some cases, the outcomes of SCFE (treated or untreated) are so poor that salvage treatment by arthrodesis or arthroplasty may be needed.

### Manipulation

The goal of manipulation is to decrease the proximal femoral deformity. In the past, use of manipulation in the case of a SCFE has been described with a variety of treatments, including spica casting and internal fixation. There is no role for any forceful manipulation in the treatment of SCFE, and many authors have long cautioned against forceful manipulation (1,128,170). In a study of four patients with SCFE and treated with manipulation, Jerre et al. noted poor results at long-term follow-up in all four; two had to undergo salvage surgery, and the other two had poor clinical hip scores (170).

Previous reports focused on the incidence of ON following the forceful manipulation/reduction of SCFE. Casey reported ON in 14% of acute cases of SCFE, with ON in 42% of those treated with only manipulation and casting and in none of those treated with traction and internal fixation, with or without supplemental reduction (95). Aadalen reported ON in 15% of the acute cases of SCFE, with a rate of 5% (1 of 19) among those treated with manipulation, epiphysiodesis, and casting; 19% (3 of 16) among those treated with manipulation and internal fixation; and 25% (3 of 12) among those treated with manipulation and epiphysiodesis 171). Hall noted ON in 5% of the cases of SCFE treated with *in situ* fixation using a Smith-Peterson nail and a 37.5% incidence among those treated with fixation using a Smith-Peterson nail following manipulation, although these results may have been influenced by selection bias (172).

Multiple authors have reported that the degree of reduction does not appear to correlate with the risk of ON (96–99,121,171,173), although others have reported a correlation between the degree of reduction and the risk of ON (174).

Forceful manipulation in cases of SCFE is never indicated because of the increased risks of complications including ON. A serendipitous reduction, which may occur with patient positioning on the operating table, does not appear to negatively affect patient outcome.

## Spica Casting

The goal of spica casting is to prevent the progression of a SCFE. Although used in the treatment of SCFE for much of the last century, spica casting is now rarely used in the treatment of SCFE. Because most children with SCFE are obese adolescents, use of a spica cast for these children holds little appeal for most patients, their families, and physicians.

Traditionally, spica casting has been associated with high rates of complications (175). Meier et al. reported complication in 14 of 17 hips in which a SCFE (82%) had been treated with spica casting, including nine cases of chondrolysis (53%), three cases of further slip after cast removal (18%), and two cases in which a total of three pressure sores developed (12%) (175). Chondrolysis has been reported in 14% to 53% of the cases of SCFE treated with spica casting, and it has also been reported in the uninvolved hip following immobilization (29,94, 175–177). ON has commonly been reported with the use of spica casting as well, although most cases of ON appear to be due to the forceful manipulation of the SCFE rather than to the spica cast itself.

Progressive slip occurs in 5% to 18% of cases of SCFE treated with spica casting (175,176). Although Betz et al.

cited only a 3% incidence (1 per 37 hips), the true rate is 5% in their study because they excluded the progression of one additional hip that had been followed up for less than 2 years (176).

The duration of casting has often been arbitrary. In the absence of any operative intervention, most proximal femoral physes do not close for a year or more following the diagnosis of SCFE. Most children treated with casting are immobilized for 3 to 4 months (175,176). Betz et al. noted that spica casts could safely be removed when the juxtaphyseal metaphyseal radiolucency was no longer visible, and that this occurred by 16 weeks in their patients (176). Although all patients were immobilized in a cast for periods ranging from 117 to 124 days, Meier reported progressive slips in 18% (3 of 17) of the hips after cast removal (175).

With the advent of current fluoroscopic imaging techniques, cannulated screw systems, and the decrease in operative morbidity, there is little role for nonsurgical treatment in children with SCFE.

## *In Situ* Fixation

The goal of *in situ* fixation of SCFE is to prevent slip progression. *In situ* fixation is currently the preferred initial treatment for most cases of SCFE, both stable and unstable, although the outcome of such treatment differs depending on the slip stability.

Over a period of more than 50 years of *in situ* fixation for SCFE, surgical techniques, implants, and imaging techniques have evolved significantly (178). Large nail-type devices gave way to pins, which have given way to cannulated screw systems in most centers. Because of the wide availability of fluoroscopic imaging, the ability to optimally position the fixation devices has improved as well. Cannulated screw systems now allow these procedures to be performed percutaneously.

The surgery may be performed on either a fracture table or a radiolucent table (178,179). Use of a fracture table allows a true lateral radiograph to be obtained, although the quality of such images in obese patients is often suboptimal and this setup requires the presence of a technician to rotate the fluoroscope. In contrast, with the patient on a radiolucent table a technician is not needed, as the fluoroscope may be left in one position and it is easy to obtain a higher quality frog lateral radiograph; however, a true lateral can only be obtained by moving the patient. In addition, the guide wire for percutaneous fixation may be bent as the hip is rotated.

Although *in situ* fixation is performed nearly universally for stable SCFE, an inadvertent reduction of an unstable SCFE sometimes occurs simply with patient positioning. This is particularly true in cases of markedly displaced, unstable SCFE. Most authors agree that such inadvertent reductions do not appear to cause ON (180,181). The risk of ON appears to be due to the disruption of the blood supply at the time of injury or with subsequent displacement prior to surgical fixation rather than to an inadvertent reduction in the operating room (128,153).

There are some important technical considerations when pinning an unstable SCFE. First, fluoroscopic imaging is helpful in assessing the degree of reduction as well as aiding in pin positioning. Gentle adjustments (such as increasing hip internal rotation) in limb positioning may be indicated in order to reduce marked displacement, if persistent, following patient positioning (182). Second, if a radiolucent table is used while an unstable SCFE is being pinned, a provisional guide wire should be placed across the physis and into the femoral head percutaneously before a lateral image is obtained, in order to prevent ongoing motion between the femoral head and neck.

Understanding the three-dimensional pathoanatomy of the SCFE is essential for understanding how to position the hardware optimally and minimize complications. As noted previously, the proximal femoral neck and shaft migrate anteriorly and rotate externally in most SCFE. As a result, a greater portion of the femoral head is located posterior to the femoral neck as the SCFE progresses. In very severe cases of SCFE, the entire femoral head is posterior to the femoral neck.

One of the significant difficulties in pinning SCFE is the three-dimensional interpretation of intraoperative radiographic images. Walters and Simon alerted the orthopaedic community to the risk of unrecognized pin penetration in cases of SCFE treated with *in situ* fixation, and the associated risk of chondrolysis (183). They demonstrated that a "blind spot" can exist radiographically, since a protruding pin may appear to be located within the femoral head on both anteroposterior and lateral views (183). Other authors have described a geometric analysis of the blind spot, although this technique is rarely used (184).

Ideally, the fixation device should be located in the center of the proximal femoral epiphysis on both the anteroposterior and lateral views and should be perpendicular to the physis in both views as well (185,186). This so-called "center-center" position of the fixation device minimizes the "blind spot," and thus the risk of pin penetration and complications (183,187).

Because of the direction of the slip, fixation should be inserted from the anterior femoral neck in most cases in order to allow fixation perpendicular to the physis and to prevent hardware penetration through the posterior femoral neck (135,188) (Fig. 26.5). In fact, in very severe cases, the hardware may need to be inserted in a directly anterior-to-posterior direction (Fig. 26.6).

Insertion of hardware from the lateral cortex (as is done in the pinning of adult hip fractures) will generally result in one or more of the following problems: poor biomechanical alignment of the hardware (very oblique rather than perpendicular to the physis), purchase of the hardware in only a small portion of the femoral head, joint penetration, hardware exiting the posterior femoral neck before entering the femoral head, and creation of

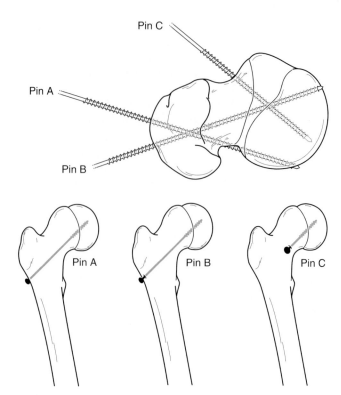

**Figure 26.5** Two common problems associated with lateral-entry pins (pins A and B) in slipped capital femoral epiphysis (SCFE) are contrasted with correct pin positioning (pin C) using an anterior entry point. **Top:** Because of their lateral starting points, pins A and B are both eccentric in the femoral head and oblique to the physis. In addition, pin A is shown exiting the posterior femoral neck before entering the epiphysis. **Bottom:** How pins A, B, and C will look on an anteroposterior radiograph, and how a potential blind spot exists in which a protruding screw may be missed radiographically. This reinforces the importance of imaging a pinned hip as the hip is rotated through a complete range of motion.

stress risers on the tension side of the proximal femur. Common sequelae with a lateral starting point are that the hardware either entirely misses or engages only a small portion of the anterior femoral head, and that such hardware also often penetrates the joint surface. If the hardware exits the posterior femoral neck before entering the femoral head, as has been reported in up to 6% of cases (97,189), the extraosseous and intraosseous blood supplies to the femoral head are at risk, thereby increasing the risk of ON.

The anatomic constraints of SCFE markedly limit the amount of space in the femoral head and neck for appropriate hardware positioning. Multiple clinical studies have confirmed increasing rates of pin penetration and complications with an increasing number of implants (27,174, 189–194). In 1984, Lehman et al. reported a 37% incidence of unrecognized pin penetration in cases of SCFE undergoing treatment with implants and noted that some areas of the head may not be well visualized fluoroscopically (195). In a 1990 study of the cases of SCFE fixed with multiple pins or screws, Riley et al. reported hardware-related complications in 26% of the treated hips, which included pin penetration in 14% (196) (Fig. 26.7).

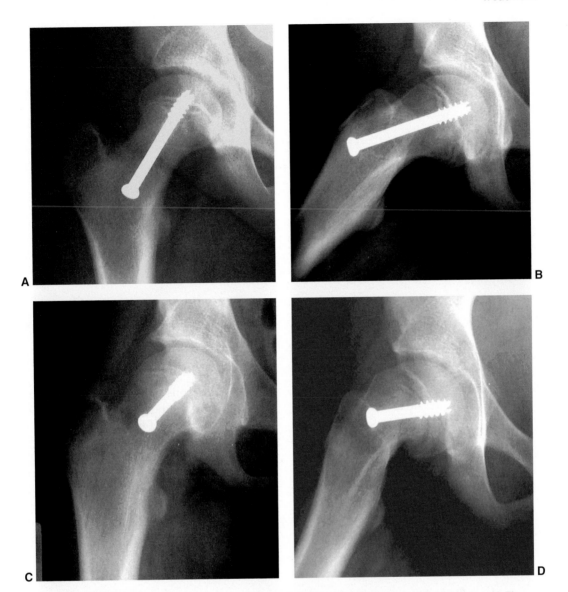

**Figure 26.6**  Proper screw locations in slips of varying severity in three different cases: **(A,B)**, **(C,D)**, and **(E,F)**. In all three cases, the screws enter the anterior femoral neck, are perpendicular to the physis, and are located in the center of the femoral head. The starting point is more proximal and the screw is angled progressively more posteriorly as the magnitude of slip progresses from least **(A,B)** to most **(E,F)** severe.

The hips are taken through a full range of motion while using fluoroscopy. This can be done throughout the procedure if a radiolucent table is used. If a fracture table is used, this can only be done following removal of traction on the operated leg. The "approach-withdraw phenomenon" described by Moseley is checked (197). This is the fluoroscopic appearance of the implanted hardware approaching the subchondral bone and then moving away from it (197). When the hardware reaches the apex of this arc and then begins to recede, the point of maximal proximity to the subchondral bone has been reached, and this distance should be measured. Center-center pins are left 5 to 6 mm from the subchondral bone (corrected for magnification) while other pins are left 10 mm from the subchondral bone (183). The posterior and superior portions of the femoral

neck should be avoided, because the hardware implanted in such locations may compromise the intraosseous blood supply to the femoral head and increase the risk of ON. Poor hardware position has been noted to correlate with poor clinical outcomes (188,193).

Injection of arthrographic dye through the hardware under fluoroscopic control and bone endoscopy are two ways that have been reported for checking for pin penetration when high-quality radiographic images cannot be obtained intraoperatively (198,199). However, imaging quality is almost always sufficient to obviate the need for either of these techniques. In addition, each of these techniques has the potential risk of flushing bone chips into the hip joint. If radiographic imaging is deemed insufficient intraoperatively, then a hip arthrogram through a

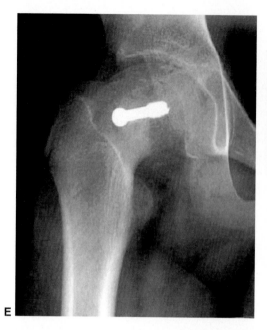
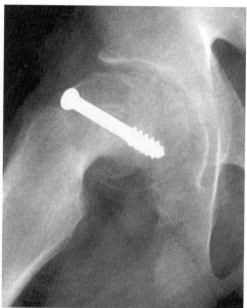

**Figure 26.6** (*continued*)

standard anterior approach may be performed to better ascertain the relation of the hardware to the femoral head.

The biomechanical properties of various fixation techniques have been studied. Two previous biomechanical studies of acute physeal disruptions in animal femora stripped of soft tissue attachments have demonstrated an increased rigidity for two-pin or two-screw constructs compared to those using only one comparable fixation device (200,201), and another found no statistically significant difference in resistance to creep in between single- and double-screw constructs in bovine femora (202). The authors of the two bovine studies stated that the biomechanical advantages of two-screw constructs were insufficient to justify the increased risk of pin penetration when two screws are used instead of one (200,202). One additional study using bovine femora with acutely created physeal disruptions indicated that compression across the physis may be obtained if screw threads do not cross the physis, although there was no significant difference in the ultimate strength or the energy absorbed or in the

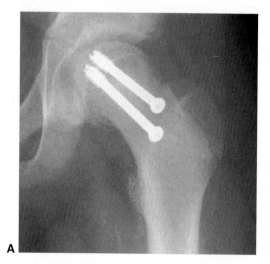
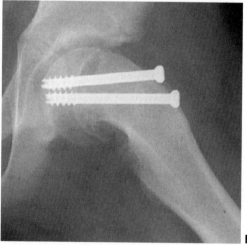

**Figure 26.7**   An 11.5-year-old boy presented with hip pain 1 month following *in situ* fixation of a stable slipped capital femoral epiphysis (SCFE). Anteroposterior radiograph **(A)** demonstrates what appears to be adequate alignment of the hardware, although the frog lateral view **(B)** is suggestive of pin penetration. The proximity of the hardware to the joint surface had not been recognized at the time of surgery, and demonstrates the importance of leaving the pin at least 5 mm from subchondral bone, even if the hip is imaged through a range of motion at the time of surgery. This case also illustrates that only one implant can be in both a center-center position and perpendicular to the physis.

degree of failure as compared to the results with a standard screw (203). Because all these studies involve acute physeal disruptions, their applicability to stable SCFE is limited. Their applicability to even acute SCFE in humans is unclear as well.

Physeal closure generally occurs within 6 to 12 months following *in situ* fixation of a SCFE (27,108,189,204–206). Physeal closure occurs in the operated hip first in most cases, and simultaneous closure occurs in fewer than 10% of cases (27,108,189,204–206). Prolonged time for closure has been associated with eccentric screw placement and increasing severity of the SCFE (205). Whether the rapid physeal closure is due to the SCFE itself or to the fixation across the physis is not known. In a young child with unilateral SCFE, rapid unilateral physeal closure has the undesired effect of causing a potential limb length discrepancy (LLD). Multiple studies carried out in Europe have touted the use of fixation devices without threads crossing the physis (including smooth wires, hook pins, and partially threaded screws) as a way to avoid physeal closure and to allow further growth of the proximal femur (207,208). In young patients with underlying causes of SCFE, some authors have noted that epiphysiodesis may be needed in combination with *in situ* fixation (36).

Recent studies of a combination of acute, acute-on-chronic, and chronic cases of SCFE (with 75% to 86% chronic cases of SCFE) reported good or excellent results in 90% to 95% of the patients (2,209). Another recent series, limited to 21 hips with acute or acute-on-chronic SCFE treated with single screws, reported 95% good to excellent results, with no cases of ON or chondrolysis (187). In series of studies with worse results, it is seen that the results are better in milder slips than in the more severe slips (188). Aronson et al. reported good or excellent results in 70% of the overall cases, with 86% good or excellent results in cases of mild SCFE, 55% in cases of moderate SCFE, and 24% in cases of severe SCFE (188).

Radiographs often demonstrate a remodeling of the SCFE following *in situ* fixation (19,26,116,206,209,210). This remodeling typically involves resorption of a portion of the prominent superior femoral neck, and has also been reported to result in changes in the proximal femoral head–neck and head–shaft angles. Studies that report proximal femoral remodeling typically report angular changes in the range of 7 degrees to 14 degrees (26,206, 209,210). Remodeling is most commonly reported in more severe slips and has been reported in 68% to 83% of moderate to severe cases of SCFE at long-term follow-up (19,116, 209,210). An open triradiate cartilage has been reported to be an indicator of more potential for such remodeling (210,211). However, some authors have even reported remodeling after proximal femoral physeal closure (194).

All of these studies on remodeling have significant limitations. One such limitation is the inherent error in radiographic measurements. Another limitation is the variability in patient positioning, especially when a painful hip with synovitis is imaged at the time of presentation and a painless hip is imaged on subsequent evaluations. Finally, significant remodeling in the slowly growing peripubertal proximal femur with a fixation device across the physis seems intuitively unlikely.

Marked improvement in the dynamic and static measures of hip motion have been noted postoperatively, especially in the first 6 months (26). Siegel et al. reported such rapid improvement prior to significant remodeling, even in hips with severe deformity (26). At 2-year follow-up, by which time the average slip angle had decreased from 44 degrees to 30 degrees, mean hip flexion had improved by 22 degrees (to 118 degrees), hip abduction by 11 degrees (to 40 degrees) and hip internal rotation in flexion by 19 degrees (to 11 degrees) (26). Other authors have noted similar improvement in the range of hip motion postoperatively, with improvements of 31 degrees for hip flexion, 25 degrees for internal rotation, 19 degrees for external rotation, and 21 degrees for abduction (193). However, a decreased range of motion was still noted relative to the unaffected hip in 40% of the patients, with flexion decreased by 15 degrees, internal rotation decreased by 17 degrees, and external rotation decreased by 10 degrees in this same study (193). O'Brien and Fahey noted painless hips in 83% (10 of 12) of moderate to severe cases of SCFE 2 to 17 years following *in situ* pinning, with seven of these ten hips having "essentially normal" motion except for a loss of 5 degrees to 20 degrees of internal rotation (210).

The range of motion at long-term follow-up (mean follow-up, 32.7 years) in cases of SCFE hips without OA was examined (212). There were no significant differences between the range of motion of normal hips and those that had not been treated for SCFE or those treated with *in situ* fixation. The only significant loss of range was the loss of external rotation of hips treated previously with osteotomy. The hips without treatment (slip angle 18.8 degrees) or treated with *in situ* fixation (slip angle 25.4 degrees) had markedly lower slip angles than did those with osteotomy (slip angle 73.7 degrees). Although this study has obvious selection bias, it does demonstrate that in cases of hips without OA, there is no inexorable loss of motion.

Complications of *in situ* fixation may be either iatrogenic or may be due to the natural history of SCFE. The two most severe complications are ON and chondrolysis. ON may be the natural sequela of an unstable SCFE or may result from pin placement problems (with superior and/or posterior femoral head placement), whereas chondrolysis may occur because of unrecognized pin penetration. Other complications include further slipping, growing off the screw, loosening or failure of screw fixation, proximal femoral fracture, and LLD.

Previous studies have repeatedly reported lower rates of ON with stable SCFE than with unstable SCFE. Many series of studies have reported 0% ON in stable SCFE, with the rates of ON in unstable SCFE ranging from 12.5% to 58%

(2,97,173,174,213). In a series of 55 acute cases of SCFE treated with internal fixation, Loder et al. reported ON in 14 cases (25%) with a rate of 47% in unstable slips (14 of 30) and 0% in stable slips ($n = 25$) (97). In another series with a 10% rate of ON in cases of acute SCFE, Dietz et al. reported a 21% incidence in unstable SCFE and none in stable SCFE (214).

Most cases of ON occur in unstable SCFE and appear to be due to the SCFE itself, although it is likely that the intraosseous blood supply to the femoral head may be disrupted if internal fixation devices are located in the superior or posterosuperior regions of the femoral head (151,152,154,180,182). Difficulty in avoiding these areas with any implants may be the reason that the rate of ON is greater when multiple implants are used to fix a SCFE (174,189).

In one previous study, preoperative angiography showed a filling of the superior retinacular artery in only two of five unstable slips (153). One of the three hips without filling of the superior retinacular artery preoperatively was studied postoperatively, at which stage postoperative restoration of the filling of the artery was evident (153). Preoperative bone scans are quite sensitive in detecting ON, although both false positives and false negatives have been reported (128). Because almost all cases of ON were noted to have abnormal tracer uptake preoperatively, the surgery does not appear to be the main cause of ON in these patients.

The impact of capsulotomy on the rate of ON following the treatment of cases of unstable SCFE is undetermined. Clinical and laboratory studies have suggested a potential benefit, with capsulotomy reducing the rate of ON in adults and children with proximal femoral fractures; studies have also shown an increase in intracapsular pressure when the hip is maintained in internal rotation (215–220). In the laboratory, Woodhouse documented ON in dogs with intracapsular pressures of at least 50 mm of mercury for at least 12 hours (220). As seen from this and other studies (221,222), the amount of pressure required to cause a significant decrease in the femoral head perfusion seems to greatly exceed the increased intracapsular pressure present in human hips with SCFE.

In clinical practice, the issue of whether or not capsulotomy is beneficial remains unresolved. Some authors have recommended capsulotomy at the time of SCFE fixation in an attempt to decrease the rate of ON (128). Such recommendations are based on inconclusive data from a small number of cases. Gordon et al. advocate the importance of performing a capsulotomy at the time of reduction and fixation of unstable SCFE, although examination of their data demonstrates that this recommendation is based on a single case of "mild" ON out of a total of five patients who underwent early reduction without capsulotomy, in comparison to no ON in six cases treated early with capsulotomy (128). Even in this case of "mild" ON, the authors reported that the child with mild ON was asymptomatic at

5-year follow-up. The supposition with recommending capsulotomy is that there is a significant hemarthrosis under pressure, which should be decompressed, although the pressures that appear necessary to cause vascular embarrassment to the proximal femur do not likely occur in most children with SCFE. At the current time, there is insufficient evidence to conclude whether capsulotomy is beneficial in reducing the rate of ON following acute/unstable SCFE.

Forceful reduction of acute/unstable SCFE has been implicated as a cause of ON (95,171). The timing of SCFE reduction has also been suggested as a causative factor for ON. Several series have reported ON in 0% to 9% of hips treated within 24 hours of symptom onset and in 18% to 20% of cases treated thereafter (99,128,171,223). Loder et al., however, did not demonstrate any benefit to early reduction in a series of 55 acute cases of SCFE, 30 of which were unstable (97).

Early evaluation for ON may be carried out by a bone scan or MRI. If ON is present, consideration may be given to free the vascularized fibular graft prior to femoral head collapse in order to maximize patient outcome (224). If vascularity of the femoral head appears normal, then the child, family, and physician may be reassured and earlier resumption of normal activities allowed.

Chondrolysis is another potentially severe complication. Aprin et al. have demonstrated that pin penetration in rabbits can lead to chondrolysis, and that the severity of chondrolysis is related to the duration of pin penetration (225). In another study carried out in rabbits, Sternlicht et al. demonstrated that pin protrusion caused mechanical destruction of the cartilage and loss of proteoglycans in the articular cartilage, but did not result in decreased joint space (226).

Chondrolysis following *in situ* pinning varies from 0% to 9% in most of the reported series and appears to be due to unrecognized pin penetration at the time of surgery (2,21,94,116,187–190,193,196,205,227,228). Multiple series of studies carried out recently, each with more than 50 cases of SCFE treated using current fixation techniques with a single screw, have reported no cases of chondrolysis (2,205,229). Rates of chondrolysis appear to be higher when multiple fixation devices are used because of the increased risk of unrecognized pin penetration with the use of multiple fixation devices (189). Pin penetration with single cannulated screws appears to be quite low. Ward et al. (205) reported pin penetration in 1.7% (1 of 59 hips) fixed with one screw, and others (187) have reported a 0% rate.

It is important to note, however, that in humans there are many cases of unrecognized pin penetration in the treatment of SCFE without any resultant chondrolysis (189,228). Previous authors have reported chondrolysis to occur in 11% to 51% of the cases with unrecognized pin penetration. In one study with pin penetrations reported in 28 cases, chondrolysis resulted in only three of these 28 hips (11%) (189). The location of pin penetration is important (193), with less apparent risk if the penetration occurs in the inferior head or fovea. Several studies have reported that if pin penetration is recognized at the time of surgery and the protruding pin is removed, there does not appear to be an increased risk of chondrolysis or other complication (230,231).

Slip progression can occur following *in situ* fixation if the progressive growth of the proximal femur results in loss of fixation across the physis, or if a properly located screw loses fixation. Slip progression following *in situ* pinning has been reported in 0% to 3% of the cases in most series (2,94,97,205,209,232,233), although one series reported a rate of 20% (234). This high rate reported by Carney et al. is likely due to femoral neck resorption and changes in patient positioning rather than to true slip progression. In another series, the proximal femur was noted to grow off 29% of hips fixed with Steinmann pins, 18% of hips fixed with Knowles pins, and 0% of hips fixed with cannulated screws (235). Growing off a screw appears much less common than growing off wires (229,236). Previous authors have noted the risk of progressive slip if hardware is removed prior to physeal closure (237).

Jerre et al. noted slip progression in 1.5% of hips (3 of 202) without any evident cause, and progression in an additional 5% of the hips after the fixation device(s) no longer engaged the epiphysis (236). By far the highest rate of progression following *in situ* fixation was recently reported by Carney et al., who found progression of SCFE in 20% of hips following *in situ* fixation with a single screw (234). In a series of seven progressive slips with appropriate hardware positioning, fixation in the epiphysis remained good, but metaphyseal loosening with "windshield wipering" was noted in each case (233).

Proximal femoral fracture is a rare, although potentially disastrous, complication associated with *in situ* pinning of SCFE, occurring in 0% to 2% of the cases (193,196,229, 238). Such fractures often follow relatively minor trauma. Many reports have focused on subtrochanteric fractures following insertion of the hardware from the lateral aspect of the femur, which is the side of the bone with more tension (193,196,229,238). Most such fractures occur through the used or unused drill holes at or distal to the lesser trochanter (238,239) (Fig. 26.8). Fracture has also been reported following hardware removal (2).

Femoral neck fractures have also been reported following appropriate placement of hardware through the anterior femoral neck (128,240,241). Previous reports have focused on the importance of minimizing the number of drill holes (and, therefore, stress risers) in the proximal femur. Local bone death due to the high temperatures associated with reaming through dense bone has been suggested as a possible etiology in some cases as well (240). Stress fracture of the femoral neck has also been reported (229). It appears that the way to minimize the risk of proximal femoral fractures is to use an anterior starting point in the femoral neck and to avoid drilling into the proximal femur until the precise insertion site is localized.

Stambough et al. reported LLD of at least 1 cm in 14%, and of at least 2 cm in 5%, of patients treated with *in situ* pinning (193). Chen et al. reported LLD of at least 1 cm in six of ten patients (60%) treated with *in situ* pinning (242). To prevent significant LLD in children with unilateral SCFE, prophylactic pinning of the contralateral hip should be considered if such children are younger than 10 years at presentation. If a projected LLD is the only concern, then an alternative would be to perform a contralateral distal femoral epiphysiodesis at a later stage.

Complications of hardware removal have been reported in 19% to 53% of hips with implants (209,243,244). Complications of hardware removal include hardware breakage, inability to retrieve the hardware, difficulties requiring extensive bone removal, and fracture. Bellemans et al. reported inability to remove the hardware in 30% of the cases and the need for major decortication to remove hardware in 20% of the cases in the same series (209). Greenough et al. reported two subtrochanteric fractures in a study of 57 hips following hardware removal, presumably due to significant bone removal at the time of hardware removal (243). Crandall et al. reported lower complication rates with cannulated screw removal compared to pin removal, although the screws were noted to be buried and difficult to remove in 36% of the cases (245). Screw breakage during attempted removal has been reported in 6% of the cases in one series (2). Removal of titanium screws has been reported to be more difficult than removal of stainless steel screws, possibly due to the significant amount of osseous integration seen with titanium screws (246).

Because of the high rate of complications with hardware removal, routine hardware removal is not recommended following *in situ* fixation in cases of SCFE. If hardware removal is necessary (for later surgery, for example), then removal of the screws with reverse-cutting threads may prove easier.

Although late OA is commonly reported after SCFE, Hagglund noted that no patient who had a hip with a mild or moderate slip in childhood or adolescence and who had been treated with *in situ* pinning developed arthritis before the age of 50 years (247). Hansson et al. reported that at 30.9 years mean follow-up, OA was seen in 22% of mild slips (30 degrees or less) and in 50% of moderate slips (30 degrees to 50 degrees) and that Harris hip scores were at least 90 in 93% of the cases with mild slips and in 78% of the cases with moderate slips (158). They also noted that radiographic findings correlated with Harris hip scores, with hips with mild OA having a mean score of 96.5 and hips with severe OA having a mean score of 74.3 (158).

Long-term follow-up studies have compared the results of various treatment modalities (94,116). These studies noted that the best long-term results were obtained with *in situ* fixation, and that SCFE reduction or realignment resulted in higher rates of complications (including ON and chondrolysis). Carney et al. also noted that Iowa hip scores decreased with the increase of every decade in follow-up

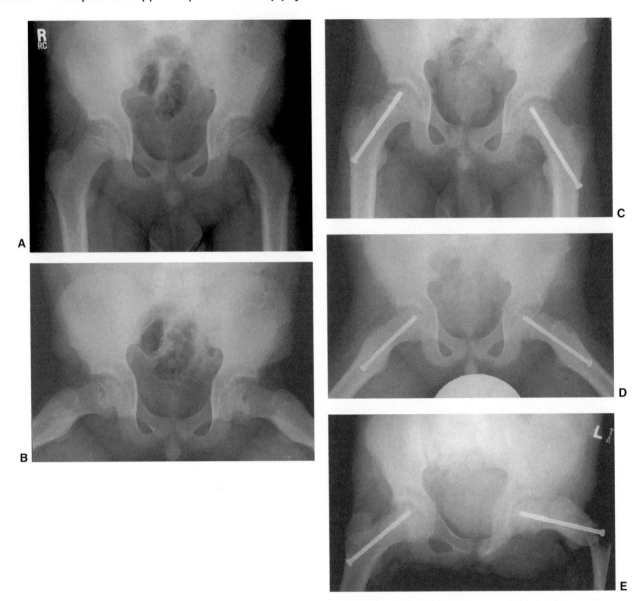

**Figure 26.8** A 12-year-old boy presented with bilateral stable slipped capital femoral epiphysis (SCFE). Anteroposterior and lateral radiographs demonstrate mild bilateral SCFE **(A,B)**. Postoperative radiographs demonstrate that both screws were inserted through the lateral cortex at or distal to the lesser trochanter **(C,D)**. Six weeks postoperatively the boy had acute onset of pain while playing baseball, due to a left subtrochanteric fracture **(E)**. Proximal femoral fractures occur most commonly when hardware enters the lateral cortex of the femur at or distal to the lesser trochanter, and may also occur through unused drill holes at this level. Because of the posterior direction of slip, an anterior femoral neck starting point would have been feasible in this case, and preferable both for biomechanical reasons and the lower risk of fracture associated with an anterior starting point.

studies (94). However, even those with late OA often function relatively well into their fifties in the absence of any significant complications of the initial treatment. Carney et al. stated that *in situ* fixation is the procedure of choice, regardless of slip magnitude, because of its long-term functional and radiographic outcomes and low risk of complications. Despite the presumed accuracy of the data, their interpretation may be incorrect because of an inherent bias involved in the selection of cases: *in situ* fixation was used to treat milder cases of SCFE and realignment procedures used to treat more severe cases of SCFE. *In situ*

fixation cannot be recommended over realignment in severe cases of SCFE unless *in situ* fixation has demonstrably better results in the treatment of such severe cases.

Other authors cite a more guarded long-term prognosis following *in situ* fixation. Ross et al. reported good or excellent results in patients without intraoperative complications at 10- to 20-year follow-up, but fair to poor results in 10 of 15 hips (67%) at more than 20-year follow-up. One potential reason for this difference, in addition to increased duration of follow-up and potential bias in selection, is that moderate and severe slips accounted for 40% of the hips followed up for less than 20 years and 53% of the hips followed up for more than 20 years. Ross et al. also noted that this deterioration seemed related to bilateral SCFE (248).

With current radiographic and surgical techniques, the complication rates following *in situ* fixation of cases with SCFE have decreased considerably. Much of this decrease is due to a reduction in the rates of ON and chondrolysis because of the recognition of the importance of proper pin or screw placement. *In situ* fixation is considered the treatment of choice for cases of SCFE of all degrees in most centers because of the relative simplicity of this extensively studied and well-documented technique (94,156,249,250).

## Author's Preferred Method

I use cannulated screw fixation for the initial treatment of all cases of SCFE, regardless of the slip stability and degree of displacement. I prefer to use a radiolucent table to pin a SCFE because I find the frog lateral image on a radiolucent table to be of superior quality to the true lateral obtained on a fracture table. I also find it easier and quicker to reposition the patient's leg (as is done with a radiolucent table) to obtain a lateral view than to move the fluoroscopy machine (as is necessary with a fracture table).

However, if a radiolucent table is used, care must be taken to rotate the affected hip internally until the patella is facing forward before obtaining an anteroposterior image of the hip when choosing a pin insertion point and directing the guide wire. Failure to do so will result in the pin being inserted with the hip in a degree of external rotation; as a result, when a true anteroposterior view is obtained, the screw will be seen to be located in the superior portion of the femoral head. Other potential disadvantages of using a radiolucent table are that obtaining a true lateral is more difficult, and that the guide wire may be bent as the hip is moved into the frog position. In order to obtain a true lateral radiograph on a radiolucent table, in addition to rotating the patient's hip, the patient's body must be tilted (rotated) toward the affected hip.

For a stable SCFE, I use one 7.3-mm cannulated screw with reverse-cutting threads. The starting point is on the anterior femoral neck, and I attempt to place the screw so that it is perpendicular to the physis on all views, is in a center-center position in the femoral head, and is 5 to 6 mm from the subchondral bone at its closest location when the hip is taken through a full range of motion intraoperatively.

Regardless of the duration of symptoms I treat a stable SCFE, as noted in the preceding text. It is important to remember, however, that there may be some differences in pin position and results depending on the duration of symptoms and the magnitude of the slip. As a rule, stable slips will be only mildly displaced in patients with only a few days or weeks of symptoms, and will be more displaced in patients with many months of symptoms. For a

mild slip, the starting point on the anterior femoral neck will be more distal and the screw will be inserted more horizontally than for a more displaced slip because of the posterior direction of the slip. Because the screw in a more severe slip has a more proximal starting point and often has to traverse a shorter distance in order to fix the physis, a more severe SCFE is often less difficult to pin than a very mild slip, if the correct starting point is used.

For an unstable SCFE (as classified in preceding text), I generally use a single, cannulated 7.3-mm screw as well. However, if a slip is noted to be markedly unstable at the time of surgery—with gross movement or a significant change in alignment—I prefer to use two screws. The decision to use two screws is arbitrary, although I believe that the added stability is worthwhile in markedly unstable slips, despite the increased risk of pin penetration.

For an unstable slip, unlike the treatment of a stable SCFE, I place a temporary guide wire across the physis before checking a lateral x-ray film in order to assess the proximal femoral alignment before definitive fixation. Frequently, simply positioning the child on the radiolucent table with the patella directed anteriorly results in satisfactory alignment. However, if there is still marked displacement following this positioning, I will return the hip to an anteroposterior position on the fracture table, back the temporary pin out the epiphysis, and apply gentle traction and internal rotation. Fluoroscopic images are checked following this repositioning. Following stabilization of the epiphysis with the guide wire, the frog view may be rechecked. Once the alignment is deemed appropriate, then two screws are inserted with avoidance of the posterosuperior head.

I do not believe that current evidence is sufficient to support hip capsulotomy, although I do attempt an aspiration of the hip joint with an 18-gauge spinal needle for markedly unstable slips, since the risks of aspiration are small, although this is an arbitrary decision. Usually, only a few milliliters of blood can be aspirated without any clear evidence of significant pressure.

I believe that an early bone scan or MRI should be considered following unstable SCFE to evaluate for ON. If ON is detected prior to radiographic evidence of collapse, then treatment with a vascularized fibula graft may be considered.

Postoperatively, I allow children with stable SCFE to bear weight as tolerated. They are given crutches that are generally discarded by the time of the 1-week postoperative office visit. Sporting activities are allowed at 3 to 6 months postoperatively. I arbitrarily preclude children with unstable SCFE from full weight bearing for 3 to 4 weeks. In the absence of any evidence of ON, they resume sporting activities at 6 months postoperatively.

Following the first 2 months (during which I obtain x-ray films at 1 week, 1 month, and 2 months postoperatively), radiographic and clinical follow-up is continued every 3 months for at least the first year, and every 3 to

6 months thereafter until both proximal femoral physes are closed.

## Bone Graft Epiphysiodesis

The goal of bone graft epiphysiodesis, as with *in situ* fixation, is the prevention of slip progression. However, the way in which this is achieved with the two methods defer. Slip progression is prevented with bone graft epiphysiodesis primarily by hastening physeal closure, whereas *in situ* fixation prevents slip progression primarily by stabilizing the physis. Indications for bone graft epiphysiodesis include acute/unstable or chronic/stable SCFE of any magnitude, although some authors have conceded that cases of mild SCFE are better treated with *in situ* fixation (251).

Bone graft epiphysiodesis, which involves drilling across the physis into the epiphysis with placement of bone graft (most commonly autologous bone pegs), was first described in 1931 by Ferguson and Howorth (252). Although reported results have often been good (213,251, 253–260), this operation has been abandoned at many institutions because of potential for morbidity and technical difficulties (261–263).

The surgery may be performed through an anterior or an anterolateral approach and may be combined with osteoplasty of the anterior femoral neck (251,260,264). A 50-year experience with bone graft epiphysiodesis in 318 cases of SCFE presents this procedure as a "reasonable alternative" for the treatment of SCFE (253). Patients with acute SCFE are placed in a spica cast or brace postoperatively and kept without bearing weight for 6 to 8 weeks. Patients with chronic slips begin touch-down weight bearing 2 to 3 days postoperatively and bear weight progressively as the physeal closure progresses. Some authors have reported the time required until full weight bearing as averaging 10 weeks (259).

As reported in most series, surgical time (excluding casting, when necessary) averages 2 hours (213,259,262). Weiner et al. have reported estimated blood loss (EBL) for autologous bone peg epiphysiodesis of at least 200 mL in 52% (25 of 48) patients (259), and other authors have reported mean EBL ranging from 426 to 800 mL (261,262,265). When allograft is used instead of autograft, mean EBL has been reported as 360 mL (213).

Physeal closure following an autograft bone peg epiphysiodesis is reported to occur at 4 to 6 months by most authors (213,254,255,261,262). In a series of bone peg epiphysiodesis with allograft, a partial physeal closure was noted radiographically after an average of 11 weeks and complete closure after an average of 28 weeks, with physeal closure occurring in the operated hip before it occurred in the unoperated hip in all of the 16 unilateral cases (213).

Complications of this procedure include graft failure, failure to achieve physeal closure, slip progression, heterotopic ossification, lateral femoral cutaneous nerve (LFCN) palsy, donor site morbidity, chondrolysis, and

ON. Heterotopic ossification has been reported in up to 69% of patients (262). Despite intraoperative protection of the nerve, Ward et al. reported LFCN palsy in 10 out of 14 patients (71%) specifically examined for this finding postoperatively (265). Rao et al. reported transient LFCN palsy in 11% of their patients (262).

Graft complications following bone peg epiphysiodesis are well described. In two large series with very good results, Adamczyk et al. reported graft resorption with failure of epiphysiodesis in a period of 1 year in 4% of cases (12 of 318 hips) (253), and Howorth reported graft resorption in 2% of cases (4 of 200 hips), with no cases of progressive slip (254). In a series of 17 cases of SCFE, Ward and Wood reported "graft insufficiency," defined as graft movement, resorption, or fracture, in eight hips (47%) (265). Protrusion of the graft into the hip joint has also been reported (261).

The rate of ON associated with bone peg epiphysiodesis has generally been low, with most reports in the range of 0% to 6%, with higher rates in acute/unstable SCFE (213,253,254,262,264,265). Adamczyk reported an overall rate of 2%, with a risk of 7% in acute slips (3 of 45 cases) and 1.5% in chronic slips (4 of 273 cases) (253). The low rate of ON in bone peg epiphysiodesis is likely due to placement of the grafts from the anterolateral neck and into the center of the epiphysis, thereby avoiding the intraosseous blood supply.

Chondrolysis is reported to occur in 0% to 6% of the cases of SCFE treated with bone peg epiphysiodesis (213, 253,254,262,265). Most cases of chondrolysis occur in acute/unstable SCFE (253,262).

Progressive slip has been reported in 0% to 19% of cases following bone peg epiphysiodesis, with the highest risk being in acute SCFE (213,253,254). Although Rao et al. noted a change in the femoral head–shaft angle of at least 5 degrees in 42% of patients (27 of 64), the angle increased in 19% and decreased in 23% of the cases (262). One presumed reason for slip progression is that the bone graft does not stabilize (and may actually destabilize) the proximal femur as well as does a screw. Another potential cause of progressive slip in these patients is the delayed or incomplete physeal closure.

Femoral neck fracture has also been reported in 0% to 5% of cases following bone peg epiphysiodesis (213,253, 261). Schmidt et al. reported two proximal femoral fractures in a series of 40 bone peg epiphysiodeses (5%) (213), in striking contrast to Adamczyk et al (253)., who reported no fractures in a series of 318 bone peg epiphysiodeses.

Bone graft epiphysiodesis does not have significant advantages relative to *in situ* fixation of SCFE, although there are significant drawbacks to its use. Children treated with bone graft epiphysiodesis have greater blood loss, increased donor site morbidity, increased risk of nerve palsy, increased risk of slip progression, and are not allowed to bear weight as early as do those children undergoing *in situ* fixation. Bone graft epiphysiodesis does not appear to have a significant role in the treatment of SCFE in the 21st century.

## Proximal Femoral Osteotomy

Osteotomy in the treatment of SCFE can be classified in both temporal and anatomic terms. Temporally, osteotomies can be thought of as either early or delayed. Early osteotomies are undertaken as part of the primary treatment of SCFE in an attempt to restore a more normal anatomy as well as to prevent further slipping. These osteotomies require fixation across the physis in order to prevent progression. Late osteotomies are generally undertaken to correct residual deformity after physeal closure. Usually these are performed at least 1 year after the initial treatment if significant symptoms persist or if the anatomic derangement is felt to be severe enough to require treatment.

Anatomically, osteotomies may be classified as subcapital, femoral neck, or intertrochanteric (Fig. 26.9). The ability to correct the deformity is greatest with a subcapital osteotomy, least with a femoral neck osteotomy, and intermediate with an intertrochanteric osteotomy. The risk of ON is inversely related to the distance from the physis to the osteotomy, with subcapital osteotomies having the highest risk and intertrochanteric osteotomies having the lowest. Frymoyer reported ON in 30% of the femoral neck osteotomies compared to 0% of intertrochanteric osteotomies (266). Interestingly, Jerre et al. reported lower short-term complications but poorer long-term outcomes with intertrochanteric osteotomies compared to subcapital osteotomies (170).

Using computer modeling, previous authors have reported lower intraarticular contact stress in femoral neck osteotomy compared to intertrochanteric osteotomy (267). Although clearly still experimental, preoperative computer simulation of osteotomies has been suggested as an option to optimize the surgical planning for patients with SCFE (268).

Previous computer modeling (136) and clinical studies (136–140) have demonstrated the potential risks of femoroacetabular impingement, with resultant cartilage damage and/or labral tears, in hips with SCFE, especially in hips with more severe slips. After remodeling, as the range of motion increases, an increasing portion of the remodeled metaphysis becomes an intraarticular weight-bearing surface, potentially contributing to late OA (136). Although theoretical reasons and indications from some medium-term clinical studies argue that restoring a more normal osseous alignment may be beneficial to the hip in the long term (269,270), there are no clinical data in the literature to prove that such realignment results in enhanced long-term hip function or durability.

### Subcapital Osteotomy

Subcapital proximal femoral osteotomies have most commonly been described as a primary treatment of moderate to severe SCFE, with the goals of deformity correction and prevention of slip progression. Because they are performed at the level of deformity, subcapital osteotomies are the

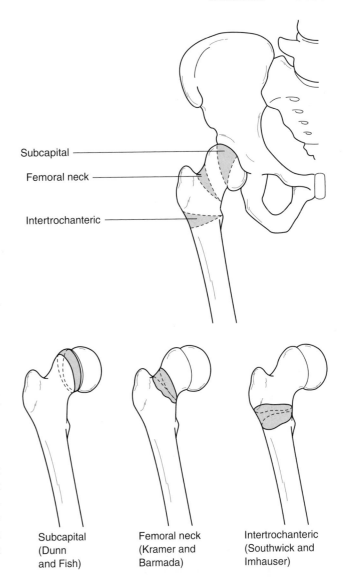

**Figure 26.9** The three levels of osteotomy to correct the proximal deformity following slipped capital femoral epiphysis (SCFE). The ability to correct the deformity is greatest with a subcapital osteotomy, least with a femoral neck osteotomy, and intermediate with an intertrochanteric osteotomy. The risk of osteonecrosis (ON) is inversely related to the distance from the physis to the osteotomy. Intertrochanteric osteotomies are currently the most commonly performed osteotomies because of the low rate of ON and the ability to obtain good correction.

most powerful osteotomies for deformity correction. These are very technically demanding operations, are associated with high rates of ON, and are rarely performed. As early as 1948, Martin noted the importance of avoiding tension on the posterior periosteal vessels in order to minimize the risk of ON (271). Subcapital osteotomies have been referred to as *orthopaedic roulette* because of their risky nature (272).

Fish has reported good to excellent results in 92% of patients following cuneiform subcapital osteotomy at a mean follow-up of 13 years (273,274). This surgery was limited to those with slips exceeding 30 degrees (273,274).

He noted the importance of removing all callus and physis in order to avoid tension on the posterior periosteum as the epiphysis is reduced onto the femoral neck, and also noted that this osteotomy should only be performed in hips with an open proximal femoral physis. He demonstrated excellent corrections with low rates of complications. Other reports of such excellent results following subcapital osteotomy are rare, although Nishiyama et al. reported 93% excellent results at a mean follow-up of 10 years in the cases of 15 patients with 18 SCFEs treated with cuneiform osteotomies (275).

Dunn (276) and Dunn and Angel (277) also described a transtrochanteric subcapital osteotomy which shortened the femoral neck and preserved the posterior blood supply to the femoral head. Even in Dunn's hands results were mixed, with good clinical results in only 55 of 73 hips (75%) and good radiographic results in only 41 (56%) of the hips at a mean follow-up of less than 9 years (277). Other authors following Dunn have reported mixed results and high rates of complications (170,263,278–281). Average EBL exceeding 500 mL has been reported (279).

Complications including ON, chondrolysis, OA, and LLD are common after subcapital femoral osteotomies (170,263,278–281). One exception is slip progression, which does not appear to have been reported following subcapital femoral osteotomy (273–277,279,282).

Chondrolysis has been reported in 3% to 42% of cases following subcapital osteotomies, with most authors reporting rates in the range of 3% to 18% (274–276,278–281,283). Dunn reported chondrolysis in 18% of his cases (13 of 73), with a rate of 17% in 24 in acute-on-chronic cases and 18% in 49 in chronic cases (276).

LLD is common following subcapital femoral osteotomy (274,275,281). Fish reported an LLD of at least 1 cm in 35% of patients (23 of 66) and of at least 2 cm in 6% (4 of 66) of patients treated with cuneiform subcapital osteotomy, with a maximum difference of 5 cm (274). Nishiyama et al. reported an average LLD of 1.5 cm in their series of subcapital osteotomies, ranging from 1 to 2 cm (275). Velasco et al. noted LLD of at least 1 cm in 6% and at least 2 cm in 3% of their patients (281).

Subcapital osteotomies are theoretically very appealing because of the powerful scope for correction they afford. However, because the learning curve is steep, complications are frequent and severe, and experience is necessary for good results, subcapital osteotomies are rarely used currently.

### Femoral Neck Osteotomy

In comparison to subcapital osteotomies, femoral neck osteotomies have less power to correct deformity but are also associated with a somewhat lower risk of ON. These osteotomies can be performed in the middle of the neck or at the base of the neck and may be performed as either a primary or a secondary treatment of SCFE. As with other proximal femoral osteotomies, the goal of femoral neck osteotomy is to restore a more normal proximal femoral alignment.

Because these osteotomies are somewhat distant from the deformity, maximum correction may be incomplete in moderate to severe slips. Despite the incomplete correction of the underlying deformity, proponents note that sufficient correction can be obtained to significantly improve hip alignment and biomechanics (284–286).

Osteotomy at the base of the femoral neck may be intracapsular or extracapsular (284–286). Care must be taken to preserve the posterior blood supply to the femoral head. Extracapsular osteotomies have the theoretical benefit of a decreased risk of ON, although they are less able to correct the underlying deformity because of their more distal location (284,285). In a series of 36 extracapsular osteotomies, Abraham et al. reported 89% good to excellent results and no cases of ON at an average follow-up of 9 years (284).

Complications of femoral neck osteotomies include unrecognized pin penetration, chondrolysis, ON, hardware failure, LLD, joint space narrowing, and OA. Gage et al. have noted decreasing rates of both ON and chondrolysis with more distal osteotomies (283). Even with attempts to preserve the blood supply, ON has been reported in up to 10% of cases following femoral neck osteotomy (283). Chondrolysis has been reported in 2% to 10% of the base-of-neck osteotomies for SCFE (284,285).

In a series of 56 intracapsular osteotomies, Kramer et al. reported two cases of pin penetration and an 11% reoperation rate (286). Barmada et al. reported one case each of loss of fixation and joint penetration by hardware in their study of a series of 20 hips (285). Joint space narrowing has been noted in 10 of 11 hips (91%) followed up for at least 13 years in one series (284).

Base-of-neck osteotomy has been reported to lead to LLD of at least 1 cm in 61% of patients and at least 2 cm in 42% (15 of 36 patients) (284). Three patients in the same series (8%) had LLD of at least 4 cm, and in male adolescents with at least 3 years of growth remaining, unilateral SCFEs were noted to lead to LLD of 3 to 5 cm (284).

Currently, the trend is away from femoral neck osteotomies and toward intertrochanteric osteotomies because of the technical difficulties of femoral neck osteotomies, their risk of complications, and the limited ability to completely correct the deformity.

### Intertrochanteric Angular Osteotomy

Intertrochanteric osteotomies are currently the most commonly performed osteotomy for SCFE. Such osteotomies are generally performed after physeal closure in patients with significant limitations in the range of motion, significant pain, and/or marked proximal femoral deformity. The most common intertrochanteric osteotomies are angular osteotomies described by Southwick and by Imhauser (115,287–290,291). These osteotomies are generally fixed with plates, but use of external fixation has also been reported (292,293).

Angular osteotomies may be uniplanar, biplanar, or triplanar. The three common components of the osteotomy are valgus, flexion, and internal rotation. The degree of correction is based on anatomic alignment, range of motion deficit, and patient complaints. The Southwick osteotomy is the most commonly performed intertrochanteric osteotomy in North America, and the Imhauser osteotomy is more popular in Europe. Southwick described a valgus and flexion osteotomy to which internal rotation of the distal fragment is generally added (115,287–290). Therefore, Southwick osteotomies are generally triplanar osteotomies. Imhauser described a biplanar flexion and internal rotation osteotomy without valgus. A "reverse" Imhauser osteotomy has been reported for the uncommon valgus SCFE (294). With either type of intertrochanteric osteotomy, significant internal rotation of the distal fragment must usually be performed in order to restore both proximal femoral anatomy and a more normal rotational arc of motion.

Recommendation for intertrochanteric osteotomy can be made on the basis of clinical signs and symptoms or on a biomechanical basis in an attempt to normalize proximal femoral anatomy with the theoretical decrease in the long-term risk of OA. Clinical indications for intertrochanteric osteotomy may include hip and/or groin pain with prolonged sitting (owing to femoral neck impingement on the acetabulum) and difficulty in performing activities because of the abnormal arc of hip motion. Lack of hip flexion and internal rotation may make routine activities such as sitting in a chair, climbing stairs, riding a bicycle or scooter, donning and doffing socks, and cutting one's toenails difficult or impossible. A significant varus deformity of the proximal femur may result in significant abductor weakness, with a persistent Trendelenburg gait and fatigue pain with ambulation. If the recommendation for intertrochanteric osteotomy is based on clinical signs and symptoms, the physician should wait at least one year following *in situ* fixation to be certain that such signs and symptoms do not spontaneously improve.

Increasingly, a recommendation for proximal femoral osteotomy is being made on a biomechanical basis regardless of the patient's symptomatology. The argument for such surgery is the increasing body of knowledge that OA is more common and more severe in the more severe cases of SCFE, even in the absence of short-term complications (94,96,116,156,158,159). In addition, biomechanical modeling studies have shown that the deformity associated with SCFE would place patients with SCFE at long-term risk of OA (136). A SCFE can result in the anterior femoral metaphysis articulating with acetabular cartilage and can also cause impingement of the femoral neck against the anterior acetabulum (136). Two recent studies have reported an apparent decrease in the expected rate of OA following a realignment at a follow-up of more than 20 years (269,270). Despite these results there are currently no long-term clinical data that conclusively demonstrate advantages of routine proximal femoral osteotomy in patients followed into middle and old age (86,295,296).

The amount of correction necessary depends on the degree of deformity and the clinical arc of motion. As a result, the amount of correction noted at follow-up may vary with patient selection criteria. In one series of Southwick osteotomies, Salvati et al. noted a mean increase in internal rotation of 33 degrees and an abduction of 17 degrees at follow-up (297).

Overall, the results of intertrochanteric osteotomies have been good, with acceptable rates of complications. At a follow-up at least 5 years after the surgery, Southwick reported excellent or good results in 93% of the patients (115), and 13 years later the long-term follow-up results were reported as good or excellent in 87%, although the precise duration of the follow-up was not specified (287). Other authors have reported good to excellent clinical results in 80% to 85% of patients who were followed up for 5 to 10 years, with good radiographic results in about 60% (298,299). Other authors who reported poor results noted that the poor results were seen in conjunction with insufficient surgical correction of the underlying deformity (300).

Similarly, good clinical results have been reported with Imhauser osteotomies, with Parsch et al. reporting good or very good results in 92% of the hips operated on from 1975 to 1982, and an average Iowa hip score exceeding 90 in patients operated on subsequently (301).

Intertrochanteric osteotomies, despite their low risk of ON, are noted to have other significant complications including chondrolysis, delayed union, need for reoperation, late arthritis, LLD, and fracture. Because these osteotomies are typically performed after physeal closure, progressive slip does not occur.

Chondrolysis has been reported in 2% to 25% of hips following intertrochanteric osteotomies, although rates up to 59% have been reported in small series (115,228,266, 287,297,298,301). Delayed unions have been reported in up to 3% or 4% of the hips following intertrochanteric osteotomy in several series (270,297,299). Loss of fixation has been reported in 4% to 6% of cases in some series 297,300). Fractures are not reported in most series following osteotomy, but were reported in 6% of 130 cases of intertrochanteric osteotomies in one series (301).

LLD following intertrochanteric osteotomy is well described. However, because a Southwick intertrochanteric osteotomy includes a valgus component, it is believed to lead to less LLD than other osteotomies. LLD following Southwick osteotomy has been reported in 19% to 26% of the cases, with a maximum LLD of 2 cm (297,299,300). The operated leg was short in 15% to 19% of patients in these series and was long in 0% to 11% (297,299,300). Schai et al. reported LLD in 81% of patients (38 of 47) following Imhauser osteotomy, with the affected leg being an average of 0.9 cm short in 35 patients and being 0.5 to 2.0 cm long in the other three patients (270).

At a mean of 24 years following Imhauser intertrochanteric osteotomy, Schai et al. reported moderate OA in 28% of the hips and severe OA in 17% (270). Jerre et al.

reported 36% good to excellent results in 11 hips at long-term follow-up averaging 36.1 years, although radiographic and surgical techniques have advanced significantly in the interim (170). One of these 11 patients (9%) was found to have undergone salvage surgery by the time of long-term follow-up (170).

Intertrochanteric osteotomies are currently the most common osteotomies performed on children with SCFE. These osteotomies can be challenging in these very large, heavy patients with significant deformity. Intertrochanteric osteotomies are also somewhat limited in their ability to correct the deformity because of their considerable distance from the site of deformity. Despite incomplete correction, there is generally sufficient correction to allow for good clinical outcomes with an acceptably low rate of complications (Fig. 26.10).

In asymptomatic patients with severely affected slips, the role of osteotomy is unclear. The real question to consider in such patients is whether they are best served by an osteotomy in adolescence, with its attendant risks, in an attempt to delay or avoid total hip arthroplasty (THA). One of the confounding variables in such an evaluation is that it is impossible to be certain what impact the advances in THA or basic science (such as gene manipulation) may have on the long-term outcomes of SCFE and OA in the coming decades.

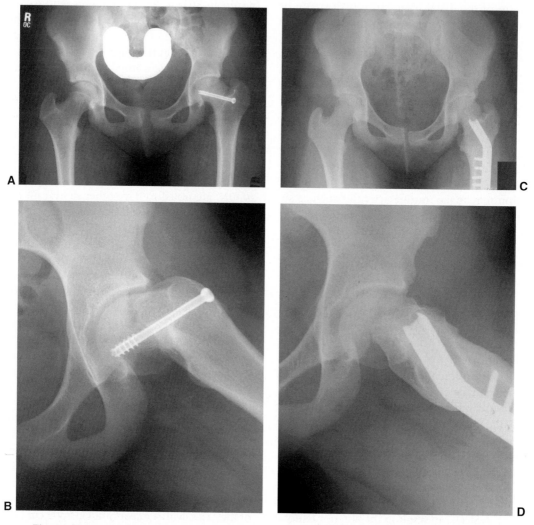

**Figure 26.10** A 13-year-old girl presented with pain on sitting and difficulty riding a bike because of external rotation of the left hip 16 months following *in situ* fixation. Anteroposterior pelvis (**A**) and lateral (**B**) radiographs of the left hip show the residual deformity 16 months following pinning. Lateral x-ray film shows the proximal femoral metaphysis articulating with the acetabulum preoperatively. Anteroposterior (**C**) and lateral (**D**) radiographs show the alignment 1 year after triplanar (flexion-valgus-internal rotation) osteotomy. Following redirectional osteotomy, there is an increased neck–shaft angle, with distal and slightly lateral translation of the greater trochanter (with a resultant increase in the articulotrochanteric distance), and the relation of the femoral head and acetabulum has changed. The metaphysis is no longer intraarticular. A downside of the surgery is that if total hip arthroplasty is necessary in the future, distortion of the proximal femoral anatomy will make such a replacement more difficult.

## *Transtrochanteric Rotational Osteotomy*

Sugioka described a rotational intertrochanteric osteotomy for correction of significant residual proximal femoral deformity following SCFE (302,303). Sugioka states that such an osteotomy is indicated for SCFE with a displacement greater than 45 degrees, based on the head–shaft angle measurement (303). Although this osteotomy has the potential to significantly enhance the anatomic alignment, it is quite demanding technically and is rarely used.

Sugioka reported 90% excellent results in 10 cases of SCFE treated with this method, with an improved range of motion of the hip in 90% of the patients (303). One case of ON was reported among these 10 hips. Sugioka noted postoperative valgus in three hips that had marked deformity preoperatively.

Another series of five hips has been described, with complications in two patients (40%) (304). One patient had ON and the other had loss of fixation. At less than 3 years mean follow-up, four hips were clinically asymptomatic. No cases of chondrolysis have been reported in the literature in the two small series (a total of 15 patients) of transtrochanteric rotational osteotomies in children with SCFE (303,304).

Although the results with this technique appear promising, the technique is demanding, complications are common, and its use has been reported in only a few centers.

## *Author's Preferred Method*

I currently reserve proximal femoral osteotomies for those patients with significant signs and/or symptoms that persist at least 1 year following *in situ* fixation. Most commonly, these include hip and/or groin pain with prolonged sitting (owing to femoral neck impingement on the acetabulum) and functional limitations due to loss of the hip range of motion. Although such signs and symptoms are common in the first few months following *in situ* fixation, they often improve within 1 year of pinning. If such limitations persist and affect a patient's quality of life, I will perform an osteotomy.

I prefer performing an intertrochanteric osteotomy, because I believe that an osteotomy at this level provides the best ratio of deformity correction to risk. I generally perform a triplanar proximal femoral osteotomy using a blade plate with correction in the planes of valgus, flexion, and internal rotation.

I do not perform prophylactic osteotomies in asymptomatic patients with moderate or severe slips. I currently think that the risks of such osteotomies in asymptomatic patients are too great relative to the uncertain potential for long-term gains, especially given the anticipated ongoing advances in the fields of orthopaedics and basic science during the lifetime of these children. In addition, asymptomatic patients who undergo proximal femoral osteotomy are generally made clinically worse for at least the first 6 months following a proximal femoral osteotomy.

## Prophylactic Pinning

Prophylactic pinning of the uninvolved hip remains an area of significant controversy in the management of children with SCFE. Recent authors have attempted to weigh the risks and benefits and their recommendations are conflicting. Proponents of prophylactic pinning cite the high rates of bilateral SCFE, the increased risk of OA in patients with SCFE at long-term follow-up, and the decreased risks of prophylactic pinning as technology and techniques improve (10,247,305,306). Schultz et al. indicated that prophylactic pinning of the contralateral hip in cases with unilateral SCFE would appear to be beneficial in terms of long-term Iowa hip scores, but cautioned that clinical judgment and patient preferences should be used on a case-by-case basis (307).

Opponents of prophylactic pinning cite the complications of prophylactic treatment, noting the potential risks of pinning numerous hips that will never slip, and also pointing out that with appropriate patient counseling and close follow-up most subsequent slips will be detected while still mild. Previous authors have reported complication rates of up to 34% with prophylactic pinning of possible SCFEs, although the techniques and results in these studies would not be considered acceptable by current standards (209,243,308). In fact, in one recent study of 94 hips treated with prophylactic pinning, there were no complications (10).

When considering the risks and benefits of prophylactic pinning in unilateral SCFE, it is important to consider the data regarding the risk of contralateral SCFE, the anticipated severity and stability of such a slip, and the risks and benefits of observation and of prophylactic treatment. An important consideration in prophylactic pinning is that because the distance the screw must traverse in an unslipped hip is much greater than the distance in a moderate to severe SCFE, there is actually less room for error in selecting the starting point and the angle of screw insertion. This geometry dictates that for every few degrees of deviation from the optimal path, the tip of the screw will be more eccentric in the epiphysis in a mild slip (or in a hip that has not slipped) than it would be in a severe slip (Fig. 26.11).

As noted earlier, in children without any evident systemic causes of SCFE, bilateral SCFE is present in approximately 20% at the time of initial presentation, is identified in another 15% to 20% in adolescence, and is present at long-term follow-up in approximately 60% (9–13,19,25, 27–30,76,94–96,101, 107,116,156,235,305,309,310). These data indicate that in the 80% of the patients who present with unilateral SCFE, 20% to 25% will develop a contralateral SCFE in adolescence, and half of the 80% will develop a second SCFE by the time of long-term follow-up. It can be inferred from these data that the probability of a contralateral slip first being recognized after adolescence is 25% to 30%. It is likely that these represent minimal, asymptomatic slips that were not recognized during adolescence.

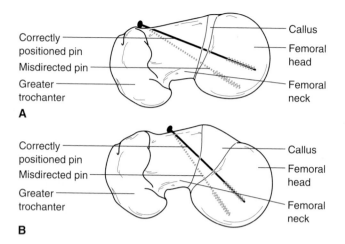

**Figure 26.11** Despite an accurate starting point on the anterior femoral neck, if the angle of insertion varies from the optimal angle, the hardware will not be perpendicular to the physis and will be eccentric in the femoral head. For a given degree of misdirection, the biomechanical alignment and eccentricity in the femoral head will be worse for a mild slip (**A**) than it will be for a more severe slip (**B**) because of the longer distance the screw must traverse in a mild slip. These problems are most pronounced for a pre-slip, or a hip that is pinned prophylactically.

Because the risk of major complications is closely tied to the stability of the SCFE, it is also important to estimate the frequency of unstable contralateral metachronous slips. Because 20% to 25% of those presenting with unilateral SCFE will develop a contralateral slip during adolescence, and because 5% to 10% of the SCFEs are unstable, the risk of a contralateral, unstable SCFE occurring during adolescence is 1% to 2%. With appropriate counseling about the risk of contralateral SCFE and potential signs and symptoms thereof, the risk of unstable contralateral SCFE may be even less.

For stable contralateral SCFE, progression to a moderate or severe contralateral SCFE during adolescence should also be low if there is no underlying systemic cause of SCFE and the child is compliant with follow-up (Fig. 26.12). Most contralateral SCFEs initially noted at the time of long-term radiographic follow-up are also quite mild.

Summarizing these data, it appears that prophylactic pinning of all hips will potentially prevent two complications: ON due to unstable SCFE and late OA. Given the data provided in preceding text, prophylactic pinning will only prevent ON in 1% or fewer of all contralateral hips even if the rate of ON in unstable SCFE is as high as 50%. Prophylactic pinning of contralateral hips in children with unilateral SCFE would potentially decrease OA by 9% in the contralateral hips of these patients, based on Hagglund's report of radiographic evidence of OA in 27% of hips (28 of 104) with SCFE compared with 9% of control hips (9 of 101) at a mean follow-up of 33 years and based on his report that the risk of metachronous contralateral SCFE is approximately 50% (28). Further, Hagglund noted that no hip with a mild or moderate slip treated with

*in situ* pinning developed arthritis before the age of 50 years. Because most patients with appropriate follow-up would likely be diagnosed before a severe contralateral slip develops, OA occurring before 50 years of age would be expected to be unusual in contralateral hips (247). Chondrolysis will not be prevented because chondrolysis occurs almost exclusively in treated hips.

These potential benefits of prophylactic fixation must be weighed against the frequency of its potential complications, including those of chondrolysis (2%), ON (1%), and proximal femoral fracture (1%). It is also important to recognize that slip progression occurs postoperatively in 0% to 3% of the cases of SCFE in most of the series of SCFE treated with *in situ* fixation (2,94,97,205,209,232,233).

Prophylactic pinning is commonly performed in certain patient groups. Prophylactic pinning should be performed for children with underlying endocrine disease because of their high rate of contralateral slip. Previous pelvic radiation, which included the contralateral hip in the field, is another indication for prophylactic pinning. Prophylactic pinning should be strongly considered in children younger than 10 years at the time of presentation because of potential LLD following unilateral pinning and the high risk of bilateral involvement in such young children (25,311). In addition, children residing in more remote areas, who do not have easy access to medical care, should be considered for prophylactic fixation of the contralateral hip. In children with renal disease, medical management rather than prophylactic pinning is recommended.

## Femoral Neck Osteoplasty

Prominence of the anterosuperior femoral neck following SCFE has been cited as a cause for decreased hip flexion, abduction, and internal rotation (312). Femoral neck osteoplasty involves removal of the prominent anterosuperior femoral neck and may be performed alone or in combination with other procedures, such as proximal femoral osteotomies (115,312,313). The goals of such treatment are to enhance hip range of motion and/or to potentially prevent anterior femoroacetabular impingement and OA (141).

A potential indication for osteoplasty is a prominent anterosuperior femoral neck which abuts the acetabulum in cases of chronic SCFE (264,313). Symptoms that may suggest the potential benefit of osteoplasty include pain on sitting caused by the impingement with hip flexion.

If performed in isolation, osteoplasty leaves unchanged the abnormal relation between the femoral head, neck, and shaft, with relative retroversion, extension, and varus. Because the anatomic relation between the femoral head, neck, and shaft are not changed by osteoplasty, isolated osteoplasty will still result in impingement of the anterior femoral neck against the acetabulum and persistent range of motion deficits. Previous authors have noted that

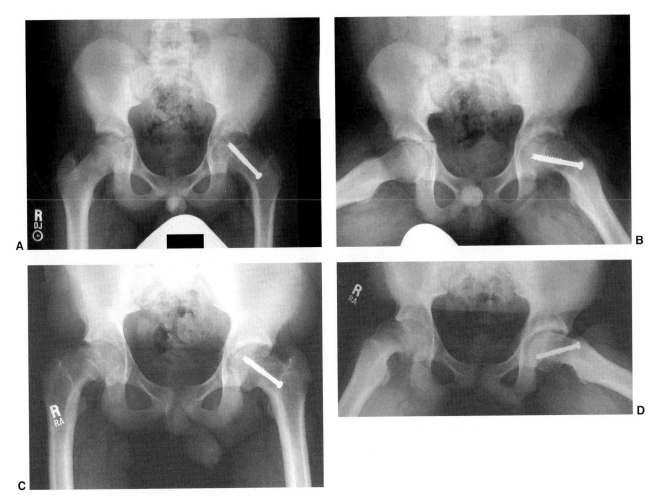

**Figure 26.12** Anteroposterior **(A)** and frog lateral **(B)** radiographs show a left slipped capital femoral epiphysis (SCFE) following *in situ* fixation with a single cannulated screw. The hardware is aligned adequately. Anterior metaphyseal prominence is evident. Right hip pain began several months later, although the child did not return to the orthopaedist for more than 1 year. At the time of re-presentation, Anteroposterior **(C)** and frog lateral **(D)** radiographs demonstrate marked slip of the previously normal right hip. Significant remodeling of the left hip (including resorption of the metaphyseal prominence) is visible, although there is no significant change in the femoral head–neck angle. This case exemplifies the importance of expert clinical and radiographic follow-up of children with SCFE until closure of the proximal femoral physes.

osteoplasty may further enhance hip range of motion following intertrochanteric osteotomies (115,312,313).

Osteoplasty is rarely performed today. If surgery is performed for patients with symptomatic anterior impingement and/or significantly distorted proximal femoral anatomy, proximal femoral osteotomies are much more commonly recommended in an attempt to restore more normal proximal femoral alignment and range of motion.

## COMPLICATIONS

The most important factor in the long-term outcome in cases of SCFE is avoidance of complications. Hall noted that complications were the only factor that seemed to lead to an early poor result (172). Previous authors have reported that the results of treated SCFE were often worse than those of untreated SCFE because of the lack of catastrophic complications in untreated hips (29,159,314).

Natural history studies confirm that most children who have an uncomplicated course following a SCFE function well until at least the 5th decade. At a mean follow-up of 41 years, Carney and Weinstein reported Iowa hip scores of at least 80 in 26 of 31 hips (84%) (157). At a mean follow-up of 37 years, Ordeberg et al. reported that, of 49 cases of SCFE, only "a few" patients had restrictions regarding their work or social lives, and that only 2 of the 49 (4%) had required surgery for arthritis (159).

Complications of SCFE may occur immediately or later. The late complications include OA, ON, and chondrolysis. OA is a nearly inevitable late sequela of SCFE whether treated or not, whereas ON and chondrolysis are often devastating complications that occur almost exclusively following treatment of SCFE.

## Osteoarthritis

OA appears to be an essentially universal sequela of both treated and untreated SCFE because any significant biomechanical derangement of the hip joint can lead to OA if the affected individual reaches old age. The prevalence and severity of OA increases with the increased time to follow-up and increased slip severity. The complications of chondrolysis and ON markedly accelerate the development of OA, with OA occurring in adolescents and young adults who have a history of these serious complications (96).

Biomechanical modeling studies have shown that the deformity associated with SCFE would place the patients with SCFE at long-term risk of OA (136). A SCFE can result in the anterior femoral metaphysis articulating with acetabular cartilage and can also cause impingement of the femoral neck against the anterior acetabulum (136). As noted earlier, in an attempt to potentially decrease this long-term risk of arthritis from such mechanical malalignment, some authors use such biomechanical studies to advocate early osteotomies in children with significant residual deformity following SCFE (86,269,270, 295,296).

Long-term studies show significantly increased rates of OA in patients with a history of SCFE (28,94,212). Many authors have also reported increasing rates of OA with increasing degrees of SCFE at long-term follow-up (94,96, 116,156,158,159). Hagglund noted that no hip with a mild or moderate slip treated with *in situ* pinning developed arthritis before 50 years of age (247).

Despite SCFE affecting between 1 in 1000 and 1 in 2000 persons, only 2% to 9% of those with end-stage OA have been reported to have a history of SCFE (160–164). Studies of adults undergoing THA have shown that up to 40% of these patients have evidence of pediatric hip disease, including SCFE, at the time of joint arthroplasty (167). Radiographic studies of adult hips also demonstrate the stigmata of pediatric hip disease in up to 40% of those with findings of OA (166). Not all authors agree with these studies, and some have noted that these radiographic findings are common in end-stage OA of various etiologies (168).

As noted previously, severe deformity following SCFE results in significant biomechanical changes in the hip because a portion of the proximal femoral metaphysis articulates with the acetabulum and leads to accelerated degenerative changes in the hip. Recent authors have sought to prevent late arthritis by restoring more normal proximal femoral anatomy by performing proximal femoral redirectional osteotomies (269,270). Although such authors report an apparent decrease in OA following realignment at follow-up beyond 20 years in each study (269,270), longer follow-up will be needed to know if these apparently superior results continue in the ensuing decades, and to decide whether such procedures are indicated in patients who are asymptomatic despite significant residual deformity.

In summary, OA appears to be an almost inevitable sequela of both treated and untreated SCFE, with earlier onset and more severe degeneration in high-degree slips. The complications of ON and chondrolysis greatly accelerate the development of OA and often lead to end-stage OA in adolescence.

## Osteonecrosis

ON is, along with chondrolysis, one of the two most serious complications encountered in the treatment of children with SCFE. ON is reported to occur in 4% to 25% of the cases of SCFE in most series and is found almost exclusively in hips classified as acute on a temporal basis or unstable (as classified by Loder). The rate of ON is most commonly reported as 10% to 15% in acute or acute-on-chronic SCFE (95,96,133,214).

There appear to be two main potential causes of ON in children with SCFE: disruption of the blood supply preoperatively and disruption of the blood supply due to the surgery itself. With current techniques, including recognition of the posterosuperior blood supply to the femoral head and the importance of accurate hardware placement, the risk of iatrogenic ON should decrease.

Whether or not the degree of slip influences the rate of ON in unstable SCFE is debated. In two series in which ON was noted to occur only in unstable SCFE, Kennedy et al. (173) reported that the degree of slip does not appear to be an independent predictor of ON, whereas Tokmakova et al. (174) reported that the degree of slip is a risk factor for developing ON. When considering this, however, the degree of displacement evident radiographically at the time of presentation may have no relation to the true amount of maximal displacement that has already occurred or will occur prior to operative stabilization.

In addition to the slip stability at presentation, the method of treatment affects the rate of ON. The incidence of ON following proximal femoral osteotomy is greatest with subcapital osteotomies and progressively decreases with more distal osteotomies (21,172,266,271,274,275, 277–280,282,283). Most authors report ON rates of 5% to 35% following subcapital osteotomy, with rates at times as high as 42% (21,271,274,275,277–280,282,283). Base-of-neck osteotomies result in ON in 0% to 5% of the cases (284–286). Most authors do not report any cases of ON following intertrochanteric osteotomy for SCFE (115,266, 298,299), although rates of up to 6% have been reported (270,297,300,301).

ON occurs in 0% to 5% of patients treated with *in situ* pinning, with rates most commonly at 2% to 3% in recent series (2,187–190,193,196,205,229,315). The rate of ON reported following bone peg epiphysiodesis is generally between 0% and 6% (213,253,254,262,264,265).

Two recent studies report no cases of ON in a total of more than 50 cases of SCFE treated in spica casts (176,175). In these two series, the overall breakdown of slips was 76% chronic, 21% acute-on-chronic, and 3% acute. Many cases of ON previously associated with spica casting were likely due to a manipulative reduction prior to cast application and/or positioning in the cast.

The prognosis of ON associated with SCFE is poor, although it is better than the prognosis attributed to ON from other causes (316). In a series of 22 patients with 24 cases of SCFE complicated by ON, who were followed an average of 31 years, nine of the hips (38%) had required salvage treatment and the other 15 hips had osteoarthritic changes that were evident radiographically (316).

If ON is diagnosed prior to femoral head collapse, treatment is aimed at maintenance of the range of motion, prevention of progressive femoral head collapse, and joint preservation when possible. The combination of antiinflammatory medications, physical therapy, and protected weight bearing may be helpful in maintaining the range of motion and preventing progressive femoral head collapse. When femoral head collapse occurs in the area of previously placed screws, the screws must often be backed out or removed in order to prevent joint penetration and chondrolysis.

Joint-preserving procedures, including redirectional osteotomies (294,317–321), vascularized fibular grafting (224), and bone grafting procedures (322), have been reported following ON in children, although no large series has been reported specifically addressing ON following SCFE.

If ON is not diagnosed until after femoral head collapse, the long-term prognosis is significantly worse. With progressive collapse and joint degeneration, salvage procedures are often necessary.

In summary, ON is one of the devastating complications of SCFE. With the passage of time, hips with ON complicating SCFE will inexorably develop arthritic changes if left untreated. Even if ON is detected early, salvage procedures are often necessary for these hips. As a result, one of the prime goals in the treatment of SCFE should be the avoidance of ON.

### Author's Preferred Method

In patients with significant risks of ON—those who present with markedly displaced, unstable slips, and those with evidence of gross instability at the time of surgery—I recommend routine MRI screening for ON approximately 1 month following operative stabilization. Following MRI, those patients without ON can be allowed to bear weight as tolerated and return to sporting activities by 3 to 6 months postoperatively, as do those children with uncomplicated stable slips. For those with ON, the distribution and extent of femoral head involvement must be determined and further treatment (such as free vascularized fibular grafting or proximal femoral osteotomy) considered.

I do not routinely screen other children for ON. However, if a child initially does well in the weeks or months immediately after surgery and then begins to have recurrent hip symptomatology, ON must be considered. Alternatively,

ON may first be evident months after fixation on routine follow-up radiographs. In either suspected or documented ON, MRI is a critical part of a thorough evaluation.

It is important to remember that, although imperfect, treatment of ON carries a better prognosis when undertaken prior to femoral head collapse. I believe that free vascularized fibular grafting, despite donor site morbidity, is the most appropriate option for a hip with segmental ON involving the weight-bearing portion of the femoral head before femoral head collapse. If ON is not detected until after femoral head collapse occurs, then I would consider a redirectional femoral osteotomy if a sufficient pillar of viable bone can be moved into a weight-bearing position.

Whenever femoral head collapse occurs, it is important to remove any hardware that is protruding into the joint and to replace screws into another area of the head so long as the physis remains open.

If surgical intervention is not undertaken in children with ON, either because it is not indicated (as with severe collapse) or because such treatment is declined by the patient's family, conservative measures should be undertaken in an attempt to delay salvage treatment. Impact activities such as running, jumping, and ball sports should be avoided, whereas swimming and bicycling may be undertaken to maintain cardiovascular fitness, strength, and range of motion. Antiinflammatory medications and ambulatory aids may be beneficial as well, although these are often rejected by otherwise healthy adolescents and young adults.

## Chondrolysis

Although first described in conjunction with SCFE in 1930, chondrolysis remains poorly understood (323). Chondrolysis involves cartilage destruction of both the femoral head and the acetabulum, and is defined as the triad of pain, decreased hip range of motion, and radiographic joint space narrowing (Fig. 26.13). Normal cartilage thickness of the pediatric hip has been reported to decrease from a mean of 6 mm in children aged 1 to 7 years, to 5 mm in those aged 8 to 12 years, and to 4 mm in those aged 13 to 17 years (324). Chondrolysis has been reported to occur in 0% to 28% of patients with SCFE (4,94,100,187,189, 228,325–328).

Chondrolysis should be suspected if synovitis and hip range of motion are not improved in the first 2 to 3 weeks following surgery, and any child with decreasing range of motion postoperatively must be suspected of having chondrolysis. Unlike many other hip maladies, chondrolysis causes the hip to be held in abduction and ultimately results in a fixed abduction contracture.

Chondrolysis is more common in the female population than in the male population (228,230,329). Previously, chondrolysis was believed to be more common in black children (70,175,193,228,326,330), although more recent studies have refuted this assertion (188,190, 228,330,331). One series reported a higher incidence of chondrolysis in those of Hawaiian descent (327).

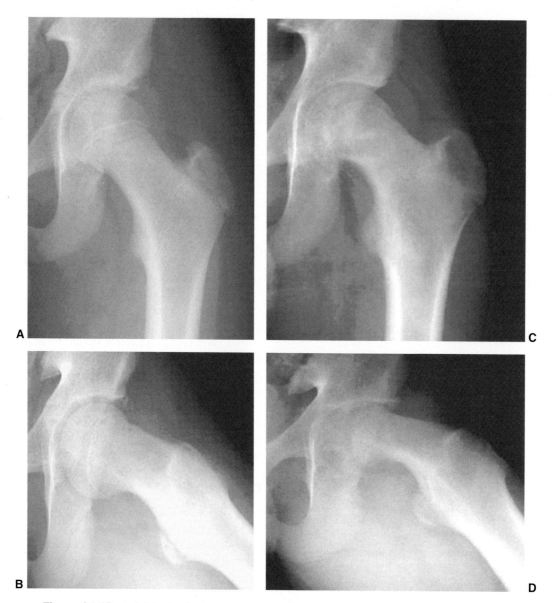

**Figure 26.13** Left hip chondrolysis in a 13-year-old boy. **A,B:** Normal joint space of the left hip when the patient presented with a right slipped capital femoral epiphysis (SCFE). Ten months later, the patient presented to the office with a one-month history of left hip pain. **C,D:** Radiographs at that time demonstrated a left SCFE and joint space narrowing. The left hip was pinned *in situ* with prompt symptom resolution. However, 2 months postoperatively the patient began to have increased hip pain, difficulty walking, and decreased hip range of motion. **E,F:** Radiographs at that time revealed mild additional joint space narrowing. This case demonstrates that joint space narrowing can occur without treatment, but that chondrolysis is not simply joint space narrowing. Rather, it is the triad of joint space narrowing, pain, and decreased range of motion.

Chondrolysis is seen following all forms of treatment and has also been reported to be present at the time of initial presentation in some patients (228,230). Maurer suggested that chondrolysis was more common with severe slips and with spica casting, open reduction, or prolonged casting (327). Ingram et al. noted that chondrolysis was more common in acute-on-chronic slips, and that the highest rates occurred with osteotomies and the lowest rates with *in situ* fixation (228). Chondrolysis

in the unaffected hip has been reported following immobilization (29,177).

Chondrolysis appears most common following treatment of SCFE with spica casting, with its incidence reported as 14% to 53% of the cases (94,175,176). Rates of chondrolysis are commonly reported as 3% to 18% following subcapital osteotomy (274–276,278–281,283), 2% to 10% following base-of-neck osteotomy (284,285), and 2% to 25% following intertrochanteric osteotomy (115,228,266,

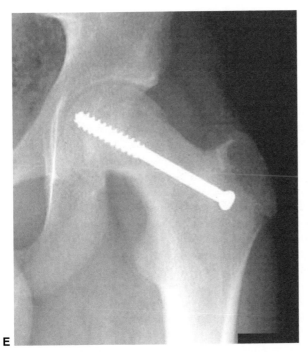

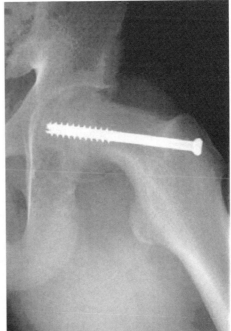

E

F

**Figure 26.13** *(continued)*

287,297,298,301). Reported rates of chondrolysis following *in situ* pinning and bone peg epiphysiodesis are most commonly less than 5% (2,21,94,116,187–190,193,196, 205,213,227,228,253,254,262,265).

In addition to narrowing of the joint space, radiographs may also reveal premature closure of the apophysis of the greater and lesser trochanters (228,332). Bone scan has been noted to demonstrate decreased activity in the apophysis of the greater trochanter in 47% of hips affected with chondrolysis, a finding that may precede radiographic changes (333). In cases with an unusual presentation, workup for a septic hip including joint aspiration may be indicated.

Chondrolysis varies from a relatively minor, self-limited condition from which full recovery may occur to the rapid destruction of a joint necessitating salvage treatment in teenagers (230,328,334). Despite decades of experience in treating children with chondrolysis, the reasons for such disparate prognoses remain unclear. When an individual patient presents with chondrolysis, it is still impossible to accurately predict the child's prognosis.

Treatment of chondrolysis is generally conservative, with a combination of protected weight bearing, physical therapy (for range of motion and attempted strengthening of the hip musculature), and oral antiinflammatory medications. Distraction of the hip joint with external fixation has been reported to be of value in selected cases (335). Failure of such conservative measures may require surgical intervention such as arthrodesis or arthroplasty.

Chondrolysis remains one of the most devastating complications of SCFE. Early recognition and treatment are indicated, but the prognosis following this complication is guarded. In patients unresponsive to conservative measures, salvage procedures may be necessary.

## SALVAGE PROCEDURES

Most hips with SCFE will function well into the 5th to 7th decades of life if the complications of chondrolysis and ON are avoided. Unfortunately, if treatment is complicated by chondrolysis and/or ON, rapid clinical deterioration may occur in adolescence or early adulthood. Significant symptomatology such as pain with sitting, with sleeping, and with activities of daily living may necessitate salvage treatment. In the child with such significant symptomatology following SCFE that has been complicated by ON, joint-preserving procedures including osteotomies, vascularized fibular grafting, and bone grafting procedures are sometimes possible, although such procedures are not beneficial in children with chondrolysis following SCFE because of their diffuse joint destruction.

If such significant symptoms are present in hips that are not good candidates for joint-sparing procedures, then salvage treatment with hip fusion or hip arthroplasty should be considered. The extent of hip disease in both hips is important in making the decision regarding hip arthrodesis versus arthroplasty. Patients can be thought of as falling into one of three categories: a unilateral salvage hip with a normal contralateral hip, a unilateral salvage hip with a mild contralateral SCFE, or bilateral salvage hips. In an adolescent with a unilateral salvage hip and either a normal contralateral hip or a mild contralateral

SCFE, either hip fusion or arthroplasty may be considered. Hip fusion should never be considered in a case with bilateral salvage hips.

Hip fusions have traditionally been the treatment of choice for a degenerated hip in adolescents with unilateral hip disease because of the poor long-term results of THA in heavy, young, active patients (336–339). Currently, many teenagers and their families are reluctant to accept the physical limitations associated with hip arthrodesis, despite the less than stellar results of hip arthroplasty in young patients.

An articulation between metal and ultrahigh-molecular-weight polyethylene has been the gold standard since the earliest total joint replacements. The long-term results in young patients have been inferior to those in older patients, with much of the loosening attributable to the generation of particulate debris and component loosening (161,338–341). New bearing surfaces such as those including highly cross-linked polymers, metal-on-metal, and ceramics have given hope to a new generation of surgeons and patients about the potential for hip arthroplasty in the young and active population. However, such promise is currently just that, and the current reality is that THA is expected to have a limited lifespan in this patient population and that multiple revisions will likely be necessary throughout adulthood.

Even with these constraints, hip fusion should only be considered if the contralateral hip is normal or has only a mild SCFE due to the increased demand that would be placed on the contralateral hip following hip fusion of the affected hip. Many procedures have been described for hip fusion including intraarticular and extraarticular fusion using a variety of fixation devices including screws, plates, and external fixation (342–347). The most common hip fusion technique in children currently is an intraarticular fusion with subtrochanteric osteotomy, which has been reported by multiple authors since it was first reported by Farkas in 1939 (344,348–350). This technique is felt to promote fusion because contact between the femoral head and acetabulum can be maximized and the long lever arm of the leg is avoided by performing the subtrochanteric osteotomy. With the typical deformity following SCFE and ON, optimizing the fit between femoral head and acetabulum would result in unacceptable positioning of the leg without subtrochanteric osteotomy. Further, the alignment of the leg can be readjusted postoperatively if needed.

The advantages of hip fusion include the durability of the fusion and the ability to return to full activity, including manual labor. Long-term results in studies with mean follow-up exceeding 35 years have been quite satisfying, although reported findings include back pain in 57% to 61%, ipsilateral knee pain in 45% to 57%, and contralateral hip pain in 17% to 27% (343,347). Conversion to total joint arthroplasty was reported in 13% to 21% in the two studies (343,347).

Other authors have reported results following the conversion of hip arthrodesis to THA (351–353). There is reliable relief of back, hip, or knee pain, although the results are not comparable to those with primary joint replacements. The results are also better in hips that have fused spontaneously than in those which have undergone surgical fusion. Technically, the conversion procedure is much easier and the results are better if the abductor musculature was not disturbed with the initial procedure.

In a child with bilateral salvage hips, arthrodesis is not an option and arthroplasty should be considered if symptoms are severe. The advantages of THA are the rapid restoration of motion and function without added stress across the contralateral hip, ipsilateral knee, and the spine. Because many of these patients are rather active, once the THA renders them essentially asymptomatic early failure is a frequent result. In a recent series of primary THA in patients 50 years and younger at implantation, THA survivorship was only 54% at 15-year follow-up (339). Others have reported actual or potential loosening in 57% of the prostheses at the 5-year follow-up in patients who had undergone THA prior to 30 years (337). One study of THA in patients aged less than 50 years reported more encouraging results, noting that the survivorship of the original prosthesis was 63% in patients living at least 25 years postoperatively (161).

If a significantly symptomatic joint that is not amenable to redirectional osteotomy needs salvage treatment, the two options that remain are THA and hip arthrodesis. Neither of these treatments has outstanding long-term results for the hip and the other joints of the lower extremity or for the spine. Currently, decisions continue to be made on a case-by-case basis to choose between THA (with better short-term hip function and less risk to other joints) and hip arthrodesis (with better long-term durability but more risk to the remainder of the lower extremities and spine). Promising technologic advances in bearing surfaces hold hope for the future of THA in young, active patients.

## Author's Preferred Method

Obviously, both hips must be considered when weighing the most appropriate salvage treatment of a given hip, as well as the current and future demands that would be placed upon the hip. As noted, hip arthrodesis or arthroplasty are both reasonable options in an adolescent with a unilateral salvage hip and no or mild contralateral hip disease, and arthroplasty is the only reasonable choice in a child with bilateral salvage hips.

I continue to be plagued by the decision between the two suboptimal options for treating a unilateral salvage hip in adolescents with SCFE. In the short term, the range of motion and rehabilitation benefits clearly favor arthroplasty. Although the patients can walk extremely well following arthrodesis, within several years of an arthrodesis they may have back and ipsilateral knee pain at the end of the day. These adolescents also often struggle with routine activities including donning and doffing socks, cutting toenails, riding a bicycle, and climbing stairs.

In the long term, the trade-offs are more difficult to define precisely. The risks of arthroplasty involve the affected hip itself, and can be marked and repetitive because of wear, loosening, and dislocation. In contrast, the complications of arthrodesis most frequently are resultant degeneration in the lumbar spine, ipsilateral knee, and contralateral hip. An additional confounding variable is the uncertainty of the future changes in orthopaedics and basic science, which may dramatically alter the implications of these long-term risks.

I am very reluctant to recommend arthroplasty in adolescents exceeding a weight of 200 pounds, given the high demands placed on such a joint. For those weighing less than 200 pounds, I discuss the options of both hip fusion and hip replacement, with the understanding that impact-type sporting activities must be avoided following either surgery. Some young women are not interested in arthrodesis because of concerns regarding sexuality and childbearing. Only the patient and family can make the ultimate decision between arthroplasty and arthrodesis.

# REFERENCES

1. Key JA. Epiphyseal coxa vara or displacement of the capital epiphysis of the femur in adolescence. *J Bone Joint Surg Am* 1926; 8:53–117.

## Epidemiology

2. Aronson DD, Carlson WE. Slipped capital femoral epiphysis. A prospective study of fixation with a single screw. *J Bone Joint Surg Am* 1992;74:810–819.
3. Bennet GC, Koreska J, Rang M. Pin placement in slipped capital femoral epiphysis. *J Pediatr Orthop* 1984;4:574–578.
4. Dreghorn CR, Knight D, Mainds CC, et al. Slipped upper femoral epiphysis—a review of 12 years of experience in Glasgow (1972–1983). *J Pediatr Orthop* 1987;7:283–287.
5. Henrikson B. The incidence of slipped capital femoral epiphysis. *Acta Orthop Scand* 1969;40:365–372.
6. Jacobs B. Diagnosis and natural history of slipped capital femoral epiphysis. *Instr Course Lect* 1972;21:167–173.
7. Jerre R, Billing L, Hansson G, et al. Bilaterality in slipped capital femoral epiphysis: importance of a reliable radiographic method. *J Pediatr Orthop B* 1996;5:80–84.
8. Kelsey JL. The incidence and distribution of slipped capital femoral epiphysis in Connecticut. *J Chronic Dis* 1971;23: 567–578.
9. Oram V. Epiphysiolysis of the head of the femur; a follow-up examination with special reference to end results and the social prognosis. *Acta Orthop Scand* 1953;23:100–120.
10. Seller K, Raab P, Wild A, et al. Risk-benefit analysis of prophylactic pinning in slipped capital femoral epiphysis. *J Pediatr Orthop* 2001;10:192–196.
11. Sorensen KH. Slipped upper femoral epiphysis. Clinical study on aetiology. *Acta Orthop Scand* 1968;39:499–517.
12. Hagglund G, Hansson LI, Ordeberg G. Epidemiology of slipped capital femoral epiphysis in southern Sweden. *Clin Orthop* 1984;191:82–94.
13. Jerre R, Karlsson J, Henrikson B. The incidence of physiolysis of the hip: a population-based study of 175 patients. *Acta Orthop Scand* 1996;67:53–56.
14. Kelsey JL, Keggi KJ, Southwick WO. The incidence and distribution of slipped capital femoral epiphysis in Connecticut and Southwestern United States. *J Bone Joint Surg Am* 1970;52: 1203–1216.
15. Loder RT. The demographics of slipped capital femoral epiphysis. An international multicenter study. *Clin Orthop* 1996;322: 8–27.
16. Loder RT, Farley FA, Herzenberg JE, et al. Narrow window of bone age in children with slipped capital femoral epiphyses. *J Pediatr Orthop* 1993;13:290–293.
17. Morsher E. Strength and morphology of growth cartilage under the hormonal influence of puberty. *Reconstr Surg Traumatol* 1968;10:3.
18. Puylaert D, Dimeglio A, Bentahar T. Staging puberty in slipped capital femoral epiphysis: importance of the triradiate cartilage. *J Pediatr Orthop* 2004;24:144–147.
19. Moreau MJ. Remodelling in slipped capital femoral epiphysis. *Can J Surg* 1987;30:440–442.
20. Wilson PD. The treatment of slipping of the upper femoral epiphysis with minimal displacement. *J Bone Joint Surg Am* 1938; 20:379–399.
21. Wilson PD, Jacobs B, Schecter L. Slipped capital femoral epiphysis: an End-Result study. *J Bone Joint Surg Am* 1965;47:1128–1145.
22. Brenkel IJ, Dias JJ, Davies TG, et al. Hormone status in patients with slipped capital femoral epiphysis. *J Bone Joint Surg Br* 1989; 71:33–38.
23. Kelsey JL, Acheson RM, Keggi KJ. The body build of patients with slipped capital femoral epiphysis. *Am J Dis Child* 1972; 124:276–281.
24. Wilcox PG, Weiner DS, Leighley B. Maturation factors in slipped capital femoral epiphysis. *J Pediatr Orthop* 1988;8:196–200.
25. Loder RT, Aronson DD, Greenfield ML. The epidemiology of bilateral slipped capital femoral epiphysis. A study of children in Michigan. *J Bone Joint Surg Am* 1993;75:1141–1147.
26. Siegel DB, Kasser JR, Sponseller P, et al. Slipped capital femoral epiphysis. A quantitative analysis of motion, gait, and femoral remodeling after in situ fixation. *J Bone Joint Surg Am* 1991;73: 659–666.
27. Blanco JS, Taylor B, Johnston CE II. Comparison of single pin versus multiple pin fixation in treatment of slipped capital femoral epiphysis. *J Pediatr Orthop* 1992;12:384–389.
28. Hagglund G, Hansson LI, Ordeberg G, et al. Bilaterality in slipped upper femoral epiphysis. *J Bone Joint Surg Br* 1988;70: 179–181.
29. Jerre T. A study in slipped upper femoral epiphysis. *Acta Orthop Scand* 1950;(Suppl. 6):1–157.
30. Billing L, Severin E. Slipping epiphysis of the hip; a roentgenological and clinical study based on a new roentgen technique. *Acta Radiol* 1959;51:1–76.
31. Brown D. Seasonal variation of slipped capital femoral epiphysis in the united states. *J Pediatr Orthop* 2004;24:139–143.
32. Loder RT. A worldwide study on the seasonal variation of slipped capital femoral epiphysis. *Clin Orthop* 1996;322:28–36.
33. Maffulli N, Douglas AS. Seasonal variation of slipped capital femoral epiphysis. *J Pediatr Orthop B* 2002;11:29–33.

## Etiology

34. Speer DP. The John Charnley Award paper. Experimental epiphysiolysis: etiologic models slipped capital femoral epiphysis. In: Nelson JP, ed. *The Hip: Proceedings of the Tenth Open Scientific Meeting of the Hip Society*. St. Louis, MO: CV Mosby Company, 1982: 68–88.
35. Loder RT, Wittenberg B, DeSilva G. Slipped capital femoral epiphysis associated with endocrine disorders. *J Pediatr Orthop* 1995;15:349–356.
36. McAfee PC, Cady RB. Endocrinologic and metabolic factors in atypical presentations of slipped capital femoral epiphysis. Report of four cases and review of the literature. *Clin Orthop* 1983;180:188–197.
37. Primiano GA, Hughston JC. Slipped capital femoral epiphysis in a true hypogonadal male (Klinefelter's mosaic XY-XXY). A case report. *J Bone Joint Surg Am* 1971;53:597–601.
38. Qadan L, Al-Quaimi M, Ahmad A. Slipped capital femoral epiphysis associated with primary hyperparathyroidism and severe hypercalcemia. *Clin Pediatr (Phila)* 2003;42:439–441.
39. Rennie W, Mitchell N. Slipped femoral capital epiphysis occurring during growth hormone therapy. Report of a case. *J Bone Joint Surg Br* 1974;56-B:703–705.
40. Zubrow AB, Lane JM, Parks JS. Slipped capital femoral epiphysis occurring during treatment for hypothyroidism. *J Bone Joint Surg Am* 1978;60:256–258.

41. Harris WR. The endocrine basis for slipping of the upper femoral epiphysis: an experimental study. *J Bone Joint Surg Br* 1950;32:5–11.

42. Hillman JW, Hunter WA Jr, Barrow JA III. Experimental epiphysiolysis in rats. *Surg Forum* 1957;8:566–571.

43. Oka M, Miki T, Hama H, et al. The mechanical strength of the growth plate under the influence of sex hormones. *Clin Orthop* 1979;145:264–272.

44. Williams JL, Vani JN, Eick JD, et al. Shear strength of the physis varies with anatomic location and is a function of modulus, inclination, and thickness. *J Orthop Res* 1999;17:214–222.

45. Benjamin B, Miller PR. Hypothyroidism as a cause of disease of the hip. *Am J Dis Child* 1938;55:1189–1211.

46. Burrow SR, Alman B, Wright JG. Short stature as a screening test for endocrinopathy in slipped capital femoral epiphysis. *J Bone Joint Surg Br* 2001;83:263–268.

47. Heatley FW, Greenwood RH, Boase DL. Slipping of the upper femoral epiphyses in patients with intracranial tumours causing hypopituitarism and chiasmal compression. *J Bone Joint Surg Br* 1976;58:169–175.

48. Heyerman W, Weiner D. Slipped epiphysis associated with hypothyroidism. *J Pediatr Orthop* 1984;4:569–573.

49. Hirano T, Stamelos S, Harris V, et al. Association of primary hypothyroidism and slipped capital femoral epiphysis. *J Pediatr* 1978;93:262–264.

50. Moorefield WG Jr, Urbaniak JR, Ogden WS, et al. Acquired hypothyroidism and slipped capital femoral epiphysis. Report of three cases. *J Bone Joint Surg Am* 1976;58:705–708.

51. Nicolai RD, Grasemann H, Oberste-Berghaus C, et al. Serum insulin-like growth factors IGF-I and IGFBP-3 in children with slipped capital femoral epiphysis. *J Pediatr Orthop B* 1999;8:103–106.

52. Wells D, King JD, Roe TF, et al. Review of slipped capital femoral epiphysis associated with endocrine disease. *J Pediatr Orthop* 1993;13:610–614.

53. Mann DC, Weddington J, Richton S. Hormonal studies in patients with slipped capital femoral epiphysis without evidence of endocrinopathy. *J Pediatr Orthop* 1988;8:543–545.

54. Razzano CD, Nelson C, Eversman J. Growth hormone levels in slipped capital femoral epiphysis. *J Bone Joint Surg Am* 1972;54:1224–1226.

55. Jingushi S, Hara T, Sugioka Y. Deficiency of a parathyroid hormone fragment containing the midportion and 1,25-dihydroxyvitamin D in serum of patients with slipped capital femoral epiphysis. *J Pediatr Orthop* 1997;17:216–219.

56. Hayes A, Batshaw ML. Down syndrome. *Pediatr Clin North Am* 1993;40:523–535.

57. Karlsson B, Gustafsson J, Hedov G, et al. Thyroid dysfunction in Down's syndrome: relation to age and thyroid autoimmunity. *Arch Dis Child* 1998;79:242–245.

58. Tuyusz B, Beker DB. Thyroid dysfunction in children with Down's syndrome. *Acta Paediatr* 2001;90:1389–1393.

59. Blethen SL, Rundle AC. Slipped capital femoral epiphysis in children treated with growth hormone. A summary of the National Cooperative Growth Study experience. *Horm Res* 1996;46:113–116.

60. Clayton PE, Cowell CT. Safety issues in children and adolescents during growth hormone therapy—a review. *Growth Horm IGF Res* 2000;10:306–317.

61. Rappaport EB, Fife D. Slipped capital femoral epiphysis in growth hormone-deficient patients. *Am J Dis Child* 1985; 139:396–399.

62. Weiner D. Pathogenesis of slipped capital femoral epiphysis: current concepts. *J Pediatr Orthop B* 1996;5:67–73.

63. Bright RW, Burstein AH, Elmore SM. Epiphyseal-plate cartilage. A biomechanical and histological analysis of failure modes. *J Bone Joint Surg Am* 1974;56:688–703.

64. Chapman JA, Deakin DP, Green JH. Slipped upper femoral epiphysis after radiotherapy. *J Bone Joint Surg Br* 1980;62:337–339.

65. Loder RT, Hensinger RN, Alburger PD, et al. Slipped capital femoral epiphysis associated with radiation therapy. *J Pediatr Orthop* 1998;18:630–636.

66. Fine RN, Ho M, Tejani A, et al. Adverse events with rhGH treatment of patients with chronic renal insufficiency and end-stage renal disease. *J Pediatr* 2003;142:539–545.

67. Loder RT, Hensinger RN. Slipped capital femoral epiphysis associated with renal failure osteodystrophy. *J Pediatr Orthop* 1997;17:205–211.

68. Mehls O, Ritz E, Krempien B, et al. Slipped epiphyses in renal osteodystrophy. *Arch Dis Child* 1975;50:545–554.

69. Oppenheim WL, Bowen RE, McDonough PW, et al. Outcome of slipped capital femoral epiphysis in renal osteodystrophy. *J Pediatr Orthop* 2003;23:169–174.

70. Eisenstein A, Rothschild S. Biochemical abnormalities in patients with slipped capital femoral epiphysis and chondrolysis. *J Bone Joint Surg Am* 1976;58:459–467.

71. Morrissy RT, Kalderon AE, Gerdes MH. Synovial immunofluorescence in patients with slipped capital femoral epiphysis. *J Pediatr Orthop* 1981;1:55–60.

72. Morrissy RT, Steele RW, Gerdes MH. Localised immune complexes and slipped upper femoral epiphysis. *J Bone Joint Surg Br* 1983;65:574–579.

73. Allen CP, Calvert PT. Simultaneous slipped upper femoral epiphysis in identical twins. *J Bone Joint Surg Br* 1990;72:928–929.

74. Burrows HJ. Slipped upper femoral epiphysis; characteristic of a hundred cases. *J Bone Joint Surg Br* 1957;39-B:641–658.

75. Gajraj HAR. Slipped capital femoral epiphysis in identical twins. *J Bone Joint Surg Br* 1986;68:653–654.

76. Green WT. Slipping of the upper femoral epiphysis: diagnostic and therapeutic considerations. *Arch Surg* 1945;50:19–33.

77. Hagglund G, Hansson LI, Sandstrom S. Familial slipped capital femoral epiphysis. *Acta Orthop Scand* 1986;57:510–512.

78. Montsko P, de Jonge T. Slipped capital femoral epiphysis in 6 of 8 first-degree relatives. *Acta Orthop Scand* 1995;66:511–512.

79. Moreira JF, Neves MC, Lopes G, et al. Slipped capital femoral epiphysis. A report of 4 cases occurring in one family. *Int Orthop* 1998;22:193–196.

80. Rennie AM. The inheritance of slipped upper femoral epiphysis. *J Bone Joint Surg Br* 1982;64:180–184.

81. Bednarz PA, Stanitski CL. Slipped capital femoral epiphysis in identical twins: HLA predisposition. *Orthopedics* 1998;21:1291–1293.

82. Diwan A, Diamond T, Clarke R, et al. Familial slipped capital femoral epiphysis: a report and considerations in management. *Aust N Z J Surg* 1998;68:647–649.

83. Gunal I, Ates E. The HLA phenotype in slipped capital femoral epiphysis. *J Pediatr Orthop* 1997;17:655–656.

84. Wong-Chung J, Al-Aali Y, Farid I, et al. A common HLA phenotype in slipped capital femoral epiphysis? *Int Orthop* 2000;24:158–159.

85. Gelberman RH, Cohen MS, Shaw BA, et al. The association of femoral retroversion with slipped capital femoral epiphysis. *J Bone Joint Surg Am* 1986;68:1000–1007.

86. Kordelle J, Millis M, Jolesz FA, et al. Three-dimensional analysis of the proximal femur in patients with slipped capital femoral epiphysis based on computed tomography. *J Pediatr Orthop* 2001;21:179–182.

87. Galbraith RT, Gelberman RH, Hajek PC, et al. Obesity and decreased femoral anteversion in adolescence. *J Orthop Res* 1987;5:523–528.

88. Mirkopulos N, Weiner DS, Askew M. The evolving slope of the proximal femoral growth plate relationship to slipped capital femoral epiphysis. *J Pediatr Orthop* 1988;8:268–273.

89. Kitadai HK, Milani C, Nery CA, et al. Wiberg's center-edge angle in patients with slipped capital femoral epiphysis. *J Pediatr Orthop* 1999;19:97–105.

90. Loder RT, Mehbod AA, Meyer C, et al. Acetabular depth and race in young adults: a potential explanation of the differences in the prevalence of slipped capital femoral epiphysis between different racial groups? *J Pediatr Orthop* 2003;23:699–702.

91. Kordelle J, Richolt JA, Millis M, et al. Development of the acetabulum in patients with slipped capital femoral epiphysis: a three-dimensional analysis based on computed tomography. *J Pediatr Orthop* 2001;21:174–178.

92. Chung SM, Batterman SC, Brighton CT. Shear strength of the human femoral capital epiphyseal plate. *J Bone Joint Surg Am* 1976;58:94–103.

93. Pritchett JW, Perdue KD. Mechanical factors in slipped capital femoral epiphysis. *J Pediatr Orthop* 1988;8:385–388.

## Clinical Features

94. Carney BT, Weinstein SL, Noble J. Long-term follow-up of slipped capital femoral epiphysis. *J Bone Joint Surg Am* 1991; 73:667–674.

95. Casey BH, Hamilton HW, Bobechko WP. Reduction of acutely slipped upper femoral epiphysis. *J Bone Joint Surg Br* 1972;54: 607–614.

96. Rattey T, Piehl F, Wright JG. Acute slipped capital femoral epiphysis. Review of outcomes and rates of avascular necrosis. *J Bone Joint Surg Am* 1996;78:398–402.

97. Loder RT, Richards BS, Shapiro PS, et al. Acute slipped capital femoral epiphysis: the importance of physeal stability. *J Bone Joint Surg Am* 1993;75:1134–1140.

98. Loder RT. Unstable slipped capital femoral epiphysis. *J Pediatr Orthop* 2001;21:694–699.

99. Peterson MD, Weiner DS, Green NE, et al. Acute slipped capital femoral epiphysis: the value and safety of urgent manipulative reduction. *J Pediatr Orthop* 1997;17:648–654.

100. Herman MJ, Dormans JP, Davidson RS, et al. Screw fixation of grade III slipped capital femoral epiphysis. *Clin Orthop* 1996; 322:77–85.

101. Cowell HR. The significance of early diagnosis and treatment of slipping of the capital femoral epiphysis. *Clin Orthop* 1966;48: 89–94.

102. Matava MJ, Patton CM, Luhmann S, et al. Knee pain as the initial symptom of slipped capital femoral epiphysis: an analysis of initial presentation and treatment. *J Pediatr Orthop* 1999;19: 455–460.

103. Ledwith CA, Fleisher GR. Slipped capital femoral epiphysis without hip pain leads to missed diagnosis. *Pediatrics* 1992;89: 660–662.

104. Skaggs DL, Roy AK, Vitale MG, et al. Quality of evaluation and management of children requiring timely orthopaedic surgery before admission to a tertiary pediatric facility. *J Pediatr Orthop* 2002;22:265–267.

105. Stanitski CL. Acute slipped capital femoral epiphysis: treatment alternatives. *J Am Acad Orthop Surg* 1994;2:96–106.

106. Loder RT, Greenfield ML. Clinical characteristics of children with atypical and idiopathic slipped capital femoral epiphysis: description of the age-weight test and implications for further diagnostic investigation. *J Pediatr Orthop* 2001;21:481–487.

## Radiographic Features

107. Klein A, Joplin RJ, Reidy JA, et al. Management of the contralateral hip in slipped capital femoral epiphysis. *J Bone Joint Surg Am* 1953;35-A:81–87.

108. Klein A, Joplin RJ, Reidy JA, et al. Roentgenographic features of slipped capital femoral epiphysis. *Am J Roentgenol* 1951;66: 361–374.

109. Steel HH. The metaphyseal blanch sign of slipped capital femoral epiphysis. *J Bone Joint Surg Am* 1986;68:920–922.

110. Billing L, Eklof O. Slip of the capital femoral epiphysis: revival of a method of assessment. *Pediatr Radiol* 1984;14:413–418.

111. Cohen MS, Gelberman RH, Griffin PP, et al. Slipped capital femoral epiphysis: assessment of epiphyseal displacement and angulation. *J Pediatr Orthop* 1986;6:259–264.

112. Loder RT. Effect of femur position on the angular measurement of slipped capital femoral epiphysis. *J Pediatr Orthop* 2001;21: 488–494.

113. Billing L, Bogren HG, Wallin J. Reliable X-ray diagnosis of slipped capital femoral epiphysis by combining the conventional and a new simplified geometrical method. *Pediatr Radiol* 2002;32:423–430.

114. Morrissy RT. General considerations. In: Morrissy RT, ed. *Slipped capital femoral epiphysis.* Rosemont, IL: American Academy of Orthopaedic Surgeons, 2002:1–18.

115. Southwick WO. Osteotomy through the lesser trochanter for slipped capital femoral epiphysis. *J Bone Joint Surg Am* 1967; 49:807–835.

116. Boyer DW, Mickelson MR, Ponseti IV. Slipped capital femoral epiphysis. Long-term follow-up study of one hundred and twenty-one patients. *J Bone Joint Surg Am* 1981;63:85–95.

117. Guzzanti V, Falciglia F. Slipped capital femoral epiphysis: comparison of a roentgenographic method and computed tomography in determining slip severity. *J Pediatr Orthop* 1991;11:6–12.

118. Umans H, Liebling MS, Moy L, et al. Slipped capital femoral epiphysis: a physeal lesion diagnosed by MRI, with radiographic and CT correlation. *Skeletal Radiol* 1998;27:139–144.

119. Castriota-Scanderbeg A, Orsi E. Slipped capital femoral epiphysis: ultrasonographic findings. *Skeletal Radiol* 1993;22:191–193.

120. Kallio PE, Lequesne GW, Paterson DC, et al. Ultrasonography in slipped capital femoral epiphysis. Diagnosis and assessment of severity. *J Bone Joint Surg Br* 1991;73:884–889.

121. Kallio PE, Mah ET, Foster BK, et al. Slipped capital femoral epiphysis. Incidence and clinical assessment of physeal instability. *J Bone Joint Surg Br* 1995;77:752–755.

122. Kallio PE, Paterson DC, Foster BK, et al. Classification in slipped capital femoral epiphysis. Sonographic assessment of stability and remodeling. *Clin Orthop* 1993;294:196–203.

123. Acosta K, Vade A, Lomasney LM, et al. Radiologic case study. Bilateral slipped capital femoral epiphysis, acute on the left and preslip on the right. *Orthopedics* 2001;24:737, 808–809, 811–812.

124. Futami T, Suzuki S, Seto Y, et al. Sequential magnetic resonance imaging in slipped capital femoral epiphysis: assessment of preslip in the contralateral hip. *J Pediatr Orthop B* 2001;10:298–303.

125. Lalaji A, Umans H, Schneider R, et al. MRI features of confirmed "pre-slip" capital femoral epiphysis: a report of two cases. *Skeletal Radiol* 2002;31:362–365.

126. Fragniere B, Chotel F, Vargas Barreto B, et al. The value of early postoperative bone scan in slipped capital femoral epiphysis. *J Pediatr Orthop B* 2001;10:51–55.

127. Rhoad RC, Davidson RS, Heyman S, et al. Pretreatment bone scan in SCFE: a predictor of ischemia and avascular necrosis. *J Pediatr Orthop* 1999;19:164–168.

128. Gordon JE, Abrahams MS, Dobbs MB, et al. Early reduction, arthrotomy, and cannulated screw fixation in unstable slipped capital femoral epiphysis treatment. *J Pediatr Orthop* 2002;22: 352–358.

## Pathoanatomy

129. Lee KE, Pelker RR, Rudicel SA, et al. Histologic patterns of capital femoral growth plate fracture in the rabbit: the effect of shear direction. *J Pediatr Orthop* 1985;5:32–39.

130. Rudicel S, Pelker RR, Lee KE, et al. Shear fractures through the capital femoral physis of the skeletally immature rabbit. *J Pediatr Orthop* 1985;5:27–31.

131. Segal LS, Weitzel PP, Davidson RS. Valgus slipped capital femoral epiphysis. Fact or fiction? *Clin Orthop* 1996;322:91–98.

132. Shanker VS, Hashemi-Nejad A, Catterall A, et al. Slipped capital femoral epiphysis: is the displacement always posterior? *J Pediatr Orthop B* 2000;9:119–121.

133. Aronson J, Tursky EA. The torsional basis for slipped capital femoral epiphysis. *Clin Orthop* 1996;322:37–42.

134. Griffith MJ. Slipping of the capital femoral epiphysis. *Ann R Coll Surg Engl* 1976;58:34–42.

135. Nguyen D, Morrissy RT. Slipped capital femoral epiphysis: rationale for the technique of percutaneous in situ fixation. *J Pediatr Orthop* 1990;10:341–346.

136. Rab GT. The geometry of slipped capital femoral epiphysis: implications for movement, impingement, and corrective osteotomy. *J Pediatr Orthop* 1999;19:419–424.

137. DeAngelis NA, Busconi BD. Hip arthroscopy in the pediatric population. *Clin Orthop* 2003;406:60–63.

138. Futami T, Kasahara Y, Suzuki S, et al. Arthroscopy for slipped capital femoral epiphysis. *J Pediatr Orthop* 1992;12:592–597.

139. McCarthy J, Noble P, Aluisio FV, et al. Anatomy, pathologic features, and treatment of acetabular labral tears. *Clin Orthop* 2003;406:38–47.

140. Leunig M, Casillas MM, Hamlet M, et al. Slipped capital femoral epiphysis: early mechanical damage to the acetabular cartilage by a prominent femoral metaphysis. *Acta Orthop Scand* 2000;71: 370–375.

141. Ganz R, Parvizi J, Beck M, et al. Femoroacetabular impingement: a cause for osteoarthritis of the hip. *Clin Orthop* 2003;417: 112–120.

142. Agamanolis DP, Weiner DS. Slipped capital femoral epiphysis: a pathologic investigation into light microscopy, histochemistry and ultrastructure. *Orthop Trans* 1985;9:496–497.

143. Agamanolis DP, Weiner DS, Lloyd JK. Slipped capital femoral epiphysis: a pathological study. I. A light microscopic and histochemical study of 21 cases. *J Pediatr Orthop* 1985;5:40–46.

144. Agamanolis DP, Weiner DS, Lloyd JK. Slipped capital femoral epiphysis: a pathological study. II. An ultrastructural study of 23 cases. *J Pediatr Orthop* 1985;5:47–58.

145. Guzzanti V, Falciglia F, Stanitski CL, et al. Slipped capital femoral epiphysis: physeal histologic features before and after fixation. *J Pediatr Orthop* 2003;23:571–577.

146. Ippolito E, Mickelson MR, Ponseti IV. A histochemical study of slipped capital femoral epiphysis. *J Bone Joint Surg Am* 1981;63:1109–1113.

147. Lacroix P, Verbrugge J. Slipping of the upper femoral epiphysis. *J Bone Joint Surg Am* 1951;33:371–381.

148. Mickelson MR, Ponseti IV, Cooper RR, et al. The ultrastructure of the growth plate in slipped capital femoral epiphysis. *J Bone Joint Surg Am* 1977;59:1076–1081.

149. Ponseti IV, McClintock R. The pathology of slipping of the upper femoral epiphysis. *J Bone Joint Surg Am* 1956;38-A:71–83.

150. Wattleworth AS, Heiple KG, Chase SW, et al. Pathology of slipped capital femoral epiphysis. *Instr Course Lect* 1972;21:174–181.

## Blood Supply

151. Chung SM. The arterial supply of the developing proximal end of the human femur. *J Bone Joint Surg Am* 1976;58:961–970.

152. Crock HV. A revision of the anatomy of the arteries supplying the upper end of the human femur. *J Anat* 1965;99:77–88.

153. Maeda S, Kita A, Funayama K, et al. Vascular supply to slipped capital femoral epiphysis. *J Pediatr Orthop* 2001;21:664–667.

154. Brodetti A. The blood supply of the femoral neck and head in relation to the damaging effects of nails and screws. *J Bone Joint Surg Br* 1960;42:794–801.

## Natural History

155. Stasikelis PJ, Sullivan CM, Phillips WA, et al. Slipped capital femoral epiphysis. Prediction of contralateral involvement. *J Bone Joint Surg Am* 1996;78:1149–1155.

156. Boero S, Brunenghi GM, Carbone M, et al. Pinning in slipped capital femoral epiphysis: long-term follow-up study. *J Pediatr Orthop B* 2003;12:372–379.

157. Carney BT, Weinstein SL. Natural history of untreated chronic slipped capital femoral epiphysis. *Clin Orthop* 1996;322:43–47.

158. Hansson G, Billing L, Hogstedt B, et al. Long-term results after nailing in situ of slipped upper femoral epiphysis. A 30-year follow-up of 59 hips. *J Bone Joint Surg Br* 1998;80:70–77.

159. Ordeberg G, Hansson LI, Sandstrom S. Slipped capital femoral epiphysis in southern Sweden. Long-term result with no treatment or symptomatic primary treatment. *Clin Orthop* 1984;191:95–104.

160. Gudmundsson G. Intertrochanteric displacement osteotomy for painful osteoarthritis of the hip. *Acta Orthop Scand* 1970;41:91–109.

161. Keener JD, Callaghan JJ, Goetz DD, et al. Twenty-five-year results after Charnley total hip arthroplasty in patients less than fifty years old: a concise follow-up of a previous report. *J Bone Joint Surg Am* 2003;85-A:1066–1072.

162. Lloyd-Roberts GC. Osteoarthritis of the hip; a study of the clinical pathology. *J Bone Joint Surg Br* 1955;37-B:8–47.

163. Ranawat CS, Atkinson RE, Salvati EA, et al. Conventional total hip arthroplasty for degenerative joint disease in patients between the ages of forty and sixty years. *J Bone Joint Surg Am* 1984;66:745–752.

164. Solomon L. Patterns of osteoarthritis of the hip. *J Bone Joint Surg Br* 1976;58:176–183.

165. Goodman DA, Feighan JE, Smith AD, et al. Subclinical slipped capital femoral epiphysis. Relationship to osteoarthrosis of the hip. *J Bone Joint Surg Am* 1997;79:1489–1497.

166. Murray RO. The etiology of primary osteoarthritis of the hip. *Br J Radiol* 1965;38:810–824.

167. Stulberg SD, Cordell LD, Harris WH, et al. Unrecognized childhood hip disease: a major cause of idiopathic osteoarthritis of the hip. In: Amstutz HC, ed. *The hip: Proceedings of the Third Open Scientific Meeting of the Hip Society*. St. Louis, MO: CV Mosby Company, 1975:212–228.

168. Resnick D. The 'tilt deformity' of the femoral head in osteoarthritis of the hip: a poor indicator of previous epiphysiolysis. *Clin Radiol* 1976;27:355–363.

## Treatment

169. Smith JT, Price C, Stevens PM, et al. Does pediatric orthopedic subspecialization affect hospital utilization and charges? *J Pediatr Orthop* 1999;19:553–555.

170. Jerre R, Hansson G, Wallin J, et al. Long-term results after realignment operations for slipped upper femoral epiphysis. *J Bone Joint Surg Br* 1996;78:745–750.

171. Aadalen RJ, Weiner DS, Hoyt W, et al. Acute slipped capital femoral epiphysis. *J Bone Joint Surg Am* 1974;56:1473–1487.

172. Hall JE. The results of treatment of slipped femoral epiphysis. *J Bone Joint Surg Br* 1957;39-B:659–673.

173. Kennedy JG, Hresko MT, Kasser JR, et al. Osteonecrosis of the femoral head associated with slipped capital femoral epiphysis. *J Pediatr Orthop* 2001;21:189–193.

174. Tokmakova KP, Stanton RP, Mason DE. Factors influencing the development of osteonecrosis in patients treated for slipped capital femoral epiphysis. *J Bone Joint Surg Am* 2003;85-A:798–801.

175. Meier MC, Meyer LC, Ferguson RL. Treatment of slipped capital femoral epiphysis with a spica cast. *J Bone Joint Surg Am* 1992;74:1522–1529.

176. Betz RR, Steel HH, Emper WD, et al. Treatment of slipped capital femoral epiphysis. Spica-cast immobilization. *J Bone Joint Surg Am* 1990;72:587–600.

177. Lowe HG. Avascular necrosis after slipping of the upper femoral epiphysis. *J Bone Joint Surg Br* 1961;43:688–699.

178. Morrissy RT. Slipped capital femoral epiphysis technique of percutaneous in situ fixation. *J Pediatr Orthop* 1990;10:347–350.

179. Lee FY, Chapman CB. In situ pinning of hip for stable slipped capital femoral epiphysis on a radiolucent operating table. *J Pediatr Orthop* 2003;23:27–29.

180. Aronsson DD, Loder RT. Treatment of the unstable (acute) slipped capital femoral epiphysis. *Clin Orthop* 1996;322:99–110.

181. Canale ST. Problems and complications of slipped capital femoral epiphysis. *Instr Course Lect* 1989;38:281–290.

182. Schmitz M. Treatment. In: Morrissy RT, ed. *Slipped capital femoral epiphysis*. Rosemont, IL: American Academy of Orthopaedic Surgeons, 2002:19–38.

183. Walters R, Simon SR. Joint destruction: a sequel of unrecognized pin penetration in patients with slipped capital femoral epiphysis. In: Riley LH Jr., ed. *The Hip: Proceedings of the Eighth Open Scientific Meeting of the Hip Society*. St. Louis, MO: CV Mosby Company, 1980:145–164

184. Orr TR, Bollinger BA, Strecker WB. Blind zone determination of the femoral head. *J Pediatr Orthop* 1989;9:417–421.

185. Morrissy RT. In situ fixation of chronic slipped capital femoral epiphysis. *Instr Course Lect* 1984;33:319–327.

186. Morrissy RT. Principles of in situ fixation in chronic slipped capital femoral epiphysis. *Instr Course Lect* 1989;38:257–262.

187. Goodman WW, Johnson JT, Robertson WW Jr. Single screw fixation for acute and acute-on-chronic slipped capital femoral epiphysis. *Clin Orthop* 1996;322:86–90.

188. Aronson DD, Peterson DA, Miller DV. Slipped capital femoral epiphysis. The case for internal fixation in situ. *Clin Orthop* 1992;281:115–122.

189. Gonzalez-Moran G, Carsi B, Abril JC, et al. Results after preoperative traction and pinning in slipped capital femoral epiphysis: K wires versus cannulated screws. *J Pediatr Orthop B* 1998;7:53–58.

190. Aronson DD, Loder RT. Slipped capital femoral epiphysis in black children. *J Pediatr Orthop* 1992;12:74–79.

191. Crawford AH. Slipped capital femoral epiphysis. *J Bone Joint Surg Am* 1988;70:1422–1427.

192. de Sanctis N, Di Gennaro G, Pempinello C, et al. Is gentle manipulative reduction and percutaneous fixation with a single screw the best management of acute and acute-on-chronic slipped capital femoral epiphysis? A report of 70 patients. *J Pediatr Orthop B* 1996;5:90–95.

193. Stambough JL, Davidson RS, Ellis RD, et al. Slipped capital femoral epiphysis: an analysis of 80 patients as to pin placement and number. *J Pediatr Orthop* 1986;6:265–273.

194. Stevens DB, Short BA, Burch JM. In situ fixation of the slipped capital femoral epiphysis with a single screw. *J Pediatr Orthop B* 1996;5:85–89.

195. Lehman WB, Menche D, Grant A, et al. The problem of evaluating in situ pinning of slipped capital femoral epiphysis: an experimental model and a review of 63 consecutive cases. *J Pediatr Orthop* 1984;4:297–303.

196. Riley PM, Weiner DS, Gillespie R, et al. Hazards of internal fixation in the treatment of slipped capital femoral epiphysis. *J Bone Joint Surg Am* 1990;72:1500–1509.

197. Moseley C. The "approach-withdraw" phenomenon in the pinning of slipped capital femoral epiphysis. *Orthop Trans* 1985; 9:497.

198. Bassett GS. Bone endoscopy: direct visual confirmation of cannulated screw placement in slipped capital femoral epiphysis. *J Pediatr Orthop* 1993;13:159–163.

199. Lehman WB, Grant A, Rose D, et al. A method of evaluating possible pin penetration in slipped capital femoral epiphysis using a cannulated internal fixation device. *Clin Orthop* 1984; 186:65–70.

200. Karol LA, Doane RM, Cornicelli SF, et al. Single versus double screw fixation for treatment of slipped capital femoral epiphysis: a biomechanical analysis. *J Pediatr Orthop* 1992;12:741–745.

201. Kruger DM, Herzenberg JE, Viviano DM, et al. Biomechanical comparison of single- and double-pin fixation for acute slipped capital femoral epiphysis. *Clin Orthop* 1990;259:277–281.

202. Kibiloski LJ, Doane RM, Karol LA, et al. Biomechanical analysis of single- versus double-screw fixation in slipped capital femoral epiphysis at physiological load levels. *J Pediatr Orthop* 1994;14:627–630.

203. Early SD, Hedman TP, Reynolds RA. Biomechanical analysis of compression screw fixation versus standard in situ pinning in slipped capital femoral epiphysis. *J Pediatr Orthop* 2001;21: 183–188.

204. Stanton RP, Shelton YA. Closure of the physis after pinning of slipped capital femoral epiphysis. *Orthopedics* 1993;16: 1099–1102; discussion 1102–1103.

205. Ward WT, Stefko J, Wood KB, et al. Fixation with a single screw for slipped capital femoral epiphysis. *J Bone Joint Surg Am* 1992; 74:799–809.

206. Wong-Chung J, Strong ML. Physeal remodeling after internal fixation of slipped capital femoral epiphyses. *J Pediatr Orthop* 1991;11:2–5.

207. Hansson LI. Osteosynthesis with the hook-pin in slipped capital femoral epiphysis. *Acta Orthop Scand* 1982;53:87–96.

208. Kumm DA, Lee SH, Hackenbroch MH, et al. Slipped capital femoral epiphysis: a prospective study of dynamic screw fixation. *Clin Orthop* 2001;384:198–207.

209. Bellemans J, Fabry G, Molenaers G, et al. Slipped capital femoral epiphysis: a long-term follow-up, with special emphasis on the capacities for remodeling. *J Pediatr Orthop B* 1996;5: 151–157.

210. O'Brien ET, Fahey JJ. Remodeling of the femoral neck after in situ pinning for slipped capital femoral epiphysis. *J Bone Joint Surg Am* 1977;59:62–68.

211. Jones JR, Paterson DC, Hillier TM, et al. Remodelling after pinning for slipped capital femoral epiphysis. *J Bone Joint Surg Br* 1990;72:568–573.

212. Jerre R, Billing L, Karlsson J. Loss of hip motion in slipped capital femoral epiphysis: a calculation from the slipping angle and the slope. *J Pediatr Orthop B* 1996;5:144–150.

213. Schmidt TL, Cimino WG, Seidel FG. Allograft epiphysiodesis for slipped capital femoral epiphysis. *Clin Orthop* 1996;322:61–76.

214. Dietz FR. Traction reduction of acute and acute-on-chronic slipped capital femoral epiphysis. *Clin Orthop* 1994;302:101–110.

215. Cheng JCY, Tang N. Decompression and stable internal fixation of femoral neck fractures in children can affect outcome. *J Pediatr Orthop* 1999;19:338–343.

216. Holmberg S, Dalen N. Intracapsular pressure and caput circulation in nondisplaced femoral neck fracture. *Clin Orthop* 1987; 219:124–126.

217. Ng GPK, Cole WG. Effect of early hip decompression on the frequency of avascular necrosis in children with fractures of the neck of the femur. *Injury* 1996;27:419–421.

218. Soto-Hall R, Johnson LH, Johnson RA. Variations in the intra-articular pressure of the hip joint in injury and disease. *J Bone Joint Surg Am* 1964;46:509–516.

219. Stromqvist B, Nilsson LT, Egund N, et al. Intracapsular pressures in undisplaced fractures of the femoral neck. *J Bone Joint Surg Br* 1988;70:192–194.

220. Woodhouse C. Dynamic influences of vascular occlusion affecting development of avascular necrosis of the femoral head. *Clin Orthop* 1964;32:119–129.

221. Swiontkowski MF, Tepic S, Perren SM, et al. Laser Doppler flowmetry for bone blood flow measurement: correlation with microsphere estimates and evaluation of the effect of intracapsular pressure on femoral head blood flow. *J Orthop Res* 1986; 4:362–371.

222. Vegter J, Klopper PJ. Effect of intracapsular hyperpressure on femoral head blood flow. *Acta Orthop Scand* 1991;62:337–341.

223. Phillips SA, Griffiths WE, Clarke NM. The timing of reduction and stabilisation of the acute, unstable, slipped upper femoral epiphysis. *J Bone Joint Surg Br* 2001;83:1046–1049.

224. Dean GS, Kime RC, Fitch RD, et al. Treatment of osteonecrosis in the hip of pediatric patients by free vascularized fibula graft. *Clin Orthop* 2001;386:106–113.

225. Aprin H, Goodman S, Kahn LB. Cartilage necrosis due to pin penetration: experimental studies in rabbits. *J Pediatr Orthop* 1991;11:623–630.

226. Sternlicht AL, Ehrlich MG, Armstrong AL, et al. Role of pin protrusion in the etiology of chondrolysis: a surgical model with radiographic, histologic, and biochemical analysis. *J Pediatr Orthop* 1992;12:428–433.

227. Bianco AJ Jr. Treatment of slipping of the capital femoral epiphysis. *Clin Orthop* 1966;48:103–110.

228. Ingram AJ, Clarke MS, Clarke CS Jr, et al. Chondrolysis complicating slipped capital femoral epiphysis. *Clin Orthop* 1982; 165:99–109.

229. Koval KJ, Lehman WB, Rose D, et al. Treatment of slipped capital femoral epiphysis with a cannulated-screw technique. *J Bone Joint Surg Am* 1989;71:1370–1377.

230. Vrettos BC, Hoffman EB. Chondrolysis in slipped upper femoral epiphysis. Long-term study of the aetiology and natural history. *J Bone Joint Surg Br* 1993;75:956–961.

231. Zionts LE, Simonian PT, Harvey JP Jr. Transient penetration of the hip joint during in situ cannulated-screw fixation of slipped capital femoral epiphysis. *J Bone Joint Surg Am* 1991;73: 1054–1060.

232. Denton JR. Progression of a slipped capital femoral epiphysis after fixation with a single cannulated screw. A case report. *J Bone Joint Surg Am* 1993;75:425–427.

233. Sanders JO, Smith WJ, Stanley EA, et al. Progressive slippage after pinning for slipped capital femoral epiphysis. *J Pediatr Orthop* 2002;22:239–243.

234. Carney BT, Birnbaum P, Minter C. Slip progression after in situ single screw fixation for stable slipped capital femoral epiphysis. *J Pediatr Orthop* 2003;23:584–589.

235. Laplaza FJ, Burke SW. Epiphyseal growth after pinning of slipped capital femoral epiphysis. *J Pediatr Orthop* 1995;15:357–361.

236. Jerre R, Karlsson J, Romanus B, et al. Does a single device prevent further slipping of the epiphysis in children with slipped capital femoral epiphysis? *Arch Orthop Trauma Surg* 1997;116:348–351.

237. Plotz GM, Prymka M, Hassenpflug J. The role of prophylactic pinning in the treatment of slipped capital femoral epiphysis— a case report. *Acta Orthop Scand* 1999;70:631–634.

238. Canale ST, Azar F, Young J, et al. Subtrochanteric fracture after fixation of slipped capital femoral epiphysis: a complication of unused drill holes. *J Pediatr Orthop* 1994;14:623–626.

239. Schmidt R, Gregg JR. Subtrochanteric fractures complicating pin fixation of slipped capital femoral epiphysis. *Orthop Trans* 1985;9:497.

240. Baynham GC, Lucie RS, Cummings RJ. Femoral neck fracture secondary to in situ pinning of slipped capital femoral epiphysis: a previously unreported complication. *J Pediatr Orthop* 1991;11:187–190.

241. Canale ST, Casillas M, Banta JV. Displaced femoral neck fractures at the bone-screw interface after in situ fixation of slipped capital femoral epiphysis. *J Pediatr Orthop* 1997;17:212–215.

242. Chen CE, Ko JY, Wang CJ. Premature closure of the physeal plate after treatment of a slipped capital femoral epiphysis. *Chang Gung Med J* 2002;25:811–818.

243. Greenough CG, Bromage JD, Jackson AM. Pinning of the slipped upper femoral epiphysis—a trouble-free procedure? *J Pediatr Orthop* 1985;5:657–660.

244. Kahle WK. The case against routine metal removal. *J Pediatr Orthop* 1994;14:229–237.

245. Crandall DG, Gabriel KR, Akbarnia BA. Second operation for slipped capital femoral epiphysis: pin removal. *J Pediatr Orthop* 1992;12:434–437.

246. Lee TK, Haynes RJ, Longo JA, et al. Pin removal in slipped capital femoral epiphysis: the unsuitability of titanium devices. *J Pediatr Orthop* 1996;16:49–52.

247. Hagglund G. The contralateral hip in slipped capital femoral epiphysis. *J Pediatr Orthop B* 1996;5:158–161.

248. Ross PM, Lyne ED, Morawa LG. Slipped capital femoral epiphysis: long-term results after 10–38 years. *Clin Orthop* 1979;141:176–180.

249. Aronsson DD, Karol LA. Stable slipped capital femoral epiphysis: evaluation and management. *J Am Acad Orthop Surg* 1996;4:173–181.

250. Givon U, Bowen JR. Chronic slipped capital femoral epiphysis: treatment by pinning in situ. *J Pediatr Orthop B* 1999;8:216–222.

251. Weiner DS. Bone graft epiphysiodesis in the treatment of slipped capital femoral epiphysis. *Instr Course Lect* 1989;38:263–272.

252. Ferguson AB, Howorth MB. Slipping of the upper femoral epiphysis. *JAMA* 1931;97:1867–1870.

253. Adamczyk MJ, Weiner DS, Hawk D. A 50-year experience with bone graft epiphysiodesis in the treatment of slipped capital femoral epiphysis. *J Pediatr Orthop* 2003;23:578–583.

254. Howorth B. The bone-pegging operation for slipping of the capital femoral epiphysis. *Clin Orthop* 1966;48:79–87.

255. Melby A, Hoyt WA Jr, Weiner DS. Treatment of chronic slipped capital femoral epiphysis by bone-grafted epiphyseodesis. *J Bone Joint Surg Am* 1980;62:119–125.

256. Weiner DS. Epiphysiodesis in slipped capital femoral epiphysis. *J Pediatr Orthop* 1986;6:754–755.

257. Weiner DS. Open bone graft epiphysiodesis for slipped capital femoral epiphysis. *J Pediatr Orthop* 1990;10:673–674.

258. Weiner DS. Use of open bone-graft epiphysiodesis in the treatment of slipped capital femoral epiphysis. *J Pediatr Orthop* 1998;18:136–137.

259. Weiner DS, Weiner S, Melby A, et al. A 30-year experience with bone graft epiphysiodesis in the treatment of slipped capital femoral epiphysis. *J Pediatr Orthop* 1984;4:145–152.

260. Weiner DS, Weiner SD, Melby A. Anterolateral approach to the hip for bone graft epiphysiodesis in the treatment of slipped capital femoral epiphysis. *J Pediatr Orthop* 1988;8:349–352.

261. Irani RN, Rosenzweig AH, Cotler HB, et al. Epiphysiodesis in slipped capital femoral epiphysis: a comparison of various surgical modalities. *J Pediatr Orthop* 1985;5:661–664.

262. Rao SB, Crawford AH, Burger RR, et al. Open bone peg epiphysiodesis for slipped capital femoral epiphysis. *J Pediatr Orthop* 1996;16:37–48.

263. Rostoucher P, Bensahel H, Pennecot GF, et al. Slipped capital femoral epiphysis: evaluation of different modes of treatment. *J Pediatr Orthop B* 1996;5:96–101.

264. Herndon CH, Heyman CH, Bell DM. Treatment of slipped capital femoral epiphysis by epiphyseodesis and osteoplasty of the femoral neck. A report of further experiences. *J Bone Joint Surg Am* 1963;45:999–1012.

265. Ward WT, Wood K. Open bone graft epiphyseodesis for slipped capital femoral epiphysis. *J Pediatr Orthop* 1990;10:14–20.

266. Frymoyer JW. Chondrolysis of the hip following Southwick osteotomy for severe slipped capital femoral epiphysis. *Clin Orthop* 1974;99:120–124.

267. Zupanc O, Antolic V, Iglic A, et al. The assessment of contact stress in the hip joint after operative treatment for severe slipped capital femoral epiphysis. *Int Orthop* 2001;25:9–12.

268. Richolt JA, Teschner M, Everett PC, et al. Impingement simulation of the hip in SCFE using 3D models. *Comput Aided Surg* 1999;4:144–151.

269. Kartenbender K, Cordier W, Katthagen BD. Long-term follow-up study after corrective Imhauser osteotomy for severe slipped capital femoral epiphysis. *J Pediatr Orthop* 2000;20:749–756.

270. Schai PA, Exner GU, Hansch O. Prevention of secondary coxarthrosis in slipped capital femoral epiphysis: a long-term follow-up study after corrective intertrochanteric osteotomy. *J Pediatr Orthop B* 1996;5:135–143.

271. Martin PH. Slipped epiphysis in the adolescent hip: a reconsideration of open reduction. *J Bone Joint Surg Am* 1948;30:9–19.

272. Crawford AH. The role of osteotomy in the treatment of slipped capital femoral epiphysis. *Instr Course Lect* 1989;38:273–279.

273. Fish JB. Cuneiform osteotomy of the femoral neck in the treatment of slipped capital femoral epiphysis. *J Bone Joint Surg Am* 1984;66:1153–1168.

274. Fish JB. Cuneiform osteotomy of the femoral neck in the treatment of slipped capital femoral epiphysis. A follow-up note. *J Bone Joint Surg Am* 1994;76:46–59.

275. Nishiyama K, Sakamaki T, Ishii Y. Follow-up study of the subcapital wedge osteotomy for severe chronic slipped capital femoral epiphysis. *J Pediatr Orthop* 1989;9:412–416.

276. Dunn D. Severe slipped capital femoral epiphysis and open replacement by cervical osteotomy. In: *The hip: Proceedings of the Third Open Scientific Meeting of the Hip Society*. St. Louis, MO: CV Mosby Company, 1975:115–126.

277. Dunn DM, Angel JC. Replacement of the femoral head by open operation in severe adolescent slipping of the upper femoral epiphysis. *J Bone Joint Surg Br* 1978;60-B:394–403.

278. Barros JW, Tukiama G, Fontoura C, et al. Trapezoid osteotomy for slipped capital femoral epiphysis. *Int Orthop* 2000;24:83–87.

279. DeRosa GP, Mullins RC, Kling TF Jr. Cuneiform osteotomy of the femoral neck in severe slipped capital femoral epiphysis. *Clin Orthop* 1996;322:48–60.

280. Fron D, Forgues D, Mayrargue E, et al. Follow-up study of severe slipped capital femoral epiphysis treated with Dunn's osteotomy. *J Pediatr Orthop* 2000;20:320–325.

281. Velasco R, Schai PA, Exner GU. Slipped capital femoral epiphysis: a long-term follow-up study after open reduction of the femoral head combined with subcapital wedge resection. *J Pediatr Orthop B* 1998;7:43–52.

282. Wiberg G. Surgical treatment of slipped epiphysis with special reference to wedge osteotomy of the femoral neck. *Clin Orthop* 1966;48:139–152.

283. Gage JR, Sundberg AB, Nolan DR, et al. Complications after cuneiform osteotomy for moderately or severely slipped capital femoral epiphysis. *J Bone Joint Surg Am* 1978;60:157–165.

284. Abraham E, Garst J, Barmada R. Treatment of moderate to severe slipped capital femoral epiphysis with extracapsular base-of-neck osteotomy. *J Pediatr Orthop* 1993;13:294–302.

285. Barmada R, Bruch RF, Gimbel JS, et al. Base of the neck extracapsular osteotomy for correction of deformity in slipped capital femoral epiphysis. *Clin Orthop* 1978;132:98–101.

286. Kramer WG, Craig WA, Noel S. Compensating osteotomy at the base of the femoral neck for slipped capital femoral epiphysis. *J Bone Joint Surg Am* 1976;58:796–800.

287. Clark CR, Southwick WO, Ogden JA. Anatomic aspects of slipped capital femoral epiphysis and correction by biplane osteotomy. *Instr Course Lect* 1980;29:90–100.

288. Southwick WO. Biplane osteotomy for very severe slipped capital femoral epiphysis. In: *The hip: Proceedings of the Third Open Scientific Meeting of the Hip Society*. St. Louis, MO: CV Mosby Company, 1975:105–114.

289. Southwick WO. Compression fixation after biplane intertrochanteric osteotomy for slipped capital femoral epiphysis. A technical improvement. *J Bone Joint Surg Am* 1973;55:1218–1224.

290. Southwick WO. Slipped capital femoral epiphysis. *J Bone Joint Surg Am* 1984;66:1151–1152.

291. Imhauser G. Pathogenese und therapie der jugendlichen huftenkopflosung. *Z orthop Ihre Grenzgeh* 1957;88:3–41.

292. Colyer RA. Compression external fixation after biplane femoral trochanteric osteotomy for severe slipped capital femoral epiphysis. *J Bone Joint Surg Am* 1980;62:557–560.

293. Ito H, Minami A, Suzuki K, et al. Three-dimensionally corrective external fixator system for proximal femoral osteotomy. *J Pediatr Orthop* 2001;21:652–656.

294. Scher MA, Sweet MB, Jakim I. Acute-on-chronic bilateral reversed slipped capital femoral epiphysis managed by Imhauser-Weber osteotomy. *Arch Orthop Trauma Surg* 1989;108:336–338.

295. Millis MB, Murphy SB, Poss R. Osteotomies about the hip for the prevention and treatment of osteoarthrosis. *Instr Course Lect* 1996;45:209–226.

296. Millis MB, Poss R, Murphy SB. Osteotomies of the hip in the prevention and treatment of osteoarthritis. *Instr Course Lect* 1992;41:145–154.

297. Salvati EA, Robinson JH Jr, O'Down TJ. Southwick osteotomy for severe chronic slipped capital femoral epiphysis: results and complications. *J Bone Joint Surg Am* 1980;62:561–570.

298. Ireland J, Newman PH. Triplane osteotomy for severely slipped upper femoral epiphysis. *J Bone Joint Surg Br* 1978;60-B:390–393.

299. Rao JP, Francis AM, Siwek CW. The treatment of chronic slipped capital femoral epiphysis by biplane osteotomy. *J Bone Joint Surg Am* 1984;66:1169–1175.

300. Merchan EC, Na CM, Munuera L. Intertrochanteric osteotomy for the treatment of chronic slipped capital femoral epiphysis. *Int Orthop* 1992;16:133–135.

301. Parsch K, Zehender H, Buhl T, et al. Intertrochanteric corrective osteotomy for moderate and severe chronic slipped capital femoral epiphysis. *J Pediatr Orthop B* 1999;8:223–230.

302. Sugioka Y. Transtrochanteric anterior rotational osteotomy of the femoral head in the treatment of osteonecrosis affecting the hip: a new osteotomy operation. *Clin Orthop* 1978;130:191–201.

303. Sugioka Y. Transtrochanteric rotational osteotomy in the treatment of idiopathic and steroid-induced femoral head necrosis, Perthes' disease, slipped capital femoral epiphysis, and osteoarthritis of the hip. Indications and results. *Clin Orthop* 1984; 184:12–23.

304. Masuda T, Matsuno T, Hasegawa I, et al. Transtrochanteric anterior rotational osteotomy for slipped capital femoral epiphysis: a report of five cases. *J Pediatr Orthop* 1986;6:18–23.

305. Castro FP Jr, Bennett JT, Doulens K. Epidemiological perspective on prophylactic pinning in patients with unilateral slipped capital femoral epiphysis. *J Pediatr Orthop* 2000;20:745–748.

306. Kumm DA, Schmidt J, Eisenburger SH, et al. Prophylactic dynamic screw fixation of the asymptomatic hip in slipped capital femoral epiphysis. *J Pediatr Orthop* 1996;16:249–253.

307. Schultz WR, Weinstein JN, Weinstein SL, et al. Prophylactic pinning of the contralateral hip in slipped capital femoral epiphysis: evaluation of long-term outcome for the contralateral hip with use of decision analysis. *J Bone Joint Surg Am* 2002;84-A:1305–1314.

308. Emery RJ, Todd RC, Dunn DM. Prophylactic pinning in slipped upper femoral epiphysis. Prevention of complications. *J Bone Joint Surg Br* 1990;72:217–219.

309. Hurley JM, Betz RR, Loder RT, et al. Slipped capital femoral epiphysis. The prevalence of late contralateral slip. *J Bone Joint Surg Am* 1996;78:226–230.

310. Sorensen KH. Slipped upper femoral epiphysis: clinical examinations concerning the aetiology. *Acta Orthop Scand* 1969; 40:686.

311. Segal LS, Davidson RS, Robertson WW Jr, et al. Growth disturbances of the proximal femur after pinning of juvenile slipped capital femoral epiphysis. *J Pediatr Orthop* 1991;11:631–637.

312. Whiteside LA, Schoenecker PL. Combined valgus derotation osteotomy and cervical osteoplasty for severely slipped capital femoral epiphysis: mechanical analysis and report of preliminary results using compression screw fixation and early weight bearing. *Clin Orthop* 1978;132:88–97.

313. Carlioz H, Vogt JC, Barba L, et al. Treatment of slipped upper femoral epiphysis: 80 cases operated on over 10 years (1968–1978). *J Pediatr Orthop* 1984;4:153–161.

## Complications

314. Howorth B. Slipping of the capital femoral epiphysis. History. *Clin Orthop* 1966;48:11–32.

315. Nonweiler B, Hoffer M, Weinert C, et al. Percutaneous in situ fixation of slipped capital femoral epiphysis using two threaded Steinmann pins. *J Pediatr Orthop* 1996;16:56–60.

316. Krahn TH, Canale ST, Beaty JH, et al. Long-term follow-up of patients with avascular necrosis after treatment of slipped capital femoral epiphysis. *J Pediatr Orthop* 1993;13:154–158.

317. Notzli HP, Chou LB, Ganz R. Open-reduction and intertrochanteric osteotomy for osteonecrosis and extrusion of the femoral head in adolescents. *J Pediatr Orthop* 1995;15:16–20.

318. Scher MA, Jakim I. Intertrochanteric osteotomy and autogenous bone-grafting for avascular necrosis of the femoral head. *J Bone Joint Surg Am* 1993;75:1119–1133.

319. Sugano N, Takaoka K, Ohzono K, et al. Rotational osteotomy for non-traumatic avascular necrosis of the femoral head. *J Bone Joint Surg Br* 1992;74:734–739.

320. Sugioka Y, Hotokebuchi T, Tsutsui H. Transtrochanteric anterior rotational osteotomy for idiopathic and steroid-induced necrosis of the femoral head. Indications and long-term results. *Clin Orthop* 1992;277:111–120.

321. Trumble SJ, Mayo KA, Mast JW. The periacetabular osteotomy. Minimum 2 year followup in more than 100 hips. *Clin Orthop* 1999;363:54–63.

322. Ko JY, Meyers MH, Wenger DR. "Trapdoor" procedure for osteonecrosis with segmental collapse of the femoral head in teenagers. *J Pediatr Orthop* 1995;15:7–15.

323. Waldenstrom H. On necrosis of the joint cartilage by epiphyseolysis capitis femoris. *Acta Chir Scand* 1930;67:936–946.

324. Hughes LO, Aronson J, Smith HS. Normal radiographic values for cartilage thickness and physeal angle in the pediatric hip. *J Pediatr Orthop* 1999;19:443–448.

325. Bellemans J, Fabry G, Molenaers G, et al. Pin removal after in-situ pinning for slipped capital femoral epiphysis. *Acta Orthop Belg* 1994;60:170–172.

326. Cruess RL. The pathology of acute necrosis of cartilage in slipping of the capital femoral epiphysis. A report of two cases with pathological sections. *J Bone Joint Surg Am* 1963;45:1013–1024.

327. Maurer RC, Larsen IJ. Acute necrosis of cartilage in slipped capital femoral epiphysis. *J Bone Joint Surg Am* 1970;52:39–50.

328. Tudisco C, Caterini R, Farsetti P, et al. Chondrolysis of the hip complicating slipped capital femoral epiphysis: long-term follow-up of nine patients. *J Pediatr Orthop B* 1999;8:107–111.

329. Mankin HJ, Sledge CB, Rothschild S, et al. Chondrolysis of the hip. In: *The hip: Proceedings of the Third Open Scientific Meeting of the Hip Society*. St. Louis, MO: CV Mosby Company, 1975:127–135.

330. Kennedy JP, Weiner DS. Results of slipped capital femoral epiphysis in the black population. *J Pediatr Orthop* 1990;10: 224–227.

331. Spero CR, Masciale JP, Tornetta P III, et al. Slipped capital femoral epiphysis in black children: incidence of chondrolysis. *J Pediatr Orthop* 1992;12:444–448.

332. El-Khoury GY, Mickelson MR. Chondrolysis following slipped capital femoral epiphysis. *Radiology* 1977;123:327–330.

333. Mandell GA, Keret D, Harcke HT, et al. Chondrolysis: detection by bone scintigraphy. *J Pediatr Orthop* 1992;12:80–85.

334. Lowe HG. Necrosis of articular cartilage after slipping of the capital femoral epiphysis. Report of six cases with recovery. *J Bone Joint Surg Br* 1970;52:108–118.

335. Kitakoji T, Hattori T, Ida K, et al. Arthrodiatasis for chondrolysis with hinge abduction: a case report. *J Pediatr Orthop B* 2000; 9:198–200.

## Salvage Procedures

336. Brinker MR, Rosenberg AG, Kull L, et al. Primary total hip arthroplasty using noncemented porous-coated femoral components in patients with osteonecrosis of the femoral head. *J Arthroplasty* 1994;9:457–468.

337. Chandler HP, Reineck FT, Wixson RL, et al. Total hip replacement in patients younger than thirty years old. A five-year follow-up study. *J Bone Joint Surg Am* 1981;63:1426–1434.

338. Duffy GP, Berry DJ, Rowland C, et al. Primary uncemented total hip arthroplasty in patients <40 years old: 10- to 14-year results using first-generation proximally porous-coated implants. *J Arthroplasty* 2001;16:140–144.

339. McAuley JP, Szuszczewicz ES, Young A, et al. Total hip arthroplasty in patients 50 years and younger. *Clin Orthop* 2004; 418:119–125.

340. Crowther JD, Lachiewicz PF. Survival and polyethylene wear of porous-coated acetabular components in patients less than fifty years old: results at nine to fourteen years. *J Bone Joint Surg Am* 2002;84-A:729–735.

341. Perez RE, Rodriguez JA, Deshmukh RG, et al. Polyethylene wear and periprosthetic osteolysis in metal-backed acetabular components with cylindrical liners. *J Arthroplasty* 1998;13:1–7.

342. Benaroch TE, Richards BS, Haideri N, et al. Intermediate follow-up of a simple method of hip arthrodesis in adolescent patients. *J Pediatr Orthop* 1996;16:30–36.

343. Callaghan JJ, Brand RA, Pedersen DR. Hip arthrodesis. A long-term follow-up. *J Bone Joint Surg Am* 1985;67:1328–1335.

344. Mowery CA, Houkom JA, Roach JW, et al. A simple method of hip arthrodesis. *J Pediatr Orthop* 1986;6:7–10.

345. Scher DM, Jeong GK, Grant AD, et al. Hip arthrodesis in adolescents using external fixation. *J Pediatr Orthop* 2001;21:194–197.

346. Schoenecker PL, Johnson LO, Martin RA, et al. Intra-articular hip arthrodesis without subtrochanteric osteotomy in adolescents: technique and short-term follow-up. *Am J Orthop* 1997; 26: 257–264.

347. Sponseller PD, McBeath AA, Perpich M. Hip arthrodesis in young patients. A long-term follow-up study. *J Bone Joint Surg Am* 1984;66:853–859.

348. Farkas A. New operative treatment of tuberculous coxitis in children. *J Bone Joint Surg Am* 1939;21:323–333.

349. Price CT, Lovell WW. Thompson arthrodesis of the hip in children. *J Bone Joint Surg Am* 1980;62:1118–1123.

350. Thompson FR. Combined hip fusion and subtrochanteric osteotomy allowing early ambulation. *J Bone Joint Surg Am* 1956;38:13–21.

351. Amstutz HC, Sakai DN. Total joint replacement for ankylosed hips. Indications, technique, and preliminary results. *J Bone Joint Surg Am* 1975;57:619–625.

352. Kilgus DJ, Amstutz HC, Wolgin MA, et al. Joint replacement for ankylosed hips. *J Bone Joint Surg Am* 1990;72:45–54.

353. Lubahn JD, Evarts CM, Feltner JB. Conversion of ankylosed hips to total hip arthroplasty. *Clin Orthop* 1980;153:146–152.

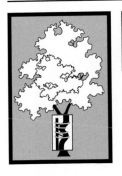

# 27

# Other Conditions of the Hip

**Matthew B. Dobbs** **José A. Morcuende**

# COXA VARA

## Definition

Coxa vara is defined as any decrease in the femoral neck-shaft angle below the normal. Coxa vara was initially classified by Elmslie (1). This classification has subsequently been modified by Fairbank and condensed into three broad categories: congenital coxa vara, acquired coxa vara, and developmental coxa vara (2) (Table 27.1).

Congenital coxa vara is characterized by a primary cartilaginous defect in the femoral neck. This can be a congenital short femur, a congenital bowed femur, or part of a proximal femoral focal deficiency (PFFD) (Fig. 27.1). The deformity is not always evident clinically at birth; however, it is usually evident on radiographs (3,4). Significant leg length inequality is often present.

Acquired coxa vara can be caused by a number of conditions including trauma (Fig. 27.2), infection, pathologic bone disorders (Fig. 27.3), slipped capital femoral epiphysis, and Legg-Calvé-Perthes disease (LCPD). The resulting coxa vara can be secondary to necrosis of the femoral head or altered physeal growth. Coxa vara can also be associated with skeletal dysplasias and, although these conditions probably should be classified separately, they are included under "acquired causes" for the sake of simplicity (5–8) (Fig. 27.4).

*Developmental coxa vara* is a term reserved for coxa vara of the proximal femur in early childhood with classical radiographic changes and no other skeletal manifestations

## TABLE 27.1

### CLASSIFICATION OF COXA VARA

Congenital coxa vara
  Congenital short femur
  Congenital bowed femur
Proximal femoral focal deficiency (PFFD)
Acquired coxa vara
  Trauma
    Femoral neck fracture
    Dislocation of femoral head
  Infection
    Septic necrosis of the femoral head
    Proximal femoral osteomyelitis
  Slipped upper femoral epiphysis
  Legg-Calvé-Perthes disease
  Pathologic bone disorders
    Osteogenesis imperfecta
  Fibrous dysplasia
  Rickets
  Osteopetrosis
  Skeletal dysplasia
    Cleidocranial dysostosis
    Metaphyseal dysostosis
    Spondylometaphyseal dysplasia
  Tumor
Developmental coxa vara

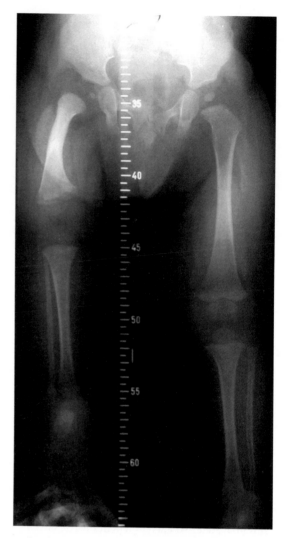

**Figure 27.1** The radiographic appearance of congenital coxa vara in an 18-month-old child with a congenital short femur. (Courtesy of Perry L. Schoenecker.)

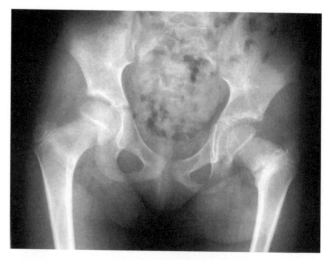

**Figure 27.2** The radiographic appearance of acquired coxa vara in a 7-year-old girl who had an intertrochanteric left hip fracture.

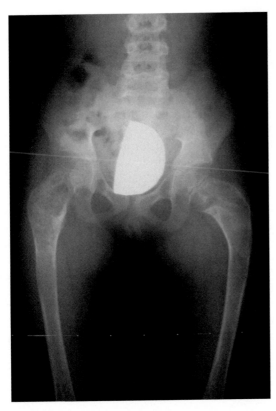

**Figure 27.3** The radiographic appearance of acquired coxa vara in an 8-year-old child who had fibrous dysplasia and a shepherd-crook deformity of the proximal femur. (Courtesy of Perry L. Schoeneker.)

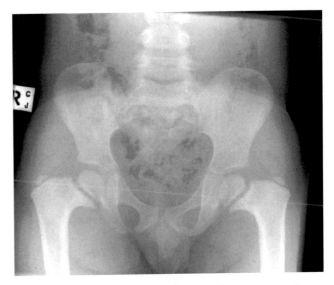

**Figure 27.5** Radiographic appearance of developmental coxa vara in a 3-year-old child.

or obvious underlying causes (9,10) (Fig. 27.5). There is associated mild limb-length inequality that develops secondary to the progressive varus deformity, but not because of a significant decrease in the length of the femoral shaft. The growth behavior and radiographic changes help differentiate this condition from the others mentioned previously.

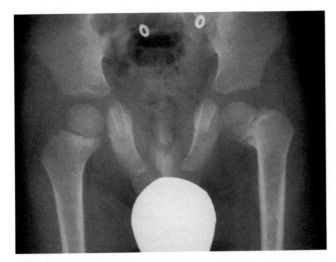

**Figure 27.4** The radiographic appearance of coxa vara associated with spondylometaphyseal dysplasia in a 4-year-old child. (Courtesy of Perry L. Schoenecker.)

## Epidemiology

Developmental coxa vara is a rare entity, with a reported incidence of 1 in 25,000 live births worldwide (10,11). The ratio of boys to girls is 1:1, and there do not seem to be any major racial predilections (12,13). The rate of occurrence in the left and right hips is also equal. The condition is bilateral in 30% to 50% of patients (10,12,14–18). Bilateral cases may more likely be associated with a skeletal dysplasia, so the examiner should investigate for this possibility during the physical and radiographic examination. There is presumed to be a genetic cause of developmental coxa vara, with several reports suggesting an autosomal dominant pattern of inheritance with incomplete penetrance (10,13,17–20).

## Etiology

The exact cause of developmental coxa vara remains unknown. The most widely accepted theory is that the deformity in the proximal femur results from a primary defect in endochondral ossification of the medial part of the femoral neck (21). This results in dystrophic bone along the medial inferior aspect of the femoral neck, which fatigues with weight bearing, resulting in the progressive varus deformity that is seen clinically. In this regard, the condition has been likened to infantile Blount disease of the proximal tibia; however, the two conditions have not been shown to coexist (22,23).

Other investigators hypothesize that the varus deformity is caused by excessive intrauterine pressure on the developing fetal hip, resulting in a depression in the neck of the femur (9). A vascular insult causing a growth arrest to the developing femoral head and neck has also been proposed as a cause of coxa vara (24). Yet another theory is that the varus deformity results from faulty maturation of the cartilage and metaphyseal bone of the femoral neck (10).

## Clinical Features

The child with developmental coxa vara usually presents after he or she has started walking and before 6 years of age (25,26). Clinically, the child presents with a painless limp that is caused by both the functional abductor muscle weakness and a relatively minor limb-length inequality in unilateral cases. When the disease is bilateral, the child presents with a waddling gait and increased lumbar lordosis as seen in bilateral developmental hip dislocation (2,10,25,27–29). Although pain is seldom reported as a symptom, older children may report a deep ache in the buttock muscles after prolonged exercise.

On physical examination, the greater trochanter will be more prominent and proximal than the contralateral normal side, thereby altering normal hip joint mechanics. With increasing coxa vara deformity, the origin and insertion of the hip abductors approach each other, resulting in functional hip abductor weakness and a positive Trendelenburg test. An associated limb-length inequality is present in unilateral cases but is rarely greater than 3 cm at skeletal maturity, even in untreated patients (13,30).

The range of motion of the hip is reduced in all planes of motion, with limitations of abduction and internal rotation being the greatest (12,25). The limitation in abduction is due to impingement of the greater trochanter on the side of the pelvis. The loss of internal rotation is due to the loss of the femoral neck anteversion that is a feature of developmental coxa vara. As part of the general clinical examination other causes of coxa vara should be ruled out, for example, skeletal dysplasias (15,31).

## Radiographic Features

The diagnosis of developmental coxa vara is confirmed with a plain anteroposterior radiograph of the affected hip. The typical radiographic findings are listed in Table 27.2. Mild acetabular dysplasia is sometimes present as well (4,10,15,16,21,26,31,32). The inverted Y pattern seen in the inferior femoral neck remains the *sine qua non* of this condition. The inverted Y pattern is formed by a triangular piece of bone in the medial femoral neck, abutting the physis and bounded by two radiolucent bands. Although

## TABLE 27.2

### RADIOGRAPHIC FEATURES OF DEVELOPMENTAL COXA VARA

1. Decreased femoral neck-shaft angle
2. Vertical position of physeal plate
3. Triangular metaphyseal fragment in inferior femoral neck with associated inverted Y appearance
4. Shortened femoral neck
5. Decrease in normal anteversion

these bands were once postulated to be two physeal plates, biopsy specimens and magnetic resonance studies have shown this to be an area of widening of the physeal plate with associated abnormal ossification (22). Kim et al. used computed tomography (CT) scanning in three patients and suggested that the triangular metaphyseal fragment is a Salter-Harris type 2 "separation" through the defective femoral neck (32).

The amount of varus deformity of an affected hip may be quantified on anteroposterior radiographs by measuring the neck-shaft angle, the head-shaft angle, or the Hilgenreiner-epiphyseal angle (H-E) (33). Neither the neck-shaft angle nor the head-shaft angle provides an accurate reflection of the severity of the deformity and its likely progression or correction (24,29). On the other hand, the H-E angle, described by Weinstein, has been shown to have good prognostic value (33). The H-E angle is the angle between the physeal plate and Hilgenreiner's line (33) (Fig. 27.6). In 100 healthy patients, this angle averaged 16 degrees. In developmental coxa vara, the angle is between 40 and 70 degrees. Using this measurement in 22 patients with coxa vara, Weinstein was able to make recommendations concerning the natural history and treatment options for this group of children. These are discussed in the subsequent text.

## Pathoanatomy

In early fetal development, the proximal femoral physis extends across the entire proximal femur. The cartilage columns that make this physis then differentiate into cervical epiphyseal and trochanteric apophyseal portions. The medial cervical portion matures first, elongating the femoral neck. The neck-shaft angle is determined by the relative amount of growth at these two sites (34–38). The mean angle of the femoral neck-shaft angle is 150 degrees at 3 weeks of age, decreasing to 120 degrees in adulthood (39) (Fig. 27.7).

A number of reports have been published on biopsies taken from both the proximal femoral physis and femoral neck in patients with developmental coxa vara (12,34,40). These have shown defects in cartilage production and secondary metaphyseal bone formation in the inferior portion of the proximal femoral physeal plate and adjacent femoral neck. The cartilage cell numbers are decreased and the remaining cells are not well organized in regular columns as seen in a healthy physis. The adjacent metaphyseal bone is osteoporotic and infiltrated with nests of cartilage cells (34,40) (Fig. 27.8). Chung and Riser reported on the postmortem findings in a 5-year-old boy with unilateral coxa vara. They noted that the acetabular volume and femoral head were smaller, the femoral neck was shorter, and the physis was wider on the affected side than on the normal contralateral side. They found that endochondral ossification was altered in the affected hip as well as in the "normal" contralateral side. They also

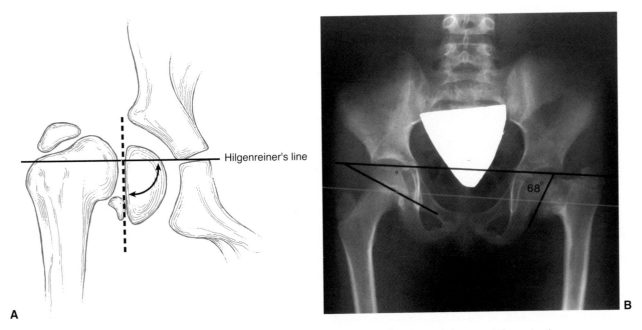

**Figure 27.6**  Hilgenreiner-epiphyseal (H-E) angle. **A:** The H-E angle is the angle between Hilgenreiner's line and a line drawn parallel to the capital femoral physis. **B:** H-E angle of 68 degrees in a patient with developmental coxa vara.

observed that there was a "reduction in the number and caliber of intraosseous arteries supplying the metaphyseal sides of the growth plates in the proximal femur and those supplying the subchondral region and extraosseous medial ascending cervical arteries on the surface of the femoral neck" (34).

The resulting deformity is a combination of the underlying pathology and the altered mechanical forces across the hip. With progressive varus deformity of the femoral neck, the force across the proximal femoral physis changes from compression to shear as it assumes a more vertical orientation. The shortened lever arm and relative proximal migration of the greater trochanter also leads to altered muscular forces in the abductor group.

## Natural History

Untreated developmental coxa vara was once viewed as a condition in which increased tensile forces on the superior femoral neck led to progressive varus deformity of the proximal femur, ultimately resulting in the development of a stress-fracture-related nonunion of the femoral neck and

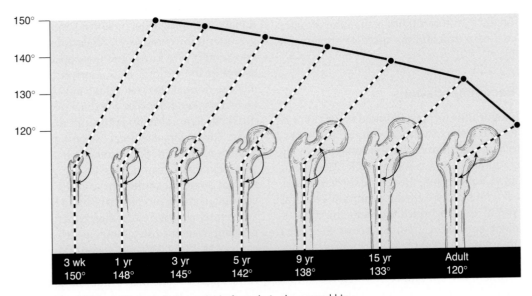

**Figure 27.7**  Evolution of the neck-shaft angle in the normal hip.

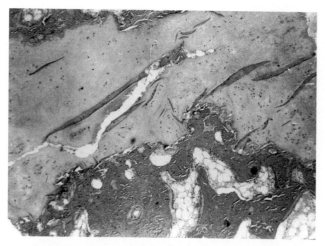

**Figure 27.8** Photomicrograph of a biopsy specimen of the proximal femoral physeal plate of a patient with developmental coxa vara demonstrates irregularly distributed germinal cells in the resting zone; an absence of normal, orderly progression of the cartilage columns; and a poorly defined zone of provisional calcification. Nests of cartilage cells reside at the margin of the metaphyseal bone.

premature degenerative arthritic changes within the hip joint in almost all the affected patients (41). Weinstein et al. (33), however, showed that not all patients with developmental coxa vara follow such a progressive course. Their study demonstrated that the determining factor for progression of the varus deformity is the H-E angle. If the H-E angle is less than 45 degrees, the condition is stable and progressive deformity is unlikely. If the H-E angle is greater than 60 degrees, surgical intervention is recommended because the deformity invariably progresses. Between 45 and 60 degrees the natural history is not as clear, and these patients must have serial radiographs to reevaluate their varus deformity (33). Serafin et al. (16), Carroll et al. (22), Cordes et al. (23), and Desai et al. (15) have all confirmed these parameters in their own patient populations. What is not clear from natural history studies is the time of onset of developmental coxa vara and the speed of progression of the deformity.

## Treatment Recommendations

The treatment algorithm for developmental coxa vara is based on the natural history studies mentioned in the preceding text. Because the cause of the abnormal pathology is not known, a biologic cure is not possible. Treatment, therefore, is aimed at preventing the secondary deformities of the proximal femur created by the condition's natural history. Borden et al. (42) identified the main objectives of current treatment approaches: correction of the varus angulation into a more normal physiologic range; changing the loading characteristics seen by the abnormal femoral neck from shear to compression; correction of limb-length inequality; and reestablishment of a proper abductor muscle length-tension relation.

### Nonsurgical

Patients who have an H-E angle of less than 45 degrees and are asymptomatic need to be assessed for limb-length inequality (in unilateral cases) and for evidence of skeletal dysplasia. These patients should also have periodic radiographic assessments to assess for progressive deformity until skeletal maturity. In patients with an H-E angle between 45 and 59 degrees, serial radiographs are essential so as to assess for progression. In those who develop a symptomatic limp, Trendelenburg gait, or progressive deformity, surgical treatment is warranted. In general, nonsurgical treatments including bed rest, traction, and hip immobilization in a spica cast have not altered the natural course of the disease (24,29,43). Zadek (21), in a review of conservative treatment of developmental coxa vara, concluded that the previously attempted nonoperative methods had universally little or no value.

### Surgical

**Indications.** Surgical intervention is recommended for hips with an H-E angle of 60 degrees or greater, a progressive decrease in the femoral neck-shaft angle to 90 to 100 degrees or less, or for patients who develop a symptomatic limp or Trendelenburg gait (25,33,44).

**Options.** A variety of surgical treatments have been recommended for developmental coxa vara over the years, many of which are of historical interest only. One such procedure is epiphysiodesis of the greater trochanter, which has been shown to be unreliable as the sole surgical treatment of this condition (12,27,45). Other historical surgical procedures included pin fixation and bone grafting of the femoral neck defect, which did not correct the varus deformity, did not prevent progression, and sometimes resulted in growth arrest of the capital femoral physis (27).

The most successful way to correct the deformity and restore more normal hip joint mechanics is with a derotational valgus-producing proximal femoral osteotomy. A valgus osteotomy converts the shear forces across the physes into compressive forces, and this appears to improve ossification in the femoral neck. Correction of the neck-shaft angle to normal also restores the muscle function to the hip abductors. Restoration of a normal neck-shaft angle allows proximal femoral remodeling and normal ossification to occur. The proximal femoral osteotomy has been performed at the level of the neck, the intertrochanteric region, and the subtrochanteric region, all with the goal of restoring the normal anatomy of the hip joint (2,12,29,42,44,46,47). Femoral neck osteotomies have had a higher morbidity rate and poorer clinical results than either the intertrochanteric or subtrochanteric osteotomies, which are the treatments of choice (14,15,22,23,31,33,48–50). Many intertrochanteric and subtrochanteric osteotomies have been described for correcting coxa vara, thereby indicating that no one method has proved to be totally satisfactory. Langenskiöld's valgus-producing osteotomy (12) (Fig. 27.9) and Pauwel Y-shaped

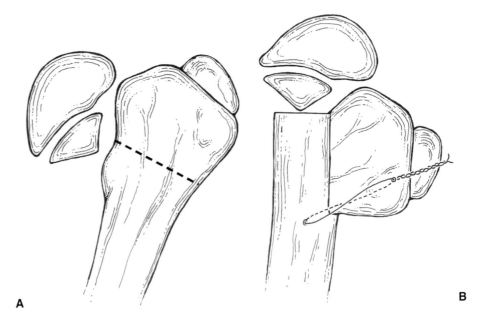

**Figure 27.9** Langenskiöld intertrochanteric osteotomy. **A:** Site of osteotomy in proximal femur. **B:** After osteotomy with fixation in place and resulting coxa valga.

osteotomy (23,51) (Fig. 27.10) are examples of intertrochanteric corrective osteotomies that have produced good results. Pauwel osteotomy is technically demanding and does not allow rotational correction of the upper femur. Borden et al. describe a subtrochanteric valgus-producing osteotomy that has been used successfully in achieving and maintaining the goals of surgical treatment (42) (Fig. 27.11). An alternative form of internal fixation suggested by Wagner is performed with a bifurcated plate driven through the intramedullary surface of the proximal fragment and secured to the distal fragment with screws (Fig. 27.12).

A difficult decision to make is the timing of the osteotomy. Some orthopaedists advocate performing the osteotomy as soon as it is clinically indicated, whereas others prefer to wait until the child is older. Pylkkanen (12), Weighill (47), and Serafin (52) recommend that the osteotomy be performed at an early age, even as young as 18 months. Weinstein et al. (33), and Duncan (10), on the other hand, recommend delaying surgery until the patient is 5 to 6 years of age. In very young children, it is difficult to obtain adequate fixation because of the mostly cartilaginous proximal femur, and this may accentuate the propensity for recurrence of the deformity in this age group. On the other hand, the amount of acetabular dysplasia associated with developmental coxa vara most likely increases with increasing age, and the capacity for acetabular remodeling decreases with increasing age. Therefore, the appropriate time for surgical intervention in indicated patients is as soon as there is adequate bone development to allow secure internal fixation.

The most secure fixation of the osteotomy is achieved with either a blade plate or sliding hip screw. A number of other devices have been used, including cerclage wire (53), hook plates (54), and external fixators (55), all of which have a higher incidence of fixation failure. The advantage

of the blade plate over the sliding hip screw is that it does not cross the proximal femoral physis, and so it can be used in very young patients. Good results have also been reported with the use of a spike osteotomy and no internal fixation (56). Stability is obtained in these cases by careful fashioning of the spike so that there is a tight fit into the cancellous bone of the metaphysis.

The goal of surgical treatment is to produce a valgus overcorrection of the neck-shaft angle of the proximal femur, regardless of the patient's age. A number of authors have reported recurrence rates of between 30% and 70% because of insufficient correction at the time of surgery, or loss of correction in the postoperative period because of inadequate fixation of the osteotomy (15,22,23). Carroll et al. (22) found that if the H-E angle is reduced to less than 38 degrees, 95% of the patients showed no evidence of recurrence (Fig. 27.13). In contrast, 93% of the osteotomies that retained a physeal angle greater than 40 degrees required revision for recurrent varus deformity.

In addition to the varus deformity being corrected by a valgus osteotomy, the femur must be internally rotated to recreate the normal femoral neck anteversion. The amount of derotation required is a clinical decision made during surgery. An adductor tenotomy performed at the time of the valgus osteotomy allows easier positioning of the proximal femur (47). In cases where it is difficult to correct the varus deformity, a proximal femoral shortening procedure at the level of the osteotomy can be used (25). Care should be taken to avoid crossing the physeal plate with the fixation device, if possible. A spica cast may be applied, depending on the stability of the internal fixation.

Successful treatment results in maintenance of the valgus correction and restoration of more normal growth of the proximal physis. By converting the shear stresses to compression, the osteotomy allows this more normal development.

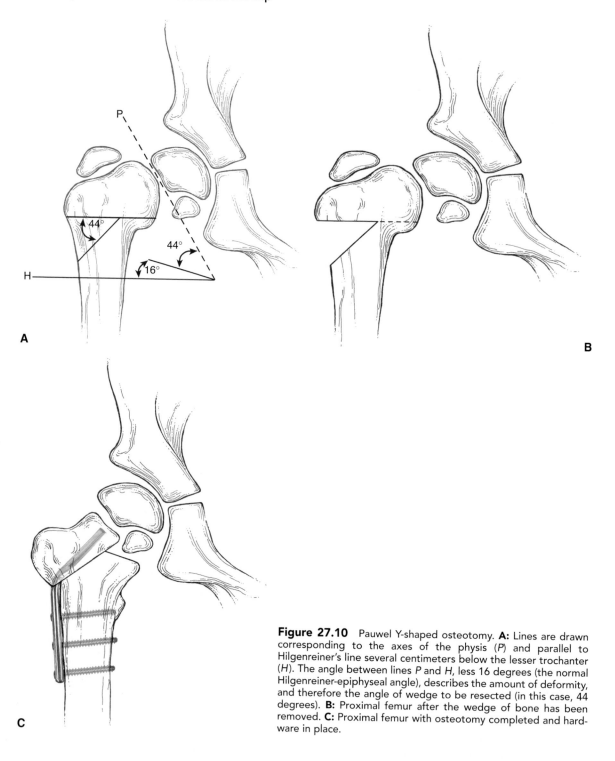

**Figure 27.10** Pauwel Y-shaped osteotomy. **A:** Lines are drawn corresponding to the axes of the physis (*P*) and parallel to Hilgenreiner's line several centimeters below the lesser trochanter (*H*). The angle between lines *P* and *H*, less 16 degrees (the normal Hilgenreiner-epiphyseal angle), describes the amount of deformity, and therefore the angle of wedge to be resected (in this case, 44 degrees). **B:** Proximal femur after the wedge of bone has been removed. **C:** Proximal femur with osteotomy completed and hardware in place.

The triangular metaphyseal defect in the femoral neck spontaneously closes within the first months postoperatively in most cases, if adequate valgus has been created (25) (Fig. 27.14). The results of most studies show that a correction of the H-E angle to less than 40 degrees will result in a good clinical outcome. The published results of valgus osteotomies for coxa vara invariably include multiple etiologies for this deformity; hence, some conclusions are not necessarily specific for developmental coxa vara. In

a review of 14 patients who had had a Pauwel Y-shaped intertrochanteric osteotomy for coxa vara, Cordes et al. (23) reported good maintenance of correction at 11 years average follow-up in patients in whom the H-E angle had been corrected to less than 40 degrees. Desai and Johnson (15) reviewed 20 hips in 12 patients for an average of 20 years and found that satisfactory results were achieved if the H-E angle was 35 degrees or less. Twelve hips had trochanteric overgrowth; however, only 5 of these patients

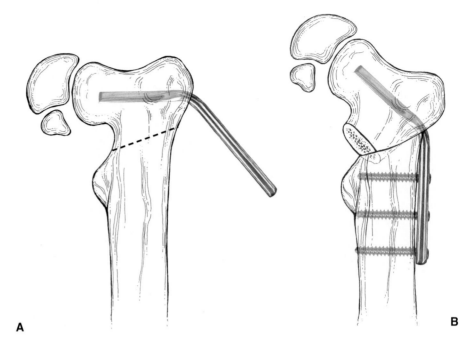

**Figure 27.11** Borden subtrochanteric osteotomy. **A:** Line of osteotomy and insertion of 140-degree angle blade plate parallel to the superior border of the femoral neck. **B:** Varus deformity corrected. Note that the lateral cortex of the proximal fragment is approximated to the upper end of the distal fragment. **A**

**B**

had weakness of the abductor. Yang and Huang (50) showed that the acetabular depth improves significantly in patients with developmental coxa vara who are treated with a valgus intertrochanteric osteotomy, especially if it is performed before the child reaches 6 years of age. Carroll et al. (22) reviewed 37 affected hips in 26 children following a valgus osteotomy for congenital or acquired coxa

vara. They reported a 50% recurrence rate that was unrelated to age at the time of surgery, the type of internal fixation, or the etiology. Of the children in whom the H-E angle was corrected to less than 38 degrees, 95% had no recurrence of the deformity. If the femoral osteotomy is performed before 10 years of age, 83% of the patients will have excellent acetabular development.

## Authors' Preferred Recommendations

The important first step in treating developmental coxa vara is to rule out any other possible cause for this condition (Table 27.1). Once diagnosed, the child should be followed up every 4 to 6 months with anteroposterior radiographs of the pelvis. Surgical intervention is recommended for hips with an H-E angle of 60 degrees or greater, a progressive decrease in the femoral neck-shaft angle of 90 to 100 degrees or less, or in patients with developmental coxa vara who develop a symptomatic limp or Trendelenburg gait. The authors prefer a subtrochanteric valgus-producing derotational osteotomy of the proximal femur. The preferred fixation device is either a blade plate or a sliding hip screw (Fig. 27.15). An adductor tenotomy is frequently used so as to facilitate correction of the deformity. Spica cast immobilization is used, in addition, for 6 to 8 weeks in most patients.

## Complications

Schmidt and Kalamchi (31) showed that 89% of hips that have had an osteotomy have premature closure of the proximal femoral physeal plate. This usually occurs in the first 12 to 24 months after surgery (Fig. 27.14). This phenomenon is probably due to an inherently abnormal

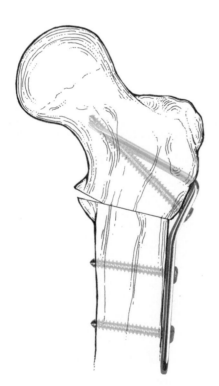

**Figure 27.12** Internal fixation of valgus osteotomy with the Wagner bifurcated plate. The bifurcated end of the plate is driven into the proximal fragment through its intramedullary surface.

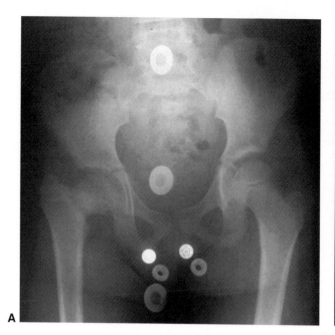
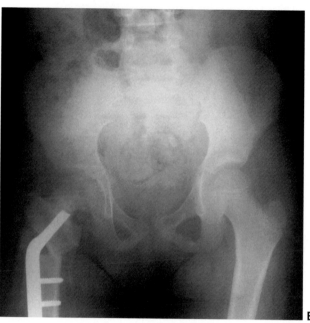

**Figure 27.13** Anteroposterior pelvic radiographs of a 4-year-old child with developmental coxa vara. **A:** Preoperative radiograph. **B:** Postoperative radiograph. A subtrochanteric derotational proximal femoral osteotomy successfully achieved the objectives of surgical correction, including correction of the varus angulation, restoring the Hilgenreiner-epiphyseal (H-E) angle to less than 30 degrees, and lateralizing the distal fragment to help reestablish the proper abductor muscle length-tension relation. (Courtesy of Perry L. Schoenecker.)

physis that has a compressive force applied across it rather than any physeal injury at the time of surgery. The surgery itself may also accelerate physeal closure. This premature closure may lead to both limb-length inequality and trochanteric overgrowth with resultant recurrent coxa vara. To prevent this recurrent deformity, it is recommended that after premature closure of the proximal femoral epiphyseal plate has been documented, an apophyseodesis of the greater trochanter or a trochanteric advancement be performed before the development of a recurrent deformity (25). If the varus deformity does recur, a repeat valgus-producing femoral osteotomy can be performed. The residual limb-length inequality is usually mild and can be addressed in most cases with a shoe lift. Contralateral epiphysiodesis around the knee can be used in more severe cases to achieve equal limb lengths.

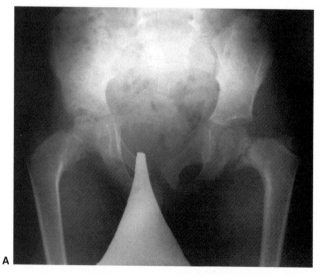
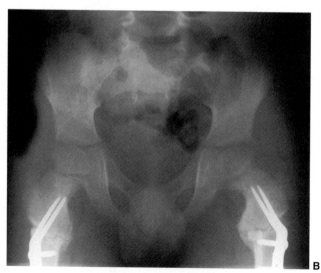

**Figure 27.14** Anteroposterior pelvic radiographs of a child with developmental coxa vara. **A:** The preoperative radiograph demonstrates a classic inferior femoral neck triangular fragment. **B:** Two months postoperatively, the radiograph demonstrates correction of the physeal angle, with spontaneous closure of the femoral neck triangular metaphyseal fragment. (Courtesy of Perry L. Schoenecker.)

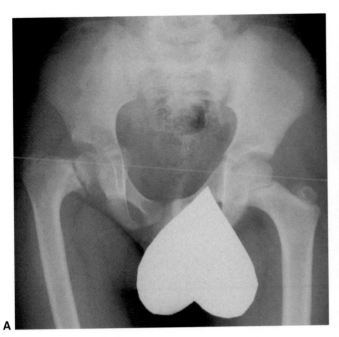
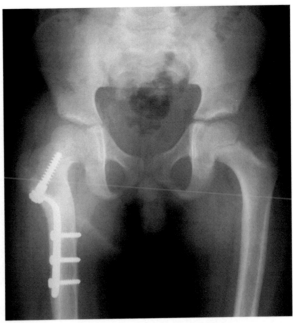

**Figure 27.15** The anteroposterior pelvic radiographs of an 8-year-old child with developmental coxa vara. **A:** Preoperative radiograph. **B:** The postoperative radiograph 11 months after the subtrochanteric proximal femoral derotational osteotomy and fixation with a sliding hip screw demonstrates spontaneous closure of the proximal femoral epiphyseal plate. The greater trochanteric apophyses remain open. (Courtesy of Perry L. Schoenecker.)

## BLADDER EXSTROPHY

### Definition

Bladder exstrophy is part of a spectrum of anomalies which may involve, to varying degrees, the bladder, pelvis, intestinal tract, and external genitalia. The prototypical and most common form is "classic" exstrophy, involving a widened pelvis with an anterior diastasis, an open bladder, and a complete epispadias (57). The most minor form of this spectrum is epispadias, which may have a closed bladder but widened pelvic symphysis. The most pronounced expression of this spectrum is cloacal exstrophy, which usually involves all of the findings discussed in the preceding text, as well as omphalocele and often, a lumbosacral neural tube defect. Although classic exstrophy is a relatively uniform anomaly, cloacal exstrophy is extremely variable from patient to patient and often includes anomalies of the spine and extremities. The orthopaedic surgeon may be consulted with questions about prognosis of the pelvic defect, for assistance during closure of the bladder, and for treatment of associated anomalies of the spine and extremities.

### Epidemiology

The incidence of bladder exstrophy is between 1 in 10,000 and 1 in 50,000 live births (57). Boys are much more commonly affected, with a gender ratio of at least 2.5:1 between boys and girls. "Classic" exstrophy is the most common type seen, with cloacal exstrophy being about one fifth as

common. When parents have a child with exstrophy, the risk of their having a subsequent child with the same defect is approximately 1:100.

### Etiology and Pathogenesis

The etiology of this disorder is not known. The pathogenesis is thought to be a failure of the cloacal membrane to get reinforced by the ingrowth of mesoderm (57). The cloacal membrane is the caudal end of the embryonic abdominal wall. It initially forms the anterior boundary of the bladder and hindgut. Mesenchymal ingrowth allows formation of the anterior part of the pelvis and the abdominal wall muscles. This defective structure leads to the development of a large open bladder and urethra. In cloacal exstrophy, the hindgut is exposed as well.

### Clinical Features

The constant finding is a midline defect in the anterior abdominal wall at the level of the pubic symphysis, exposing an open bladder and urethra. This usually measures at least 3 to 4 cm at birth in classic exstrophy (Fig. 27.16). The bladder itself is a flat plate instead of a closed sac. In classic exstrophy, the innervation is normal, the hips are usually stable, and the extremities are functional. In cloacal exstrophy, the abdominal wall defect is much larger and the lower intestinal tract is variably exposed (Fig. 27.17). A spinal exam and a neurologic exam of the lower extremities should be performed. Often, in patients with cloacal

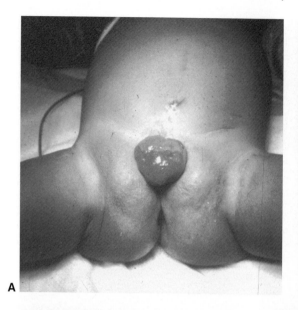

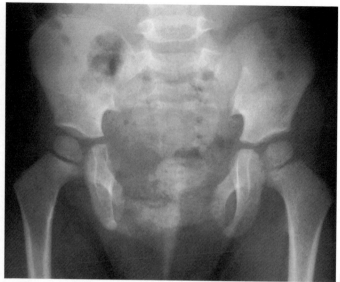

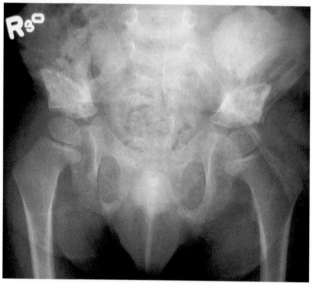

**Figure 27.16** Patient with classic exstrophy before closure. **A:** Clinical photo. **B:** Radiograph prior to closure. **C:** Radiograph after closure. (Courtesy of Paul Sponseller.)

exstrophy, there is a lower lumbar neurologic deficit caused by lipomeningocele or myelomeningocele. Hip dislocation, foot deformity, and hemisacral agenesis are not uncommon. Other anomalies that may coexist with cloacal exstrophy include partial failures of formation of the lower extremity or a distal duplication of the spine.

## Radiographic Features

There is separation of two paired pubic bones, which are usually symmetrically formed in patients with classic exstrophy. This separation is typically approximately 4 to 5 cm at birth and increases steadily with age (58) (Fig. 27.16B). In normal persons, this separation is constant at approximately 1 cm throughout life. The iliac wings are externally rotated by approximately 15 degrees each, and assume a "flattened" or "flared" shape. The anterior (ischiopubic) portions of the pelvis are slightly underdeveloped, having a decreased transverse diameter. The

hips themselves, apart from being in a retroverted position, rarely show dysplasia. In cloacal exstrophy, the diastasis is much larger (Fig. 27.17B) and many other spinopelvic anomalies exist: posterior laminar defects, vertebral body anomalies, sacroiliac asymmetry, and hip dysplasia (Fig. 27.18).

## Other Imaging Studies

Other studies are rarely needed in classic exstrophy. In cloacal exstrophy, CT scan may show the sacroiliac and pelvic malformations more completely. Magnetic resonance imaging (MRI) of the spine may be valuable in patients with cloacal exstrophy for the purpose of assessing anomalies.

## Pathoanatomy

Studies of the pelvis by CT scan, MRI, and dissection of anatomic specimens of classic exstrophy have established

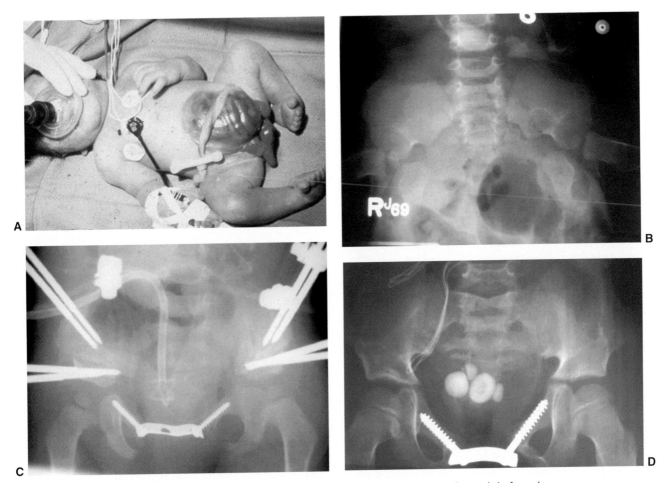

**Figure 27.17** Patient with cloacal exstrophy. **A:** Clinical photo. **B:** Radiograph before closure. **C:** Radiograph 2 months after closure. **D:** Radiograph 6 years after closure. (Courtesy of Paul Sponseller.)

the following (59–61) (Fig. 27.19):

1. The pubic bones are foreshortened by about one third in transverse length.
2. The ilia are normal in size but externally rotated approximately 13 degrees.
3. The acetabulae are retroverted but femoral version is normal. Biomechanical modeling has shown that the total stress on the hip joint is increased by approximately 30% above normal, mainly because of the increased transverse distance of the center of hip rotation from the center of body mass, as well as the change in orientation of the trochanter and acetabulum.
4. The sacroiliac joints are also externally rotated and the pelvis is angled caudally.
5. The muscles of the pelvic floor are divergent, causing a risk of prolapse.
6. The bladder itself is opened into the shape of a flat plate, small and fibrotic. The external genitalia are hypoplastic.
7. In cloacal exstrophy, there may be absence, hypoplasia, or asymmetry of the sacroiliac joint, as well as a dislocation of the hip(s). In these patients, the bone density is usually diminished. The genitalia may be severely anomalous.

## Natural History

The function of the pelvis and hips is generally quite good in the untreated patient with classic bladder exstrophy. Children learn to walk at a normal age, although they

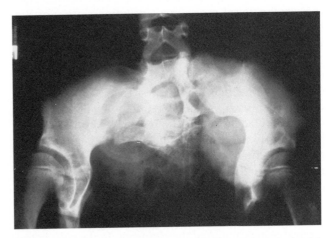

**Figure 27.18** Patient with severe multiple neurologic and pelvic anomalies associated with cloacal exstrophy. (Courtesy of Paul Sponseller.)

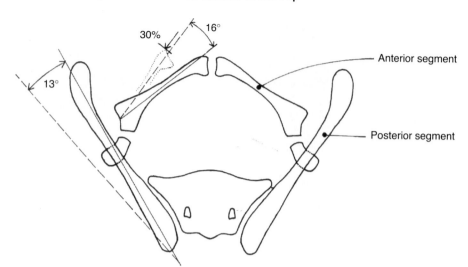

30%    16°

13°

— Anterior segment

— Posterior segment

**Figure 27.19** Schematic representation of pelvic differences in classic exstrophy versus normal in the transverse plane. (Courtesy of Paul Sponseller.)

have an increased external foot-progression angle. This becomes less pronounced over time (58). Athletic ability is not impaired. Adults with exstrophy seem to have an increased incidence of pain in the region of the sacroiliac joints. One natural history study suggested that there is an increased incidence of degenerative disease of the hip in patients with uncorrected exstrophy (61). However, the number of patients in the study was small, and the affected patients appeared to have a degree of acetabular dysplasia that is not commonly seen in most patients with classic exstrophy. It is not currently established that osteotomy of the pelvis for exstrophy is necessary to protect against premature osteoarthritis of the hip in a patient with no associated acetabular dysplasia. There are some reports of uterine prolapse in adult women with exstrophy, but the frequency of this is not known. Both men and women patients with exstrophy are usually fertile, and a number of women have successfully given birth, usually by cesarean section.

## Treatment Recommendations

The pediatric urologist usually performs the reconstruction in several surgical procedures, including closure of the bladder and lower abdominal wall soon after birth, followed by epispadias closure at a later date. Surgery for achieving continence is commonly performed after the age at which children normally become continent and may consist of bladder neck suspension and/or collagen injections. Patients who are unable to become continent are offered a bladder augmentation and a catheterizable umbilical stoma. Finally, in the older child, occasionally plastic surgery is an option to optimize the appearance of the perineum. In general, orthopaedic surgery of the pelvic deformity is indicated as part of one of these procedures only if it is needed for achieving urologic goals. These goals include achieving a closed bladder, urinary continence, and acceptable appearance of the perineum. In the past, it was most common for boys with cloacal exstrophy to be reconstructed as girls with appropriate endocrine supplementation

because of the extreme abnormalities of the external genitalia. However, long-term studies have shown that psychological distress at maturity is not uncommon after this procedure, so families are given both gender options.

### Nonsurgical

Patients with an exstrophy that has been successfully managed without osteotomy may not need any procedures to be done on the pelvic bones. These are patients who may have been managed without bladder closure or had closure done in the newborn period without osteotomy. They may have had closures with soft-tissue rotational procedures to manage a mild-to-moderate sized exstrophy defect.

Neonates whose bladders are closed at birth can usually have their pubic symphysis closed down by manually approximating the two halves of the pelvis and placing a strong suture between the pubic bones. The lower extremities are immobilized in traction or a cast or splint. The mobility to allow the approximation of the pubis probably occurs by plastic deformation of the sacral ala and by the laxity of the sacroiliac joints. Although the pelvis gradually assumes its original diastasis over time, the tissue relaxation achieved by this sequence of events lasts long enough for the midline closure to become mature in most patients.

### Surgical

*Indications.* The most common indication for orthopaedic surgery on the pelvis is a bladder and lower urinary tract that cannot be closed without approximation of the pubic bones. This is usually the case in a patient who presents for closure after about the first month of age, or in whom a prior closure without osteotomy has failed. Another indication is in an older patient with a closed bladder who requires osteotomy and pubic reapproximation to achieve continence. The final, and least common, indication is in an older child in whom perineal reconstruction is aided by bringing the pelvis closer together. This decreases the width of the perineum and restores a more normal appearance to the external genital structures. Patients who have acetabular dysplasia with classic exstrophy should undergo osteotomy.

**Options.** The benefit of approximating the divergent urogenital structures with the aid of pelvic osteotomy was first described by Shultz and O'Phelan in Minneapolis nearly half a century ago (62). They employed bilateral vertical iliac osteotomies through a posterior approach, with a midline wire to hold the pubic bones together (63). This necessitated turning the patient from prone to supine in the middle of the procedure. Although the original procedure remains popular, other approaches have been developed. Transverse supra-acetabular iliac osteotomies from an anterior approach were described in the 1980s by several surgeons. A group in Toronto has also described an oblique osteotomy of the ilium, midway between the two approaches discussed earlier, which can help bring the wings of the ilium together (64). Anterior pubic ramotomy is a simple procedure that can aid in the approximation of the two pubic bones, although the effect is not as pronounced as iliac osteotomy.

The osteotomized pelvis may be immobilized using bed rest and a cast, traction, external fixation, or internal fixation. A combination of external and internal fixation provides the most consistent results.

## Authors' Preferred Recommendations

The authors' preference is to assist the urologist in closing all classic exstrophy within a few days after birth, when the relaxin is maximal and the pelvic bones are soft. In most babies, the exstrophy can be successfully closed without osteotomy. We prefer to immobilize these patients in modified Bryant traction with the legs suspended vertically so that the pelvis is slightly off the bed (Fig. 23.29 in Chapter 23 of Lovell and Winter's Pediatric Orthopaedics 5th Edition). This maintains an anterior closing force to the anterior pelvis while the closure heals. Other surgeons employ casts or splints to adduct or internally rotate the hips, cutting out the surgical site for urologic access.

For those whose bladders reopen, who present late, or in whom simpler procedures to achieve continence fail, the authors prefer anterior supraacetabular iliac osteotomies. In children older than 1 year, an additional closing-wedge greenstick osteotomy is added lateral to the sacroiliac joints to rotate the iliac wings together. Pins are inserted for external fixation, and the urologist closes the bladder, perineum, and abdomen. The external fixator is then assembled.

In patients with cloacal exstrophy, the diastasis is much larger and the bone is softer. An anterior plate is especially helpful in maintaining the closure. For this reason, we prefer to defer cloacal closure until the child is at least 6 to 12 months of age and plating is feasible.

All children have some recurrence of the diastasis as they grow after an osteotomy, although it is less than it would have been without closure. The patients who have osteotomy at the youngest ages have greatest recurrence. The goal of maintaining pelvic approximation while the urologic reconstruction heals appears to be successful in most cases.

## Complications

In one large series, the complication rate of orthopaedic treatment of exstrophy was 4% (65). These were classified as bony or neurologic complications at the osteotomy site, complications of traction, and infection. Bony complications included vertical migration or nonunion after posterior iliac osteotomies, as well as inadvertent osteotomy through the sacroiliac joints because the procedure does allow visualization of these joints. The most frequent neurologic complication was femoral nerve palsy after anterior osteotomy. This appears to be caused by medial pressure and tension on the nerve, and resolves spontaneously within 3 months. There were two reports of sciatic palsy, by mechanisms unknown. Complications of immobilization include skin breakdown from wrapping the two legs tightly adducted together. Deep infection at the osteotomy site does not occur with more frequency than in other elective surgeries, despite the proximity to the incontinent bladder.

# ILIOPSOAS SNAPPING HIP

## Definition

Coxa saltans, or snapping hip, is characterized by an audible snapping that usually occurs with flexion and extension of the hip. This snapping can be accompanied by pain and often occurs during physical activity. It can be divided into three types: external, intraarticular, and internal, with the external type being by far the most common (66). The external type is caused by snapping of either the posterior border of the iliotibial band or the anterior border of the gluteus maximus over the greater trochanter when the hip is flexed from an extended position (66–69). The internal type, which is still the most poorly understood, has a variety of presumed etiologies, with snapping of the iliopsoas tendon over the iliopectineal eminence (70) or over the femoral head (69) being the most common. The intraarticular type is caused by a loose body in the joint, such as a fracture fragment or a torn piece of labrum. It usually has a distinctive presentation and, unlike the other types of snapping, almost always requires surgery for symptomatic relief (71,72).

## Epidemiology

The incidence of coxa saltans of the internal type is unknown because snapping of the iliopsoas tendon is often unrecognized or misdiagnosed. In addition, internal snapping can be asymptomatic and therefore not reported, making it difficult to assess the true incidence (73,74). One study demonstrated that only 14 of 26 (54%) sonographically diagnosed snapping hips were clinically painful (75). From the few reports in the literature, patients of both sexes are affected equally (66,67,74,76). In the adolescent population, symptomatic internal snapping is most common among teenagers (aged 14 to 17 years) who are engaged in sports activities that involve running (74,76). There is no evidence in support of a genetic basis for this condition.

## Etiology and Pathogenesis

The internal type of coxa saltans is a poorly recognized entity that was first reported in 1951 (70). The cause of this condition was believed to be snapping of the iliopsoas tendon over the iliopectineal eminence. Two of the three patients in the initial report had good relief after iliopsoas lengthening. Other reported causes of internal snapping include snapping of the iliopsoas over an exostosis of the lesser trochanter (69), snapping attributed to the iliopsoas bursa (77), and snapping caused by habitual dislocation of the hip (78). Slipping of the iliofemoral ligaments over the femoral head and slipping of the long head of the biceps femoris tendon over the ischial tuberosity have also been proposed as causes of snapping, but no pathologic or surgical basis has yet been identified (79). The pain associated with iliopsoas snapping hip is generally believed to be caused by the sudden movement of the iliopsoas tendon over the pelvic pectineal eminence, femoral head, or lesser trochanter.

## Clinical Features

The history and physical examination are usually diagnostic of the internal type of coxa saltans, with the patient describing a painful snapping sensation localized to the anterior part of the groin. However, because of its rarity, this type of snapping hip can present a formidable diagnostic challenge. The snapping can often be reproduced at will by the patient in either the supine or standing position. In addition, the examiner can frequently reproduce the snapping by having the patient lie supine and bringing the hip from a flexed and abducted position to an extended and adducted position (Fig. 27.20). This is due to the iliopsoas tendon shifting from lateral to medial over the iliopectineal eminence (70,74) and/or the femoral head (69) when the hip is brought from flexion into extension. If the snapping occurs with these motions, blocking the snapping by applying finger pressure over the iliopsoas tendon at the level of the femoral head and/or iliopectineal eminence will corroborate the diagnosis.

The average duration of symptoms before presentation to the orthopaedist is 2 years (74). A specific event typically precipitates the symptoms; the most common precipitating activities are sprinting and long-distance running (74). The snapping gradually increases in frequency and intensity so that it occurs with daily activities and inhibits participation in sports activities.

## Radiographic Features

Plain radiographs can be used to rule out other causes of hip pain, such as osteitis pubis, pubic ramus fracture, avascular

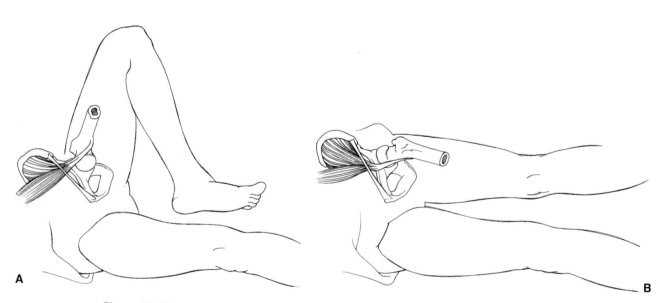

**A**                                                                  **B**

**Figure 27.20**    A schematic demonstrating the snapping iliopsoas tendon. **A:** The iliopsoas tendon is lateral to the pelvic brim with the hip in flexion and abduction. **B:** Snapping is produced as the tendon moves to a more medial position on the pelvic brim with extension and adduction of the hip.

necrosis of the femoral head, and synovial chondromatosis, but are not helpful in diagnosing a snapping iliopsoas tendon.

## Other Imaging Studies

If the diagnosis remains uncertain, a magnetic resonance arthrogram may be useful for ruling out labral tears and intraarticular loose bodies. Bursography, tenography, and ultrasonography have been recommended for evaluating snapping of the iliopsoas tendon, but each modality has its limitations, and they are generally unnecessary for the diagnosis (69,75,80). Bursography involves injecting contrast material into the iliopsoas bursa whereas tenography involves injecting into the iliopsoas tendon itself. Both are performed under fluoroscopic guidance with the use of a local anesthetic. One limitation of bursography is that the tendon itself is not injected and is therefore only visualized indirectly as a negative defect impressing upon the bursa. Tenography allows direct observation of the iliopsoas tendon's movement under fluoroscopic examination. Unlike bursography, this technique allows direct visualization of the tendon. Although tenography has been useful in furthering our understanding of the etiology of the snapping, it is not necessary for clinical diagnosis. Recently, dynamic sonography has emerged as a noninvasive technique for examining a snapping iliopsoas tendon (75). This has the advantage of being noninvasive and can be used in cases in which the clinical diagnosis is not obvious.

## Natural History

The natural history of iliopsoas snapping hip is poorly understood. Although iliopsoas tendon snapping can occur without pain, symptomatic iliopsoas tendon snapping in adolescence follows a somewhat predictable course (74). A specific event typically precipitates the symptoms; the most common precipitating activities are sports that involve running. The snapping initially occurs only rarely and does not inhibit participation in sports. Over a period of months to a few years, the snapping increases in severity to a point that participation in sports is no longer possible. The snapping often begins to occur even with daily activities. It is often at this point that the individual seeks medical attention.

## Treatment Recommendations

### Nonsurgical

Only patients who are symptomatic warrant treatment. Initial treatment includes rest, avoidance of activities that produced the snapping, nonsteroidal antiinflammatory medications, and a 3-month physical therapy program emphasizing stretching of the iliopsoas tendon (74).

### Surgical

**Indications.** The indication for surgical lengthening of the iliopsoas tendon is continued snapping of the iliopsoas tendon with resulting pain despite an intensive 3-month supervised physical therapy program. The snapping and pain at this stage often occur with daily activities but, occasionally, are present only during physical exertion.

**Options.** Over the last 50 years, various surgical techniques have evolved for the treatment of refractory cases of the iliopsoas snapping tendon. In 1984, Schaberg et al. (69) reviewed six patients treated with lengthening of the iliopsoas tendon, performed through a modified anterior approach to the hip, with the tendon being partially divided near its insertion on the lesser trochanter. Two of the patients had an exostosis removed from the anteromedial aspect of the lesser trochanter; these exostoses were believed to have been contributing to the symptomatic snapping. In 1990, Jacobson et al. (67) reviewed these 6 patients and also reported on an additional 14 patients who had undergone lengthening of the iliopsoas tendon as a treatment for internal snapping hip. The authors noted that their skin incision changed from an anterior vertical incision to a more cosmetically appealing incision running just distal to the inguinal crease in the last 14 patients. In all the patients, the tendon was partially divided below the pelvic brim near its insertion onto the lesser trochanter. Of the 20 patients in the series, 6 (30%) had recurrent snapping, 3 (15%) reported weakness in hip flexion, and 2 (10%) required reoperation. In addition, 10 of 20 patients (50%) reported periincisional loss of sensation.

Taylor et al. (81), in 1995, reported on 14 patients with internal snapping treated by partial iliopsoas tendon release. They described a medial approach through a horizontal incision several centimeters below the inguinal skin crease. As with previously reported approaches, the tendon lengthening was performed below the pelvic brim, close to the insertion of the tendon on the lesser trochanter. Of the 14 patients, 2 reported postoperative hip-flexion weakness. Six patients continued to have snapping after surgery.

Gruen et al. (76), in 2002, described 11 patients with internal snapping hip treated with iliopsoas tendon lengthening above the pelvic brim through an ilioinguinal approach. Of the 11 patients, 5 reported postoperative hip-flexion weakness. No patients experienced continued snapping postoperatively, but two patients reported continued hip pain.

In the only study to address internal snapping hip in the adolescent population, Dobbs et al. (74), describe 11 hips in 9 patients. These internal snapping hips were unresponsive to conservative measures. All the hips were treated with a fractional iliopsoas tendon lengthening above the pelvic brim through a modified iliofemoral approach. This approach allows excellent visualization of the iliopsoas musculotendinous junction and facilitates complete transection of all tendon fibers at this level. One patient in this study described recurrent snapping in one operatively treated hip, but stated that the symptoms were much less frequent and severe than they had been preoperatively. All patients returned to their preoperative level of activity. No patient had a detectable loss of hip-flexion strength. Two patients had a transient decrease in sensation that was localized to the anterolateral aspect of the thigh.

### Authors' Preferred Recommendations

Treatment is necessary only for patients with a painful and symptomatic iliopsoas snapping hip. A supervised physical therapy program emphasizing iliopsoas stretching for a minimum of 3 months is the first line of treatment. For patients with continued pain and popping that limits activities, a fractional iliopsoas tendon lengthening through a modified iliofemoral approach is recommended (74). This approach has been effective in relieving symptoms and allowing patients to return to their preoperative level of functioning while preserving hip-flexion strength.

### Complications

Both the anterior and medial approaches to the hip allow the surgeon to partially divide the iliopsoas tendon just above its insertion on the lesser trochanter. The advantages of these two approaches include good visualization of the tendon insertion and direct access to any contributing exostoses on the lesser trochanter and femoral head. The major problem with these two surgical approaches that attempt to lengthen the tendon below the pelvic brim lies in judging the amount of tendon to release. Insufficient lengthening results in recurrent snapping, whereas overlengthening results in hip-flexion weakness (67,69,81). Other problems include the potential for a cosmetically unappealing scar resulting from an anterior vertical incision (67), and the frequent periincisional loss of sensation with the medial approach through a horizontal incision below the inguinal crease (81).

Approaches that lengthen the tendon above the pelvic brim have better reported maintenance of hip-flexion strength and less recurrence of snapping than those that lengthen the tendon below the pelvic brim (74,76). A disadvantage of the ilioinguinal approach for this condition is the relative unfamiliarity of this approach to many pediatric orthopaedic surgeons. The modified iliofemoral approach (74), on the other hand, is used frequently by pediatric orthopaedists in performing pelvic osteotomies. Extreme care should be taken to correctly identify the tendon before transection because the femoral nerve lies nearby. To minimize risk of injury of the femoral nerve, the authors recommend that the patient have no paralyzing agents administered during the procedure and the surgeon

use very low-level electrocautery to stimulate the tendon before cutting its fibers so as to ensure that nerve fibers are not included. Care should also be taken to avoid injury to the lateral femoral cutaneous nerve. The nerve should be identified on the sartorius side of the sartorius-tensor muscle interval and retracted medially.

## TRANSIENT SYNOVITIS OF THE HIP

### Definition

Transient synovitis of the hip is the most common source of pain in the young child. Transient synovitis is characterized by an acute onset of hip pain associated with a limp in a child that has no other musculoskeletal or constitutional symptoms. This clinical problem has been often referred to as *irritable hip, observation hip, toxic synovitis, transitory coxitis, coxitis serosa, coxalgia fugax,* and *phantom hip. Transient synovitis* is the term most commonly used because it aptly describes the short duration of this benign condition.

### Epidemiology

Affected children range in age from 3 to 12 years, with the average patient being between 5 and 6 years of age. However, the condition has been reported in children as young as 3 months. The annual hospital admissions for the diagnosis of transient synovitis is 0.4% to 0.9% , but the actual incidence of the condition may be higher because many patients never seek medical attention and only a few patients are hospitalized when the diagnosis is made. Landin et al. (82) reported that the risk that a child will be affected by at least one episode of acute transient synovitis of the hip is 3%. They also reported a seasonal variation, with more cases in the fall than in the winter. Boys are twice as often affected than girls, and there is a much lower incidence among African Americans (83). Right and left hips are affected equally. Ninety-five percent of the cases are unilateral. After a child has had an episode of transient synovitis of the hip, the annual risk of recurrence for that child is 4% (82,84).

### Etiology

Lovett (85) first described this condition as a *short-lived and ephemeral form of hip disease,* and differentiated it from tuberculosis. Since then, many investigators have described a similar painful condition that is self-limiting and rapidly resolving, and that is now considered as transient synovitis of the hip. However, its cause still remains unknown.

Because a high percentage of the children with transient synovitis present with a recent history of an upper respiratory tract infection, a viral etiology has been suggested. Leibowitz et al. (86) found that blood interferon levels were significantly raised in 40% of patients with acute transient synovitis of the hip. In healthy subjects, these levels are usually not measurable, but various viral diseases cause significantly raised concentrations. They concluded that a viral infection was the cause. Tolat et al. (87) evaluated 80 children who were admitted with acute transient synovitis of the hip. Their management protocol included a clinical examination, venous samples, synovial fluid samples taken when ultrasonography had detected an effusion, and recall after 3 or 4 weeks for clinical examination and procurement of samples for convalescent viral titers. Twenty-eight of 65 patients (43%) had raised blood interferon levels. Fifteen of the 16 patients with an effusion that was successfully aspirated showed raised levels of interferon in the synovial fluid. Bacterial and viral cultures of all synovial fluid samples were negative. Viral serology in 67 patients showed raised antibody titers to viruses including rubella, enterovirus, and Epstein-Barr. Other investigators have evaluated different viruses including parvovirus B-19 and herpes virus-6, and were unable to confirm any correlation between transient synovitis and infection with these specific viruses (88–90).

Upper respiratory bacterial infections, pharyngitis, otitis media, and gastrointestinal problems have also been associated with transient synovitis of the hip in up to 70% of the patients. Spock (91) reported a higher incidence of nose and throat β-hemolytic streptococci in patients with transient synovitis when compared to asymptomatic patients. However, Hardinge (92) did not find any correlation between infection sources and transient synovitis.

Allergic predisposition has also been associated with transient synovitis of the hip in up to 25% of patients. In 1952, Edwards reported that patients with transient synovitis recovered in a few days with the use of antihistamines, and Rothschild et al. found a rapid clinical improvement when steroid injections were given intramuscularly. However, Nachemson and Scheller (93) did not find any association between allergic hypersensitivity and transient synovitis in a group of 73 patients, compared to the general population.

In the early part of the 20th century, some investigators proposed trauma as a cause of transient synovitis, with local trauma to the involved hip being present in up to 30% of the cases (91,94–97). However, as with most childhood musculoskeletal conditions, a significant number of patients may relate an episode of trauma to the onset of symptoms, but this may not be the actual cause of this condition. No other studies have reported on this association.

Finally, some investigators have suggested that growth abnormalities are associated with transient synovitis of the hip. Spock (91) found a three times greater incidence of transient synovitis in obese, stocky children compared with a randomly selected, age-matched control group. Vila-Verde and da Silva (98) evaluated children with LCPD and transient synovitis, and found that in the active stage of both diseases there was a bone age delay that persisted after healing, but became normal by puberty.

## Clinical Features

The usual clinical presentation is a fairly rapid onset of limping, unilateral hip pain, and subsequent refusal to bear weight on the involved extremity in an otherwise healthy child. The pain is usually unilateral, with fewer than 5% of cases being bilateral. The pain is usually located in the groin and hip area, with referred pain to the anteromedial aspect of the thigh and knee. The pain is acute in about half of the patients, with symptoms being present for 1 to 3 days before presentation. In other patients, the symptoms may be more chronic, with symptoms being present for several weeks in some cases. The pain is usually mild, but in some children, mostly very young ones, it can be severe enough to awaken them at night. Because the symptoms sometimes follow a recent upper respiratory tract infection, the patient may have a low-grade fever at presentation (rarely greater than 38°C).

Physical examination demonstrates a child in mild distress who will not bear weight or walk, or who does so reluctantly and with an antalgic limp. The extremity is held in flexion and external rotation, and there is decreased range of motion, especially for hip abduction and internal rotation. The irritability of the hip is usually mild or moderate. If it is severe, a diagnosis of septic arthritis should be considered. Ipsilateral muscle atrophy may be present, and this implies a longstanding duration of the symptoms, although this is not very common. In this situation, a diagnosis other than transient synovitis should be considered.

## Radiographic Features

Radiographs of the pelvis and affected hip are usually normal or may demonstrate slightly widened joint space medially. The main purpose of the radiograph is to exclude other conditions that may involve the hip joint such as LCPD, eosinophilic granuloma, osteomyelitis, osteoid osteoma, and so on. Bone density is normal in all cases. Loss of the hip capsular shadow has been reported in cases of transient synovitis; however, this sign is not specific and it is related to holding the hip in abduction and external rotation.

Rosenborg and Mortensson (99) evaluated the diagnostic significance of some radiographic signs (abnormal hip "joint space" and periarticular fat layers) as indicators of hip joint effusion or hip complaints without effusion. These indicators were studied with ultrasonography and radiography in 47 children (58 examinations), of whom 40 had acute unilateral transient synovitis. It was found that "joint depth" was not influenced by presence of intra-articular fluid collections; blurring and/or displacement of the periarticular fat pads medial and lateral to the hip joint occurred more frequently when joint effusion was present than in symptom-free hips or in painful hips without effusion. However, the radiographic signs provided too low a diagnostic accuracy to be of practical value (100). It is suggested that ultrasonography is a valuable means of obtaining a better definition of the hip joint, thereby aiding in the diagnosis of transient synovitis.

## Other Imaging Studies

### Ultrasonography

Ultrasonography can be very useful in documenting the presence of an effusion in the hip joint, and it is usually performed prior to hip aspiration to be certain that an effusion accompanies the clinical findings (101–106) (Fig. 27.21). Although ultrasonography cannot identify the cause of an effusion in the joint, a negative result directs attention to other causes of hip pain.

Bickerstaff et al. (107) made a prospective study of 111 children with acute hip pain to assess whether ultrasonography can replace traditional radiography. An effusion was diagnosed in 71% of the cases by ultrasonography but in only 15% by radiography. This effusion persisted for a mean of 9 days; symptoms lasted for 5 days. Interestingly, in patients without an effusion there was no obvious factor that could be causing their pain, so the pressure of an effusion from a transient synovitis does not account for all patients with irritable hips. Patients with an effusion persisting for over 24 days had more symptoms, a significantly larger effusion, and greater limitation of movement. The investigators proposed a protocol of management for irritable hip, using ultrasonography at the first presentation of certain categories of patients, thereby reducing the number of early radiographs by 75%.

Fink et al. (108) assessed a protocol for the management of irritable hip with the aim of avoiding hospital admissions while identifying all other serious causes of hip pain, in particular, septic arthritis. Fifty children with painful hips were studied prospectively with immediate ultrasonographically guided aspiration and Gram stain of all hip effusions. Bone scintigraphy at an early stage was reserved for patients with unremitting symptoms. Thirty-six hips were aspirated. Only two patients were admitted to hospital. The final diagnoses were transient synovitis (45 patients), Perthes disease (3 patients), fracture (1 patient), and septic arthritis (1 patient). The single case of hip sepsis was diagnosed on presentation.

Miralles et al. (109) prospectively evaluated 500 children with painful hips or limps by using plain films and ultrasonography. The clinical, radiographic, and ultrasonographic findings were correlated with the final diagnoses. Ultrasonography disclosed hip effusion in 235 patients, and plain films were abnormal in 58 of these 235 patients and in 4 others. Both ultrasonography and plain films were normal in 261 patients. There were no ultrasonographic signs that were useful in differentiating sterile, purulent, or hemorrhagic effusion. Ultrasonography showed that 73% of patients with presumed transient synovitis had no effusion 2 weeks after diagnosis. Patients with hip disorders other than transient synovitis had persistent effusion for more than 2 weeks; however, this was also observed in 27% of the patients with presumed transient synovitis. Ultrasonography was more sensitive than plain films in detecting hip effusion, but ultrasonographic detection of effusion changed the therapeutic approach in only six patients. Therefore, although ultrasonography can be useful in documenting and following a hip effusion, it is not

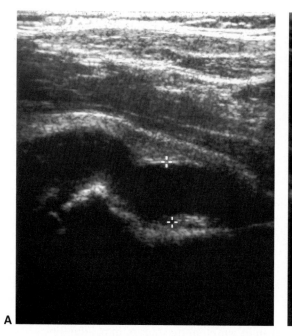 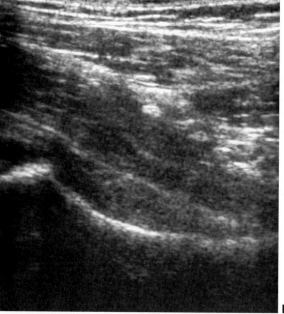

**Figure 27.21**    Longitudinal linear ultrasonographic view of the hips in a girl 6 years and 6 months of age. **A:** Ultrasonographic scan of the symptomatic right hip demonstrates a large effusion in the joint, as indicated between the cursor markings. **B:** Ultrasonographic scan of asymptomatic left hip, for comparison, demonstrates no effusion.

in and of itself diagnostic of this condition, and is not routinely required in making the diagnosis.

### Bone Scintigraphy

Skeletal scintigraphy is frequently used in the clinical investigation of young children who present with limping as their only or predominant symptom. In cases of transient synovitis, it usually demonstrates a variety of possible patterns of isotope uptake, including those showing normal, increased, or decreased activity of the femoral epiphysis (110–115).

Hasegawa et al. (116) evaluated 55 consecutive children presenting with transient synovitis of the hip, using $^{99m}$Tc-MDP scintigraphy and pinhole collimator technique. A decrease in isotope uptake in the proximal femoral epiphysis was observed in 13 children. This was correlated with a reduced uptake in the growth plate, indicating a disturbance of blood supply to these regions. A characteristic pattern of isotope uptake relating to the duration of symptoms was observed, with a decrease in uptake during the first week followed by rebound hyperemia within 1 month. The significance of this finding is uncertain, but there has been a report of coxa magna following transient synovitis of the hip, which may be caused by this increase in blood supply (117).

Royle and Galasko (118) reported on a 4-year study during which 192 patients with a typical transient synovitis syndrome underwent radionuclide scintigraphy shortly after presentation. Three different patterns were found, suggesting that not all the cases may have shared the same etiology. Fifteen patients had evidence of ischemia of the femoral head, but only four patients went on to develop the typical radiographic features of Perthes disease. The other 11 patients are thought to represent a minor, radiographically silent form of Perthes disease.

The results of these studies demonstrate that there can be an early, transient decrease in vascular perfusion of the proximal femoral epiphysis, but it will resolve spontaneously. The role of bone scintigraphy in the diagnosis of transient synovitis and in the decision-making about the management of the condition remains undetermined, and its routine use is not recommended.

### Magnetic Resonance Imaging

With the advent of MRI and, subsequently, magnetic resonance arthrography, the imaging algorithm for hip pain is evolving. Toby et al. (119) reported the use of MRI in the assessment of pediatric hip disease (24 children, 8 of them with transient synovitis). MRI accurately showed articular cartilage thickening and effusion in the joint in two of the patients with transient synovitis. The images in the other six patients were unremarkable.

Ranner et al. (120) used conventional radiography, radioisotope bone scan, and MRI for evaluating 45 children who presented with acute hip pain. The final diagnoses were transient synovitis ($n = 17$), septic arthritis ($n = 2$), LCPD ($n = 13$), epiphyseal dysplasia ($n = 2$),

other conditions ($n = 4$), and normal findings ($n = 7$). In the workup, MRI provided more morphologic information than other techniques and enlarged the diagnostic possibilities. MRI is extremely sensitive to alterations in the bone marrow that may represent pathology that remains occult to plain radiography and bone scintigraphy of the hips. For diagnosis and treatment planning, MRI of the hips should be performed early in patients with persistent pain and negative radiography findings.

Lee et al. (121) evaluated differences in MRI findings between septic arthritis (7 patients) and transient synovitis (14 patients). The diagnoses were made by means of aspiration of the joint, bacteriologic study, arthrotomy, and clinical evaluation. MRI findings were analyzed with emphasis on the grade of effusion and alterations in signal intensity in the soft tissue and bone marrow of the affected hip joint. Alterations in the signal intensity in bone marrow (i.e., low signal intensity on fat-suppressed gadolinium-enhanced T1-weighted spin-echo images and high signal intensity on fat-suppressed T2-weighted fast spin-echo images) were seen in 8 of 9 patients with septic arthritis. Such alterations in signal intensity were not seen in the 14 patients with transient synovitis. The investigators concluded that signal intensity alterations in the bone marrow of the affected hip joint are useful in differentiating septic arthritis from transient synovitis.

## Other Diagnostic Studies

The laboratory evaluation may show normal or mild elevation in the white blood cell (WBC) count (10,000 to 14,000 cells per mm$^3$), erythrocyte sedimentation rate (ESR) (range 1 to 63 mm/h) and C-reactive protein (CRP) level (less than 0.5). Urinalysis, serum electrophoresis, rheumatoid factor, blood culture, and tuberculin skin test results are usually within normal limits.

Aspiration of the hip joint should be performed if septic arthritis is suspected. Gram stain of the aspirated fluid will confirm the diagnosis of septic arthritis in 30% to 50% of the patients. The cell count of the fluid in the joint can vary, but it is usually less than 25,000 cells per mm$^3$. The glucose concentration of the aspirate is normal in transient synovitis. Zawin et al. (122) found that ESR and the WBC count of the synovial fluid were significantly higher in patients with septic arthritis than in those with transient synovitis.

## Differential Diagnosis

Transient synovitis should be distinguished from septic arthritis, which requires emergent treatment to prevent proximal femoral destruction and subsequent permanent deformity leading to early degenerative arthritis of the hip. Because of these disabling possibilities, many institutions have a policy of hospital admissions and workup investigations for all patients who present with an acutely painful hip.

Because similar symptoms are present in these two diseases at the early stages, the differential diagnosis should remain one of exclusion. Classically, septic arthritis presents with more severe pain and marked limitation of motion of the hip because of the pain. However, low-grade septic arthritis in an older child or in a child who has received antibiotics for another problem (such as upper respiratory infection) may have a less acute presentation. Many investigators agree that if the diagnosis is not clear from the history, physical examination, and radiography, hip aspiration should be performed, preferably with fluoroscopy or ultrasonography guidance. If the initial attempt is "dry" during fluoroscopy, dye should be injected to confirm that the needle has entered the joint.

Several investigators have evaluated clinical prediction algorithms that are designed to help differentiate septic arthritis from transient synovitis (122–128). However, there are different opinions about the parameters to be used for this indication. It has been suggested that aspiration should be performed in patients with a temperature higher that 37.5°C (99.5°F) or an ESR greater than 20 mm/h. With the use of these two criteria, 97% of the patients with septic arthritis would have been identified as requiring a hip aspiration. On the other hand, 50% of the patients with transient synovitis would have undergone an unnecessary aspiration (123).

Taylor and Clarke (124) evaluated 97 patients with transient synovitis and 27 patients with septic arthritis. Plain radiographs showed a displacement or blurring of periarticular fat pads in all patients with acute septic arthritis, and multivariate regression analysis showed that body temperature greater than 37°C, ESR higher than 20 mm/h, CRP greater than 1 mg/dL, WBC count greater than 11,000 per mL, and an increased hip joint space of more than 2 mm were independent multivariate predictors of acute septic arthritis. Eich et al. (129) found that all children with septic arthritis had hip effusion detectable by ultrasonography, and at least two of the following criteria: fever, elevation of ESR and elevation of CRP.

Kocher et al. (125,128) identified four independent multivariate clinical predictors to differentiate between septic arthritis and transient synovitis: history of fever, non–weight bearing, ESR greater than 40 mm per hour, and serum WBC greater than 12,000 cells per mL. However, Luhmann et al. (127) found that this algorithm was not as useful in their institution. Given the devastating effects of a missed septic arthritis, the surgeons should rule out this possibility by setting a very low threshold to indicate the need for aspiration of the joint.

Other infections that should also be considered include femoral or pelvic bacterial osteomyelitis and tuberculosis. These conditions may present with very similar manifestations including hip pain, limited range of motion and effusion in the joint. Some patients may demonstrate minimal elevation of body temperature and of laboratory values (WBC, ESR, and CRP). MRI and bone scintigraphy are very useful in differentiating between these conditions and can demonstrate characteristic bone marrow changes. Skin testing will be diagnostic for tuberculous arthritis.

Synovitis associated with acute rheumatic fever and group A streptococcal infections usually occurs 2 to 4 weeks postinfection. The joint is usually warm, erythematous, and exquisitely painful to any range of motion, and there may be an associated skin rash. Several joints can become affected over time (migratory arthritis). In addition, juvenile rheumatoid arthritis or one of the seronegative spondyloarthropathies should also be considered in the differential diagnosis. In these cases, the arthritis is more insidious in onset and will persist beyond the 2 weeks that are typical for transient synovitis. A careful examination of other joints and serology analysis will help clarify the diagnosis.

LCPD often presents in a similar manner and occurs in the same age range, but it has a slightly greater male predominance. Pain is usually more insidious in onset, and more protracted in duration. Hip motion at the onset of symptoms tends to be limited to a lesser degree than in transient synovitis. Radiographs may show joint space widening and a smaller femoral ossified nucleus on the affected side. Bone scintigraphy and MRI in the early stages of LCPD may show a decreased uptake of the femoral head, and bone marrow abnormalities, respectively.

Finally, tumors, particularly osteoid osteoma of the proximal femur, must also be included in the differential diagnosis. Osteoid osteoma is usually associated with night pain that is relieved by aspirin.

## Pathoanatomy

Finder (130) first described the pathoanatomy of this condition. Biopsy material demonstrated nonspecific inflammatory changes and synovial hypertrophy without pyogenic-related abnormalities. Aspiration of the hip joint has shown culture-negative synovial effusion, usually measuring between 1 and 5 mL (83,117,131–133).

It has been proposed that transient synovitis of the hip could cause ischemia of the proximal femoral epiphysis by a tamponade effect from increased intraarticular pressure. However, many other studies have shown little or no evidence of such a causative association. One of the reasons for this confusion is the fact that many cases of LCPD may initially present as synovitis of the hip before any changes can be seen in radiograms; therefore, subsequent proximal femoral epiphyseal changes may be misdiagnosed as transient synovitis.

## Natural History

As the term implies, transient synovitis of the hip is a self-limiting condition that resolves spontaneously. Most short-term studies of patients with transient synovitis usually demonstrate a limited duration of the symptoms with no evidence of residual clinical or radiographic abnormalities (134). However, longer follow-up studies have demonstrated some abnormalities in the proximal femur. Sequelae or conditions associated with transient synovitis of the hip include coxa magna, LCPD, and mild degenerative cystic changes of the femoral neck.

Coxa magna, defined as an enlargement of 2 mm or more of the proximal femoral epiphysis, has been noted in up to 32% of patients (93,117,135). The reason for this increase in size is not clear, but it has been suggested that a reactive increase in the blood supply to the femur or an increased growth of the articular cartilage secondary to the transient inflammation may be associated with this finding (102). De Valderrama (135) reported a 21-year follow-up of patients who had transient synovitis of the hip. He found a 50% incidence of radiographic changes including coxa magna, widening of the femoral neck, and changes consistent with degenerative arthritis of the hip. However, Nachemson and Scheller (93) did not find any abnormalities of the hip joint. The full importance of these radiographic changes remains unknown, and whether these patients will develop degenerative arthritis over the long term remains uncertain.

The reported incidence of LCPD following transient synovitis of the hip ranges from 1% to 3%. A direct correlation between transient synovitis of the hip and the development of LCPD has, however, never been documented. Therefore, it is reasonable to conclude that there is no association between these two conditions and many of the reported instances of correlation undoubtedly represent an initial misdiagnosis of early LCPD.

## Treatment

Patients with transient synovitis of the hip present frequently at the emergency department. The main aim of the treatment is to resolve the underlying synovitis with its associated symptomatology. Bed rest and non–weight bearing on the affected side is the primary method of treatment of this condition. Light skin traction can be applied for comfort in patients with recalcitrant or recurrent symptoms. On the basis of ultrasonographic studies and intraarticular pressure recording it was found that the best position is with the hip in 30 to 45 degrees of flexion and some abduction (133,136,137). For patients in whom the diagnosis is uncertain, hospital admission is often necessary. Close observation is essential in these cases, and worsening of the symptoms suggests septic arthritis.

Antiinflammatory medications can be used for a short period of time, and this often results in rapid improvement. Kermond et al. (138) performed a randomized, double-blind, placebo-controlled trial using ibuprofen syrup (10 mg per kg three times a day for 5 days). They found that ibuprofen shortened the duration of the symptoms to 2 days compared to 4.5 days in the placebo group. Because many children may have an associated upper respiratory tract viral infection, the use of aspirin should be avoided so as to prevent Reye syndrome. There is no indication for the use of antibiotics if the diagnosis is certain.

Protected weight bearing with crutches can begin when full range of motion of the hip is reestablished and the pain has improved. Most patients will have resolution of their symptoms in 5 to 7 days. Recurrences are uncommon unless the child returns to full activities prematurely (96). Patients should be reevaluated if significant residual symptoms persist 7 to 10 days after the initial presentation, so as to rule out other pathologies. In some cases, however, low-grade symptoms can last up to several weeks.

# IDIOPATHIC CHONDROLYSIS OF THE HIP

## Definition

Idiopathic chondrolysis of the hip is a very rare disorder that occurs during adolescence. It is characterized by pain and a limp, with a rapid loss of the articular cartilage of the hip joint resulting in narrowing of the joint space and consequent stiffness in the joint. This condition should be differentiated from chondrolysis secondary to prolonged immobilization, trauma, severe burns, infection, juvenile idiopathic arthritis, Marfan syndrome, or slipped capital femoral epiphysis (139–142).

It was first described by Jones (143) in 1971. He reported a series of nine adolescent girls who spontaneously developed symptoms and signs similar to the description of chondrolysis secondary to slipped capital femoral epiphysis. Since then several investigators have documented the pathology, clinical presentation, natural history, prognosis, and treatment of idiopathic chondrolysis of the hip (139,144–149).

## Epidemiology and Etiopathogenesis

The true incidence of idiopathic chondrolysis of the hip remains unclear. Although there are fewer than 100 patients recorded in the literature to date with idiopathic chondrolysis of the hip, it may be more common than was once thought. In fact, Kozlowski and Scougall (150) believe that it is probably one of the most common causes of degenerative arthritis of the hip in women.

Idiopathic chondrolysis of the hip is more common unilaterally than bilaterally (144–146,149,151). The right hip is involved at a slightly higher rate of occurrence than the left (152). There is an approximately sixfold predominance among girls. Onset is most frequently around the age of 11 to 12 years of age, but it may occur until the age of 20 years. When first described it appeared to be more common among individuals of African descent, but it has since been documented as occurring ubiquitously in African, Asian, Indian, Australian, Hispanic, American, and European populations (143,145,147,148,150–157).

Various theories have been suggested to account for the origin of this process. These include nutritionally based abnormalities in the joint because of abnormal synovium (140,142); mechanical insult to the articular cartilage, resulting in a release of chondrolytic enzymes (158); abnormal intracapsular pressure (159); and intrinsic abnormal chondrocyte metabolism that can be triggered by an unknown environmental event (145,150,160).

The most widely accepted theory is that the articular cartilage resorption seen in idiopathic chondrolysis of the hip is caused by an autoimmune response within the hip joint in genetically susceptible individuals (159,161). This theory is supported by the fact that microscopic evaluation of the synovial tissue from affected joints shows an increase in chronic inflammatory cells, and these patients have serologic abnormalities as well (143,147,162,163).

In the early stages of the disease, the synovium is edematous and demonstrates villous formation, nodular lymphoid hyperplasia of the subsynovium, and perivascular infiltrates of lymphocytes, plasma cells, and monocytes (160). No fibrinoid necrosis or granuloma formation is seen. There is minimal synovial fluid in the joint. The changes to the articular cartilage include loss and thinning of the superficial areas on both sides of the joint, with more significant destruction on the femoral side. There may be complete loss of articular cartilage in the weight-bearing areas of the femoral head. Thickening of the joint capsule is common. The adjacent bone is osteopenic without evidence of necrosis, but there may be cysts filled with synovium.

Microscopic studies demonstrate a nonspecific chronic inflammation. The articular cartilage is fragmented, with the superficial zone I missing and with necrotic chondrocytes. However, the basal zone II shows abnormalities in the organization and size of the collagen fibrils, with viable chondrocytes interspersed with necrosis and debris (Fig. 27.22). These chondrocytes are important for the subsequent regeneration of the articular cartilage in some cases (162,164).

Van der Hoeven et al. (165) demonstrated deposition of IgM and the C3 component of the complement in the synovium in patients with idiopathic chondrolysis. However, other investigators reported normal levels of serum immunoglobulins and normal immunofluorescence studies of the synovium and cartilage (144,156).

## Clinical and Laboratory Features

The typical presentation of idiopathic chondrolysis of the hip is that of an adolescent girl (mean age 11 years, range 6 to 15 years) with a 2- to 3-month history of unexplained hip pain, stiffness, and a limp. Pain is usually insidious in onset, and is located in the hip, anterior thigh, or knee area. There is a distinct absence of systemic symptoms. Physical examination demonstrates significant restriction of the range of motion in all planes with associated muscle spasm.

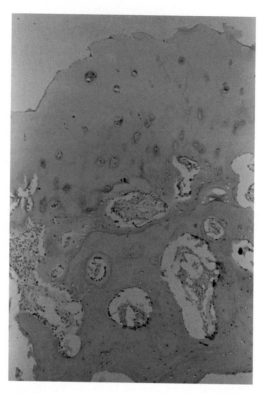

**Figure 27.22**  The photomicrograph of a biopsy specimen of the femoral head from a patient with idiopathic chondrolysis demonstrates a frayed and fragmented superficial layer of articular cartilage, with viable chondrocytes remaining in the more basal layers. The subchondral bone appears histologically normal.

If presentation for orthopaedic treatment is delayed, many patients will demonstrate fixed contractures about the hip, the most common being in the flexed, abducted, and externally rotated position (143–145,149,152). Contractures about the hip can result in secondary leg-length inequality, pelvic obliquity caused by an adduction contracture, and increased lumbar lordosis.

Laboratory studies including complete blood count, urinalysis, rheumatoid factor, human leucocyte antigen HLA-B27, antinuclear antibody, blood cultures, and tuberculin skin test are usually within normal limits. The ESR is usually normal although in some cases it can be slightly elevated (less than 30 mm per hour) (146,150,152,165).

The differential diagnosis for idiopathic chondrolysis of the hip includes trauma, slipped capital femoral epiphysis, LCPD, juvenile rheumatoid arthritis, septic arthritis, tuberculosis, migratory or transitory osteoporosis, idiopathic protrusio acetabuli, reflex sympathetic dystrophy, pigmented villonodular synovitis, and synovioma. Septic arthritis of the hip is one of the most important entities that should be examined for and excluded on presentation because this condition requires urgent surgical treatment. Although the findings of the physical examination can be similar in the acute stages of both clinical entities, the history, and laboratory results are usually quite different. Septic arthritis usually has a more acute onset and the patient may by systemically ill with high fever. Laboratory studies in septic

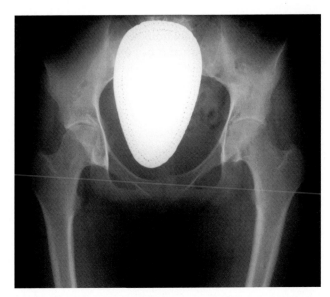

**Figure 27.23** Anteroposterior hip radiograph of a girl 13 years and 6 months of age. Radiographic findings in this case of bilateral idiopathic chondrolysis of the hip include a narrowing of the joint space to less than 3 mm and diffuse osteopenia.

arthritis typically show a significant elevation in the WBC count and ESR, which is not the norm for idiopathic chondrolysis (166).

## Radiographic Features

Radiographs of the pelvis and hip joints performed early in the course of the disease are often normal, but are important to exclude other causes of hip pain. Early features of cartilage destruction include periarticular osteopenia, narrowing of the joint space, and small subchondral bone erosions. Concentric diminution of the articular space to less than 3 mm is considered to be a diagnostic criterion of chondrolysis (normal space measures between 3.5 and 7 mm) (144,145) (Fig. 27.23). There may be slight overgrowth of the proximal femur, seen as widening and altered angulation of the epiphysis and femoral neck.

Later characteristics are obliteration of the joint space, subchondral bone cysts, protrusio acetabuli, and narrowing or early closing of the growth plate (Fig. 27.24A). This early closing of the growth plate rarely results in any major growth abnormality or significant change in the proximal femur. Protrusio acetabuli has been reported in as many as 50% of the patients and is thought to be caused by a softening of the acetabular floor, paralleling the loss of joint space seen radiographically (167) (Fig. 27.25). Widening of the symphysis pubis has also been noted. With resolution of the disease, there will be up to 2 mm restoration of the joint space in as many as 50% of the patients. Long-term radiographic results demonstrate osteopenia with degenerative changes, osteophytes, and cavities in the two articular surfaces, leading to complete ankylosis of the joint (144,149).

## Other Imaging Studies

Isotopic bone scan demonstrates normal flow and blood pool, but delayed scans demonstrate periarticular increase in uptake within the femoral head and the acetabulum

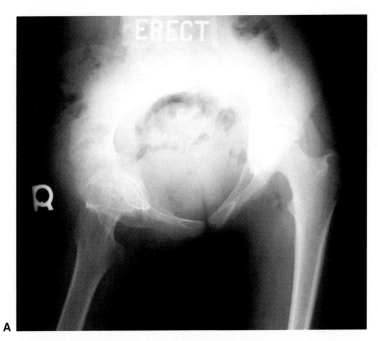
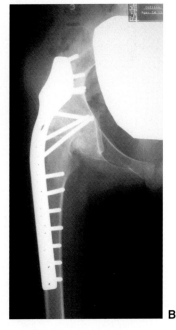

**Figure 27.24** **A:** Anteroposterior radiograph of the pelvis of a girl, 12 years and 4 months of age, with idiopathic chondrolysis of the right hip. Late radiographic signs shown here include obliteration of the joint space, subchondral bone cysts, narrowing or early closing of the growth plate, and pelvic obliquity. **B:** Anteroposterior radiograph of the same patient 1 year after a hip arthrodesis.

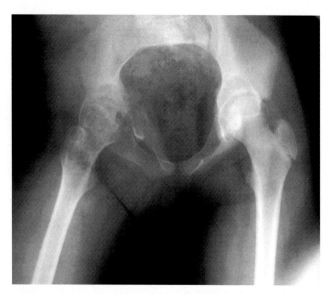

**Figure 27.25** Anteroposterior radiograph of the pelvis of a girl 13 years and 2 months of age, with idiopathic chondrolysis of the right hip. This radiograph reveals complete loss of the joint space with resultant acetabuli protrusio.

(Fig. 27.26) (168). MRI is used in children with severe symptoms or unusual presentation, or where there is doubt about the diagnosis. In idiopathic chondrolysis, there may be a small effusion in the joint, without synovial enhancement, and with cartilage loss being confined initially to areas of focal irregularity with deeper erosions.

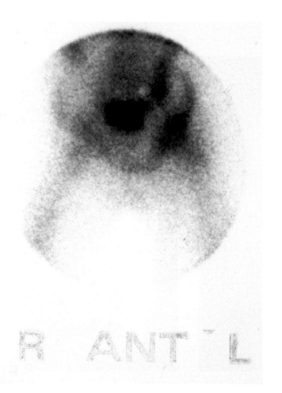

**Figure 27.26** The technetium bone scan of the pelvis of a patient with idiopathic chondrolysis demonstrating a diffuse uptake of the isotope by both sides of the affected left hip.

Interestingly, on serial examinations the cartilage loss was seen to extend peripherally from the center. Some degree of bone marrow edema and bone remodeling can be observed, with progressive protrusio acetabuli. Profound muscle wasting around the affected hip can be observed in most cases (169).

## Natural History

The natural history of idiopathic chondrolysis with or without treatment is unpredictable. Outcomes vary from spontaneous resolution to ankylosis of the hip joint, avascular necrosis, and long-term hip deformity. It was originally thought that idiopathic chondrolysis of the hip always followed the same progressive downhill course resulting in pain and a dramatic loss of range of motion and function in the affected hip. In 1971, Jones (143) in his original description of idiopathic chondrolysis of the hip, described nine cases, all of which had poor outcomes. All nine patients developed progressive loss of motion of the involved hip, leading to complete ankylosis in eight of them. Sparks and Dall (155) in 1982 reported a follow-up of Jones's original nine patients and included nine additional patients. Of Jones's original nine patients, two had an arthrodesis, one had a cup arthroplasty, one had a femoral head resection, two had complete spontaneous ankylosis, and two had what was described as severe limitation in hip motion. The additional nine patients also displayed the same natural history, which consisted of progressive stiffening and malposition of the affected hips. The authors concluded that idiopathic chondrolysis inevitably results in the development of a malpositioned fibrous ankylosis of the involved hip joint.

Bleck (144) in 1983 reported a more favorable outcome for patients affected with idiopathic chondrolysis of the hip. At a mean follow-up of 6.2 years, six of the nine patients had either no symptoms or only minor intermittent discomfort in the hip, with an improved range of hip motion and a partial restoration of joint space width. Roy et al. (170) in 1988 published the results for three patients with idiopathic chondrolysis followed for a mean of 3 years after onset of symptoms. All three patients had improved range of motion and reconstitution of the joint space at latest follow-up. Similarly, Daluga and Millar (145) in 1989 reported 14 patients (16 hips) with idiopathic chondrolysis of the hip, after a mean follow-up of 84 months. Partial restoration of the joint space occurred in eight hips. Nine hips demonstrated improved range of motion, and five of these hips had a full restoration of motion.

Despite the fact that the outcomes for patients with idiopathic chondrolysis of the hip vary, the disease process appears to have two distinct stages in most patients. The acute stage commences with the onset of the condition and typically lasts for 6 to 16 months. The patient presents with an insidious onset of pain and decreased motion of the hip caused by an inflammatory response. Radiographically, there is concentric narrowing of the articular space, caused by loss of articular cartilage in the femoral head and acetabulum. As the synovial inflammation decreases toward the end of the acute stage, there is an increase in fibrous tissue deposition. The acute stage is followed by the chronic stage, which lasts from 3 to 5 years and follows a less predictable course than the acute stage. At the end of the chronic stage, the affected hip will manifest one of three possible outcomes: (a) the involved hip may continue to deteriorate to a painful and malpositioned ankylosis; (b) the involved hip may become stiff and ankylosed in a position that limits function but causes minimal pain; and (c) the involved hip may show resolution of pain, improved motion, and partial or complete return of joint space, as evidenced by radiographs (Fig. 27.27).

Further investigation is necessary to better elucidate the etiology of idiopathic chondrolysis of the hip and improve the understanding of its natural history.

## Treatment

Treatment recommendations have changed over the years and are still in evolution as more information is collected concerning the natural history of idiopathic chondrolysis of the hip. Historically, the prognosis of idiopathic chondrolysis was viewed as universally poor. Therefore, early definitive surgical intervention was routinely practiced, including hip fusion, joint arthroplasty, and corrective osteotomies. This form of early definitive treatment has been largely abandoned because of reports that as many as 50% to 60% of affected hips in some series achieve satisfactory function, motion, and improved joint space, as seen radiographically, because of various management strategies (144,145,152,170).

### Nonsurgical

Duncan et al. reported five cases of idiopathic chondrolysis in 1975 (147) and nine hips in eight patients in 1979 (146). Mild cases, defined as those without severe pain or contractures, were treated with physical therapy, non–weight bearing, and analgesics. Joint space improved radiographically in four hips, and range of motion was reported as approximately two thirds of normal. More severely involved hips were treated with prolonged spica casting until fibrous ankylosis was achieved. These patients were reported to be functioning well at latest evaluation with an ankylosed pain-free hip and satisfactory gait.

A treatment protocol including nonsteroidal antiinflammatory medications, aggressive physical therapy, periodic traction with bed rest, and prolonged protected weight bearing for the involved hip was reported on by two different groups in the 1980s for the treatment of idiopathic chondrolysis of the hip (144,145). In both groups, 50% to 60% of the patients showed clinical improvement in the range of motion of the involved joint, and improved radiographic appearance of the joint space. In 1985, Hughes (152) reported the use of continuous passive motion in the acute stage of idiopathic chondrolysis of the hip in one patient, in whom a good range of hip motion was maintained even during the acute stage.

### Surgical

Aggressive surgical treatment during the acute stage, to try to maintain hip motion, has also been investigated. Bleck (144) reported one patient who underwent surgical release of tendon contractures as well as an anterior capsulotomy. This patient at final follow-up was pain-free, with functional range of motion of the hip and improved joint space radiographically. In 1988, Roy and Crawford (170) reported on

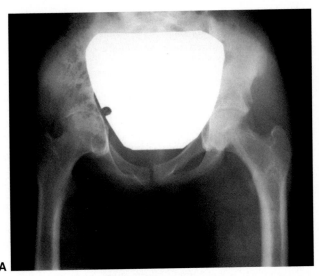
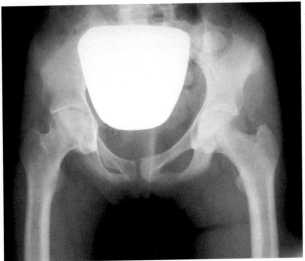

**Figure 27.27** Anteroposterior pelvic radiographs of a girl 13 years and 3 months of age, with idiopathic chondrolysis of the right hip. **A:** A radiograph made at the time of diagnosis demonstrates significant loss of joint space and osteopenia at the involved hip. **B:** A radiograph of the same patient 18 months after diagnosis demonstrates partial regeneration of the joint space width in the affected hip. (Courtesy of Perry L. Schoenecker.)

three patients with idiopathic chondrolysis of the hip, who were treated with a subtotal circumferential capsulectomy of the involved hip. Concomitant muscle releases were performed as necessary to relieve joint contractures. Surgery was followed by a period of traction as well as aggressive physical therapy emphasizing non–weight bearing range-of-motion exercises. Continuous passive motion was also tried in some patients. At an average follow-up of 3 years, all the patients were reported to be symptom-free, with full return of hip motion and an improved joint space radiographically. Del Couz Garcia et al. (149) reported on eight hips in seven patients with idiopathic chondrolysis of the hip treated by capsulectomy and tenotomy of the iliopsoas and adductor muscles with an average 13.2-year follow-up. Postoperative skin traction was used for 3 weeks, followed by an aggressive range-of-motion rehabilitation program. Although there was some initial improvement in the range of motion of the affected hips postoperatively, long-term follow-up showed progressive degeneration of the joint with resultant stiffness and pain.

## Authors' Preferred Recommendations

The current recommendations for treatment of idiopathic chondrolysis of the hip include controlling inflammation and maintaining hip motion during the acute stage. This is accomplished in most patients with the use of antiinflammatory medications, periodic skin traction and bed rest during the time of acute exacerbation of pain and loss of motion, surgical release of unresolved contractures, and an aggressive physical therapy program that emphasizes both passive and active range of motion. During the acute stage the patient is also maintained on non–weight bearing or limited–weight bearing status for the involved hip, until all pain has resolved and progressive joint space loss has ceased as shown radiographically. Although the initial results of aggressive subtotal capsulectomy and tendon release were favorable, more recent long-term follow-up indicates that the improvements achieved may deteriorate with time. For this reason, the routine use of this procedure for the treatment of idiopathic chondrolysis of the hip cannot yet be recommended. In patients with hips that are painful, despite nonoperative measures, or are malaligned, a hip arthrodesis is the preferred operative intervention (Fig. 27.24B).

## REFERENCES

### Coxa Vara

1. Elmslie RC. Injury and deformity of the epiphysis of the head of the femur—coxa vara. *Lancet* 1907;1:410.
2. Fairbank H. Coxa vara due to congenital defect of the neck of the femur. *J Anat* 1928;62:232.
3. Almond HG. Familial infantile coxa vara. *J Bone Joint Surg Br* 1956;38-B:539–544.
4. Amstutz HC. Developmental (infantile) coxa vara—a distinct entity. Report of two patients with previously normal roentgenograms. *Clin Orthop* 1970;72:242–247.
5. Cooper RR, Ponseti IV. Metaphyseal dysotosis: description of an ultrastructural defect in the epiphyseal plate chondrocytes. *J Bone Joint Surg Am* 1973;55:485–495.
6. Felman AH, Frias JL, Rennert OM. Spondylometaphyseal dysplasia: a variant form. *Radiology* 1974;113:409–415.
7. Kozlowski K, Bellemore MC. Spondylo-metaphyseal dysplasia of Sutcliffe type. *Br J Radiol* 1989;62:862–864.
8. Kozlowski K, Napiontek M, Beim ER. Spondylometaphyseal dysplasia, sutcliffe type: a rediscovered entity. *Can Assoc Radiol J* 1992; 43:364–368.
9. Hoffa A. Die angeborenen coxa vara. *Dtsch Med Wochenschr* 1905; 31:1257.
10. Duncan GA. Congenital coxa vara occurring in identical twins. *Am J Surg* 1937;37:112.
11. Johanning K. Coxa vara infantum. I. Clinical appearance and aetiological problems. *Acta Orthop Scand* 1951;21:273–299.
12. Pylkkanen PV. Coxa vara infantum. *Acta Orthop Scand* 1960; 48(Suppl. 48):1–120.
13. Letts RM, Shokeir MH. Mirror-image coxa vara in identical twins. *J Bone Joint Surg Am* 1975;57:117–118.
14. Magnusson R. Coxa vara infantum. *Acta Orthop Scand* 1954; 23:284–308.
15. Desai SS, Johnson LO. Long-term results of valgus osteotomy for congenital coxa vara. *Clin Orthop* 1993;294:204–210.
16. Serafin J, Szulc W. Coxa vara infantum, hip growth disturbances, etiopathogenesis, and long-term results of treatment. *Clin Orthop* 1991;272:103–113.
17. Atasu M, Taysi K, Say B. Dermatoglyphic findings in familial coxa vara with dominant inheritance. *Turk J Pediatr* 1974;16:15–20.
18. Barrington-Ward LE. Double coxa vara with other deformities occurring in brother and sister. *Lancet* 1912;1:157.
19. Fisher RL, Waskowitz WJ. Familial developmental coxa vara. *Clin Orthop* 1972;86:2–5.
20. Say B, Tuncbilek E, Pirnar T, et al. Hereditary congenital coxa vara with dominant inheritance? *Humangenetik* 1971;11:266–268.
21. Zadek I. Congenital coxa vara. *Arch Surg* 1935;30:62.
22. Carroll K, Coleman S, Stevens PM. Coxa vara: surgical outcomes of valgus osteotomies. *J Pediatr Orthop* 1997;17:220–224.
23. Cordes S, Dickens DR, Cole WG. Correction of coxa vara in childhood. The use of Pauwels' Y-shaped osteotomy. *J Bone Joint Surg Br* 1991;73:3–6.
24. Nilsonne H. On congenital coxa vara. *Acta Chir Scand* 1929; 64:217.
25. Kehl DK, LaGrone M, Lovell WW. Developmental coxa vara. *Orthop Trans* 1983;7:475.
26. Pavlov H, Goldman AB, Freiberger RH. Infantile coxa vara. *Radiology* 1980;135:631–640.
27. Langenskiold A. Femur remodelled during growth after osteomyelitis causing coxa vara and shaft necrosis. *J Pediatr Orthop* 1982;2:289–294.
28. Blockey NJ. Observations on infantile coxa vara. *J Bone Joint Surg Br* 1969;51:106–111.
29. Le Mesurier AB. Developmental coxa vara. *J Bone Joint Surg Br* 1951;33-B:478–482.
30. Say B, Taysi K, Pirnar T, et al. Dominant congenital coxa vara. *J Bone Joint Surg Br* 1974;56:78–85.
31. Schmidt TL, Kalamchi A. The fate of the capital femoral physis and acetabular development in developmental coxa vara. *J Pediatr Orthop* 1982;2:534–538.
32. Kim HT, Chambers HG, Mubarak SJ, et al. Congenital coxa vara: computed tomographic analysis of femoral retroversion and the triangular metaphyseal fragment. *J Pediatr Orthop* 2000;20: 551–556.
33. Weinstein JN, Kuo KN, Millar EA. Congenital coxa vara. A retrospective review. *J Pediatr Orthop* 1984;4:70–77.
34. Chung SM, Riser WH. The histological characteristics of congenital coxa vara: a case report of a five year old boy. *Clin Orthop* 1978;132:71–81.
35. Morsy HA. Complications of fracture of the neck of the femur in children. A long-term follow-up study. *Injury* 2001;32:45–51.
36. Morgan JD, Somerville EW. Normal and abnormal growth at the upper end of the femur. *J Bone Joint Surg Br* 1960;42:2264.
37. Salenius P, Videman T. Growth disturbances of the proximal end of the femur: an animal experimental study with tetracycline. *Acta Orthop Scand* 1970;41:199.

38. Savastano AA, Bliss TF. Contribution of the epiphyses of the greater trochanter to the growth of the femur. *Int Surg* 1975;60: 280–281.

39. Von Lanz T, Wachsmuth W. *Praktische anatomie.* Berlin: Springer-Verlag, 1938.

40. Bos CF, Sakkers RJ, Bloem JL, et al. Histological, biochemical, and MRI studies of the growth plate in congenital coxa vara. *J Pediatr Orthop* 1989;9:660–665.

41. Babb FS, Ghormley RK, Chatterton CC. Congenital coxa vara. *J Bone Joint Surg Am* 1949;31:115.

42. Borden J, Spencer GE Jr, Herndon CH. Treatment of coxa vara in children by means of a modified osteotomy. *J Bone Joint Surg Am* 1966;48:1106–1110.

43. Barr JS. Congenital coxa vara. *Arch Surg* 1929;18:1909.

44. Amstutz HC, Wilson PD Jr. Dysgenesis of the proximal femur (coxa vara) and its surgical management. *Am J Orthop* 1962; 44-A:1–24.

45. Mau H. Juvenile epiphyseolysis of the femoral head—coxa vara development and treatment. *Z Orthop Ihre Grenzgeb* 1990;128: 531–535.

46. Horwitz T. The treatment of congenital (or developmental) coxa vara. *Surg Gynecol Obstet* 1948;87:71.

47. Weighill FJ. The treatment of developmental coxa vara by abduction subtrochanteric and intertrochanteric femoral osteotomy with special reference to the role of adductor tenotomy. *Clin Orthop* 1976;116:116–124.

48. Hamilton CD, DeLuca PA. Valgus osteotomy in the treatment of developmental coxa vara. *Orthop Trans* 1994;18:1111.

49. Jorring K, Movin R. Experience with 79 subtrochanteric valgus osteotomies of the hip. *Acta Orthop Scand* 1973;44:467.

50. Yang SH, Huang SC. Valgus osteotomy for congenital coxa vara. *J Formos Med Assoc* 1997;96:36–42.

51. Von Bormann PFB, Erken EHW. Pauwels' osteotomy for coxa vara in childhood. *J Bone Joint Surg Br* 1982;64:144.

52. Serafin J. Coxa vara infantum, growth disorders of the hip, their etiopathogenesis and remote results of treatment. *Chir Narzadow Ruchu Ortop Pol* 1985;50:196–200.

53. Pauwels F. *Biomechanics of the normal and diseased hip.* New York: Springer-Verlag, 1976.

54. Muller ME, Allgower M, Willenegger H. *Manual of internal fixation: techniques recommended by the AO group.* New York: Springer-Verlag, 1979.

55. Galante VN, Caiaffa V, Franchin F, et al. The treatment of infantile coxa vara with the external circular fixator. *Ital J Orthop Traumatol* 1990;16:491–500.

56. Dietz FR, Weinstein SL. Spike osteotomy for angular deformities of the long bones in children. *J Bone Joint Surg Am* 1988;70:848–852.

## Bladder Exstrophy

57. Gearhart JP. Exstrophy, epispadias and other bladder anomalies. In: Walsh PC, ed. *Campbell's urology.* Philadelphia, PA: WB Saunders, 2001:2136–2195.

58. Sponseller PD, Bisson LJ, Gearhart JP, et al. The anatomy of the pelvis in the exstrophy complex. *J Bone Joint Surg Am* 1995;77: 177–189.

59. Sponseller PD, Jani MM, Jeffs RD, et al. Anterior innominate osteotomy in repair of bladder exstrophy. *J Bone Joint Surg Am* 2001;83-A:184–193.

60. Stec AA, Pannu HK, Tadros YE, et al. Pelvic floor anatomy in classic bladder exstrophy using 3-dimensional computerized tomography: initial insights. *J Urol* 2001;166:1444–1449.

61. Jani MM, Sponseller PD, Gearhart JP. The hip in adults with classic bladder exostrophy: a biomechanical study. *J Pediatr Orthop* 2000;20:296–301.

62. O'Phelan EH. Iliac Osteotomy in Exstrophy of the bladder. *J Bone Joint Surg Am* 1963;45:1409–1422.

63. Aadalen RJ, O'Phelan EH, Chisholm TC, et al. Exstrophy of the bladder: long-term results of bilateral posterior iliac osteotomies and two-stage anatomic repair. *Clin Orthop* 1980;151:193–200.

64. McKenna PH, Khoury AE, McLorie GA, et al. Iliac osteotomy: a model to compare the options in bladder and cloacal exstrophy reconstruction. *J Urol* 1994;151:182–186; discussion 186–187.

65. Okubadejo GO, Sponseller PD, Gearhart JP. Complications in orthopedic management of exstrophy. *J Pediatr Orthop* 2003; 23:522–528.

## Iliopsoas Snapping Hip

66. Allen WC, Cope R. Coxa saltans: the snapping hip revisited. *J Am Acad Orthop Surg* 1995;3:303–308.

67. Jacobson T, Allen WC. Surgical correction of the snapping iliopsoas tendon. *Am J Sports Med* 1990;18:470–474.

68. Mayer L. Snapping hip. *Surg Gynecol Obstet* 1919;29:425–428.

69. Schaberg JE, Harper MC, Allen WC. The snapping hip syndrome. *Am J Sports Med* 1984;12:361–365.

70. Nunziata A, Blumenfeld I. Snapping hip; note on a variety. *Prensa Med Argent* 1951;38:1997–2001.

71. Ikeda T, Awaya G, Suzuki S, et al. Torn acetabular labrum in young patients. Arthroscopic diagnosis and management. *J Bone Joint Surg Br* 1988;70:13–16.

72. Suzuki S, Awaya G, Okada Y, et al. Arthroscopic diagnosis of ruptured acetabular labrum. *Acta Orthop Scand* 1986;57:513–515.

73. Lyons JC, Peterson LF. The snapping iliopsoas tendon. *Mayo Clin Proc* 1984;59:327–329.

74. Dobbs MB, Gordon JE, Luhmann SJ, et al. Surgical correction of the snapping iliopsoas tendon in adolescents. *J Bone Joint Surg Am* 2002;84-A:420–424.

75. Janzen DL, Partridge E, Logan PM, et al. The snapping hip: clinical and imaging findings in transient subluxation of the iliopsoas tendon. *Can Assoc Radiol J* 1996;47:202–208.

76. Gruen GS, Scioscia TN, Lowenstein JE. The surgical treatment of internal snapping hip. *Am J Sports Med* 2002;30:607–613.

77. Harper MC, Schaberg JE, Allen WC. Primary iliopsoas bursography in the diagnosis of disorders of the hip. *Clin Orthop* 1987; 221:238–241.

78. Stuart PR, Epstein HP. Habitual hip dislocation. *J Pediatr Orthop* 1991;11:541–542.

79. Hughes LO, Aronson J, Smith HS. Normal radiographic values for cartilage thickness and physeal angle in the pediatric hip. *J Pediatr Orthop* 1999;19:443–448.

80. Staple TW, Jung D, Mork A. Snapping tendon syndrome: hip tenography with fluoroscopic monitoring. *Radiology* 1988;166: 873–874.

81. Taylor GR, Clarke NM. Surgical release of the 'snapping iliopsoas tendon'. *J Bone Joint Surg Br* 1995;77:881–883.

## Transient Synovitis of the Hip

82. Landin LA, Danielsson LG, Wattsgard C. Transient synovitis of the hip. Its incidence, epidemiology and relation to Perthes' disease. *J Bone Joint Surg Br* 1987;69:238–242.

83. Haueisen DC, Weiner DS, Weiner SD. The characterization of "transient synovitis of the hip" in children. *J Pediatr Orthop* 1986;6:11–17.

84. Illingworth CM. Recurrences of transient synovitis of the hip. *Arch Dis Child* 1983;58:620–623.

85. Lovett RW. A transient or ephemeral form of hip disease. *Boston Med Surg J* 1892;127:161.

86. Leibowitz E, Levin S, Torten J, et al. Interferon system in acute transient synovitis. *Arch Dis Child* 1985;60:959–962.

87. Tolat V, Carty H, Klenerman L, et al. Evidence for a viral aetiology of transient synovitis of the hip. *J Bone Joint Surg Br* 1993; 75:973–974.

88. Blockey NJ, Porter BB. Transient synovitis of hip. A virological investigation. *Br Med J* 1968;4:557–558.

89. Zeharia A, Reif S, Ashkenazi S. Lack of association of transient synovitis of the hip joint with human parvovirus B19 infection in children. *Pediatr Infect Dis J* 1998;17:843–844.

90. Lockhart GR, Longobardi YL, Ehrlich M. Transient synovitis: lack of serologic evidence for acute parvovirus B-19 or human herpesvirus-6 infection. *J Pediatr Orthop* 1999;19:185–187.

91. Spock A. Transient synovitis of the hip joint in children. *Pediatrics* 1959;24:1042–1049.

92. Hardinge K. The etiology of transient synovitis of the hip in childhood. *J Bone Joint Surg Br* 1970;52:100–107.

93. Nachemson A, Scheller S. A clinical and radiological follow-study of transient synovitis of the hip. *Acta Orthop Scand* 1969; 40:479–500.

94. Todd AH. Discussion on the differential diagnosis of nontuberculous coxitis in children and adolescents. *Proc R Soc Med* 1925; 18:31.

95. Rauch S. Transitory synovitis of the hip joint in children. *Am J Dis Child* 1940;59:1245.

96. Hermel MB, Albert SM. Transient synovitis of the hip. *Clin Orthop* 1962;22:21–26.

97. Gledhill RB, McIntyre JM. Transient synovitis and Legg-Calve-Perthes disease: a comparative study. *Can Med Assoc J* 1969; 100:311–320.

98. Vila-Verde VM, da Silva KC. Bone age delay in Perthes disease and transient synovitis of the hip. *Clin Orthop* 2001;385:118–123.

99. Rosenborg M, Mortensson W. The validity of radiographic assessment of childhood transient synovitis of the hip. *Acta Radiol Diagn (Stockh)* 1986;27:85–89.

100. Shih TT, Su CT, Chiu LC, et al. Evaluation of hip disorders by radiography, radionuclide scanning and magnetic resonance imaging. *J Formos Med Assoc* 1993;92:737–744.

101. Kallio P, Ryoppy S, Jappinen S, et al. Ultrasonography in hip disease in children. *Acta Orthop Scand* 1985;56:367–371.

102. Wingstrand H. Transient synovitis of the hip in the child. *Acta Orthop Scand Suppl* 1986;219:1–61.

103. McGoldrick F, Bourke T, Blake N, et al. Accuracy of sonography in transient synovitis. *J Pediatr Orthop* 1990;10:501–503.

104. Futami T, Kasahara Y, Suzuki S, et al. Ultrasonography in transient synovitis and early Perthes' disease. *J Bone Joint Surg Br* 1991;73:635–639.

105. Terjesen T, Osthus P. Ultrasound in the diagnosis and follow-up of transient synovitis of the hip. *J Pediatr Orthop* 1991;11:608–613.

106. Strouse PJ, DiPietro MA, Adler RS. Pediatric hip effusions: evaluation with power Doppler sonography. *Radiology* 1998;206:731–735.

107. Bickerstaff DR, Neal LM, Booth AJ, et al. Ultrasound examination of the irritable hip. *J Bone Joint Surg Br* 1990;72:549–553.

108. Fink AM, Berman L, Edwards D, et al. The irritable hip: immediate ultrasound guided aspiration and prevention of hospital admission. *Arch Dis Child* 1995;72:110–113; discussion 113–114.

109. Miralles M, Gonzalez G, Pulpeiro JR, et al. Sonography of the painful hip in children: 500 consecutive cases. *AJR Am J Roentgenol* 1989;152:579–582.

110. Kloiber R, Pavlosky W, Portner O, et al. Bone scintigraphy of hip joint effusions in children. *AJR Am J Roentgenol* 1983;140:995–999.

111. Bower GD, Sprague P, Geijsel H, et al. Isotope bone scans in the assessment of children with hip pain or limp. *Pediatr Radiol* 1985;15:319–323.

112. Wingstrand H, Bauer GC, Brismar J, et al. Transient ischaemia of the proximal femoral epiphysis in the child. Interpretation of bone scintimetry for diagnosis in hip pain. *Acta Orthop Scand* 1985;56:197–203.

113. Paterson D, Savage JP. The nuclide bone scan in the diagnosis of Perthes' disease. *Clin Orthop* 1986;209:23–29.

114. Connolly LP, Treves ST. Assessing the limping child with skeletal scintigraphy. *J Nucl Med* 1998;39:1056–1061.

115. Connolly LP, Connolly SA. Skeletal scintigraphy in the multimodality assessment of young children with acute skeletal symptoms. *Clin Nucl Med* 2003;28:746–754.

116. Hasegawa Y, Wingstrand H, Gustafson T. Scintimetry in transient synovitis of the hip in the child. *Acta Orthop Scand* 1988;59:520–525.

117. Kallio PE. Coxa magna following transient synovitis of the hip. *Clin Orthop* 1988;228:49–56.

118. Royle SG, Galasko CS. The irritable hip. Scintigraphy in 192 children. *Acta Orthop Scand* 1992;63:25–28.

119. Toby EB, Koman LA, Bechtold RE. Magnetic resonance imaging of pediatric hip disease. *J Pediatr Orthop* 1985;5:665–671.

120. Ranner G, Ebner F, Fotter R, et al. Magnetic resonance imaging in children with acute hip pain. *Pediatr Radiol* 1989;20:67–71.

121. Lee SK, Suh KJ, Kim YW, et al. Septic arthritis versus transient synovitis at MR imaging: preliminary assessment with signal intensity alterations in bone marrow. *Radiology* 1999;211:459–465.

122. Zawin JK, Hoffer FA, Rand FF, et al. Joint effusion in children with an irritable hip: US diagnosis and aspiration. *Radiology* 1993;187:459–463.

123. Del Beccaro MA, Champoux AN, Bockers T, et al. Septic arthritis versus transient synovitis of the hip: the value of screening laboratory tests. *Ann Emerg Med* 1992;21:1418–1422.

124. Taylor GR, Clarke NM. Management of irritable hip: a review of hospital admission policy. *Arch Dis Child* 1994;71:59–63.

125. Kocher MS, Zurakowski D, Kasser JR. Differentiating between septic arthritis and transient synovitis of the hip in children: an evidence-based clinical prediction algorithm. *J Bone Joint Surg Am* 1999;81:1662–1670.

126. Jung ST, Rowe SM, Moon ES, et al. Significance of laboratory and radiologic findings for differentiating between septic arthritis and transient synovitis of the hip. *J Pediatr Orthop* 2003;23:368–372.

127. Luhmann SJ, Jones A, Schootman M, et al. Differentiation between septic arthritis and transient synovitis of the hip in children with clinical prediction algorithms. *J Bone Joint Surg Am* 2004;86-A:956–962.

128. Kocher MS, Mandiga R, Zurakowski D, et al. Validation of a clinical prediction rule for the differentiation between septic arthritis and transient synovitis of the hip in children. *J Bone Joint Surg Am* 2004;86-A:1629–1635.

129. Eich GF, Superti-Furga A, Umbricht FS, et al. The painful hip: evaluation of criteria for clinical decision-making. *Eur J Pediatr* 1999;158:923–928.

130. Finder JG. Transitory synovitis of the hip in children. *JAMA* 1936;148:30.

131. Adams JA. Transient synovitis of the hip joint in children. *J Bone Joint Surg Br* 1963;45:471–476.

132. Jacobs BW. Synovitis of the hip in children and its significance. *Pediatrics* 1971;47:558–566.

133. Kesteris U, Wingstrand H, Forsberg L, et al. The effect of arthrocentesis in transient synovitis of the hip in the child: a longitudinal sonographic study. *J Pediatr Orthop* 1996;16:24–29.

134. Mattick A, Turner A, Ferguson J, et al. Seven year follow up of children presenting to the accident and emergency department with irritable hip. *J Accid Emerg Med* 1999;16:345–347.

135. De Valderrama JAF. The "observation hip" syndrome and its late sequelae. *J Bone Joint Surg Br* 1963;45:462.

136. Wingstrand H, Egund N, Carlin NO, et al. Intracapsular pressure in transient synovitis of the hip. *Acta Orthop Scand* 1985;56:204–210.

137. Kallio P, Ryoppy S. Hyperpressure in juvenile hip disease. *Acta Orthop Scand* 1985;56:211–214.

138. Kermond S, Fink M, Graham K, et al. A randomized clinical trial: should the child with transient synovitis of the hip be treated with nonsteroidal anti-inflammatory drugs? *Ann Emerg Med* 2002;40:294–299.

## Idiopathic Chondrolysis of the Hip

139. Heppenstall RB, Marvel JP Jr, Chung SM, et al. Chondrolysis of the hip. *Clin Orthop* 1974:136–142.

140. Waldenstrom H. On necrosis of the joint cartilage by epiphyseolysis capitis femoris. *Acta Chir Scand* 1930;67:936.

141. Pellicci PM, Wilson PD Jr. Chondrolysis of the hips associated with severe burns. A case report. *J Bone Joint Surg Am* 1979;61:592–596.

142. Cruess RL. The pathology of acute necrosis of cartilage in slipping of the capital femoral epiphysis. A report of two cases with pathological sections. *J Bone Joint Surg Am* 1963;45:1013–1024.

143. Jones BS. Adolescent chondrolysis of the hip joint. *S Afr Med J* 1971;45:196–202.

144. Bleck EE. Idiopathic chondrolysis of the hip. *J Bone Joint Surg Am* 1983;65:1266–1275.

145. Daluga DJ, Millar EA. Idiopathic chondrolysis of the hip. *J Pediatr Orthop* 1989;9:405–411.

146. Duncan JW, Nasca R, Schrantz J. Idiopathic chondrolysis of the hip. *J Bone Joint Surg Am* 1979;61:1024–1028.

147. Duncan JW, Schrantz JL, Nasca RJ. The bizarre stiff hip. Possible idiopathic chondrolysis. *JAMA* 1975;231:382–385.

148. Wenger DR, Mickelson MR, Ponseti IV. Idiopathic chondrolysis of the hip. Report of two cases. *J Bone Joint Surg Am* 1975;57:268–271.

149. del Couz Garcia A, Fernandez PL, Gonzalez MP, et al. Idiopathic chondrolysis of the hip: long-term evolution. *J Pediatr Orthop* 1999;19:449–454.

150. Kozlowski K, Scougall J. Idiopathic chondrolysis—diagnostic difficulties. Report of four cases. *Pediatr Radiol* 1984;14:314–317.

151. Rowe LJ, Ho EK. Idiopathic chondrolysis of the hip. *Skeletal Radiol* 1996;25:178–182.
152. Hughes AW. Idiopathic chondrolysis of the hip: a case report and review of the literature. *Ann Rheum Dis* 1985;44:268–272.
153. Donnan L, Einoder B. Idiopathic chondrolysis of the hip. *Aust N Z J Surg* 1996;66:569–571.
154. Sivanantham M, Kutty MK. Idiopathic chondrolysis of the hip: case report with a review of the literature. *Aust N Z J Surg* 1977; 47:229–231.
155. Sparks LT, Dall G. Idiopathic chondrolysis of the hip joint in adolescents. Case reports. *S Afr Med J* 1982;61:883–886.
156. Smith EJ, Ninin DT, Keays AC. Idiopathic chondrolysis of the hip. A case report. *S Afr Med J* 1983;63:88–90.
157. Rachinsky I, Boguslavsky L, Cohen E, et al. Bilateral idiopathic chondrolysis of the hip: a case report. *Clin Nucl Med* 2000;25: 1007–1009.
158. Jacobs B. Chondrolysis after epiphyseolysis. *Instr Course Lect* 1972;21:224.
159. Eisenstein A, Rothschild S. Biochemical abnormalities in patients with slipped capital femoral epiphysis and chondrolysis. *J Bone Joint Surg Am* 1976;58:459–467.
160. Herman JH, Herzig EB, Crissman JD, et al. Idiopathic chondrolysis—an immunopathologic study. *J Rheumatol* 1980;7: 694–705.
161. Mankin H. Chondrolysis of the hip. *Proceedings of the third open scientific meeting of the hip society.* Saint Louis, MO: CV Mosby, 1975:127.
162. Ippolito E, Ricciardi-Pollini PT. Chondrolysis of the hip (idiopathic and secondary forms). *Ital J Orthop Traumatol* 1981;7: 335–344.
163. Morrissy RT, Kalderon AE, Gerdes MH. Synovial immunofluorescence in patients with slipped capital femoral epiphysis. *J Pediatr Orthop* 1981;1:55–60.
164. Ippolito E, Bellocci M, Santori FS, et al. Idiopathic chondrolysis of the hip: an ultrastructural study of the articular cartilage of the femoral head. *Orthopedics* 1986;9:1383–1387.
165. van der Hoeven H, Keessen W, Kuis W. Idiopathic chondrolysis of the hip: A distinct clinical entity? *Acta Orthop Scand* 1989; 60:661–663.
166. Green NE, Edwards K. Bone and joint infections in children. *Orthop Clin North Am* 1987;18:555–576.
167. Shore A, Macauley D, Ansell BM. Idiopathic protrusio acetabuli in juveniles. *Rheumatol Rehabil* 1981;20:1–10.
168. Mandall, GA; Keret, D; Harcke, HT; Bowen, JR. Chondrolysis: detention by bone scintography. *J Pediatr Orthop* 1992;12: 80–85.
169. Johnson K, Haigh SF, Ehtisham S, et al. Childhood idiopathic chondrolysis of the hip: MRI features. *Pediatr Radiol* 2003;33: 194–199.
170. Roy DR, Crawford AH. Idiopathic chondrolysis of the hip: management by subtotal capsulectomy and aggressive rehabilitation. *J Pediatr Orthop* 1988;8:203–207.

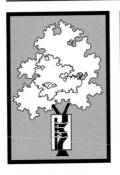

# 28 The Lower Extremity

*Perry L. Schoenecker*    *Margaret M. Rich*

# ROTATIONAL VARIATION

## Definition

Rotational profiles vary widely among healthy children (1–3). Differences in appearance related to foot position during walking or running are most often just that, differences, not pathologic conditions. Foot position during walking is described by the direction of the foot relative to the body's line of progression during the gait cycle (internal, external, or neutral). This is *torsion*. It results from the summation of several factors that include version of the bones, capsular pliability, and muscle control (1,3–5). *Version* is tilt or inclination within a bone, such as the relation of the femoral head/neck to the shaft of the femur. Contracture of a joint capsule may restrict rotation. Similarly, capsular laxity may allow a greater than normal arc of motion. Arthrosis or incongruity may also restrict motion. The balance between opposing muscle groups is also a determinant of foot position and may introduce a significant, dynamic component to the rotational profile. Age is another important variable because version, soft-tissue pliability, and muscle coordination change as the child matures (1–8).

## Assessment

Assessment of rotational alignment includes static and dynamic components. The static examination describes the available range of rotational motion. The dynamic examination displays the effect of various torsional forces at play during the walking cycle (Fig. 28.1). The static examination is best performed on a firm examining table, with the child in comfortable, loose clothing such as shorts or a diaper. Rotation is best assessed with the child in the prone position, keeping the pelvis flat and level on the examination table (3–5). Flexion of the knee to 90 degrees allows the leg to be used like a goniometer relative to the thigh. Some children will not allow examination other than on a parent's lap. This is usually adequate although not as controlled as in the prone position. The arc of rotation may be more generous if measured with the hip flexed as in a sitting position (5).

Rotation of the foot laterally or medially is used to assess the degree of available hip rotation. When there is a greater degree of internal or medial rotation (outward movement of the foot in the prone position) than external or lateral

rotation, a toed-in gait is more likely to be observed. Similarly, if there is greater external rotation than internal rotation, the gait pattern is usually toed-out. A greater ability to rotate the thigh internally than externally is frequently referred to as *anteversion*. It should correctly be called *antetorsion* because hip rotation is the combined effect of version of the femur, joint mobility, and muscle function (1,3,5).

Medial hip rotation is generally greater in girls than in boys (Fig. 28.2). Variability is greater in younger children. Static medial hip rotation averages 40 degrees in infants, but can range from 10 to 60 degrees. It increases slightly by the age of 10 years and then decreases gradually in adulthood. Lateral hip rotation is greater than medial rotation in infants; it averages 65 degrees (range, 45 to 90 degrees), compared to children over the age of 10 years who average 40 degrees (range, 20 to 55 degrees) (1–3,5,9,10). It increases slightly in adults.

Observation of the alignment of the sole of the foot relative to the thigh, which is held in neutral rotation, determines the thigh-foot angle (TFA), as shown in Figure 28.1B. This relation also describes the contribution of the leg segment or the degree of tibial torsion. Foot deformity, which may contribute to rotational abnormalities, can easily be assessed in this position. Forefoot adduction or abduction and hindfoot varus or valgus is noted. Many young children have significant rotational laxity through the knee. Internal and external rotation of the tibia with the knee flexed demonstrates the degree of knee joint laxity. This may contribute to variation in foot position. Average TFA is 5 degrees internal in infants (range, −30 to +20 degrees) and 10 degrees external by 8 years of age (range, −5 to +30 degrees) (1–3,5). TFA changes very little after 12 years of age.

Correlation between the static examination and the dynamic examination is important. The child's walking pattern should be observed in an area large enough to allow comfortable and safe walking and running. The child should be able to walk alone (i.e., not holding someone's hand). It is often helpful to observe the child in shoes as well as barefoot. Often the in-toeing is more apparent with shoes on, presumably because the weight of the shoe may be more taxing on the muscle control of foot position. An oversized shoe may also compound the appearance of in-toeing. Variations are common with change in speed or direction of walking. Foot and knee position should be observed over several cycles of gait. The relation of foot position to an imaginary line along the path being walked describes the foot-progression angle (FPA). Variability is considerable in children up to 5 years of age. Out-toed position predominates in older children. Once a mature gait pattern is established, usually by 5 years of age, FPA changes very little (1–6,9,10).

The child's rotational profile includes the contribution of each of these components to the gait pattern. The FPA, TFA, and position of the knee relative to the body (femoral torsion), all contribute to the sum of rotational factors.

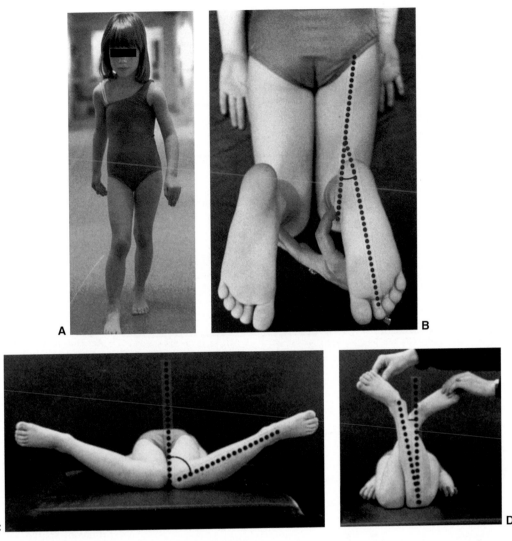

**Figure 28.1** How the rotational profile measurements are made. **A:** The foot-progression angle (FPA) is estimated by observing the child's gait. It is defined as the angular difference between the axis of the foot and the line of progression. This child's FPA is 0 degrees. **B:** The thigh-foot angle (TFA) is the angular difference between the axis of the foot and thigh as viewed from above. The TFA in this child is 18 degrees. From this view the shape of the foot is apparent. **C:** Medial hip rotation is the maximum angular difference between the vertical and the axis of the tibia. In these hips, this measurement is 70 degrees. **D:** Lateral hip rotation is the corresponding measurement. On this child, the angle is 10 degrees.

Each area needs to be assessed along with its contribution, either positive (internal rotation) or negative (external rotation), to the overall gait pattern. Those children whose rotational profiles are beyond two standard deviations of the mean are considered abnormal according to Staheli's criteria (3,4) (Fig. 28.2).

## Differential Diagnosis

Infrequently, pathologic conditions will cause a rotational abnormality. Residual foot deformities, disorders of the hip, and neuromuscular diseases are the most common causes of pathologic in-toeing or out-toeing. In-toeing may be caused by residual foot deformity from metatarsus adductus, clubfoot, or skewfoot (1,4,5). These conditions

are discussed in detail elsewhere in this text (see Chapter 29). In-toeing, which is only apparent during swing phase, may be the result of overpull of the posterior tibial tendon, often seen in spastic hemiplegia (11,12).

Femoral antetorsion is often seen in spastic diplegia or quadriplegia. This may be a combination of excess femoral anteversion with contracture of the adductor and medial hamstring muscles (4,5,13). Excess valgus and pronation of the foot, which contribute to an out-toed foot progression, may also be seen (13). For some children with spasticity, extremes in rotational posture are a compensatory mechanism for limited hip, knee, or ankle motion. The combination of excess internal femoral rotation and external tibial rotation (malicious malalignment) is often observed in children with spasticity. Children with diplegia

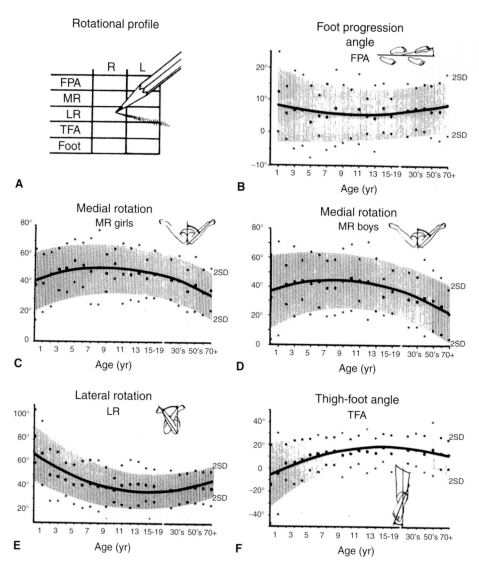

**Figure 28.2** The rotational profile. **A:** The method of recording the degree measurements for each element of the profile is depicted. This simple chart includes the vital information necessary to establish the diagnosis and to document severity. **B–F:** Normative values for the profile based on 1000 healthy limbs are shown. In each figure the age is listed on the abscissa on a logarithmic scale and the degrees are shown on the ordinate scale. Mean values are shown by the solid line with ±2 standard deviations; reference range is shown in shaded areas. A sex difference was found to affect the values for medial rotation, so the values are shown independently.

and quadriplegia often have heel cord tightness. To maintain foot contact with the floor, the calcaneus tends to rotate laterally beneath the talus, which allows the talar head to drop plantarward, producing a valgus deformity (14). If the peroneal tendons are also spastic, the forefoot will also be pulled into an abducted position creating a planovalgus deformity. If the child is unable to clear the foot during swing phase, the foot is repeatedly dragged along the floor, adding to the external torsional force applied to the foot. This produces a malalignment, with the foot externally rotated from the planovalgus deformity and the knee internally rotated from femoral antetorsion.

Pathologic out-toeing may result from the severe pes planovalgus often associated with external tibial torsion (15) (Fig. 28.3). This may be secondary to tarsal coalition, but may also be seen in adolescents with rigid flat feet without a coalition. It is unclear whether the out-toed position is an adaptation to a rigid flat foot, or whether the lack of foot flexibility promotes the development of external rotation. The combination of femoral retrotorsion, external tibial torsion, and pes planovalgus can also be seen, particularly in large adolescents, which produces a

striking out-toed gait. Slipped capital femoral epiphysis (SCFE) should be considered in a differential diagnosis of out-toeing, particularly when the deviation is asymmetric or of recent onset (4,16). Hip dysplasia can alter rotation, but its effect is highly variable (7). An asymmetric hip may be apparent upon examination, but is not reliable in detecting hip dysplasia. In such instances, further evaluation with radiographic hip examination is warranted (3,4). Coxa vara may also present as an out-toed gait.

## Radiographic Evaluation

It is recommended that any child who presents to an orthopaedic surgeon with concerns of a gait abnormality have an anteroposterior pelvis radiograph. Children older than 8 years with a recent change in gait or with complaints of pain should also have a lateral radiograph of the hips (3,4,16). A cross-table lateral film is optimal to detect a minimally displaced SCFE. Although the incidence of otherwise occult pathology is low, the consequence of a missed diagnosis, such as hip dysplasia or an SCFE, is significant for the child.

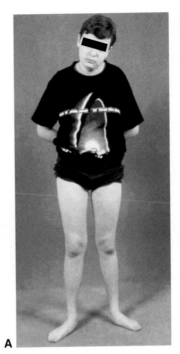
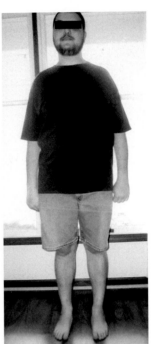

**Figure 28.3**  **A:** Excess external rotational deformity may not resolve. It may be associated with symptomatic flatfoot, with or without tarsal coalition. The use of medial support orthotics may reduce symptoms, but will not alter rotation. **B:** Alignment at 18 years of age following tibial internal rotation osteotomy to correct excessive external tibial rotation.     **A**     **B**

It is not necessary to obtain serial radiographs of the hips or lower extremities to follow the course of normal rotational development (4,5). Special views to quantify version of the femur or tibia are not indicated in the routine evaluation of rotation (3–5). Three-dimensional imaging studies [computed tomography (CT) and magnetic resonance imaging (MRI)] are rarely indicated in the assessment or follow-up of rotational variations, but are more accurate in quantifying rotation than clinical or biplane radiography (17).

## Natural History

Most children brought in for concerns of in-toeing or out-toeing are normal. Rotational profiles are highly variable, particularly in toddlers who have not mastered the basic skills needed for normal walking, which includes just about every child younger than 2 years and many of those who are 2 to 5 years of age (1,2,6,10). Internal and external rotational variations should be considered just that, variations of normal, not a pathologic condition. The natural history of rotational variations is gradual normalization, usually accomplished by 5 to 6 years of age. There are no conclusive studies to show that any nonsurgical intervention speeds up or assures the normalization of gait (4,5,18).

Internal tibial torsion is more common than external tibial torsion in toddlers (4,5) (Fig. 28.4). It is often associated with physiologic bowlegs and decreases 1 to 2 years after resolution of the bowing. Occasionally, it will persist into preadolescence. External tibial torsion is less common, but is more likely to persist through adolescence (4,5).

The assessment of hip range of motion in newborns and infants is highly variable (2,3,5,7). Most healthy infants have an external rotation contracture about the hip, which is likely to be a result of intrauterine positioning. This may not fully resolve until they become established walkers at 18 to 24 months of age. An in-toed gait may then be more apparent. Lateral hip rotation gradually decreases as medial rotation increases. Paradoxically, anteversion in the femoral neck typically decreases from 30 degrees (range, 15 to 50 degrees) at birth to 20 degrees (range, 10 to 35 degrees) by 10 years of age (1–5,7,8). A decrease in anteversion of the femoral neck would be expected to produce greater external rotation of the hip; however, changes in muscle balance and hip capsule pliability appear to have greater influence on gait. By 8 years of age, a child who toes in while walking, but has at least 20 degrees of hip external rotation, is within normal limits as defined by the mean plus or minus two standard deviations. Similarly, one who toes out while walking, but has at least 20 degrees of hip internal rotation, has motion within a normal range (4,5,10).

Variations in rotation have not been linked directly to the risk of degenerative joint disease (9,10,19–22). Several authors have tried to correlate the degree of femoral anteversion with the presence of osteoarthritis of the hip using postmortem studies or by preoperative CT scan. Most studies have shown a similar measure of anteversion in hips with and without arthritic changes (20–24). One study measured anteversion in hips of patients undergoing proximal femoral osteotomy or total hip replacement. Patients with bilateral disease had an average 9 degrees greater anteversion than patients with healthy hips. Patients with unilateral arthritis averaged 4 degrees more anteversion in the arthritic hip than in the healthy hip (24). Some authors have demonstrated a relation of anteversion with degenerative changes in the knee, presumably from increased shear loads (25). Hip pain is rarely a complaint in children with increased femoral anteversion alone (19,21,26). Anterior knee pain may be associated with increased medial rotation

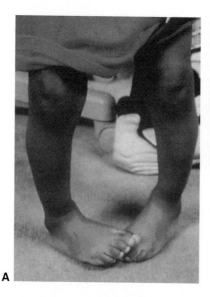
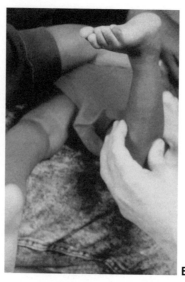

**Figure 28.4** **A:** Internal tibial torsion is often seen in toddlers in association with physiologic bowlegs and results in an in-toed gait. **B:** The thigh-foot angle is best assessed in the prone position.

of the femur, but not generally with patellofemoral changes (21,22,26). Although some recent publications have suggested that torsional variations may increase the risk of osteoarthritis, anatomic studies have not conclusively shown a causal relation between femoral anteversion and osteoarthritis. A subset of patients exists in whom the limits of tolerance in hip or knee range of motion is exceeded and for whom the risk for early degenerative changes may be increased (25,27,28). In these patients, the alteration in rotation places increased stress across the hip or knee, which can promote the development of osteoarthritic changes. The precise limit of tolerance remains undefined. However, the presence of hip or knee pain should be considered as indications for osteotomy.

Although the presence of hip's external rotation may augment posterior shear loads, an increased incidence of slipped epiphysis has not been found in patients with femoral retroversion without other contributory factors being present (16). Athletic ability does not correlate with the position assumed during normal walking, although some activities may be hindered by rotational variations, particularly hip or tibial external rotation (29–31). High-performance sprinters, however, tend to adopt a toed-in position during running regardless of their walking style (31). Functional impairments such as tripping, clumsiness, or lack of running ability, although often attributed to rotational differences, have not been shown to correlate with rotational profile (29).

There are some children with such extreme variation in rotation that their appearance is unacceptable to them or their parents. The natural history of rotational variation, the lack of evidence for musculoskeletal sequelae, and the absence of objective functional disability must be kept in mind and the family educated in this regard (1,3–5). The natural history of rotational variation should be clearly communicated to the parents and understood by them prior to any recommendation for active treatment.

## Treatment

The natural history of rotational variations is gradual normalization. No treatment is necessary in most children who present with concerns of in-toeing or out-toeing. The use of shoe modifications, orthotics, or positioning devices is ineffective (5,16). Although these measures are not harmful, there are few data to show any positive effect. Their use reinforces the errant notion that in-toeing or out-toeing is an abnormal condition or disorder that requires treatment. The cost of orthopaedic shoes and orthotics can be considerable. Muscle-strengthening exercises or activities may diminish the dynamic component that produces variation in gait; however, no studies have addressed this specific topic. Treatment options for foot and ankle abnormalities are covered in Chapter 29.

Rotational osteotomy may be considered for those otherwise healthy children who have persistent rotational abnormality into later childhood and adolescence and find the appearance of their gait or their function unacceptable (4,5,25,32,33). An awkward gait may appear less following osteotomy. Patients and their parents often express satisfaction with the change in appearance following osteotomy. Improvement in function is variable and less predictable. Those with in-toeing typically note less tripping. Those with out-toeing are more likely to notice an improvement in running ability.

Pain, although rarely a complaint, may be improved following surgical treatment (25). Most often, this occurs in patients with malicious malalignment or the combination of femoral internal rotation with tibial external rotation (25,34). These patients may experience knee symptoms preoperatively, likely related to the increased shear forces through the knee. This combination of rotational abnormalities has been associated with some risk of patellofemoral arthritis (35,36).

Supramalleolar rotational osteotomy of the tibia and fibula has less potential for serious neurovascular complication than does proximal tibial osteotomy (32,37). The authors' preferred technique uses fixation with crossed Kirschner wires (K-wires), supplemented with a long-leg cast. Alternatively, a small fragment T-plate supplemented with a short-leg cast can be used. The tibia should be cut 2 to 3 cm above the physis and parallel to the ankle. Rotation through an oblique cut will tilt the articular surface of the tibia. Sectioning of the fibula also allows easier rotation of the tibia without displacement. The degree of correction is determined by aligning the foot and ankle, such that the second toe is in line with the tibial tubercle and the center of the patella. As the foot is dorsiflexed and knee bent, the foot should remain in line with the lateral thigh. Two or three stainless steel wires of appropriate size are inserted, one from proximal medial to distal lateral and another from distal medial to proximal lateral, avoiding the growth plate of the distal tibia. A third wire is used if rotational stability does not seem adequate with two wires. A long-leg, bent-knee cast is used for 6 weeks. Healing is usually sufficient at that time for pin removal and application of a short-leg weight-bearing cast for an additional 4 to 6 weeks.

Alternatively, a small fragment T-plate may be used along with a short-leg non–weight-bearing cast for 6 to 8 weeks. The T-plate may be preferable in older patients. Plate removal may be necessitated by the subcutaneous position of the plate.

Correction of excess femoral internal or external rotation is obtained by equalizing the degree of internal versus external rotation. The amount to be rotated can be estimated during the prone examination, comparing internal and external hip rotation, preoperatively (5). Femoral osteotomy may be performed proximally or distally depending on the surgeon's preference and the type of fixation to be used (33,38,39). Proximal femoral osteotomy is preferred if there is also varus, valgus, flexion, or extension deformity of the hip. Similarly, angular deformities about the knee are better addressed by a distal femoral osteotomy. A standard lateral approach to the femur is used, whether proximal or distal. In proximal osteotomy, a pediatric or adolescent blade plate is used for fixation. If a distal femoral osteotomy is performed in a skeletally immature patient, a small straight compression or 95-degree condylar (adolescent) blade plate fixation may be used. Use of cast or orthotic immobilization is at the discretion of the surgeon. Alternatively, a medial approach can be used along with K-wire fixation (33). This latter technique should be reserved for smaller children, and must be supplemented with a spica cast. The desired amount of rotational correction is typically that which achieves an equal amount of internal and external rotation.

Intramedullary fixation can be used for either the tibia or the femur (39). Locking screws or similar mechanisms are needed proximal and distal to the osteotomy because the osteotomy has no intrinsic stability. In the skeletally immature and in those with a relatively narrow medullary canal, the osteotomy is generally performed by a limited open technique. The proximal femur entry site is made lateral and distal to the tip of the greater trochanter. Great care is taken to avoid any dissection (including penetration) on the medial side of the trochanter. A recent modification in femoral nail design (proximally angulated 15 degrees) facilitates correct nail placement. This lateral trochanter entry site is necessary to avoid injury to the medial portion of the trochanteric growth plate and injury to the terminal branches of the medial circumflex artery in the trochanteric fossa. Neither coxa valga nor avascular necrosis has occurred in the early experiences with this approach (40). An intramedullary saw can be used to section the femur in skeletally mature patients who have a larger medullary canal. Fixation with an intramedullary rod does not allow for any concomitant correction of varus, valgus, flexion, or extension. However, intramedullary fixation does allow for early weight bearing, a particular advantage if bilateral procedures are performed.

A unilateral frame can be used for acute correction. Manipulation may be hindered by the pull of the soft tissues, particularly in large adolescents (41,42). Pins should be inserted, taking into account the rotation to be accomplished. The amount of change in rotation can be reassessed in the early postoperative period and adjusted if needed.

Increased femoral internal rotation and tibial external rotation may coexist, producing a rotational malalignment (25,34) (Fig. 28.5). Knee pain, which is usually diffuse, may be present. Patellar mal-tracking usually is not present. Because the deformities are complementary, foot progression may be normal, but the static examination will demonstrate the abnormality. Combined osteotomy of the femur and tibia may be necessary to correct symptomatic malrotation (4,25,34). Femoral rotation is corrected as the first step of the procedure. The foot is then aligned with a tibial osteotomy completing the correction. Correction of bilateral deformities can be performed as staged unilateral procedures 6 to 12 months apart.

## Complications

The risks and complications of in-toeing and out-toeing are related to its treatment, not its presence (3–5,17, 19,20,29). Because most patients who have surgical alteration of their rotation do so to effect a change in the appearance of their gait, the surgical procedure must accomplish the desired change in rotation. Functional change is noted in some children, but not consistently.

Complications of rotational osteotomy are the same as for other osteotomies. Problems related to nonunion, infection, blood loss, joint stiffness, scarring, and anesthesia are the most serious (25,32,33,37). Distal tibial osteotomy has less risk of compartment syndrome and peroneal nerve injury than proximal osteotomy. Whether performed proximally or distally, the use of a blade plate for fixation of a femoral osteotomy may inadvertently produce undesirable frontal or sagittal plane deformity.

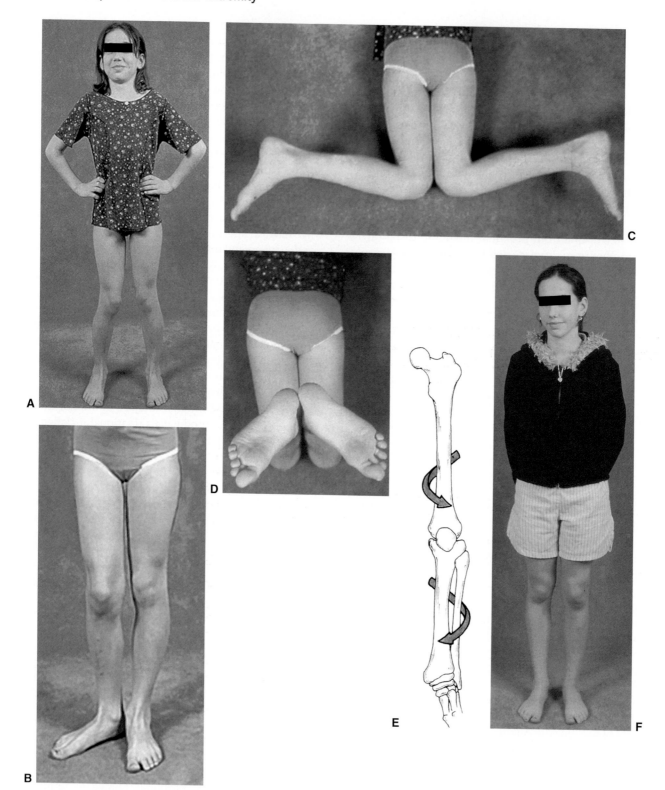

**Figure 28.5    A:** This 10-year-old girl is attempting to stand with her feet directly forward. The patellae face medially, and with effort she can direct the feet straight ahead. **B:** When the limb is positioned with the patella facing forward, the outward rotation of the foot becomes apparent. **C:** Examination in the prone position demonstrates approximately 80 degrees of internal rotation of the thigh, or medial femoral torsion. **D:** With knees flexed, the outward direction of the foot can also be appreciated. If the rotational deformities are complementary, foot progression may be deceptively normal. **E:** The combination of increased medial thigh rotation and external rotation of the lower leg segment may result in symptomatic torsional malalignment. This deformity may be a cause of nonspecific knee pain in adolescents because of the increased shear forces through the knee. **F:** Combined femoral external rotation and tibial internal rotation osteotomies correct the malicious malalignment. Knee symptoms are predictably improved.

Similarly, inadvertent deformity can be produced in the distal tibia if an oblique osteotomy is made, rather than a transverse cut, in performing a distal tibial osteotomy. The distal tibial physis should not be violated when using K-wires to fix a supramalleolar tibial osteotomy. The authors have observed distal tibial physeal growth arrest and deformity following K-wire penetration of the medial tibial physis. Asymmetric growth arrest can occur from periosteal stripping and injury to the lateral distal femoral physis. Injury to the greater trochanteric apophysis can produce valgus deformity in the proximal femur. Scars may be less visible with proximal osteotomy, a consideration for a procedure that is largely cosmetic.

Angular deformity may be less problematic when a locked intramedullary fixation device is used; however, adjustments in position can be difficult once the rod is locked. Use of a lateral entry point helps minimize the risk of avascular necrosis to the femoral head and potential disruption of normal growth of the proximal femur (39,40,42–44). Recent changes in pediatric intramedullary nail design permit safer entry through the lateral aspect of the greater trochanter, minimizing both the potential for avascular necrosis and the disruption of normal growth of the proximal femur (40). In the skeletally immature patient, use of this lateral entry site is imperative.

## PHYSIOLOGIC BOWING AND GENU VARUM

### Physiologic Bowing

#### Definition

Infants and children frequently present to the orthopaedic surgeon for evaluation of bowleg deformity (45). Typically, these children are early walkers, achieving independent ambulation before the first year of life (46–48). The normal knee alignment at birth is 10 to 15 degrees of varus, which remodels to a neutral femoral-tibial alignment at approximately 14 months of age (1,49,50) (Fig. 28.6). Levine and Drennan (51) have defined physiologic bowing radiographically as more than 10 degrees of bilateral femoral-tibial varus noted after the age of 18 months.

#### Clinical Features

Parents are concerned with both the cosmetic appearance of the bowing deformity and the associated problems of excessive tripping. A family history of bowleg deformity is common (45,52). Examination typically reveals bowing of both the lower extremities with in-toeing (Fig. 28.7). Although the bowing deformity is bilateral, its severity in the left versus right extremities can vary. Despite their bowlegged, toed-in gait, these young children are characteristically very agile walkers. The child should be observed walking, both toward and away from the examiner, to assess the severity of the dynamic varus and associated internal rotation deformity. Internal rotation of the extremity permits contact of the foot with the floor as the child stands. This also maintains the body center over the midline as the child walks. The presence of a lateral thrust should be noted. This is a brief, dynamic, lateral, knee joint protrusion that occurs in stance. It represents a lateral subluxation or shifting of the femur on the depressed medial tibia and is accentuated by ligamentous laxity. It is characteristic of pathologic bowlegs.

The degree of varus deformity of the lower extremity is measured with a goniometer with the knees extended and patella facing forward. Photographs are helpful in documenting the deformity. Angular and rotational alignment and joint range of motion of the entire lower extremity are assessed. Knee joint laxity typically is not present in physiologic bowing.

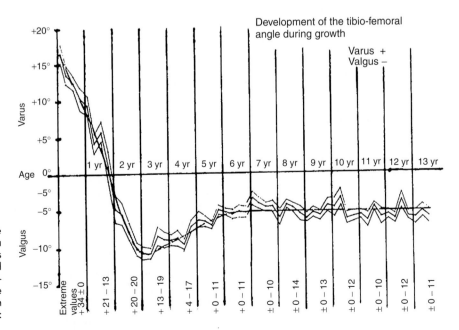

**Figure 28.6** The graph depicts the expected change in genu varum and genu valgum with age. Children with bowlegs after 2 years of age are outside the normal range and should be thoroughly evaluated. (From Salenius P, Vankka E. The development of the tibiofemoral angle in children. *J Bone Joint Surg Am* 1975;57: 259, with permission.)

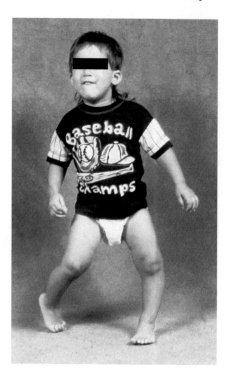

**Figure 28.7** Examination of the child with physiologic bowing shows symmetric bowing throughout the tibia and internal tibial torsion which is often more noticeable with walking.

In younger children, those less than 18 months of age, radiographs can document the degree and location of the varus deformity, but usually will not distinguish between physiologic bowing and early Blount disease. Radiographs are an essential part of the evaluation in the older child (over 18 months of age), for those with more pronounced deformities (greater than 20 degrees), when a lateral thrust is observed, if the child is of short stature (below fifth percentile), or if a metabolic bone disease is suspected (Fig. 28.8). The radiograph is taken with the patient standing, if possible, and the patella pointing straight ahead. The relative degree of varus deformity is noted by observing the shaft-to-shaft angle of the femur and tibia (51,52). More importantly, the distribution of bowing deformity is noted (53). When physiologic, the bowing occurs throughout the distal femur, proximal tibia, and distal tibia (54). In contrast, early Blount disease has more focal deformity limited to the proximal tibia.

### Differential Diagnosis

The differential diagnosis of bowing in the young child includes physiologic bowing and pathologic bowing (Table 28.1). Pathologic bowing occurs in infantile tibia vara (Blount disease), metabolic bone disease, and skeletal dysplasias (Fig. 28.8 B–D). The clinical and radiographic features associated with metabolic bone disease or skeletal dysplasia readily differentiate these pathologic conditions from physiologic bowing. Most often, the differentiation is between physiologic bowing and infantile Blount disease. If the bowing is physiologic, the entire lower extremity will

## TABLE 28.1
### DIFFERENTIAL DIAGNOSIS OF BOWED LEGS

Physiologic bowing
Blount disease
   Metabolic bone disease
   X-linked hypophosphatemic rickets
Nutritional rickets
   Skeletal dysplasia
   Achondroplasia
   Pseudoachondroplasia
   Metaphyseal chondrodysplasia
Neoplastic disease

appear to be bowed. If the varus results from a relatively greater deformity of the proximal tibia, infantile tibia vara or Blount disease may be present (54–56). Children with either physiologic bowing or Blount disease usually are early walkers and typically present for evaluation at 15 to 18 months of age. Often, there is a positive family history of bowing deformity (in siblings, parents, uncles, and aunts) (45,46,52,53). Physiologic bowing and Blount disease ought to be perceived as two points within the same spectrum, with Blount disease being the pathologic result of unresolved infantile bowing (46,51,55). Frequently, one extremity will have physiologic bowing with Blount disease affecting the contralateral tibia.

***Radiographic Evaluation.*** Radiographic distinction between physiologic bowing and Blount disease is not obvious in very young children. The Langenskiöld changes, diagnostic of Blount disease, are not always distinct before 2 to 3 years of age (47,50,51,53,56). Measuring the metaphyseal-diaphyseal (MD) angle of both the proximal tibia and distal femur further helps to identify the specific location and relative severity of varus deformity (51,56,57). Although an absolute MD angle is not diagnostic, it does serve as a guide in differentiating Langenskiöld stage I infantile Blount disease from physiologic bowing (50,53) (Fig. 28.9). Measurement can be affected by limb position (58). A study of the proximal tibial MD angle in patients with bowing (physiologic bowing or Blount disease) identified two distinct populations with considerable overlap (56) (Fig. 28.10). On the basis of this study by Feldman and Schoenecker, when the MD angle is less than 10 degrees, there is a 95% probability that the diagnosis is physiologic bowing. Conversely, if the MD angle is greater than 16 degrees, then there is a 95% probability that the diagnosis is Blount disease. For those patients with an MD angle between 10 and 16 degrees, follow-up for at least 1 to 2 years is necessary to determine whether the metaphyseal changes resolve (physiologic bowing) or progress (Blount disease). In a recent report, Bowen et al. (54) noted that all children with a tibial MD angle greater than 16 degrees showed progression of the varus deformity.

The ratio of the distal femoral MD angle relative to that of the proximal tibia can be helpful in differentiating

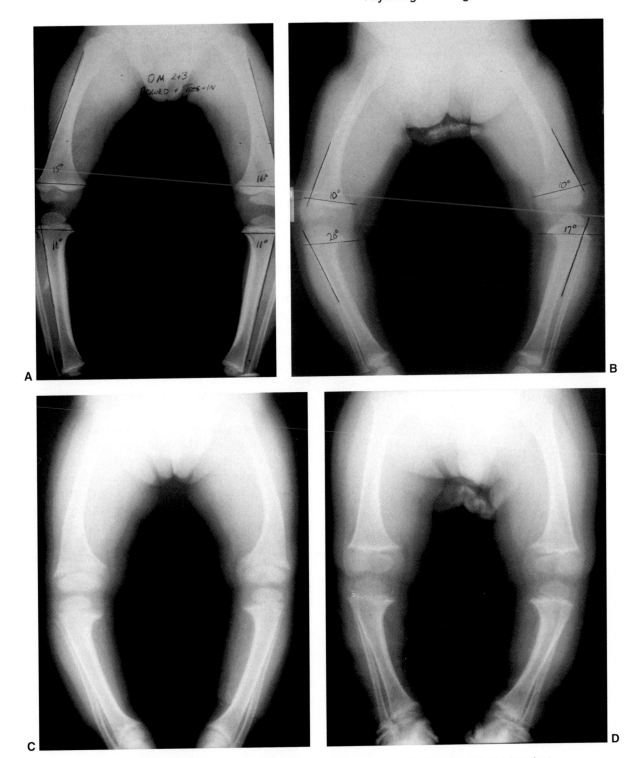

**Figure 28.8** Standing anteroposterior films of both lower extremities help distinguish physiologic bowing from pathologic causes. **A:** Tibial metaphyseal-diaphyseal (MD) angles are typically 11 degrees or less. A similar angle constructed in the distal femur is the same or greater, indicating that the femur and tibia contribute similarly to the bowing. The ratio of femoral to tibial MD angle is greater than 1. **B:** Early Blount disease may be difficult to distinguish from severe physiologic bowing. The MD angle in Blount disease is usually greater than 16 degrees and the ratio of femur to tibia is less than 1. Fragmentation of the medial tibial metaphysis may not be evident. **C:** This patient with X-linked hypophosphatemic rickets (XLH) has multiple widened physes. Osteopenia is evident in the adjacent metaphysis, which is also flared. Bowing tends to be more diffuse throughout the bone rather than focal in the proximal tibia. **D:** Skeletal dysplasia, such as chondrometaphyseal dysplasia, may cause genu varus. These children are usually of short stature. Skeletal abnormalities are multifocal as in this example of Schmid metaphyseal chondrodysplasia. The proximal and distal metaphyses of the femur and tibia are all abnormal. The epiphyses, physes, and bone density are normal.

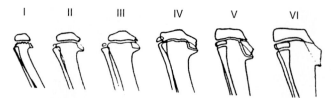

**Figure 28.9** Depiction of the six stages of radiographic changes seen in Langenskiöld classification of tibia vara. (From Langenskiöld A. Tibia vara, A critical review. *Clin Orthop Relat Res* 1989;246:195, with permission.)

physiologic bowing from early Blount disease. This is measured on the anteroposterior lower extremity x-ray film by constructing a distal femoral MD angle similar to that measured in the proximal tibia. This angle represents the contribution of varus in the distal femur to the overall measure of femoral-tibial varus in the limb. The distal femoral MD angle is divided by the proximal tibial MD angle. This quotient represents the proportion of varus found in the femur relative to the tibia. A ratio of greater than one suggests the bowing is physiologic, that is the femur contributes as much as the proximal tibia to the varus, and resolution is expected

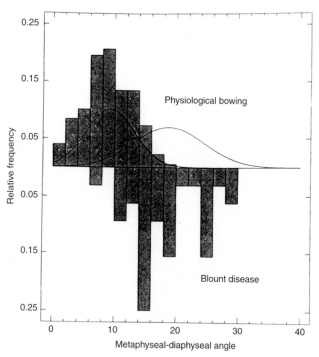

**Figure 28.10** The relative frequency of metaphyseal-diaphyseal (MD) angle measured in children with physiologic and Blount disease is presented. MD angle in physiologic bowing is graphed above the horizontal line; similar measurements in Blount disease are graphed below. The bell curve to the left shows the distribution in physiologic bowing. The bell curve to the right is the distribution in Blount disease. Although peak distributions are clearly separate, there is significant overlap between MD angles of 10 and 16 degrees. Below 10 degrees, there is a 95% probability that the bowing is physiologic. Above 16 degrees, there is a 95% probability that the bowing observed is in fact Blount disease. Angles in between are indeterminate. Additional risk factors such as obesity, instability (lateral thrust), and family history must be considered.

to occur (57). A ratio of less than one indicates that the bowing is predominantly within the tibia and is more likely to evolve into Blount disease.

Less often, physiologic bowing must also be differentiated from the pathologic bowing associated with metabolic bone disease or skeletal dysplasia (Fig. 28.8). Rickets [usually X-linked hypophosphatemic rickets (XLH)] is the most likely metabolic bone disease to present as a bowed leg deformity in a toddler (59,60). Nutritional rickets should be suspected if the child was breast-fed and did not receive supplemental vitamin D. Infants presenting with rickets are short; the measured height is often below the tenth percentile. Radiographs of infants with bowing deformity secondary to rickets should not be mistaken for physiologic bowing (53). In patients with XLH, the physis appears abnormally wide, and the metaphysis is flared and curves like a trumpet around the physis. Similar changes are found within all growth plates. Bone density will be diminished overall, including thinned diaphyseal and metaphyseal cortices. The severity of changes in bone morphology and the degree of osteomalacia is variable. The diagnosis of XLH is made by analyzing calcium and phosphate in serum and in urine (59,60). Patients suspected of having rickets should be referred to an endocrinologist for a thorough metabolic workup.

Skeletal dysplasias can present as a bowing deformity of the lower extremity. The child who presents with bowing deformity in association with a skeletal dysplasia will be short, typically below the fifth percentile. The radiographic changes for each skeletal dysplasia vary with the site of involvement, which may be principally epiphyseal, physeal, metaphyseal, or diaphyseal or may involve multiple sites and may include the spine. Achondroplasia often presents with bowing. Distinctive physical findings, including a knee-centered varus deformity with an elongated fibula, are characteristic of achondroplasia. Patients with pseudoachondroplasia may present with a varus deformity (although valgus is sometimes present) in association with ligamentous laxity. Metaphyseal chondrodysplasia (Schmid or McKusick type) typically presents with persistent bowing and short stature in an otherwise normal-appearing child (Fig. 28.8D). The radiographic changes about the physis and metaphysis are not those associated with osteomalacia, and bone density will appear normal.

Focal fibrocartilaginous dysplasia is a very uncommon, but progressive, unilateral, focal deformity that can occur either in the proximal tibial metaphysis or distal femoral metaphysis (61–66) (Fig. 28.11). The clinical presentation is similar to unilateral infantile Blount disease. The lesion consists of a focus of fibroblastic and cartilaginous tissue, usually below the insertion of the pes anserinus on the tibia. This produces an acute angulation below the metaphysis. The diagnosis is made radiographically. A characteristic indentation is noted in the medial cortex at the junction of the metaphysis and diaphysis, and a focal varus

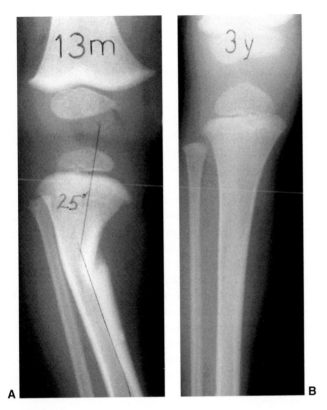

### Natural History of Physiologic Bowing

Parents should be informed that spontaneous correction of physiologic bowing is anticipated as predicted by the data of Salenius and Vankka (1,49) (Fig. 28.6). Salenius and Vankka followed the changes in frontal plane alignment of the lower extremities over time. Bowing, although present in infants, may not be noticed until the child begins weight bearing. The bowing resolves, typically by 2 years of age, and physiologic valgus develops between 3 to 4 years of age (Fig. 28.12). Nonoperative treatment (orthotic insert, shoe modification, or nighttime splinting) is ineffective. Follow-up visits may not be necessary in these physiologic, mild deformities because the bowing and its associated internal tibial torsion predictably resolve. For those with more pronounced or persistent deformities, follow-up visits are scheduled at 4- to 6-month intervals. Correction or progression of the varus that occurs with growth can be documented by subsequent physical examination. Serial photos can be compared with the initial image to determine the degree of resolution or progression of the bowing deformity. Serial radiographs should be obtained if the initial tibial MD angle was greater than 10 degrees, or if the varus does not appear improved on clinical appearance or by serial goniometric measurement. Uncommonly, physiologic varus may persist into late childhood, warranting longer follow-up and the possible need for treatment with hemiepiphyseal stapling.

## Infantile Blount Disease

### Definition

In 1937, Walter Blount (67) published his classic review of tibia vara or osteochondrosis deformans of the proximal tibia, noting the progressive course of both the clinical deformity and the correlative radiographic pathology. The distal femur is typically normal, but occasionally it will develop a valgus deformity (46,49,68). These changes

**Figure 28.11** Focal fibrocartilaginous dysplasia. **A:** Initial radiograph of a patient at 13 months of age shows anterior and lateral bowing of the tibia, but bowing is more proximal than in congenital pseudarthrosis. **B:** The deformity resolved spontaneously, as seen in a radiograph made at 3 years of age.

deformity is associated with it. The lesion is radiolucent and well circumscribed, often with a rim of reactive bone. The physis and epiphysis are normal. An identical process has also been observed in a corresponding location in the distal medial femur (66). Some authors have reported spontaneous improvement in angulation.

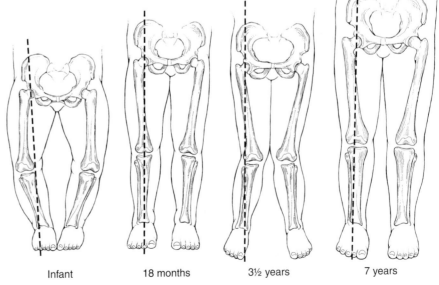

**Figure 28.12** Lower-limb alignment follows a predictable pattern. Infants typically have a gentle varus bow throughout the femur and tibia. By 18 to 24 months, the lower leg is nearly straight with a neutral mechanical axis. Valgus gradually develops and is most apparent between 3 and 4 years of age. By 7 years of age, the lower limb is in slight valgus and changes very little thereafter. Varus should not recur nor should valgus increase.

Infant          18 months          3½ years          7 years described by Blount and histopathologic changes described by Langenskiöld (47,69–71) were felt to be secondary to a disruption of normal growth of cartilage and bone caused by excessive pressure on the proximal medial tibial growth plate and adjacent bone from abnormal weight bearing. Avascular necrosis of bone in Blount disease has not been observed (71). Progression of this developmental, pathologic tibia vara can be corrected with treatment (67,70,72–74).

### Etiology

Like physiologic bowing, infantile Blount disease is usually bilateral (46,48,52). Infants with physiologic bowleg deformity cannot be clearly distinguished from those with infantile Blount disease (46,48,52,55,75–78). Physiologic bowing is a continuum with Blount disease. When unilateral infantile Blount disease is noted, often the contralateral extremity is bowed physiologically, and this can be indistinguishable from early infantile Blount disease (Fig. 28.13A,B). These children typically are early walkers and often are overweight. As with physiologic bowing, there may be a family history of bowing deformity, (46–48,50,51,53,55,67,69,79–81).

Cook et al. (82), using finite element analysis, calculated that the compressive force resultant from weight-bearing stresses on a bowed leg were sufficient to cause growth disturbance. Obesity increases the potential for growth-plate injury. In some extremities, the bowing resolves through remodelling (46,50), but in others, the focal pathologic changes in the proximal medial tibia growth plate cause clinical varus to progress (Blount disease). The chronic growth disturbance results in the osteochondrosis of the medial proximal tibial physis and adjacent epiphysis and metaphysis as described by Blount (46,52,55,67,77,80,81). Inevitably, the proximal medial tibia fails to grow normally, and tibia vara of variable severity develops. This results in extremity shortening and intraarticular depression of the medial tibial condyle.

### Pathoanatomy and Radiographic Features

In 1952, Langenskiöld identified six distinct radiographic stages of development of the proximal tibia depicting the natural progression of untreated infantile Blount disease (69) (Fig. 28.9). The stage and the age at which it occurs has prognostic significance (50,52,53,69,71). In stages I and II, the irregular metaphyseal ossification changes are often indistinguishable from physiologic bowing. These changes may be reversible. Clear-cut stage I or stage II changes of Blount disease are typically not apparent until the patient is 2 to 2$\frac{1}{2}$ years of age. Stage III shows definite deformity in the proximal tibial physis, often with some fragmentation. Stage IV lesions can be associated with early bar formation across the deformed physis, as it assumes a vertical orientation (50,53). These physeal bars are often difficult to detect.

There is profound disruption of the physeal cartilage and abnormal growth in the adjacent bone as stage V develops, usually in children older than 8 years. Eventually this process results in severe depression of the articular surface and stage VI disease (47).

In North America, advanced stages often occur at a much younger age than Langenskiöld reported. All of Langenskiöld's patients were whites from Finland, whereas in the United States, a high proportion of patients with infantile Blount disease are African American. The greater severity of disease may also be attributed to a higher proportion of overweight children in North America. These children tend to show more rapid progression with more severe, irreversible changes at an earlier age than their European counterparts. Stage IV changes are seen in 4- to 5-year-old children in the United States compared to 7- to 8-year-old children in Finland.

The distal femur in infantile Blount disease is usually normal. Although distal femoral varus does not occur in infantile Blount disease, valgus does occur in some children with more advanced tibial changes. It may be a response to the asymmetric load across the knee, allowing relative overgrowth of the distal medial femur (46,68,77,83).

### Nonoperative Treatment

Brace treatment should be considered in all patients less than 2$\frac{1}{2}$ years of age with early Blount disease changes (Langenskiöld stages I, II) and in patients older than 2 years who have persistent bowing and risk factors for Blount disease. A tibial MD angle of greater than 16 degrees is a radiographic sign of significant risk for Blount disease (50,53,56). A sign of relative risk is an MD angle between 10 and 16 degrees along with the clinical appearance of a varus deformity or progression of varus. Additional risk factors include obesity, ligamentous instability, or the presence of a lateral thrust, any of which may potentiate a varus deformity (53,56). Improvement in the tibial MD angle should be apparent within 12 months of brace treatment.

Recent studies have demonstrated that brace treatment can correct both the varus deformity and the pathologic proximal-medial tibial growth disturbance (72–74). In three studies that were reported, 79 extremities were treated using a brace. The best results were obtained with unilateral deformity, where brace treatment was successful in 22 of 23 patients. In contrast, brace treatment was less successful for treating bilateral deformities, with only 18 of 28 patients noted to be successfully treated. Compliance was much more difficult to achieve for the child with bilateral deformity, as is understandable. It is also less effective in obese patients. Bracing should not be initiated after 3 years of age, nor should brace treatment be continued if Langenskiöld stage III changes develop (72–74).

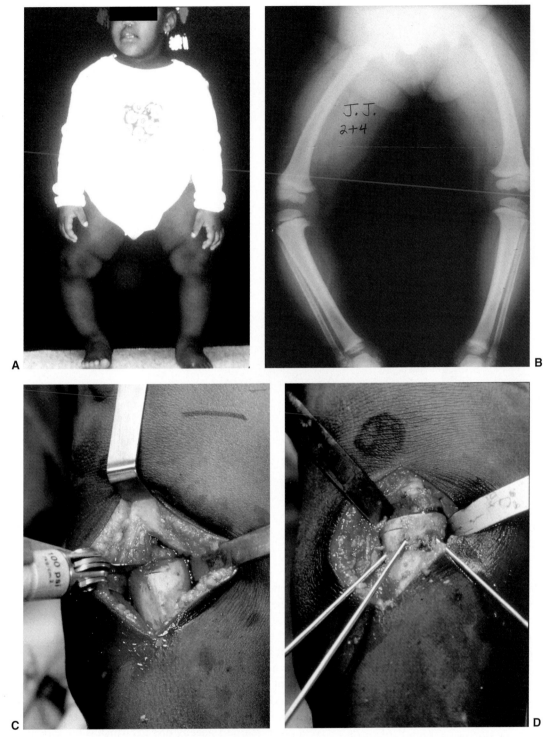

**Figure 28.13** **A:** This 30-month-old girl shows clinically asymmetric bowing. She is large for her age ( >95% weight). **B:** The metaphyseal-diaphyseal (MD) angle on the right is 20 degrees, compared to 10 degrees on the left. This is consistent with stage II changes of Blount disease on the right and physiologic bowing on the left. **C:** A transverse osteotomy is performed distal to the tibial apophysis. An appropriately sized wedge is removed to allow slight overcorrection. **D:** Smooth Kirschner (K) wires are used for fixation, supplemented with cast immobilization. **E:** Clinical alignment can be assessed using a bovie cord, which is visualized radiographically. The leg should be allowed to rest in its neutral position. **F:** Intraoperative films of a right proximal tibial osteotomy show slight overcorrection to valgus. A bovie cord centered over the hip and ankle is an easy method to assess mechanical axis intraoperatively. **G:** A clinical photo taken 2 years later shows maintenance of correction on the right. Spontaneous correction of physiologic bowing has occurred on the left.

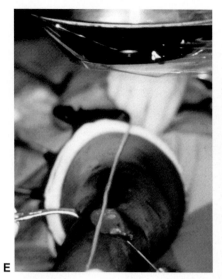

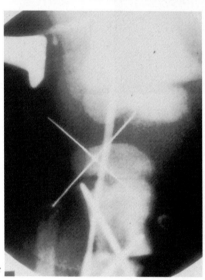

E

F

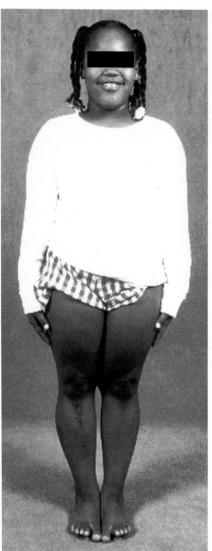

G    **Figure 28.13** (continued)

We have used a modified knee-ankle-foot orthosis (KAFO) that prevents knee flexion. It is worn for 23 of 24 hours (52,56,84) (Fig. 28.14). The locked KAFO counteracts the pathologic medial compressive forces, allowing resumption of more normal growth and correction of the genu varum. The bowleg deformity typically improves over the ensuing months. The pathologic radiographic changes at the proximal medial tibial metaphysis, physis, and epiphysis are slow to remodel. Brace treatment is continued until the bony changes in the proximal medial tibia resolve; typically, this takes $1\frac{1}{2}$ to 2 years of brace treatment (72–74). Sustained, successful correction with nonoperative treatment requires that correction be achieved before 4 years of age. Appropriate alignment means that the mechanical axis of the lower extremity passes through the center of the knee (28,48–50,53).

### Operative Treatment

Children older than 3 years with Blount disease, who are either noncompliant or not good candidates for brace treatment because of obesity or bilateral involvement, should be treated with a varus-correcting osteotomy (50,72). The proximal tibial varus should decrease within 12 months in those children who are compliant with bracing. The radiographic appearance of the medial epiphysis and metaphysis should normalize by 5 years of age. If such improvement does not occur, varus-correcting osteotomy should be recommended. Early surgery to realign the leg (that is, osteotomy performed by 4 years of age) is necessary to prevent progression to stage IV disease, which is the formation of a physeal bar. The osteotomy unloads the medial compartment of the knee and facilitates growth of the proximal medial physis. Restoration of normal growth in the medial tibial physis is less likely to occur if surgery is delayed (50,52,53,71,76) (Fig. 28.13A,B). Simple osteotomy after 5 years of age does not assure permanent correction and carries a higher risk of recurrent deformity because of the greater pathologic change and potential for physeal bar formation.

The proximal tibia osteotomy is performed with attention to the risks related to osteotomy in the upper tibia and the need for obtaining adequate correction of the

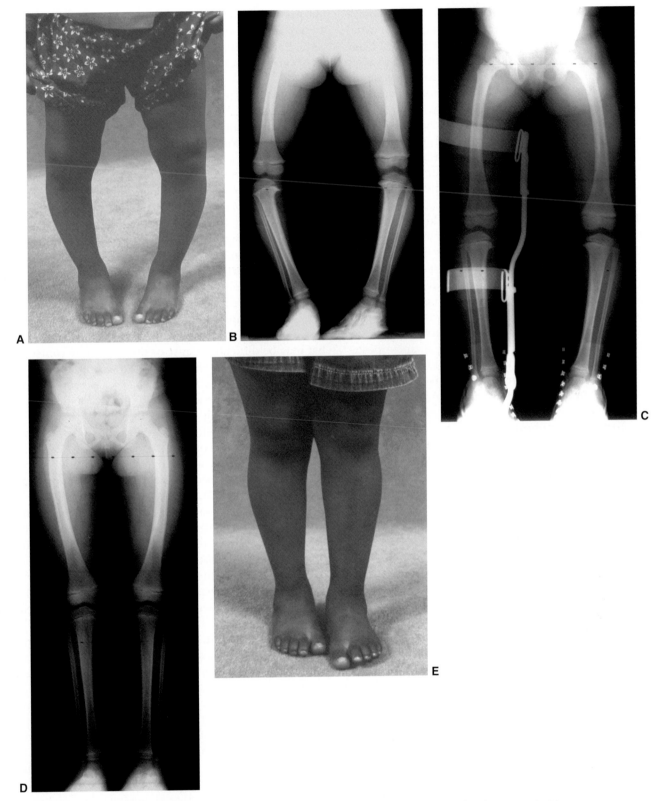

**Figure 28.14** Orthotic treatment of Blount disease. **A:** This 2-year-old girl presented with asymmetric bowing. **B:** Lower limb radiographs show an increased metaphyseal-diaphyseal (MD) angle with changes of stage II Blount disease. **C:** A locked knee-ankle-foot orthosis (KAFO) was worn full time. **D:** Radiographic appearance improved following 18 months of orthotic use. **E:** Clinical appearance at 4 years of age.

deformity (50,53,85,86). The fibula is osteotomized through a separate lateral incision, taking care to avoid injury to the deep motor branches of the peroneal nerve (37). The tibial osteotomy can be accomplished in a variety of ways (50,53,71,87–90). A straight transverse osteotomy optimally allows for necessary adjustment in correction of frontal, sagittal, and rotational deformity. The fragments are stabilized with smooth K-wires (Fig. 28.13C,D). Alternatively, Price et al. (91) have effectively utilized monolateral external fixation to stabilize the tibial osteotomy. A slight "overcorrection" into valgus with or without translation of the distal fragment laterally is desirable (50,52,53,92). This places the mechanical axis of the leg within the lateral compartment of the knee, optimally unloading the medial proximal tibia. The mechanical axis of the leg can be assessed intraoperatively using the bovie cord. The cord is stretched from the center of the hip and across the center of the ankle with the leg resting on a radiolucent table. The leg should not be held, but simply allowed to rest on the table. The wire within the bovie cord, which is visible on the C-arm, is used to verify the position of the mechanical axis by taking an anteroposterior spot radiograph of the knee (Fig. 28.13E,F). This simple technique provides a reproducible method to verify that the mechanical axis has actually been transferred lateral to the center of the knee joint (91). Alternatively, an intraoperative anteroposterior x-ray film of the entire lower extremity can be taken to assess the correction obtained. If a unilateral deformity is present, clinical comparison to the normal extremity is helpful in determining whether adequate correction has been obtained. A subcutaneous fasciotomy of the anterior compartment is performed prior to wound closure. Suction drains are also routinely used.

Postoperatively, the extremity is immobilized in a non–weight-bearing long-leg, bent-knee cast. Alternatively, a spica cast is used for the child with relatively short, fat extremities. On occasion, a KAFO is used following cast removal if the preoperative deformity was severe and associated with ligamentous laxity. Following corrective osteotomy, the pathologic changes in the proximal medial tibia must be carefully monitored. These bony changes are not always reversible, and further progression in their development may be associated with a recurrence of deformity (47,50,53). It is essential to document that valgus alignment has been obtained and maintained by using long cassette radiographs and comparing serial examinations until skeletal maturity (Fig. 28.13G).

*Complications.* Neurovascular complications are risks associated with a proximal tibia osteotomy (37,52,85, 93–96). A careful subperiosteal exposure minimizes direct nerve and vessel trauma. Prophylactic limited fasciotomy and the use of drains help prevent increased compartment pressure (37,52,53). If a compartment syndrome is suspected postoperatively, immediate fasciotomy should be performed. On the basis of our recent clinical experience, an acute traction or impingement injury to the peroneal nerve may also occur (37). Prompt surgical release of any peroneal nerve compression has typically resulted in a satisfactory outcome.

### Worsening Varus Deformity and Physeal Bar Formation

The risk for recurrent deformity is greater in black females, children with Langenskiöld stage III or stage IV disease, marked obesity ( >95th percentile weight), or ligamentous laxity (50,52,53,76) (Fig. 28.15). Worsening varus deformity or persistent pathologic radiographic changes can occur despite restorative osteotomy performed prior to 4 or 5 years of age (52,53,76). Advanced changes in Langenskiöld stage IV or V can occur even in these young patients, independent of race or body habitus. If patients present with advanced pathologic changes or with recurrent deformity following brace or surgical treatment, MRI, CT scan, or conventional tomography should be utilized to search for the presence of a physeal bar within the distorted proximal medial tibia anatomy. Identification of a bar may be difficult because of the serpentine course of this abnormal physis, which takes on a vertical slope as the deformity worsens. Early bridging across the physis typically occurs at the inferior aspect of the vertical limb of the distorted medial physis (Fig. 28.15B).

Worsening varus deformity may occur without an obvious bony bar (Langenskiöld III or early IV) (50). This occurs rather subtly because of a relatively decreased growth rate of the proximal medial tibial physis and can occur any time prior to skeletal maturity. Careful observation is needed to detect this change early in the course of treatment. Children need regular follow-up until skeletal maturity. Premature closure of the medial tibial physis frequently occurs because of persistent abnormal growth in the medial physis. If this occurs, the varus deformity can be controlled with temporary hemiepiphyseal stapling (50,97,98). The staples are removed after a slight overcorrection is obtained.

*Operative Treatment.* If an osseous bar is identified, appropriate restorative surgery is indicated. Left untreated, progression of bar formation will result in complete arrest of the medial physis (Langenskiöld stage VI). Physeal bar resection in conjunction with a varus-correcting osteotomy will be most effective if the patient is younger than 10 years, the bar is relatively small, and the patient is not excessively overweight (50,53,71,76,99–101).

The proximal tibia is approached through an anteromedial longitudinal incision and the physeal bar is resected first. Often the bar is not discreet, but is a collection of several small punctate foci of bone that coalesce and function as a tether. The medial edge of the normal physis is often difficult to locate. Excision of the bony bridge is done cautiously, preserving as much normal physeal tissue as possible. However, resection must be complete so that an intact physeal line coursing 180 degrees from the posteromedial

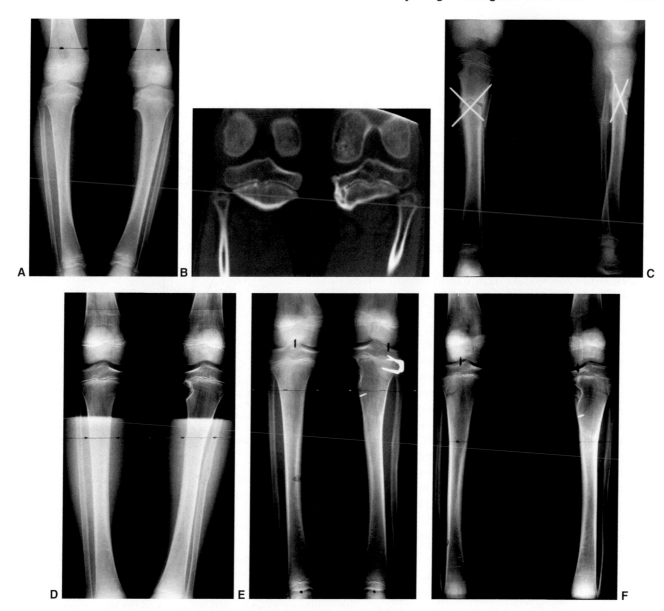

**Figure 28.15**   **A:** These anteroposterior radiographs show focal changes of unilateral stage IV Blount disease. The medial tibial physis is indistinct. These changes are suggestive of physeal bar formation. **B:** A computed tomography (CT) scan shows the deformity in the medial physis. The growth plate has a vertical rather than horizontal orientation. A bridge of bone is clearly evident here. Varus will rapidly recur following osteotomy if the physeal bar is not recognized and treated. **C:** These postoperative films show correction of the varus and resection of the bar. The defect created by excision is filled with radiolucent methylmethacrylate (Cranioplast). **D:** Subsequent films show recurrent bar formation with gradual loss of correction over 2 years. **E:** A second excision of the physeal bar along with lateral physeal stapling has resulted in improved alignment. **F:** Following removal of the staples, varus has gradually recurred. The abnormal medial physis tends to close prematurely.

to the anteromedial cortical edge of the tibia is defined. The C-arm can be helpful in monitoring the procedure. Methylmethacrylate (Cranioplast) is used to fill the void to inhibit formation of another osseous tether. Varus-correcting osteotomies of the tibia and fibula are then performed (Fig. 28.15C). Alternatively, a temporary lateral hemiepiphyseal staple can be used in conjunction with the medial epiphysiolysis. This is most applicable if the varus deformity is mild, the patient is not obese, and there is no lateral thrust of the knee.

Most patients experience resumption of medial physeal growth, but to varying degrees (99,102). Continued normal growth in the medial physis generally does not equal growth of the lateral physis. There is a risk of retethering or premature medial physeal closure. A second bar resection and varus corrective osteotomy can be performed for small recurrent bars in younger patients (Fig. 28.15D). If lateral hemiepiphyseal stapling has been done, the patient requires close follow-up for the appropriate timing of staple removal (Fig. 28.15E and F).

For relatively large osseous bars or recurrent deformity in obese or older patients, a permanent lateral epiphysiodesis of the tibia and fibula is indicated, and is performed in conjunction with osteotomies to correct depression of the medial plateau and any residual varus, as described in the next section (50,53,71,76). A potential for leg-length inequality exists with any of the above approaches. If anticipated, it often can be corrected with an appropriately timed contralateral epiphysiodesis or with lengthening of the tibia.

### Severe Varus Deformity with Medial Joint Depression

Patients with Langenskiöld stage V or VI deformity have irreversible changes in the medial tibial physis. The architecture of the proximal tibia is distorted, including the medial tibial condylar surface (Fig. 28.16). Typically, they are seen in children older than 10 years, yet these changes may be seen as in patients as young as 6 years. The proximal tibial varus deformity is characterized by severe depression of the medial tibial plateau, often with ligamentous laxity. Compensatory distal femoral valgus deformity may develop (68,83,90). In severe cases, the tibia will be subluxed medially on the femur. Left untreated, degenerative arthritis is likely to occur early in life (103,104). For a lasting satisfactory outcome, the surgical goal is to correct both the abnormal limb alignment and the pathologic depression of the medial tibial plateau (Fig. 28.17). This deformity occurs because the medial physis is closed or so extensively involved that epiphysiolysis, as in stage IV disease, will not restore proximal tibial growth (71).

***Operative Treatment.*** The preferred approach to correct this complex deformity is a combination of medial tibial plateau elevation and realignment osteotomy of the proximal tibia (Fig. 28.18A,B). If significant distal femoral valgus is present, osteotomy of the distal femur is performed

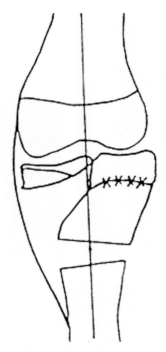

**Figure 28.17** Restoration of normal limb alignment requires complex reconstruction. An arcuate osteotomy is performed to restore the tibial condyle to its normal position. A proximal lateral hemiepiphysiodesis is performed to prevent recurrent deformity because the medial physis is no longer functional. A valgus osteotomy of the proximal tibia is also usually needed to restore a normal mechanical axis and orientation of the proximal tibia.

as well (47,68,71,92,105–107). The proximal medial tibia should not be approached subperiosteally. Rather, soft-tissue attachments to the proximal medial tibia need to be preserved to minimize devascularization of the medial tibial condyle following the plateau-elevating osteotomy. A medial parapatellar arthrotomy is usually performed to visualize the articular surface of the tibia. The posterior neurovascular structures are at risk and are protected by placing a curved retractor between the neurovascular structures and the tibia. A drill bit or osteotomes are used to complete the curved osteotomy (Fig. 28.18C). The osteotomy is begun distally, starting at the apex of angulation in the proximal medial metaphysis, and curves proximally toward the tibial eminence. Intraoperative radiography or fluoroscopy is used to assure that the plane of the osteotomy is directed superolaterally in order to bisect the tibia intercondylar eminence. The depressed tibial condyle must be sufficiently elevated to restore the articular surface. A smooth laminar spreader is helpful in maintaining elevation of the medial tibial plateau while the bone grafting and internal fixation is completed. Autogenous graft is preferred. A segment of fibula obtained at the time of fibular osteotomy or adjacent tibial cortex can be used. Alternatively, a cortical iliac crest graft may be used. Fixation may be difficult. The elevated fragment is small, and fixation must not disturb the articular cartilage (Fig. 28.18D). The correction obtained following plateau elevation typically restores the tibial condylar angle to a near normal value

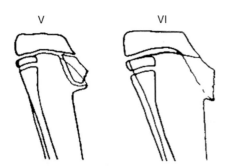

**Figure 28.16** Stage V and stage VI Blount disease are complicated by depression of the medial tibial condyle. The physis has a vertical orientation. This marked growth disturbance is the result of physeal bar formation seen at the junction of the normal horizontal physis and the depressed medial plateau. Insufficient normal physis remains for growth of the medial physis to be restored by resection of these large physeal bars.

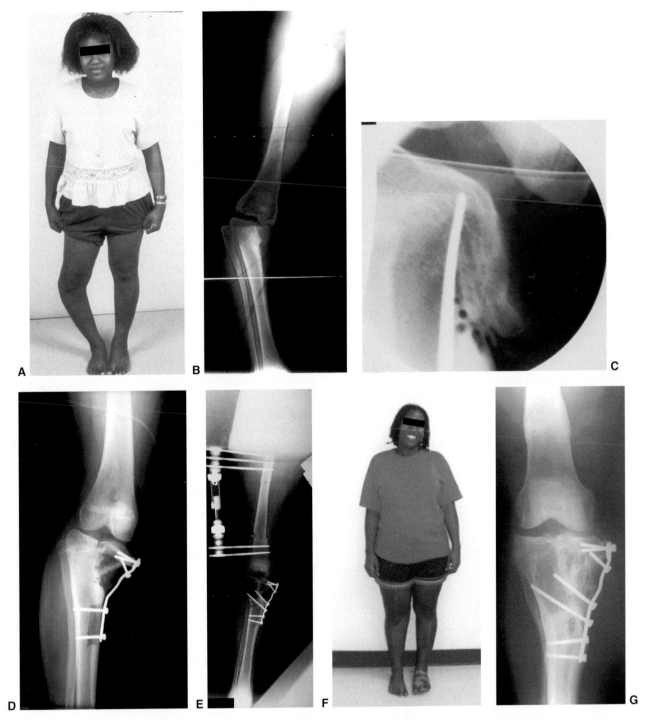

**Figure 28.18** Treatment of stage V Blount disease. **A:** Severe deformity and a lateral thrust are noted clinically. **B:** Blount disease that progresses to physeal bar formation results in severe depression of the medial metaphysis. Valgus may develop in the distal femur because of overgrowth of the medial femoral condyle. Restoration of medial physeal growth is not possible. **C:** Image intensification is useful to control the direction of the medial elevation osteotomy. The cut begins at the apex of deformity in the medial cortex and is completed between the tibial spines. **D:** A cortical strut is used to support the elevated plateau. **E:** Osteotomy of the tibia or femur, or both, is performed to correct residual tibial varus or femoral valgus. **F:** Normal anatomic and mechanical alignment can be achieved with this approach. Residual limb-length inequality can be managed by contralateral epiphysiodesis if needed. **G:** Radiographic appearance after healing of the osteotomies shows restoration of joint orientation and mechanical alignment.

(105). A concomitant epiphysiodesis of the lateral proximal tibia and proximal fibula is always done because there is no growth potential remaining in the medial physis.

Tibial plateau elevation alone will produce a marked correction of the preoperative varus deformity. However, correction may be incomplete, and a proximal tibial varus-correcting osteotomy is often needed to restore normal alignment to the tibia. Occasionally a distal femoral osteotomy may also be required to correct valgus deformity. Alternatively, a hemiepiphyseal stapling of the distal lateral femur can be used for gradual correction. The surgical goal of this comprehensive approach is correction of all components of the deformity, including medial tibial plateau depression, asymmetric proximal tibial growth, varus of the tibia, and valgus of the distal femur (Fig. 28.18E). By addressing all aspects of the deformity, both joint orientation (relation of the knee and the ankle) and alignment of the extremity (mechanical axis of the limb bisects the center of the knee joint) can be normalized (Fig. 28.18F,G).

After correction of the angular deformity, significant limb-length inequality may remain. This may be managed by epiphysiodesis of the contralateral limb, or in the case of a more severe discrepancy, a combination of lengthening and shortening may be required to equalize limb length. Davidson (92) has utilized a circular external fixator to stabilize the elevated plateau fragment and perform a gradual correcting osteotomy of the proximal tibia. Use of the external fixator provides the option of lengthening, in addition to deformity correction of the proximal tibia.

*Complications.* Extensive soft-tissue and bony dissection is necessary to concomitantly elevate the medial tibial plateau and perform a varus-correcting proximal tibial osteotomy. The medial proximal tibia is more prominent and elongated following the plateau elevation. Wound closure may be compromised and needs to be performed as a delayed closure. In a series by Schoenecker et al. (105), 3 of 22 patients treated by this comprehensive approach experienced wound healing complications. In two patients, eventual wound healing occurred with local care, and one required operative repair with subsequent satisfactory secondary wound healing.

The extensive soft-tissue and bony dissection necessary to perform a tibial plateau elevation also increases the risk of avascular necrosis of the medial tibial condyle. This occurred in 1 of 22 tibial plateau elevations. Satisfactory revascularization and reossification occurred in this morbidly obese 8-year-old child following a 1-year period of non–weight bearing.

## Late-Onset Juvenile and Adolescent Blount Disease

### Definition

Blount (67) identified a second group of patients who developed varus deformity of the tibia in later childhood or early adolescence. He described this deformity as adolescent tibia vara (Fig. 28.19). Typically, these children present for evaluation of bowlegged deformity that develops later in childhood. They are usually overweight, sometimes morbidly so (108–111). The varus deformity in this group of patients with late-onset or adolescent Blount disease typically involves both the proximal medial tibia and the distal femur. In contrast, children with deformity from persistent early–onset or

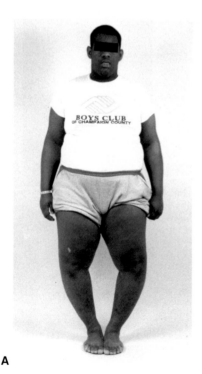
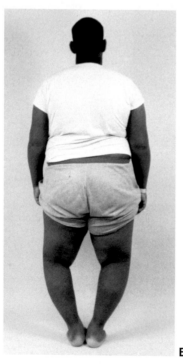

**A**    **B**

**Figure 28.19** A 13-year-old boy with adolescent Blount disease. As is often seen in this group of patients, he is morbidly obese. The large thigh circumference in such patients contributes to the deformity and increased load across the medial distal femur and proximal tibia.

infantile Blount disease have varus of the proximal tibia only. There should be no confusion in differentiating patients who present as adolescents with Blount-like changes from those who have had varus deformity since infancy. Patients in this latter group will typically have advanced pathologic changes involving the proximal medial tibia by later childhood. Children with infantile Blount disease develop advanced pathologic changes in the proximal medial tibia, as described by Langenskiöld, whereas those with juvenile or adolescent Blount disease develop varus without medial joint depression. Distal femoral deformity is also more common in these older children (68).

### Etiology

Classically, adolescent Blount disease occurs in obese patients with characteristically wide thighs; however, there are exceptions (77,78,108–110,112). Obesity potentiates the occurrence of adolescent Blount disease because of the increased load across the medial compartment of the knee (108,109,112,113). The varus develops after 9 to 10 years of age and often involves both the proximal tibia and distal femur. Increased thigh circumference makes it difficult for these children to keep their center of mass over the weight-bearing foot during the single stance phase of gait. Their extreme weight adds to an already increased load on the medial knee joint and promotes development of the varus deformity.

Adolescent tibia vara and SCFE occur in association with each other (110,114,115). Davids et al. (108) examined the gait deviations that compensate for the increased thigh girth associated with obesity. During ambulation, individuals tend to minimize the horizontal displacement of their center of mass by positioning the foot during single leg stance as centrally as possible along the line of progression. This optimizes energy expenditure during normal gait. An obese individual, with large thighs, has difficulty adducting the hip adequately in order to allow placement of the foot along the line of progression. Davids speculated that this "fat thigh syndrome" produces a varus moment on the knee that leads to increased pressure on the medial proximal tibial physis and inhibits growth in accordance with the Hueter-Volkmann principle (77). This work supports the observation that preexisting varus of the knee is not necessary to initiate the pathologic mechanical changes that result in adolescent tibia vara. The incidence of adolescent Blount disease has markedly increased in the past 20 years corresponding to the development of earlier and more severe adolescent obesity (109,116).

A second, smaller group of patients present with genu varus. They are older than those with infantile Blount disease and generally are not morbidly obese. In retrospect, these are children with mild bowing that never resolved. They do not develop the pathologic changes seen in infantile Blount disease. The varus deformity in these children becomes more apparent during the rapid growth of early adolescence (108–111).

### Pathoanatomy

An affected growth plate will have histologic aberrations throughout the entire physis; however, the medial physis is more affected than the lateral physis (110). The histologic changes are very similar to those found in infantile Blount disease and SCFE (110,111). In adolescent Blount disease, the radiographic changes in the epiphysis and metaphysis are less apparent compared to infantile Blount disease, because the secondary ossification center is larger and better established in these older patients (92,93).

The growth inhibition present in the proximal tibia affects the posteromedial physis and initially produces varus, followed by progressive procurvation of the proximal tibia (50,83,110). Although the name adolescent tibia vara would suggest that varus of the proximal tibia is the only deformity present, distal femoral varus deformity is common, because that physis can also undergo excessive loading (83,110,116) (Fig. 28.20A–C). This is in contradistinction to infantile tibia vara in which the distal femur is either normal or in valgus. The in-toeing noted in adolescent Blount disease is generally less severe than it is in infantile tibia vara. The combination of varus, procurvatum, and internal rotation results in a complex three-dimensional deformity of the proximal tibia. As the proximal tibial and distal femoral varus deformities increase, there is a significant strain placed on the lateral collateral ligament of the knee, which leads to laxity and varus deformity within the knee joint. In some very severe cases, compensatory distal tibial valgus develops to allow the patient to place the foot flat on the floor (Fig. 28.20D). Although the natural progression of advanced infantile Blount disease is the formation of a medial proximal tibial physeal bar, discreet physeal bar formation is not noted in adolescent Blount disease. However, early closure of all lower extremity physes can occur, perhaps because of overload related to obesity.

### Clinical Features

The typical patient with adolescent tibia vara is an obese male who presents with complaints of bowing, often with knee pain and/or instability (109,110,112,117,118). The patient should be assessed while walking both toward and away from the examiner, who should note gait mechanics and, specifically, the presence of a limp or lateral thrust to one or both knees. Although unilateral complaints are more common, attention should be paid to both limbs because the patient's obesity can mask mild bowing on the contralateral limb (108,112,117). Knee stability is assessed because lateral collateral ligament laxity can occur. Proximal tibia procurvatum deformity may occur, producing a relative knee flexion deformity. The patient may have anterior knee pain secondary to holding the knee in a flexed position during gait. Patients complain of medial knee pain secondary to medial knee joint stress. The hips should also be examined for evidence of SCFE (110,114,115). Morbidly obese patients presenting with adolescent Blount disease may have varying amounts of respiratory distress. The walk

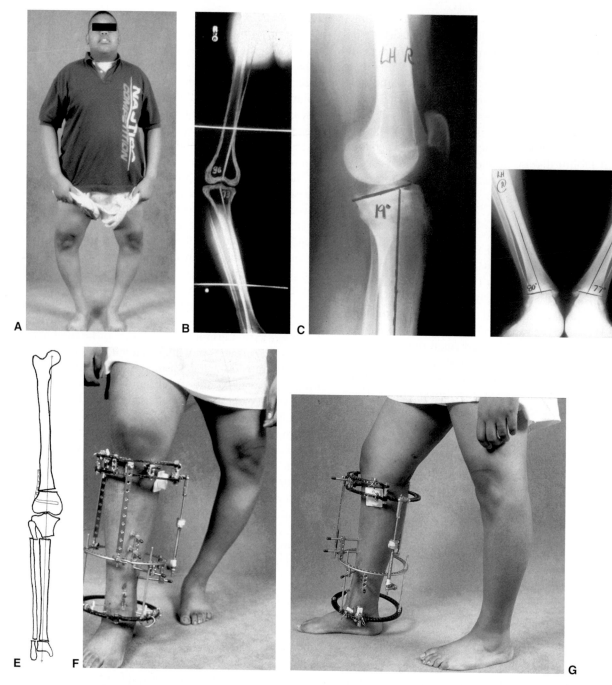

**Figure 28.20**   **A:** Adolescent Blount disease frequently occurs in very large teenagers. The deformity is often bilateral. **B:** Long cassette films are used to assess mechanical alignment as well as the anatomic axes of the femur and tibia. Distal femoral deformity is often present as well as proximal tibial varus. **C:** Procurvatum of the proximal tibia develops, with increased posterior slope of the proximal tibia. **D:** Distal tibial valgus develops to allow the foot to have flat contact with the floor. **E:** Restoration of normal alignment may include multilevel osteotomies. Preoperative templates are useful for planning operative strategies. **F:** In this example, the plan included immediate correction of distal femoral varus using a blade plate and gradual correction of proximal tibial varus and distal tibial valgus using a circular small wire frame. **G:** Multiplane correction is facilitated with this technique. Adjustments can also be made to correct the procurvatum that may be present. **H:** The circular frame provides flexibility. It also allows lengthening as needed in cases of unilateral or asymmetric deformity. **I:** Radiographs confirm the restoration of alignment. Correction is generally well maintained. **J:** Clinical photo after bilateral treatment shows satisfactory clinical correction compared to the preoperative photo. **K:** Correction of procurvatum restores normal orientation of the knee.

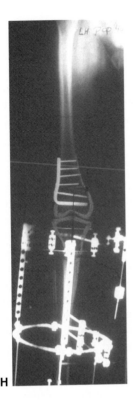
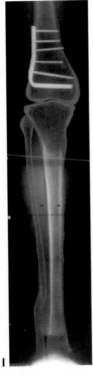
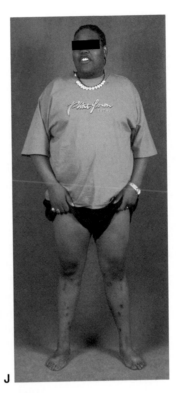
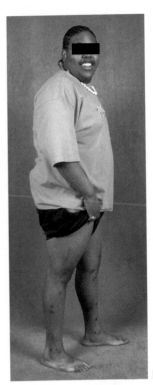

H          I          J          K

**Figure 28.20** (continued)

from the waiting room to the examination area can be quite taxing to these patients. Sleep disorders related to apnea are also common.

### Radiographic Features

A standing long cassette radiograph of both lower extremities is essential for evaluating the patient with adolescent tibia vara (Fig. 28.20B). Most adolescent patients require a 51-in (129.5 cm) cassette. Simultaneous satisfactory visualization of the hips through an abundance of soft tissue as well as the ankles through a relative paucity of soft tissue can be difficult. Care should be taken when positioning the patient to ensure that the knees are straight ahead with the patella centered. This is particularly difficult in large patients in whom the palpation of bony landmarks is uncertain. Radiology technicians who are not experienced in obtaining these radiographs frequently compensate for the inability to identify the patella by simply turning the feet straight ahead. Because of the internal tibial torsion, this produces external rotation of the knees and an inadequate radiograph for accurate assessment of bony deformity. Occasionally, because of the width of the patient or the patient's inability to sufficiently rotate the hip internally, it may be necessary to obtain separate standing radiographs of each lower extremity. A true lateral supine radiograph of the proximal tibia is obtained to evaluate the magnitude of the procurvatum deformity. The radiograph should be centered on the knee and the film positioned so that a significant portion of the tibial diaphysis can be visualized. Finally, with the feet positioned straight ahead, a standing anteroposterior radiograph of both ankles is obtained.

The radiographs should be assessed according to the method described by Paley and Tetsworth (28,119,120). Initially, the mechanical axis deviation should be measured using a line drawn from the center of the femoral head to the center of the ankle (Fig. 28.21). The surgeon should also look for a limb-length discrepancy at this point. Both the lateral distal femoral angle and the medial proximal tibial angle should be measured to evaluate the frontal plane deformity of both the distal femur and the proximal tibia. It is incorrect to assume that the distal femur is normal because the knee joint appears to be parallel to the floor (28,68). The genu varum produces relative abduction at the hip and can mask a significant femoral deformity. The radiograph of the knee in the weight-bearing position must be examined to assess the presence of significant lateral collateral laxity and an increased joint line congruency angle (the angle formed by an intersect of two lines, one drawn parallel to the distal articular surface of the femur and one parallel to the proximal articular surface of the tibia). Likewise, the lateral view of the knee should be evaluated to assess the size and location of the procurvatum deformity (Fig. 28.20C). The presence of compensatory distal tibial valgus is assessed on the anteroposterior ankle film (28,68,121)

### Operative Treatment Goals

The problems that must be addressed are varus deformity of the proximal tibia and distal femur and, occasionally, a secondary valgus deformity of the distal tibia. The goal of surgery is to restore normal anatomical orientation of the knee and ankle joint and a normal mechanical axis of the

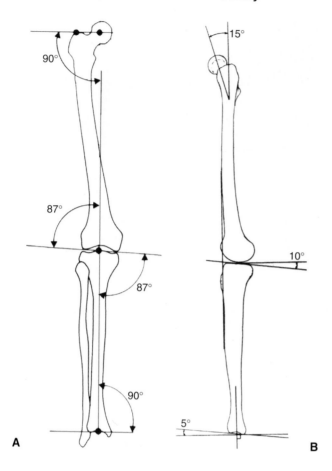

**Figure 28.21   A:** Frontal plane mechanical axis of the lower extremity consists of two components: colinear centers of the femoral head, knee joint, and ankle joint; and an almost perpendicular relation of the hip, knee, and ankle joints' orientation lines to the mechanical axis. **B:** Normal sagittal plane mechanical axis and joint orientation lines.

leg (91,95,112,116,117,119–121). For a unilateral deformity, leg-length inequality also needs to be addressed. Osteotomy is the definitive treatment of adolescent Blount disease. However, depending on the patient's age, limb realignment can be attained on occasion by staple hemiepiphysiodesis or, more likely, by a combination of hemiepiphysiodesis and osteotomy.

**Preoperative Evaluation.** Prior to proceeding with operative intervention, an appropriate, detailed, preoperative plan is essential to the hope of obtaining a mechanically well-aligned limb (Fig. 28.20E). The magnitude and location of the various bony deformities, the presence of soft-tissue laxity at the lateral collateral ligament, and the presence of joint contractures and leg-length discrepancy should all be assessed and incorporated into an overall plan for addressing the deformity.

Because these patients are often obese or morbidly obese, a thorough evaluation of their cardiopulmonary system is essential prior to any consideration of operative treatment. The extreme size of these patients can lead to

nocturnal hypoxia with significant decreases in sleeping $O_2$ levels and accompanying hypercarbia (122). If these changes are prolonged, significant pulmonary hypertension can result, leading to right-heart hypertrophy (122). If symptoms such as marked snoring or irregular breathing patterns at night are present, sleep studies with pulmonary and cardiology evaluations may be indicated prior to a general anesthesia.

**Hemiepiphysiodesis.** Hemiepiphysiodesis by any of several techniques is indicated if the growth plates are still open and the varus deformity is not too severe (69,117,123) (Fig. 28.22A,B). Staple hemiepiphysiodesis is preferred. Two to three "Blount staples" (Zimmer, Inc., Warsaw, IN, USA) with reinforced corners are placed extraperiosteally at the lateral distal femoral physis, the lateral proximal tibial physis, or the medial distal tibial physis depending on the site of deformity (50,97). Once hemiepiphyseal stapling is performed, it is critical to follow up the patients closely with clinical and radiographic examinations to monitor the correction obtained and possible staple displacement and/or breakage. If complete deformity correction is obtained, staple removal may be necessary to prevent overcorrection. Relative rebound varus growth is unpredictable in this clinical setting (97). Complete epiphyseodesis may be preferred to avoid loss of correction by rebound. Hemiepiphyseal stapling has resulted in reduction of deformity or arrest of progression of the proximal tibial or distal femoral deformities in some of the patients who had at least 15 to 18 months of growth remaining. This simple technique may obviate the need for subsequent femoral and sometimes tibial varus-correcting osteotomy (Fig. 28.22C,D). The adolescent who may not be a good candidate for staple hemiepiphysiodesis is one with a history of progressive varus deformity and knee joint pain. A dynamic lateral thrust is usually present in the patients who have knee joint laxity. Hemiepiphyseal stapling does not allow rapid enough resolution of the bony deformity or correction of the ligamentous laxity that is present.

**Osteotomy.** Most patients with moderate to severe adolescent Blount disease will require an osteotomy of the proximal tibia, and sometimes the distal femur as well, to achieve restoration of a normal mechanical axis and joint orientation. In skeletally mature or nearly mature patients, osteotomy is indicated if the mechanical axis of the lower extremity is deviated medially to the center third of the knee joint. The extent of deformity in both the proximal tibia medial angle (PTMA) and distal femur lateral angle (DFLA) is determined (28,124). In addition, the sagittal plane alignment is assessed and procurvatum deformity noted. All patients will require a proximal tibial varus-correcting osteotomy, ideally restoring a normal anatomical alignment of the proximal tibia. Regardless of the method chosen, the proximal tibial deformity should be completely corrected by the redirectional osteotomy including varus, procurvatum, and internal rotation.

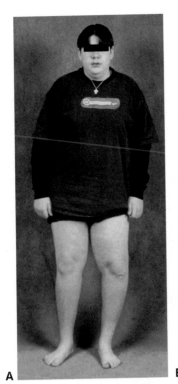
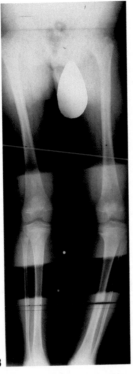
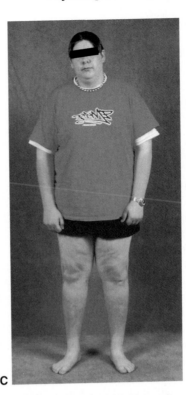
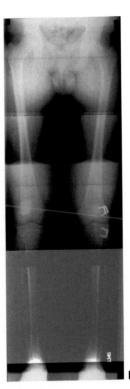

A    B    C    D

**Figure 28.22    A:** Clinical photo of a teenager with unilateral adolescent Blount disease. **B:** Long cassette radiograph demonstrates varus deformity in the distal femur and proximal tibia in a skeletally immature individual. **C:** Clinical appearance following correction. **D:** Hemiepiphyseal stapling was used. Correction is noted 1 year after staple insertion in the lateral distal femur and proximal tibia. This technique is optimal in mild to moderate deformities where 1 to 2 years of growth remain.

Similarly, restoration of the distal femoral alignment with a concomitant femoral varus-correcting osteotomy is indicated if the DFLA measures more than 5 degrees varus (normal DFLA is 87 degrees) (68,121). If there is sufficient growth remaining, the distal femoral deformity may be amenable to hemiepiphyseal stapling. If a distal femoral osteotomy is performed, the transverse cut can be made through the physeal scar in skeletally mature patients or proximal to the physis as in the skeletally immature. This allows correction closest to the anatomic site of the deformity. A blade plate is used for fixation.

Compensatory valgus may be present in the distal tibia and is assessed on the anteroposterior ankle radiograph. Hemiepiphyseal stapling is used if there are 5 degrees or more of distal tibial valgus and the physis is open. If the physis is closed and more than 8 degrees of valgus is present, an osteotomy is performed.

*Limited Internal Fixation.* Osteotomy with limited internal fixation, the mainstay of treatment of infantile Blount disease, is generally not recommended in adolescent Blount disease. A supplemental long-leg cast often adds minimal additional protection for these extraordinarily large patients. The difficulties associated with non–weight bearing on the affected extremity make ambulation difficult in these patients. Outcome of treatment with this approach has far too often been unsatisfactory (112).

*Stable Internal Fixation.* Osteotomy, with acute correction and more stable internal fixation, can be effectively utilized in patients with mild-to-moderate varus and procurvatum deformity (50,125,126). Because the deformity occurs at the level of the physis, a transverse osteotomy of the tibia in the metaphysis distal to the tubercle must be translated laterally, sometimes as much as the entire diameter of the tibia in order to prevent creating an offsetting deformity. To circumvent this deformity, Millis (125) has utilized an oblique, laterally based, closing wedge osteotomy in skeletally mature patients which hinges at the intact cortex just distal to the proximal tibial physeal scar (127) (Fig. 28.23). Fixation is achieved using a laterally placed compression plate that serves as a tension band and permits weight bearing without external immobilization. As the hinge point is near the physeal scar, the correction is achieved at the level of the deformity and a translational deformity is not created.

*Monolateral External Fixation.* External fixation of the tibia can be used for correction of severe deformities. The dynamic axial monolateral fixator has the advantages of ease of achieving an acute correction, adjustability after the initial surgical correction, and relative patient acceptance (127). Price et al. obtained satisfactory stability of the osteotomy fragments even in heavier patients (91). In applying a monolateral fixator of any type, pin placement parallel to the knee and ankle joint aids in obtaining a satisfactory acute correction of deformity (127). Similarly, Gaudinez et al. and Stanitski et al. have effectively incorporated the Garche clamp when utilizing a monolateral fixation in the treatment of Blount disease in adolescents (128,129). The Garche external fixator optimizes fixation and allows for postoperative frontal plane adjustment and lengthening. It is, however, not conducive to postoperative adjustments in the sagittal plane or in rotation (129).

*Circular External Fixation.*   Circular external fixation is the preferred approach for gradual correction of the proximal tibia; it allows for the maximal adjustability of the alignment in all planes and is ideally applicable in the most severe deformities and more obese patients (95,121,130). Advantages include stable fixation with improved patient mobility, the ability to evaluate alignment in a functional, standing position, and the ability to correct accurately all of the tibial deformities including proximal tibial varus and procurvatum, internal tibial torsion, and distal tibial valgus (121, 129,130). A hybrid circular fixator such as an Ilizarov or Taylor spatial frame can be used. The latter device is our preferred method of fixation (Fig. 28.20F,G).

Ideally, all of the deformities are addressed in a single surgical procedure. If indicated, the distal femoral varus is acutely corrected first. The distal femoral deformity may be addressed by supracondylar osteotomy and stable fixation of the distal femur using a blade plate to maintain alignment. This may be performed through a medial or lateral approach, with an opening or closing wedge osteotomy technique. A lateral approach is preferred for performing an opening wedge osteotomy of the distal femur; the fragments are fixed with an adult 95-degree condylar blade plate.

Next, a fibular osteotomy is performed through a posterolateral incision over the midshaft of the fibula at least 10 cm distal to the fibular head. Great care should be taken in obtaining subperiosteal exposure of the fibula to avoid injury to the branches of the deep peroneal nerve, the extensor hallucis longus, or the peroneal vessels, which lie just medial to the fibula. A 1-cm section of the fibula is removed and used as bone graft for the distal femoral osteotomy if needed.

The preconstructed circular fixator is placed over the leg and applied with a combination of transfixing wires and half-pins. Ring strategy and placement of transfixing wire vary depending on the presence of open growth plates, the need for fibular transfer to correct ligamentous laxity, and the need for distal tibial valgus-correcting osteotomy (121,129). The proximal tibial osteotomy is performed through a limited incision, using drill bits and osteotomes. If indicated, a distal tibial osteotomy is created in an identical fashion.

Gradual correction is begun on postoperative day two or three, and serial radiographs are obtained to monitor the correction and bone formation (Fig. 28.20H). The patient is encouraged to undertake full weight bearing as early as possible, and vigorous physical therapy is instituted to maintain mobility and joint range of motion. Adjustments in the circular frame are made as necessary to correct all planes of the deformity. The fixator is left in place and progressively dynamized until consolidation and cortication of the osteotomy site is complete. Bilateral deformities are corrected one side at a time. Correction of the second extremity is usually planned within 6 months of completion of the first side. This comprehensive approach has provided very satisfactory results in this most difficult group of patients and has been a marked improvement over traditional methods of treatment (112,129,131) (Fig. 28.20I–K). There have been very few surgical complications in these patients despite their extremely large size (121,130). All osteotomies, including those that included lengthening, have healed without delay. The knee and ankle joints have been realigned and the normal mechanical axis of the leg restored. Knee pain has resolved. Patients are satisfied with their more normal lower-extremity alignment.

# KNOCK-KNEES AND GENU VALGUM

## Definition

Parental concerns regarding knock-knees are far less common than those regarding bowed legs (5,132,133). Physiologic knock-knee generally becomes a concern when the child is between 3 and 5 years of age, and the normal femoral-tibial angle is at its maximum valgus angle (5,132,133) (Fig. 28.24). Parents often notice the flat appearance of the foot before the valgus knee position is noted. There may be occasional complaints of medial foot or medial knee pain.

Typically, valgus knee position becomes apparent after 2 years of age, reaching a maximum femoral-tibial angle of 8 to 10 degrees at approximately 3 to 4 years of age, a time when it is most noticeable (2,5,49). As demonstrated by Salenius and Vankka, valgus gradually decreases to a stable "adult" level of 5 degrees to 7 degrees of femoral-tibial valgus angulation by 6 to 7 years of age (Fig. 28.6). There is, however, wide variation among normal children, that is, those who fall within two standard deviations of the mean. This range includes measurements of ±8 to 10 degrees, which means that normal femoral-tibial angles may range from 2 degrees of varus to 20 degrees of valgus at 3 to 4 years of age and neutral to 12 degrees of valgus after 7 years of age (49,132,133).

Physiologic knock-knees are typically symmetric (5,132). The severity of the deformity can easily be assessed and documented by standing photographs. Radiographic evaluation is indicated in those children with clinically excessive femoral-tibial angles, those who present outside of typical age range for physiologic valgus, those with asymmetric deformity, or those who fall below the tenth percentile of height.

Genu valgum is a pathologic condition that may result from persistent knock-knee in a young child, but more often develops during early adolescence (Fig. 28.25). Typically, the deformity arises from asymmetric growth in the distal femur and does not spontaneously resolve. In some cases, the proximal tibia is also abnormal.

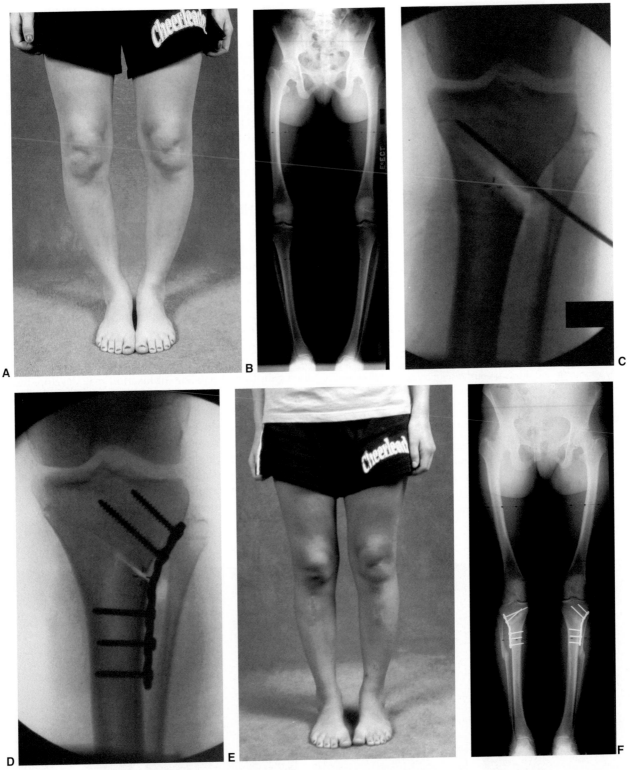

**Figure 28.23**  **A:** There is a subgroup of patients with adolescent Blount disease who are not obese. Deformity is typically bilateral and mild to moderate. **B:** Radiographs in this nearly skeletally mature girl demonstrate deformity only in the proximal tibia. **C:** The oblique osteotomy directed toward the physeal scar. **D:** A laterally based wedge is removed, and the osteotomy fixed with a "tension band" plate. **E:** Clinical photo after bilateral correction. **F:** Bilateral lower extremity radiographs following osteotomy.

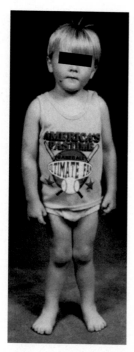

**Figure 28.24** Physiologic genu valgus peaks between 3 and 4 years of age. It may be associated with asymptomatic flat feet. It is typically symmetric and shows gradual resolution by 8 years of age.

## Differential Diagnosis

Most children younger than 6 years who present with a concern of knock-knees are normal (49). The differential diagnosis includes metabolic bone disease such as rickets, posttraumatic valgus, or skeletal dysplasia (134–137) (Table 28.2). If the onset of rickets (osteomalacia) occurs

when physiologic valgus is present, a knock-knee deformity is more likely to develop. Valgus may result from overgrowth of the proximal medial tibia following a proximal tibia fracture (Cozen fracture) or from an injury to the distal lateral femoral physis (137–139). Skeletal dysplasias most typically associated with genu valgum are chondroectodermal dysplasia (Ellis–van Creveld), mucopolysaccharidosis type IV, and spondyloepiphyseal dysplasia tarda (136). Benign neoplastic processes such as multiple hereditary exostoses and focal fibrocartilaginous dysplasia may also produce a valgus deformity (140).

## Natural History

Physiologic knock-knee predictably remodels to normal alignment (slight valgus) by 7 years of age (2,5,49,132,133). No treatment is necessary for this type of knock-knees (Fig. 28.12). Minimal, if any, change in femoral-tibial angle should occur through adolescent growth.

In contrast, genu valgum occurs in older childhood or early adolescence. Knee pain is a common feature. The clinical deformity is often more striking than the radiographic appearance. It may be associated with an out-toed gait. Lateral patellar subluxation may develop, but is uncommon. Many of these children are above the 90th percentile in height and weight. Walking may become awkward because of the knees rubbing or hitting together as the child tries to narrow the base of support. This degree of deformity is not physiologic and typically does not resolve on its own. Valgus of the knee which increases after 7 years of age is not physiologic. This genu valgum is a pathologic state and often requires surgical treatment (140,141).

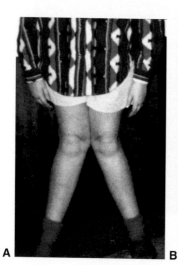
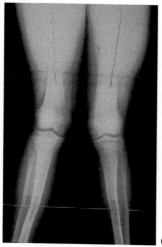
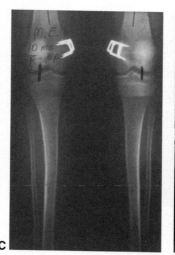
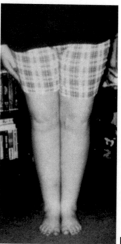

**Figure 28.25**   **A:** Lower limb valgus that persists past 8 years of age is not physiologic. It may cause an awkward gait, in addition to concerns about appearance. **B:** These long cassette films of a 12-year-old girl confirm the presence of valgus in both the femur and tibia. She is not skeletally mature, making hemiepiphyseal stapling a treatment option. **C:** Stapling of the medial physis of both distal femurs and tibiae in a growing adolescent results in rapid correction. Correction of the mechanical axis is achieved in this patient within a year. **D:** There is marked clinical improvement in alignment. Correction is generally well maintained.

## TABLE 28.2
### DIFFERENTIAL DIAGNOSIS OF KNOCK-KNEES

Developmental
   Physiologic
   Genu valgum
   Skeletal dysplasia
      Ellis–van Creveld
      Pseudoachondroplasia
      Morquio MPS IV
Acquired
   Metabolic
   Posttraumatic
   Neoplastic
      Multiple hereditary exostoses
      Focal fibrocartilaginous dysplasia

MPS, mucopolysaccharidosis.

## Assessment

An anteroposterior, standing, long cassette radiograph of both lower extremities, which includes the hips, knees, and ankles, is best for assessing the mechanical axis and any deviation in joint alignment. The lower extremities should be placed so that the kneecaps are facing directly forward. This must be done without regard to foot position. This technique produces the truest anteroposterior x-ray film of the knees and allows for reliable serial comparisons if needed. The mechanical axis of the lower extremity is drawn from the center of the hip through the center of the ankle. A normal mechanical axis passes through the central third of the knee, roughly defined by the tibial spines, or through zones $+1$ to $-1$ where positive values represent valgus and negative values are varus (28,98,141,142).

Lateral deviation of the mechanical axis, beyond the mid portion of the lateral tibial plateau (zone $+2$ or $+3$), can result in relative overload of the lateral compartment (28,142) (Figs. 28.26 and 28.27). The severity of deformity sufficient to produce premature degenerative changes in the lateral compartment of the knee, is not known. Genu valgum that results in mechanical axis deviation beyond the lateral margin of the tibia is pathologic and warrants correction. In addition to improving the appearance of lower limb alignment, correction can restore a normal mechanical axis (138,141,143). Gait analysis has demonstrated abnormal moments about the hip and knee in proportion to the deviation from normal.

## Treatment of Physiologic Knock-Knees

Treatment of knock-knees consists of education of the parents regarding the natural history of this physiologic condition, which is anticipation of spontaneous correction by 7 years of age (133). Lower-extremity bracing is not indicated (133). Long-leg bracing is poorly tolerated in these children, who are typically older than 4 years. Unlike Blount disease, the deformity may be present above and below the knee, making bracing less effective.

The inherited metabolic bone disease XLH requires medical management of the osteomalacia. Genu valgum associated with bone diseases such as XLH and skeletal dysplasias may worsen with time, necessitating surgical treatment (see Chapters 7 and 8). Postfracture valgus deformity also may require treatment, as spontaneous correction does not always occur. Observation is the appropriate initial management; however, if the valgus deformity does not resolve, hemiepiphyseal stapling or proximal tibial osteotomy is recommended to restore normal limb alignment.

## Treatment of Genu Valgum

Surgical treatment of genu valgum is indicated if the mechanical axis passes through zone 3, that is to say, at or beyond the lateral cortex of the tibial plateau, or if it passes through zone 2 and knee pain is present. In most cases, surgery can be deferred until the child is 10 to 11 years of age.

### Hemiepiphysiodesis
Correction in the skeletally immature child with 1 to 2 years of growth remaining can be accomplished with

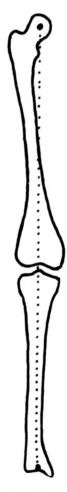

**Figure 28.26** The mechanical axis is assessed on a standing, anteroposterior, long cassette radiograph that includes the hips and ankles. A line is constructed from the center of the femoral head to the center of the ankle. For consistent serial measurements, the knees are positioned with the patellae facing forward.

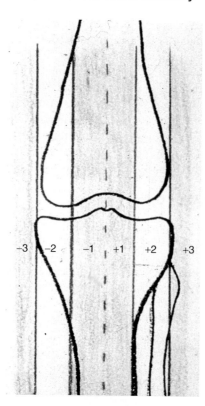

**Figure 28.27** To determine the mechanical axis of the tibia, the proximal tibia is longitudinally divided into four parts. Positive values are lateral to the midline or valgus. Negative values are medial to the midline or varus. Zone 1 is centered over the tibial spines, zone 2 is within the tibial condyle, and zone 3 is beyond the cortex. A normal mechanical axis falls within zone 1.

hemiepiphysiodesis, preferably by hemiepiphyseal stapling (97,98,123,141,143–147) (Fig. 28.25C). Whether medial physeal stapling is performed in the distal femur, proximal tibia, or both will depend on the location of the deformity and the amount of growth remaining (123,138,147). Most often valgus deformity arises primarily from the femur. The mechanical axis of the femur and tibia and the relative abnormality in the distal lateral femoral and proximal medial tibial angles should be utilized to determine the appropriate site for hemiepiphysiodesis (28,125,141). The technique of stapling, although simple, requires attention to a few important details to maximize its effectiveness and minimize the potential for growth-plate injury (97,98,138,144,145).

The staples are carefully placed extraperiosteally. Use of C-arm image intensification is critical in assuring optimal staple placement. On the anteroposterior or frontal view, the staple prongs should both span and be parallel to the physis. This may require a slightly oblique orientation to the cortex. On the lateral view the staples should be placed centrally (equidistant from the anterior and posterior edges of the physis) to avoid inadvertent creation of a sagittal plane deformity. Two staples per location are generally sufficient. Three may be used if the bone is unusually large. We use staples made of cobalt-chrome alloy (Zimmer, Inc.,

Warsaw, IN, USA) that have reenforced corners and are less likely to break or be ineffective (143,144).

Patients selected for hemiepiphyseal stapling, particularly those with more than 2 years of growth remaining, must have reliable follow-up. Overcorrection to a varus position can occur and is not desirable. Long cassette radiographs of the lower extremities should be obtained at 3-month intervals. Some improvement in the lower extremity mechanical axis should be apparent 3 to 6 months after stapling. Once the mechanical axis passes through the central third of the knee joint, the staples should be removed to avoid overcorrection into varus unless the lateral physis is closed (Fig. 28.25D). Following staple removal, rebound medial overgrowth can occur resulting in some loss of correction. This is more common in children who are younger than 10 years when stapling is performed (97,143–145). It is unclear how long extraperiosteal staples can safely span a growth plate without affecting future growth. It has been our practice to remove staples within 18 to 24 months if resumption of growth is desired. Stevens has reported resumption of growth following removal of staples that were across the physis for more than 2 years in patients with a variety of deformities (98,141). It has been our experience that in children with XLH or skeletal dysplasia, staples can safely remain for more than 2 years, and growth will resume following removal. If rebound overgrowth is a concern and the possibility of another surgical procedure is not acceptable, a complete epiphysiodesis can be performed; however, this will result in limb shortening in proportion to the amount of growth remaining. As the procedure is usually bilateral and performed close to skeletal maturity, the absolute amount of shortening is usually not significant.

### Osteotomy

Osteotomy is indicated when immediate correction of the deformity is desired (148,149). It may be preferred in very young children with severe deformity such as valgus associated with a skeletal dysplasia or in those who are skeletally mature. The site of deformity correction is dependent on the anatomic deviations present in the tibia and/or femur, just as in the determination for hemiepiphyseal stapling (125,150–152). The femur is more often the primary site of valgus deformity. In young children, valgus is corrected using a transverse osteotomy in the distal femur. Appropriately sized K-wires or a small fragment plate can be used for fixation and supplemented with a long-leg cast. Immediate correction of femoral valgus using internal fixation with a 95 degree condylar blade plate is preferred for older children and adolescents. A lateral approach to the distal femur is preferred. It also allows exploration and release of the peroneal nerve, which is sometimes necessary in severe deformities.

External fixation with immediate correction can also be used (148). Gradual correction using external fixation may also be considered for children with severe deformity, in whom it reduces the risk of peroneal nerve neurapraxia, and for those with limb-length inequality when lengthening is also needed (42,125,149). Circular frame fixation may facilitate angulatory correction in combination with lengthening (42,148,149). A unilateral frame may be considered when external fixation is used with immediate correction.

Similar techniques can be used for valgus correction in the tibia. In young children, correction can be accomplished by simple, closing wedge technique in the proximal tibia, using two or three crossed stainless steel wires as described regarding rotational variation earlier in this chapter (148). In adolescents and young adults, tibial valgus deformity can be corrected by a proximal tibial osteotomy that uses a medially based oblique wedge osteotomy and hinges proximally and laterally near the physeal scar, analogous to that described in Figure 28.23. The wedge is carefully removed and the distal medial cortex is compressed together utilizing a short compression plate to produce a controlled fracture of the lateral cortex.

### Complications

When placing staples around the growth plate, there is potential for injury to the involved growth plate. Errors in technique can lead to failure with hemiepiphyseal stapling. Poor fixation and inadequate design or number of staples will compromise results (97,98,144). Timing of placement, follow-up, and removal are sources of error (123,143). If the stapling is performed too late, there will not be adequate growth remaining to correct the deformity. Lack of appropriate and timely evaluation poststapling, resulting in overcorrection, is the most common serious complication of hemiepiphyseal stapling. The resultant varus alignment produces greater mechanical loads across the medial compartment of the knee than the same degree of valgus would produce over the lateral compartment (50). Increased medial compartment load can accelerate degenerative changes.

Overcorrection can also occur because of unrecognized premature physeal closure beneath the staple. The length of time extraperiosteal staples can be left across a growth plate without permanently affecting growth is unclear. We have used 18 to 24 months as the upper limit if resumption of growth is desired. The actual limit may be dependent on the patient's age at the time of stapling and the number of staples and their design. In a recent report by Stevens (141), none of his patients had premature growth arrest or rebound when treated with temporary physeal stapling for genu valgum.

Complications related to osteotomy include failures of union or fixation, infection, blood loss, knee stiffness, and scar formation. None of these is unique to distal femoral or tibial osteotomy for valgus correction. Peroneal nerve injury is a serious concern in the process of valgus correction. Mobility of the peroneal nerve is limited above the knee as it passes around the distal femur and across the lateral edge of the biceps femoris tendon and below the knee as it curves around the proximal fibula and through the crural fascia (37). More severe deformities may require release of one or more of these sites to reduce the risk of permanent injury. Closing wedge technique for immediate correction is less likely to stretch the peroneal nerve than opening wedge. Gradual correction of severe deformities may allow the nerve to accommodate to these changes more safely than does acute correction. Injury to the nerve must be avoided during pin placement, however.

## BOWING OF THE TIBIA

### Congenital Pseudarthrosis of the Tibia

#### Definition

Bowing of the tibia that presents at birth typically is either anterior, anterolateral, or posterior medial. Anterior tibial bowing that occurs in association with a deficient or absent fibula is diagnostic of fibular hemimelia. Posterior medial bowing occurs in association with calcaneovalgus foot deformity and has a relatively excellent prognosis. In contrast, anterolateral bowing, which usually presents soon after birth, is typically a progressive deformity which often results in a pseudarthrosis. Anterolateral bowing associated with congenital pseudarthrosis of the tibia is rare (1:140,000), yet it is the most common type of congenital pseudarthrosis (153,154). Neurofibromatosis occurs in more than 50% of patients with anterolateral bowing, with or without pseudarthrosis of the tibia (153–157). This bowing may be the first clinical manifestation of neurofibromatosis (155,156).

#### Natural History

Spontaneous resolution is uncommon (158). Rather, the tibia with an anterolateral bow appears dysplastic, with failure of tubulation, cystic prefracture, or frank pseudarthrosis, or a combination of these features, with narrowing of the fragments (153,155). Fracture with resultant pseudarthrosis typically occurs in the first 4 to 5 years of life (Fig. 28.28). Once established, the natural history of a pseudarthrosis is that of persistent instability and progressive deformity. Numerous classification systems have been proposed in an attempt to prognosticate the natural history and outcome of treatment. In reality, there has been very little correlation with initial radiograph classification and eventual outcome of treatment (155,159–162). The radiographic appearance of congenital pseudarthrosis of the tibia has been classified by Boyd and by Crawford (153, 155). Both noted the variable natural history and prognosis of each of the types they described (Table 28.3). Consolidation of the pseudarthrosis was most difficult to obtain in the Boyd type II or Crawford dysplastic type II-C (Fig. 28.29).

## Nonoperative Treatment

Once the diagnosis of anterolateral bowing is made, full-time brace treatment is indicated. An ankle-foot orthosis (AFO) is appropriate protection prior to walking, and a KAFO is fit as the infant begins walking. Orthotic support is continued indefinitely during the growing years with or without surgical reconstruction of a pseudarthrosis. Although very uncommon, some forms of anterolateral bowing, such as Boyd type IV, occasionally do not progress (158). These unusual patients present with a bowed tibia, with or without a previous fracture that consolidates with immobilization (158). Supplemental bone grafting may be beneficial (163). These unique patients seem to carry less chance of progression and fracture following the bone graft procedure.

## Operative Treatment

Despite a gradual improvement in the outcome of treatment in the past 100 years, congenital pseudarthrosis of the tibia remains one of the most challenging problems in pediatric orthopaedics. Even with consolidation, the tenuous status of the atrophic bone markedly limits functional potential (156–158). A major improvement in outcome can be traced to Boyd's use of dual onlay grafts, Moore's use of staged bone graft and external fixator, McFarland's bypass graft, and Sofield and Millar's innovative use of intramedullary rod stabilization (164–170). Less invasive technical innovations were developed by Brighton and Bassett (171,172) utilizing implanted cathode leads or pulsed electromagnetic current, either alone or in combination with surgical stabilization.

Currently, three surgical approaches are being used successfully in the treatment of pseudarthrosis of the tibia (Fig. 28.30). All techniques include excision of the pseudarthrosis site. Techniques used to achieve union of the pseudarthrosis include intramedullary fixation with autogenous iliac crest bone graft, circular ring fixation with bone transport, and vascularized fibular graft. However, even after obtaining consolidation with any of these techniques, long-term follow-up is critical to address associated deformities that frequently occur later in the course of the disease. These include refracture, persistent or increasing valgus deformity, and limb-length inequality.

*Solid Intramedullary Rod Fixation.* Charnley is credited with the first reported innovative use of an intramedullary rod that both stabilized the pseudarthrosis site and transfixed the ankle joint (173). In a similar technique, Umber et al. (174) popularized the use of the two-part Peter Williams intramedullary (IM) solid rod in North America (175). This IM rod technique, in conjunction with pseudarthrosis excision and iliac crest bone grafting, has been further refined in dealing with all aspects of the deformity (176–179). It is our approach of choice in treating congenital pseudarthrosis of the tibia. A posterior iliac bone graft is obtained consisting of adequate corticocancellous strips and cancellous bone graft. The pseudarthrosis is excised and the bone fragments stabilized with a Williams rod (177,179). The entire rod assembly is inserted at the pseudarthrosis site into the medullary canal of the distal fragment and is advanced in an antegrade direction through the distal tibia and across the

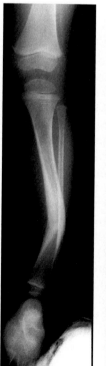
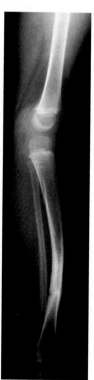
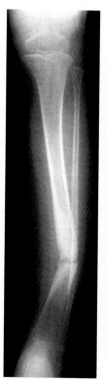
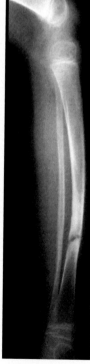

**Figure 28.28** **A:** Anterolateral bowing of the tibia may be apparent at birth or may progress with weight bearing. Bowing usually occurs between the middle and distal thirds of the tibia. The adjacent bone may appear sclerotic, with increased density, or it may be atrophic and spindle shaped. Once the deformity is recognized, the leg should be protected with a total-contact orthosis. Although fracture is not likely to be avoided, it may be delayed until the child is bigger. **B:** Fracture occurs at the apex of the bow, usually without prodromal symptoms and with minimal or no trauma. Once fracture occurs, surgical management begins.

A

B

**TABLE 28.3**

**CLASSIFICATION OF CONGENITAL PSEUDARTHROSIS OF THE TIBIA**

| Boyd Classification | | Crawford Classification | |
|---|---|---|---|
| I | Fracture present at birth | I | Nondysplastic type |
| II | Hourglass constriction of tibia | | –Anterolateral bowing with increased density |
| III | Bone cysts | | –Sclerosis of medullary canal |
| IV | Sclerotic segment of tibia, no constriction, stress fracture results | | –May convert to dysplastic type following osteotomy |
| V | Dysplastic fibula | II | Dysplastic type—Anterolateral bowing |
| VI | Intraosseous neurofibroma | | A–With failure of tubulation |
| | | | B–Cystic prefracture or canal enlargement from prior fracture |
| | | | C–Frank pseudarthrosis with atrophy "sucked candy" narrowing of ends |

talus and calcaneus as it exits through the heel pad (Fig. 28.31A,B). During the passage of the rod across the ankle joint, it is imperative that the foot be positioned to correct the calcaneus position of the foot and valgus deformity of the distal tibia. The desired foot position is neutral dorsiflexion/plantar flexion verified clinically and with the C-arm. The tibial fragments are anatomically reduced at the pseudarthrosis site, and the rod is driven retrograde into the proximal fragment (Fig. 28.31C). In selecting an appropriately sized rod, consideration should be given to the desired length of rod based on the need to transfix the

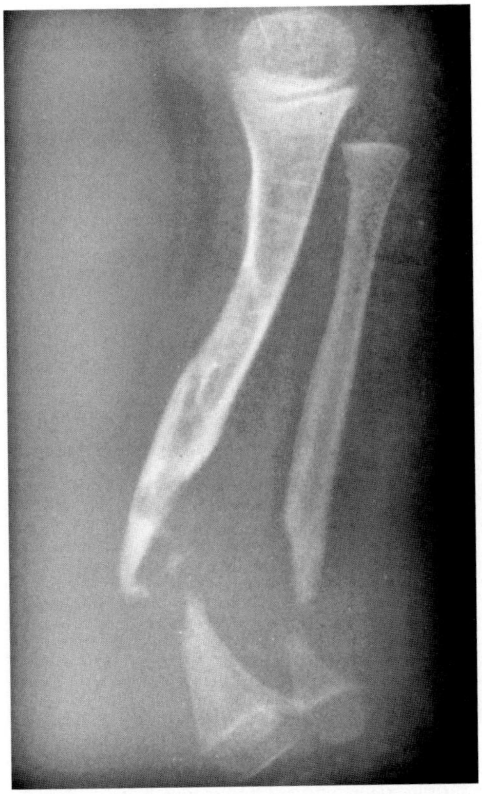

**Figure 28.29** Early (Boyd type II, Crawford II-C) congenital pseudarthrosis of the tibia and fibula in a patient with neurofibromatosis.

ankle joint and the amount of growth remaining in the distal tibia (Fig. 28.32A–E). In smaller children and with distal defects, ankle-joint fixation for 1 to 2 years may be desirable to minimize stress on the pseudarthrosis site, which facilitates consolidation. Distally, the rod should extend into the talus, calcaneus, or both. Proximally, the rod should remain within the proximal tibia metaphysis and not cross the physis. The rod may be advanced across the ankle joint once the defect has united (at least 1 to 2 years following placement) to allow ankle motion. Ideally, there will have been sufficient growth in the proximal tibia so that the rod can be advanced into the tibia and not cross the proximal tibial physis. Occasionally, the presence of deformity in the proximal tibia necessitates an additional osteotomy in the proximal tibia to assure intramedullary passage of the rod and anatomic alignment of the tibia. An intact fibula is not osteotomized unless it distracts the tibial fragments. If the fibula is not intact, it may be possible to stabilize it with an intramedullary rod. A small-diameter K-wire is used for fibular fixation and is placed into the distal fragment through a separate incision. The wire is directed antegrade and out the of distal tip of the fibula, then in a retrograde direction into the proximal fragment. Fibular fixation adds stability to the construct (178,179).

With longitudinal growth of the distal tibia, the distal end of the rod "migrates" proximally. Therefore, the anticipated remaining growth determines the appropriate placement of the distal end of the rod at the time of surgery. The previously harvested iliac bone graft strips are then placed circumferentially around the pseudarthrosis site and secured with absorbable suture as a barrel-stave construction. By protocol for children 6 years and younger, a one and one-half spica cast is applied to assure minimal rotational stress at the pseudarthrosis site. The spica cast is replaced with a long-leg cast after 6 to 8 weeks, and cast immobilization is discontinued after approximately 4 months. Older children are treated with long-leg casts for the entire 4 months. Once cast protection is discontinued, the involved extremity is protected with a custom-fabricated KAFO with a locked ankle joint and free

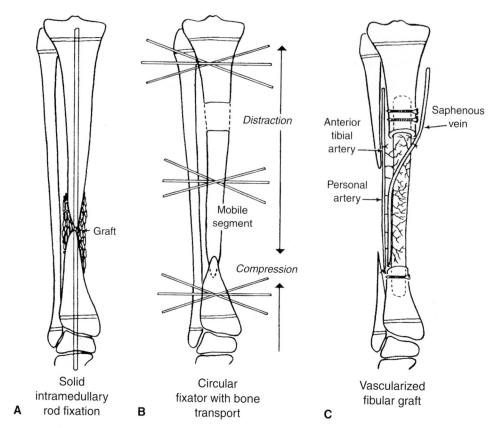

**Figure 28.30**  Operative options for pseudarthrosis of the tibia. **A:** Solid intramedullary rod fixation. **B:** Circular fixation with bone transport and compression. **C:** Vascularized fibula graft.

knee joint (Fig. 28.32F). The presence of the rod across the ankle joint and in the hindfoot has a considerable advantage in providing optimal immobilization and protection of the consolidating pseudarthrosis. Refracture may occur; although spontaneous healing with plaster immobilization may occur it is not always assured, and repeat grafting, with or without rerodding, may be required. With longitudinal growth of the tibia, the distal end of the rod "migrates" more proximally and eventually will be positioned in the distal tibia. As the tip of the rod crosses the ankle joint, the potential

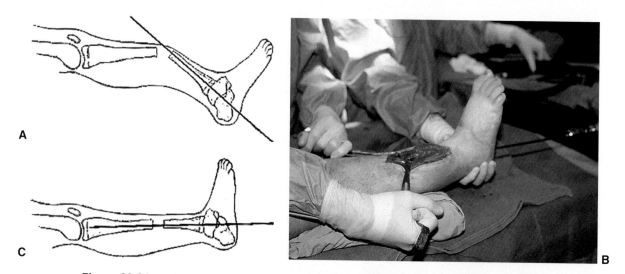

**Figure 28.31**  Technique of solid intramedullary rod fixation. **A:** After excision of the pseudarthrosis, the Williams rod is inserted, antegrade, through the distal tibia, talus, and calcaneus and exits through the heel pad. Care is taken to maintain the foot in a neutral, plantigrade position as the rod passes across the ankle and subtalar joints. **B:** The tibial surfaces are opposed. **C:** The rod is then passed into the proximal fragment, just below the proximal tibial physis. If the tibia is distracted, a fibular osteotomy is performed to allow contact across the tibia.

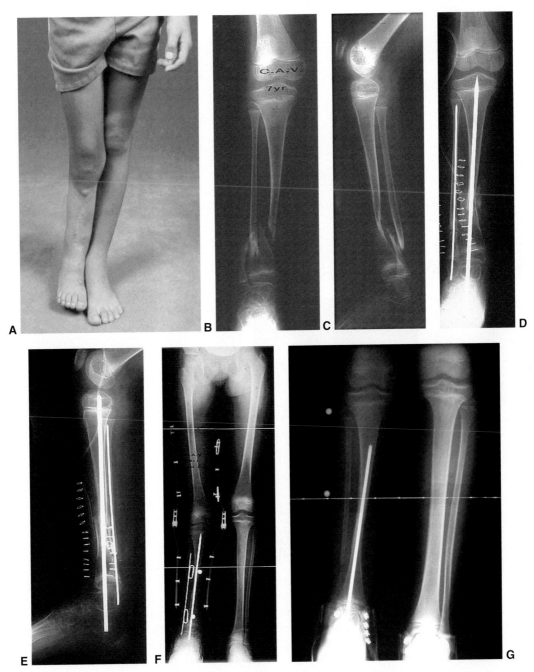

**Figure 28.32** **A:** This is another example of a tibial pseudarthrosis. Treatment includes stabilization of the fracture, establishment of a source of healthy bone, and maintenance of alignment. **B:** Atrophic pseudarthrosis of the tibia and fibula. **C:** Boyd type II or Crawford II-C dysplasia. **D:** The pathologic bone was resected; a Williams rod was used in the tibia and a Steinman pin in the fibula. Iliac crest graft was packed around the pseudarthrosis. **E:** The ankle and foot are held in a neutral position during placement of the rod. Transfixing the ankle and subtalar joint increases stabilization of the pseudarthrosis. **F:** A spica cast is applied postoperatively and a total contact orthosis used once union is established. Ankle motion is prohibited as long as the rod remains across the subtalar and ankle joints. A KAFO is used in smaller children. A patellar-tendon-bearing (PTB) orthosis can be used in most children over 7 years of age. **G:** With growth, the rod typically is drawn proximally and comes to lie within the tibia. In this case, the rod has remained with the distal fragment and continues to cross the ankle. Note the increased distance from the rod tip to the proximal tibial physis. **H:** A second rod can be used to push the Williams rod across the ankle. Image intensification is helpful in guiding placement. **I:** A syndesmosis screw was added to stabilize the persistent fibular pseudarthrosis. **J:** Hemiepiphyseal stapling of the proximal and/or distal medial tibia is used to correct valgus. **K:** This comprehensive treatment has resulted in a stable, healed pseudarthrosis. **L:** Satisfactory tibial alignment and stabilization of the pseudarthrosis have been achieved. Limb-length inequality can be managed with contralateral epiphysiodesis. Lengthening of the affected leg may be complicated by delayed bone formation and healing.

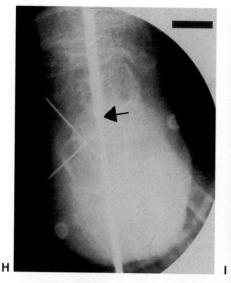

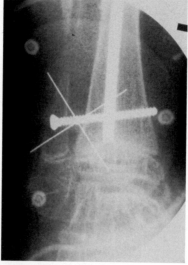

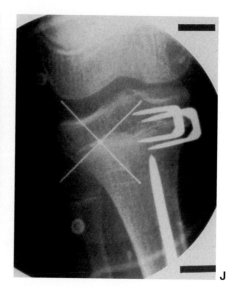

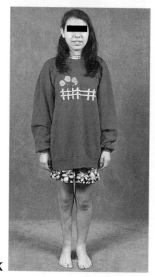

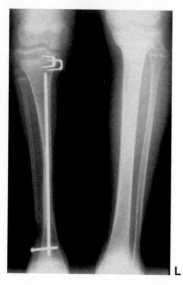

**Figure 28.32** (continued)

for disruption of articular cartilage exists. To minimize such an occurrence, the rod can be surgically pushed across the ankle joint as the tip approaches the articular surface of the talus. This adjustment is easily accomplished with a slightly larger diameter, concave-tipped, IM pusher rod inserted through the calcaneus and guided with C-arm assistance (Fig. 28.32G–I). On occasion, despite consolidation of the pseudarthrosis and growth of the tibia, the rod does not migrate. If this occurs, the rod should be replaced, with or without repeat grafting. In the case of failure of rod migration, the replacement rod should be secured proximally with methylmethacrylate (176,177,179).

Valgus deformity of the tibia or the ankle is common and can compromise the functional result. This valgus deformity is part of the natural history of the pseudarthrosis that has a deficient fibula and therefore lacks lateral support. It is not a result of traversing the physis with the rod. Long-term bracing protects the distal tibia and ankle and is mandatory during growth to minimize the risk of valgus

deformity. This is particularly true once the rod no longer crosses the distal tibial physis. Valgus has been satisfactorily treated by placement of staples across the medial tibial physis, either proximally, distally, or across both (Fig. 28.32J). The valgus deformity usually improves over a 1- to 2-year period. Once correction is achieved, the staples are removed. A transverse tibiofibular syndesmosis screw is inserted at the time of staple insertion or removal if the distal fibula remains nonunited or has migrated proximally, compromising ankle stability. With this approach, symmetric growth of the distal tibia has generally continued and the valgus deformity has not recurred.

Leg-length inequality secondary to pseudarthrosis of the tibia is often significant (177,179). In a recently reported review of our congenital pseudarthrosis of the tibia (CPT) treatment experience, 11 of 21 patients had a significant limb-length inequality (179). The average discrepancy in these 11 patients was 5 cm and ranged from 2 to 9 cm. Six of these patients were treated by epiphysiodesis for an average predicted leg-length discrepancy at maturity of 4 cm. Two patients underwent a proximal tibial leg lengthening. Two patients with leg-length discrepancies of 6 cm and 9 cm underwent amputations at parental request, one at 8 years of age and the other at 15 years of age.

A satisfactory functional outcome has been achieved in 16 of the 21 patients who were followed up for an average of 14 years (179) (Fig. 28.32K,L). The remaining five patients have had an amputation because of limb-length inequality (two patients), refracture with persistent nonunion (two patients), or significant residual angulatory deformity (one patient). The quality of ankle motion and of gait has varied considerably. The best results have been noted in those patients in whom the tibia is anatomically aligned and the foot is plantigrade.

Two recent reports document the outcome for a total of 44 patients utilizing the Williams rod technique (178,179); results were generally satisfactory. More recently treated patients fared better than those patients treated earlier in the series. This is likely because of modifications made in techniques based on earlier experience. One recommendation that has improved outcome is stabilization of the fibula. This enhances stability of the pseudarthrosis and reduces the risk of valgus deformity in the distal tibia and ankle. Second, advancement of the rod across the ankle minimizes the effect on ankle range of motion and function. A third lesson learned is that secondary deformities such as refracture, valgus, and leg-length discrepancy must be more aggressively managed.

A recent gait analysis assessment of the outcome of treatments of CPT cited relatively poor push-off following IM rod treatment (180). Gait analysis of our more recently treated patients has shown a better outcome concerning push-off ability. We now utilize an active ankle-strengthening program once the rod is positioned within the tibia.

*Circular External Fixation and Bone Transport.* Ilizarov pioneered the use of a circular external fixator that used a combination of compression, distraction, resection of the pseudarthrosis, and bone transfer (Fig. 28.33). Subsequently, numerous authors have refined this technique (181–184). The report by Paley et al. (183) on their initial experience with 16 patients cited a primary union rate of 94% after one procedure and 100% after two. The mean age at treatment was 8 years. Five refractures occurred, and all were successfully treated with additional procedures. Paley now incorporates the use of an intramedullary rod along with the frame assembly in the treatment of pseudarthrosis. The rod is left in place at the time of fixator removal, providing additional protection against refracture and recurrent deformity.

In a recent multicenter study, Boero et al. (185) reported failures in 33% of patients with CPT managed by Ilizarov technique. In their study, all 21 patients had neurofibromatosis. The best results were obtained with sclerotic and normotrophic bone where all six tibias had early consolidation (10 to 12 months) and did not refracture. In contrast, only 5 of 11 tibias with an hourglass appearance

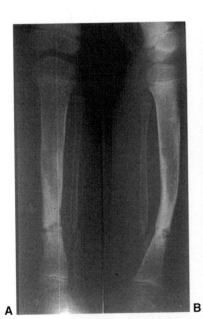
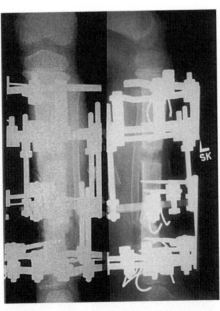
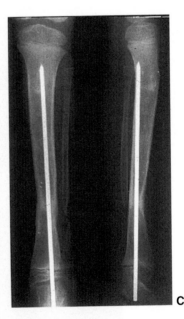

**A**      **B**      **C**

**Figure 28.33** **A:** Tibial pseudarthrosis recurred following multiple bone graft procedures and intramedullary pinning in this 6-year-old with neurofibromatosis. **B:** The pseudarthrosis was resected. The circular frame was used to apply compression across the distal site and to lengthen proximally. **C:** Subsequently, an intramedullary rod was placed across both osteotomy sites in the tibia and the ankle. A solid AFO has also been used. Alignment and bone union have been maintained as shown in these radiographs 2 years later.

eventually healed. In the same series, consolidation was obtained in 86% of those patients who were older than 5 years at the time of operation and only 14% of those younger than 5 years.

Dahl (186) reported on 21 of his surgical patients, followed up to maturity. To date he has observed a satisfactory outcome of treatment, that is, sustained consolidation and independent ambulation in 87% of 20 of these patients. One patient had an amputation. The average age at the time of treatment was 11 years (range, 8 months to 29 years), and 18 of 21 patients had multiple prior surgical procedures. Dahl (186) noted refractures in 33% of the first 12 patients he treated. Refinements in his techniques led to fewer fractures. To achieve prompt and lasting union, he made the following recommendations: (a) resection of the pseudarthrosis and pathologic periosteum, (b) creation of a stable intrinsic fit of the bone end, (c) bone graft of the pseudarthrosis to maximize the cross-sectional area, (d) ideal axial alignment to eliminate bending forces, (e) judicious correction of length and angulatory deformity through the proximal tibia, and (f) prophylactic intramedullary pinning after fixator removal (186). The intramedullary rod is placed 8 weeks after fixator removal to reduce the risk of contamination.

### Vascularized Fibula Graft.

Vascularized composite donor tissue transfers have been utilized for the past 100 years in the surgical treatment of congenital pseudarthrosis of the tibia (187–189). In the last 25 years, refinements in microsurgical techniques have been developed that allow for successful transfer of vascularized bone from a variety of donor sites to remote bony defects (190,191) (Fig. 28.34). Early reports demonstrated that a free vascularized fibular graft could successfully be used as a biologic bridge across a congenital pseudarthrosis of the tibia (192–197). Tolo's (192) current indications for the use of a vascularized graft in the treatment of pseudarthrosis of the tibia are lesions with marked bony atrophy or measurable gap at the pseudarthrosis site. His recommended technique for implanting a free vascularized fibular graft for a congenital pseudarthrosis of the tibia includes the following essential steps. Preoperative arteriography of both legs is obtained. Two surgical teams are used to facilitate treatment by allowing simultaneous harvest of an autologous bone graft from the contralateral fibula and preparation of the pseudarthrosis site. The distal fibula on the involved side is stabilized with a screw into the tibia. The pseudarthrosis is resected extraperiosteally to normal bone. Next, the harvested fibula is dowel fitted into the host tibia and fixed with a plate or an external fixator. Vessels are anastomosed, and a skin paddle is used to monitor blood flow. A spica cast is used for 2 to 3 months and a clamshell orthosis for several years.

Using a similar protocol, Weiland et al. (193) was able to achieve union in 18 of 19 pseudarthroses, observed at an average follow-up of 6.3 years. Several recent series (194–197) have reported on treatment of CPT by a vascularized fibular graft. Combination of this data allowed review of 65 cases with sufficient follow-up to assess outcome. Fifty-six cases eventually healed. Often a second bone graft was necessary to achieve union (195). As with

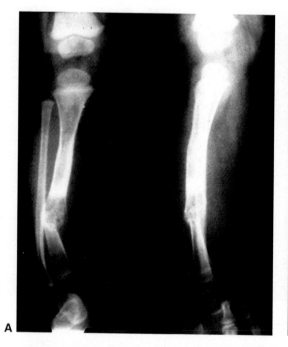
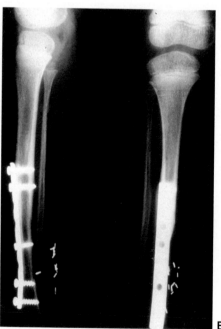

**Figure 28.34** **A:** This film shows another fracture resulting from anterolateral bowing. Note the quality of the bone at the pseudarthrosis site. **B:** A contralateral vascularized fibular graft has been used to bridge the pseudarthrosis. Healing proximally and distally has occurred.

intramedullary rod and external fixation techniques, sequelae may have to be addressed including refracture, nonunion at one end of the graft site, and recurrent pseudarthrosis with failure of the fibular graft (195–197). Subsequent additional surgical treatment was often necessary, with variable success in achieving a functional consolidation. Anterior bowing and valgus deformity were also problems (193). The angulatory deformity did not remodel and was often progressive (190,193). Fourteen of Weiland's patients were noted to have residual angular deformity. In a recent report of six patients with Crawford type IV atrophic pseudarthrosis, Dimeglio et al. (198) added an intramedullary rod to his technique of fibular transfer to maintain length and improve stability of the reconstruction.

Donor site morbidity consisting of progressive valgus with proximal migration of the distal fibula on the normal side can occur following harvest of the fibula (191). The occurrence of this most concerning deformity has not consistently been addressed (190,191,193–197). Prophylactic stabilization of the donor site distal tibiafibular syndesmosis was done by Weiland and Kanaya and was not done by Dormans or Simonis (190,193,194, 196). In follow-up, Dormans and Simonis both noted minimal donor site morbidity such as progressive valgus deformity.

Congenital pseudarthrosis of the tibia has been and will continue to be a very challenging problem. A stable consolidation is essential for a long-term satisfactory functional outcome. Each case is unique, and as such, the treatment plan must often be modified. The newer techniques of intramedullary stabilization, external fixation with bone transport, and vascularized fibular graft have been refined and successfully used by a few. All of these authors have had considerable experience in learning how to apply and adapt their particular surgical technique to the variables of each individual case. Early results demonstrate satisfactory outcomes with these refined surgical techniques and are encouraging. However, as Boyd and Sage (199) suggested years ago, the true success of treatment of CPT in the growing child can only be known by following up these patients until maturity.

*Amputation.* Amputation can be a viable and prudent alternative. Amputation should be considered when there is failure to obtain consolidation despite application of these described surgical techniques, or if the outcome is otherwise unsatisfactory for the patient as in those with poor limb function or severe limb-length inequality. Traditionally, a below-knee amputation is performed. Crawford and Jacobsen et al. (155,200) recommended preserving the hindfoot with a Boyd or Syme procedure, which preserves length of the residual limb and uses a prosthesis to stabilize and protect the pseudarthrosis. These authors suggest that a longer lever may enhance prosthetic fitting and minimize increased energy expenditure,

compared to a below-knee amputee. We have not had the same success with a Syme procedure performed in two patients and have found the need to revise both of them to a below knee level because of residual limb instability and problems related to prosthetic fit.

## Congenital Pseudarthrosis of the Fibula

### Definition

Congenital pseudarthrosis of the fibula usually occurs in association with congenital pseudarthrosis of the tibia. It rarely occurs as an isolated entity. Only 21 cases of isolated fibular pseudarthrosis have been reported in the literature (201–207). Congenital pseudarthrosis of the fibula presents later in life than congenital pseudarthrosis of the tibia (Fig. 28.35). This entity typically presents because of an abnormal gait or because a valgus deformity of the leg and a prominent fibula are noted (201,202,205,206). The condition is frequently linked to neurofibromatosis. The tibia is not normal. The deformity is variable and represents a prepseudarthrosis (201).

### Pathoanatomy

As with congenital pseudarthrosis of the tibia, congenital pseudarthrosis of the fibula may occur after a fracture

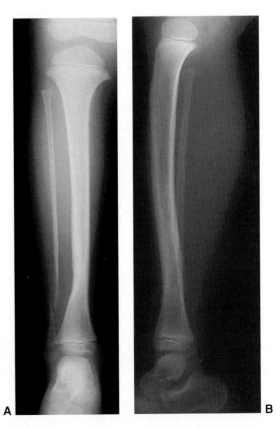

**Figure 28.35  A:** Rare presentation of a fibular pseudarthrosis. **B:** The tibia is also abnormal. Most are associated with neurofibromatosis.

through pathologic bone or through an area of mesodermal maldevelopment (202). Dooley et al. (202) outlined a gradation in the severity of the condition: (a) fibular bowing without pseudarthrosis, (b) fibular pseudarthrosis without ankle deformity, (c) fibular pseudarthrosis with ankle deformity, and (d) fibular pseudarthrosis with late development of tibial pseudarthrosis.

### Treatment

Bowing of a congenitally abnormal fibula does not require treatment if the ankle and tibia are unaffected (201,202). Isolated pseudarthrosis of the fibula in a growing child does not always potentiate ankle valgus deformity (202,203). Dooley et al. (202) suggested observation if no ankle deformity is noted. In contrast, Hsu et al. (203) felt that the potential for ankle valgus was significant without an intact fibula and suggested interpositional bone graft to reconstitute the fibula. If pseudarthrosis of the fibula is associated with ankle valgus, it should be treated. Langenskiöld recommended synostosis of the fibula to the tibia to prevent progression of valgus deformity in the growing child (201,202,204). If there is associated significant distal tibial valgus deformity, it should be surgically addressed. In less severe deformities and in skeletally immature patients, this can be accomplished with medial tibial staple hemiepiphysiodesis, either proximal or distal. In severe deformities or in skeletally mature patients, this is best done with a supramalleolar valgus-correcting osteotomy.

## Posterior Medial Bow of the Tibia

### Definition

Posterior medial bow of the tibia is a congenital anomaly, associated with a calcaneovalgus foot deformity (208). Unlike its counterpart, anterior lateral bowing, posterior medial bowing is not associated with pathologic fracture or pseudarthrosis of the tibia, and has generally been considered a relatively benign condition. Although the severity of the bow does diminish, considerable leg-length discrepancy develops (208,209). This residual deformity presents the greatest need for orthopaedic management.

### Etiology

The pathogenesis of posterior medial bowing is unclear. Mechanical forces (the dorsiflexed foot against the tibia) and embryologic vagaries of tibial development (circulatory or limb bud anomaly) have been suggested as causes but remain unproven. The rapid decrease of bow in the tibia in the first 6 to 12 months supports mechanical factors as a cause of bowing (208,210). However, it cannot account for the growth inhibition.

### Assessment

What is obvious at birth is the extreme dorsiflexed position of the foot against the tibia (Fig. 28.36). Plantar flexion of the foot may be limited. The bow is most easily felt by palpation of the anterior border of the tibia. A normal infant has an anterior bow, which is distinct from the posterior defect palpated in infants with posterior medial bow. A skin dimple is often present over the posterior apex of the bow. Shortening of the affected tibia may not be readily apparent in newborns, but is expected to increase as the child grows.

Evaluation should include anteroposterior and lateral radiographs of both tibias. The severity of the posterior and medial deformity can be measured and a percent inhibition of tibial growth calculated. Serial measurement of tibial length in infants is more accurate when the lateral tibial radiograph is used. Orthoradiographs or similar radiographic techniques can be used for serial assessments of limb-length inequality. The posterior angulation usually remodels, often producing a mildly "S-shaped" tibia (Fig. 28.37). The medial angulation is less likely to resolve completely, and significant residual valgus may remain.

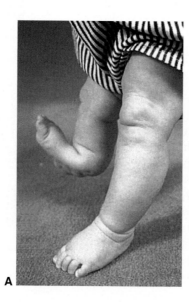
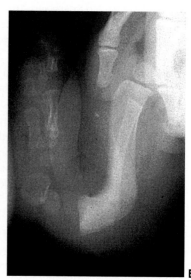

**Figure 28.36** **A:** Infants with posteromedial bowing usually present because the foot is in an abnormal, severely dorsiflexed position. The bow can be palpated along the subcutaneous border of the tibia. A skin dimple is usually present over the apex of the bow. Shortening of the leg may not be as obvious as the bowing deformity. **B:** This infant's lateral radiograph shows how the foot seems to nestle against the curve of the tibia. The bone appears normal or may show signs of remodeling with thickening of the anterior cortex and smoothing posteriorly. **A** **B**

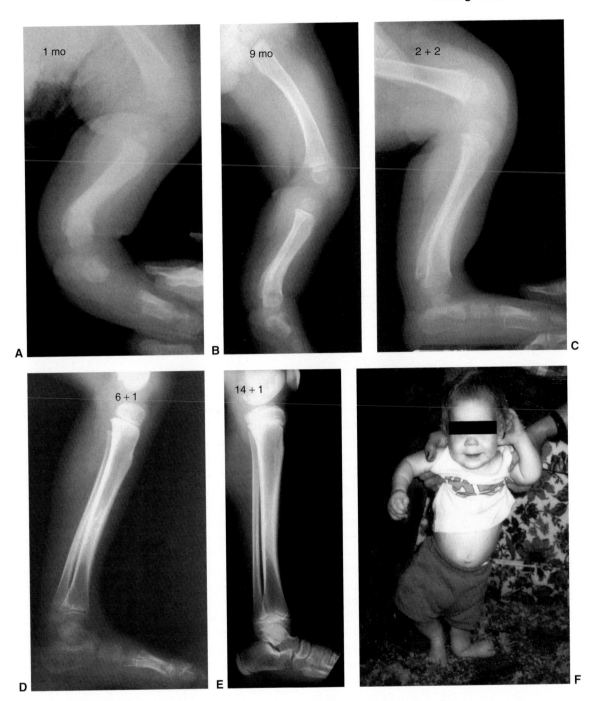

**Figure 28.37** **A–E:** Composite serial lateral radiographs show the degree of spontaneous resolution of the posterior bow. Improvement is often very dramatic within the first year. Similarly, there is improvement in the medial component; however, this bow may not fully resolve, resulting in residual valgus. Posteromedial bow is not associated with risk of pathologic fracture. **F–H:** Shortening of the involved tibia is expected and increases with growth as seen in these serial photographs. The percent inhibition remains fairly constant after 3 years of age.

Growth inhibition is constant as the absolute leg-length difference increases with growth (209).

### Differential Diagnosis
There is little to consider in the differential diagnosis of posterior medial bowing. Its direction is clearly different from the more serious pathology of anterolateral bowing.

Posterior medial bowing may initially be overlooked in the presence of severe calcaneovalgus foot deformity. Occasionally, adolescents will present with limb inequality and mild valgus, the result of previously unrecognized posterior medial bowing. Metabolic bone disease such as osteogenesis imperfecta rarely results in this type of bowing deformity.

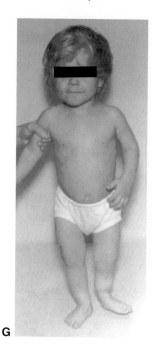

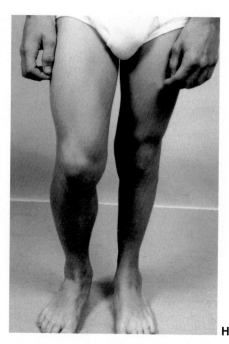

G · · · H · · · **Figure 28.37** (continued)

### Treatment

Initial treatment of infants is primarily passive stretching of the foot. Serial cast application may be used for severe deformities. The bowing generally corrects rapidly in the first few years (208–210). Rarely, extreme dorsiflexion and valgus persist such that plantigrade weight bearing cannot be accomplished. In such cases, a solid AFO may facilitate weight bearing for walking-aged children (211,212). As tibial length inequality increases, a shoe lift may be needed to balance the pelvis. Gradual contracture of the plantarflexors may occur as a compensation for leg-length discrepancy. Passive stretching is usually adequate treatment in young children.

Recently 43 patients with posterior medial bowing of the tibia were reviewed at the Shriners Hospital for Children in St. Louis. All had some degree of limb-length inequality. The minimum discrepancy was 1.4 cm at 1 month of age, and the projected difference at maturity ranged from 3 to 8 cm. Pes planovalgus that was seen in some children resulted in decreased foot height as well. This degree of inequality is best managed by surgical equalization, either by shortening the long tibia by epiphyseodesis or lengthening the short tibia. Residual valgus deformity can also be corrected. In the past 10 years, most patients have chosen lengthening and about half have had bi-level osteotomies to allow lengthening proximally and deformity correction distally. The others have been treated with epiphyseodesis, often preceded by proximal medial tibia hemiepiphyseal stapling to correct residual valgus deformity (209).

Appropriately timed epiphyseodesis has been used for differences as great as 4 to 5 cm. Shortening is usually confined to the tibia. Epiphyseodesis of the proximal tibia is usually sufficient. There are several techniques that can be employed. A staged hemiepiphysiodesis may be used to correct residual angulation prior to completion of the epiphyseodesis.

Lengthening techniques have been used for those children with projected discrepancies greater than 4 cm and for those with residual valgus angulation (Fig. 28.38). Lengthening alone in this group can exaggerate a valgus deformity, particularly when unilateral frames are used. Circular frame fixation allows better control of valgus (42,124). Bi-level osteotomies in the tibia (lengthening proximally, deformity correction distally) provide optimum management of both length and angulation. The foot may assume a varus position to compensate for residual tibial valgus and require modification of the frame if the foot deformity is rigid. Lengthening and deformity correction in our patients with posterior medial bowing has been successful, with few complications compared to procedures in children with other forms of congenital shortening.

## CONGENITAL DISLOCATION OF THE KNEE

### Definition

Congenital dislocation of the knee (CDK) is a relatively rare deformity that varies from simple hyperextension to anterior dislocation of the tibia on the femur. The spectrum of deformity in CDK has been classified as recurvatum, subluxation, and dislocation (213,214) (Fig. 28.39). The incidence of CDK is estimated at 1 per 100,000 live births,

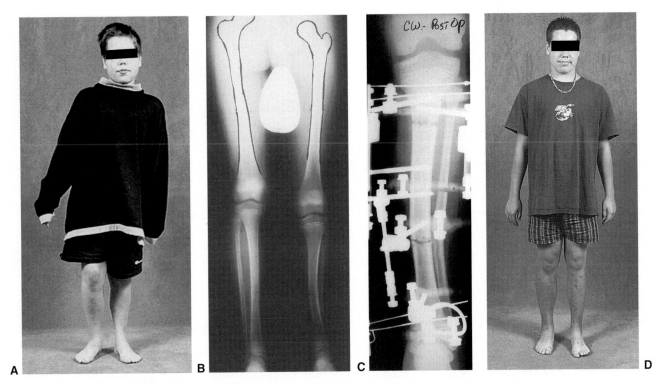

**Figure 28.38    A:** This 10-year-old boy had posteromedial bowing of the left tibia. He had 4.3 cm shortening and a 13% growth inhibition in the tibia. **B:** A long cassette radiograph demonstrates the limb-length inequality as well as the residual valgus in the distal tibia. **C:** A bi-level tibial osteotomy was performed. Residual valgus was corrected through the distal tibia, and limb-length equalization was accomplished with proximal lengthening. **D:** Valgus has been corrected and the pelvis balanced as shown in this follow-up photograph at 16 years of age.

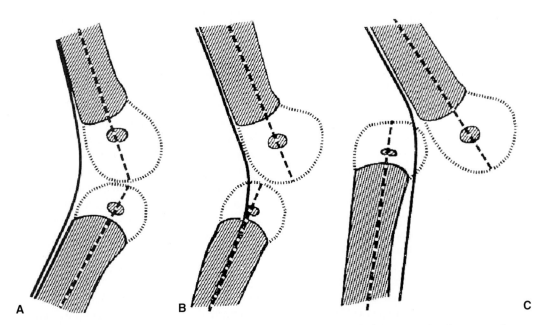

**Figure 28.39**    Congenital knee dislocation can range from simple hyperextension (recurvatum) **(A)** to subluxation to **(B)** complete anterior dislocation of the tibia on the femur **(C)**.

that is, 1% of the incidence of developmental hip dysplasia (215–217). Although there are some reports of occurrence within families, most cases are sporadic (218–220). The deformity may be unilateral or bilateral.

## Etiology

Several etiologic factors have been proposed for CDK. The familial occurrence suggests a possible genetic basis. CDK has also been seen in association with developmental hip dysplasia, idiopathic clubfoot, and congenital vertical talus (213–215,221). All of these have a genetic basis or polygenic mode of inheritance, which suggests a genetic link for CDK as well (213,215,222).

Milder forms of CDK occur in association with breech position *in utero*. In one study, 41% of otherwise healthy newborns with CDK were of breech presentation. These are generally believed to be positional, not pathologic deformities (215). Severe CDK often occurs in the presence of muscle imbalance and/or ligamentous laxity, such as that occurring in myelodysplasia, arthrogryposis, Larsen syndrome, and oligohydramnios (213,215,221,223).

Imbalance about the knee created by a relatively strong or contracted quadriceps muscle can, along with deficient hamstrings, lead to anterior dislocation of the knee. These infants typically have severe hyperextension *in utero* and, presumably, decreased fetal mobility. Chronic knee hyperextension results in anterior subluxation of the hamstrings, allowing them to function as knee extensors (224). The quadriceps muscle is short and contracted. Uhthoff and Ogata (225) were able to study a $19\frac{1}{2}$–week-old fetus with such a deformity. They found fibrosis of the quadriceps, absence of the suprapatellar pouch, and incomplete patellofemoral cavitation. The authors suggest that knee subluxation resulted from these abnormalities, intrinsic to the extensor mechanism, rather than from some secondary, extrinsic cause. The pathologic findings in this fetus are the same as those found in patients treated surgically.

## Clinical Presentation

The hyperextended knee deformity is obvious, but of variable severity (Fig. 28.40). In cases of subluxation, passive flexion is limited, but improves with splinting and gentle stretching. Milder forms, such as hyperextension or recurvatum, are usually isolated abnormalities. In the case of dislocation, there is inability to flex the knee actively or passively. The quadriceps tendon is often severely contracted. A dimple or deep crease may be present over the anterior aspect of the knee. The patella is difficult to palpate and often laterally displaced. Those with a more severe variant of CDK are more likely to have hip dysplasia and congenital foot deformities. When it occurs in association with a neuromuscular or genetic syndrome, CDK is typically very severe and difficult

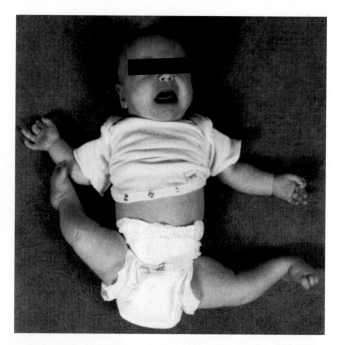

**Figure 28.40** This infant has bilateral anterior knee subluxation and clubfoot deformities. These deformities are often associated with intrauterine breech position. Deep skin creases are often found across the front of the knee. The skin may be dimpled posteriorly.

to manage (213,214,226,227). Radiographs help to differentiate the mild hyperextension deformity from the more severe type with fixed anterior dislocation of the tibia on the distal femur (Fig. 28.41).

## Nonoperative Treatment

Treatment begins with gentle stretching. The tibia is easily manipulated over the femoral condyle as flexion increases. Serial casts are used to hold the knee in flexion. They are changed every few days in neonates and then weekly as the knee position improves. This is followed by the use of removable splints to maintain flexion. Mild deformities may be treated with splinting alone. These knees often show rapid improvement in flexion. A Pavlik harness is useful for maintaining knee flexion achieved by stretching, splinting, or casting (228–230). The femoral condyles should be easily palpable once flexion beyond 90 degrees is achieved. Once this degree of flexion is obtained, it is unlikely that additional treatment will be needed. A lateral radiograph or ultrasound image of the knee can be obtained to document anatomic restoration of the femoral-tibial articulation.

In contrast, knees with more severe subluxation or dislocation do not respond to passive stretching or splinting. Traction has been suggested as a means to achieve gradual reduction (213,227,231). During attempted closed treatment, it is particularly important to document restoration of a normal relation of the tibia on the femur with a lateral knee radiograph. Ultrasound can also be used. It is possible to create an iatrogenic physeal separation of the distal femur or to deform the proximal tibia plastically. Rather,

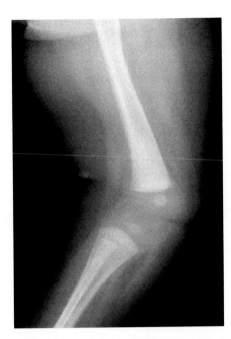

**Figure 28.41** A lateral radiograph differentiates among simple hyperextension, subluxation, and anterior dislocation. The anterior aspect of the knee is to the left. Note the deep skin crease anteriorly. The ossification center of the proximal tibial epiphysis is anterior to that of the distal femur. Serial lateral radiographs should be used to document anatomic reduction of the knee. Failure to achieve anatomic reduction by closed manipulation or inability to flex the knee more than 45 degrees are indications for surgical treatment.

the correction obtained must occur through the knee joint, allowing the tibia to translate on the femur. Closed treatment should be abandoned if appropriate reduction of the tibia cannot be confirmed.

## Operative Treatment

For infants whose knees fail to gain reduction of the anteriorly dislocated tibia on the end of the femur and therefore lack flexion, early surgical treatment at 1 to 2 months of age should be considered (217). As suggested by Roy and Crawford (221) this release is done through a variable limited incision in the distal thigh. The quadriceps tendon and adjacent medial and lateral retinaculum are transected as necessary to obtain both reduction and flexion of the tibia on the femur, followed by serial casting. Range-of-motion exercises, along with intermittent splinting in flexion or extension as needed, are used to maintain the reduction and knee mobility. These authors have reported favorable outcome from surgical treatment in these infants; however, our experience with this limited approach has been less satisfactory.

If left untreated, the quadriceps contracture rapidly becomes more severe and requires a more extensive release as the infant grows. Some authors have had success correcting moderate contractures using a simple V-Y advancement of the quadriceps tendon (213,214). This is insufficient for more severe dislocations that require greater lengthening of the quadriceps mechanism and release of contractures.

An extensile exposure from the distal half of the quadriceps mechanism to the patella is recommended to allow correction of this complex deformity. A serpentine incision extends from the proximal thigh to slightly past the tibial tubercle. This incision, rather than a straight incision, facilitates wound closure and results in fewer problems related to wound healing. Subcutaneous flaps are raised to expose the quadriceps mechanism. In these cases of severe contracture, fibrosis and scarring of the muscle is more extensive. It may be adherent to the periosteum of the femur. The patella is usually very small and often laterally displaced. The extensor mechanism is usually malrotated and pulls the tibia into valgus. The quadriceps mechanism requires considerable lengthening, yet it must remain attached both proximally and distally. The release requires extensive dissection through fibrotic tissue. The quadriceps tendon is lengthened using a long Z-plasty or V-Y advancement, depending on the degree of quadriceps contracture present (213,214). The capsule of the anterior knee joint is released transversely to the collateral ligaments, which often must be reflected and/or partially released. The knee can usually be flexed to 90 degrees following this release. Occasionally the medial hamstrings, iliotibial band, and the lateral intermuscular septum must be released to correct valgus and external rotational deformity (217). The cruciate ligaments are typically present but may be attenuated (213,214,222,224). The authors have not found it necessary to release the cruciates to gain flexion. The elongated quadriceps mechanism, which may be tenuous in these infants, is repaired with the knee in approximately 30 degrees of flexion (213,217,224). A spica cast is used for immobilization, with the knee placed in enough flexion (approximately 45 degrees) to prevent recurrent tibial subluxation (215,217). Too much flexion jeopardizes the quadriceps mechanism repair and potentiates necrosis of the skin and subcutaneous tissue (213). Long-term orthotic splinting and range-of-motion exercises are essential to maintain maximal flexion and minimize loss of extension. A knee flexion contracture can be more debilitating than a lack of full flexion.

Treatment of an ipsilateral hip dislocation is performed either at the time of reduction of the knee dislocation or later as a staged procedure. Following release of the contracted quadriceps mechanism, the knee can be flexed, facilitating treatment of the hip (213–215,217). Mild hip dysplasia, which is amenable to simple closed reduction or limited open reduction using a medial approach, can be treated concurrently with the spica cast utilized to immobilize a surgically reduced CDK. More severe hip dysplasia, which requires open reduction by an anterior approach, should be done later. If a coexisting foot deformity requires operative treatment, this can be staged or done in conjunction with the knee reconstruction. Knee flexion facilitates cast application necessary for the treatment of associated foot deformities.

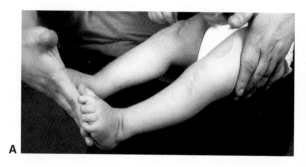
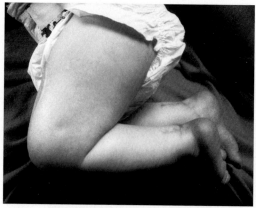

**Figure 28.42   A:** The upper photo shows knee extension following open reduction of these bilateral knee deformities. Hyperextension is no longer evident. **B:** Knee flexion greater than 90 degrees has been accomplished. Range-of-motion exercises and intermittent use of orthotics may be needed to maintain this correction.

The long-term outcome of treatment is generally good. Those who have had hyperextension or mild dislocation and required only stretching and minimal intervention as infants have the best results. They do not report problems later on. Function is excellent and radiographs appear nearly normal (216,226,229,230). Children with more severe dislocation who required an open reduction, but do not have any other musculoskeletal problems, generally do well (Fig. 28.42). In these patients knee range of motion includes full to nearly full extension and flexion that averages 80 to 120 degrees. This allows very functional, independent ambulation, and participation in most normal play activities; however, activities such as running or bicycling, which requires flexion beyond 90 degrees, may be limited. Radiographic abnormalities are found in some, but not all knees. This usually consists of flattening of the femoral and tibial articular contours (213,215).

Those with bilateral deformity do not do as well as those with unilateral deformity. These also tend to be children with associated neuromuscular disorders. Early repair generally has a more satisfactory functional result than late repair (213,215,221). Recurrent hyperextension deformity is not likely. However, loss of flexion, particularly that gained at surgery, can be a late complication. Similarly, the development of a flexion contracture can compromise long-term function.

## IDIOPATHIC TOE-WALKING

### Definition

Children may present at any age with a history of toe-walking. The habit of doing so is not that uncommon or abnormal in 2- to 3-year-old children. Typically, the habitual toe-walkers, with coaxing, can walk plantar grade. By the age of three, children should walk with a heel strike (6,232,233). Persistent toe-walking beyond this age is abnormal.

### Etiology

A toe-toe gait is often observed in children when they first begin weight bearing. If the toe-walking persists, a contracture develops and worsens over time. In the child who is otherwise neurologically normal, toe-walking may be associated with a shortened heel cord; however, this is generally not recognized at birth or within the first year (234–236).

### Natural History

Very little is known about the natural history of idiopathic toe-walking (ITW). Stricker and Angulo (236) retrospectively reviewed 80 patients who were evaluated and treated for ITW. Forty-eight of the 80 patients, generally those with the mildest deformity, were observed without treatment from ages 3 years to 6 years. The degree of heel cord contracture was mild and remained essentially unchanged in these patients. Only 25% of parents noted a spontaneous improvement; that is, appreciably less toe-walking. For the children with more than 5 degrees of passive dorsiflexion, persistent toe-walking is not a functional problem and does not result in any foot deformity or pain. For many patients, toe-walking either diminishes or ceases with time. This may occur as the body mass becomes too large to be supported by the triceps surae or as a result of secondary development of external tibial torsion (235). The development of a mid-foot break to permit foot contact with the floor is frequently seen in neuromuscular conditions, but is not typically seen in ITW (14).

### Clinical Features

Patients typically present to the orthopaedist for evaluation of ITW at 3 to 4 years of age (236). The condition predominates in the male sex, and the family history (siblings and generation to generation) is often positive for similar ITW persisting into adulthood (234,236,237).

The suggested inheritance pattern is autosomal dominant with variable penetrance (238,239). Although Stricker et al. (236) noted a frequent history of both prematurity and developmental delay, walking was not delayed. On examination, ITW occurs bilaterally and is best seen when the child is walking barefoot (Fig. 28.43). When the child stands still, the feet may be flat on the ground. With time, toeing-out and splaying of the forefoot frequently occur. Idiopathic toe-walkers, in contrast to children with spastic diplegia, do not have a tendency to walk with a back-knee thrust in order to achieve foot flat position.

On bench examination, the range of passive ankle plantar flexion will be normal and dorsiflexion will be limited, secondary to a variable degree of true shortening of the heel cord (234). The posterior calf muscles are typically very well developed; in fact, they may appear to be enlarged. However, the muscle texture will feel normal on examination and there will be no evidence of any weakness, proximal or distal, in the upper or lower extremities. Importantly, no spasticity is present and clonus will not be elicited by a rapid stretch of the triceps surae. The diagnosis of ITW is a diagnosis of exclusion, and typically can be made from the child's history and physical examination (234,237,240–242).

## Differential Diagnosis

The differential diagnosis of early-onset toe-walking includes neuromuscular etiologies such as spastic diplegia (236,237,243). ITW that develops in a child with a previously normal gait must be differentiated from primary muscle diseases such as muscular dystrophy, myotonic dystrophy, dystonia, and tethered cord syndrome, and from central nervous system (CNS) neoplastic processes (236,237). Further evaluation by a neurologist may be indicated to exclude such consequential neuromuscular diagnoses.

Usually, the diagnosis of ITW is made without computerized gait analysis or dynamic electromyograph (EMG);

however, an EMG may be helpful if it is essential to differentiate between ITW and spastic diplegia (235,240–243). Children with mild cerebral palsy who walk on their toes often have out-of-phase gastrocnemius soleus muscle activity, whereas idiopathic toe-walkers will be in phase (242,243). Both groups show lack of heel strike. Children with mild diplegia show greater sustained knee flexion at terminal swing. Maximal knee extension occurs at ground contact for idiopathic toe-walkers and at mid-to-late stance for diplegics (240). In the ITW gait, ankle dorsiflexion occurs early in maximal swing, followed by plantar flexion. Ankle dorsiflexion occurs throughout swing in diplegics.

## Nonoperative Treatment

The treatment of ITW begins with instructions given to the parents regarding the importance of a long-term commitment to assisting the child with both heel cord stretching and dorsiflexion strengthening exercises. This is particularly true in early childhood, when stretching exercises are more likely to make a difference. It is important to maintain inversion of the hindfoot to optimize stretch of the heel cord. If the calcaneus is allowed to evert, the forefoot will be allowed to dorsiflex independent of the hindfoot and create a mid-foot break without effectively stretching the heel cord. A 3- to 4-month course of twice daily dorsiflexion manipulations may be effective in obtaining increased dorsiflexion. The response to treatment varies with the duration and severity of the equinus deformity and compliance with the exercise regimen. Clinical improvement will be sustained with continued daily heel cord stretching exercises and active dorsiflexion strengthening exercises supplemented with orthotics. An articulated AFO with a plantar-flexion stop and free dorsiflexion is used to maintain position.

If toe-walking persists, serial heel cord dorsiflexion casts should be considered. Predictably, stretching casts will be more effective when there is a "springy" rather than a firm

**Figure 28.43** **A:** Children with idiopathic toe-walking assume an externally rotated posture to facilitate a foot flat position. They typically do not hyperextend the knee. **B:** While up on their toes, the heel moves to a varus position. Chronic toe-walking can cause the forefoot to splay because of the overload of the intermetatarsal ligaments. Forefoot splay and tibial external rotation typically do not resolve after heel cord lengthening.

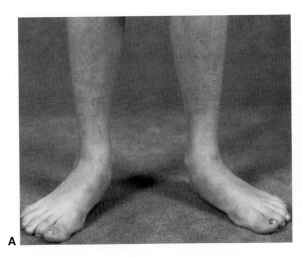
**A**

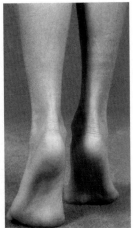
**B**

feel of maximal heel cord stretch during foot dorsiflexion. The casts are applied with the foot maximally dorsiflexed and the heel in a neutral position or slightly inverted. Flexing the knee or prone positioning facilitates placement of the cast. A series of two or three sets of short-leg casts will often elongate the heel cord and result in greater passive dorsiflexion. This immobilization also produces short-term weakness. The combination of stretch and slight weakness usually produces a marked decrease in the tendency to toe-walk. After casting, articulated AFOs with plantar-flexion stops are used full time, and the heel cord stretching and dorsiflexion-strengthening regimen is resumed. If dorsiflexion can be maintained for 3 to 6 months, the children are weaned from daytime use. Nighttime splinting can be discontinued if there is no recurrence of the toe-walking. Although serial casting and subsequent orthotic usage is widely recommended, very little is known of its long-term effectiveness (241). This approach will often be successful in younger patients (younger than 4 years), and even in some of the older patients. However, relapse is common due to lack of compliance, often requiring repeat serial casting, AFO use, or surgical treatment. Compliance with a comprehensive program of heel cord stretching, dorsiflexor strengthening, and bracing is essential for long-term success.

## Operative Treatment

If the use of serial stretching casts does not realize a satisfactory clinical improvement in the tendency to toe-walk, then heel cord lengthening procedures will be necessary to effect a change in gait (234,236). Age also becomes an important determinant in treatment recommendations. The authors feel that by 6 to 7 years of age, children should have improved sufficiently to consistently demonstrate a normal heel-toe, rather than toe-heel or toe-toe gait. Far too often, parents are inappropriately advised that ITW will resolve on its own. In fact, toe-walking after 6 years of age often does not improve, and the heel cord contracture slowly worsens.

Persistent toe-walking secondary to a heel cord contracture can potentiate both forefoot splay and a disproportionately wide forefoot compared to the heel. Standard footwear may not accommodate the wide forefoot and narrow heel. External tibial torsion frequently develops to compensate for the lack of foot flat contact. This external tibial torsion deformity becomes more obvious once the heel cord has been lengthened. It may be severe enough to warrant corrective osteotomy.

The heel cord lengthening can be done by a variety of techniques. The authors prefer performing a fractional lengthening at the junction of the middle and distal thirds of the triceps surae complex if the foot can be brought to neutral with the knee flexed. Lengthening is performed sufficient to obtain 10 degrees of dorsiflexion with the knee

extended. In some, release of the posterior ankle capsule may be necessary. Short-leg walking casts are used for 5 to 6 weeks, then the child is fitted with AFOs, which are used 22 of 24 hours for 4 to 6 weeks, then gradually weaned during daytime but used at night for up to 6 months postoperatively. Heel cord stretching and ankle strengthening exercises are performed twice daily.

Surgical correction predictably has a satisfactory outcome. Generally, parents are very satisfied with the improved gait following heel cord lengthening; however, the parents need to be well informed as to the anticipated postoperative course. The child's postoperative gait (relatively weak plantar flexor power) will be considerably different from the preoperative gait (relatively strong plantar flexion power). The predominately equinus gait is replaced by a gait with relatively weak push off. Quick cadence is replaced by a slower cadence gait. It takes time for the push-off power to recover to near normal levels (234). Younger children regain a relatively normal gait pattern soon after weaning from orthotics, whereas those older than 8 years at the time of surgical treatment may take a year or more to normalize their gait. Hall et al. (234), at an average length of follow-up of 3 years following heel cord lengthening, reported a satisfactory outcome for all 20 patients. In a review of all treatment methods, Stricker and Angulo (236) noted that surgical lengthening of the heel cord was the only treatment that permanently improved ankle dorsiflexion. Although 33 of 56 patients still exhibited some degree of toe-walking, most parents were satisfied with the outcome of heel cord lengthening. A study by Stott et al. (244) of toe-walkers evaluated at skeletal maturity concluded that, although kinematic studies continued to demonstrate some gait abnormalities, no abnormalities were apparent clinically.

## REFERENCES

### Rotational Variation

1. Engel GM, Staheli LT. The natural history of torsion and other factors influencing gait in childhood. *Clin Orthop Relat Res* 1974;99:12.
2. Hensinger RN. *Standards in orthopedics*. New York: Raven Press, 1986.
3. Staheli LT, Corbett M, Wyss C, et al. Lower-extremity rotational problems in children. Normal values to guide management. *J Bone Joint Surg Am* 1985;67:39.
4. Staheli LT. Rotational problems in children. In: Schafer M, ed. *AAOS Instructional Course Lecture Volume 43*. Rosemont, IL: American Academy of Orthopaedic Surgeons, 1994:199.
5. Kling TF, Hensinger RN. Angular and torsional deformities of the lower limbs in children. *Clin Orthop Relat Res* 1983;176:136.
6. Sutherland DH, Olshen R, Cooper L, et al. The development of mature gait. *J Bone Joint Surg Am* 1980;62:336.
7. Walker JM. Comparison of normal and abnormal human fetal hip joints: a quantitative study with significance to congenital hip disease. *J Pediatr Orthop* 1983;3:173.
8. Watanabe RS. Embryology of the human hip. *Clin Orthop Relat Res* 1974;98:8.
9. Fabry G, MacEwen GD, Shands AR Jr. Torsion of the femur. A follow-up study in normal and abnormal conditions. *J Bone Joint Surg Am* 1973;55:1726.

10. Fabry G, Cheng LX, Molenaers G. Normal and abnormal torsional development in children. *Clin Orthop Relat Res* 1994; 302:22.

11. Sutherland DH. Varus foot in cerebral palsy: an overview. In: Heckman JD, ed. *AAOS Instructional Course Lecture Volume 42*. Rosemont, IL: American Academy of Orthopaedic Surgeons, 1993:539.

12. Vaughan CL, Nashman JH, Murr MS. What is the normal function of tibialis posterior in human gait. In: Sussman MD, ed. *The Diplegic Child Shriners Hospitals for Crippled Children Symposium*. Rosemont, IL: American Academy of Orthopaedic Surgeons, 1992:397.

13. Stefko RM, deSwart RJ, Dodgin DA, et al. Kinematic and kinetic analysis of distal derotational osteotomy of the leg in children with cerebral palsy. *J Pediatr Orthop* 1998;18:81.

14. Mazur JM, Shanks DE, Cummings RJ. Nonsurgical treatment of tight Achilles tendon. In: Sussman MD, ed. The Diplegic Child Shriners Hospitals for Crippled Children Symposium. Rosemont, IL: American Academy of Orthopaedic Surgeons, 1992:343.

15. Luhmann SJ, Rich MM, Schoenecker PL. Painful idiopathic rigid flatfoot in children and adolescents. *Foot Ankle Int* 2000; 21:59.

16. Pritchett JW, Perdue KD. Mechanical factors in slipped capital femoral epiphysis. *J Pediatr Orthop* 1988;8:385.

17. Murphy SB, Simon SR, Kijewski PK, et al. Femoral anteversion. *J Bone Joint Surg Am* 1987;69:1169.

18. Staheli LT. Footwear for children. In: Schafer M, ed. *AAOS Instructional Course Lecture Volume 43*. Rosemont, IL: American Academy of Orthopaedic Surgeons, 1994:193.

19. Hubbard DD, Staheli LT, Chew DE, et al. Medial femoral torsion and osteoarthritis. *J Pediatr Orthop* 1988;8:540.

20. Wedge JH, Munkacsi I, Loback D. Anteversion of the femur and idiopathic osteoarthrosis of the hip. *J Bone Joint Surg Am* 1989; 71:1040.

21. Eckhoff DG, Montgomery WK, Kilcoyne RF, et al. Femoral morphometry and anterior knee pain. *Clin Orthop Relat Res* 1994; 302:64.

22. Tonnis D, Heinecke A. Diminished femoral antetorsion syndrome: a cause of pain and osteoarthritis. *J Pediatr Orthop* 1991; 11:419.

23. Kiaoka HB, Weiner DS, Cook AJ, et al. Relationship between femoral anteversion and osteoarthritis of the hip. *J Pediatr Orthop* 1989;9:396.

24. Reikeras O, Hoiseth A. Femoral neck angles in osteoarthritis of the hip. *Acta Orthop Scand* 1982;53:781.

25. Eckhoff DE, Kramer RC, Alongi CA, et al. Femoral anteversion and arthritis of the knee. *J Pediatr Orthop* 1994;14:608.

26. Delgado ED, Schoenecker PL, Rich MM, et al. Treatment of severe torsional malalignment syndrome. *J Pediatr Orthop* 1996; 255:184.

27. Eckhoff DG. Effect of limb malrotation on malalignment and osteoarthritis. *Orthop Clin North Am* 1994;25:405.

28. Paley D. *Principles of Deformity Correction*. New York: Springer-Verlag, 2002.

29. Staheli LT, Lippert F, Denotter P. Femoral anteversion and physical performance in adolescent and adult life. *Clin Orthop Relat Res* 1977;129:213.

30. Bauman PA, Singson R, Hamilton WG. Femoral neck anteversion in ballerinas. *Clin Orthop Relat Res* 1994;302:57.

31. Fuchs R, Staheli LT. Sprinting and intoeing. *J Pediatr Orthop* 1996;16:489.

32. Dodgin DA, deSwart RJ, Stefko RM, et al. Distal tibial/fibular derotation osteotomy for correction of tibial torsion: review of technique and results in 63 cases. *J Pediatr Orthop* 1998; 18:95.

33. Payne LZ, DeLuca PA. Intertrochanteric versus supracondylar osteotomy for severe femoral anteversion. *J Pediatr Orthop* 1994; 14:39.

34. Bruce WD, Stevens PM. Surgical correction of miserable malalignment syndrome. *J Pediatr Orthop* 2004;24:392.

35. Takai S, Sakakida F, Yamashita F, et al. Rotational alignment of the lower limb in osteoarthritis of the knee. *Int Orthop* 1985;9: 209.

36. Turner MS, Smillie IS. The effect of tibial torsion on the pathology of the knee. *J Bone Joint Surg Br* 1981;63:396.

37. Slawski DP, Schoenecker PL, Rich MM. Peroneal nerve injury as a complication of pediatric tibial osteotomies: a review of 345 osteotomies. *J Pediatr Orthop* 1994;14:166.

38. Staheli LT. The lower limb. In: Morrissy RT, ed. *Lovell and Winter's Pediatric Orthopedics*, 3rd ed. Philadelphia, PA: JB Lippincott, 1990:741.

39. Winquist RA. Closed intramedullary osteotomies of the femur. *Clin Orthop Relat Res* 1986;212:155.

40. Gordon JE, Goldfarb CA, Luhmann SJ, et al. Femoral lengthening over a humeral intramedullary nail in preadolescent children. *J Bone Joint Surg Am* 2002;84:930.

41. Herzenberg JE, Smith JD, Paley D. Correcting torsional deformities with Ilizarov's apparatus. *Clin Orthop Relat Res* 1994; 302:36.

42. Catagni MA. Current trends in the treatment of simple and complex bone deformities using the Ilizarov method. In: Eilert RE, ed. *AAOS Instructional Course Lecture Volume 41*. Rosemont, IL: American Academy of Orthopaedic Surgeons, 1992:423.

43. Greene WB. Displaced fractures of the femoral shaft in children. Unique features and therapeutic options. *Clin Orthop Relat Res* 1998;353:86.

44. Beaty JH, Austin SM, Warner WC, et al. Interlocking intramedullary nailing of femoral-shaft fractures in adolescents: preliminary results and complications. *J Pediatr Orthop* 1994; 14:178.

## Physiologic Bowing and Genu Varum

45. Reinker K. Etiology of Blount's disease. The Pediatric Orthopaedic Society of North America 28th Annual Meeting, Orlando, FL, May 16, 1999.

46. Golding JSR, McNeil-Smith JDG. Observations on the etiology of tibia vara. *J Bone Joint Surg Br* 1963;45:320.

47. Langenskiold A, Riska EB. Tibia vara (osteochondrosis deformans tibiae) a survey of seventy-one cases. *J Bone Joint Surg Am* 1964;46: 1405.

48. Bathfield CA, Beighton PH. Blount's disease. A review of etiological factors in 110 patients. *Clin Orthop Relat Res* 1978;135:29.

49. Salenius P, Vankka E. The development of the tibiofemoral angle in children. *J Bone Joint Surg Am* 1975;57:259.

50. Greene WB. Infantile tibia vara. *J Bone Joint Surg Am* 1993;75:130.

51. Levine AM, Drennan JC. Physiological bowing and tibia vara. The metaphyseal-diaphyseal angle in the measurement of bowleg deformities. *J Bone Joint Surg Am* 1982;64:1158.

52. Schoenecker PL, Meade WC, Pierron RL, et al. Blount's disease: a retrospective review and recommendations for treatment. *J Pediatr Orthop* 1985;5:181.

53. Johnston CE II. Infantile tibia vara. *Clin Orthop Relat Res* 1990; 255:13.

54. Bowen RE, Dorey FJ, Moseley CF. Relative tibial and femoral varus as a predictor of progression of varus deformities of the lower limbs in young children. *J Pediatr Orthop* 2002;22:105.

55. Bateson EM. The relationship between Blount's disease and bow legs. *Brit J Radio* 1968;41:107.

56. Feldman MD, Schoenecker PL. Use of the metaphyseal-diaphyseal angle in the evaluation of bowed legs. *J Bone Joint Surg Am* 1993;75:1602.

57. Bashner BC, Israelite CL, Betz RR, et al. Reliable early radiographic differentiation of infantile Blount's disease and physiologic bowing: utilizing the ratio of the femoral and tibial metaphyseal-diaphyseal angles. *Ortho Trans* 1991;15:27.

58. Auerbach JD, Radomisli TE, Simoncini J, et al. Variability of the metaphyseal-diaphyseal angle in tibia vara. A comparison of two methods. *J Pediatr Orthop* 2004;24:75.

59. Glorieux FH. Hypophosphatemic vitamin D-resistant rickets. In: Favus MJ, ed. *Primer on the metabolic bone disease and disorders of mineral metabolism*, 4th ed. Philadelphia, PA: Lippincott Williams & Wilkins, 1999:328.

60. Petersen DJ, Boniface AM, Schranck FW, et al. X-linked hypophosphatemic rickets: a study (with literature review) of linear growth response to calcitriol and phosphate therapy. *J Bone Miner Res* 1992;7:583.

61. Kugler JL, Schoenecker PL. A 19-month-old female with unilateral bowed leg. *Orthop Rev* 1993;22:108.
62. Bell SN, Campbell PE, Cole WG, et al. Tibia vara caused by focal Fibrocartilaginous dysplasia, three case reports. *J Bone Joint Surg Br* 1985;67:780.
63. Bradish CF, Davies SJM, Malone M. Tibia vara due to focal fibrocartilaginous dysplasia, the natural history. *J Bone Joint Surg Br* 1988;70:106.
64. Olney BW, Cole WG, Menelaus MB. Case report, three additional case of focal fibrocartilaginous dysplasia causing tibia vara. *J Pediatr Orthop* 1990;10:405.
65. Ozonoff MB. *The lower extremity in pediatric orthopedic radiology*, 2nd ed. Philadelphia, PA: WB Saunders, 1992.
66. Beatty JH, Barrett IR. Unilateral angular deformity of the distal end of the femur secondary to a focal fibrous tether: a report of four cases. *J Bone Joint Surg Am* 1989;71:440.
67. Blount WP. Tibia vara, osteochondrosis deformans tibiae. *J Bone Joint Surg* 1937;19:1.
68. Gordon JE, Schoenecker PL, Luhmann SE, Rich MM. Distal femoral deformity in children with tibia vara. American Association for Orthopaedic Surgeons' Annual Meeting, San Francisco, CA, March, 2004.
69. Langenskiold A. Tibia vara (osteochondrosis deformans tibiae) a survey of 23 cases. *Acta Chir Scand* 1952;103:1.
70. Langenskiold A. Tibia vara: osteochondrosis deformans tibiae Blount's disease. *Clin Orthop Relat Res* 1981;158:77.
71. Langenskiold A. Tibia vara, A critical review. *Clin Orthop Relat Res* 1989;246:195.
72. Richards BS, Katz DE, Sims JB. Effectiveness of brace treatment in early infantile Blount's disease. *J Pediatr Orthop* 1998;18:374.
73. Zionts LE, Shean CJ. Brace treatment of early infantile tibia vara. *J Pediatr Orthop* 1998;18:102.
74. Raney EM, Topoleski TA, Yaghoubian R, et al. Orthotic treatment of infantile tibia vara. *J Pediatr Orthop* 1998;18:670.
75. Hansson LI, Zayer M. Physiological genu varum. *Acta Orthop Scand* 1975;46:221.
76. Ferriter P, Shapiro F. Infantile tibia vara: Factors affecting outcome following proximal tibial osteotomy. *J Pediatr Orthop* 1987;7:1.
77. Arkin AM, Katz JF. The effects of pressure on epiphyseal growth. The mechanism of plasticity of growing bone. *J Bone Joint Surg Am* 1956;38:1056.
78. Smith CF. Current concepts review tibia vara (Blount's disease). *J Bone Joint Surg Am* 1982;64:630.
79. Cook SD, Lavernia CJ, Burke SW, et al. A biomechanical analysis of the etiology of tibia vara. *J Pediatr Orthop* 1983;3:449.
80. Kessel L. Annotations on the etiology and treatment of tibia vara. *J Bone Joint Surg Br* 1970;52:93.
81. Evensen A, Steffensen J. Tibia vara (osteochondrosis deformans tibiae). *Acta Orthop Scand* 1957;26:200.
82. Sibert JR, Bray PT. Probable dominant inheritance in Blount's disease. *Clin Genet* 1977;11:394.
83. Kline SC, Bostrum M, Griffin PP. Femoral varus: An important component in late-onset Blount's disease. *J Pediatr Orthop* 1992;12:197.
84. Supant M. Orthotic correction of Blount's. *Clin Orth Prosth* 1985;9:3.
85. Steel HH, Sandrow RE, Sullivan PD. Complications of tibial osteotomy in children for genu varum or valgum. *J Bone Joint Surg Am* 1971;53:1629.
86. Schrock RD. Peroneal nerve palsy following derotation osteotomies for tibial torsion. *Clin Orthop Relat Res* 1969;62:172.
87. Dietz FR, Weinstein SL. Spike osteotomy for angular deformities of the long bones in children. *J Bone Joint Surg Am* 1988;70:848.
88. Morrissy RT. *Atlas of pediatric orthopaedic surgery.* Philadelphia, PA: JB Lippincott, 1992.
89. Rab GT. Technique, oblique tibial osteotomy for Blount's disease (tibia vara). *J Pediatr Orthop* 1988;8:715.
90. Accadbled F, Laville J-M, Harper L. One-step treatment for evolved Blount's disease. Four cases and review of the literature. *J Pediatr Orthop* 2003;23:747.
91. Price CT, Scott DS, Greenberg DA. Dynamic axial external fixation in the surgical treatment of tibia vara. *J Pediatr Orthop* 1995;15:236.
92. Davidson RS. Epiphyseal deformity of infantile Blount's disease. The Pediatric Orthopaedic Society of North America 28th Annual Meeting, Orlando, FL, May 16, 1999.
93. Matsen FA, Staheli LT. Neurovascular complication following tibial osteotomy in children, a case report. *Clin Orthop Relat Res* 1975;110:210.
94. Van Olm JMJ, Gillespie R. Proximal tibial osteotomy for angular knee deformities in children. *J Bone Joint Surg Br* 1984;66:301.
95. Stanitski DF, Dahl MT, Louie K, et al. Management of late-onset tibia vara in the obese patient by using circular external fixation. *J Pediatr Orthop* 1997;17:691.
96. Matsen FA, Veith RG. Compartmental syndrome in children. *J Pediatr Orthop* 1981;1:33.
97. Zuege RC, Kempken TG, Blount WP. Epiphyseal stapling for angular deformity at the knee. *J Bone Joint Surg Am* 1979;61:320.
98. Mielke CH, Stevens PM. Hemiepiphyseal stapling for knee deformities in children younger than 10 years: a preliminary report. *J Pediatr Orthop* 1996;16:423.
99. Birch JG. Surgical technique of physeal bar resection. In: Eilert R, ed. *AAOS Instructional Course Lecture Volume 41.* Rosemont, IL: American Academy of Orthopaedic Surgeons, 1992;445.
100. Birch JG, Lapinsky AS. Results of partial physeal bar resection in patients with Langenskiold stage VI infantile Blount's disease, POSNA, Memphis, Tennessee 1994.
101. Herring JA. Instructional case, Blount disease. *J Pediatr Orthop* 1987;7:601.
102. Beck CL, Burke SW, Roberts JM, Johnston CE. Physeal bridge resection in infantile Blount disease. *J Pediatr Orthop* 1987;7:161.
103. Doyle BS, Vok AG, Smith CF. Infantile Blount disease: long-term follow-up of surgically treated patients at skeletal maturity. *J Pediatr Orthop* 1996;16:469.
104. Hoffman A, Jones RE, Herring JA. Blount's disease after skeletal maturity. *J Bone Joint Surg Am* 1982;64:1004.
105. Schoenecker PL, Johnston R, Rich MM, et al. Elevation of the medial plateau of the tibia in the treatment of Blount disease. *J Bone Joint Surg Am* 1992;74:351.
106. Gregosiewicz A, Wosko I, Kandzierski G, et al. Double elevating osteotomy of tibia in the treatment of severe cases of Blount's disease. *J Pediatr Orthop* 1989;9:178.
107. Siffert R. Intraepiphyseal osteotomy for progressive tibia vara: case report and rationale of management. *J Pediatr Orthop* 1982;2:81.
108. Davids JR, Huskamp M, Bagley AM. A dynamic biomechanical analysis of the etiology of adolescent tibia vara. *J Pediatr Orthop* 1996;16:461.
109. Henderson RC, Greene WB. Etiology of late-onset tibia vara: is varus alignment a prerequisite? *J Pediatr Orthop* 1994;14:143.
110. Thompson GH, Carter JR. Late-onset tibia vara (Blount's disease) current concepts. *Clin Orthop Relat Res* 1990;255:24.
111. Wenger DR, Mickelson M, Maynard JA. The evolution and histopathology of adolescent tibia vara. *J Pediatr Orthop* 1984;4:78.
112. Loder RT, Schaffer JJ, Bardenstein MB. Late-onset tibia vara. *J Pediatr Orthop* 1991;11:162.
113. Beskin JL, Burke SW, Johnston CE II, et al. Clinical basis for a mechanical etiology in adolescent Blount's disease. *Orthopedics* 1986;9:365.
114. Carter JR, Leeson MC, Thompson GH, et al. Late-onset tibia vara: a histopathologic analysis. A comparative evaluation with infantile tibia vara and slipped capital femoral epiphysis. *J Pediatr Orthop* 1988;8:187.
115. Lovejoy JF, Lovell WW. Adolescent tibia vara associated with slipped capital femoral epiphysis. *J Bone Joint Surg Am* 1970;52:361.
116. Dietz WH, Gross WL, Kirkpatrick JA Jr. Blount's disease (tibia vara): another skeletal disorder. *J Pediatr* 1982;101:735.
117. Henderson RC, Kemp GJ, Greene WB. Adolescent tibia vara: alternatives for operative treatment. *J Bone Joint Surg Am* 1992;74-A:342.
118. Henderson RC, Kemp GJ, Hayes PR. Prevalence of late-onset tibia vara. *J Pediatr Orthop* 1993;13:255.
119. Paley D, Tetsworth K. Mechanical axis deviation of the lower limbs. Preoperative planning of multiapical frontal plane angular and bowing deformities of the tibia or femur. *Clin Orthop Relat Res* 1992;280:65.
120. Paley D, Herzenberg J, Tetsworth K. Deformity planning for frontal and sagittal plane corrective osteotomies. *Orthop Clin North Am* 1994;25:425.

121. Gordon JE, Heidenreich FP, Comprehensive treatment of late onset tibia vara. *J Bone Joint Surg Am* 2005; 87:1561..

122. Taussig & Landau. *Textbook of pediatric medicine*. St. Louis, MO: Mosby, 1999.

123. Ferrick MR, Birch JG, Albright M. Correction of non-Blount's angular knee deformity by permanent hemiepiphyseodesis. *J Pediatr Orthop* 2004;24:397.

124. Paley D, Tetsworth K. Mechanical axis deviation of the lower limbs. Preoperative planning of uniapical angular deformities of the tibia or femur. *Clin Orthop Relat Res* 1992;280:65.

125. Millis MB. Juvenile/adolescent Blount's disease: treatment with osteotomy and internal fixation. The Pediatric Orthopaedic Society North America 28th Annual Meeting, Orlando, FL May 16, 1999.

126. Martin SD, Moran MC, Martin TL, et al. Proximal tibial osteotomy with compression plate fixation for tibia vara. *J Pediatr Orthop* 1994;14:619.

127. Jakob RP, Murphy SB. Tibial osteotomy for varus gonarthrosis: indication, planning, and operative technique. In: Eilert R, ed. *AAOS Instructional Course Lecture*, Vol. 41. Rosemont, IL: American Academy of Orthopaedic Surgeons, 1992;87.

128. Gaudinez R, Adar U. Use of orthofix T-garche fixator in late-onset tibia vara. *J Pediatr Orthop* 1996;16:455.

129. Stanitski DF, Srivastava P, Stanitski CL. Correction of proximal tibial deformities in adolescents with the T-garche external fixator. *J Pediatr Orthop* 1998;18:512.

130. Gordon JE. Treatment of Blount's disease using the Taylor spatial frame. The Pediatric Orthopaedic Society of North America 28th Annual Meeting, Orlando, FL May 16, 1999.

131. Coogan PG, Fox JA, Fitch RD. Treatment of adolescent Blount disease with the circular external fixation device and distraction osteogenesis. *J Pediatr Orthop* 1996;16:450.

## Knock-Knees and Genu Valgum

132. Heath CH, Staheli LT. Normal limits of knee angle in white children. *J Pediatr Orthop* 1993;13:259.

133. Green WB. Genu varum and genu valgum in children. In: Schafer M, ed. *AAOS Instructional Course Lectures*, Vol. 43. Rosemont, IL: American Academy of Orthopaedic Surgeons, 1994;151.

134. White GR, Mencio GA. Genu valgum in children. Diagnostic and therapeutic alternatives. *J Am Acad Orthop Surg* 1995;3:275.

135. Shim JS, Kim HT, Mubarak SJ, et al. Genu valgum in children with coxa vara resulting from hip disease. *J Pediatr Orthop* 1997; 17:225.

136. Kopits SE. Orthopedic complications of dwarfism. *Clin Orthop Relat Res* 1976;114:153.

137. Herring JA, Moseley C. Posttraumatic valgus deformity of the tibia. *J Pediatr Orthop* 1981;1:435.

138. Herring JA, Kling TF. Genu valgus. *J Pediatr Orthop* 1985;5:236.

139. McCarthy JJ, Kim DH, Eilert RE. Posttraumatic genu valgum: operative versus nonoperative treatment. *J Pediatr Orthop* 1998;18:518.

140. Ruchelsman DE, Madan SS, Feldman DS. Genu valgum secondary to focal fibrocartilaginous dysplasia of the distal femur. *J Pediatr Orthop* 2004;24:408.

141. Stevens PM, MacWilliams B, Mohr RA. Gait analysis of stapling for genu valgum. *J Pediatr Orthop* 2004;24:70.

142. Stevens PM, Maguire M, Dales MD, et al. Physeal stapling for idiopathic genu valgum. *J Pediatr Orthop* 1999;19:645–649.

143. Bartel DL. Unicompartmental arthritis: biomechanics and treatment alternatives. In: Eilert RE, ed. *AAOS Instructional Course*, Vol. 41. Rosemont, IL: American Academy of Orthopaedic Surgeons, 1992;73.

144. Frantz CH. Epiphyseal stapling: a comprehensive review. *Clin Orthop Relat Res* 1971;77:149.

145. Blount WP, Clarke GR. Control of bone growth by epiphyseal stapling. A preliminary report. *Clin Orthop Relat Res* 1971;77:4.

146. Johnston CE, Bueche MJ, Williamson B. Epiphysiodesis for management of lower limb deformities. In: Eilert RE, ed. *AAOS Instructional Course*, Vol. 41. Rosemont, IL: American Academy of Orthopaedic Surgeons, 1992:437.

147. Bowen JR, Torres RR, Forlin E. Partial epiphysiodesis to address genu varum or genu valgum. *J Pediatr Orthop* 1992;12:359.

148. Davis CA, Maranji K, Frederick N, et al. Comparison of crossed pins and external fixation for correction of angular deformities about the knee in children. *J Pediatr Orthop* 1998;18:502.

149. Rajacich N, Bell DF, Armstrong PF. Pediatric applications of the Ilizarov method. *Clin Orthop Relat Res* 1992;280:72.

150. Healy WL, Anglen JO, Wasilewski SA, et al. Distal femoral varus osteotomy. *J Bone Joint Surg Am* 1988;70:102.

151. McDermott AGP, Finklestein JA, Farine I, et al. Distal femoral varus osteotomy for valgus deformity of the knee. *J Bone Joint Surg Am* 1988;70:110.

152. Morrey BF, Edgerton BC. Distal femoral osteotomy for lateral gonarthrosis. In: Eilert RE, ed. *AAOS Instructional Course*, Vol. 41. Rosemont, IL: American Academy of Orthopaedic Surgeons, 1992:77.

## Bowing of the Tibia

153. Boyd HB. Pathology and natural history of congenital pseudarthrosis of the tibia. *Clin Orthop Relat Res* 1982;166:5.

154. Anderson KS. Congenital angulation of the lower leg and congenital pseudarthrosis of the tibia in Denmark. *Acta Orthop Scand* 1972;43:539.

155. Crawford AH. Anterolateral bowing, POSNA One Day Course, Orlando, FL, May 16, 1999.

156. Crawford AH. Neurofibromatosis in childhood. In: Murray D, ed. *AAOS Instructional Course Lecture*, Vol. 30. St. Louis, MO: CV Mosby, 1981:56.

157. Morrissy RT. Congenital pseudarthrosis of the tibia. *Clin Orthop Relat Res* 1982;166:21.

158. Tuncay IC, Johnston CE II, Birch JG. Spontaneous resolution of congenital anterolateral bowing of the tibia. *J Pediatr Orthop* 1994;14:599.

159. Masserman RL, Peterson HA, Bianco AJ. Congenital pseudarthrosis of the tibia. *Clin Orthop Relat Res* 1974;99:140.

160. Andersen KS. Radiological classification of congenital pseudarthrosis of the tibia. *Acta Orthop Scand* 1973;44:719.

161. Hardinge K. Congenital anterior bowing of the tibia. *Ann R Coll Surg Engl* 1972;51:17.

162. Rathgeb JM, Ramsey PL, Cowell HR. Congenital kyphoscoliosis of the tibia. *Clin Orthop Relat Res* 1974;103:178.

163. Strong ML, Wong-Chung J. Prophylactic bypass grafting of the prepseudarthrotic tibia in neurofibromatosis. *J Pediatr Orthop* 1991;11:757.

164. Leung PC. Congenital pseudarthrosis of the tibia. *Clin Orthop Relat Res* 1983;175:45.

165. Henderson MS. Congenital pseudarthrosis of the tibia. *J Bone Joint Surg* 1928;10:483.

166. Boyd HB. Congenital pseudarthrosis. Treatment by dual bone grafts. *J Bone Joint Surg* 1941;23:497.

167. Boyd HB, Fox KW. Congenital pseudarthrosis. Follow-up study after massive bone grafting. *J Bone Joint Surg Am* 1948; 30:274.

168. Moore JR. Delayed autogenous bone graft in the treatment of congenital pseudarthrosis. *J Bone Joint Surg Am* 1949;31:23.

169. McFarland B. Pseudarthrosis of the tibia in childhood. *J Bone Joint Surg Br* 1951;33:36.

170. Sofield HA, Millar EA. Fragmentation, realignment and intramedullary rod fixation of deformities of the long bones in children. *J Bone Joint Surg Am* 1959;41:1371.

171. Brighton CT, Friedenberg ZB, Mitchell EI, et al. Treatment of nonunion with constant direct current. *Clin Orthop Relat Res* 1977;124:106.

172. Bassett CAL, Caulo N, Kort J. Congenital "pseudarthroses" of the tibia: treatment with pulsing electromagnetic fields. *Clin Orthop Relat Res* 1981;154:136.

173. Charnley J. Congenital pseudoarthrosis of the tibia treated by the intramedullary nail. *J Bone Joint Surg Am* 1956;38:283.

174. Umber JS, Moss SW, Coleman SS. Surgical treatment of congenital pseudarthrosis of the tibia. *Clin Orthop Relat Res* 1982;166:28.

175. Williams PF. Fragmentation and rodding in osteogenesis imperfecta. *J Bone Joint Surg Br* 1965;47:23.

176. Schoenecker PLS. Treatment of pseudoarthrosis of tibia with intramedullary rod. POSNA One Day Course, Orlando, FL, May 16, 1999.

177. Anderson DJ, Schoenecker PL, Sheridan JJ, et al. Use of an IM rod in treatment of congenital pseudarthrosis of the tibia. *J Bone Joint Surg Am* 1992;74:161.

178. Johnston CE II. Congenital pseudarthrosis of the tibia. Results of technical variations in the Charnley-Williams procedure. *J Bone Joint Surg Am* 2002;84:1799.

179. Dobbs MB, Rich MM, Gordon JE, et al. Use of an intramedullary rod for treatment of congenital pseudarthrosis of the tibia. A long-term follow-up study. *J Bone Joint Surg Am* 2004;86:1186.
180. Karol LA, Haideri NF, Halliday SE, Johnson CE, et al. Gait analysis and muscle strength in children with congenital pseudarthrosis of the tibia: The effect of treatment. *J Pediatr Orthop* 1998;18:381.
181. Fabry G, Lammens J, Melkebeek JV, et al. Treatment of congenital pseudarthrosis with the Ilizarov technique. *J Pediatr Orthop* 1988;8:67.
182. Plawecki S, Carpentier E, Lascombes P, et al. Treatment of congenital pseudarthrosis of the tibia by the Ilizarov method. *J Pediatr Orthop* 1990;10:786.
183. Paley D, Catagni M, Argnani F, et al. Treatment of congenital pseudoarthrosis of the tibia using the Ilizarov technique. *Clin Orthop Relat Res* 1992;280:81.
184. Grill F. Treatment of congenital pseudarthrosis of tibia with the circular frame technique. *J Pediatr Orthop* 1996;5:6.
185. Boero S, Catagni M, Donzelli O, et al. Congenital pseudarthrosis of the tibia associated with neurofibromatosis-1: treatment with Ilizarov's device. *J Pediatr Orthop* 1997;17:675.
186. Dahl MT. Congenital pseudarthrosis of the tibia treated with circular external fixation. POSNA One Day Course, Orlando, FL, May 16, 1999.
187. Farmer AW. The use of a composite pedicle graft for pseudarthrosis of the tibia. *J Bone Joint Surg Am* 1952;34:591.
188. Hagan KF, Buncke HJ. Treatment of congenital pseudarthrosis of the tibia with free vascularized bone graft. *Clin Orthop Relat Res* 1982;166:34.
189. Gordon L, Weulker N, Jergesen H. Vascularized fibular grafting for the treatment of congenital pseudarthrosis of the tibia. *Orthopedics* 1986;9:825.
190. Kanaya F, Tsai TM, Harkess J. Vascularized bone grafts for congenital pseudarthrosis of the tibia. *Microsurgery* 1997;17:459.
191. Minami A, Kaneda K, Igota H, et al. Free vascularized fibular grafts. *J Reconstr Microsurg* 1989;5(1):37.
192. Tolo VT. The role of free vascularized fibular grafts in congenital tibial pseudoarthrosis treatment. POSNA One Day Course, Orlando, FL, May 16, 1999.
193. Weiland AJ, Weiss APC, Moore JR, et al. Vascularized fibular grafts in the treatment of congenital pseudarthrosis of the tibia. *J Bone Joint Surg Am* 1990;72:654.
194. Dormans JP, Krajbich JI, Zucker R, et al. Congenital pseudarthrosis of the tibia: treatment with free vascularized fibular grafts. *J Pediatr Orthop* 1990;10:623.
195. deBoer HH, Verbout AJ, Nielsen HKL, et al. Free vascularized fibular graft for tibial pseudarthrosis in neurofibromatosis. *Acta Orthop Scand* 1988;59(4):425.
196. Simonis RB, Shirali HR, Mayou B. Free vascularized fibular grafts for congenital pseudarthrosis of the tibia. *J Bone Joint Surg Br* 1991;73:211.
197. Coleman SS, Coleman DA. Congenital pseudarthrosis of the tibia—treatment by transfer of the ipsilateral fibular with vascular pedicle. *J Pediatr Orthop* 1994;14:156.
198. Dimeglio A, Moukoko D, Chammas M. Treatment of severe congenital pseudarthrosis of the tibia: A combined method associating intramedullary nailing and free folded vascularized fibular transfer. The Pediatric Orthopaedic Society of North America Annual Meeting, Amelia Island, FL 2003.
199. Boyd HB, Sage FP. Congenital pseudarthrosis of the tibia. *J Bone Joint Surg Am* 1958;40:1245.
200. Jacobsen ST, Crawford AH, Millar EA, et al. The Syme amputation in patients with congenital pseudarthrosis of the tibia. *J Bone Joint Surg Am* 1983;65:533.
201. DalMonte A, Donzelli O, Sudanese A, et al. Congenital pseudarthrosis of the fibula. *J Pediatr Orthop* 1987;7:14.
202. Dooley BJ, Menelaus MB, Paterson DC. Congenital pseudarthrosis and bowing of the fibula. *J Bone Joint Surg Br* 1974;56:739.
203. Hsu LCS, O'Brien JP, Yau ACMC, et al. Valgus deformity of the ankle in children with fibular pseudarthrosis. *J Bone Joint Surg Am* 1974;56:503.
204. Langenskiold A. Pseudarthrosis of the fibula and progressive valgus deformity of the ankle in children: treatment by fusion of the distal tibial and fibular metaphyses. *J Bone Joint Surg Am* 1967;49:463.
205. Merkel KD, Peterson HA. Isolated congenital pseudarthrosis of the fibula: report of a case and review of the literature. *J Pediatr Orthop* 1984;4:100.
206. Younge D, Arford C. Congenital pseudarthrosis of the forearm and fibula. *Clin Orthop Relat Res* 1991;256:277.
207. DiGiovanni CW, Ehrlich MG. Treatment of congenital pseudarthrosis of the fibula with interposition allograft. *Orthopedics* 1998;21:1225.
208. Hofmann A, Wenger DR. Posteromedial bowing of the tibia. Progression in leg lengths. *J Bone Joint Surg Am* 1981;63:384.
209. Rich MM. Posterior medial bowing of the tibia. Shriners Hospitals for Children experience. POSNA One Day Course, Orlando, FL, May 16, 1999.
210. Pappas AM. Congenital posteromedial bowing of the tibia and fibula. *J Pediatr Orthop* 1984;4:525.
211. Heyman CH, Herndon CH. Congenital posterior angulation of the tibia. *J Bone Joint Surg Am* 1949;31:571.
212. Heyman CH, Herndon CH, Heiple KG. Congenital posterior angulation of the tibia with talipes calcaneus. A long-term report of eleven patients. *J Bone Joint Surg Am* 1959;41:476.

## Congential Dislocation of the Knee

213. Curtis BH, Fisher RL. Heritable congenital tibiofemoral subluxation. Clinical features and surgical treatment. *J Bone Joint Surg Am* 1970;52:1104.
214. Johnston CE II. Complex congenital knee deformities, POSNA Specialty Day, San Francisco, CA, Mar. 13, 2004.
215. Johnson E, Audell R, Oppenheim WL. Congenital dislocation of the knee. *J Pediatr Orthop* 1987;7:194.
216. Ko JY, Shih CH, Wenger DR. Congenital dislocation of the knee. *J Pediatr Orthop* 1999;19:252.
217. Drennan JC. Congenital dislocation of the knee and patella. In: Heckman JD, ed. *AAOS Instructional Course Lecture 42* Rosemont, IL, American Academy of Orthopaedic Surgeons 1993:517.
218. Curtis BH, Fisher RL. Congenital hyperextension with anterior subluxation of the knee. *J Bone Joint Surg Am* 1969;51:255.
219. McFarland BL. Congenital dislocation of the knee. *J Bone Joint Surg* 1929;11:281.
220. Provenzano RW. Congenital dislocation of the knee. A case report. *N Engl J Med* 1947;236:360.
221. Roy DR, Crawford AH. Percutaneous quadriceps recession: a technique for management of congenital hyperextension deformities of the knee in the neonate. *J Pediatr Orthop* 1989;9:717.
222. Katz MP, Grogono BJS, Soper KC. The etiology and treatment of congenital dislocation of the knee. *J Bone Joint Surg Br* 1967;49:112.
223. Vedantam R, Douglas DL. Congenital dislocation of the knee as a consequence of persistent amniotic fluid leakage. *Br J Clin Pract* 1994;48:342.
224. Bell MJ, Atkins RM, Sharrard WJW. Irreducible congenital dislocation of the knee, aetiology and management. *J Bone Joint Surg Br* 1987;69:403.
225. Uhthoff HK, Ogata S. Early intrauterine presence of congenital dislocation of the knee. *J Pediatr Orthop* 1994;14:245.
226. Ferris B, Aiclroth P. The treatment of congenital dislocation of the knee. A review of 19 knees. *Clin Orthop Relat Res* 1987;216:135.
227. Laurence M. Genu recurvatum congenitum. *J Bone Joint Surg Br* 1967;49:121.
228. Iwaya T, Sakaguchi R, Tsuyama W. The treatment of congenital dislocation of the knee with the Pavlik harness. *Int Orthop* 1988;7:25.
229. Bensahel H, DalMonte A, Hjelmstedt A, et al. Congenital dislocation of the knee. *J Pediatr Orthop* 1989;9:174.
230. Nogi J, MacEwen GD. Congenital dislocation of the knee. *J Pediatr Orthop* 1982;2:609.
231. Neibauer JJ, King DE. Congenital dislocation of the knee. *J Bone Joint Surg Am* 1960;42:207.

## Idiopathic Toe-Walking

232. Preis S, Klemms A, Muller K. Gait analysis by measuring ground reaction forces in children: changes to an adaptive gait pattern between the ages of one and five years. *Dev Med Child Neurol* 1997;39:228.
233. Statham L, Murray MP. Early walking patterns of normal children. *Clin Orthop Relat Res* 1971;79:8.

234. Hall JE, Salter RB, Bhalla SK. Congenital short tendo calcaneus. *J Bone Joint Surg Br* 1967;49:695.

235. Hicks R, Durinick N, Gage JR. Differentiation of idiopathic toe-walking and cerebral palsy. *J Pediatr Orthop* 1988;8:160.

236. Stricker SJ, Angulo JC. Idiopathic toe walking: a comparison of treatment methods. *J Pediatr Orthop* 1998;18:289.

237. Kalen V, Adler N, Bleck EE. Electromyography of idiopathic toe walking. *J Pediatr Orthop* 1986;6:31.

238. Katz MM, Mubarak SJ. Hereditary tendo achillis contractures. *J Pediatr Orthop* 1984;4:711.

239. Levine MS. Congenital short tendo calcaneus: report of a family. *Am J Dis Child* 1973;125:858.

240. Kelly IP, Jenkinson A, Stephens M, et al. The kinematic patterns of toe-walkers. *J Pediatr Orthop* 1997;17:478.

241. Griffin PP, Wheelhouse WW, Shiavi R, et al. Habitual toe-walkers: a clinical and electromyographic gait analysis. *J Bone Joint Surg Am* 1977;59:97.

242. Papariello SG, Skinner SR. Dynamic electromyography analysis of habitual toe-walkers. *J Pediatr Orthop* 1985;5:171.

243. Policy JF, Torburn L, Rinsky LA, et al. Electromyographic test to differentiate mild diplegic cerebral palsy and idiopathic toe-walking. *J Pediatr Orthop* 2001;21:784.

244. Stott NS, Walt SE, Lobb GA, et al. Treatment for idiopathic toe-walking. Results at skeletal maturity. *J Pediatr Orthop* 2004;24:63.

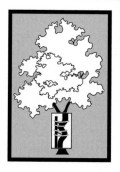

# 29

# Leg-Length Discrepancy

*Colin F. Moseley*

Cases of leg-length discrepancy frequently present challenges to the orthopaedic surgeon, who must understand the mechanisms and concepts of growth, including the relations among age, maturity, and leg length. Because the patient usually presents during the growing years, the orthopaedic surgeon must understand the need to correct the discrepancy as it will exist at maturity and not the discrepancy that is present in the growing child. The surgeon must be familiar with the methods used to analyze growth and to predict future growth and the effects of surgery. The techniques of leg lengthening evolve rapidly, and the orthopaedic surgeon must consider these new techniques in choosing the most appropriate management. As surgeons become more confident in their ability to utilize leg-lengthening procedures, they accept discrepancies of greater magnitude for correction, and they must be confident that the improvements in their abilities outweigh the increased risks. The final challenge facing the orthopaedic surgeon is to maintain a holistic perspective and to resist the temptation to direct attention solely toward the lengths of the legs, thereby neglecting the other factors that are important in the patient's overall function and appearance.

The treatment of leg-length discrepancy must be preceded by careful and sometimes difficult education of the patient and parents. In the case of epiphysiodesis, parents frequently find it difficult to understand why a problem in one leg requires an operation on the normal leg, and they are not pleased at the thought that it will make their child shorter. In the case of leg lengthening, the parents and the patients must understand that a fairly high morbidity is associated with this procedure even if things go well because the child must wear an external device for many months and must restrict his or her recreation and athletics. They also must understand that the risk of complications is high and that these complications can compromise the final result. The orthopaedic surgeon knows that surgery is necessary to correct leg-length discrepancy, but parents are often anxious to find some nonsurgical method of stimulating the growth of the short leg. If risks were equal, it would certainly be better to correct the leg-length discrepancy by lengthening the abnormally short leg than to compensate for the discrepancy by shortening the normal long leg.

## EFFECTS

The mechanical and functional effects of leg-length discrepancy are immediately apparent. The long-term effects, however, are less understood. Despite a consensus in the orthopaedic and lay communities that leg-length discrepancy does have deleterious effects on the spine and the hips, good documentation to support that consensus is lacking.

## Mechanisms of Compensation

The child with leg-length discrepancy usually compensates better than the adult, probably because of a higher strength-to-weight ratio. The child can compensate for minor degrees of leg-length discrepancy by walking on the toes of the short leg with the heel never touching the ground. This can result in a smooth, symmetrical gait that shows no abnormality except for the lack of heel strike on the short side.

The adult, on the other hand, seldom compensates in that manner but tends to walk with a heel-to-toe gait even on the short side and to vault over the long leg. This action produces excessive up-and-down motion of the pelvis and trunk (Fig. 29.1). Although it is theoretically possible to compensate for the leg-length discrepancy by flexing the knee on the long side, this is almost never done by either adults or children, probably because it would require too much of the quadriceps mechanism.

## Gait

Despite evidence to suggest that discrepancies of less than 2.5 cm are not significant in the adult (1), postural sway has been shown to increase when simulated discrepancies are as small as 1 cm (2). Liu et al. proposed the "symmetry index" (SI) as a measure of the quality of gait and found that correction of discrepancy by a heel lift considerably improves the SI (3).

Patients are usually able to compensate extremely well for their discrepancies. The movements about the lower limb joints with simulated and real leg-length discrepancies have been found to be essentially unchanged with small discrepancies (4). Song found that discrepancies greater than 5.5% of the long extremity increased the mechanical work performed by the long limb and increased the vertical displacement of the center of body mass, with consequent

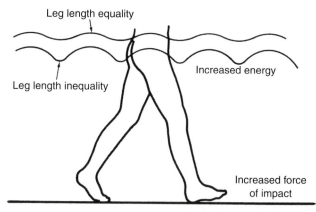

**Figure 29.1** Motion of pelvis during gait. The amplitude of vertical pelvic motion is increased by leg-length discrepancy. The patient vaults over the long leg and descends to plant the heel of the short leg.

energy penalty. Children with lesser discrepancies were able to normalize the work performed by the two extremities.

## Hip

Degenerative arthritis of the hip that is termed *idiopathic* in the elderly patient may actually be the result of some previously unrecognized minor problem, such as mild dysplasia, slipping of the capital femoral epiphysis, or, possibly, leg-length discrepancy. In two-legged stance with the legs straight, the patient with leg-length discrepancy has a pelvic obliquity, with respect to the floor, that relatively uncovers the hip of the long leg and that increases the coverage of the hip of the short leg (Fig. 29.2).

As the leg-length discrepancy increases, the uncovering on the high side also increases, with a decrease in the center-edge (CE) angle. This relation is illustrated in Figure 29.3.

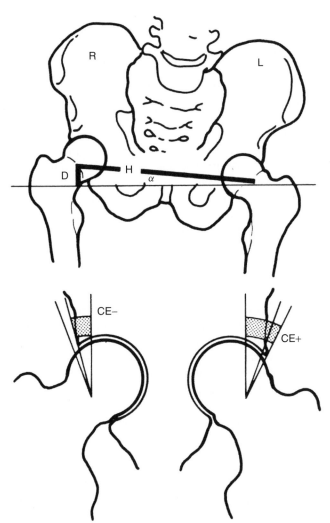

**Figure 29.2** Decrease in center-edge (CE) angle with pelvic obliquity. The CE angle is decreased on the side of the long leg. Coverage is decreased and the resulting decrease in the load-bearing area causes an increase in pressure. Such a hip may be susceptible to late degenerative arthritis (*L*, left; *R*, right; *H*, Hilgenrine's line; *D*, leg-length discrepancy). (From Morscher E. Etiology and pathophysiology of leg length discrepancies. *Prog Orthop Surg* 1977;1:9.)

It is reasonable to suspect that the patient with a leg-length discrepancy throughout his or her life may be subject to an increased risk of developing degenerative arthritis in the hip of the long leg (5), however, there is no documentation to prove this hypothesis. The effect of the leg-length discrepancy in decreasing coverage is present only during two-legged stance and perhaps during gait if the pelvis is lowered on the short side during swing phase as a compensatory mechanism. When the patient is in one-legged stance, sitting, or lying down, as is the case most of the time, this effect disappears.

## Knee

Leg-length discrepancy appears to increase the incidence of knee pain in athletes, although the nature of the relation has not been elucidated (6).

## Spine

The effects of leg-length discrepancy on the spine are also not clearly established. The parents of young children with leg-length discrepancy worry about the children developing degenerative arthritis of the spine, low back pain, and scoliosis. Contradictory evidence exists about the possibility that leg-length discrepancy causes low back pain in the long term (7–9). Low back pain is unusual in the younger child and is more common in the adolescent, but there is no evidence that low back pain and leg-length discrepancy are related in this age-group. Froh et al. (10) studied whether leg-length discrepancy had any effect on the orientation of the facet joints in adults and found none, whereas Giles and Taylor (11) found changes in the facet joints of cadavers with leg-length discrepancy. It is not clear whether the incidence of back pain is higher in patients with leg-length discrepancy than it is in the general population. Radiographs of the spine should be examined carefully to rule out anomalous development of the vertebrae.

Several studies have been performed to determine whether leg-length discrepancy leads to scoliosis. Gibson et al. assessed 15 patients with leg-length discrepancy following femoral fractures and found that after 10 years none had structural scoliosis (12), but minor structural changes have been reported in such patients (13). Studies have demonstrated an increased incidence of structural scoliosis in patients with leg-length discrepancy when compared with the general population (14), but the leg-length discrepancy has not been established as being the cause of scoliosis. If leg-length discrepancy were the cause, the scoliosis would have been expected to be in the direction that would compensate for the leg-length discrepancy, but in up to one third of the cases in these studies, the scoliosis was in the opposite direction (Fig. 29.4). Because the leg-length discrepancy affects the spine only during two-legged stance, and to some extent while walking, some of the skepticism toward the cause-and-effect

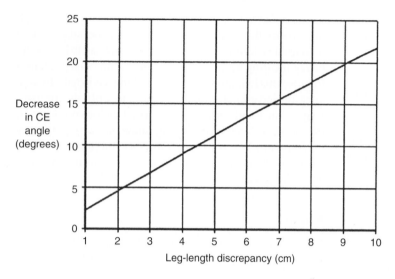

**Figure 29.3** Relation between leg-length discrepancy and center-edge (CE) angle. The CE angle and coverage decrease with increasing leg-length discrepancy. For every centimeter of leg-length discrepancy, there is a decrease of approximately 2.6 degrees in the CE angle. (From Morscher E. Etiology and pathophysiology of leg length discrepancies. *Prog Orthop Surg* 1977;1:9.)

hypothesis seems justified. It has been suggested, however, that scoliosis develops more as the result of the dynamic forces of walking and not the static forces of standing (15).

If leg-length discrepancy has long-term effects on the spine or hips, it is reasonable to suspect that the severity of the problem is related to the severity of the discrepancy, the degree to which it remains uncompensated or uncorrected, and the age of the patient at onset.

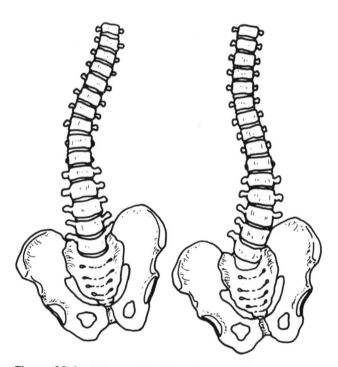

**Figure 29.4** Oblique pelvis with scoliosis in compensatory and noncompensatory directions. If leg-length discrepancy causes scoliosis, the direction of the spinal curvature is expected to be in the direction that is compensatory for the scoliosis. When scoliosis occurs in the other direction, it must be concluded that the leg-length discrepancy is not responsible.

## GROWTH

An understanding of growth is an essential prerequisite to the treatment of patients with leg-length discrepancy. The mechanisms of growth are discussed in Chapter 1. In the study of leg-length discrepancy, we are concerned with the rates and patterns of growth. Growth of the leg is the result of both growth at the four physeal plates at the proximal and distal ends of the tibia and femur and an increase in size of the four adjacent epiphyses. The growth of the epiphyses contributes only 5% to the total growth of the legs, and this is usually ignored in treating patients with leg-length discrepancy.

The only good studies relating growth of the legs to age were performed by Anderson and Green (16). Their first study involved populations of girls and boys at various ages, from 5 years to the age of physeal closure (16). Their second study was longitudinal in that a single group of children was followed up until maturity. They published their data in two forms. The first form related the lengths of the femur and the tibia of boys and girls to their ages (from 1 to 18 years) (17). These data can be combined to show the total leg lengths rather than the lengths of the individual bones. The total leg-length data are shown here in tabular (Table 29.1) and in graphic forms (Figs. 29.5 and 29.6). The graph showing leg lengths related to age is a useful tool in the analysis of leg-length data. They later published their data in the form of a graph showing the growth remaining at the distal femoral and proximal tibial physes of boys and girls as a function of skeletal age (Fig. 29.7) (18).

Most of the growth of the lower extremity occurs in the physes near the knee, as opposed to the upper extremity where most of the growth is contributed by the physes farthest from the elbow. The four growth plates of the lower limb contribute consistent proportions of growth to their individual bones and to the entire lower extremity (Fig. 29.8) (19). These percentages are worth remembering

**TABLE 29.1**

## LENGTH AS A FUNCTION OF SKELETAL AGE

| Age (yr) | Total Leg Length (cm) | | | | | Age (yr) | Total Leg Length (cm) | | | | |
|---|---|---|---|---|---|---|---|---|---|---|---|
| | + 2 SD | + 1 SD | Mean | − 1 SD | − 2 SD | | + 2 SD | + 1 SD | Mean | − 1 SD | − 2 SD |
| Boys | | | | | | Girls | | | | | |
| 1 | 28.58 | 27.33 | 26.08 | 24.83 | 23.58 | 1 | 29.02 | 27.70 | 26.38 | 25.06 | 23.74 |
| 2 | 36.06 | 34.37 | 32.69 | 31.01 | 29.32 | 2 | 36.00 | 34.37 | 32.74 | 31.11 | 29.48 |
| 3 | 41.81 | 39.84 | 37.88 | 35.92 | 33.95 | 3 | 42.09 | 40.09 | 38.10 | 36.11 | 34.11 |
| 4 | 46.89 | 44.61 | 42.32 | 40.03 | 37.75 | 4 | 47.75 | 45.26 | 42.78 | 40.30 | 37.81 |
| 5 | 51.55 | 48.97 | 46.38 | 43.79 | 41.21 | 5 | 52.56 | 49.83 | 47.09 | 44.35 | 41.62 |
| 6 | 56.06 | 53.14 | 50.21 | 47.45 | 44.54 | 6 | 57.20 | 54.04 | 51.05 | 47.97 | 44.90 |
| 7 | 60.63 | 57.32 | 54.01 | 50.70 | 47.39 | 7 | 61.75 | 58.29 | 54.82 | 51.35 | 47.89 |
| 8 | 64.83 | 61.25 | 57.66 | 54.07 | 50.49 | 8 | 66.05 | 62.34 | 58.61 | 54.88 | 51.17 |
| 9 | 69.14 | 65.24 | 61.35 | 57.45 | 53.55 | 9 | 70.49 | 66.38 | 62.27 | 58.16 | 54.05 |
| 10 | 73.16 | 68.99 | 64.82 | 60.65 | 56.48 | 10 | 74.99 | 70.49 | 66.00 | 61.51 | 57.01 |
| 11 | 77.33 | 72.80 | 68.26 | 63.72 | 59.19 | 11 | 79.52 | 74.66 | 69.81 | 64.96 | 60.10 |
| 12 | 81.83 | 76.86 | 71.87 | 66.88 | 61.91 | 12 | 85.21 | 78.28 | 73.35 | 68.42 | 63.49 |
| 13 | 86.86 | 81.27 | 75.66 | 70.06 | 64.46 | 13 | 85.75 | 80.94 | 76.14 | 71.34 | 66.53 |
| 14 | 90.71 | 85.03 | 79.36 | 73.69 | 68.01 | 14 | 86.57 | 82.07 | 77.57 | 73.07 | 68.57 |
| 15 | 92.32 | 87.20 | 82.07 | 76.95 | 71.82 | 15 | 86.80 | 82.43 | 78.06 | 73.69 | 69.32 |
| 16 | 93.01 | 88.35 | 83.70 | 79.05 | 74.39 | 16 | 86.90 | 82.55 | 78.21 | 73.87 | 69.52 |
| 17 | 93.02 | 88.66 | 84.29 | 79.92 | 75.56 | 17 | 86.95 | 82.60 | 78.25 | 73.90 | 69.55 |
| 18 | 92.95 | 88.73 | 84.52 | 80.31 | 76.09 | 18 | 86.99 | 82.63 | 78.28 | 73.93 | 69.57 |

SD, standard deviation.
From Anderson M, Messner M, Green W. Distribution of lengths of the normal femur and tibia in children from one to eighteen years of age. *J Bone Joint Surg* 1964;46-A(6):1197–1202.

because they can be useful in clinical situations. For example, a child with avascular necrosis of the femoral head in infancy cannot lose more than 15% of future growth of the affected leg, and a child whose distal femoral growth plate was destroyed because of infection will loose at the most 38% of future growth. Also noteworthy is that the femur is longer than the tibia, comprising 54% of the total length of the leg.

The study of growth, as it pertains to leg-length discrepancy, involves relations among three factors: leg length,

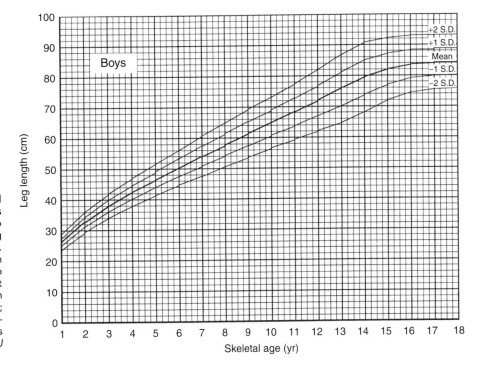

**Figure 29.5** Graph showing total leg length versus skeletal age for boys allows a specific boy to be related to the population by plotting his leg length as a function of his skeletal age. It is useful in the analysis of leg-length data because it allows a projection into the future on the basis of the present situation. (From Anderson M, Green WT. Lengths of the femur and tibia; norms derived from orthoroentgenograms of children from five years of age until epiphyseal closure. *Am J Dis Child* 1948;75:279–290.)

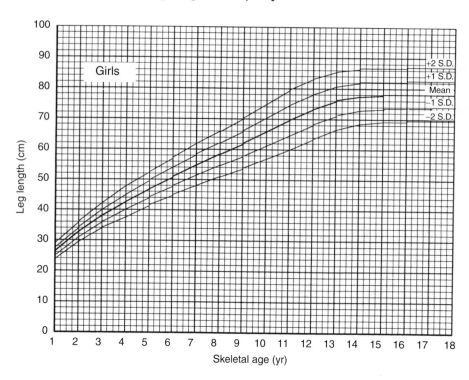

**Figure 29.6** Graph showing total leg length versus skeletal age for girls serves the same purpose for girls that Figure 29.5 serves for boys. (From Anderson M, Green WT. Lengths of the femur and tibia; norms derived from orthoroentgenograms of children from five years of age until epiphyseal closure. *Am J Dis Child* 1948;75:279–290.)

Means and standard deviations derived from longitudinal series 50 girls and 50 boys

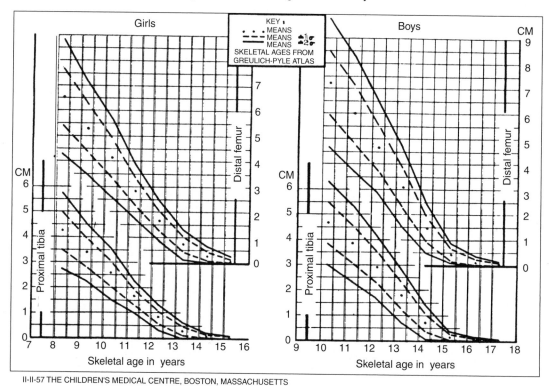

II-II-57 THE CHILDREN'S MEDICAL CENTRE, BOSTON, MASSACHUSETTS

**Figure 29.7** Green and Anderson growth-remaining graph. This graph shows the amount of growth potential remaining in the growth plates of the distal femur and the proximal tibia of boys and girls as functions of skeletal age. The graph is useful in determining the amount of shortening that will result from epiphysiodesis. (From Anderson M, Messner M, Green W. Distribution of lengths of the normal femur and tibia in children from one to eighteen years of age. *J Bone Joint Surg* 1964;46-A(6):1197–1202.)

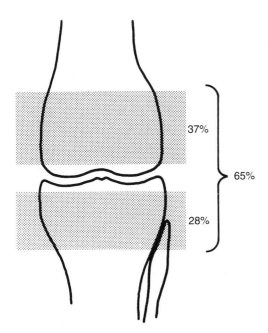

**Figure 29.8** The growth plates of the lower limb contribute definite and constant proportions to the growth of the long bones of the leg and the total growth of the limb. These contributions determine the slopes of the reference lines of the straight-line graph method and are therefore automatically taken into account by it.

maturity, and chronologic age (Fig. 29.9). Although these relations are familiar, some aspects deserve elaboration.

It is evident to all physicians who deal with children that maturation and aging are only weakly related. Some children mature rapidly and go through their growth spurts early. These children appear tall during the growing years not because they are of a taller growth percentile but because they are of advanced maturity. Many of these children who are tall for their chronologic age during early adolescence who mature early stop growing at a younger age than usual, and are shorter than the mean height at maturity. Pediatricians, in their studies of stature, and orthopaedic surgeons, in their studies of leg lengths, need a measure of maturity rather than a measure of age. Although

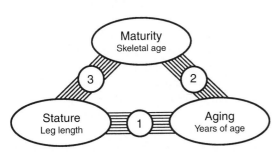

**Figure 29.9** Leg length, maturity, and age change with time, but the way they do so is not identical in every child. The three relations among these factors can be examined individually, and it is important to do so to understand parents' perceptions and to predict the patient's future growth. Relation 2 is about maturation, whereas relations 1 and 3 are both about growth but from different perspectives.

leg lengths and chronologic age can be measured accurately and easily, maturity cannot be.

The most useful measure of maturity has been the development of the bones of the skeleton as seen on radiographs. By comparing the radiographs of a patient with standard radiographs in an atlas (20), it is possible to derive a number known as the *skeletal age*. The skeletal age is actually the most likely age of a person with the given radiograph, but orthopaedic surgeons use it as a measure of maturity. It correlates well with menarche and other signs of maturation such as the appearance of secondary sexual characteristics and also correlates more closely with the growth of the legs than chronologic age does. Because the skeletal age standards represent an average of the general population, it should be apparent that for a random group of children, the mean skeletal age should be equal to the mean chronologic age.

The three relations seen among chronologic age, skeletal age, and leg length (Fig. 29.9) can be examined individually, and it is instructive to do so. First, consider the relation between growth and chronologic age. This relation is obvious to parents. The parent who is concerned about his or her child being too short or too tall repeatedly compares the child to classmates and other children of the same age. In this relation, there is steady growth throughout life, with a growth spurt in early adolescence and cessation of growth at the age of 16 to 17 years in boys and 14 to 15 years in girls (Fig. 29.10) (21). Although this relation is the most obvious, it is virtually meaningless without a consideration of maturity, and its variability from child to child presents problems for the treating doctor. A more consistent relation must be used.

Although the relation between chronologic age and skeletal age is extremely variable within the population, children tend to pass the various landmarks of maturity in the same orderly and consistent manner. The child who develops secondary sexual characteristics early also goes through the growth spurt early, reaches menarche early, and has advanced skeletal age. The implication is that children who mature more quickly or slowly than the average rate do so throughout their growing years, but this is not necessarily so. Some children appear to be going through a maturation spurt, during which they mature faster than they age. This maturity spurt tends to coincide with the growth spurt, and the orthopaedic surgeon who is waiting for just the right time to do an epiphysiodesis can be caught unawares. It is as if these children deal with their rapid growth rate by turning the pages of the skeletal age atlas at a faster rate.

The third relation, that between maturity and growth, correlates more closely than the relation between chronologic age and skeletal age and is of most interest to the orthopaedic surgeon. This is the relation shown in the data of Green and Anderson (Figs. 29.5 and 29.6), and it has interesting properties. The first property is that growth is never faster as the child becomes older, in either absolute

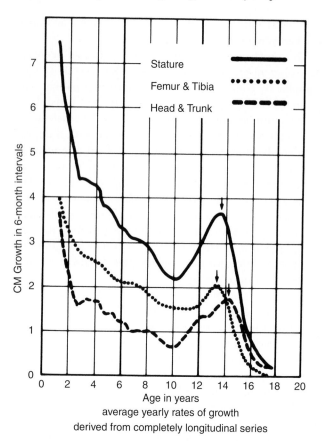

**Figure 29.10** Green and Anderson growth curve. The examination of growth rate as a function of chronologic age shows a major growth spurt during adolescence. Interestingly, no such spurt appears in the growth curve of Figures 29.6 and 29.7. (From Green W, Anderson M. Skeletal age and the control of bone growth. *Instr Lect Am Acad Orthop Surg* 1960;17:199–217.)

or relative terms, than it was when he or she was a newborn. The growth rate continually slows down until it stops completely at maturity. There is no inflection point in the curve, which means that the growth spurt that is obvious when growth is correlated with chronologic age disappears when growth is correlated to skeletal age. The absence of the growth spurt has two possible explanations. The first is that these curves are derived from averages of a number of patients and that averaging data tends to minimize individual variations that occur at different times. The second, more interesting, explanation is that the growth spurt may actually represent a maturation spurt in which growth maintains its customary relation to skeletal age.

The Green and Anderson study provides good documentation of the relation between skeletal age and leg length for the population studied, but there is no guarantee that these data hold for children of other races or of other genetic stocks from within the same race. Indeed, there is one report that shows that Dutch children are taller than those described by Green and Anderson (22). It is not clear, however, that these children actually follow a pattern of growth that is different from that described by Green and Anderson. They may just behave like children taller than Green and Anderson's mean. Indeed, Paley supported

this concept by reporting an extensive review of published growth patterns of children of varied races and by concluding that they all share the same pattern of growth (23).

## ETIOLOGY

Leg-length discrepancy can be classified purely by etiology, but the concepts involved in understanding the disorder and in treating patients suggest a more logical approach. Leg-length discrepancy can result from two types of processes: those that change the length of the leg directly and those that alter its growth. A fracture that heals with overriding is an obvious example of an alteration in length with no effect on growth, and injury to the growth plate from osteomyelitis is an example of an alteration in growth rate with no immediate effect on length. These two effects determine whether a discrepancy is static or dynamic and, therefore, greatly influence the choice of treatment. The causes of leg-length discrepancy can be classified according to their effect on length or growth, but the classification system breaks down because certain causes can affect different patients differently, and some causes affect both length and growth. A fracture, for example, can cause leg shortening in one patient and overgrowth in another, and a congenitally short femur can be thought of as being both short and retarded in its growth. Such a classification is shown in Table 29.2.

Some patients with asymmetry above or below the legs present as having leg-length discrepancy and may be treated in the same manner as for leg-length discrepancy, although their legs may be of equal length. Examples include high-riding congenital dislocation of the hip (Fig. 29.11) and fixed pelvic obliquity secondary to scoliosis, both of which illustrate the difference between functional and anatomic leg-length discrepancy.

### Interference with Length

By definition, the only processes that can acutely affect the length of the leg are fractures and dislocations. Whether a congenitally short bone has suffered direct interference with its length is a moot point, because this interference occurred before birth, and it is the inhibition growth that is the important factor. The terminal deletions and proximal focal femoral deficiency and its variants can be thought of as growth inhibition superimposed on a short limb.

Fractures can result in short bones either by overriding or by angular deformity. In the latter case, the shortening often disappears when the angulation is corrected (24). Sugi and Cole have shown that shortening of up to 10% of the femoral length can be accepted in the treatment of femoral fractures by early spica without causing considerable discrepancy (25). Overgrowth frequently accompanies healing of fractures and can spontaneously correct the shortening (26). Excessive length can result when excessive force is applied in traction.

## TABLE 29.2

### CLASSIFICATION OF CAUSES OF LEG-LENGTH DISCREPANCY

| Classification | By Growth Retardation | By Growth Stimulation |
| --- | --- | --- |
| I. Congenital | Congenital hemiatrophy with skeletal anomalies (e.g., fibular aplasia, femoral aplasia, and coxa vara), dyschondroplasia (Ollier disease), dysplasia epiphysealis punctata, multiple exostoses, congenital dislocated hip, clubfoot | Partial giantism with vascular abnormalities (Klippel-Trenaunay and Parkes Weber syndromes) Hemarthrosis due to hemophila |
| II. Infection | Epiphyseal plate destruction due to osteomyelitis (e.g., in femur and tibia), tuberculosis (e.g., in hip, knee joint, and foot), septic arthritis | Diaphyseal osteomyelitis of femur or tibia, Brodie abscess Metaphyseal tuberculosis of femur or tibia (tumor albus) Septic arthritis Syphilis of femuror tibia Elephantiasis as a result of soft tissue infections |
| III. Paralysis | Poliomyelitis, other paralysis (spastic) | Thrombosis of femora or iliac veins |
| IV. Tumors | Osteochondroma (solitary exostosis) Giant cell tumors Osteitis fibrosa cystica generalisata Neurofibromatosis (Recklinghausen disease of the bone) | Hemangioma, lymphangioma Giant cell tumors Osteitis fibrosa cystica generalisata Neurofibromatosis (Recklinghausen disease of the bone) Fibrous dysplasia (Jaffe-Lichtenstein disease) |
| V. Trauma | Damage of the epiphyseal plate (e.g., dislocation, operation) Diaphyseal fractures with marked overriding of fragments Severe burns | Diaphyseal and metaphyseal fractures of femur or tibi (osteosynthesis) Diaphyseal operations (e.g., stripping of periosteum, bone graft removal osteotomy) |
| VI. Mechanical | Immobilization of long duration by weight-relieving braces | Traumatic arteriovenous aneurysms |
| VII. Others | Legg-Calvé-Perthes disease Slipped upper femoral epiphysis Damage to femoral or tibial epiphyseal plates due to radiation therapy | |

From Taillard W, Morscher E. *Beinlangenunterschiede*, Basel: Karger, 1965.

Dislocations have a direct effect on length only if they are unreduced.

### Interference with Growth

The growth of the physis can be slowed by three mechanisms. First, congenital short bones grow more slowly than normal bones because of abnormal programming of the genetic mechanism that determines growth rate. Second, the growth plate can be injured in such a way that a part or all of it is no longer able to grow, and it eventually gets converted to solid bone in the form of a physeal bridge or a prematurely closed plate. Any part of the plate that has retained its ability to grow cannot do so effectively because of tethering by the fused part. Third, a change in the environment of the plate can influence its growth rate. Unusual vascular malformations can stimulate or inhibit growth (27,28). Children with paralysis usually have shortening of the more severely affected leg, presumably because the growth rate of the plate responds to the decreased compressive forces across it. The concept that pressure might change the direction of the growth of the plate is commonly known as the *Heuter-Volkmann law* (29,30), but this concept was first proposed by Delpech

(31,32). Delpech treated an angular deformity of the ankle with casting that caused the distal tibial plate to change its direction of growth.

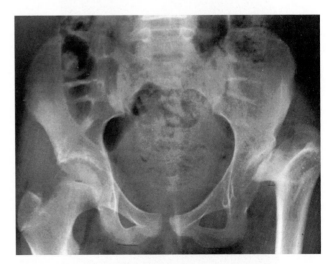

**Figure 29.11**  High-riding dislocation of hip. This patient has a functional leg-length discrepancy that is greater than the actual discrepancy in the lengths of the legs because of the adduction of the short leg.

## Congenital Shortening

When a patient is born with legs of unequal length that are otherwise normal, it is often impossible to know which leg is the abnormal one. Because the more severe cases clearly involve shortening, it is appropriate to think of these cases as hemiatrophy rather than hemihypertrophy. Beals has stated that hemiatrophy and hemihypertrophy are distinct clinical syndromes, partly because of their associated anomalies (33). The dysplasia usually involves the entire limb, with some shortening of all components, and usually is accompanied by a diminution in girth. Each leg appears to be genetically programmed to be of a different size (34).

Congenitally short bones frequently show qualitative, as well as quantitative, changes (Fig. 29.12) (35). The congenitally short femur also can show coxa vara, bowing, hypoplasia of the lateral condyle (Fig. 29.13), and external torsion (36). It can be associated with anterior cruciate insufficiency (37–40), a short or missing fibula (41,42), and absence of the lateral rays of the foot. Indeed, the congenital short femur is thought by some to be a variant of proximal focal femoral deficiency (43).

Congenitally bowed tibias are frequently accompanied by leg-length discrepancy and hypoplastic feet (44–46). Askins and Ger (47) found that 24% of patients with congenital constriction bands have leg-length discrepancy; and Garbarino et al. (48) reported short tibias in association with congenital diastasis of the inferior tibio-fibular joint.

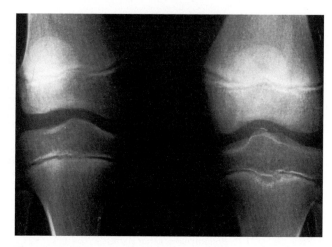

**Figure 29.13** Hypoplasia of femoral condyle is frequently found in association with congenital shortening of the femur.

## Trauma

A trauma that injures the physeal plate can slow its rate of growth either by direct injury to the cells responsible for growth or by formation of a bony bridge that tethers the epiphysis to the metaphysis. Salter and Harris provided a classification of fractures of the physeal plate that is useful in anticipating the effect of fractures on future growth (49). This classification is shown diagrammatically in Figure 29.14. Fractures can wander through all zones of the plate, but tend to pass through the zone of cell hypertrophy where the material is weakest and the amount of material is least. The material in that zone is cartilage, which is weaker than bone, and because the cells there are large, the ratio of matrix volume to cell volume is low (Fig. 29.15). It is important to note that this part of the plate is the site of conversion of cartilage to bone, but it is not primarily responsible for growth that occurs by virtue of cell multiplication and matrix production in the zones nearer the epiphysis.

Because type I and type II fractures do not pass through the growth zone, they are less likely to interfere with growth than other fractures are. Both types of fractures, however, may be associated with a crush injury, which injures the cells by compression. This mechanism may account for the higher than expected incidence of growth disturbance in type II fractures of the weight-bearing bones, such as the distal femur, where growth arrest is found in more than one third of patients (50). Type III and IV fractures do, however, cross the growth zone and are therefore more likely to result in growth arrest. The type IV fracture, in particular, can result in a bony bridge when the fracture fragment displaces in the diaphyseal direction (Fig. 29.14). This is one reason why these fractures must be anatomically reduced. Type V fractures can occur in isolation or can accompany any of the other types of fractures. Type V fractures are insidious because they are not initially recognizable on radiographs and they always demonstrate their presence by a disturbance of growth, either a shortening or

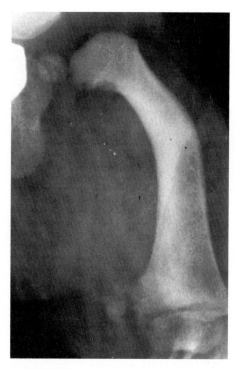

**Figure 29.12** In proximal focal femoral deficiency, the leg-length discrepancy is accompanied by qualitative changes, including coxa vara and bowing.

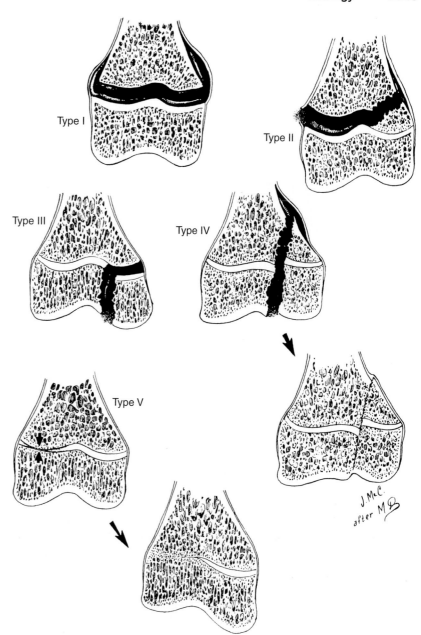

**Figure 29.14** Salter-Harris classification of epiphyseal fractures. Fractures of types I and II do not cross the part of the growth plate that is responsible for growth, whereas those of types III and IV do. In the type IV fracture, approximation of epiphyseal bone to metaphyseal bone can result in formation of a bony bridge. (From Salter R, Harris W. Injuries involving the epiphyseal plate. *J Bone Joint Surg* 1963;45A: 587–622.)

a combination of shortening and angulation, usually in the first year after the occurrence of the fracture. Although the fracture classifications provide guidelines about the likelihood of growth arrest, the orthopaedic surgeon must be wary of giving a definite prognosis for a given epiphyseal fracture until enough time has elapsed to rule out a type V injury.

The bony bridge that causes a growth disturbance following physeal fractures usually is discrete and well defined and lends itself to excision if the fractures are small and peripheral. Bridge resections usually are limited to those that involve less than 50% of the plate in patients who have at least 2 years of growth remaining. Even more extensive resections can be considered in very young children because, if successful, difficult treatment of severe leg-length discrepancy might be avoided. Resection of a bony bridge always

should be considered if there is significant growth remaining, even if leg-length discrepancy is already present. The angular deformity that may also be present because of the bridge can influence treatment of the discrepancy because both deformities can be corrected at once.

### Infection

Osteomyelitis adjacent to the plate can result in the destruction of physeal cells and disturbance of growth if not treated early (51). The infection is usually hematogenous osteomyelitis of the metaphysis, but it can be epiphyseal in infants and can follow or precede septic arthritis of the joint. The bony bridge that results from infection is more difficult to treat than that following trauma because it is not so amenable to resection. The bridge tends to be larger,

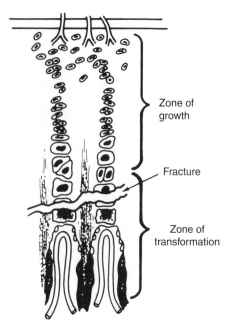

**Figure 29.15** Location of fractures in the growth plate. Fractures tend to occur through the part of the growth plate where the matrix is least, although individual fractures may wander from zone to zone.

more central, and less discrete than that following trauma and can even consist of multiple small bridges. It is difficult to define by radiograph, is usually more extensive than it appears, and is more difficult to define during resection. There is the danger that minor components of the bridge can be left behind because the usual end point of resection, a continuous line of physis around the resection tunnel, can be achieved despite incomplete resection of all components of the bridge.

Infection tends to produce more serious leg-length discrepancy problems than trauma does because it occurs commonly in younger children with much growth ahead of them. As with trauma, angular deformity and leg-length discrepancy can coexist.

### Paralysis

Inhibition of growth commonly accompanies weakness or paralysis of the leg, but the mechanism of this inhibition is not clear. It may be true that blood flow to the limb is reduced because of the reduced muscle mass, but this does not necessarily mean that flow to the plate is also reduced. Venous return results partly from muscle activity and, therefore, it is conceivable that reduced muscle activity and decreased pumping effect could reduce blood flow to the limb and perhaps to the plate. Alternatively, abnormal vasomotor control from the neurologic abnormality could affect blood flow.

Paralysis and reduced muscle activity may have a more direct effect on the growth rate. The Heuter-Volkmann law (29) suggests that the growth rate of the physis responds to the compression forces across it, and this law is frequently used to explain how a spontaneous reorientation of the physis occurs while contributing to the remodeling of angular deformities in the immature child. This mechanism also can explain the decrease in the overall growth rate that occurs in children with muscle weakness.

The parents of children with cerebral palsy are frequently concerned about leg-length discrepancy, and minor degrees of discrepancy can be seen in this condition. More often, however, the discrepancy is more apparent than real and occurs because of pelvic obliquity due to hip contractures or asymmetric posturing due to asymmetric spasticity. It is likely that serious discrepancies do not occur more often because even dysfunctional spasticity can be effective, through the Heuter-Volkmann law, in stimulating the physis to grow.

### Tumors

Leg-length discrepancy can be related to tumors in several ways. The first way involves destruction of the plate by direct tumor invasion, the mechanism of invasion in this instance being similar to that of infection.

The second way involves damage to the plate by irradiation that is used to treat the tumor (52). Irradiation has a particularly harmful effect because the osteocytes of the neighboring bone also are killed, and the bone can take many years to become revascularized and repopulated with healthy osteocytes. The absence of healthy osteoblasts and precursors can complicate the treatment of the ensuing leg-length discrepancy by precluding lengthening procedures through the affected bone. Radiation damage to regional soft tissues also complicates lengthening procedures (53,54).

The third way that tumors produce leg-length discrepancy involves the diversion of cartilage cells of the physis into the tumor, thereby stealing growth potential from the plate. Examples of this are enchondromatosis, Ollier disease (55), and osteochondromatosis, all of which are derived from chondrocytes of the growth plate. Although unicameral cysts usually do not result in significant leg-length discrepancy, some of the growth disturbances can result from aggressive attempts to remove the cyst wall when the cyst is active and immediately adjacent to the plate. Unicameral cysts and fibrous dysplasia cause leg-length discrepancy because of both growth inhibition and repeated fractures with minimal displacement that produce progressive varus.

### Avascular Necrosis

Because the circulation of the physis is derived from the epiphyseal circulation, avascular necrosis of the epiphysis frequently involves the growth plate as well, resulting in leg-length discrepancy. This may be seen in Legg-Perthes disease and in avascular necrosis following treatment of developmental dislocation of the hip. Peterson has reported a case in which a discrepancy resulted from a temporary but substantial episode of vascular insufficiency during surgery in an infant (56). In the case of congenital dislocation of the hip, the effect is maximized by onset at an early age and by the years of future growth that are affected but is moderated by the fact that the growth plate of the proximal femur contributes only approximately 15% of the growth of the limb. The likelihood of substantial discrepancy has been correlated with the pattern of ischemic damage to the head and increases with increasing involvement (57). The fact that the vascular damage to the epiphysis does not always significantly affect the physis is indicated by the observation that patients with Legg-Perthes disease do not usually develop substantial deformity (58). Leg-length discrepancy also has been reported as a complication of catheterization of the umbilical or femoral artery (59), presumably because of impairment of the arterial supply to the physis.

## Stimulation of Growth

Certain conditions are known to stimulate growth. Although increased circulation is thought to be the mechanism of growth stimulation, there is only circumstantial evidence to support this theory. Attempts to stimulate growth in the treatment of leg-length discrepancy have been made by numerous means, including sympathectomy to increase blood flow, insertion of foreign materials next to the physis, stripping and elevation of the periosteum (60–62), surgical establishment of an arteriovenous fistula (63), shortwave diathermy (64), and electrical stimulation (65). None of these methods has consistently produced sufficient growth stimulation to be clinically useful (66,67), but the fact that the arteriovenous fistula does produce stimulation at all supports the hypothesis that increased circulation can be a final common pathway for the conditions that stimulate growth.

### Tumor

Vascular malformations, particularly when they involve large portions of the limb, produce growth stimulation that often involves all growth plates of the limb and not just the ones in proximity to the tumor or the plates of the involved bone. This stimulation is seen with hemangiomatosis and Klippel-Trenaunay-Weber syndrome (68). Stimulation is also seen with certain nonvascular tumors, such as neurofibromatosis, fibrous dysplasia, and Wilms tumor, although an increase in circulation could be the final common pathway to growth stimulation.

### Inflammation

Overgrowth of the involved bone is a common feature of chronic osteomyelitis, presumably because of the increased blood flow to the limb as part of the inflammation. Infection, therefore, can both inhibit and stimulate growth. Overgrowth of the affected limb can be seen in pauciarticular juvenile rheumatoid arthritis (69), particularly in those cases with onset before the age of 3 years (70), and has also been

reported in a patient with hemophilia and with chronic knee synovitis (71).

### Fracture

Overgrowth usually is seen following fractures of long bones in children and also is believed to result from the increased blood flow to the limb that is part of the healing process (72). One particularly pernicious example of this effect is the overgrowth of the tibia and valgus deformity that can follow minimally displaced proximal metaphyseal fractures (73). The mechanism involves overgrowth of the medial side of the tibial growth plate (74), possibly because of tethering by the fibula or by release of the torn medial periosteum (75–78).

Overgrowth most commonly occurs following femoral fractures in young children (79,80). Some studies have reported that the stimulatory effect can last for years, but it is believed to occur principally during the healing and remodeling periods in the first 2 years after the fracture (81). The stimulation has been reported variously to be the greatest in fractures in the proximal third of the femur, the middle third of the femur (82), and in those fractures with greater degrees of overriding (83); it can be accompanied by overgrowth of the fractured tibia on the same side. Conversely, Meals (84) found that the patient's age and the type and location of the fracture did not influence the extent of overgrowth, although, inexplicably, handedness did.

## PATIENT ASSESSMENT

There is a tendency when dealing with patients with leg-length discrepancy to concentrate attention on the lengths of the legs and the discrepancy and to ignore other factors that are important in the patient's function and the ultimate outcome of treatment. When the process of choosing treatment goals is discussed later in this chapter, the importance of a complete and thorough assessment of the patient is emphasized.

## History of Discrepancy

A complete history of the patient, the discrepancy, and its previous treatment should be obtained. The cause of the leg-length discrepancy is important because knowledge of whether length, growth, or both is affected is essential to understanding the growth pattern. Also important is knowledge of the affected physeal plates, because this permits an estimation of the future increase in the discrepancy. Parents of patients expect this kind of information on the first visit, and it is important in establishing a good parent-patient-surgeon relationship to be as knowledgeable as possible about the condition and its future. The history of surgery, including surgery to correct angular deformity, is needed because the numeric data about leg lengths can be misinterpreted if the examiner is unaware of previous surgery that might have affected the leg lengths.

The history, which delineates the cause, associated deformity, and neuromuscular deficits, is referred to during selection of the treatment goal. The fact that a patient's discrepancy is of congenital origin suggests increased risk and indicates that certain precautionary steps to avoid complications must be taken in conjunction with lengthening. Instability of an adjacent joint can preclude lengthening. Weakness of the leg suggests that the weak leg should be left a little short to facilitate floor clearance during swing phase.

## Clinical Assessment

The accuracy and ease of obtaining radiologic measurements of the patient should not blind the physician to the necessity of conducting a careful and complete physical examination. There are two reasons for this. First, the radiographic measurements can be wrong because of artifacts caused by angular deformity, positioning, or patient movement. Second, there are important factors that are not measured by routine radiographs but that can be crucial to the outcome of the treatment. The second point is discussed in the section on goal selection. After assessment of the patient is complete, the clinical assessment must be consistent with the radiologic assessment, or else an explanation must be sought. Additional radiographs or reexamination can be necessary to determine the reason for the inconsistency. In the final analysis, it is the functional leg-length discrepancy that must be treated, and that cannot be determined by radiographs.

### Leg Length

A tape measure is used to measure the real length of each leg from the anterior superior iliac spine to the tip of the medial malleolus. The apparent length is measured from the umbilicus to the tip of the medial malleolus. These two measurements of the leg-length discrepancy may yield different results, because the apparent length is affected by pelvic obliquity and hip position. The leg on the side of the adducted hip appears shorter, but the real length is minimally affected (Fig. 29.16). The patient should be undressed completely for this measurement to avoid tenting of the tape over the clothes. In any case, the tape often tents over or around the knee, impairing the accuracy of the measurement. Because different landmarks are used, the lengths of the legs measured in this way are not the same as those measured by radiograph, but the discrepancies should correspond closely.

The medial aspect of the joint line of the knee can be used as a landmark for measuring the segment lengths of the tibia and femur. Although this method is less accurate than the radiologic measurement, it is useful for comparison to prevent errors. If the relative heights of the knees will be a strategy factor, then the lengths of the individual bones can be determined as well.

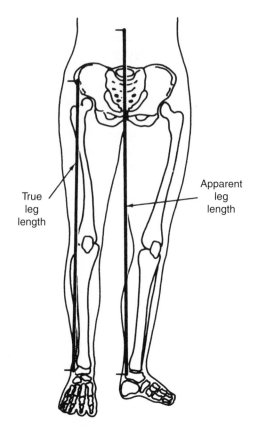

**Figure 29.16**  The measurement of real length is relatively immune from error because of pelvic obliquity. Measurement of apparent length is susceptible to error.

It is useful to place blocks under the foot on the short side to lengthen the short leg effectively (Fig. 29.17). The block height required to produce a level pelvis should correspond to the measured discrepancy. Blocks also can be used to estimate the extent of correction that feels best to the patient and provides him or her with the best correction. This amount can be different from the radiographic measurement, and it may indicate that the goal of treatment should not be exact correction of leg length. This assessment is most useful in the mature patient whose discrepancy will not be changing with growth. Although it only measures the present length and does not indicate the desired amount of correction, it can be helpful in immature patients to indicate that exact correction is not the best goal. Carrying this idea further, the patient can be provided with a temporary shoe lift and can be assessed after a period of ambulation. These techniques are especially useful for patients with complex deformities, because they take into account the combined effects of asymmetric feet, angular deformities, contractures, pelvic obliquity, and spinal balance.

### Other Factors

Several factors other than leg length must be assessed because they affect the measurement of leg length or influence the final outcome of the patient's treatment.

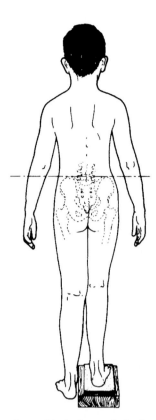

**Figure 29.17** Placing blocks beneath the heel of the short leg allows assessment of the combined effect of all factors that produce functional leg-length discrepancy.

The examiner must remain aware that knee and hip flexion contractures tend to shorten the leg, an equinus contracture of the ankle tends to lengthen it, and pelvic obliquity also tends to affect apparent length. The term pelvic obliquity has a broader meaning here than when used by spinal surgeons, who use it to refer to the relation of the position of the pelvis to that of the spine (85). In the context of leg-length discrepancy, it refers to the relation of the position of the pelvis to that of the legs, and it is affected both by adduction and abduction contractures of the hips and by spinal deformity. An adduction contracture of the hip causes the leg on the affected side to appear short and to be functionally short, whereas an abduction contracture has the opposite effect (86). This situation is common in patients with cerebral palsy and those with the residuals of poliomyelitis. A difference between the measured real and apparent discrepancies indicates that pelvic obliquity is present.

Hip contractures are particularly important because adduction contractures produce a functionally short leg and abduction contractures produce a functionally long leg (87). These effects occur even in the absence of an actual discrepancy as measured by a scanogram. Conversely, in a patient with true shortening, a limitation of ipsilateral hip abduction or other side hip abduction will prevent him or her from compensating easily and will exaggerate the effect of the discrepancy.

Angular deformity must be assessed because it affects the measurements of leg length and influences the final outcome if it is to be corrected later. Joint stability must be assessed because it pertains particularly to the risks of leg lengthening. Femoral lengthening is contraindicated in the presence of hip instability. Congenitally short femurs always are associated with laxity of the anterior cruciate ligament (37) and with hypoplasia of the lateral femoral condyle (Fig. 29.13) that predisposes to posterolateral subluxation of the tibial plateau. Lengthening of the tibia can be contraindicated in the presence of an unstable ankle or a useless foot which might be better handled by amputation and prosthetic fitting.

Spinal deformity and balance should be assessed. If there is stiff suprapelvic obliquity such that the axis of the trunk cannot be made perpendicular to the transverse axis of the pelvis, an equalization of leg lengths will cause an imbalance of the trunk, and some modification of that goal will be necessary. Adduction and abduction contractures of the hips produce infrapelvic obliquity, with apparent and functional leg-length discrepancy (88).

Weakness and the need for bracing must be assessed because leg-length discrepancy in patients with paralysis or weakness is usually best handled by undercorrection, leaving the weak leg short to facilitate swing-through, particularly if the leg is braced with the knee locked in extension. Patients who require bracing of the short leg to walk can have their leg-length discrepancy corrected in the brace and may not require surgical correction at all.

Finally, the concerns, compliance, and emotional state of the parents and patient must be taken into account. This aspect is particularly important when lengthening is being considered, because this is a long and difficult process requiring understanding and cooperation by all involved. Despite excellent education and preparation, parents and patients always underestimate the challenge of dealing with the duration of lengthening and the later restriction of activities. If there is a lack of understanding or a suggestion of poor compliance, then another approach may be more appropriate. The surgeon constantly must be aware that patients frequently express concerns about function when they are actually concerned about cosmetic effect, which may be less important when compared with the risks of surgery.

## Radiologic Assessment

### Leg Lengths

Several methods exist for the radiologic measurement of leg length. These methods are more accurate than clinical methods, but each has its advantages and disadvantages. The nonexistent, ideal method would allow the hip and ankle to be viewed, minimize radiation, use only one exposure, use a film of convenient size, demonstrate angular deformity, have no magnification, give true readings from a scale on the film, and be inexpensive.

The bony landmarks used are the top of the femoral head, the medial femoral condyle, and the ankle. The ankle mortise is slightly saddle shaped, and the midpoint of the saddle can be easily identified. Although these techniques allow the measurement of the femur and tibia individually, these values are not required in analyzing and predicting growth, and the length of the entire leg suffices.

The surgeon cannot rely on measurements recorded in the patient's record but must review all radiographs before performing surgery to check their accuracy and reliability. There is the possibility that radiographs taken over the years have been read by different individuals using different techniques and landmarks. It is also possible that the scales have been misread or that arithmetic errors have been made in determining lengths and discrepancies.

There are four radiologic techniques that measure leg lengths directly and others that provide useful information. The terminology is confusing because names used for these techniques are inconsistent in the literature and in use. The term "scanogram," for example, was derived from the technique of split scanography, in which the x-ray beam was tightly collimated to a thin transverse slit that exposed the film as the x-ray tube was moved from one end of the leg to the other. The principles are more important than the terminology.

The teleoradiograph (Fig. 29.18) is a single exposure of both legs on a long, 35 cm × 90 cm (14 in × 36 in) film. It is taken from a 2-m (6-ft) distance, usually with the patient standing and with a radiopaque ruler placed on the cassette. It has the advantage of showing angular deformities and of using a single exposure, but it produces a radiographic film that is inconvenient to handle and measurements that are subject to magnification because of parallax of the x-ray beam. There is no significant difference between measurements of the leg taken supine and those taken standing (89).

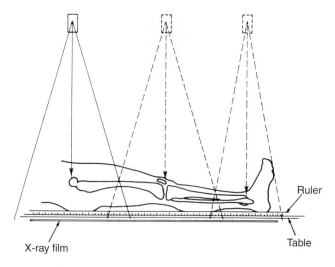

**Figure 29.19** The orthoradiograph technique exposes each joint individually, thereby ensuring that the x-ray beam through each joint is perpendicular to the x-ray film, thereby avoiding errors of magnification.

The orthoradiograph (Fig. 29.19) avoids the magnification factor by taking separate exposures of the hip, knee, and ankle so that the central x-ray beam passes through the joints, giving true readings from the scale (90). However, the orthoradiographic film is still cumbersome, and the need for multiple exposures introduces the risk of error if the patient moves.

The scanogram (Figs. 29.20 and 29.21) avoids magnification in the same way but reduces the size of the resulting film by moving the film cassette beneath the patient between exposures (91). This technique is preferred in children older than 5 or 6 years who can be compliant with instructions not to move, because it gives true measurements without

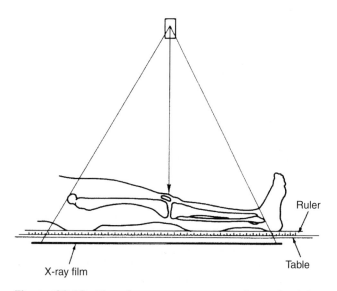

**Figure 29.18** The teleoroentgenogram reveals angular deformity but is subject to errors of magnification. It is probably the best technique for children who cannot reliably comply with instructions to remain still for multiple exposures.

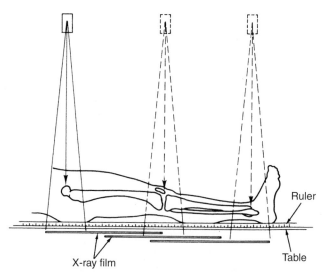

**Figure 29.20** The scanogram technique avoids magnification error in the same manner as the orthoroentgenogram does and is the preferred technique for children who can remain still for three exposures.

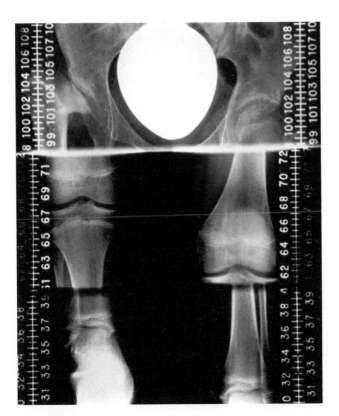

**Figure 29.21** Scanogram technique allows the images of the three joints to be captured on a film of convenient size by moving the film beneath the patient between exposures.

magnification, but younger children are better assessed using the teleoradiograph.

Positioning for the scanogram must be modified for patients with contractures of the hip or knee. Patients with hip flexion contractures can have accurate measurements taken in the reclining position. In those with only knee contractures, the femur can be measured in either the lateral or the prone position, and the tibia can be measured in the lateral position. Assessment of both bones can be made on one x-ray film in the lateral position if two rulers are used, one parallel to each bone. If a hip contracture is also present, the femur must be assessed in the lateral position. The scanogram of both femur and tibia can be done in the lateral position.

Digital radiography can be used to measure leg length (92,93). Computed tomography scan can be used to measure the distances between points on the radiographic film, reducing errors from angular deformity (94). If the examination is done specifically for this purpose, the cost is comparable with more traditional techniques (95–97), multiple sections are unnecessary, and the radiation exposure is less, especially with microdose techniques (98).

Whatever technique is used, it is important to be consistent and to not mix true and magnified measurements when analyzing data to determine the timing of surgery. Because errors are possible with all of these techniques, the resulting measurements should be compared with, and should correspond with, the clinical measurements.

An anteroposterior film of the pelvis and hips, taken with the patient standing and the legs straight (on blocks if necessary), is occasionally useful in assessing the combined effect of leg-length discrepancy, angular deformity, and asymmetry of the foot and pelvis because it more closely approximates the functional discrepancy. The leg-length discrepancy is calculated from the heights of the femoral heads from the floor, by taking into account the height of the blocks. This assessment can supplement the clinical examination done with blocks.

It is important for the surgeon to integrate all the information from the various methods of measuring leg length while preparing a treatment strategy.

### Skeletal Age

All methods of estimating skeletal age involve comparing radiographs of the patient with standards in an atlas. Methods have been described using the bones of the pelvis and hip, the knee, and the hand and wrist (99,100). The estimation of skeletal age is only moderately accurate and is the weak link in the techniques of analysis and prediction of growth.

The Greulich and Pyle method is used universally in this context. Their atlas (20) consists of reproductions of radiographs of the left hand and wrists of boys and girls that the authors considered typical for the stated skeletal age. To estimate the skeletal age of the patient, a radiograph of the left hand and wrist is taken according to the technique described in the atlas, and this film is then compared with the standard radiographs of the appropriate gender according to qualitative (e.g., the visibility of the hook of the hamate) and quantitative (e.g., the degree of conformity of an epiphysis to its metaphysis) criteria. The standard that most closely matches the patient's radiograph is taken as the skeletal age.

This technique has certain deficiencies. The first is that in some parts of the atlas the standards represent skeletal ages that are far apart, with a gap as great as 14 months. There is therefore a large standard error built into the technique. With practice, it is possible to interpolate between standards, but this practice is difficult, and studies have shown significant interobserver and intraobserver errors (101). A second problem is that some children do not follow the same orderly succession of maturity indicators shown in the atlas, and an arbitrary choice must be made in assigning a skeletal age. Third, some children with leg-length discrepancy of congenital origin also have congenital anomalies of the hand and wrist, making it impossible to reliably compare their radiographs with the standards. Finally, one of the features of almost all atlases of skeletal ages is that the mean skeletal age of a sample of similarly aged children is equal to their chronologic age so that the skeletal age is, in fact, the best possible predictor of chronologic age. That is, of a random sampling of boys or girls of the stated chronologic age, half would be more developed and half would be less developed than the standard radiograph. Greulich and Pyle, however, in selecting standards

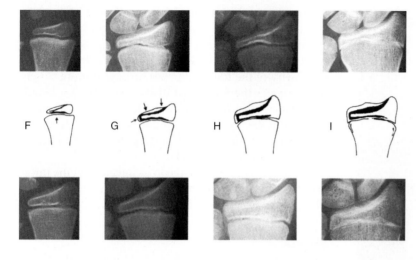

**Figure 29.22** The Tanner-Whitehouse atlas provides standards such as this for 20 different landmarks in the hand and wrist. This technique allows the determination of skeletal age to an accuracy of months but is not consistent with the Greulich-Pyle atlas. (From Tanner J, Whitehouse R, Marshall W, et al. *Assessment of skeletal maturity and prediction of adult height (TW2 method)*, London: Academic Press, 1975.)

for their atlas, did not follow this principle exactly, and in some cases they selected radiographs that they believed were more representative.

The Tanner-Whitehouse method (102) is similar in that it uses radiographs of the hand and wrist but was developed using modern computerized mathematical procedures. It adds a level of refinement and accuracy to the Greulich-Pyle technique by defining and showing examples of successive stages of development of 20 specific bony landmarks in the hand and wrist (Fig. 29.22). The same standards are used for boys and girls. The patient's radiograph is compared with the standards, and a letter score is assigned to each of the 20 landmarks. The letter score then is converted to a numeric score by consulting a table for the appropriate gender. The sum of these 20 scores represents the level of skeletal maturity attained by the patient, and it can be converted to years and months with a much smaller standard error than with the Greulich-Pyle technique. Of special interest in dealing with leg-length discrepancy is that the bony landmarks can be divided into two groups. Tanner and Whitehouse provide tables for including either the 12 long bone standards of the hand or the eight cuboid bone standards of the wrist in the assessment. When these two approaches give different results, it is reasonable to assume that the long bone standards give a skeletal age that is more pertinent to the growth of the long bones of the leg. The concept that the long bones are more important than the cuboid bones in the context of leg-length discrepancy can be useful, even with the Greulich-Pyle atlas, in allowing the resolution of difficulty in selecting the appropriate standard for a given radiograph.

This method is more cumbersome and time consuming than the Greulich-Pyle method. Its use in the context of leg-length discrepancy is problematic because this method and the Greulich-Pyle method can produce different skeletal ages from the same x-ray. This is surprising and probably is related in part to the fact that different populations and different techniques were used to develop the standards.

The relation between skeletal age and leg length is not as reliable as we would like it to be, and we must accept the relative inaccuracy of skeletal age estimation. It is still possible to make acceptably accurate predictions.

## DATA ANALYSIS

The adult with leg-length discrepancy, who has no future growth and no possibility of a changing discrepancy, presents with no need of analyzing data. The growing child, on the other hand, whose legs may be growing at different rates and whose discrepancy may be changing, presents another level of difficulty. The treatment goal must be chosen by considering the discrepancy that would be present at maturity and not the present discrepancy, and therefore, before performing surgery, the orthopaedic surgeon must be able to predict the situation at maturity. The importance of proper data analysis cannot be overemphasized. Blair et al. (103) reviewed 67 epiphysiodeses and found that correction to within 1 cm had been achieved in only 22 cases, and 35 failures had occurred because of incorrect use of the Green and Anderson data.

Four methods are useful in analyzing leg-length data: the arithmetic method, the growth-remaining method, the multiplier method, and the straight-line graph method. These methods differ significantly in their convenience, complexity, and accuracy, but the analysis moves through the same stages in all four. The first stage is the analysis of past growth, including the determination of the present discrepancy, and, depending on the method, the growth percentile and the growth inhibition. The second stage involves the prediction of future growth, including the lengths of the legs and discrepancy at maturity. The third stage is the prediction of the effects of corrective surgery.

All four methods have their place in the armamentarium of the orthopaedic surgeon. To be used properly and without error, all require a good understanding of the methodologies and the principles of growth. The four methods are discussed here in general terms, and step-by-step instructions for their use are shown in Figures 29.23, 29.24, and 29.25. The charts depicted in these figures are examples

# Determining leg-length discrepancy: The arithmetic method

## Leg-length data

(for examples for all three methods):

Sex: Female

| Age (yr) | Skeletal age (yr) | Right leg length (cm) | Left leg length (cm) |
|----------|-------------------|----------------------|---------------------|
| 7 + 10 | 8 + 10 | 60.0 | 58.2 |
| 8 + 4 | 9 + 4 | 64.4 | 61.9 |
| 9 + 3 | 10 + 3 | 70.0 | 66.2 |

## Prerequisite growth information

Distal femoral plate grows 10 mm/yr.
Proximal tibial plate grows 6 mm/yr.

Girls stop growing at 14 years of age.
Boys stop growing at 16 years of age.

## A Assessment of past growth

**1.** Longest time interval for data
= age at last visit – age at first

**2.** Years of growth remaining
= 14 (16 for boys) – age at last visit

**3.** Past growth of legs
= present length – first measured length

**4.** Growth rate of long leg
$= \dfrac{\text{past growth}}{\text{time interval}}$

**5.** Growth inhibition
$= \dfrac{(\text{growth of long leg} - \text{growth of short leg})}{\text{growth of long leg}}$

**1.** Longest time interval for data
= 9 yr 3 mo – 7 yr 10 mo = 1 yr 5 mo
= 1.42 yr

**2.** Years of growth remaining
= 14 yr – 9 yr 3 mo = 4 yr 9 mo = 4.75 yr

**3.** Past growth of:
long leg = 70.0 – 60.0 = 10.0 cm
short leg = 66.2 – 58.2 = 8.0 cm

**4.** Growth rate of long leg
$= \dfrac{10.0}{1.42} = 7.04$ cm/yr

**5.** Inhibition
$= \dfrac{(10.0 - 8.0)}{10.0} = 0.2$ cm

## B Prediction of future growth

**1.** Future growth of long leg
= years remaining × growth rate

**2.** Future increase in discrepancy
= future growth of long leg × inhibition

**3.** Discrepancy at maturity .
= present discrepancy + future increase

**1.** Future growth of long leg
= 4.75 × 7.04 = 33.4 cm

**2.** Future increase in discrepancy
= 33.4 × 0.2 = 6.7 cm

**3.** Discrepancy at maturity
= (70.0 – 66.2) + 6.7 = 10.5 cm

## C Prediction of effect of surgery

Effect of epiphysiodesis
= growth rate × years remaining

Effect of epiphysiodesis
Femoral = 1.0 × 4.75 = 4.75 cm
Tibial = 0.6 × 4.75 = 2.85 cm
Both = 1.6 × 4.75 = 7.6 cm

**Figure 29.23** Step-by-step instructions for use of the arithmetic method. The method presented here is modified from that presented by Menelaus and Westh, in that the future increase in discrepancy is calculated from growth acquired in the past instead of being assumed to be 0.3175 cm per year of growth remaining. An example is shown in the panels in the right column.

# Determing leg-length discrepancy: The growth-remaining method

## A Assessment of past growth

**1.** Growth of both legs
   = present length – first length

**1.** Growth of long leg
   = 70.0 – 60.0 = 10.0 cm

**1.** Growth of short leg
   = 66.2 – 58.2 = 8.0 cm

**2.** Present discrepancy
   = length of long leg – length of short leg

**2.** Present discrepancy
   = 70.0 – 66.2 = 3.8 cm

**3.** Growth inhibition
$$= \frac{(\text{growth of long leg} - \text{growth of short leg})}{\text{growth of long leg}}$$

**3.** Growth inhibition
$$= \frac{(10.0 - 8.0)}{10.0} = 0.2 \text{ cm}$$

## B Prediction of future growth

**1.** Plot present length of long leg on Green-Anderson leg length graph for appropriate sex

**1.**

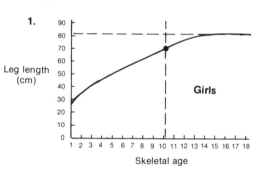

**2.** Project to right parallel to standard deviation lines until maturity to determine mature length of long leg

**2.** Length of long leg at maturity = 81.1 cm

**3.** Future growth of long leg
   = mature length – present length

**3.** Future growth of long leg
   = 81.1 – 70.0 = 11.1 cm

**4.** Future increase in discrepancy
   = future growth long × inhibition

**4.** Future increase in discrepancy
   = 11.1 × 0.2 = 2.2 cm

**5.** Predicted discrepancy at maturity
   = present discrepancy + future increase

**5.** Discrepancy at maturity
   = 3.8 + 2.2 = 6.0 cm

## C Prediction of effect of surgery

**1.** The effect of epiphysiodesis of the distal femoral and proximal tibial plates for a given sex and skeletal age can be determined by the Green-Anderson growth = remaining graph.

**1.** Correction from proximal tibial arrest
   = 2.7 cm

Correction from distal femoral arrest
   = 4.1 cm

Correction from combined arrest
   = 2.7 + 4.1 = 6.8 cm

**2.** The effect of lengthening is not affected by growth.

**Figure 29.24** Step-by-step instructions for use of the growth-remaining method. An example, shown in the right column, uses the same data as in the example in Figure 29.23.

# Determining leg-length discrepancy: The straight line graph method

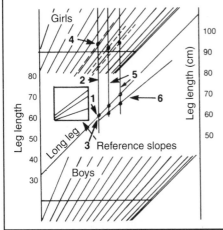

## A Assessment of past growth

1. Plot the point for the long leg on the sloping line labeled "LONG LEG" at the appropriate length.

2. Draw a vertical line through that point representing the current assessment.

3. Plot the point for the short leg on the vertical line.

4. Plot the point for skeletal age with reference to the sloping lines in the nomogram.

5. Plot successive visits in the same fashion.

6. Draw a straight line through the short leg points to represent the growth of the short leg.

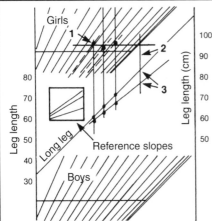

## B Prediction of future growth

1. Draw the horizontal straight line that best fits the points previously plotted for skeletal age. The fit to later points is more important than to earlier points. This is the growth percentile line.

2. From the intersection of the growth percentile line with the maturity skeletal age line, draw a vertical line to intersect the growth lines of the two legs. This line represents the end of growth.

3. The points of intersection of the vertical line with the two growth lines indicate the predicted lengths of the legs at maturity.

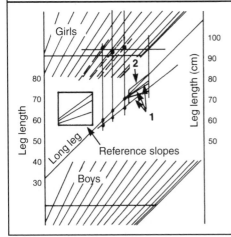

## C Prediction of effect of surgery

1. To predict the outcome after epiphysiodesis, draw three lines to the right from the last point for the long leg parallel to the three reference slopes. The intersections of these lines with the vertical line representing the end of growth indicates the predicted lengths of the long leg after the three possible types of epiphysiodesis.

2. To predict the outcome after leg lengthening, draw a line parallel to the growth line of the short leg but elevated above it by the amount of length gained.

**Figure 29.25**   Step-by-step instructions for use of the straight-line graph method. The data used are the same as in the example in Figure 29.24.

of the use of these methods in a specific case. It should be noted that the arithmetic method, the growth-remaining method, and the multiplier method are designed solely to arrive at the correct timing of epiphysiodesis. The straight-line graph method, on the other hand, provides a visualization of the child's entire pattern of growth and also provides for the prediction of future growth.

The accuracy of all methods depends to a degree on the nature of available data. The calculation of growth inhibition, for example, is more accurate with data over longer intervals. It is the interval over which data is collected and not the number of visits that is important, and data should be gathered for at least 1 or, preferably, 2 years. Minor errors in measurement over a short time can lead to major errors in estimating the growth inhibition and, consequently, to major errors in predicting the discrepancy at maturity. In the straight-line graph method, a greater number of visits can be useful in recognizing values that are in error, because they do not fit the pattern established by other visits. For example, one erroneous radiographic reading can be noticed in a group of other valid points, but can be missed if the patient makes only one or two visits. The straight-line graph is the only one of the three methods that uses all available skeletal ages, and the accumulation of more skeletal age estimates diminishes the errors in single estimates.

Some physicians, concerned with the inaccuracy of skeletal age estimation, have suggested that the use of chronologic age is just as accurate and have reported on series in which that appears to be true (104). The validity of that suggestion is difficult to accept, however, when one considers that it would lead to treating a 14-year-old boy with a skeletal age of 16 years in the same manner as a 14-year-old boy with a skeletal age of 12 years. Indeed, although Menelaus is frequently reported as using chronologic and not skeletal age, he said that his method should not be used if the difference was more than 1 year.

## Arithmetic Method

The arithmetic method was first described by White and, more recently, was evaluated by Menelaus and Westh (105,106). It is a method designed solely to manage discrepancy and to determine the timing of epiphysiodesis and is not a general method to describe growth. Menelaus intended the method to be based on measurements of discrepancy by blocks and not on measurements of leg length (Menelaus M, *Personal communication*, 1997). Although the method uses calendar age and not skeletal age, Menelaus suggests that it be used only in children whose skeletal and chronologic ages are less than a year apart, rendering moot the question of calendar versus skeletal age (Menelaus M, *Personal communication*, 1997).

The arithmetic method depends on the following statements, all of which are first approximations of the true growth pattern described by Green and Anderson.

Girls stop growing at the age of 14 years.
Boys stop growing at the age of 16 years.
The distal femoral plate grows 3/8 in. (10 mm) per year.
The proximal tibial plate grows 1/4 in. (6 mm) per year.
The discrepancy increases by 1/8 in. (3 mm) per year.

These approximations are reasonably good during the last years of growth but are inaccurate in young children. The statement that the discrepancy increases by 1/8 in. per year is obviously not true in all cases. It is, however, fairly accurate in those children who are in the last few years of growth, whose discrepancies began at birth, whose maturation is not considerably advanced or delayed relative to their chronologic ages, and whose discrepancies are within the clinical range for epiphysiodesis.

The most important advantage of the arithmetic method is its convenience, because no special tools are needed for its use. Menelaus recommended using English measure rather than metric measure because the arithmetic required to deal with one eighths of inches is elementary. There are several disadvantages of this method. It uses chronologic age rather than skeletal age and is therefore subject to error in children who grow and mature very early or very late. It uses an approximation of the growth curve rather than the growth curve itself and is only accurate in children approaching skeletal maturity. If, however, its use is restricted to determining the timing of epiphysiodesis and is applied only to the patients described earlier, then good results can be anticipated as have been reported by Menelaus et al. (106). Step-by-step instructions for the use of this method are shown in Figure 29.23.

Fries also has published straight-line approximations to the growth-remaining graph, in which the remaining growth in the epiphyses of boys and girls is determined by first-order equations using skeletal age, but this approach lacks the simplicity of the arithmetic method (107).

## Growth-remaining Method

The growth-remaining method is based on the data and tables of growth that Green and Anderson published in their two studies (16,17). These studies are to my knowledge the only good studies published that relate leg lengths to chronologic and skeletal age and that serve as the foundations of the more accurate methods of analyzing growth. Their graphs describing the lengths of the legs of boys and girls as a function of age can be used to determine the growth percentile of the child and the future growth of the long leg. Their graph showing the growth remaining in the distal femur and proximal tibia can be used to predict the effects of epiphysiodesis (108) (Fig. 29.7).

The advantages of this method are that it uses skeletal age, is based on an accurate description of the growth pattern, takes into account the child's growth percentile in predicting future growth, and has been demonstrated to be accurate over decades of use. The disadvantages are that it requires the availability of the two sets of graphs, does not take into account the growth percentile in predicting the effect of epiphysiodesis, and, because it uses only the most recent skeletal age estimation, it will be in error to the extent that the skeletal age estimate is in error. An inherent hazard of this method is that the growth-remaining graph is so familiar and easy to use that unwary physicians are tempted to correct the present discrepancy in a growing child, neglecting the steps that involve the prediction of future change. Step-by-step instructions for the use of this method are shown in Figure 29.24.

## Multiplier Method

The Green and Anderson data, as presented in Table 29.1, show the leg lengths achieved at various ages. By simple division, this data can be used to determine the proportion of adult leg length achieved by any specific age. Assuming that congenital discrepancies increase in proportion to leg length, it follows that the proportion of ultimate discrepancy achieved is the same as the proportion of adult length achieved. Paley et al. have calculated these proportions and, by inverting them, have provided a table of multipliers that can be used to predict the discrepancy at maturity given the present discrepancy and age of the child (23). These multipliers are shown in Table 29.3. The Green and Anderson data, for example, show that a boy has achieved 50% of his adult leg length by the age of 4 years. The multiplier for 4-year-old boys is 2, that is, a 4-year-old boy with a congenital discrepancy of 3 cm can be expected to have a $2 \times 3 = 6$ cm discrepancy at maturity.

## TABLE 29.3

### MULTIPLIERS

| Age (yr) | Boys | | Girls | |
|---|---|---|---|---|
| | **Femur** | **Tibia** | **Femur** | **Tibia** |
| 0 | 5.90 | 5.40 | 4.64 | 4.76 |
| 1 | 3.26 | 3.21 | 2.94 | 2.99 |
| 2 | 2.60 | 2.56 | 2.39 | 2.39 |
| 3 | 2.24 | 2.22 | 2.05 | 2.06 |
| 4 | 2.00 | 2.00 | 1.82 | 1.84 |
| 5 | 1.82 | 1.82 | 1.66 | 1.67 |
| 6 | 1.68 | 1.69 | 1.53 | 1.54 |
| 7 | 1.56 | 1.57 | 1.42 | 1.43 |
| 8 | 1.46 | 1.47 | 1.33 | 1.34 |
| 9 | 1.37 | 1.38 | 1.26 | 1.26 |
| 10 | 1.30 | 1.31 | 1.19 | 1.18 |
| 11 | 1.24 | 1.24 | 1.12 | 1.12 |
| 12 | 1.18 | 1.17 | 1.07 | 1.06 |
| 13 | 1.12 | 1.11 | 1.03 | 1.02 |
| 14 | 1.07 | 1.06 | 1.00 | 1.00 |
| 15 | 1.03 | 1.03 | — | — |
| 16 | 1.01 | 1.01 | — | — |
| 17 | 1.00 | 1.00 | — | — |

From Paley D, Bhave A, Herzenberg J, et al. Multiplier method for predicting limb-length discrepancies. *J Bone Joint Surg* 2000;59A: 1432–1446.

The use of this method to determine the timing of epiphysiodesis becomes more complex and requires calculations according to formulas provided by Paley et al. (23). This is particularly the case in developmental discrepancies where the discrepancy does not increase in proportion to leg length. Paley et al. have shown that the accuracy of this method is similar to that of other methods (23).

## Straight-line Graph Method

The straight-line graph method initially was devised as a method of presenting the relative growth of the legs in a clear, graphic manner (Fig. 29.26). By incorporating the data of Green and Anderson (17), it evolved into a method of recording, analyzing, and predicting growth (109,110). The method is based on two principles: the growth of the legs can be represented graphically by straight lines, and a nomogram can be used to determine the growth percentile from the skeletal age and leg length.

The representation of leg growth by straight lines appears to contradict the Green and Anderson description of growth, in which the growth lines of the legs are clearly curved. It is accomplished by manipulating the scale of the abscissa (x-axis) in strict accordance with the Green and Anderson data so that the curve that disappears from the growth lines reappears as an irregularity of that scale. This curve actually appears on the straight-line graph as a variable distance between the skeletal age lines. The important fact is that the straight line is not an approximation of the Green and Anderson data but represents the data just as accurately as their original graphs did. In the absence of active disease or treatment, the relative rates of growth of the two legs stay constant, with the result that the growth line of the short leg also follows a straight line on the graph. This means that the length of the leg is represented on the graph by the vertical position of its growth line, and its growth rate by the slope of the growth line. The discrepancy, therefore, is represented by the vertical distance between the two growth lines and the inhibition by the difference in slope.

The nomogram for skeletal age allows the plotting of points in a way that relates the length of the patient's long leg to the population and, in a sense, depicts the growth percentile. The nomogram is constructed so that all points for the child whose growth pattern exactly follows the pattern described by Green and Anderson lie on a horizontal straight line. In practice, this is rarely the case, partly because of the inaccuracy of estimation of skeletal age, and also in part because of the possibility that children of other races or other genetic stock have different patterns of growth. It is likely that the plotting of every skeletal age point on the nomogram before drawing the horizontal line representing the growth percentile "averages out" the inaccuracies of individual determinations of skeletal age. Similarly, the risk of error due to single estimates of skeletal age is likely to decrease with an increasing number of estimates.

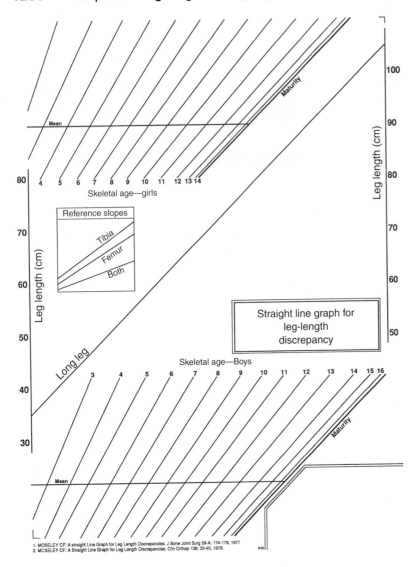

1. MOSELEY CF: A straight Line Graph for Leg Length Discrepancies. J Bone Joint Surg 59-A: 174-179, 1977
2. MCSELEY CF: A Straight Line Graph for Leg Length Discrepancies. Clin Orthop 136: 33-40, 1978.

**Figure 29.26** The straight-line graph comprises three parts: the leg-length area with the predefined line for the growth of the long leg, the areas of sloping lines for plotting skeletal ages, and reference slopes to predict growth following epiphysiodesis.

The straight-line graph facilitates the prediction of the effect of surgery. Lengthening or shortening will be represented on the graph by a vertical shift of its growth line either upward or downward to the appropriate extent without any change in its rate of growth. Conversely, the effect of an epiphysiodesis will be to decrease the slope of the growth line of the long leg. This is a strict mathematical relation, and because the contributions of the individual growth plates to the overall growth of the leg are known, the future slope of the growth line can be predicted accurately. Reference slopes on the graph depict the slopes to be followed after each of the three possible types of epiphysiodeses: distal femoral, proximal tibial, or both. For example, the slope of the growth line of the leg following a proximal tibial epiphysiodesis will be reduced to 73%, having lost the 27% normally contributed by that epiphysis. Because the unoperated long leg is defined on the graph as having a slope of 1.0, the slope following that surgery would be 0.73.

The advantages of this method are that it (i) uses skeletal age and the actual growth pattern described by Green and Anderson; (ii) takes into account the growth percentile in predicting future growth and the effect of surgery; (iii) minimizes errors due to the inaccuracy of skeletal age estimation; (iv) facilitates the flagging of erroneous values; and (v) avoids arithmetic errors (111). It is a general tool for analysis, illustration, and prediction in leg-length discrepancy and can be used in children with large discrepancies and inhibitions, extreme growth percentiles, and marked delay or advancement of maturation. Step-by-step instructions for the use of this method are shown in Figure 29.25.[1]

## Patterns of Inhibition

In all three of the preceding methods, the growth inhibition is determined on the basis of past growth and is then used to predict future growth. Evidence supports the

---

[1]A color version of the straight-line graph in PDF format suitable for printing is available at the author's web site, *www.pedipod.com*.

assumption that the growth inhibition will remain constant throughout the growing years (112). Indeed, in my study of patients who went on to have epiphysiodeses, the linear correlation coefficient between the lengths of the two legs was greater than 0.955 in every case (109,110). This is an extremely close fit and suggests that growth inhibition does indeed remain constant. It should be noted, however, that none of the children in this group had active disease or were under treatment that could affect growth.

Shapiro has reported different patterns and has also reported that the growth rate of the femur tends to increase, and that of the tibia to decrease, following a lengthening procedure (113). This effect is relatively short-lived and is not of sufficient magnitude to affect clinical decisions. Koman et al. have demonstrated constant inhibition in unilateral and bilateral proximal focal femoral deficiency (114), and Hootnick et al. have shown constant inhibition in congenitally short tibias (115).

The important question for the orthopaedic surgeon concerns the possibility of errors in correction due to changing inhibition. Does changing inhibition cause clinically significant errors in clinical judgment? A partial answer can be derived from my study mentioned earlier, in which the inhibition did not appear to change, and the straight-line graph predicted the final outcome within 1 cm in all cases. This suggests that whatever effect the changing inhibition has, it is not sufficient to prevent reaching predictions of future growth that are sufficiently accurate for good clinical results.

### Inadequate Data

There are certain situations in which patients present late, it is suspected that the time for epiphysiodesis is imminent, and there is insufficient time to accumulate data required for accurate assessment and prediction. In some cases, it is still possible to make reliable assumptions about the growth pattern that allow accurate prediction and confident treatment planning.

Consider the situation in which a child presents without any prior data, and the only information available is from that particular visit. The difficulty here is that it is impossible to calculate the growth inhibition and predict the discrepancy at maturity. If, however, the onset of the growth inhibition can be determined, it can be assumed that the legs were of equal length at that time. The length of the long (and therefore the short) leg at that time can be estimated using either the Green and Anderson growth graph or the straight-line graph, and the growth inhibition can then be calculated in the usual way. Likewise, in the case of a congenital discrepancy with inhibition beginning before birth, it can be assumed that there was a time before birth when the length of both legs was zero or, in other words, that the growth inhibition is equal to the percentage difference in the length of the legs. This assumption is consistent with the conclusion of Herron et al. (116).

At times, an opinion is sought on the basis of leg-length measurements without skeletal age when the patient is not immediately available to obtain them. In this case, the child's chronologic age can be used in place of the skeletal age, and this approach is validated if the development of secondary sexual characteristics and menarche are consistent with the chronologic age. Little et al. have suggested, in fact, that chronologic age is as accurate as skeletal age in determining the timing of epiphysiodesis, but his study eliminated several patients on the basis of skeletal age and dealt with a select population (104). In my view, a surgeon should not base his timing for epiphysiodesis on chronologic age and should take this approach only as a rough guideline.

In certain patients with remote disease that is no longer active, there exists no continuing growth inhibition or accentuation. Patients with leg-length discrepancy caused by stimulation from fracture healing or osteomyelitis, or with shortening caused by fracture malunion that occurred more than 2 years earlier, can confidently be assumed to have a static discrepancy. The discrepancy at maturity therefore will be the same as that at present, and attention can be directed at correcting the present discrepancy.

Patients with complete destruction of one physis because of trauma or infection can present with an early minimal discrepancy, but significant inhibition that, with growth, will certainly lead to a greater discrepancy requiring treatment. In select cases, these children can be treated with an epiphysiodesis of the corresponding plate of the other limb. This plan does not correct the discrepancy but ensures equal inhibition in both legs and an unchanging discrepancy throughout the growth period.

Sometimes no such assumptions are reasonable, and a decision reliable enough to undertake surgery cannot be made. In these cases, it is best to abandon the possibility of epiphysiodesis and wait until maturity, when the discrepancy can be corrected without error by shortening or lengthening.

## DETERMINATION OF TREATMENT GOALS

The choice of the treatment goal and the choice of the treatment method are two different and independent steps in the treatment of patients with leg-length discrepancy and are discussed separately here. The selection of the treatment goal depends on the careful and thorough assessment of the patient, both clinically and radiologically, and the reader is referred back to the earlier sections on patient assessment.

### Equal Leg Length

Many patients who have leg-length discrepancy as an isolated problem, such as those with hemiatrophy, present no difficulty in the choice of treatment goal. Leg-length equality at maturity is the appropriate goal.

## Unequal Leg Length

Many patients do best with incomplete correction. Undercorrection of 1 or 2 cm is best for patients with paralysis of the short leg. The residual discrepancy facilitates clearing of the floor by the weak short leg during the swing phase of gait, and this is even more important in patients who wear braces and have the knee locked in extension to ambulate. In patients who cannot walk without braces, the leg-length discrepancy usually can be made up in the brace, and corrective surgery may not be indicated.

## Level Pelvis

Patients with leg-length discrepancy often have asymmetry that extends beyond the legs. Patients with congenital shortening, for example, may have a small foot or hemipelvis, and in these cases perfectly equal leg-lengths result in residual pelvic obliquity and tilting of the lumbosacral joint. A similar situation can arise in patients who have leg-length discrepancy from avascular necrosis of the femoral head following treatment of congenital dislocation of the hip and who have also had an innominate osteotomy. These patients should be examined in the standing position, with blocks beneath the short leg to relate the desired correction to the leg-length discrepancy. The treatment goal can be modified as required.

## Vertical Lumbar Spine

Patients with fixed obliquity of the lumbosacral junction cannot achieve a level pelvis and a vertical lumbar spine at the same time. Usually, a vertical lumbar spine and good balance of the spine are more important than a level pelvis, and treatment of the leg-length discrepancy should be consistent with these more important goals. It is interesting to consider the possibility that such a patient could benefit from lengthening of the already long leg if the pelvic obliquity were greater than the leg-length discrepancy.

## Equalization by Prosthetic Fitting

Some discrepancies are too great to be considered for correction. The traditional guideline has been that a femur that is less than half of the length of the femur of the other side and legs that eventually grow to be shorter than 15 cm are candidates for prosthetic fitting. This is often done in conjunction with other procedures, including knee fusion, Syme amputation, and Van Nes rotationplasty. Modern advances in lengthening have led us to hope that we are more proficient at correcting very large discrepancies with acceptable morbidity (117–119). It is my opinion that some discrepancies up to 20 cm are reasonable candidates

for correction by a variety of combined simultaneous or staged shortening and lengthening procedures, but there is no reason why the traditional guideline should be abandoned.

## Correction of Coexisting Problems

The treatment plan must include those intermediate goals that are prerequisites to surgical treatment of the leg-length discrepancy itself. These intermediate goals can include stabilization of unstable joints, release of contractures, correction of angular deformity, correction of spinal deformity, completion of partial growth arrests causing angular deformity, and excision of bony bridges in an attempt to restore growth.

# TREATMENT

## General Principles

It is sometimes advisable to correct coexisting deformities before correcting leg-length discrepancy, because the correction of some deformities changes the treatment goal. For example, the correction of angular deformity of the limb usually increases the length of the leg, and the correction of spinal imbalance often changes pelvic obliquity and the desired amount of correction of leg length.

The choice of treatment method depends more on the magnitude of the predicted discrepancy at maturity than on the etiology. Fairly straightforward guidelines expressed in terms of the magnitude of the predicted discrepancy can be used to choose from among the major treatment categories:

| | |
|---|---|
| 0 to 2 cm: | No treatment |
| 2 to 6 cm: | Shoe lift, epiphysiodesis, shortening |
| 6 to 20 cm: | Lengthening, which may or may not be combined with other procedures |
| >20 cm: | Prosthetic fitting |

There is some flexibility in these guidelines to account for factors such as environment, motivation, intelligence, compliance, emotional stability, patient's and parents' wishes, and associated pathology in the limbs.

There are good reasons for the values of these thresholds. It has been shown that discrepancies of less than 2 cm are of no functional or clinical consequence in adults and that these discrepancies do not require treatment (120). Indeed, Rush and Steiner found leg-length discrepancy in 71% of new recruits into the United States Armed Forces (121). Because there is some advantage to being tall (122–125), lengthening procedures are often preferred by parents and patients, but lengthening is not generally done for discrepancies less than 6 cm because there are other alternatives. Because of the high morbidity and complication rate of lengthening, this procedure should be avoided in favor of epiphysiodesis or shortening whenever possible.

Because these alternatives are reasonable for corrections of up to 6 cm, they are the procedures of choice. Shortening procedures are usually not appropriate for correction of greater than 6 cm, because a disproportionate appearance results that is not pleasing to the patient. Epiphysiodesis can be performed to correct a discrepancy of any magnitude when the long leg is clearly the abnormal one, because this procedure corrects the abnormally long leg and does not result in abnormal proportions in these cases. Patient preference for lengthening over shortening is considered only in the 5- to 6-cm range of correction because there are overriding considerations outside that range.

The site of correction is chosen with the ultimate goal of making the patient's body as symmetrical as possible, with knees being as level as possible. This involves lengthening the shortest bone or shortening the bone corresponding to the shortest bone on the other side leg. This principle can be ignored in some cases of correction by epiphysiodesis in which a single plate is arrested to reduce the magnitude of surgery and risk of problems, although a combined femoral and tibial epiphysiodesis might produce the most symmetrical result. It also can be ignored if more time for data gathering allows a more confident prediction of future growth and a more dependable treatment plan. Symmetry of knee height is a secondary consideration to equality of leg length. Knee height is not a factor in function or comfort and is not very important in cosmesis.

## Shoe Lift

A shoe lift is an excellent treatment for discrepancies up to 6 cm. Though believed to be less desirable than surgical correction of the discrepancy, it is a satisfactory answer for those patients who do not wish or are not appropriate for surgery. The shoe lift is only effective when the patient is walking or is in two-legged stance and is only prescribed for its benefit on gait.

No lift is required for discrepancies less than 2 cm. For larger discrepancies, the height of the lift should be less than the discrepancy. For reasons of cosmesis, up to 2 cm of the lift can be put inside the shoe with the remainder, if necessary, on the outside. Lifts higher than 5 cm are poorly tolerated because the muscles controlling the subtalar joint are not strong enough to resist inversion stress and frequent ankle strains result. If a higher lift is required, an orthotic extension up the posterior calf can be added for stability. The optimum height of the lift can be determined by clinical trials in which the lift height is temporarily modified to suit the patient. Liu found that the benefit provided by a heel lift, although it affects the SI, is unpredictable (3).

## Prosthetic Fitting

Prosthetic fitting, often in association with amputation, is a treatment of last resort but is useful for those patients with very large discrepancies and for those with deformed and functionally useless feet (126,127). Discrepancies anticipated to become greater than 15 to 20 cm and those involving a femoral length less than 50% of the other side femur should be treated in this way (38). This approach has the advantage of involving only one hospitalization and one definitive operation. Patients with fibular hemimelia and an unstable ankle do better with this approach than with multiple hospitalizations and surgical procedures in a futile attempt to conserve the foot; the latter situation usually results in late amputation, which is more difficult to accept.

Children with below-knee amputations, such as those amputated for fibular hemimelia, do very well functionally. They have an almost normal walking gait and can participate in recreational and sporting activities. Children who are treated for proximal focal femoral deficiency require above-knee prostheses and they function well, although not as well as the children who have undergone below-knee amputations. Some of the above-the-knee prostheses can function as below-the-knee prostheses following a Van Nes rotationplasty, in which the reversed ankle functions as a knee, which provides active control and motor power to the prosthetic knee (128).

Although it is difficult for the parents to decide on an amputation on young children, the children who undergo surgery and prosthetic fitting early in life show the best results. The optimal time for performing the Syme amputation is toward the end of the first year of life and for performing the rotationplasty is at approximately 3 years of age. It is helpful for parents of children who are candidates for these procedures to meet older children who have undergone the same procedure and to talk with their parents.

## Epiphysiodesis

Epiphysiodesis has very low morbidity, a very low complication rate, and is the treatment of choice for the surgical correction of leg-length discrepancy (19,105,129,130). The operation is effective by slowing the growth rate of the long leg and by allowing the short leg to catch up. In planning for this procedure, therefore, it is necessary to take into account the ability of the short leg to catch up; this is done using the growth inhibition to predict the discrepancy at maturity. For all surgical treatments of leg-length discrepancy, it is the discrepancy at maturity that should be corrected and not the present discrepancy in a growing child. Epiphysiodesis is a highly acceptable procedure because it is straightforward, does not require postoperative immobilization, and disables the child minimally and for a short duration. It is only suitable for those children who have sufficient leg-length data to enable a confident prediction of the discrepancy at maturity and for those whose discrepancies require correction of 2 to 6 cm (131).

Epiphysiodesis is an all-or-nothing procedure that completely and permanently arrests physeal growth. Thereafter, the leg grows at a slower rate, having lost the contribution of the operated physis toward the process of growth. The loss is 27% for the proximal tibial, 38% for the distal femoral, and 65% for combined epiphysiodesis of both plates. The surgeon therefore induces a known degree of growth inhibition and has before him not a continuous spectrum of shortenings but only three discrete choices. The exact amount of desired shortening can be achieved only by performing the surgery at exactly the correct time. Performing the operation too late results in undercorrection, and performing it too early results in overcorrection. This is in contrast to shortening and lengthening procedures that can be performed at any time.

The prediction of the effect of surgery can be made accurately within 1 cm in almost all cases (109). Because there is an advantage to being tall (122–125), it is better to err on the side of undercorrection than overcorrection. Because slight discrepancies are well tolerated, it is best to aim for 0.5 to 1.0 cm of undercorrection by doing the epiphysiodesis slightly later than the time for perfect correction. To improve symmetry, the procedure is best done in the bone that is opposite the shortest one on the other-side leg, although this principle may have to be compromised if future growth is insufficient for such an epiphysiodesis to be effective.

The principle of the surgery is to produce a symmetrical bony bridge that tethers the physis and prevents future growth. The traditional open techniques involve removing a block of bone from the medial and lateral aspects of the plate, extirpating the plate with a curette, and replacing the block of bone in such a manner as to produce a bony bridge. Phemister described removal of a rectangular block, two-thirds on the metaphyseal side and one-third on the epiphyseal side of the plate, and its replacement in the reversed position (132) (Fig. 29.27). White and Stubbins used a special chisel to remove a square block that was later rotated 90 degrees before replacement (130), and Blount used a circular trephine to remove a cylindrical block that was rotated in the same way. Macnicol and Gupta have reported a percutaneous version of the Blount technique (133). All these procedures serve to bridge the physis medially and laterally with solid bone.

Blount produced physeal arrest by placing three staples across the physis, both medially and laterally, thereby producing a tethering effect resulting in arrest of growth (134–136) (Fig. 29.28). The rationale was that the arrest was temporary and that growth would resume after removal of the staples (137,138). This concept was attractive because it alleviated the need to make accurate predictions of future growth. In certain patients, however, the physes fused while the staples were in place; on the removal of the staples, growth did not resume, resulting in overcorrection of the discrepancies (139,140). Stapling therefore lost proponents and was considered to be a permanent form of growth arrest. Staples caused problems by extruding, entering the adjacent joint, or causing overlying

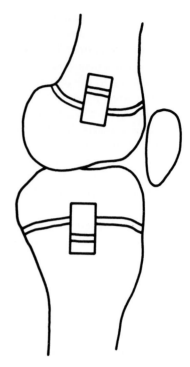

**Figure 29.27** Epiphysiodesis by the Phemister technique. A rectangular bone block is replaced in reverse position to produce a bar across the growth plate.

bursitis (141). Growth arrest was occasionally asymmetrical, and a second operation was sometimes necessary to remove the staples.

There have been reports that it is possible to perform stapling in such a way that normal growth resumes when the staples are removed (142–144). Technical details are important, among them, remaining extraperiosteal and not directly exposing the growth plate.

Traditional epiphysiodesis requires incisions on both the medial and lateral aspects of the knee, a total of four incisions if both tibial and femoral epiphysiodeses are performed. Several authors have reported percutaneous

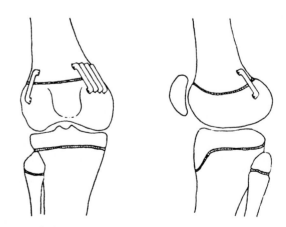

**Figure 29.28** Epiphysiodesis by stapling. Growth arrest can be accomplished by careful placement of three extraperiosteal staples over the medial and lateral aspects of the plate.

techniques developed to avoid unsightly scarring (133, 145,146). They are done with a drill or burr through small medial and lateral incisions under image intensifier control. This technique has gained wide acceptance and is considered by most to be the technique of choice. Great care must be taken to line up the image intensifier beam perfectly to ensure that the tool is in the plate.

Percutaneous epiphysiodesis is usually performed through two incisions, one medial and one lateral. Because the growth plates, particularly the distal femoral plate, are not perfectly flat, there is a significant technical challenge in making sure that the tip of the tool is in the plate and that it stays there. Scott, for example, reported a rate of continued growth of the physis of 12% (147). In the distal femur, the intercondylar notch intrudes into the posterior aspect of the plate, and the surgeon must be careful not to inadvertently enter the notch by being sensitive to the feel of the tool touching cortical bone. The operator might not notice the tool entering the notch because it is not obvious on the anteroposterior view of the image intensifier.

Approximately 50% of the area of the plate should be removed in the pattern shown in Fig. 29.29. This extent of removal is sufficient to ensure arrest of the physis and maintains enough bone strength through residual plate and surrounding periosteum and perichondral ring to make postoperative immobilization unnecessary. Tibial epiphysiodesis should be accompanied by arrest of the proximal fibular physis if the tibial shortening is greater than 2.5 cm (148). The fibular epiphysiodesis can be performed through the same skin incision as the lateral aspect of the tibia, but the surgeon must approach the fibula from the anterior aspect to avoid the peroneal nerve.

Epiphysiodesis has considerable advantages over other approaches because of its low morbidity and low complication rate, but there are minor disadvantages (149,150). It is a compensatory and not a corrective operation, in that it makes the normal leg abnormal. Compared to lengthening,

it results in a decrease in the patient's stature that may be undesirable.

## Femoral Shortening

Shortening of the femur has the same indications as epiphysiodesis but is offered to patients who do not meet the prerequisites for epiphysiodesis either because they are too old or because their conditions are such that the extent of the discrepancy at maturity cannot be confidently predicted. The advantage of this procedure over epiphysiodesis is that it can be done in the mature patient, when the discrepancy is known and unchanging and the desired degree of correction can be obtained precisely.

Shortening of the tibia also has been performed but is very rarely done except in cases in which the femur does not lend itself to shortening. Although shortening of 7.5 cm in the femur and 5 cm in the tibia have been reported with no loss of function (151), it is believed that no more than 3 cm of shortening can safely be achieved in the tibia, and it is unusual to perform shortenings of more than 5 cm in the femur. The risk of neurovascular complications is higher in the tibia because of the proximity and the tethering of neurovascular structures, as is the risk of delayed union and nonunion. Fasciotomy is advisable to reduce the risk of compartment syndrome. Internal fixation is more difficult in the tibia; closed techniques cannot be used because the bone is subcutaneous, and the muscles of the leg are slower to recover strength than those of the thigh.

It is interesting to contemplate the reason for the muscles of the leg recovering strength more slowly than those of the thigh. The ability of a muscle to adjust to shortening of the underlying bone rests on its ability to remove sarcomeres from the ends of its fibers until the average length of the remaining sarcomeres returns to normal, which is relatively constant throughout the body. The lengths of the hamstring and quadriceps muscles, crossing two joints, are approximately twice as long as the soleus, but more importantly, there is an even greater difference in the lengths of the fibers within those muscles. The soleus muscle, requiring high strength and short excursion, has a high number of short fibers oriented obliquely, whereas the hamstrings, requiring excursion more than strength, have a smaller number of longer fibers oriented longitudinally. The fiber lengths in any one muscle are relatively equal, and the fiber length in the hamstrings is much longer than the 4-cm length of fibers in the soleus muscle (152). It is not difficult to imagine that a shortening of the tibia by more than 3 cm might completely overwhelm the ability of the fibers of the soleus muscle to accommodate.

The early techniques of shortening involved making step cuts or other complex cuts in the diaphysis of the bone, using interfragmentary screws or intramedullary rods for fixation (153,154). These techniques are only of historical interest, because better techniques with more secure fixation are now available (155). The two principal techniques in use

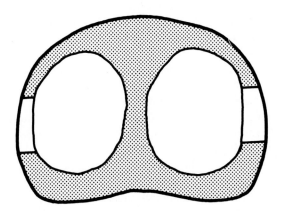

**Figure 29.29**  Area of plate to be removed in epiphysiodesis. Obliteration of medial and lateral circular segments of the plate, leaving the central part and the strong periphery, successfully stops growth, yet the bone retains sufficient strength to forego immobilization.

today are proximal shortening with blade plate fixation and middiaphyseal shortening, open or closed, with intramedullary rod fixation. Both approaches provide secure fixation and neither requires postoperative immobilization.

### Proximal Shortening

Shortening through the proximal femur at the level of the lesser trochanter with blade plate fixation has the advantage of being proximal to most of the quadriceps origin and therefore not as disadvantageous to the knee as shortening in the midshaft is. Patients recover strength and the ability to climb stairs more quickly. This approach leaves a large scar on the lateral thigh and requires a second later operation of moderate magnitude to remove the plate.

### Closed Femoral Shortening

Winquist (156) and Winquist and Hansen (157) pioneered a technique that involves the use of a special set of instruments designed to allow the procedure to be performed entirely from within the medullary cavity and without any direct approach to the shaft of the femur. The bone is cut by a special eccentric cam saw that is passed down the shaft and cuts through the cortex from within. The size of the saw required is determined by the outside diameter of the bone, and the femoral shaft is first reamed to an internal diameter that is sufficiently large to accept it. The distal cut is made first, and a second cut is then made more proximally at the precise location to give the desired amount of correction. The cuts should be placed so that the cylindrical fragment is removed from the isthmus of the femur where the internal diameter is least, because this site provides the best fixation to the rod both proximally and distally. The cylindrical piece of bone can be cut into two sections using a special hook-shaped reverse-cutting osteotome, and the pieces are pushed aside. The gap can then be closed over an intramedullary rod to provide rigid internal fixation. Locking at both ends maintains shortening and rotation. A second operation is later required to remove the rod.

The technical complications of this procedure usually result from less than rigid fixation of the fragments, usually due to inadequate reaming without locking. It is apparent, in using an unlocked nail, that if a 5-cm segment of bone is to be removed and 2.5 cm of fixation is desired both proximally and distally, then the bone has to be reamed until 10 cm of the shaft is reamed to the minimum diameter. This in itself can be a problem because the cortex can become very thin at the level of the osteotomies, especially because the reaming is usually eccentric, and can lead to fracture of the shaft. Less than rigid fixation can lead to loss of rotational control and opening of the shortening gap, two problems that are difficult to control without locking. Less reaming is necessary for a locked nail, but in this case, the reduced internal diameter of the canal may not allow passage of a cam saw large enough to cut completely through the cortex, and a percutaneous osteotomy may be required to complete the cut. Nevertheless, the benefits of control of position with the locked nail far outweigh this disadvantage, and locking is desirable in such situations.

Acute respiratory distress syndrome has been reported during or following closed intramedullary shortening and has been believed to be the result of fat embolization caused by reaming (158). Possible preventative measures include venting of the distal metaphysis and use of reamers with flutes sufficiently deep to allow the unimpeded egress of reamed material, but the effectiveness of these measures has not been demonstrated. It is not advisable to use this technique until this serious complication can be avoided with certainty.

Although this is an appealing technique, it requires familiarity with the instruments, is technically demanding, and has best results in experienced hands. The major disadvantages are the technical complications and risk of respiratory distress syndrome, as noted in the preceding text, and the significant quadriceps weakness that results. Patients with greater shortening require 6 to 12 months to regain normal knee control and function (159). It leaves a small, cosmetically acceptable scar, and the later procedure to remove the rod is of lesser magnitude than that required to remove a blade plate.

### Growth Stimulation

The best solution for a child discovered early to have growth inhibition would be to stimulate his growth to achieve a normal level. Many techniques have been used in attempts to accomplish this, but none has been successful enough to be clinically useful. On the basis of the concept that the periosteum acts as a tether inhibiting growth, circumferential release of the periosteum has been assessed both clinically and experimentally and has been found to stimulate growth (160,161). A variety of foreign materials have been implanted next to the growth plate (162), but the stimulation, if it occurred, was too little and too short-lived to be of use. Sympathectomy (163,164) and surgically constructed arteriovenous fistulae (165,166) temporarily stimulate growth, presumably by altering the circulation to the physis, as does stripping and lifting the periosteum by packing bone beneath it (60,61,167). However, these techniques have little or no clinical significance. Electrical stimulation inconsistently stimulates physeal growth, but even the maximum effect is insufficient to correct clinical discrepancies (65).

As desirable as this approach might appear, there is no method of growth stimulation available at this time that is useful in the treatment of leg-length discrepancy.

### Leg Lengthening

Lengthening an abnormally short leg would, at first glance, appear to be the preferable method of dealing with leg-length discrepancy because it is a corrective procedure. It involves operating on the abnormal leg to correct its abnormality, as opposed to epiphysiodesis and shortening, which make the normal leg abnormal and only compensate for the discrepancy.

Lengthening was first mentioned in the 18th century, in an account of injuries sustained in battle by Ignatius of Loyola. It was next reported by Codivilla at the beginning of the 20th century (168). A number of advances have been made in the surgical technique, or the lengthening apparatus, or both, and each change has been greeted with hopes that it would solve the problems associated with lengthening (169).

Lengthening is a procedure of last resort and is reserved for those situations in which other methods of correction are inappropriate. Lengthening is usually not appropriate for patients requiring correction of less than 6 cm because in these cases other procedures of lesser risk and morbidity can be used. A reasonable goal of lengthening for most patients is less than 10 cm for the femur and 7 cm for the tibia. Patients requiring large corrections may require simultaneous lengthenings of femur and tibia, repeated staged lengthenings of the same bone (170), or supplementary shortening procedures on the long leg. There is a threshold, at approximately 15 to 20 cm, where the risks outweigh the benefits, and lengthening is abandoned in favor of amputation and prosthetic fitting.

Since Codivilla's report, there have been many techniques described for lengthening the leg. These have included step

cuts (171), periosteal sleeves (172), onlay cortical grafts (173), slotted plates (174), intramedullary rods (175), and other internal and external devices for gradual controlled lengthening (176–179). Transiliac lengthening has been performed (180) and may be indicated in cases with both infrapelvic asymmetry and decompensated scoliosis cases requiring concurrent hip stabilization (181,182). Techniques of instantaneous lengthening of the femur (116,155, 183,184) and tibia (185) have been reported but have not gained widespread support because the amount of length to be gained is limited. Simultaneous shortening of one femur and lengthening of the other with the excised bone segment from the other-side leg has been recommended (186,187). The Anderson device, using large pins and an external fixator with threaded rods for lengthening, became widely used but confined the patient to bed (Fig. 29.30). Some of the older methods persist in nonindustrialized nations (e.g., double oblique osteotomy followed by elongation by balanced skeletal traction) (188). Many of these methods became obsolete with the introduction of the Wagner device and, later, the Ilizarov and Orthofix devices.

Historically, new lengthening technology has been adopted enthusiastically by the orthopaedic community and has been used extensively with great optimism. However, the complication rate has remained high, and the patient's course difficult, leading to the realization that the human leg has not made similar advances and that lengthening is still a difficult matter for both the surgeon and the patient.

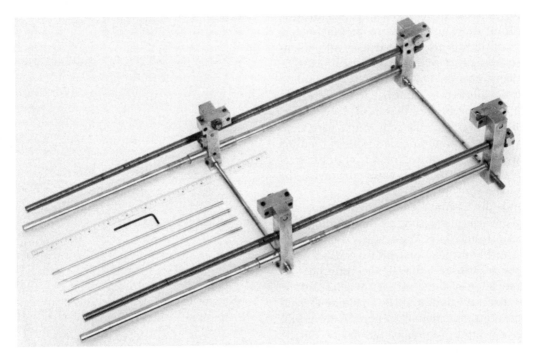

**Figure 29.30** The Anderson lengthening device was commonly used until it was superseded by the Wagner device and later by the Ilizarov and Orthofix devices. It accomplished stable fixation and gradual lengthening, but it was not appropriate for application to the femur, and it confined the patient to bed.

For two weeks following the application of the lengthening device the patient will require intensive education and observation. This allows time for the initial delay and for the patient and parents to understand and become comfortable with the lengthening mechanism, pin site care, an exercise program to maintain mobility and to attain ambulation with weight bearing. Inpatients undergoing lengthening should be examined daily for blood pressure, neurologic status, and range of motion. The reading from the scale of the lengthener should be recorded daily and should be checked to be sure that the lengthening process is going according to plan. These assessments also should be made at weekly or biweekly visits after discharge. Radiographs are taken at intervals of 2 to 4 weeks to evaluate alignment and the quality of bone in the lengthening gap (i.e., the regenerate). Ultrasonography can be used instead of radiographs to measure the lengthening gap (189,190). The rate of distraction can be modified according to clinical progress or radiologic appearance.

Maintaining motion is extremely important during the lengthening procedure. Patients and parents should be instructed in a home exercise program, and the patient's range of motion should be monitored regularly. Stopping the lengthening should be considered if limitation of motion that is resistant to a more intensive motion program develops. Wagner recommended that distraction should not be performed on any given day if the patient cannot achieve 60 degrees of flexion (191). My personal guidelines are to discontinue lengthening of the femur when a knee flexion contracture is greater than 10 degrees or knee flexion is less than 30 degrees. Lengthening can be started again if those guidelines are later met before consolidation of the regenerate prevents it. All patients regain flexion in the first year after lengthening (192), and it appears that maintaining extension is more important. Patients are allowed to ambulate with full weight bearing, with aids if necessary. The pin sites are cleaned twice daily and, if necessary, the stab wounds are elongated weekly under local anesthesia to prevent tenting and ischemia of the skin, which could lead to pin tract infection. Cutting pins and small wires circumvent the need to release pin sites.

Distraction is discontinued either when the goal has been achieved or when an unresolvable complication, usually loss of motion, supervenes. The device is retained until radiographs show consolidation and suggest adequate strength of the regenerate bone. In the consolidation period, dynamization of the device is considered to be important to subject the bone to cyclic longitudinal loading to stimulate bone formation. If the bone in the lengthening gap is slow to consolidate, the device can be shortened to put the bone under longitudinal compression, either leaving it somewhat shortened or lengthening it once again when the regenerate responds. Valid objective guidelines for what constitutes adequate consolidation for

removal of the lengthening device have not been established. Findings such as corticalization with three cortices visible on two radiographs and the appearance of a medullary cavity are considered to be signs of adequate strength, but the decision to remove the device is still empiric.

It is possible to protect the tibia externally with a cast or brace after device removal, allowing removal from the tibia earlier than from the femur. In addition, the mechanical and anatomic axes of the tibia are collinear, and the bone is subject mainly to compressive forces. This is not the case for the femur, in which the regenerate bone, especially for proximal lengthenings, is eccentric and is subject to bending loads. Patients should be restricted from violent body-contact sports for a long time, and perhaps until the bone is radiologically normal, because fractures through the lengthening gap have been reported years later.

### Wagner Technique
Wagner developed a lengthening device that was first used in North America in 1973 (Fig. 29.31) and appeared to offer several advantages over older devices, such as the Anderson device (Fig. 29.30) (54,191,193–195). It is unilateral and uses half-pins instead of through-and-through pins, thereby facilitating application to the femur. It is small and light, and it was the first device to allow the patient to be ambulatory, whereas older devices required confinement to bed. The patient can perform the lengthening procedure simply by turning a knob at one end. It is adjustable in varus-valgus and anteroposterior angulation but not in rotation (Fig. 29.31), so that minor angulation

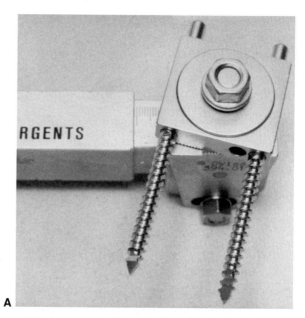

A

**Figure 29.31** The Wagner device. The device can be adjusted in two planes, but not in rotation. It allows correction of angulation that develops during lengthening but does not allow simultaneous lengthening and gradual correction of angular deformity.

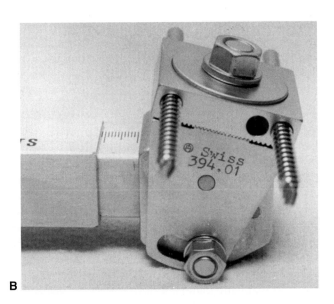

**Figure 29.31** (*continued*)

that occurs during lengthening can be corrected without removing the pins.

The Wagner technique involves at least three surgical procedures. The first involves performing an osteotomy, releasing soft tissues if necessary, and applying the device. At the end of the lengthening phase, a second procedure involves bone grafting the lengthening gap, plating the bone, and removal of the lengthener. Months or years later, when the bone has achieved sufficient strength, a third procedure is done to remove the plate. There is a prolonged period of restriction of activities to protect the bone and to avoid late fracture.

Although the Wagner device retains its simplicity and utility, it has become clear that it is ill-advised to plate the bone in the presence of contaminated pin tracts. Therefore, the technique has largely been replaced by newer methods that involve neither plating nor grafting and appear to reduce the complication rate. The device, however, remains simple and satisfactory and can be used with the newer biologic principles.

### Orthofix Technique

De Bastiani et al. have developed a lengthening device, the Orthofix device (Fig. 29.32), which is applied to the bone with two sets of conical screws (196,197). It has evolved into a lengthener in which pin blocks move along a rail placed beside the pins (Fig. 29.32). This arrangement allows the pin sets to start close together and provides long excursion. It allows the use of up to three screws in each set, which is an advantage, especially in the proximal femur. It is technically similar in operation to the Wagner device but, although it offers more stable fixation to bone, it has a more cumbersome method of elongation and is not easily adjustable once in place. Encouraging results

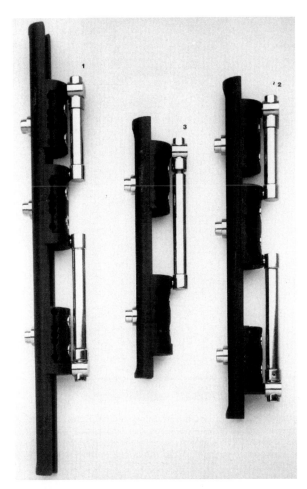

**Figure 29.32** The Orthofix track lengthening device. This device places the lengthening mechanism beside the pins instead of between them, thereby increasing the excursion and obviating device exchange during lengthening. Like the standard device, it is not adjustable once the pins are in place.

have been reported with this method, with a complication rate similar to that of other techniques (198).

### Distraction Epiphysiolysis

Distraction epiphysiolysis was pioneered by Ring and more recently reassessed by Monticelli, Spinelli, and others (199–205). It is achieved by applying a distraction force across the physis until it fractures. Lengthening can then be obtained by gradual distraction. This method has the disadvantages that the lysis is sudden, painful, and not well tolerated and that the physis can be injured, thereby compounding the leg length inequality (206,207). The complication rate is high (208) and, if it is to be used at all, it should be reserved for children who are very near the end of growth to minimize the consequences of physeal damage.

### Ilizarov Technique

Ring fixators have been developed (203,205,209–212) (Figs. 29.33 and 29.34). They are more complex than the

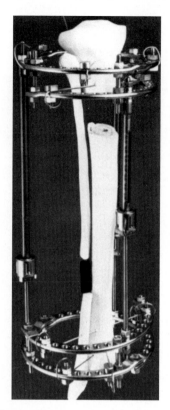

**Figure 29.33** Ilizarov lengthening device. External fixation is accomplished by tensioned wires fixed to circumferential rings. (From Ilizarov G, Deviatov A. Surgical lengthening of the shin with simultaneous correction of deformities. *Ortop Travmatol Protez* 1969;30:32–37.)

Wagner and Orthofix devices but are also more versatile in that they lend themselves to the correction of complex deformities. They can control more than two segments (213), can extend across joints, and can be used to translate segments of bone in the treatment of congenital pseudarthrosis and acquired absences (209). Fixation is accomplished by tensioned through-and-through wires attached to complete or partial rings. Unwillingness to use through-and-through wires in the proximal femur has led to the development of half-pins, which are now gaining favor at all levels.

### Lengthening Over an Intramedullary Rod

In the traditional application of any of the external lengthening devices, the device is responsible for both maintaining alignment and achieving distraction. Numerous unsightly scars result because of the multiple percutaneous pins or wires used to achieve sufficient stability and because they must be left in place for a prolonged period until the bone is strong. In 1956, Bost and Larsen introduced the concept of lengthening over an intramedullary rod (175). The rod serves to maintain alignment during both the distraction and the consolidation phases, and the external device serves only to achieve length (214). In this way, the number of percutaneous tracts can be reduced, the external device can be removed at the conclusion of lengthening, and the complication rate, particularly the rate of regenerate fracture, may be reduced (215). Lin described two cases of 15 cases of lengthening over a rod that required bone grafting (216), so the effect of rodding on osteogenesis remains unclear.

Lengthening over the rod has the disadvantages, compared with other lengthening techniques, that alignment of the anatomic axis of the femur cannot be changed and that the mechanical axis of the leg cannot be controlled. Because the anatomic axes of the femur and tibia are not collinear, elongation in this manner increases valgus of the mechanical axis of the leg. Whether or not this is a problem depends on the initial configuration of the leg. The correction, if necessary, of preexisting angular deformity or

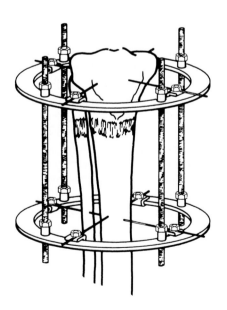

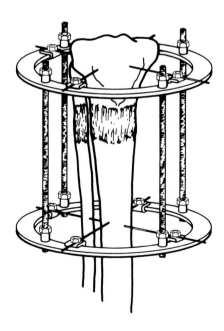

**Figure 29.34** Metaphyseal lengthening. Elongation through the metaphysis promotes osteogenesis in the lengthening gap because metaphyseal bone is so active, and it promotes strength by the large cross-sectional area.

the valgus produced by the lengthening must be performed at another time, when the rod is no longer in place.

There has been reasonable hesitation in using this approach because of the fear of producing a serious intramedullary infection with the intramedullary foreign material in continuity with the exterior through the pin tracts. Early experience with this technique is varied. Some studies report a low infection rate and recommend the technique (217,218), but others are less enthusiastic, mainly because of a significant rate of infection (219–221). Paley studied a series of 29 cases with case-matched controls and reported a reduction of time in the external lengthener by 50% and a 2.2 times faster recovery of knee motion. There were no infections and no fractures, compared to six regenerate fractures in the control group (218).

Wu et al. performed acute lengthenings over a locking rod but achieved a mean lengthening of only 2.8 cm (222).

The application of this technique is limited to bones that are straight enough to accept the rod and to children who are old enough not to be at risk for avascular necrosis of the femoral head.

### Intramedullary Distraction

Because most of the serious complications of lengthening have to do with infection resulting from pins that traverse the skin and fractures through the regenerate, there has been much interest in the development of an elongating intramedullary rod that would avoid both of these types of complication. Lengthening by motorization (223) and by electronically induced shape memory actuation (224) have been used experimentally, but reports of mechanical ratcheting devices are starting to appear in the clinical literature (225–228). Rotational movement of the distal femoral segment in relation to the proximal segment operates an internal ratcheting mechanism and, in the case of the Albizzia nail, 15 such movements achieve 1 mm of lengthening. Significant complications have been reported, especially in the form of mechanical problems with the lengthening (226,227), but the concept is promising.

### Biologic Factors

Several groups have been working in parallel over the last 3 decades to develop not only improved devices but also improved concepts and methods of lengthening. In particular, Ilizarov and De Bastiani have contributed new concepts and a new understanding of the biology of lengthening that are more important contributions than the devices themselves (196,197,209–211). Because the biologic principles are not device-specific, they are considered here in principle. Then, with that foundation, technologic issues are considered.

*Minimal Disturbance of the Bone.* Ilizarov recommended corticotomy, a technique in which the cortex is cut but care is taken that the medullary contents are not disturbed (Fig. 29.35). He felt it was important to preserve the

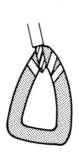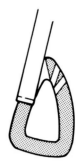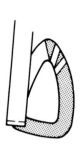

**Figure 29.35** The corticotomy technique. In this technique, care is taken to preserve the contents of the medullary cavity of the bone so that they may make their greatest contribution to osteogenesis during lengthening. Drill holes of controlled depth are made through the anterior cortex; the lateral cortices are cut with a narrow osteotome to avoid entering the medullary cavity; and the posterior cortex is cracked by bending.

intramedullary blood supply of the bone. It is difficult, however, even with careful technique, to avoid disturbing intramedullary contents, and it has been demonstrated that the intramedullary circulation reconstitutes very quickly, even if interrupted (229). The current consensus is that it is not necessary to perform a corticotomy, but care should be taken to avoid burning the bone with a saw so as to preserve the periosteum.

In contrast to the principle of minimal bone disturbance, massive bone production in the lengthening gap following peripheral decortication near the osteotomy has been reported (230).

*Location of Lengthening.* Whenever appropriate, the lengthening is done in the metaphysis, where the bone is more active and there are greater numbers of active osteoblasts to participate in the process of regeneration (Fig. 29.34) (231). A second benefit of this location is purely mechanical and is based on the principle that the strength of a structure in bending varies with the fourth power of its diameter. Because the diameter of the metaphysis is so much greater than that of the diaphysis, the bone is stronger at any stage of healing. This allows earlier removal of the fixator and decreased risk of fracture when the bone is subjected to bending loads.

*Number of Lengthening Sites.* Devices that lend themselves to fixation of more than two segments of the same bone make it possible to lengthen a single bone both proximally and distally at the same time. Although this theoretically doubles the rate of bone elongation, the soft tissues do not easily double their elongation rate, and articular cartilage has been shown experimentally in animals to suffer with rapid elongation (232); this concept has therefore been abandoned clinically.

*Delay Before Distraction.* It appears beneficial to delay the onset of distraction after the bone-sectioning procedure to allow the osteogenic process to become established. Osteogenesis can then keep up with the elongating gap. Delays of several days for young children, 1 week for adolescents, and 10 days for adults appear appropriate without risking premature consolidation, which would prevent distraction.

***Rate of Distraction.*** Ilizarov (209) recommends distraction of 1 mm per day, a rate that exceeds the ability of the regenerating bone in the gap to effect union but is not so fast that it inhibits bone formation. The rate may have to be slowed if radiographs show inadequate regeneration and a widening lucency in the regenerating bone. Faster rates often induce ischemia and considerably slow the rate of osteogenesis, but some patients who show excellent regeneration radiologically can have their distraction rate increased. The rate of 1 mm per day also appears to be appropriate for the soft tissues that must grow in length in tandem with the bone (233).

***Rhythm of Distraction.*** Increasing the frequency of lengthenings without changing the rate promotes faster consolidation experimentally and reduces the tension stress on the regenerating bone. Lengthening by 0.25 mm four times per day is better than lengthening by 1 mm one time per day, and it appears that gradual, continuous elongation, perhaps by a motorized device as suggested by Ilizarov, is ideal.

***Quality of Regenerate Bone.*** Osteogenesis in the gap begins first in the medulla and expands to fill the gap. Multipotential cells become osteoblasts and form bone without a cartilage foundation in a manner somewhat like membranous bone formation. Microscopic examination of the regenerating bone, elongated according to modern concepts, shows that it has a longitudinal orientation, probably because its formation is guided carefully by the architecture of the osteotomy surface (234). The architecture of the regenerate resembles haversian bone and is said to be stronger than woven bone and to remodel and calcify faster.

***Thin Wires.*** The ring fixators allow the use of thin (1 to 2 mm) wires instead of large screws. The wires cause less reaction of surrounding skin and bone, move through the skin more easily, and allow some axial dynamization of the bone fragments.

***Amount of Lengthening.*** It is not known whether there is an upper limit to lengthening. Reports on the new techniques suggest that greater lengthening may be possible than was formerly thought. Carroll et al. have shown that permanent changes occur in muscle and joint cartilage with tibial lengthening greater than 11% (235), and Bell has shown effects on the adjacent joints in animal experiments (232). These effects may be related more to the rate

than the magnitude of lengthening, and the degree to which they occur in human patients is uncertain.

***Activity Level.*** Patients can be encouraged to be active and to undertake full weight bearing from the start, and they should participate in vigorous calisthenics and physical therapy to maintain normal joint motion and muscle strength. Weight bearing takes advantage of the flexibility of the devices to apply dynamic compression, which is believed to stimulate bone formation.

***Dynamization.*** Cyclic loading of the regenerate is thought to promote osteogenesis. The ring fixators have the advantage of allowing dynamic loading of the lengthening gap throughout the period of fixation while they simultaneously control length. Their construct of thin wires and circumferential rings provides rigidity against bending in the sagittal and coronal planes but is not so rigid in the axial direction, allowing slight axial movement in response to applied loads. The Orthofix device can be dynamized by the application of an elastic buttress; when the regenerate bone appears strong enough to resist shortening, the buttress can be removed. The device then maintains alignment but not length, thereby allowing dynamization. All of the devices allow some dynamization by virtue of their elasticity and can be made less rigid by the removal of wires or pins in a staged manner.

***Lengthening Index.*** This quantity is the number of months of external fixation required per centimeter of lengthening. It is generally between 1 and 1.5 months per cm and tends to be greater for lesser lengthenings because one component of this time, the interval from the arrest of elongation to the removal, tends to be constant. This number is a very rough guideline to predict the duration of fixation prior to undergo lengthening but is of little clinical importance (236).

***Factors Affecting the Choice of Lengthening Hardware.*** The biologic factors discussed in the preceding text are, for the most part, independent of the device used. The choice of lengthening device is not, however, completely arbitrary. The devices have certain characteristics that affect their ease of use in specific situations. Because deformity correction often goes hand in hand with lengthening, this discussion includes some aspects of device selection and use in the correction of angular deformity.

***Gradual Versus Acute Correction.*** Not all deformities need to be corrected gradually. There is a long and successful history of acute correction of deformity by osteotomy with internal or external fixation, or no fixation at all. Although there can be advantages in the use of external fixation, in some cases Ilizarov's technique of gradual correction appears to offer little benefit (237,238).

The question then arises as to the possible advantages or disadvantages of gradual correction if an external fixator is already required to accomplish lengthening. There is good evidence to suggest that, if an external device is already in place for lengthening, either gradual or acute correction of coexisting deformity can achieve good results (238). Acute correction has the effect of simplifying the lengthening and widens the selection of devices, whereas gradual correction with the Ilizarov or another ring fixator allows the physician to monitor and modify the correction on an ongoing basis.

If the surgeon wishes to perform a gradual deformity correction, then the Ilizarov device or another ring fixator, or the Orthofix device with the Garches clamp, can be used. Using the Ilizarov apparatus to perform gradual angular correction, with or without lengthening, requires attention to the geometric principles of hinge placement as described by Herzenberg and Waanders (239). Careful hinge placement can control both translation and angular correction. Placing hinges so that the axis of rotation is outside the bone can accomplish lengthening and angular correction simultaneously.

**Thin Wires Versus Half-Pins.** The Wagner and Orthofix devices require thick half-pins, whereas the Ilizarov device can be used with either thin wires or half-pins. Thin wires appear to pass through the skin more easily, but they leave twice as many unsightly scars in the skin and tether the muscles in twice as many locations, thereby interfering with joint motion (231).

Thin wires, however, do not lend themselves to fixation of the proximal femur, and most orthopaedic surgeons prefer half-pins and partial rings at that level. There is a growing trend of using half-pins at other levels as well. Wires must be tensioned to close to their elastic limit, and it does not take much additional force to stretch the wires plastically, thereby compromising the rigidity of the frame.

**Conical Screws.** The Orthofix device uses 6 mm pins that taper slightly toward the tip. If the pins loosen, they can be tightened by advancing them slightly. Conversely, if the pins are inserted too far, they cannot be retracted without loosening. Hydroxyapatite coatings of the pins provide better adherence to bone and correspondingly greater resistance to their removal.

**Ease of Replacement of Pins and Wires.** Because the Ilizarov device allows pins and wires to be placed at almost any level and angle, there is no problem in removing troublesome wires and in inserting new ones. The monolateral fixators, on the other hand, are more limited in that the pin clamps have predesignated locations and that all the pins in one cluster are in the same plane. Replacement of one pin may require replacement of all pins of that cluster.

**Number of Pins in Each Segment.** The Orthofix allows three pins in each cluster, and the Ilizarov device sets no limits on the number of pins or wires. There can be an advantage to using more than two pins to fix the proximal femur, especially if the lengthening is through the proximal part of the shaft, and the pins must be placed proximally. In this configuration, the loading is eccentric and three pins provide better fixation with less risk of loosening.

**Ability to Fix More Than One Segment.** The Orthofix lengthener can be assembled to fix more than two segments, although with some difficulty, and with special clamps and hinges it can traverse joints. The Ilizarov device can easily be extended to provide fixation of as many segments as are required and can be extended across joints with or without hinges.

**Complex Deformities with Multiple Axes of Correction.** Only the ring fixators can accomplish gradual correction of deformities in more than one plane. Not only can multiple segments be controlled and multiple hinges incorporated, but the system can also be modified as correction progresses to meet emerging demands.

**Ability to Adjust Device While in Place.** The Orthofix lengthener is adjustable only in the plane of the pins, and the procedure requires general anesthesia and special pin clamps. The Ilizarov method is well suited for continual modification of its configuration by differential lengthening of the individual rods. In addition, its components can be changed and the hinges realigned repeatedly if required. This can be done without the patient returning to the operating room for anesthesia.

**Ease of Adjusting the Lengthening Mechanism.** Adjusting the lengthening mechanism is of no concern while patients are hospitalized under the care of trained personnel, but it becomes an issue when they are discharged home. A simple mechanism results in less anxiety and fewer errors. The Wagner mechanism is the simplest requiring only the turn of a single knob. The Orthofix devices require use of a special extender that is advanced with a wrench. The Ilizarov device requires elongation of up to three or four rods individually, perhaps by different amounts.

### Conclusion

Simple lengthenings can be accomplished by a number of devices, none of which has a clear advantage over another, except that it might be argued that the simplest device capable of solving the problem is preferable. Gradual correction of complex deformities can present demands that can only be met by a more versatile device such as the Ilizarov device.

### Complications of Lengthening

All studies of leg lengthening, regardless of technique, have reported high complication rates (165,236,240–251).

Most studies report more complications than there are patients, and many patients do not reach their anticipated lengthening goals with uncompromised function. The complication rate, however, is related to the amount of lengthening (245), and if the goal is modest the rate is reduced and the proportion of patients reaching their preoperative goals is increased (117). Ghoneem et al. found that all of the studied children who had undergone lengthening had a normal psychological score; 92% had no limitations in daily activities, and 81% were satisfied with the overall result (118).

Deformity due to soft tissue tension can occur during lengthening, and angular deformity of the tibia has been related to the degree of elongation (252). The Ilizarov technique has been proposed to supplant amputation and prosthetic fitting in fibular hemimelia, but Cheng et al. report that uncontrollable deformity of the tibia and ankle joint was encountered (253). Ultimate alignment may be improved by using arthrography to delineate the joint surfaces when applying the lengthening device (254).

Hypertension can be seen during lengthening and can occur suddenly (255–257). The mechanism is not clear, but it resolves dependably with shortening of the lengthening gap and may not recur when lengthening is resumed.

Pin tract inflammation is common and is of little consequence in itself. True pin tract infection usually responds well to local care and systemic antibiotics. It can, however, be elevated to a serious complication if the pin tract infection contaminates a surgical procedure.

Mechanical failure can occur in several ways. Pins can break or loosen and require replacement. Fractures through the lengthening gap (or deformation of the bone in the lengthening gap) can occur early or late in the procedure. It can occur soon after removal of the device, indicating that it was removed too soon, or can occur late, while the bone is still remodeling and has not yet regained its normal strength (258). In my series of Wagner lengthenings, there was one fracture 8 years after the lengthening, which suggests that the bone is extremely slow to remodel and regain full strength and is probably weak even after it looks normal radiologically. Long-term follow-up is important in assessing the results of leg lengthening because complications can occur late.

Nakamura et al. have examined the diameter of the bone in the lengthening gap and concluded that axial loading while the device is in place may not be enough to increase the diameter but that the diameter increases dependably after removal of the device (259). This finding has profound implications for the strength of the bone because strength in bending varies as the fourth power of the diameter. Indeed, there is a report substantiating this conclusion (260).

Subluxation of the knee can occur during femoral lengthening, especially in patients with congenital shortening (261,262). The subluxation appears to be a posterior subluxation of the lateral tibial plateau and is always preceded by a loss of extension of the knee. Dysplasia or absence of the anterior cruciate ligament and hypoplasia of the lateral femoral condyle are usually found in association with congenitally short femurs (263,264) and contribute to this complication. Routine lengthening of the lateral structures (the biceps tendon and iliotibial band), determined maintenance of knee extension, and avoidance of continued distraction in the face of a knee flexion contracture will prevent knee subluxation.

Dislocation of the hip has been reported; it can occur even in the early stages of distraction and tends to be associated with previous hip surgery and residual instability (265).

Delayed union is difficult to define in the context of lengthening, but there is no doubt that certain cases take significantly longer to consolidate than others. True nonunion occurs and is similar in appearance and treatment to posttraumatic nonunion, except that it can occur in narrowed and spindle-shaped regenerate so that it is fragile even when united.

It appears that the complication rate is affected by the quality of the underlying bone, but inconsistently so. For example Naudie et al. showed that the complication rate is higher in patients with an underlying bone disorder (266), but patients with achondroplasia seem to have a lower complication rate. Reasonable lengthening expectations in femoral hypoplasia are unclear (267).

Nerve or artery damage during lengthening can result from stretching, entrapment by tense tissues, movement of wires or pins through the tissues, or direct trauma (268). Nerve conduction is affected in one third or more of patients undergoing lengthening (269,270).

Karger et al. found that femoral lengthenings were more prone to complications than were tibias and that the complication rate increased with lengthenings exceeding 25% of the initial bone length (271). We found that the complication rate is significantly higher in children younger than 8 years than in older children, and this may reflect the inability of younger children to understand, or remain motivated to comply with, the instructions therapists and surgeons (262). Conversely, Noonan et al. found that the complication rate in both femoral and tibial lengthening increased in patients older than 14 years (236). To some extent, the amount of possible lengthening depends on the length of the bone to start with, and this is another reason to perform lengthening only in older children whose bones are nearing mature length.

Lengthening affects the subsequent growth of the limb. Price and Carantzas have reported a case of severe growth retardation in the lengthened limb (272). Viehweger has found that lengthening the tibia by more than 14% slows down its growth but that this has a negligible effect on the ultimate clinical result because it is compensated for by femoral overgrowth (273).

Because of the frequency of concerns, questions, problems, and complications that surround the care of patients undergoing lengthening, it facilitates their management to form a lengthening team in a program with shared responsibilities. A nurse, physical therapist, social worker, and a skilled technician are important members of the

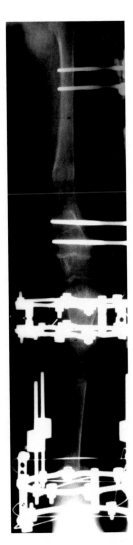

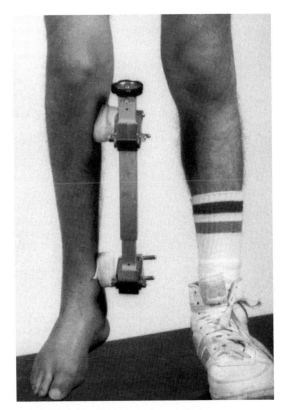

**Figure 29.37** Patients with the Wagner, Orthofix, and Ilizarov devices can be mobile and undertake partial to full weight bearing.

**Figure 29.36** The course of Ilizarov and Orthofix lengthening. This patient had complex deformities resulting from meningococcemia. The femur was managed by an acute correction of the distal femoral varus deformity and subsequent lengthening, using the Orthofix rail lengthener. The distal pins were placed carefully, before the osteotomy was performed. The tibial deformity required valgus osteotomies both distally and proximally. Because fixation of three fragments was required, the more versatile Ilizarov device was used.

team and should join the surgeon in preparing patients and families for the lengthening procedure. The team can respond to ongoing needs and offer support during the lengthening procedure. Families and patients never fully appreciate the depth and breadth of the hardship they will face, and they will require more support than is needed for most orthopaedic cases.

There is reason to believe that the complication rate from lengthening is improving with modern techniques and understanding (Figs. 29.36 and 29.37) (274,275).

## CONCLUSION

Excellent and continually improving care of patients with leg-length discrepancy requires comfortable familiarity with the techniques for patient assessment, the methods

for prediction of future growth and discrepancy, the factors important in the selection of treatment goals, and the approaches to treatment. Maintaining familiarity with up-to-date techniques and philosophies of surgical treatment is challenging, but the improvement in our capabilities should be an adequate reward.

## REFERENCES

### Effects

1. Murrell P, Cornwall M, Doucet S. Leg-length discrepancy: effect on the amplitude of postural sway. *Arch Phys Med Rehabil* 1992; 73:401–402.
2. Mahar R, Kirby R, MacLeod D. Simulated leg-length discrepancy: its effect on mean center-of-pressure position and postural sway. *Arch Phys Med Rehabil* 1985;66:822–824.
3. Liu X, Fabry G, Molenaers G, et al. Kinematic and kinetic asymmetry in patients with leg-length discrepancy. *J Pediatr Orthop* 1998;18(2):187–189.
4. Goel A, Loudon J, Nazare A, et al. Joint moments in minor limb length discrepancy: a pilot study. *Am J Orthop* 1997;26(12): 852–856.
5. Gofton J, Trueman G. Studies in osteoarthritis of the hip. II. Osteoarthritis of the hip and leg length disparity. *Can Med Assoc J* 1971;104:791–799.
6. Kujala U, Friberg O, Aalto T, et al. Lower limb asymmetry and patellofemoral joint incongruence in the etiology of knee exertion injuries in athletes. *Int J Sports Med* 1987;8:214–220.
7. Gofton J. Persistent low back pain and leg length disparity. *J Rheumatol* 1985;12:747–750.
8. Grundy P, Roberts C. Does unequal leg length cause back pain? A case-control study. *Lancet* 1984;2(8397):256–258.
9. Soukka A, Alaranta H, Tallroth K, et al. Leg-length inequality in people of working age. The association between mild inequality and low-back pain is questionable. *Spine* 1991;16:429–431.

10. Froh R, Yong-Hing K, Cassidy J, et al. The relationship between leg length discrepancy and lumbar facet otientation. *Spine* 1988; 13:325–327.
11. Giles L, Taylor J. The effect of postural scoliosis on lumbar apophyseal joints. *Scand J Rheumatol* 1984;13:209–220.
12. Gibson P, Papaioannou T, Kenwright J. The influence on the spine of leg-length discrepancy after femoral fracture. *J Bone Joint Surg* 1983;65B:584–587.
13. Papaioannou T, Stokes I, Kenwright J. Scoliosis associated with limb-length inequality. *J Bone Joint Surg* 1982;64A:59–62.
14. Scheller M. *Uber den Einfluss der Beinverkurzung auf die Wirbelsaule.* Inaug. Diss. Koln, 1964.
15. Taillard W, Morscher E. *Beinlangenunterschiede,* Basel: Karger, 1965.

## Growth

16. Anderson M, Green WT. Lengths of the femur and tibia; norms derived from orthoroentgenograms of children from five years of age until epiphyseal closure. *Am J Dis Child* 1948;75:279–290.
17. Anderson M, Messner M, Green W. Distribution of lengths of the normal femur and tibia in children from one to eighteen years of age. *J Bone Joint Surg* 1964;46-A(6):1197–1202.
18. Anderson M, Green W, Messner M. Growth and predictions of growth in the lower extremities. *J Bone Joint Surg* 1963;45-A:1.
19. Green W, Anderson M. Experiences with epiphyseal arrest in correcting discrepancies in length of the lower extremities in infantile paralysis. *J Bone Joint Surg* 1947;29:659–675.
20. Greulich W, Pyle S. *Radiographic atlas of the skeletal development of the hand and wrist,* Stanford, CA: Stanford University Press, 1959.
21. Bayley N. Individual patterns of development. *Child Dev* 1956; 27:45–74.
22. Beumer A, Lampe H, Swierstra B, et al. The straight line graph in limb length inequality. A new design based on 182 Dutch children. *Acta Orthop Scand* 1997;68(4):355–360.
23. Paley D, Bhave A, Herzenberg J, et al. Multiplier method for predicting limb-length discrepancies. *J Bone Joint Surg* 2000;59A: 1432–1446.

## Etiology

24. Harper M, Canale S. Angulation osteotomy. A trigonometric analysis. *Clin Orthop* 1982;166:173–181.
25. Sugi M, Cole W. Early plaster treatment for fractures of the femoral shaft in childhood. *J Bone Joint Surg* 1987;69B:743–745.
26. Shannak A. Tibial fractures in children: follow-up study. *J Pediatr Orthop* 1988;8:306–310.
27. Beals R, Lovrein E. Diffuse capillary hemangiomas associated with skeletal hypotrophy. *J Pediatr Orthop* 1992;12:401–402.
28. Dutkowsky J, Kasser J, Kaplan L. Leg length discrepancy associated with vivid cutis marmorata. *J Pediatr Orthop* 1993;13: 456–458.
29. Heuter C. Anatomische studien an den extremitatengelenken neugeborener und erwachsener. *Virchows Arch* 1862;25:572–599.
30. Volkmann R. Chirurgische erfahrungen uber knochenverbiegungen und knochenwachsthum. *Arch Pathol Anat* 1862;24: 512–540.
31. Arkin AM, Katz JF. The effects of pressure on epiphyseal growth. The mechanism of plasticity of growing bone. *J Bone Joint Surg* 1956;38A:1056–1076.
32. Delpech J. *De l'orthomorphie, par rapport a l'espece humaine,* Paris: Gabon, 1829.
33. Beals RK. Hemihypertophy and hemiatrophy. *Clin Orthop* 1982; 166:199–203.
34. Pappas A, Nehme A. Leg length discrepancy associated with hypertrophy. *Clin Orthop* 1979;144:198–211.
35. Pappas A. Congenital abnormalities of the femur and related lower extremity malformations: classification and treaatment. *J Pediatr Orthop* 1983;3:45–60.
36. Stanitski D, Kassab S. Rotational deformity in congenital hypoplasia of the femur. *J Pediatr Orthop* 1997;17(4):525–527.
37. Cuervo M, Albinana J, Cebrian J, et al. Congenital hypoplasia of the fibula: clinical manifestations. *J Pediatr Orthop B* 1996; 5(1):35–38.

38. Gillespie R, Torode I. Classification and management of congenital abnormalities of the femur. *J Bone Joint Surg* 1983;65B: 557–568.
39. Johansson E, Aparisi T. Missing cruciate ligament in congenital short femur. *J Bone Joint Surg* 1983;65A:1109–1115.
40. Kaelin A, Hulin P, Carlioz H. Congenital aplasia of the cruciate ligaments. A report of six cases. *J Bone Joint Surg* 1986;68B:827–828.
41. Gekeler J, Dietz J, Schuler T. Prognosis of leg loength difference in congenital fibula defect. *Z Orthop* 1982;120:729–734.
42. Westin G, Sakai D, Wood W. Congenital longitudinal deficiency of the fibula: follow-up of treatment by syme amputation. *J Bone Joint Surg* 1976;58A:492–496.
43. Kalamchi A, Cowell H, Kim K. Congenital deficiency of the femur. *J Pediatr Orthop* 1985;5:129–134.
44. Grimes J, Blair V, Gilula L. Roentgen rounds #81. Posteromedial bowing of the tibia. *Orthop Rev* 1986;15:249–255.
45. Hofmann A, Wenger D. Posteromedial bowing of the tibia. Progression of discrepancy in leg lengths. *J Bone Joint Surg* 1981;63A:384–388.
46. Pappas A. Congenital posteromedial bowing of the tibia and fibula. *J Pediatr Orthop* 1984;4:525–531.
47. Askins G, Ger E. Congenital constriction band syndrome. *J Pediatr Orthop* 1988;8:461–466.
48. Garbarino J, Clancy M, Harcke H, et al. Congenital diastasis of the inferior tibiofibular joint: a review of the literature and report of two cases. *J Pediatr Orthop* 1985;5:225–228.
49. Salter R, Harris W. Injuries involving the epiphyseal plate. *J Bone Joint Surg* 1963;45A:587–622.
50. Robert H, Moulies D, Longis B, et al. Traumatic separation of the lower end of the femur. *Rev Chir Orthop Reparatrice Appar Mot* 1988;74:69–78.
51. Roberts P. Disturbed epiphyseal growth at the knee after osteomyelitis in infancy. *J Bone Joint Surg* 1970;52B:692–703.
52. Robertson W, Butler M, D'Angio G, et al. Leg length discrepancy following irradiation for childhood tumors. *J Pediatr Orthop* 1991;11:284–287.
53. Wagner H. Radiation injuries of the locomotor system. *Langenbecks Arch Chir* 1981;355:181–185.
54. Wagner H. Surgical lengthening or shortening of femur and tibia; technique and indications. *Prog Orthop Surg* 1977;1:71–94.
55. Shapiro F. Ollier's disease. An assessment of angular deformity, shortening, and pathological fractures in twenty-one patients. *J Bone Joint Surg* 1982;64A:95–103.
56. Peterson H. Premature physeal arrest of the distal tibia associated with temporary arterial insufficiency. *J Pediatr Orthop* 1993; 13:672–675.
57. Thomas C, Gage J, Ogden J. Treatment concepts for proximal femoral ischemic necrosis complicating congenital hip disease. *J Bone Joint Surg* 1982;64A:817–828.
58. Shapiro F. Legg-Calve-Perthes disease: a study of lower extremity length discrepancies and skeletal maturation. *Acta Orthop Scand* 1982;53:437–444.
59. Rosenthal A, Anderson M, Thomson S, et al. Superficial femoral artery catheterization. Effect on extremity length. *Am J Dis Child* 1972;124:240–242.
60. Jenkins D, Cheng D, Hodgson A, Stimulation of growth by periosteal stripping. A clinical study. *J Bone Joint Surg* 1975;57B: 482–484.
61. Khoury S, Silberman F, Cabrine R. Stimulation of the longitudinal growth of long bones by periosteal stripping. *J Bone Joint Surg* 1963;45A:1679–1684.
62. Sola C, Silberman F, Cabrini R. Stimulation of the longitidinal growth of long bones by periosteal stripping. *J Bone Joint Surg* 1963;45A:1679.
63. Trueta J. Stimulation of bone growth by redistribution of the intra-osseous circulation. *J Bone Joint Surg* 1951;33B:476.
64. Doyle J. Stimulation of bone growth by short-wave diathermy. *J Bone Joint Surg* 1963;45A:15.
65. Armstrong P. Attempts to accelerate longitudinal bone growth. In: Uthhoff H, Wiley J, eds. *Behaviour of the growth plate.* New York: Raven Press, 1988:237–242.
66. Groves E. Stimulation of bone growth. *Am J Surg* 1958;95:125.
67. Tupman G. Treatment of inequality of the lower limbs. The results of operations for stimulation of growth. *J Bone Joint Surg* 1960;42B:489.

68. Peixinho M, Arakaki T, Toledo C. Correction of leg inequality in the Klippel-Trenaunay-Weber syndrome. *Int Orthop* 1982;6:45–47.

69. Simon S, Whiffen J, Shapiro F. Leg-length discrepancies in monoarticular and pauciarticular juvenile rheumatoid arthritis. *J Bone Joint Surg* 1981;63A:209–215.

70. Vostrejs M, Hollister J. Muscle atrophy and leg length discrepancies in pauciarticular juvenile rheumatoid arthritis. *Am J Dis Child* 1988;142:343–345.

71. Heim M, Horszowski H, Martinowitz U. Leg length inequality in hemophilia. An interesting case report. *Clin Pediatr* 1985;24:600–602.

72. Compere E, Adams C. Studies of the longitudinal growth of long bones: the influence of trauma to the diaphysis. *J Bone Joint Surg* 1937;19:922–936.

73. Jackson D, Cozen L. Genu valgum as a complication of proximal tibial metaphyseal fractures in children. *J Bone Joint Surg* 1971;53A:1571–1578.

74. Herring J, Moseley C. Posttraumatic valgus deformity of the tibia. *J Pediatr Orthop* 1981;1:435–440.

75. Rooker G. The effect of division of the periosteum on the rate of longitudinal bone growth: an experimental study in the rabbit. *Orthop Trans* 1980;4(3):400–401.

76. Salter R, Best T. Pathogenesis and prevention of valgus deformity following fractures of the proximal metaphyseal region of the tibia in children. *J Bone Joint Surg* 1972;54B:767.

77. Taylor J, Warrell E, Evans R. Response of the growth plates to tibial osteotomy in rats. *J Bone Joint Surg* 1987;69-B:664–669.

78. Taylor S. Tibial overgrowth: a cause of genu valgum. *J Bone Joint Surg* 1963;45A:659.

79. Aitken A, Blackett CW, Ciacotti JJ. Overgrowth of the femoral shaft following fractures in childhood. *J Bone Joint Surg* 1939;21:334–338.

80. Holschneider A, Vogl D, Dietz H. Differences in leg length following femoral shaft fractures in childhood. *Z Kinderchir* 1985;40:341–350.

81. Parrini L, Paleari M, Biggi F. Growth disturbances following fractures of the femur and tibia in children. *Ital J Orthop Traumatol* 1985;11:139–145.

82. Lorenzi G, Rossi P, Quaglia F, et al. Growth disturbances following fractures of the femur and tibia in children. *Ital J Orthop Traumatol* 1985;11:133–137.

83. Kohan L, Cumming W. Femoral shaft fractures in children: the effect of initial shortening on subsequent limb overgrowth. *Aust N Z J Surg* 1982;52:141–144.

84. Meals R. Overgrowth of the femur following fractures in children: influence of handedness. *J Bone Joint Surg* 1979;61A:381–384.

## Patient Assessment

85. Winter R, Pinto W. Pelvic obliquity. Its causes and its treatment. *Spine* 1986;11:225–234.

86. Ireland J, Kessel L. Hip adduction/abduction deformity and apparent leg-length inequality. *Clin Orthop* 1980;153:156–157.

87. Lee D, Choi I, Chung C, et al. Fixed pelvic obliquity after poliomyelitis: classification and management. *J Bone Joint Surg Br* 1997;79(2):190–196.

88. Green N, Griffin P. Hip dysplasia associated with abduction contracture of the contralateral hip. *J Bone Joint Surg* 1982;64A:1273–1281.

89. Cleveland R, Kushner D, Ogden M, et al. Determination of leg length discrepancy. A comparison of weight-bearing and supine imaging. *Invest Radiol* 1988;23:301–304.

90. Green W, Wyatt G, Anderson M. Orthoroentgenography as a method of measuring the bones of the lower extremity. *J Bone Joint Surg* 1946;28:60–65.

91. Bell JS, Thompson WAL. Modified spot scanography. *AJR Am J Roentgenol* 1950;63:915–916.

92. Aaron A, Weinstein D, Thickman D, et al. Comparison of orthoroentgenography and computed tomography in the measurement of limb-length discrepancy. *J Bone Joint Surg* 1992;74A:897–902.

93. Helms C, McCarthy S. CT scanograms for measuring leg length discrepancy. *Radiology* 1984;151:802.

94. Glass R, Poznanski A. Leg-length determination with biplanar CT scanograms. *Radiology* 1985;156:833–834.

95. Huurman W, Jacobsen F, Anderson J, et al. Limb-length discrepancy measured with computerized axial tomographic equipment. *J Bone Joint Surg* 1987;69-A(5):699–705.

96. O'Connor K, Grady J, Hollander M. CT scanography for limb length determination. *Clin Podiatr Med Surg* 1988;5:267–274.

97. Temme J, Chu W, Anderson J. CT scanograms compared with conventional orthoroentgenograms in long bone measurement. *Skeletal Radiol* 1987;16:442–446.

98. Altongy J, Harcke H, Bowen J. Measurement of leg length inequalities by micro-dose digital radiographs. *J Pediatr Orthop* 1987;7(3):311–316.

99. Acheson RM. The Oxford method of assessing skeletal maturity. *Clin Orthop* 1957;10:19–39.

100. Todd T. *Atlas of skeletal maturation*, St. Louis, MO: CV Mosby Co, 1937.

101. Carpenter C, Lester E. Skeletal age determination in young children: analysis of three regions of the hand/wrist film. *J Pediatr Orthop* 1993;13:76–79.

102. Tanner J, Whitehouse R, Marshall W, et al. *Assessment of skeletal maturity and prediction of adult height (TW2 method)*, London: Academic Press, 1975.

## Data Analysis

103. Blair V, Walker S, Sheridan J, et al. Epiphysiodesis: a problem of timing. *J Pediatr Orthop* 1982;2:281–284.

104. Little D, Nigo L, Aiona M. Deficiencies of current methods for the timing of epiphysiodesis. *J Pediatr Orthop* 1996;16(2):173–179.

105. Menelaus M. Correction of leg length discrepancy by epiphyseal arrest. *J Bone Joint Surg* 1966;48B:336–339.

106. Westh R, Menelaus M. A simple calculation for the timing of epiphyseal arrest: a further report. *J Bone Joint Surg* 1981;63B:117–119.

107. Fries J. Growth following epiphyseal arrest. A simple method of calculation. *Clin Orthop* 1976;114:316–318.

108. Green W, Anderson M. Skeletal age and the control of bone growth. *Instr Lect Am Acad Orthop Surg* 1960;17:199–217.

109. Moseley C. A straight-line graph for leg-length discrepancies. *J Bone Joint Surg* 1977;59-A(2):174–178.

110. Moseley C. A straight-line graph for leg length discrepancies. *Clin Orthop Relat Res* 1978;136:33–40.

111. Porat S, Peyser A, Robin G. Equalization of lower limbs by epiphysiodesis: results of treatment. *J Pediatr Orthop* 1991;11:442–448.

112. Bellier G, Carlioz H. The prediction of growth in long bones in poliomyelitis. *Rev Chir Orthop Reparatric Appar Mot* 1979;65:373–375.

113. Shapiro F. Longitudinal growth of the femur and tibia after diaphyseal lengthening. *J Bone Joint Surg* 1987;69A:684–690.

114. Koman L, Meyer L, Warren F. Proximal femoral focal deficiency: a 50-year experience. *Dev Med Child Neurol* 1982;24:344–355.

115. Hootnick D, Boyd N, Fixsen J, et al. The natural history and management of congenital short tibia with dysplasia or absence of the fibula. *J Bone Joint Surg* 1977;59B:267–271.

116. Herron L, Amstutz H, Sakai D. One stage femoral lengthening in the adult. *Clin Orthop* 1978;136:74–82.

## Determination of Treatment Goals

117. Bassett G, Morris J. The use of the Ilizatov technique in the correction of lower extremity deformities in children. *Orthopaedics* 1997;20(7):623–627.

118. Ghoneem H, Wright J, Cole W, et al. The Ilizarov method for correction of complex deformities. Psychological and functional outcomes. *J Bone Joint Surg Am* 1996;78(10):1480–1485.

119. Paley D. Current techniques of limb lengthening. *J Pediatr Orthop* 1988;8:73–92.

## Treatment

120. Gross R. Leg length discrepancy – how much is too much? *Scientific exhibit. Annual meeting of the American academy of orthopaedic surgeons*. Dallas, TX, 1978.

121. Rush W, Steiner H. A study of lower extremity length inequality. *AJR Am J Roentgenol* 1946;56:616.

122. Gillis J. *Too tall, too small*, Champagne, CA: Institute for personality and ability testing, 1982:9–25.

123. Grumbach M. Growth hormone therapy and the short end of the stick. *N Eng J Med* 1988;319(4):238–240.

124. Mayer-Bahlburg H. Psychosocial management of short stature. In: Shaffer D, Ehrhardt A, Greenhill L, eds. *The clinical guide to child psychiatry*. New York: Free Press, 1985:110–144.

125. Sandberg D, Brook A, Campos S. Short stature: a psychosocial burden requiring growth hormone therapy? *J Pediatr* 1994; 94(6):832–840.

126. Anderson L, Westin GW, Oppenheim WL. Syme amputation in children: indications, results, and long-term follow-up. *J Pediatr Orthop* 1984;4:550–554.

127. Mallet J, Rigault P, Padovani J, et al. Braces for congenital leg length inequality in children. *Rev Chir Orthop Reparatrice Appar Mot* 1986;72:63–71.

128. Setoguchi Y. Comparison of gait patterns and energy efficiency of unilateral PFFD in patients treated by symes amputation and by knee fusion and rotational osteotomy. In: *ACPOC Annual Meeting*. Minneapolis, MN, 1994.

129. Stephens D, Herrick W, MacEwen G. Epiphyseodesis for limb length inequality: results and indications. *Clin Orthop* 1978; 136:41–48.

130. White J, Stubbins SJ. Growth arrest for equalizing leg lengths. *JAMA* 1944;126:1146–1149.

131. Straub L, Thompson T, Wilson P. The results of epiphyseodesis and femoral shortening in relation to equalization of leg length. *J Bone Joint Surg* 1945;27:254–266.

132. Phemister D. Operative arrestment of longitudinal growth of bones in the treatment of deformities. *J Bone Joint Surg* 1933;15: 1–15.

133. Macnicol M, Gupta M. Epiphysiodesis using a cannulated tubesaw. *J Bone Joint Surg Br* 1997;79(2):307–309.

134. Anders G, Stachon I. Experience with temporary epiphyseodesis after blount. *Z Orthop Ihre Grenzgeb* 1979;117:922–927.

135. Blount WP. A mature look at epiphyseal stapling. *Clin Orthop* 1971;77:149–157.

136. Blount WP, Clarke GR. Control of bone growth by epiphyseal stapling. A preliminary report. *J Bone Joint Surg* 1949;31:464–478.

137. Hass S. Mechanical retardation of bone growth. *J Bone Joint Surg* 1948;30A:506–512.

138. McGibbon K, Deacon A, Raisbeck C. Experiences in growth retardation with heavy Vitallium staples. *J Bone Joint Surg* 1962; 44B:86–92.

139. Brockway A, Craig WA, Cockrell BRJ. End result of 62 stapling operations. *J Bone Joint Surg* 1954;36A:1063–1070.

140. Frantz C. Epiphyseal stapling. *Clin Orthop* 1971;77:149–157.

141. Bylander B, Hansson LI, Selvik G. Pattern of growth retardation after blount stapling: a roentgen stereophotogrammetric analysis. *J Pediatr Orthop* 1983;3:63–72.

142. Mielke C, Stevens P. Hemiepiphyseal stapling for knee deformities in children younger than 10 years: a preliminary report. *J Pediatr Orthop* 1996;16(4):423–429.

143. Stevens PM, MacWilliams B, Mohr RA. Gait analysis of stapling for genu valgum. *J Pediatr Orthop* 2004;24(1):70–74.

144. Stevens PM, Maguire M, Dales MD, et al. Physeal stapling for idiopathic genu valgum. *J Pediatr Orthop* 1999;19(5):645–649.

145. Canale S, Russell T, Holcomb R. Percutaneous epiphysiodesis: experimental study and preliminary clinical results. *J Pediatr Orthop* 1986;6:150–156.

146. Ogilvie J. Epiphysiodesis: evaluation of a new technique. *J Pediatr Orthop* 1986;6:147–149.

147. Scott A, Urquart B, TE C. Percutaneous vs modified phemister epiphysiodesis of the lower extremity. *Orthopedics* 1996;19(10): 857–861.

148. Canale S, Christian C. Techniques for epiphysiodesis about the knee. *Clin Orthop Relat Res* 1990;255:81–85.

149. Atar D, Lehman W, Grant A, et al. Percutaneous epiphysiodesis. *J Bone Joint Surg* 1991;73-B:173.

150. Timperlake R, Bowen J, Guille J, et al. Prospective evaluation of fifty-three consecutive percutaneous epiphysiodeses of the distal femur and proximal tibia and fibula. *J Pediatr Orthop* 1991; 11:350–357.

151. Kenwright J, Albinana J. Problems encountered in leg shortening. *J Bone Joint Surg* 1991;73B:671–675.

152. Silver R, de la Garza J, Rang M. The myth of muscle balance. *J Bone Joint Surg* 1985;67B:432–437.

153. Coppola C, Maffulli N. Limb shortening for the management of leg length discrepancy. *J R Coll Surg Edinb* 1999;44(1):46–54.

154. Merle D'Aubigne R, Dubousset J. Surgical correction of large length discrepancies in the lower extremities of children and adults. *J Bone Joint Surg* 1971;53A:411–430.

155. Kempf I, Grosse A, Abalo C. Locked intramedullary nailing. Its application to femoral and tibial axial, rotational, lengthening and shortening osteotomies. *Clin Orthop* 1986;212:165–173.

156. Winquist R. Closed intramedullary osteotomies of the femur. *Clin Orthop Relat Res* 1986;212:155–164.

157. Winquist R, Hansen S, Pearson R. Closed intramedullary shortening of the femur. *Clin Orthop Relat Res* 1978;136:54–61.

158. Edwards K, Cummings R. Fat embolism as a complication of closed femoral shortening. *J Pediatr Orthop* 1992;12:542–543.

159. Chapman M, Duwelius P, Bray T, et al. Closed intramedullary femoral osteotomy. Shortening and derotation procedures. *Clin Orthop* 1993;287:245–251.

160. Lynch M, Taylor J. Periosteal division and longitudinal growth in the tibia of the rat. *J Bone Joint Surg* 1987;69B:812–816.

161. Wilde G, Baker G. Circumferential periosteal release in the treatment of children with leg length inequality. *J Bone Joint Surg* 1987;69B:817–821.

162. Bohlman HR. Experiments with foreign materials in the region of the epiphyseal cartilage plate of growing bones to increase their longitudinal growth. *J Bone Joint Surg* 1929;11:365–384.

163. Bisgard JD. Longitudinal bone growth, the influence of sympathetic deinnervation. *Ann Surg* 1973;97:374–380.

164. Harris R, McDonald J. The effect of lumbar sympathectomy upon the growth of legs paralysed by anterior poliomyelitis. *J Bone Joint Surg* 1936;18:35–45.

165. Manning C. Leg lengthening. *Clin Orthop* 1978;136:105–110.

166. Petty W, Winter R, Felder D. Arteriovenous fistula for treatment of discrepancy in leg length. *J Bone Joint Surg* 1974;56A:581–586.

167. Yabsley R, Harris W. The effect of shaft fractures and periosteal stripping on the vascular supply to epiphyseal plates. *J Bone Joint Surg* 1965;47A:551–566.

168. Codivilla A. On the means of lengthening in the lower limbs the muscles and tissues which are shortened through deformity. *Am J Orthop Surg* 1905;2:353.

169. Magnuson P. Lengthening of shortened bones of the leg by operation. Ivory screws with removable heads as a means of holding the two bone fragments. *Surg Gynecol Obstet* 1913;16:63–71.

170. Coleman S. Simultaneous femoral and tibial lengthening for limb length discrepancies. *Arch Orthop Trauma Surg* 1985;103: 359–366.

171. Agerholm J. The zig-zag osteotomy. *Acta Orthop Scand* 1959;29: 63–70.

172. Westin G. Femoral lengthening using a periosteal sleeve. Report of twenty-six cases. *J Bone Joint Surg* 1967;49A:836–854.

173. Compere E. Indications for and against the leg lengthening operation. *J Bone Joint Surg* 1936;18:692–705.

174. McCarroll H. Trials and tribulations in attempted femoral lengthening. *J Bone Joint Surg* 1950;32A:132–142.

175. Bost FC, Larson LJ. Experiences with lengthening of the femur over an intramedullary rod. *J Bone Joint Surg* 1956;38A:567–584.

176. Gotz J, Schellerman W. Continuous lengthening of the femur with intramedullary stabilisation. *Arch Orthop Unfallchir* 1975; 82:305–310.

177. Kawamura B. Limb lengthening. *Orthop Clin North Am* 1978; 9:155–169.

178. Malhis T, Bowen J. Tibial and femoral lengthening. A report of 54 cases. *J Pediatr Orthop* 1982;2:487–491.

179. Rezaian S. Tibial lengthening using a new external extension device. Report of thirty-two cases. *J Bone Joint Surg* 1976;58A: 239–243.

180. Millis M, Hall J. Transiliac lengthening of the lower extremity. A modified innominate osteotomy for the treatment of postural imbalance. *J Bone Joint Surg* 1979;61A:1182–1194.

181. Barry K, McManus F, O'Brien T. Leg lengthening by the transiliac method. *J Bone Joint Surg* 1992;74B:275–278.

182. Lee D, Choi I, Ahn J, et al. Triple innominate osteotomy for hip stabilisation and transiliac leg lengthening after poliomyelitis. *J Bone Joint Surg* 1993;75B:858–864.

183. Cauchoix J, Morel G. One-stage femoral lengthening. *Clin Orthop Relat Res* 1978;136:66–73.

184. Morel G, Morin C. Simplified technique of extemporaneous lengthening of the femur in children. *Chir Pediatr* 1986;27:326–328.

185. Rezaian S, Abtahi M. A simple and safe technique for tibial lengthening. *Clin Orthop* 1986;207:216–222.

186. Bianco AJ Jr. Femoral shortening. *Clin Orthop* 1978;136:49–53.

187. Zanasi R. Surgical equalisation of leg length: shortening of the long femur and lengthening of the short in one operation. *Ital J Orthop Traumatol* 1982;8:265–270.

188. Yadav S. Double oblique diaphyseal osteotomy. A new technique for lengthening deformed and short lower limbs. *J Bone Joint Surg* 1993;75B:962–966.

189. Hughes T, Maffulli N, Fixsen J. Ultrasonographic appearance of regenerate bone in limb lengthening. *J R Soc Med* 1993;86:18–20.

190. Maffulli N, Hughes T, Fixen J. Ultrasonographic monitoring of limb lengthening. *J Bone Joint Surg* 1992;74-B(1):130–132.

191. Wagner H. Operative lengthening of the femur. *Clin Orthop* 1978;136:125–142.

192. Anderson WV. Leg lengthening. *J Bone Joint Surg* 1952;34B:150.

193. Wagner H. Operative Beinverlangerung. (Surgical leg prolongation). *Chirurgie* 1971;42:260–266.

194. Wagner H. Operative correction of leg length discrepancy. *Langenbecks Arch Chir* 1977;345:147–154.

195. Wagner H. Surgical lengthening of the femur. Report of fifty-eight cases. *Ann Chir* 1980;34:263–275.

196. De Bastiani G, Aldegheri R, Renzi-Brivio L, et al. Chondrodiatasis—controlled symmetrical distraction of the epiphyseal plate. Limb lengthening in children. *J Bone Joint Surg* 1986;68B:550–556.

197. De Bastiani G, Aldegheri R, Renzi-Brivio L, et al. Limb lengthening by callus distraction (callotasis). *J Pediatr Orthop* 1987;7:129–134.

198. Guidera K, Hess W, Highhouse K, et al. Extremity lengthening: results and complications with the orthofix system. *J Pediatr Orthop* 1991;11:90–94.

199. Bensahel H, Huguenin P, Briard JL. Transepiphyseal lengthening of the tibia. *Rev Chir Orthop Reparatrice Appar Mot* 1983;69:245–247.

200. Monticelli G, Spinelli R. Distraction epiphyseolysis as a method of limb lengthening. II. Morphologic investigations. *Clin Orthop* 1981;154:262–273.

201. Monticelli G, Spinelli R. Distraction epiphyseolysis as a method of limb lengthening. III. Clinical applications. *Clin Orthop* 1981;154:274–285.

202. Monticelli G, Spinelli R. Distraction epiphysiolysis as a method of limb lengthening. I. Experimental study. *Clin Orthop* 1981;154:254–261.

203. Monticelli G, Spinelli R. Limb lengthening by epiphyseal distraction. *Int Orthop* 1981;5:85–90.

204. Ring P. Experimental bone lengthening by epiphyseal distraction. *Br J Surg* 1958;46:169–173.

205. Wasserstein I, Correll J, Niethard F. Closed distraction epiphyseolysis for leg lengthening and axis correction of the leg in children. *Z Orthop Ihre Grenzgeb* 1986;124:743–750.

206. Connolly J, Huurman W, Lippiello L, et al. Epiphyseal traction to correct acquired growth deformities. An animal and clinical investigation. *Clin Orthop* 1986;202:258–268.

207. Hamanishi C, Tanaka S, Tamura K. Early physeal closure after femoral chondrodiatasis. Loss of length gain in 5 cases. *Acta Orthop Scand* 1992;63:146–149.

208. Morel G, Servant J, Valle A, et al. Extemporaneous femoral lengthening by the cauchoix technic in children and adolescents. *Rev Chir Orthop Reparatrice Appar Mot* 1983;69:195–200.

209. Ilizarov G, Deviatov A. Surgical elongation of the leg. *Ortop Travmatol Protez* 1971;32:20–25.

210. Ilizarov G, Deviatov A, Trokhova V. Surgical lengthening of the shortened lower extremities. *Vestn Khir* 1972;107:100–103.

211. Ilizarov G, Trokhova V. Surgical lengthening of the femur. *Ortop Travmatol Protez* 1973;34:73–74.

212. Monticelli G, Spinelli R. Leg lengthening by closed metaphyseal corticotomy. *Ital J Orthop Traumatol* 1983;9:139–150.

213. Ilizarov G, Deviatov A. Surgical lengthening of the shin with simultaneous correction of deformities. *Ortop Travmatol Protez* 1969;30:32–37.

214. Raschke M, Mann J, Oedekoven G, et al. Segmental transport after unreamed intramedullary nailing. Preliminary report of a monorail system. *Clin Orthop* 1992;282:233–240.

215. Huang S. Leg lengthening by the Ilizarov technique for patients with sequelae of poliomyelitis. *J Formos Med Assoc* 1997;96(4):258–265.

216. Lin C, Huang S, Liu T, et al. Limb lengthening over an intramedullary nail. An animal study and clinical report. *Clin Orthop* 1996;330:208–216.

217. Lee WH, Huang SC. Femoral lengthening: callotasis with Ilizarov external fixator alone and with intramedullary locking nail. *J Formos Med Assoc* 1997;96(2):98–102.

218. Paley D, Herzenberg JE, Paremain G, et al. Femoral lengthening over an intramedullary nail. A matched-case comparison with Ilizarov femoral lengthening. *J Bone Joint Surg Am* 1997;79(10):1464–1480.

219. Gordon JE, Goldfarb CA, Luhmann SJ, et al. Femoral lengthening over a humeral intramedullary nail in preadolescent children. *J Bone Joint Surg Am* 2002;84-A(6):930–937.

220. Kristiansen LP, Steen H. Lengthening of the tibia over an intramedullary nail, using the Ilizarov external fixator. Major complications and slow consolidation in 9 lengthenings. *Acta Orthop Scand* 1999;70(3):271–274.

221. Simpson AH, Cole AS, Kenwright J. Leg lengthening over an intramedullary nail. *J Bone Joint Surg Br* 1999;81(6):1041–1045.

222. Wu C, Shih C, Chen W. Nonunion and shortening after femoral fracture treated with one-stage lengthening using locked nailing teechnique. Good results in 48/51 patients. *Acta Orthop Scand* 1999;70(1):33–36.

223. Baumgart R, Betz A, Schweiberer L. A fully implantable motorized intramedullary nail for limb lengthening and bone transport. *Clin Orthop* 1997;343:135–143.

224. Aalsma AM, Hekman EE, Stapert J, et al. Design of an intramedullary leg lengthening device with a shape memory actuator. *Technol Health Care* 1999;7(6):461–467.

225. Cole JD, Justin D, Kasparis T, et al. The intramedullary skeletal kinetic distractor (ISKD): first clinical results of a new intramedullary nail for lengthening of the femur and tibia. *Injury* 2001;32(Suppl. 4):SD129–SD139.

226. Garcia-Cimbrelo E, Curto de la Mano A, Garcia-Rey E, et al. The intramedullary elongation nail for femoral lengthening. *J Bone Joint Surg Br* 2002;84(7):971–977.

227. Guichet JM, Deromedis B, Donnan LT, et al. Gradual femoral lengthening with the Albizzia intramedullary nail. *J Bone Joint Surg Am* 2003;85-A(5):838–848.

228. Hankemeier S, Pape HC, Gosling T, et al. Improved comfort in lower limb lengthening with the intramedullary skeletal kinetic distractor. Principles and preliminary clinical experiences. *Arch Orthop Trauma Surg* 2004;124(2):129–133.

229. Yasui N, Kojimoto H, Sasaki K, et al. Factors affecting callus distraction in limb lengthening. *Clin Orthop* 1993;293:55–60.

230. Lokietek W, Legaye J, Lokietek J-C. Contributing factors for osteogenesis in children's limb lengthening. *J Pediatr Orthop* 1991;11:452–458.

231. Bowen J, Levy E, Donohue M. Comparison of knee motion and callous formation in femoral lengthening with the wagner or monolateral-ring device. *J Pediatr Orthop* 1993;13:467–472.

232. Bell D. The effect of limb lengthening on articular cartilage: an experimental study. In: *Annual meeting of the Pediatric Orthopaedic Society of North America*. Newport, RI, 1992.

233. Ilizarov G, Irianov I, Migalkin N, et al. Ultrastructural characteristics of elastogenesis in the major arteries of the canine hindlimb during lengthening. *Arkh Anat Gistol Embriol* 1987;93:94–98.

234. Ilizarov G, Palienko L, Shreiner A. Bone marrow hematopoietic function and its relationship to osteogenesis activity during reparative regeneration in leg lengthening in the dog. *Ontogenez* 1984;15:146–152.

235. Carroll N, Grant C, Hudson R, et al. Experimental observations on the effects of leg lengthening by the Wagner method. *Clin Orthop* 1981;160:250–257.

236. Noonan K, Leyes M, Forriol F, et al. Distraction osteogenesis of the lower extremity with use of monolateral external fixation. A study of two hundred and sixty-one femora and tibiae. *J Bone Joint Surg Am* 1998;80-A(6):793–806.

237. Noonan K, Price C, Sproul J, et al. Acute correction and distraction osteogensis for the malaligned and shortened lower extremity. *J Pediatr Orthop* 1998;18(2):178–186.

238. Price C. Unilateral fixators and mechanical axis realignment. *Orthop Clin North Am* 1994;25(3):499–508.

239. Herzenberg J, Waanders N. Calculating rate and duration of distraction for deformity correction with the Ilizarov technique. *Orthop Clin North Am* 1991;22(4):601–611.

240. Bjerkreim I, Hellum C. Femur lengthening using the wagner technique. *Acta Orthop Scand* 1983;54:263–266.

241. Brockway A, Fowler SB. Experience with 105 leg-lengthening operations. *Surg Gynecol Obstet* 1942;75:252–256.

242. Chandler D, King J, Bernstein S, et al. Results of 21 Wagner limb lengthenings in 20 patients. *Clin Orthop Relat Res* 1988;230:214–222.

243. Coleman S, Stevens P. Tibial lengthening. *Clin Orthop* 1978;136:92–104.

244. Glorion C, Pouliquen J, Langlais J, et al. Femoral lengthening using the callotasis method: study of the complications in a series of 70 cases in children and adolescents. *J Pediatr Orthop* 1996;16(2):161–167.

245. Hantes ME, Malizos KN, Xenakis TA, et al. Complications in limb-lengthening procedures: a review of 49 cases. *Am J Orthop* 2001;30(6):479–483.

246. Hood R, Riseborough E. Lengthening of the lower extremity by the Wagner method. *J Bone Joint Surg* 1981;63-A(7):1122–1131.

247. Kawamura B, Mosona S, Takahashi T, et al. Limb lengthening by means of subcutaneous osteotomy. *J Bone Joint Surg* 1968;50A:851–878.

248. Rigault P, Dolz G, Padovani J, et al. Progressive tibial lengthening in children. *Rev Chir Orthop* 1981;67:461–472.

249. Seitz D, Yancey H. A review of tibial lengthening procedures. *South Med J* 1976;69:1349–1355.

250. Stanitski D, Shahcheraghi H, Nicker D, et al. Results of tibial lengthening with the Ilizarov technique. *J Pediatr Orthop A* 1996;16(2):168–172.

251. Stephens D. Femoral and tibial lengthening. *J Pediatr Orthop* 1983;3:424–430.

252. Leyes M, Noonan K, Forriol F, et al. Statistical analysis of axial deformity during distraction osteogenesis of the tibia. *J Pediatr Orthop* 1998;18(2):190–197.

253. Cheng J, Cheung K, Ng B. Severe progressive deformities after limb lengtheining in type-II fibular hemimelia. *J Bone Joint Surg* 1998;80(5):772–776.

254. Haddad F, Harper G, Hill R. Introperative arthrography and the Ilizarov technique. Role in the correction of paediatric deformity and leg lengthening. *J Bone Joint Surg Br* 1997;79(5):731–733.

255. Axer A, Elkon A, Eliahu H. Hypertension as a complication of limb lengthening. *J Bone Joint Surg* 1966;48-A:520–522.

256. Miller A, Rosman M. Hypertensive encephalopathy as a complication of femoral lengthening. *Can Med Assoc J* 1981;124:296–297.

257. Yosipovich Z, Palti Y. Alterations in blood pressure during leg-lengthening. A clinical and experimental investigation. *J Bone Joint Surg* 1967;49A:1352–1358.

258. Luke D, Schoenecker P, Blair V, et al. Fractures after Wagner limb lengthening. *J Pediatr Orthop* 1992;12:20–24.

259. Nakamura K, Matsushita T, Mamada K, et al. Changes of callus diameter during axial loading and after fixator removal in leg lengthening. *Arch Orthop Trauma Surg* 1998;117(8):464–467.

260. Mamada K, Nakamura K, Matsushita T, et al. The diameter of callus in leg lengtheining: 28 tibial lengthenings in 14 patients with achondroplasia. *Acta Orthop Scand* 1998;9(3):306–310.

261. Jones D, Moseley C. Subluxation of the knee as a complication of femoral lengthening by the Wagner technique. *J Bone Joint Surg* 1985;67B:33–35.

262. Mosca V, Moseley C. Results of limb lengthening using the Wagner device. *Ortho Trans* 1987;11:52.

263. Torode I, Gillespie R. Anteroposterior instability of the knee: a sign of congenital limb deficiency. *J Pediatr Orthop* 1983;3:467–470.

264. Torode I, Gillespie R. The classification and treatment of proximal femoral deficiencies. *Prosthet Orthot Int* 1991;15:117–126.

265. Salai M, Chechick A, Ganel A, et al. Subluxation of the hip joint during femoral lengthening. *J Pediatr Orthop* 1985;5:642–644.

266. Naudie D, Hamdy R, Fassier F, et al. Complications of limb lengthening in children who have an underlying bone disorder. *J Bone Joint Surg Am* 1998;80-A(1):18–24.

267. Herzenberg J, Paley D. Leg lengthening in children. *Curr Opin Pediatr* 1998;10(1):95–97.

268. Waldhausen J, Mosca V, Johansen K, et al. Delayed presentation of popliteal artery injury during Ilizarov limb lengthening. *Orthopedics* 1998;21(4):477–478.

269. Polo A, Aldegheri R, Zambito A, et al. Lower-limb lengthening in short stature. An electrophysiological and clinical assessment of peripheral nerve function. *J Bone Joint Surg Br* 1997;79(6):1014–1018.

270. Young N, Davis R, Bell D, et al. Electromyographic and nerve conduction changes after tibial lengthening by the Ilizarov method. *J Pediatr Orthop* 1993;13:473–477.

271. Karger C, Guille J, Bowen J. Lengthening of congenital lower limb deficiencies. *Clin Orthop* 1993;291:236–245.

272. Price C, Carantzas A. Severe growth retardation following limb lengthening: a case report. *Iowa Orthop J* 1996;16:139–146.

273. Viehweger, E, et al, Bone growth after lengthening of the lower limb in children. *J Pediatr Orthop B* 1998.7(2):154–157.

274. Aaron A, Eilert R. Results of the Wagner and Ilizarov methods of limb-lengthening. *J Bone Joint Surg Am* 1996;78(1):20–29.

275. Maffulli N, Lombari C, Matarazzo L, et al. A review of 240 patients undergoing distraction osteogenesis for congenital, post-traumatic or postinfective lower limb length discrepancy. *J Am Coll Surg* 1996;182(5):394–402.

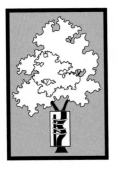

# 30

# The Foot

*James R. Kasser*

■ ACQUIRED CONDITIONS 1311

In this chapter, structural deformities of the foot as well as localized afflictions will be analyzed. To understand pathologic states and to institute treatment, it is first necessary to have a firm grasp of growth and development, as well as normal functional anatomy of the foot. The healthy foot at birth is generally flexible and well aligned. Having said this, contractures are common, involving all manner of deformity, but usually they resolve with exercises, observation, or both. The longitudinal arch is generally absent at birth but slowly and spontaneously develops (1). Commonly, there is medial deviation of the forefoot that resolves spontaneously in over 90% of cases. Even in cases with moderate residual deformity (2–4), there is little long-term disability.

Healthy development of the foot occurs in the absence of specialized footwear, including shoes and arch supports. Numerous studies in populations that use shoes suggest that adaptations to footwear are not generally required. Sim-Fook and Hodgson (5), and Rao and Joseph (6) found a higher incidence of flatfoot among children who wore shoes than those who grew up barefoot. Staheli et al. have documented the progressive development of the longitudinal arch in healthy children as measured by the ratio of midfoot to hindfoot width (1).

The appearance of foot deformity is complicated by valgus or varus alignment of the leg. In a case where valgus deformity of the knee is present, there will be increased weight bearing on the medial side of the foot and the appearance of a flatfoot. Salenius and Vankka (7) documented the progressive increase in genu valgum to 4 years of age, followed by spontaneous resolution. In addition to angular deformity, one should be aware that rotational deformity of the femoral and tibial shaft will result in apparent foot deformity as well, with altered push-off (8).

The foot grows continuously with the growth of the child, but this growth accelerates ahead of the adolescent growth spurt. Distal epiphyses tend to close first, followed by diminished growth through the midfoot and cessation of growth 1 to 2 years before the growth in height ends. Metatarsal growth plates are located proximally on the first metatarsal and distally on metatarsals 2 through 5. The tuberosity of the calcaneus grows through the calcaneal apophysis. A group led by Green (9) documented the growth of the foot with age and produced a chart as shown in Figure 30.1. Foot growth decelerates at 12 to 13 years of age in girls and 14 to 15 years of age in boys.

## ANATOMY

One must understand the anatomy of the foot in the healthy state to comprehend and treat pathologic structural conditions. The structure of the foot is based upon its constituent parts, including proper alignment of seven tarsal bones, five metatarsals, and five digits. Each tarsal bone has a defined shape with complex articular surfaces, variable ossification pattern, centripetal growth, and links to adjacent bones through thick ligaments. The complex articular surfaces allow only limited gliding transplanar

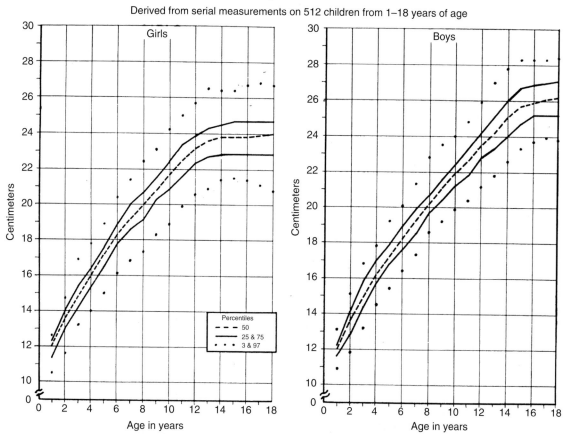

**Figure 30.1** In 1956, a group led by Green documented the growth curves for the foot in boys and in girls. Growth of the foot tends to decelerate before the longitudinal growth of the child. (From Anderson M, Blais MM, Green WT. Lengths of the growing foot. *J Bone Joint Surg Am* 1956;38-A:998–1000, with permission.)

motion. An example of this is the motion of the subtalar joint. Figure 30.2 shows the dorsal surface of the calcaneus with three articular surfaces—the posterior, middle, and anterior facets. Motion through this complex joint is best thought of as a gliding, rotational translation of the calcaneus under a fixed talus. Subtalar motion, therefore, is not pure inversion or eversion of the calcaneus under the talus. To understand the foot, rather than thinking of articular motion about a single axis, one should consider foot motion, whether inversion, eversion, or pronation and supination, as the sum of the gliding motion involving multiple joints. Restriction of any joint in the hindfoot or midfoot will result in restricted motion throughout all structures. In a cadaver study, Wulker et al. (10) showed the effect of selective fusion in the hindfoot and midfoot. Motion of the subtalar joint was not significantly affected by fusion of the calcaneocuboid joint, but reduced to 25% of its normal range by fusion of both the talonavicular joint and calcaneocuboid joint. Talonavicular motion was decreased by subtalar fusion but was not affected by calcaneocuboid fusion. It was concluded that the talonavicular joint was the key articulation for hindfoot motion.

The bones of the foot are held in position by ligaments, as the joints of the foot have no intrinsic stability. Major ligaments within the foot are the interosseous ligament, the plantar calcaneonavicular ligament, the plantar calcaneocuboid ligament, and the bifurcated or internal calcaneocuboid ligament (11). The interosseous ligament is a condensation of the articular capsules between the talus and the calcaneus, involving the posterior, middle, and anterior facets of the subtalar joint. The plantar calcaneonavicular ligament, or spring ligament, is a broad, thick band connecting the anterior margin of the sustentaculum talae of the calcaneus to the plantar surface of the navicular. This ligament connects the calcaneus to the navicular and supports the head of the talus. The spring ligament is reinforced by the posterior tibial tendon on its plantar medial surface. The interosseous ligament forms the axis of rotation of the subtalar joint, whereas the spring ligament supports the head of the talus in stance. The calcaneocuboid and the spring ligaments stabilize the articulation between the hindfoot and midfoot, known as the Chopart joint. The three cuneiforms and metatarsals are connected by a series of plantar and dorsal ligaments, which are strong, flat bands. Metatarsals are stabilized by the intermetatarsal ligament proximally. Distally, the metatarsals are connected by a transverse fibrous band between the metatarsal heads, known as the *transverse metatarsal ligament*.

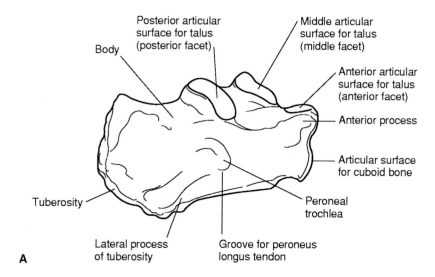

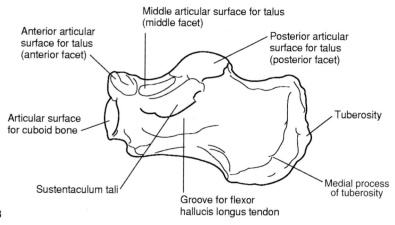

**Figure 30.2** The calcaneus has three articular surfaces that compose the subtalar joint. Motion of the calcaneus relative to the talus is a rotational translation, rather than pure inversion or eversion. **A:** Lateral surface. **B:** Medial surface.

The longitudinal arch of the foot is formed by the combination of all tarsal and metatarsal bones. The structure distributes weight evenly across the foot in stance, allowing weight distribution on the calcaneus, as well as across the metatarsal heads. Little force is required in the tibialis posterior tendon to maintain position in stance. Basmajian and Stecko (12) demonstrated that there was almost no electromyographic activity in the muscles of the foot and ankle when physiologic loads were applied to the plantigrade foot in stance. They concluded that the bone-ligament complex determines the height of the longitudinal arch, whereas muscles maintain balance, accommodate the foot on uneven terrain, protect the ligaments from stress, and propel the body forward. Mann and Inman (13) confirmed this theory.

The toes are composed of phalanges stabilized by ligaments, allowing only flexion and extension across joints. Each of the joints has a proximal cylindrical surface with a concave distal surface. Tendons inserting on the mid and distal phalanx, with intrinsic muscles acting to flex the metatarsal phalangeal (MP) joint, function well in the healthy state. This alignment, however, creates an unstable position of the MP joint in dorsiflexion, once the intrinsic muscles are unable to flex the proximal phalanx, leading to claw toes.

The relation between the bones of the foot is measured both clinically and radiographically in order to define healthy and pathologic states. Radiographically, images are always taken in the standing position, except in the case of infants, for whom position should be specified. In standing anteroposterior and lateral views of the foot, the following angles should be determined (Fig. 30.3):

1. The lateral talocalcaneal angle (A) (lateral view) is measured as the angle subtended by the long axis of the talus and the plantar surface of the calcaneus. Normally, it is in the 30 to 45-degree range. It is decreased in the varus foot and increased in the valgus foot (Fig. 30.3B).
2. The anterior talocalcaneal angle (B) (anteroposterior view) is measured as the angle subtended by the long axis of the talus and the long axis of the calcaneus. Normally, it is 30 to 45 degrees, decreased in a varus foot and increased in a valgus hindfoot (Fig. 30.3A).
3. Meary angle (lateral view) is the measurement of the angle subtended by the long axis of the talus and the long axis of the first metatarsal on a standing lateral view. Normally, these lines are colinear. In cases where the apex is directed dorsally, a cavus foot is present. Cases where apex is angled plantarward are valgus or flatfeet (Fig. 30.3B).
4. Intermetatarsal angle (C) (anteroposterior view) is the measurement of the angle subtended by the long axis of the first and second metatarsal. This angle is generally less than 5 degrees but is increased in deformities associated with bunion formation (Fig. 30.3A).
5. The longitudinal arch (D) (Hibb angle, lateral view) is generally measured as an angle between the plantar surface of the calcaneus and the first metatarsal. It is decreased in cavus feet, particularly with a "calcaneus" deformity in which the longitudinal axis of the calcaneus is increasingly vertical (Fig. 30.3B).
6. Calcaneal pitch (E) (lateral view) is measured as the angle between the horizontal and the plantar surface of the calcaneus. It is an indicator of the position of the calcaneus in stance and is particularly important in evaluating a cavus foot or clubfoot (Fig. 30.3B).

*Clinical Measurement of Foot Position*

1. Hindfoot varus and valgus: This position is measured in stance as the angle between the long axis of the tibia and the long axis of the hindfoot, either in varus, valgus, or neutral (Fig. 30.4A and B).
2. Normal hindfoot mobility. This is measured by looking for the hindfoot to tip into mild varus as the patient rises on the toes (Fig. 30.4C).
3. Longitudinal arch. Observe the normal longitudinal arch as the space under the medial side of the foot in stance. An increase in longitudinal arch in a non-weight-bearing position as well as when a person rises on the toes in stance is normal.
4. Heel bisector. The long axis of the heel should intersect the second metatarsal head in the normal state (Fig. 30.5).
5. Thigh-foot angle. With the patient in a prone position, the long axis of the foot, defined by the center of the heel to second metatarsal head, should be aligned with the long axis of the thigh. Medial and lateral deviations from this should be recorded as an angular measurement.

In addition to the bony and ligamentous structure of the foot that we have defined, one must consider both the intrinsic and the extrinsic muscles affecting this complex. The extrinsic muscles have their origin above the ankle and include the anterior tibialis, the posterior tibialis, the extensor hallucis longus, the extensor digitorum communis, the flexor hallucis longus, the flexor digitorum communis, two peroneal muscles, and the gastrocsoleus complex. The intrinsic muscles of the foot primarily are plantar and can be divided into four layers. The most superficial layer includes the abductor hallucis, the flexor digitorum brevis, and the abductor digiti minimi. The second layer is the quadratus plante and the lumbricals. The third layer is the flexor hallucis brevis, the adductor hallucis, and the flexor digiti minimi brevis. The fourth layer includes the interossei. The intrinsic dorsal musculature is the extensor digitorum brevis muscle that arises from the distal lateral calcaneus and ligaments of adjacent joints. The balance among all of these muscles is critical for proper function as well as avoidance of cavus deformity. The gastrocsoleus complex acts as a powerful plantar flexor muscle. It is opposed by the anterior tibialis

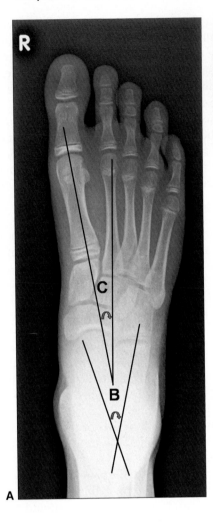

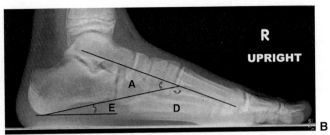

**Figure 30.3** The standard radiographs of the foot are taken in the standing position, anteroposterior and lateral views. **A:** On the antero-posterior view (*A*), the intermetatarsal angle (*C*) between the first and second metatarsal and the talocalcaneal angle (*B*) can be measured. **B:** On the lateral view of the foot, the lateral talocalcaneal angle, the Meary angle, the Hibb angle (*D*), and the calcaneal pitch (*E*) should be determined.

muscle and toe extensors. The anterior tibialis muscle is, however, a supinator of the forefoot, and unless it is counteracted by the peroneus longus, the anterior tibialis will create a deformity with forefoot supination and a dorsal bunion. The posterior tibialis muscle produces hindfoot varus and medial deviation of the forefoot unless balanced by the peroneal muscles. The complex symphony of muscle function produces coordinated, efficient activity in the healthy state. However, imbalance due to pathologic states results in deformity. Under standing the static and dynamic healthy state of the foot is necessary to approach and treat foot pathology.

# CONGENITAL DEFORMITIES AND MALFORMATIONS OF THE FOOT (NATURAL HISTORY THROUGH TREATMENT)

## Clubfoot (Congenital Talipes, Equinovarus)

### Definition

The term "clubfoot" refers to a congenital foot deformity characterized by equinus of the hindfoot and adduction of the midfoot and forefoot with varus through the subtalar joint complex (Fig. 30.6). There is also a cavus deformity

Posterior view

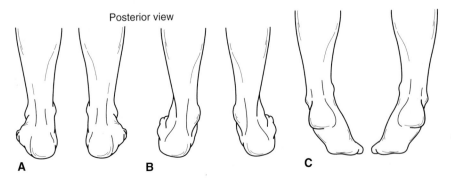

**Figure 30.4** **A,B:** Hindfoot position is measured as varus or valgus, on the basis of the angle subtended by the longitudinal axis of the tibia and the longitudinal axis of the hindfoot. **C:** With normal hindfoot mobility as the patient rises on the toes, the calcaneus tips into varus position.

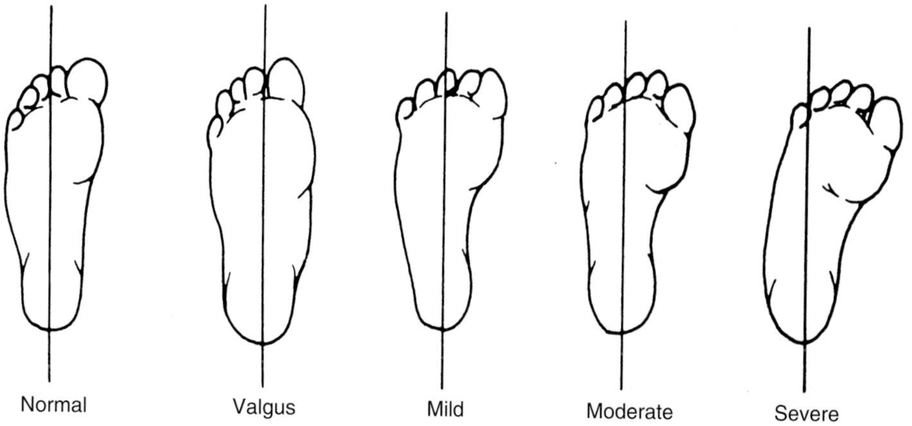

**Figure 30.5** The heel bisector method. The severity of metatarsus adductus is determined by the relation between the toes and the distal end of the line bisecting the heel. The severity does not correlate with prognosis. (From Bleck EE. Developmental orthopaedics. III. Toddlers. *Dev Med Child Neurol* 1982;24:533.)

Normal    Valgus    Mild    Moderate    Severe

through the midfoot, which accompanies most clubfeet. In identifying the pathologic tissue in a clubfoot, Irani and Sherman (14) found the talus to be uniformly abnormal, and a group led by Clarke (15) demonstrated malformation of the calcaneus. In addition, however, those who have looked at the tissue surrounding the bones have identified vascular abnormalities, muscle lesions, abnormal muscle insertions, and retracting fibrosis to be associated pathologic abnormalities in clubfoot deformity. The pathology clearly is not limited to the osseous structures. Clubfeet in general are "idiopathic," occurring in otherwise healthy children. Some are positional, with rapid correction and requiring little by way of treatment. On the other extreme of the spectrum of clubfeet are those associated with syndromes such as Freeman-Sheldon syndrome and arthrogryposis, in which there is a rigid clubfoot with fibrotic muscles and little in the way of active muscle function. Idiopathic clubfoot bridges the spectrum between these two conditions.

### Epidemiology

The incidence of clubfoot varies from a baseline occurrence of 0.6 per 1000 in Asian populations (16–18) and 0.9 per 1000 births in western Australia (19) to a high of 6.8 per 1000 in Hawaiians, Polynesians, and Maoris (20). Boys are affected more than girls in all studies, varying from a twofold increased incidence to a high of 4:1, depending on the population studied. Bilateral involvement is present in approximately 50% of cases (17,21).

Wynne-Davies (17,18) determined that the occurrence rate was 17 times higher than in the normal population for first-degree relatives and six times higher for second-degree relatives. Unaffected parents with an affected son have a 2.5% chance of another child having the disorder. If the affected child is a girl, then there is a 6.5% chance of a son having clubfoot and a 2.5% chance of a subsequent daughter being affected. Wynne-Davies proposed dominant inheritance with reduced penetrance or multifactorial inheritance to describe this pattern of occurrence.

Cowell and Wein's data (21) suggested multifactorial inheritance. Skelly et al. (22) demonstrated the effect of maternal smoking during pregnancy in increasing the risk of clubfoot. Honein et al. (23) also identified maternal smoking as a significant factor in etiology. The joint effect of family history of clubfoot and maternal smoking during pregnancy was more than additive, suggesting a genetic-environmental interaction. Rebbeck et al. (24), using a complex mathematical model, concluded that the inheritance of clubfoot could be explained as a single-gene defect.

### Pathology

In a clubfoot, the navicular is subluxated medially and plantarward on the head of the talus. In severe cases, the navicular may actually articulate with the medial malleolus. The talus is shortened, with medial deviation of its head and deformity of the talar neck, but the long axis is actually laterally deviated in the mortise, as shown by Carroll and Hertzenberg (25). The sheath of the posterior tibial tendon and the calcaneonavicular ligament are shortened and thick, contributing to medial deformity. Posterolaterally, the calcaneofibular ligament is also shortened and thickened, causing medial spin of the calcaneus in clubfoot. Deep posterior and medial skin creases are universally present in a clubfoot (Fig. 30.7).

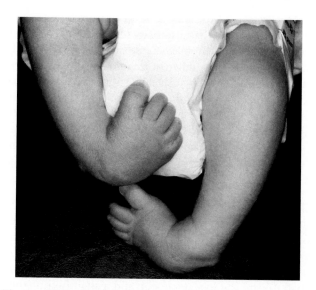

**Figure 30.6** Clubfoot deformity is associated with forefoot supination, deep medial creases, and equinovarus of the hindfoot.

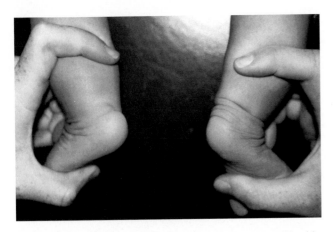

**Figure 30.7** Clubfoot (**left**) with single heel crease and healthy foot (**right**) with multiple heel creases.

The muscles are abnormal both in anatomical insertion and intrinsic structure (26,27). Muscles in clubfoot are smaller than normal and there is an increase in intracellular connective tissue within the gastrocsoleus and posterior tibial muscles. A predominance of type I muscle fiber has been seen in posterior and medial muscle groups. Electron microscopic studies have shown loss of myofibrils and atrophic fibers, suggesting a regional neuronal abnormality as well (25).

The ligaments are thick, with increased collagen fibers and increased cellularity (28). This is particularly true of the calcaneonavicular ligament or spring ligament and the posterior tibial tendon sheath (29). An electron microscopic study of medial ligaments in clubfoot identified myofibroblasts, which could be responsible for fibroblastic contracture in the postoperative clubfoot. Fukuhara et al. (30) showed myofibroblastlike cells in the deltoid and spring ligaments. Together, the thickened and shortened ligaments with contractile fibroblasts may produce a significant component of the clubfoot pathology. Sano et al. (31) confirmed these findings, showing that cells of the medial ligamentous structures contained vimentin uniformly and myofibroblasts in some cases. More recently, Khan et al. (32) were unable to show myofibroblastlike cells in clubfeet, and van der Sluijs and Pruys (33) demonstrated normal collagen cross-linking in clubfeet.

Finally, abnormal vasculature in the foot is frequently present (34). The dorsalis pedis artery in a number of cases is absent or altered. Katz et al. (35) showed deficient dorsalis pedis flow in 45% of clubfeet compared to 8% of normal controls. In the more severely affected feet requiring surgery, the incidence of dorsalis pedis abnormality was 54%, whereas those successfully treated with cast therapy had an abnormality in dorsalis pedis flow in only 20% of cases. This data suggests that the severity of clubfoot may in some way relate to the vascular abnormality frequently seen in this condition.

### Radiographic Features

There is no consensus on the role of radiography in the diagnosis and management of clubfoot (36,37). The diagnosis is made in the newborn child based on clinical findings of equinus of the hindfoot with some degree of varus and medial deviation. There is little ossification in the bones of the healthy foot of the newborn, whereas delay in ossification in the clubfoot has been documented (38). The ossific nucleus of the talus is not centrally located, further compromising the validity of x-ray evaluation of clubfoot (39,40). Ossification of the navicular does not occur until the age of 3 to 4 years in children with clubfoot and may be eccentric. Brennan et al. (41) documented poor reproducibility of x-ray films in a child with clubfoot because of problems with positioning, in addition to the unusual shape of the ossification center as it develops.

Despite these limitations, x-ray evaluation of clubfeet is helpful in determining surgical planning (42–44). The anterioposterior view is obtained with the foot pressed against a radiographic plate. In taking this view, the foot is dorsiflexed maximally and held in a position of external rotation (37,45) (Fig. 30.8). The talus to first metatarsal angle is measured on both the anteroposterior and lateral views, with increasing angles indicating more severe deformity. As the navicular is not ossified, there is no direct measurement of the position of this bone relative to the long axis of the talus (46). The axis of the talus and the calcaneus usually converge, and the axis of the talus and the first metatarsal form a straight line in the healthy state. The degree of divergence from this linear alignment represents the intrinsic deformity of the clubfoot (46). With dorsiflexion, the long axis of the talus and the calcaneus remain parallel, and the calcaneus remains plantar-flexed relative to the long axis of the talus (Fig. 30.8). The alignment of the calcaneus and the cuboid is assessed on the anterioposterior view.

Radiography may also be helpful in the intraoperative evaluation of the correction of clubfoot deformity. The difficulty in the intraoperative measurement is in reproducibly holding the foot in the right position for imaging. Intraoperative radiography remains controversial in the management of clubfoot deformity.

### Other Imaging Studies

Clubfoot deformity has also been measured by computed tomography (CT) scan, magnetic resonance imaging (MRI), and ultrasound. These different techniques of measurement have demonstrated conclusively a shortened longitudinal axis with medial deviation of the talar neck. However, the longitudinal axis of the talus is laterally rotated within the mortise. The calcaneus is internally rotated with decreased space between the calcaneus and the fibula posteriorly. The navicular is dislocated plantarward and medially on the head of the talus, as shown by ultrasound and MRI evaluation.

### Clinical Classification of Clubfoot

An examination of the patient with clubfoot should include looking for spinal pathology, neurologic abnormality, and any syndrome or associated condition in which clubfeet is frequently found (Table 30.1). Clubfoot is associated with a small calf on the ipsilateral side and a slightly shortened tibia. A minimal tibial length discrepancy is present at birth, but Spiegel and Loder (47) found it to be greater than

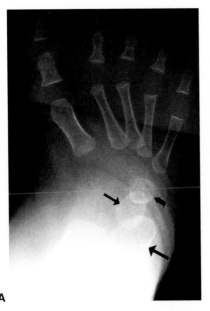
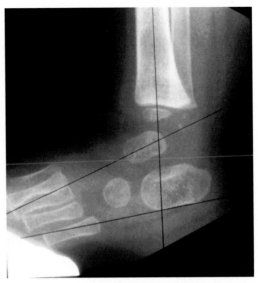

**A**    **B**

**Figure 30.8**  **A:** Simulated weight-bearing anteroposterior radiograph of clubfoot. The talus (*small straight arrow*) and calcaneus (*large straight arrow*) are parallel, rather than divergent. The metatarsals are markedly adducted in relation to the talus. The cuboid ossification center (*curved arrow*) is medially aligned on the end of the calcaneus, rather than in the normal straight alignment. **B:** Maximum dorsiflexion lateral radiograph of clubfoot. The talus and calcaneus are somewhat parallel to each other and plantar-flexed in relation to the tibia.

0.5 cm in 32 of 47 patients who were affected at maturity. Along with a shortened tibia, internal tibial torsion is occasionally associated with clubfoot deformity.

Muscle testing and sensory examination should be part of the initial examination in all patients, as clubfoot has been found to be associated with absent anterior compartment muscles and lesions involving the innervation to the anterior and lateral compartment muscles.

With respect to classification of clubfeet, important clinical features must be documented. Included in these features are:

1. The rigidity and degree of the deformity.
2. Depth of skin creases (Fig. 30.7).
3. Tightness and contractility of muscles.

Although there are a number of classification systems in use, the author finds two of them to be of particular value in

## TABLE 30.1

### SYNDROMES WITH WHICH CLUBFOOT IS COMMONLY ASSOCIATED

Arthrogryposis
Constriction bands (Streeter dysplasia)
Prune belly
Tibial hemimella
Möbius syndrome
Freeman-Sheldon syndrome (whistling face) (autosomal dominant)
Diastrophic dwarfism (autosomal recessive)
Larsen syndrome (autosomal recessive)
Opitz syndrome (autosomal recessive)
Pierre Robin syndrome (X-linked recessive)

attempting to classify clubfeet at the initiation of treatment. One of these classification systems was defined by Dimeglio et al. (48) and the second by Pirani (49). The classification systems apply a point score to a number of physical findings, which when totaled leads to a "grade of involvement." Flynn et al. (50) have shown a good correspondence between the classification systems of Pirani and Dimeglio. Flynn and MacKenzie (50) showed a correlation coefficient of 0.9 with the Pirani system and 0.83 with the Dimeglio system when applied by three individuals. The correlation improved in both systems after the initial 15 feet were scored. Wainwright et al. (51) compared four classification systems: Dimeglio, Catteral, Harold and Walker, and Ponseti and Smoley, determining that the Dimeglio system was the most reproducible. Both the Dimeglio and the Pirani point systems attempt to differentiate between mildly affected feet requiring little treatment and those that are extremely severe. If outcome of treatment is to be compared, a valid classification system at the onset of therapy must be developed.

The author uses the Dimeglio system in everyday practice. One should create a checklist with either of the systems and attempt to score feet at the initiation of treatment. Either of the scoring systems can be applied in less than 5 minutes. In the Pirani system, isolated physical findings such as space between the medial malleolus and navicular, and space between the calcaneus and the fibula, are identified and given scores on a 0, 0.5 or 1.0 basis. In the Dimeglio system (Fig. 30.9), the position of the foot deviation—whether equinus, varus, or medial—is scored based on the degree of deformity, as well as muscle function and depth of skin creases. The author

Classification

| Classification grade | Type | Frequency (%) | Score |
|---|---|---|---|
| I | Benign | 20 | (<5) |
| II | Moderate | 33 | (= 5<10) |
| III | Severe | 35 | (= 10<15) |
| IV | Very severe | 12 | (= 15<20) |

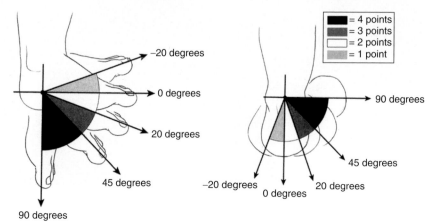

Sagittal plane evaluation of equinus.

Frontal plane evaluation of varus.

Horizontal plane evaluation of derotation of the calcaneopedal block.

Horizontal plane evaluation of forefoot relative to hindfoot.

ASSESSMENT of CLUBFOOT by SEVERITY SCALE

| Characteristics: Reproducibility | Points | Characteristics: Other parameters | Points |
|---|---|---|---|
| 90–45 degrees | 4 | Posterior crease | 1 |
| 45–20 degrees | 3 | Medial crease | 1 |
| 20–0 degrees | 2 | Cavus | 1 |
| <0 to –20 degrees | 1 | Poor muscle condition | 1 |

**Figure 30.9**  Dimeglio's classification system for clubfoot deformity rates the position of the foot relative to equinus, varus, foot rotation, and forefoot medial deviation. These are scored from 0 to 4 on the basis of severity. Finally, the depth of posterior crease, medial crease, cavus, and muscle condition are each assigned a 0 or 1 point score. Total score ranges from 0 to 20 points, correlating with the severity of the clubfoot deformity. (From Dimeglio A, Bonnet F, Mazeau P, et al. Orthopaedic treatment and passive motion machine: consequences for the surgical treatment of clubfoot. *J Pediatr Orthop B* 1996;5:173–180, with permission.)

believes that the isolated physical findings in the Pirani classification will correlate directly with the gross foot position data in the Dimeglio classification, leading to the correlation found by Flynn and others in applying these systems. Choose one and attempt to grade clubfeet, on the basis of these clinical criteria.

### Intrauterine Diagnosis

With the routine use of ultrasonography during pregnancy, intrauterine diagnosis of clubfoot has become increasingly frequent. This has implications, requiring the orthopaedist to be able to provide informed consultation concerning the long-term outcome of the deformity, as well as its proposed treatment. The orthopaedist must possess knowledge of the accuracy of diagnosis, its relation to syndromes, and the treatment regimes need in order to have an informed discussion with the prospective parents. It appears that the earliest that a clubfoot can be diagnosed by ultrasound with accuracy is 12 weeks of gestational age. With sequential studies, there is an increased ability to visualize the deformity, relating either to the progressive development of a clubfoot deformity or perhaps the accuracy with which it can be seen. According to Keret et al. (52), the clubfoot deformity has been detected in routine studies in approximately 60% of cases, which is indicative of some degree of false negative assessment. In 86% of cases, the deformity is identified by 23 weeks of gestational age, but still others are recognized up to 33 weeks. The diagnosis is made on ultrasound by the fixed position of the foot in an equinovarus position, not deviating from this on sequential observations (Fig. 30.10). Three-dimensional ultrasound may provide a more accurate diagnosis than standard ultrasound studies (53).

In studies of large populations using routine *in utero* ultrasound (54), the recognition of clubfoot deformity varies from 0.1% to 0.4% (55). Because postnatal studies suggest an occurrence rate at birth between 0.1% and 0.6%, one can assume a rather low false negative rate. The false-positive rate for diagnosis of clubfoot *in utero* using ultrasound varies from 30% to 40%, depending on series and criteria (55–58). A term *functional false-positive rate* has been used in cases in which a foot may have the appearance of remaining in a plantar flexed, varus and medially deviated position but can passively be corrected to neutral during exam just following birth. The foot is characterized with a score of 0, 1, or 2, using the Dimeglio classification system. Such a foot requires only parent-administered exercise, and no long-term deformity results. With the advancement of ultrasound and increase in experience, the accuracy of diagnosis will steadily increase.

The ability to recognize syndromes associated with skeletal malformations is also increasing with time (53,59). The combination of technologic advances and improved expertise in obtaining and interpreting images will certainly lead to further progress in recognizing fetal structural abnormalities. This brings one to the question of the need for amniocentesis and karyotyping if an isolated clubfoot deformity is found. In 1998 Shipp and Benacerraf (60) and Rijhsinghani et al. (55) suggested that amniocentesis and karyotyping were necessary to identify associated syndromes when clubfoot was identified. In 2000, Malone et al. (61) showed that in 57 cases of isolated clubfoot deformity out of 27,000 prenatal exams, there were no unrecognized associated abnormalities. Therefore, the recommendation is that karyotyping not be done in cases where a diagnosis of isolated clubfoot deformity was made. This still appears controversial, and a geneticist should be consulted about the need for amniocentesis if the question arises.

There is no attempt to provide any therapeutic intervention once an intrauterine diagnosis of clubfoot is made. The orthopaedist is only involved in counseling the family and providing treatment following birth. The author has found that this information allows for an informed discussion with the pregnant mother and interested father about the treatment and outcome in clubfoot deformity. The parents can be comforted by being shown the successful outcome after treatment of patients with this deformity. Myths about the crippling effect of clubfoot deformity can be dispelled. Accurate information about treatment and outcome allow the parents to make a personal decision concerning pregnancy and allows for an improved emotional state for the family during the delivery of their child.

### Treatment of Clubfoot

*Initial Management.* Throughout history clubfeet have been recognized as a significant deformity, with treatment consisting of some form of positional correction. The most extreme of these, perhaps, used a Thomas wrench to achieve correction. The viscoelastic properties of ligaments and tendons were recognized by Atlee as early as 1868, allowing for the correction of this deformity. In response to the traumatic methods of management of clubfoot, Kite (62,63), in 1939, presented his method of cast correction with a plea for conservative management. In Kite's method, the forefoot is distracted and laterally deviated while holding the back of the heel with the opposite hand. Pressure was placed over the calcaneocuboid joint laterally to facilitate correction, and the cast was applied. The cast was applied in two phases: first with a slipper holding the foot to prevent breech through the midfoot, and second with correction of the equinus and medial deviation deformity.

Kite's method of cast treatment required a lengthy period of immobilization, often greater than $1\frac{1}{2}$ to 2 years. Lovell et al. reported results using the Kite method in 1979 with long-term follow-up. In 47 patients with 67 affected feet, the average duration of casting was 20.4 months, while the improvement of 43 feet was rated to be good, 12 feet were rated fair, and 12 feet were rated poor (64,65). Because of this rather negative experience as well as increasingly popular methods of surgical management, use

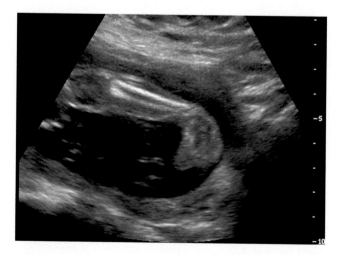

**Figure 30.10** The clubfoot is diagnosed by ultrasound *in utero* when there is persistent medial deviation and equinus of the foot relative to the tibia.

of corrective cast treatment was deemphasized through the 1970s, 1980s, and 1990s.

During this period of increased enthusiasm for surgery, Ponseti (65) developed and utilized a method for treatment of clubfoot using a combination of casting, manipulation, heel cord tenotomy, and prolonged splinting. As this method was begun as early as the 1940s, long-term follow-up of this technique is available and the results suggest that there should be new enthusiasm for the use of casts or conservative management of clubfoot deformity. The basis of Ponseti's treatment (66,67) was the knowledge of the pathoanatomy of clubfoot deformity based on the studies done on affected stillborn infants, as well as extensive experience. Using weekly manipulations and casting for a period of 5 to 8 weeks, the deformity is corrected. In over 95% of cases, extensive surgical release can be avoided in the case of idiopathic clubfoot. The Ponseti method has recently been accepted as the standard for

conservative management of clubfoot in the United States with increasing enthusiasm for it worldwide.

In the Ponseti method, the clubfoot is corrected by sequential manipulation and cast application. The foot can be thought of as having three components of deformity to be corrected sequentially: cavus, adduction, and varus equinus (2,7,68).

The cavus deformity in the clubfoot primarily involves the first ray. One needs to address this in the initial phase of correction. In order to correct cavus, the inner part of the forefoot is dorsiflexed, placing the foot in a supinated position (Fig. 30.11). Erroneously attempting to correct supination of the forefoot initially results in actually pronating the foot and increasing the cavus deformity. Whereas Carroll et al., and Carroll in 1988 (69,70), stated that cavus can only be corrected by plantar fascia release and intrinsic lengthening, Ponseti has shown the ability to alter this deformity by his casting technique. In only 6 of

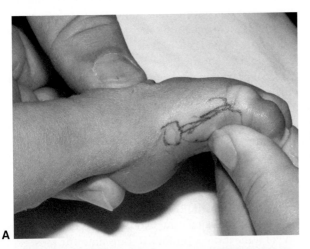

A

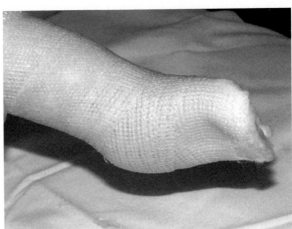

B

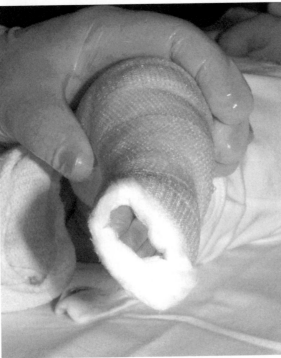

C

**Figure 30.11** **A:** At the time of initial casting of a clubfoot, the cavus deformity is treated with elevation of the first metatarsal head. **B,C:** A cast is applied with the foot in equinus and the forefoot supinated with pressure under the first metatarsal head and counterpressure over the head of the talus laterally.

104 feet was there persistent cavus in a series reported by Laaveg and Ponseti (36) in 1980 (Fig. 30.12).

At the first cast application, the forefoot is abducted with counterpressure applied laterally over the head of the talus. Pressure is placed under the first metatarsal head.

Correction of the cavus brings the metatarsals, cuneiform, navicular, and cuboid into the same plane (Fig. 30.11C). The lateral shift of the navicular and cuboid occurs as the tight joint capsule and ligaments yield to the pressure of manipulation (65). Several minutes of manipulation are required at each cast change to slowly stretch ligaments prior to cast application. A series of casts is applied on a weekly basis for the next 4 to 6 weeks to achieve midfoot (primarily talonavicular) correction. Simultaneously with the correction of the talonavicular joint, the calcaneus rotates under the talus, and the posterior aspect of the calcaneus moves away from the fibula with stretching of the calcaneofibular ligament. Care needs to be taken not to pronate the foot in this process and to maintain the forefoot in neutral position with respect to pronation and supination. The equinus is the last component corrected once the forefoot and midfoot are aligned.

During cast correction, the foot is externally rotated under the talus relative to the axis of the leg. The external rotation and abduction of the foot is steadily increased up to 70 degrees in the last cast. This is a very different position from the one generally used in traditional methods of clubfoot casting. Clearly, the only way that this position can be achieved is with a long leg cast. There is *no* role for short leg casts in the correction of clubfoot deformity.

Finally, equinus is corrected after the midfoot and forefoot deformity is addressed and completely resolved. The mechanism of correction is a combination of upward pressure under the entire foot while pulling down on the heel

with the other hand. One needs to achieve 15 degrees of dorsiflexion while holding the foot in 70 degrees of external rotation/abduction. In nearly all cases, a percutaneous tenotomy of the Achilles tendon is required to achieve this position without midfoot breech. Following a tenotomy, the foot can be dorsiflexed to a position well above neutral without midfoot breech. The heel cord reconstitutes rapidly following its lengthening, as has been documented both by clinical experience as well as by observation at the time of revision surgery. The final cast following tenotomy is left in place for 2 weeks. In this cast, the foot is held in a position of 15 degrees of dorsiflexion with 70 degrees of external rotation of the foot relative to the leg. After removal of the final cast, a Dennis-Brown bar is applied. The Dennis-Brown bar is positioned with the feet in slight dorsiflexion created by a bend in the mid-part of the bar, and 70 degrees of abduction or external rotation of the shoes. Padding over the heel in the shoe can help in providing relief for the calcaneus so that blistering does not occur, and this padding will also prevent the foot from rising out of the shoe. Dorsiflexion cannot be achieved adequately without splinting the foot in a position of severe external rotation and abduction. The author also supplements the treatment at this point with physical therapy to stimulate firing of the peroneal and anterior tibial muscles, and to maintain the range of motion of the foot.

The bar is maintained for 3 months full time, followed by night splinting. The night splinting is used until at least 18 months of age. Recurrences can be dealt with by return to corrective casting in select cases. Surgical therapy may be required in some cases with failure of this method of management. Ponseti (65) believes that in the absence of a good splinting program, a recurrence rate of 70% may occur. In

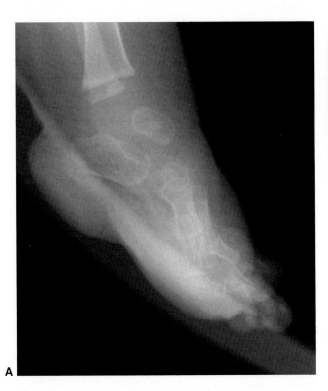

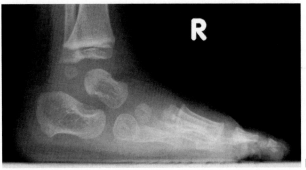

**Figure 30.12  A:** This patient had severe cavus deformity as a component of his clubfoot deformity. **B:** Following Ponseti management, x-ray films indicate resolution of his cavus deformity with sequential casting and no plantar release.

such cases, it may be difficult to reinstitute this method of management, and surgical therapy may be required.

It is therefore clear that the affected child's parents' acceptance of the need for night splinting and "buying into" this method of management is critical. With the proper approach and coaching, and support from the nursing and physical therapy staff as well as from the treating orthopaedic surgeon, acceptance of this treatment by the parents and child can be achieved.

While Ponseti recommends plaster casts for his method of clubfoot correction, advocates of semirigid fiberglass have had good success with this alternative material. Coss and Hennrikus (71) have shown that semirigid fiberglass is superior to plaster of paris in durability, convenience, performance, and ease of removal. Parents can remove semirigid casts without soaking. Molding of the cast is a bit more difficult with fiberglass than with plaster of paris.

In 1995, Cooper and Dietz (72) reviewed 45 patients, ranging in age from 25 to 42 years, with 71 clubfeet. Thirty of the patients had tibialis anterior transfers, of which 25 were rated at 5/5 strength. In the remaining 5 patients, the strength of the transfer was rated as 4+/5. Only 2 patients in the entire group had osteoarthritic changes. While the degree of dorsiflexion, inversion, and eversion were less in the patient with clubfoot than in the healthy individual, plantar flexion was normal. Improvement in 62% of clubfeet was excellent, with 16% good, and 22% poor. Fifty-four percent of the patients participated in sports, compared to 40% of age-matched controls. Twenty-six percent of patients could walk unlimited distances. There was a distinct lack of correlation between radiographs and clinical outcome. Significantly, the lateral talocalcaneal angle was not a predictor of normal function. Following the recognition of the results achieved by Ponseti, a number of individuals have tried to reproduce his results. Hertzenberg et al. (73) in 2002 compared a group of 27 patients treated with the Ponseti method to 27 patients treated with traditional casting techniques. One of the patients in the Ponseti group required posteromedial release, whereas 91% of patients in Hertzenberg's control group required surgical therapy. Foot abduction splinting with a Dennis-Brown bar was crucial to the success of this method of treatment, just as Ponseti had shown. A percutaneous heel cord lengthening was done in 31 of 34 patients in Hertzenberg's series.

Lehman et al. (74) reported their experience with the Ponseti method of management with similar results. Ninety-two percent of patients had initial success within the first year of life after using the Ponseti method. Hattori et al. (75) showed the positive effect of the Dennis-Brown bar in the postcasting management of clubfoot, particularly if applied in the first months of life. In evaluating the positive effects of the Ponseti method, Kuhns et al. (76) used ultrasound to document the progressive movement of the navicular around the head of the talus as treatment continued. Pirani et al. (77) has similarly documented the successful correlation of correction of the chondroosseous defects in clubfoot using ultrasound.

The author's experience with the Ponseti method has been positive, similar to that of Lehman and Hertzenberg. The combination of corrective casting through the specific methods of management of Ponseti has resulted in excellent reduction of the midfoot deformity, specifically the talonavicular joint. A midfoot breech is prevented by liberal use of heel cord lengthening at the time of dorsiflexion. The necessity of postoperative splinting using a Dennis-Brown bar cannot be overstated. Much effort must be used in convincing parents of affected children that the value of splinting far outweighs the inconvenience endured. As some patients have recurrent deformity postcasting, splinting must be augmented by return to casting as well as physical therapy. With long-term follow-up, one can expect some recurrence of deformity or relapse. Dobbs and Ponseti (78) have documented relapse in an 8-year-old child who was previously fully corrected. Long-term follow-up is mandatory in clubfeet managed by the Ponseti method, just as in any other technique.

***The French, or Functional, Method of Treatment of Clubfoot.*** The French, or functional, method of treatment of clubfoot was developed in the 1970s by Masse (79) and Bensahel et al. (80). It has been popularized and further developed by Dimeglio (81) in France and by Richards and Johnson in the United States (82). This is a dynamic method of management, utilizing exercise for correction with supplementation by taping and continuous passive motion (CPM) in some cases.

Exercise is begun immediately after birth to stretch the tight medial structures, including the posterior tibial tendon and plantar soft tissue. An attempt is also made to strengthen the peroneal muscles by stimulation. Adhesive taping (Fig. 30.13) is applied to supplement the exercise and maintain correction that is gained by stretching. Daily treatments are continued for 2 months. The treatment frequency in this program is then decreased to 3 sessions per week until 6 months of age. After that time, the child is continued on a physical therapy program, and night splinting is used for 2 to 3 years.

In the early 1990s, CPM was added to this regimen. Use of a CPM machine at night was advised, and this resulted in fewer patients requiring surgical treatment for residual clubfoot deformity. The CPM machine may be valuable in the first 12 weeks of life, according to Dimeglio. Using this technique, Bensahel et al. (80) achieved good results in 48% of 338 patients, as reported in 1990. With resorting to surgery to complete the treatment in half of the patients, an overall success rate of 86% in the good and excellent category was achieved. Dimeglio et al. (42) reported that 74% of patients were successfully treated with exercise and CPM, without the need for surgical therapy. In 2001, a group led by Richards and Johnson (83) from the Scottish Rite Hospital in Texas reported their initial results with this technique. In their treatment of the first 30 clubfeet, 54% required some surgery with 18% having a limited posterior release and 28% needing a traditional posterior medial clubfoot release. Just as Dimeglio saw improvement with CPM, these investigators found a small, incremental advantage to the use of CPM at

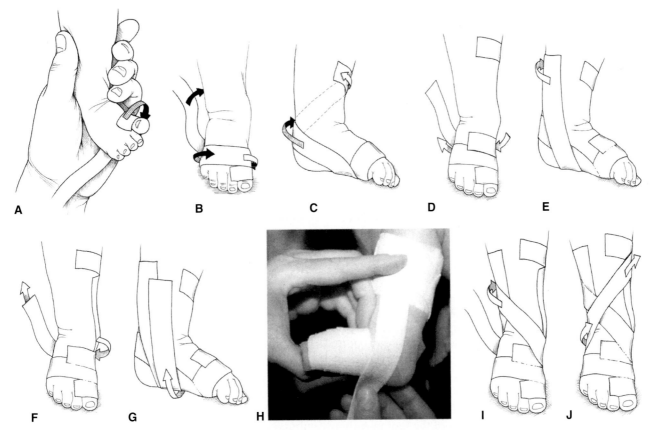

**Figure 30.13** Taping is used to maintain the passive range of motion achieved during manipulation sessions when clubfeet are managed by the French method. As the tape is applied sequentially in Steps **A** to **J** as pictured, the foot can be derotated with correction of the forefoot, midfoot, and hindfoot deformity, including equinus. (From Noonan KJ, Richards BS. Nonsurgical management of idiopathic clubfoot. *J Am Acad Orthop Surg* 2003;11:392–402, with permission.)

night. In the French method, effort is concentrated on gentle stretching of plantar and medial structures, as well as taping to hold the foot but allow motion, rather than the rigid nature of clubfoot casting. Recognizing that peroneal weakness is a significant problem in clubfoot deformity, effort is made to maintain mobility and strengthening, rather than immobilization. The author does not have personal experience with this technique, beyond taping and a gentle exercise program in mild clubfeet but believes that the results speak for themselves, and satisfactory outcome can certainly be achieved with this technique. Dimeglio and Bensahel have clearly documented the value of this method of management. One disadvantage in the functional (French) method of management of clubfoot is the added personal input with physical therapy and taping that is required. Where a cast remains in place for 1 week following manipulation and application, taping and exercise tend to require more maintenance and continuous care. The cost of application of this method is significant, both in dollars expended and interference with parental work and family functioning. These issues need to be considered while making a choice of therapy for clubfoot.

Van Campenhout et al. (84), in applying the "functional treatment of clubfoot," found that 75% of feet treated in this manner required surgical therapy. A coauthor, Fabry,

felt that there was greater benefit to the treatment of clubfoot with exercise in the Dimeglio grade 1 and 2 feet, than in the mild and moderate foot. With a Dimeglio score less than 10, he found consistent success, whereas in higher grades, surgical treatment was required.

***Surgical Correction.*** Having just read about the methods of cast and management with physical therapy of clubfoot, one might logically wonder whether there is still a role for the management of clubfoot with surgery. Clearly, less extensive clubfoot surgery and fewer clubfoot surgeries, in absolute numbers, are done now because of improved conservative methods of clubfoot management as described. In more severe clubfeet, Dimeglio grades 3 and 4, and in the syndromic or neuropathic clubfoot, surgical treatment remains necessary in a number of cases. Fabray achieved success with the physical therapy method of clubfoot management in only 25% of cases. As documented in a paper by Cohen-Sobel et al. (85), the long-term follow-up of clubfeet treated surgically is consistent with an excellent level of function in most cases despite some anatomical and radiologic imperfections. Gait studies have documented a weakness in push-off in general, but reasonable function in most series treated surgically. The negative results of surgical therapy are due to persistent deformity, weakness, stiffness, and pain.

In considering surgical management of clubfoot deformity, one must look at the indications, timing of procedure, technique, and postoperative management. The results of the various procedures should be compared, allowing the surgeon to make an educated choice of what procedure to use for primary clubfoot release, as there are a number of procedures with some variation in joints released, tendons lengthened or transferred, and bones osteotomized.

The first indication for surgical management of clubfoot is failure to correct the deformity by conservative methods within the first year of life. The author would attempt the Ponseti method in a child up to 1 year of age with a foot not previously treated or not optimally treated, as there has been a high rate of success with this technique, even in older patients. However, in the case of the foot that has failed to respond to cast correction with good application of cast technique or exercise, surgical management is certainly indicated.

With respect to timing of surgery, most choose to perform surgery when the child is between 4 and 9 months of age. Prolonged casting, once a decision that surgical therapy is necessary, is generally not indicated. The neonatal surgery recommended by Ryoppy and Sairanen (86) and Pous and Dimeglio (87) has not met with general enthusiasm and is not consistent with the general understanding of clubfoot deformity, in which an effort is made to avoid surgery, recognizing the amount of scarring that relates to the contractile fibrosis on the medial side of the foot in early infancy. Ponseti has documented the high cellular nature of medial ligaments in the infant clubfoot, and Zimny and others (2) have documented the presence of myofibroblasts that might well be stimulated by early surgery, leading to a more rigid foot and unsatisfactory outcome.

In the 1970s, Turco (88,89) recommended the first comprehensive, single-stage surgical therapy for clubfoot. The emphasis in this procedure was on the correction of the medial subtalar joint and ankle joint; medial release of the talonavicular joint was done as well. The deformity at the posterolateral corner of the foot or calcaneofibular ligament was not addressed in this procedure. Whereas many feet achieved satisfactory correction with this technique, one of the major complications that occurred was hindfoot lateral translation with persistent medial spin of the foot and valgus hindfoot. Hudson and Catterall (43) published a paper suggesting that the release of the tissue at the posterolateral corner or calcaneofibular ligament along with posterior release could be done without need for extensive medial release, yielding satisfactory results in clubfoot surgery. Their method, although not subjected to a common grading system as is true of most clubfoot surgery, resulted in satisfactory outcome in a vast majority of cases. Through the 1980s and 1990s, a number of surgical procedures for correction of clubfoot were recommended, with strong advocates for each technique. Such surgical procedures were attributed to Simons (90), McKay (91,92), Goldner and Fitch (93), and Carroll (70). This article will attempt to briefly describe each of these procedures and identify how each one is unique. When the procedures are actually compared and commonality is

searched for, one finds that there is much in common in these procedures, yet each has a distinctive feature with which an individual's name has been and continues to be associated.

In Goldner's procedure (93,94), a posterior ankle release is done without opening the subtalar joint. The extension of the release medially through the deltoid is significant, focusing on the deltoid as a major pathologic structure responsible for medial deviation of the talus. Correction involves lengthening of the deltoid with extensive medial release and reconstruction of the talonavicular joint medially and laterally, avoiding the subtalar joint.

Carroll and his colleagues documented the external rotation of the talus within the mortise (69,70,95). His procedure is based upon a concept of achieving proper rotation of the calcaneus under the talus. The interosseous ligament remains intact, but a limited release of the subtalar joint as well as ankle joint, concentrating on the posterolateral corner, is performed. The plantar fascia is always released as well as intrinsic toe flexors, and the calcaneocuboid joint is addressed to achieve satisfactory alignment of the lateral column.

Simons (90,96) espoused the concept of correction of clubfoot deformity by complete subtalar release dividing the interosseous ligament. The application of this extensive procedure has resulted, even in Simons' own series, in significant overcorrection in some feet. Most surgeons and authors have cautioned against division of the interosseous ligament because of overcorrection and severe deformity because of this procedure. Simons (97) also described the concept of correction of the calcaneocuboid joint in clubfoot; this has resulted in recognition of the contribution of lateral column deformity to the overall unsatisfactory surgical results in clubfoot correction.

The incisions used for clubfoot surgery vary from a medial incision advocated by Turco (88,89), to a circumferential (Cincinnati) (98) incision around the posterior aspect of the foot several millimeters above the posterior crease, to a two-incision Carroll approach (70) with a posterolateral incision and a zigzag medial incision. In cases in which the wound cannot be closed following clubfoot correction (Cincinnati), researchers have found that the wound can be left open, and it closes spontaneously during a period of healing without negatively affecting outcome (99).

At present, clubfoot surgery is primarily used in syndromic and severe clubfoot deformity based on Dimeglio classification. The accepted procedure for clubfoot surgery at this time might be described as the "a la carte" procedure (44). In this procedure, pathologic structures leading to deformity are released in order to properly align the foot. Common features in an "a la carte" release are heel cord lengthening and posterior release of the ankle and subtalar joint with extension to the calcaneofibular ligament. The medial release is a judicious one, with lengthening of the posterior tibial tendon as needed. In doing the midfoot release, attention is paid both to the medial and lateral columns to ensure that the long axis of the talus is properly aligned with the first ray and the long axis of the calcaneus is properly aligned with the fourth and fifth ray. The interosseous ligament is always left intact. In cases where the heel cord can be lengthened in a fractional rather than a Z technique, this is done. Supramalleolar lengthenings of the flexor hallucis longus and flexor digitorum longus tendons are preferable, if they can be done. Cavus deformity is corrected with a plantar fascia release if needed. Finally, the tendons are generally repaired tight to avoid postoperative weakness. The author prefers repairing the heel cord with the proximal tendon at half-tension with the foot at neutral.

Postoperative management of clubfoot varies from early motion advocated by McKay (91) to casting for a period of time until healing has occurred and exercises begun. Kirschner-wire (K-wire) stabilization of the foot with one or two wires following surgery has been generally advocated. Generally, wire stabilization of the talonavicular joint is done to prevent talonavicular subluxation. The residual deformity or increasing postoperative deformity from subluxation of the navicular is severe and has prompted most surgeons to stabilize the talonavicular joint following release. A second wire may be placed through the subtalar joint to prevent lateral translation of the calcaneus, particularly if the interosseous ligament is divided. Finally a wire may be placed across the calcaneocuboid joint in cases where marked deformity of the lateral column is documented and surgical correction required.

Postoperative management of the clubfoot has changed little over recent years. Cast immobilization is universal, in recognition of the need for holding the foot in a corrected position to allow for ligament and tendon healing as well as bone remodeling. Attempts to stimulate early motion (91,92) have not been widely utilized. Postoperative casting is generally done for 2 to 3 months, followed by a prolonged period of observation, physical therapy, and postoperative splinting. Generally, special shoes are not required, but the use of arch supports or simple shoe modifications may be of benefit in selected cases.

Despite the wide variation in clubfoot surgical procedures as described in the preceding text, the results in most reports document 60% to 80% good or excellent results (43,89,90,92,94,95), with improvement of residual deformity in a number of cases and failure in approximately 10%. This general distribution of outcome is reflective of much in the surgical literature. Researchers who have studied patients with clubfoot deformity, however, find consistent abnormalities in all feet that have been corrected surgically. The most prominent of these abnormalities is weakness in the gastrocsoleus and difficulty with push-off (100). Others have found some element of foot drop and a tendency to externally rotate from the hip to compensate for some of the persistent internal rotation deformity of the foot (101). Despite these weaknesses, function is generally good and compatible with normal shoe wear and full activity. There are, however, a group of residual deformities that are consistent across all methods of management, and this article will consider each of these.

Postoperative problems or complications are commonly seen because a clubfoot, with its diffuse spectrum of pathology, is not rendered healthy by a single operation. The individual problems are not seen in isolation but in combination. It will, however, be beneficial to consider each of these deformities or problems separately in order to understand the diagnosis and management of postoperative clubfoot deformity.

*Valgus Hindfoot.* This may result from a number of causes including insufficient release of the calcaneofibular ligament (43), overrelease of the interosseous ligament between talus and calcaneus (85), or posterior tibial muscle insufficiency (Fig. 30.14). The inadequate release of the calcaneofibular ligament or the posterior lateral corner is probably one of the most common causes of valgus hindfoot. As the foot is dorsiflexed, the posterior lateral tether draws the calcaneus laterally toward the fibula. As Ponseti

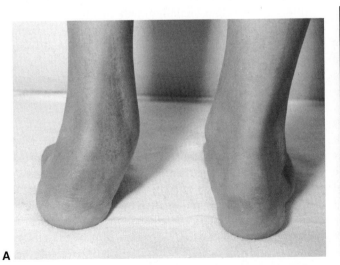
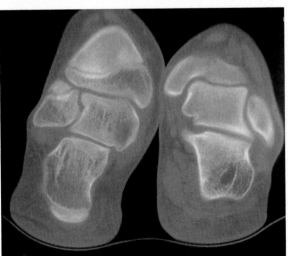

**Figure 30.14** **A:** Valgus deformity of the hindfoot is a complication of clubfoot management resulting in weak push-off and pain. **B:** Computed tomography (CT) scan is used to evaluate the deformity and the subtalar joint.

(65) has shown, this ligament is shortened and thickened in the clubfoot in the absence of treatment. Although it may seem counterintuitive that a release at the posterior lateral corner will prevent hindfoot valgus, a surgeon can prove it to him- or herself by doing sequential ligament release at the time of surgery. Catterall (43) has demonstrated the importance of posterior lateral release.

A second cause of valgus hindfoot is subtalar instability, in which division of the interosseous ligament as well as release of the subtalar joint may result in lateral translation of the calcaneus under the talus, as shown by Simons (90). Although complete subtalar release has been recommended by some, overcorrection of the hindfoot into a valgus position is one of the complications that can result from this procedure.

Supination of the forefoot in a rigid position may produce hindfoot valgus, in that as a patient bears weight, the forefoot will rotate into a position in which it is flat on the ground, forcing the hindfoot into valgus. Therefore, a rigid forefoot and midfoot malalignment may contribute to hindfoot valgus. Posterior tibial insufficiency may also lead to valgus hindfoot over time.

The problem with valgus malalignment of the hindfoot is that it produces a poor mechanical situation in which the gastrocsoleus complex is compromised. With the insertion of the gastrocsoleus displaced laterally relative to the axis of rotation of the ankle joint, push-off is diminished and a deforming moment is applied to the hindfoot with activity. This leads to both poor push-off and pain. Lateral impingement between the calcaneus and fibula may also result from lateral displacement of the calcaneus. With time, progressive lateralization of the hindfoot associated with midfoot collapse will lead to an unsatisfactory result.

In the evaluation of the valgus hindfoot deformity, look for rigid forefoot supination that may drive the hindfoot deformity. Also evaluate the muscle strength in all groups, including the posterior tibial muscles. With the patient rising on the toes, look for evidence of subtalar motion, with normal mechanics representing a slight tip of the hindfoot into varus with plantar flexion. Standing anteroposterior and lateral radiographs of the foot underestimate the deformity of hindfoot valgus in general. A CT scan will allow evaluation of the subtalar joint as well as the alignment of the hindfoot deformity. Also, be aware that valgus may result from the tilting of the distal tibial articular surface.

The manner in which one may deal with hindfoot valgus includes both conservative and surgical measures. An arch support or University of California Berkeley (UCB) insert may improve hindfoot position to a point where symptoms are relieved and progressive deformity does not occur. Physical therapy to strengthen the posterior tibial muscle may be of value. Mild hindfoot valgus may follow operative management, but also may be a complication of conservative or cast treatment for clubfoot.

Surgical options for correcting hindfoot valgus include calcaneal translational osteotomy as well as calcaneal lengthening, and finally, subtalar arthrodesis. In severe cases, triple arthrodesis may be necessary. In a calcaneal slide osteotomy, the tuberosity of the calcaneus is shifted medially, generally from the lateral approach, with the calcaneal osteotomy just posterior to the posterior facet of the subtalar joint. In order for the procedure to work, a competent subtalar joint must be present and is best evaluated using a CT scan (Fig. 30.14B). The axis of alignment of the foot in weight-bearing may be corrected with a translational osteotomy, and the pull of the gastrocsoleus complex may be shifted into proper alignment with the tibial talar joint. The calcaneal slide osteotomy will not affect the midfoot and forefoot deformity. It also will not affect the longitudinal arch of the foot nor the talonavicular relation.

Another possible procedure for the valgus hindfoot is the calcaneal lengthening osteotomy as described by Mosca (102). In this procedure, the hindfoot is corrected by distraction of the calcaneus with a secondary improvement in the talocalcaneal as well as the talonavicular alignment. The negative effect of calcaneal lengthening on the foot is forefoot supination, which is a frequent pathologic state in clubfoot deformity. An intact peroneus longus muscle may decrease forefoot supination, but one should be aware that with the calcaneal lengthening osteotomy forefoot supination may be increased. In cases where significant supination is the result of calcaneal lengthening, a plantar flexion osteotomy done through the first and second cuneiform will restore medial column sagittal plane alignment. The goal of this procedure is to restore proper foot balance, with the healthy tripod sharing weight bearing between the first and fifth metatarsal and the tuberosity of the calcaneus. A preoperative requirement for calcaneal lengthening osteotomy in the postoperative clubfoot is flexibility of the foot such that the lengthening osteotomy will produce the desired midfoot effect. In a rigid clubfoot deformity, translational osteotomy may be of more benefit.

If the hindfoot is translated in severe valgus with an incompetent subtalar joint as judged by CT scan, subtalar arthrodesis can be considered. In such a case, the correction of the valgus malalignment of the hindfoot will require an iliac crest graft in order to improve the weight-bearing axis through the subtalar joint. Internal fixation with either screw or staple is required as well. In cases where the distal articular surface of the tibia is the cause of valgus deformity, an appropriately timed medial epiphyseodesis may correct the problem (103,104).

*Hindfoot Varus.* Hindfoot varus is associated with medial deviation of the forefoot, lateral weight bearing in stance, and persistent medial rotation of the foot. Functionally, the patients tend to push off over the lateral border of the foot without normal weight-bearing and have foot pain with recurrent ankle sprains. In general, this is a persistent foot position that relates to undercorrection of the clubfoot. Mechanically, it may be better in push-off strength than a persistent valgus foot deformity. Persistent hindfoot varus deformity may result from undercorrection after surgical or casting treatment of clubfoot deformity. A Coleman block

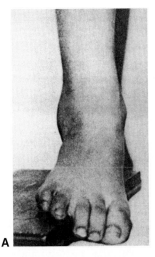
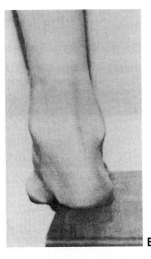

**Figure 30.15** The Coleman block test for determination of hindfoot flexibility. The flexible varus deformity of the hindfoot will correct to valgus when the plantar-flexed first metatarsal is allowed to drop down off the edge of the block of wood. Failure to correct to valgus indicates the need for surgical correction of the hindfoot, in addition to the procedures on the forefoot. (From Coleman SS, Chesnut WJ. A simple test for hindfoot flexibility in the cavovarus foot. *Clin Orthop* 1977;123:60–62, with permission.)

test (Fig. 30.15) may be used to demonstrate the degree of flexibility of the hindfoot. In the block test that is commonly used for cavus foot deformity, hindfoot varus secondary to medial column plantar flexion can be differentiated from a rigid hindfoot deformity. In the clubfoot, the rigid hindfoot deformity is generally, but not always, present. Remember that forefoot pronation or plantar flexion of the first ray may contribute to hindfoot varus and must be identified by physical examination in order to properly manage this condition. By motor testing, one should evaluate the strength or competence of the peroneals, as well as the strength of all muscle groups within the foot.

Treatment of persistent varus of the hindfoot depends upon its cause and the extent of the associated foot deformity.

In the young child with undercorrection of the entire clubfoot after surgical release, a revision surgery addressing forefoot medial deviation, cavus, and hindfoot varus may be required. In the older child with persistent hindfoot varus, a calcaneal osteotomy as a combination of lateral closing wedge and translation is generally the treatment of choice.

Clubfoot release in the older child, between 1 and 4 years of age, with secondary deformity of the bones, may require osteotomy in addition to capsular release in order to achieve correction. Use of lateral column wedge osteotomy for shortening, either through the cuboid or calcaneus should be considered in order to achieve satisfactory alignment. Calcaneocuboid fusion, as described by Evans (105), has been used in selected cases in achieving lateral column alignment. Loss of calcanecuboid motion produces little effect on subtalar motion (10).

Calcaneal osteotomy to realign the hindfoot may be done as a combination of sliding of the tuberosity as well as lateral closing wedge. If the entire deformity is corrected by lateral closing wedge of the calcaneus, the heel height is significantly decreased, making shoe fitting with impingement on the lateral malleolus more difficult. The combination osteotomy using lateral shift as well as closing wedge gives a better functional result. Stabilization of the osteotomy is done with screw or threaded K-wire fixation.

*Calcaneus Deformity.* Occasionally the hindfoot deformity is one of calcaneus with increased calcaneal pitch (Fig. 30.16). This may result from overlengthening of the heel cord and mimic the foot deformities seen in poliomyelitis and other neurologic conditions. The moment arm for pull of the gastrocsoleus is decreased, further compromising push-off that is at first weakened simply by the overlengthening of the heel cord. Coleman (106) has described an osteotomy of the calcaneus in which the tuberosity is translated posteriorly. The

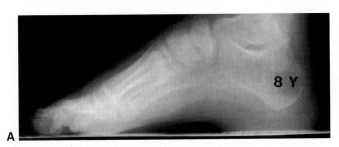
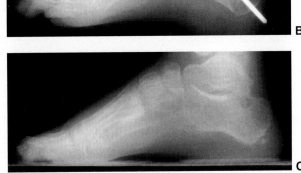

**Figure 30.16** **A:** A weak gastrocsoleus complex may result in a "calcaneus" deformity in which the calcaneal pitch is significantly increased and the mechanical advantage of the gastrocsoleus complex significantly decreased. **B,C:** A calcaneal lengthening osteotomy improves foot alignment and lengthens the gastroc moment arm.

combined effect of this osteotomy is to decrease the calcaneal pitch while increasing the moment arm for pull of the gastrocsoleus complex. Clinically, patients with foot pain and weak push-off may be improved by this operation. The author has no data on the increased strength of the gastrocsoleus that is associated with such an osteotomy, but it does decrease the elevation of the longitudinal arch and does relieve some of the symptoms associated with the short cavus foot.

*Dorsolateral Navicular Dislocation.* Given that a clubfoot is a deformity with a plantar medial displacement of the navicular on the head of the talus, it is clear that this deformity represents a postsurgical complication. Kuo and Jansen (107) have described this navicular displacement as having an occurrence rate of about 8% in their series regardless of the type of incision used. The actual deformity is one of rotation of the navicular on the head of the talus, mimicking dorsal and lateral translation of the navicular. Once the navicular is displaced, its shape becomes altered from a bean-shaped bone with a concave articular surface opposing the talar head to a wedge-shaped bone that is nearly impossible to replace in its anatomic location and maintain alignment. Recurrent deformity following attempted reduction of the talonavicular joint therefore has been somewhat distressing. A group led by Davidson (108) has recommended talonavicular fusion as a definitive procedure to treat severe cases of talonavicular subluxation requiring surgery. While this decreases midfoot and hindfoot mobility, the trade-off for improvement in alignment is at times necessary.

Left untreated, mild talonavicular subluxation is compatible with a quite reasonable outcome. The foot tends to be short with a relatively short plantar flexed medial column compared to the lateral. Asymptomatic talonavicular subluxation should be managed with observation and adaptive footwear as needed. The midfoot tends to be a bit elevated and the foot a bit wider through the midfoot. At times, arch supports or cushioning of the shoe may relieve pain. If symptoms continue unabated, attempts to realign the foot surgically as discussed in the preceding text are required.

*Decrease in Longitudinal Arch.* In postsurgical or, much less frequently, postcasting treatment of clubfoot, the longitudinal arch is decreased with weight bearing and the head of the talus is plantar-flexed. This is usually associated with a valgus hindfoot and probably results from incompetence of the spring ligament or calcaneonavicular ligament, posterior tibial muscle insufficiency, or malalignment at the time of surgery (2,7,68).

The spring ligament along with the navicular and anterior facet of the calcaneus provide a stable articulation for the head of the talus. When the ligament is overly stretched by casting or divided with overlengthening at the time of surgery, malalignment of the talonavicular joint will result. Pinning of the medial column postsurgery is done in an attempt to maintain the proper talonavicular joint relationship and avoid sagging of the longitudinal arch. The force of

the posterior tibial tendon is always decreased postlengthening, and this may aggravate midfoot collapse postsurgery.

The deformity may be prevented by avoiding excessive dorsiflexion against a tight heel cord when casting. The use of a percutaneous heel cord tenotomy using the Ponseti method of clubfoot casting will prevent midfoot breech and decrease the incidence of this problem after conservative management of clubfeet. Pinning of the talonavicular joint may prevent this deformity at the time of surgery; finally, overlengthening of the posterior tibial tendon should be avoided.

Treatment of the deformity itself may simply be an arch support in mild cases associated with mild symptoms. If the decrease in the longitudinal arch is accompanied by symptoms unrelieved by arch supports, treatment with surgical reconstruction may be indicated. This may be best handled with a calcaneal lengthening and medial reefing if a flexible foot with competent subtalar joint is present (102).

*Convex Lateral Border of the Foot.* This may be rigid or flexible and is secondary to undercorrection of the clubfoot deformity. In the flexible deformity in which the navicular can be properly aligned on the head of the talus, peroneal weakness and relative overpull of the posterior tibial muscle is often present. In the young child, this is managed with exercise, stimulation of the peroneal muscles, and prolonged night splinting to maintain position and flexibility of the foot until peroneal strength increases to a point that the foot will be stabilized. Attempts at electrical stimulation have been tried with variable benefit. In the older child, aged 3 or 4 years, addressing persistent lateral weakness with an anterior tibial tendon transfer, either split or whole, is the treatment of choice (discussed in the following text regarding forefoot supination) (109,110).

In the rigid foot, the convex lateral border muscle transfer and muscle strengthening will not be sufficient. Corrective casting or exercise can be utilized first, in order to achieve realignment of the foot if possible. In the absence of success with conservative management, either shortening of the lateral column or lengthening of the medial column is required. The lateral column may be shortened either through the cuboid, the calcaneus, or a combination with calcaneocuboid joint fusion as described by Evans (105). It has been shown that the calcaneocuboid joint fusion has little effect on subtalar and hindfoot motion and may be a beneficial procedure in neglected or recurrent clubfoot deformity. Osteotomies, however, with maintenance of joint motion, are in general preferable to fusions if satisfactory alignment can be achieved. In the very young child less than 12 months of age, a "Lichtblau" (111) procedure, which is a resection of a portion of the cartilaginous articular surfaces of the calcaneus, allows correction of lateral column deformity. This is only used for infants at the time of the primary clubfoot procedure.

*Supination of the Forefoot and Dorsal Bunion.* A common deformity in clubfoot is persistent supination of the forefoot;

this results from relative overpull of the anterior tibial tendon with weak peroneus longus or simply from undercorrection of forefoot supination, as a component of the original clubfoot deformity. In the initial cast treatment, great care is taken *not* to pronate the foot in the Ponseti method of management. Once the cavus deformity is treated and the talonavicular joint reduction achieved, the forefoot is placed in neutral, but care is always taken not to pronate the first ray, as this may increase the underlying cavus foot deformity. After proper technique of casting or clubfoot release, it is noted, however, that some cases have persistent supination of the forefoot with dorsal bunion. Long-term muscle imbalance is probably the most common cause of a dorsal bunion. The muscle imbalance that commonly leads to this is a weak gastrocnemius, compensated by increased overpull of the great toe flexor and weak peroneals countered by overpull of the anterior tibial tendon. McKay (112) has suggested that the flexor hallucis brevis is responsible for the toe flexion deformity of the great toe in a number of cases. The first treatment for this deformity is exercise, stretching the toe flexor and increasing the strength of the peroneal muscles. Surgery is required for persistent deformity, with transfer of the anterior tibial tendon, either whole or in part, to the second cuneiform or the cuboid (109,110). Studies suggest that both of these transfers have a positive effect in balancing the foot. Treatment for the dorsal bunion may involve flexor transfer to the first metatarsal, as shown by McKay (112).

The anterior tibial transfer is beneficial for the treatment of dynamic supination (113). It appears that results of split transfer and complete transfer are equivalent. If a split transfer is used, the lateral limb must be sufficiently tight to hold the foot in a slightly everted position following insertion.

*Severe Residual Clubfoot Deformity.* If the patient is rather asymptomatic but has significant degree of deformity, surgery should be delayed or limited to osteotomy rather than arthrodesis. Symptomatic, severely deformed feet may be improved by proper alignment despite the need for arthrodesis, multiple osteotomies, or Ilizarov correction. Triple arthrodesis is not generally indicated in patients younger than 10 years, as foot growth will be severely compromised. The stiff, deformed foot can only be improved by triple arthrodesis if a stiff, plantigrade foot is achieved. There is no question that a foot with intact subtalar motion is less symptomatic with vigorous activity than one in which fusion has occurred (114). Accepting this, the role for arthrodesis is limited to a rigid foot in which deformity compromises ability to stand and walk. In the preoperative evaluation, be sure to look for opportunities to correct a foot by osteotomies, and always be certain to manage deformities conservatively with arch supports, pads, and braces prior to embarking on surgical correction.

Be certain to look for angular deformity of the ankle and knee contributing to the apparent foot deformity prior to surgery. In general, the techniques of triple arthrodesis applied to varus deformities are much more successful than those applied to valgus deformities. Correction with closing lateral wedge osteotomy to correct a varus deformity is much easier to achieve a plantigrade foot. The techniques of a Beak triple arthrodesis described by Siffert et al. (115), or Lambrinudi triple arthrodesis as modified by Hall and Calvert (116), are beneficial and highly successful. In cases of valgus triple arthrodesis, a bone graft is often required in order to create a satisfactory hindfoot alignment.

Bennett et al. (117) have shown a high patient satisfaction with triple arthrodesis in adults for correction of deformity and eliminating hindfoot pain. However, the objective data of their series on patient performance is less positive than patient perception of improvement. Ilizarov management of the relapsed clubfoot was popularized by Grill and Franke (118); in 1990, he reported the use of this apparatus for correcting relapsed clubfeet to a plantigrade position in which normal shoe wear was possible. At the time of the report, deformity had recurred in 2 of 13 affected feet operated on in the initial series. Wallander et al. (119), Choi et al. (120), Bradish and Noor (121), and Steinwender et al. (122) have shown the value of Ilizarov management of severe clubfoot deformity. Synthesizing the available literature, it appears that a patient with a severe relapsed clubfoot will generally benefit from a combination of soft-tissue releases and osteotomies with Ilizarov frame distraction. Hutchinson has documented the benefit of Ilizarov management using pedobarography, showing a more normal pressure distribution of the foot following Ilizarov correction.

*Persistent Internal Rotation Gait.* If the foot is reasonably aligned but internally rotated, supramalleolar osteotomy may be of value. Internal tibial torsion is generally associated with clubfoot deformity; however, internal rotation gait is highly associated with clubfoot deformity and has been identified in postoperative patients in 8% to 48% of cases. This may result from either weak peroneal musculature, internal tibial torsion, persistent medial spin of the foot in the mortise, or persistent foot deformity with metatarsus adductus. Use of a distal tibial osteotomy to correct the internal rotation component of the deformity, which results from internal tibial torsion, has been recommended by Goldner and Fitch (123). It also may be used as a compromise in realigning a foot that has internal rotation deformities from all of the above possible etiologies. The distal tibial osteotomy may be done without fibular osteotomy. If rotational correction cannot be achieved without unacceptable translation, a fibular osteotomy at approximately the same level should be done. The osteotomy can be held in place by 2 crossed K-wires or a small plate. In Goldner's series, 2 of 66 patients required change in position because of vascular compromise at the time of rotational correction. In general, rotational osteotomy through the tibia results in excellent alignment of the foot and improved gait.

## Metatarsus Abductus

### Definition

Metatarsus adductus is the most common foot deformity of infancy and is characterized by medial deviation of the forefoot on the hindfoot (Fig. 30.17). The deformity in its mildest form resolves spontaneously, has no rigidity, and is of little clinical significance. In its more severe form, it may be associated with pain and difficulty wearing shoes, and hence requires treatment.

### Epidemiology

Wynne-Davies (17) reported the incidence of metatarsus adductus to be 1 per 1000 live births, with an increased incidence with positive family history. This is a significant variation from the data of Hunziker et al. (124), who found an overall frequency of metatarsus adductus at 12%, with even higher incidence in twin births. As there is increased awareness of this condition and increased reporting, higher frequencies are recorded (125–127). Although historically this has been associated with hip dysplasia (128,129), recently no association between hip dysplasia and metatarsus adductus has been found (130,131). Therefore, there is no indication for ultrasound screening of hips in infants when this deformity exists.

### Pathogenesis

The true cause of metatarsus adductus remains unknown. Fetal studies by Morcuende and Ponseti (132) have documented an alteration in the medial cuneiform in association with metatarsus adductus without joint subluxation or tendon abnormalities. Reimann and Werner (133) suggested that the primary abnormality in metatarsus adductus was subluxation of the tarsal metatarsal joints in addition to cuneiform abnormality (133). The possibility of muscle contracture, with imbalance between the anterior and posterior tibial tendons and abnormal insertion of the anterior tibial tendon, has been suggested (126,134–136). An abnormally shaped cuneiform (137) may play a role in persistent metatarsus adductus (Fig. 30.18).

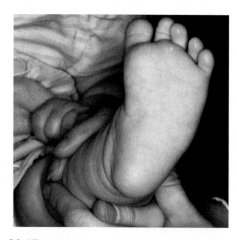

**Figure 30.17** Metatarsus adductus in an infant. Note convex lateral border and neutral hindfoot alignment.

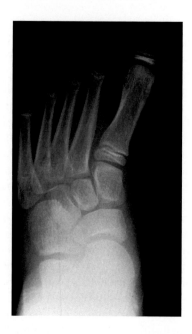

**Figure 30.18** Metatarsus adductus in an older child with trapezoidal-shaped medial cuneiform. (From Cappello T, Mosca VS. Metatarsus adductus and skewfoot. *Foot Ankle Clin* 1998:683, with permission.)

### Clinical Features

Medial deviation of the forefoot in metatarsus adductus is the hallmark of this condition. There is prominence of the proximal fifth metatarsal laterally. The hindfoot is generally in neutral and forefoot slightly supinated. A deep medial crease is usually present.

There are two clinical classification systems published by Bleck (138,139) to define this condition. One is known as the *heel bisector* (Fig. 30.5) in which the feet are placed on a photocopy machine and the axis of the heel is projected through the forefoot or a similar line is drawn on the plantar surface of the foot. The heel bisector moves laterally across the toes with increasing severity of the condition. The second classification (Fig. 30.19) (138) defines metatarsus adductus based on flexibility. By holding the heel with a thumb providing a fulcrum over the fifth metatarsal head, pressure is applied laterally to the forefoot. The degree to which the lateral border of the foot can be corrected determines the flexibility of the foot.

### Radiographic Features

Radiographs are in general not necessary in classification and treatment of metatarsus adductus. Although Berg (140) developed a classification system for metatarsus adductus and skewfoot based on radiographs in a small group of children, Cook et al. (141) found that classification system to have high interobserved and intraobserver error. Given that the natural history of this condition is one of spontaneous resolution, simply documenting the clinical deformity and observing for spontaneous resolution is a generally accepted routine. Radiographs are indicated for patients with persistent deformity. A standing or simulated weight-bearing view will demonstrate a trapezoidal shape to the medial cuneiform

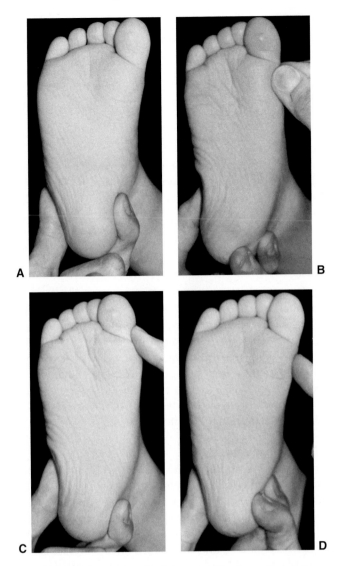

**Figure 30.19** Bleck's flexibility classification of metatarsus adductus. **A:** Metatarsus adductus in an infant. **B:** A flexible foot can be passively overcorrected into abduction with little effort. **C:** A partly flexible foot can be passively corrected only to the midline. **D:** An inflexible foot cannot be passively corrected to the midline. (From Bleck EE. Developmental orthopaedics. III. Toddlers. *Dev Med Child Neurol* 1982;24:533.)

and medial deviation of the metatarsals (Fig. 30.18). This can be differentiated from skewfoot, in which lateral subluxation of the navicular is a hallmark on the anteroposterior view. When the navicular is not ossified, the long axis of the first metatarsal is translated laterally relative to the talus.

As internal rotation gait is a common parental complaint in the older child, a contribution of internal tibial torsion and femoral anteversion in addition to metatarsus adductus should be noted on physical examination and clearly documented. The natural history of each of these deformities will then contribute to the spontaneous resolution or persistence of the intoeing deformity.

### Treatment

The prognosis for spontaneous correction in flexible metatarsus adductus is excellent (2,3,134). Although passive

stretching exercises are commonly recommended, their efficacy has not been clearly demonstrated. Ponseti and Becker (3) noted potential harm in increasing hindfoot deformity by overzealous treatment.

Bleck (138), Berg (140) and Ponseti have demonstrated efficacy in manipulation and serial casting in resolution of metatarsus adductus that is either partially flexible or inflexible. Best results from corrective casting occur in patients younger than 1 year at initiation of therapy (3,138,140). In the use of corrective casting, there is some risk of increasing hindfoot valgus or producing an iatrogenic skewfoot (3,126). One way in which the risk of hindfoot valgus can be decreased in corrective casting for metatarsus adductus is by plantar-flexing the foot slightly to lock the subtalar joint. Postcast splinting may be used to decrease the rate of recurrence, which has been reported as occurring in between 8% and 37% of cases (126,138,142).

The role for casting tends to be in children between 6 months and 1 year of age. In children younger than 6 months, gentle exercises are advocated with use of a reverse-last shoe or Bebax shoe at times to maintain correction.

Surgical treatment of persistent metatarsus adductus is rarely indicated (2). Spontaneous resolution of minor residual deformity may occur until 3 or 4 years of age (2,3). It should also be noted that minor residual deformity carries with it no significant disability in most cases (2,4). In select cases in which the deformity has a primary component of medial deviation of the great toe, release of the abductor hallucis has been advocated; it should be noted that this may result in the development of hallux valgus (143). Medial capsulotomies have been reported in treatment of this deformity (144). Heyman et al. (145) described treatment using forefoot capsulotomy of the tarsometatarsal joints with release of intermetatarsal ligaments. Long-term studies (146,147), however, have shown a 41% failure rate, with complications including skin slough and pain with prominence of the tarsal metatarsal joints.

Osteotomies of the base of the metatarsals have been used as a beneficial extraarticular alternative, avoiding the complications of capsulotomies (148,149). The greatest risk in this procedure, however, is growth arrest of the first metatarsal from physeal injury, noted in a significant number of patients treated in this manner (148,150,151).

In the rare situation of an older child with significant disability from metatarsus adductus, a combination osteotomy including closing wedge of the cuboid and opening wedge of the first cuneiform has been advocated (152) (Fig. 30.20). As the primary deformity in metatarsus adductus is a trapezoid-shaped first cuneiform in most cases, this procedure is most appealing. It treats the deformity where the pathology is, and carries no risk of growth arrest to the first metatarsal. It has been described with removal of a lateral wedge from the cuboid with insertion into the first cuneiform. The author has found the wedge from the cuboid to be of insufficient substance to provide sufficient strength as a spacer in the opening wedge of the cuneiform; allograft appears to be a

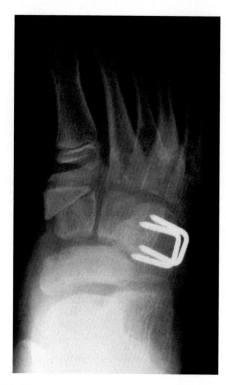

**Figure 30.20** Correction of symptomatic metatarsus adductus in an older child with an opening-wedge osteotomy of the medial cuneiform and a closing-wedge osteotomy of the cuboid.

better choice. In severe cases, the cuboid-closing osteotomy and cuneiform-opening osteotomy can be combined with osteotomies of the second, third, and fourth metatarsals at their bases, to provide better correction (153–156).

## Skewfoot

### Definition

Skewfoot is a term indicative of a complex foot deformity combining medial deviation of the forefoot, lateral translation of the midfoot, and valgus hindfoot into one condition (Fig. 30.21). The recognition of the multiplanar abnormalities in this deformity is critical to its appropriate treatment. In the past, inconsistent terminology has been applied to this, including congenital metatarsus varus (136) or serpentine metatarsus adductus (125). Mosca (102,157,158) defined the skewfoot with a significant valgus hindfoot (Fig. 30.22) as a major component of this deformity.

### Epidemiology

Given the lack of definition and complexity of terminology relative to this deformity, not to mention its rarity, the pathogenesis, natural history, and treatment remain a bit confusing. Researchers have stated that the deformity may result from improper cast technique applied to metatarsus adductus and/or clubfoot, but there clearly are a number of idiopathic cases.

### Pathogenesis

Although the deformity can result from improper casting of metatarsus adductus with iatrogenic lateral subluxation of the navicular and creation of valgus hindfoot (3), its cause generally remains unknown. Most cases occur spontaneously with a trapezoid-shaped medial cuneiform as seen in metatarsus adductus (157,159), but the hallmark of the condition is medial deviation of the forefoot with lateral translation of the midfoot.

### Clinical Features

It is difficult to differentiate metatarsus adductus from skewfoot in the infant, in whom no calcification of the navicular or first cuneiform is present. However, clinically one may note a significant valgus deformity in association with metatarsus adductus and the ability to palpate the head of the talus in the longitudinal arch. By direct observation (Fig. 30.21), a deep concavity in the medial aspect of the foot, created by a step-off between the head of the talus and the base of the first metatarsal, is palpable. This is seen in association with adduction of the first ray and valgus hindfoot. The deformity is generally flexible with

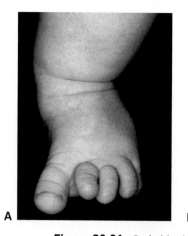
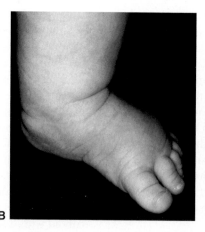
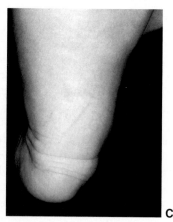

**Figure 30.21** Probable skewfoot in an infant. Apparent metatarsus adductus, but with the head of the talus visible and palpable medially. This indicates coexistent eversion of the subtalar joint with abduction of the navicular on the head of the talus. (From Mosca VS. Flexible flatfoot and skewfoot. In: Drennan JC, ed. *The child's foot and ankle.* New York: Raven Press, 1992:355, with permission.)

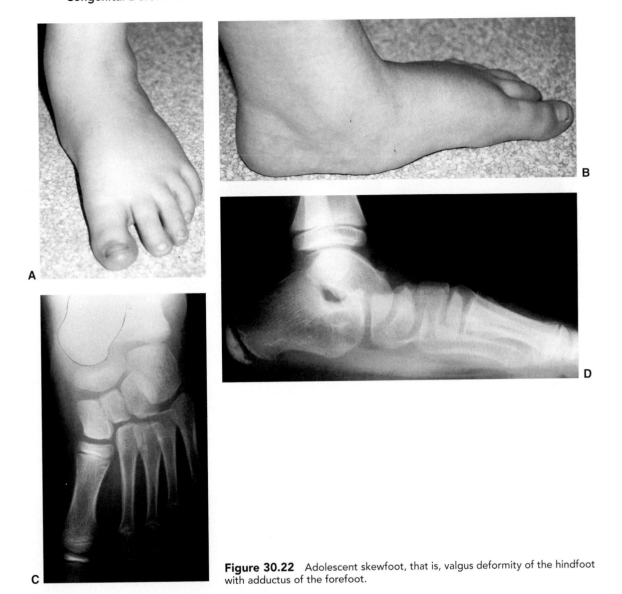

**Figure 30.22**  Adolescent skewfoot, that is, valgus deformity of the hindfoot with adductus of the forefoot.

respect to subtalar motion but somewhat rigid with respect to correction of the forefoot. Callusing may be present under the head of the talus (Fig. 30.23) and at the base of the fifth metatarsal, as seen in severe metatarsus adductus (102,157,159). Tightness of the heel cord may cause symptoms of pain, as it often does in the flatfoot.

### Radiographic Features

Because of lack of ossification of the bones of the midfoot, radiographs taken at birth are difficult to interpret in differentiating metatarsus adductus from skewfoot. It is, however, noted that in metatarsus adductus, there is generally medial deviation of the first ray, but that the proximal portion of the first metatarsal is aligned with the head of the talus, whereas in the skewfoot (Fig. 30.24), the first ray is translated relative to the long axis of the talus, and may actually be parallel to it, and yet appear to be significantly medially deviated. Attempts by Berg (140) to radiographically differentiate metatarsus adductus from skewfoot in

the infant have been unrewarding because of poor interobserver and intraobserver reliability (141).

Standing anteroposterior and lateral radiographs in the older child and adolescent are indicated in order to

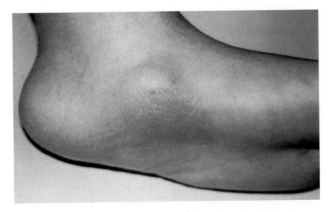

**Figure 30.23**  Painful callus that developed under the head of the talus in a skewfoot with contracted Achilles tendon.

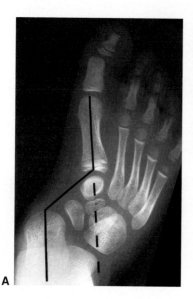

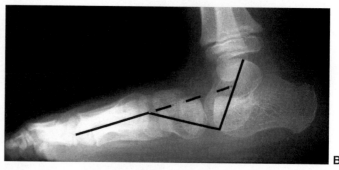

**Figure 30.24** Anteroposterior **(A)** and lateral **(B)** radiographs of a skewfoot demonstrating skew, or zigzag, deformities in both planes. (From Mosca VS. Calcaneal lengthening for valgus deformity of the hindfoot. Results in children who had severe, symptomatic flatfoot and skewfoot. *J Bone Joint Surg Am* 1995;77:500–512, with permission.)

determine the degree of deformity, both in the anteroposterior and lateral projections.

### Natural History

The natural history of skewfoot is unknown, but it seems that many cases of mild skewfoot undergo spontaneous correction, as happens with metatarsus adductus (3,4) and flexible flatfoot (1,46). The long-term disability attributed to this deformity remains difficult to estimate, but treatment is clearly required in some cases because of pain and difficulty with wearing shoes at the end of the first decade of life (102,125–127,136,157–160).

### Treatment

Treatment with cast correction for skewfoot in infancy is difficult. In applying cast treatment to the forefoot deformity in skewfoot, the risk is of increasing the valgus deformity in the hindfoot and the lateral translation of the midfoot. Therefore, when corrective casting is applied to skewfoot in early childhood, the foot should be placed in a plantar-flexed position with slight varus to lock the hindfoot and gentle pressure applied to the forefoot. Overaggressive casting should not be undertaken (3,125–127,138,140). Dennis-Brown bars are not indicated in this condition.

Some older children and adolescents with skewfoot deformity have pain and callusing under the head of the talus as well as over the fifth metatarsal and the first metatarsal head medially (102,157–159). Tight heel cord is often associated with painful skewfoot, as is present in a painful flatfoot. Stretching of the Achilles tendon is indicated as part of conservative management. A soft orthosis to support the talar head and the longitudinal arch and decrease the deformity in the hindfoot may be of value. Use of a rigid orthosis in this condition may cause increased pain and should be used cautiously.

Surgery is indicated if nonoperative treatment fails to relieve pain and callosities. Operative management should be directed at the specific deformity that appears to be associated with symptoms in a given case; that is, if the lateral translation through the midfoot and forefoot deformity is most prominent, treatment may include closing-wedge osteotomy of the cuboid and lengthening of the first cuneiform (Fig. 30.25), similar to metatarsus adductus. If, however, the deformity has a major component of hindfoot valgus (Fig. 30.26), it must be treated. Historical recommendations have included osteotomies at the base of the

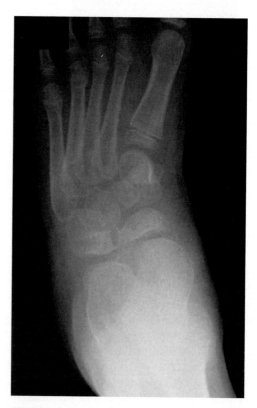

**Figure 30.25** In the skewfoot without severe hindfoot valgus deformity, appropriate management may be first cuneiform lengthening with lateral closing wedge of the cuboid, similar to treatment of metatarsus adductus.

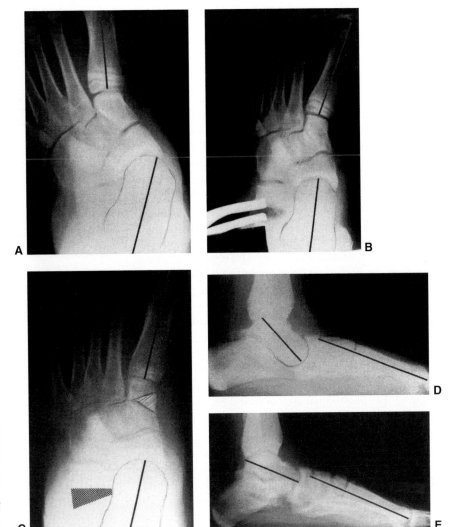

**Figure 30.26** Preoperative, intraoperative, and postoperative radiographs of a painful skewfoot in a 13-year-old adolescent. **A:** Preoperative anteroposterior view. **B:** Intraoperative distraction of calcaneal osteotomy. **C:** Corrected deformity on anteroposterior radiographs with grafts in place. **D:** Preoperative lateral view. **E:** Postoperative correction. Calcaneal lengthening osteotomy, medial cuneiform opening-wedge osteotomy, and Achilles tendon lengthening were used. (From Mosca VS. Flexible flatfoot and skewfoot. In: Drennan JC, ed. *The child's foot and ankle.* New York: Raven Press, 1992:355, with permission.)

metatarsals (136) and subtalar and triple arthrodesis of the hindfoot (147,148,160). The use of arthrodesis in this condition should be avoided and attempts at correction through osteotomy encouraged. Complications of triple arthrodesis and subtalar arthrodesis are enumerated in the section on flatfoot in this chapter. Mosca (157) proposed correction of symptomatic skewfoot by combining individual osteotomies of the forefoot and hindfoot to result in the correction of this foot deformity (Fig. 30.26). The combination of a calcaneal lengthening to correct hindfoot valgus as well as a first cuneiform lengthening to correct forefoot deformity is warranted. This is done according to the modified technique of Evans (102,161); it is always associated with lengthening of the heel cord and generally associated with medial reefing of the talonavicular joint. In Mosca's series (157), 9 of 10 patients with severe skewfoot achieved satisfactory clinical and radiographic corrections of skewfoot deformity.

## Flexible Flatfoot

Flexible flatfoot refers to an exceedingly common condition in which a decrease in the healthy longitudinal arch of the foot is present in stance, associated with valgus alignment of the hindfoot. Although this deformity is often referred to as "pronation," it should be noted that the actual deformity is a valgus hindfoot associated with a relative supination of the forefoot. The term flexibility refers to mobility about the subtalar joint, which differentiates this from the rigid flatfoot or peroneal spastic flatfoot indicative of an underlying pathologic state. A "flexible" flatfoot indicates a variation of a normal, which is occasionally associated with symptoms in its pathologic state.

### Epidemiology

The incidence of flatfoot deformity is unknown but clearly decreases with age, as described by Staheli (1,46). According to Harris (162), flatfoot was present in 23% of 3619 adults. They classified them into flexible, or hypermobile, flatfoot, which was generally asymptomatic and accounted for at least two thirds of the flatfeet. In 25% of cases, the flatfoot was associated with a tight heel cord and was much more likely to be associated with symptoms (162,163). According to a study by Reimers et al. carried out in Danish schoolchildren (164), the proportion of feet with decreased longitudinal arch declined from 42% in the 3- to 5-year age group to 6% in the teenagers. They found a strong relation between short Achilles tendon and persistence of deformity in the teenagers.

### Pathogenesis

Flexible flatfoot is a normal variation of foot alignment in early childhood, with spontaneous resolution in the vast majority of cases. Although muscle weakness has been proposed as a possible etiology, Basmajian and Stecko (12) demonstrated that little or no electromyographic activity of the muscles of the foot and ankle is present when physiologic loads are applied to a standing subject with the foot in plantigrade position. They, therefore, concluded that the bone-ligament complex, and not muscle contraction, determines the height of the longitudinal arch. Mann and Inman (13) confirmed this theory. The effects of extrinsic factors on the shape and development of the longitudinal arch is suggested by studies from developing countries, including those of Sim-Fook and Hodgson (5) and Rau and Joseph (6), finding a higher incidence of flatfoot in children wearing shoes than those who did not. Echarri and Forriol (165), in applying Staheli's index of arch development, found boys to have a higher tendency for flatfoot than girls, and wearing of shoes to have no influence on the height of the longitudinal arch or morphology of the foot.

### Clinical Features

Recognizing the nearly universal presence of decreased longitudinal arch in early infancy and its spontaneous resolution with growth, one may be hard pressed to call this, in general, a pathologic condition. However, in a number of cases, spontaneous resolution does not occur and symptoms become quite significant. The difficulty is in isolating the pathologic form of flatfoot deformity from the normal developmental form. The general examination should include assessment of ligamentous laxity as well as torsional and angular deformities. It is noted that flatfoot deformity has a higher presence in association with valgus deformities of the knees and generalized ligamentous laxity. In the presence of external tibial torsion or external rotatory deformity of the hip, the push-off in gait is compromised and the deformity of flatfoot increased. In general, a flexible flatfoot will revert to a normal position with the presence of a longitudinal arch in a non–weight-bearing or sitting position. When rising on the toes, the longitudinal arch will form and the hindfoot tip into the varus with plantar flexion of the hindfoot and simultaneous development of a longitudinal arch (Fig. 30.27).

Observation of the foot in a non–weight-bearing position with the patient kneeling on a chair will often demonstrate the hindfoot to be in neutral with an associated supination deformity of the forefoot. In stance, the elevation of the great toe (in the Jack toe-raise test) (Fig. 30.28) will produce an elevation in the longitudinal arch by using the windlass effect of the plantar fascia (159,166). Dorsiflexion of the foot with knee extended and hindfoot slightly inverted should be done to test for

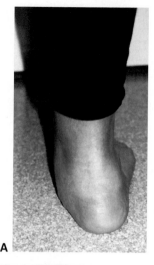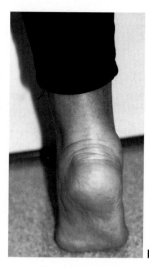

**Figure 30.27**    The arch elevates and the heel corrects from valgus to varus in a flexible flatfoot during toe standing, because of the windlass effect of the plantar fascia. (From Mosca VS. Flexible flatfoot and skewfoot. In: Drennan JC, ed. *The child's foot and ankle.* New York: Raven Press, 1992:355, with permission.)

Achilles tendon tightness, as this is the common pathologic state associated with painful flatfoot deformity. Finally, the skin pattern on the plantar aspect of the foot should be viewed, as callosities over the head of the talus are associated with symptoms and greater severity of flatfoot deformity. Sequential footprint measurements can be done in order to determine severity of the foot deformity. Kanatli et al. (167) have shown an excellent correlation between footprint and radiographic analysis in flexible flatfeet in children. Lin (168) showed that subjects with flatfoot deformity tended to perform physical tasks poorly and walked more slowly than controls with healthy feet. They also found that flatfoot deformity was associated with valgus knees and generalized ligamentous laxity to some degree. They cautioned against regarding flatfoot deformity as a static problem and encouraged analysis of its effect on activity. Cowan et al. (169) reported a study of prospective Army recruits, indicating that low-arched individuals had no increase in the risk of injury, whereas Kaufman et al. (170) reported an increased risk of overuse injuries in patients with dynamic pes planus, particularly with restricted ankle dorsiflexion.

In summary, in evaluating a patient with flatfoot deformity, a complete physical examination must be done, testing muscle strength of all lower extremity muscles and ruling out spinal pathology by physical examination. Range of motion and alignment as well as muscle strength and sensation should be evaluated in the lower extremities. Tightness of the Achilles tendon and flexibility of the foot deformity must be emphasized.

### Radiologic Findings

Radiographs of the flatfoot deformity are not generally needed for routine evaluation. In severe cases, however, a series of sequential lateral radiographs may be helpful in

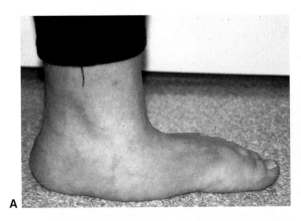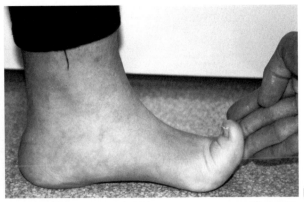

A                                                                                                              B

**Figure 30.28**    The arch elevates in a flexible flatfoot with the Jack toe-raise test because of the windlass effect of the plantar fascia. (From Mosca VS. Flexible flatfoot and skewfoot. In: Drennan JC, ed. *The child's foot and ankle*. New York: Raven Press, 1992:355, with permission.)

determining the course of the deformity. Radiographs, however, define only a static position and cannot be used as an indication for treatment (46,171).

The lateral radiograph of the flatfoot reveals the *Meary angle* (172) as measured between the long axis of the talus and the first metatarsal and the calcaneal pitch, which are indicative of the severity of the flatfoot deformity (Fig. 30.29). One may also look for localized sag between the navicular and first cuneiform rather than at the talonavicular joint, as this may have significant implications for treatment. A tarsal coalition may also be evaluated radiographically by standing anteroposterior, lateral, and oblique radiographs. Brown et al. (173) found that the C-sign on the lateral radiograph was more specific for flatfoot than for subtalar coalition. Although some have felt that the C-sign (Fig. 30.30) was diagnostic of middle facet talocalcaneal coalition, it appears not to be so.

In the young child, a severe flexible flatfoot at times must be differentiated from a vertical talus. In doing this, a plantar-flexion lateral view of the foot is obtained in order to show that the long axis of the first metatarsal becomes colinear with the long axis of the talus on a lateral view (Fig. 30.30).

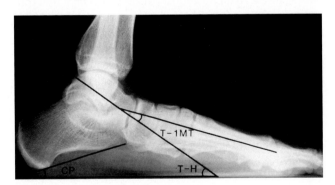

**Figure 30.29**    Weight-bearing lateral radiograph. The calcaneal pitch (CP) and the talus-horizontal angle (*T-H*) are the best measurements to assess valgus deformity of the hindfoot. The talus-first-metatarsal angle (*T-1MT*) is known as the Meary angle. A plantar flexed apex is seen in a valgus foot. (From Mosca VS. Calcaneal lengthening for valgus deformity of the hindfoot. Results in children who had severe, symptomatic flatfoot and skewfoot. *J Bone Joint Surg Am* 1995;77:500–512, with permission.)

## Natural History

Flatfeet are ubiquitous in infants and spontaneously resolve in most cases, as has been shown by Staheli and others. Shoeing has no effect on the development of the longitudinal arch and may actually be detrimental to it (165). There appears to be a wide range of arch height at all ages, but in general, there is consistent development of a healthy longitudinal arch during childhood (Fig. 30.31). There are no long-term prospective studies on the natural history of flatfoot deformity related to symptoms. It does appear, however, that in select cases, particularly in association with a tight heel cord, unresolved flatfoot deformity may be associated with an increase in foot pain and stress injuries in the lower extremities. Most authorities agree that flexible flatfoot is an anatomic variant and not a disabling deformity (159,162,171). Nevertheless, it may be associated with symptoms in its unresolved state. Uncontrolled studies indicate some efficacy of orthotic devices and shoe modifications in the development of the longitudinal arch in a child's foot (174). More recently, randomized control studies reveal no benefit from shoe modifications and inserts compared to normal development (175–177). In a study by Garcia-Rodriguez et al. (178), the prevalence of flexible flatfoot was evaluated in school children between the ages of 4 and 13 years. They found the prevalence of flatfoot deformity to be 2.6%. However, 14.2% of the children were receiving orthopaedic treatment, despite the diagnostic criteria for flatfeet being satisfied in only 2.7% of the children. More surprisingly, the children meeting the diagnostic criteria for flatfoot deformity were only being treated in 28.1% of the cases. Overweight children were found to be at greater risk of flatfoot deformity. Caution against the rate and expense of overtreatment of a physiologic, self-limiting deformity was raised.

Having said this, it should be noted that some children with flexible flatfoot deformity may have activity-related pain. The pain is usually diffuse or may be focal over the longitudinal arch. An exam should be done to evaluate muscle tightness as well as the foot deformity and flexibility of the flatfoot. If a tight heel cord is found, a stretching

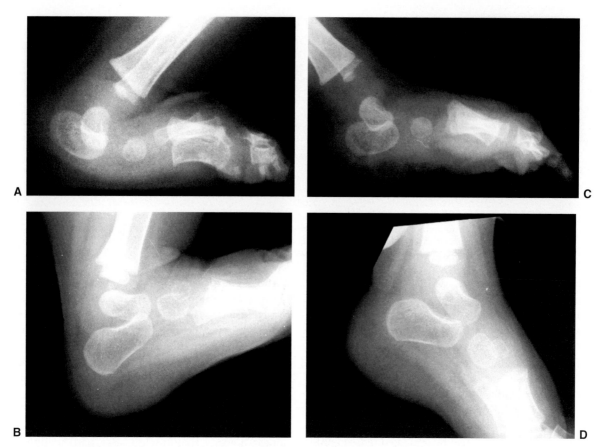

**Figure 30.30   A:** Lateral dorsiflexion radiograph of congenital vertical talus, showing persistent plantar flexion of the talus and calcaneus. **B:** Lateral dorsiflexion radiograph of a healthy foot, showing full dorsiflexion of the talus and calcaneus. **C:** Lateral plantar-flexion radiograph of the congenital vertical talus, showing persistent dorsal translation of the forefoot on the hindfoot. **D:** Lateral plantar-flexion radiograph of a healthy foot, showing good alignment of the forefoot on the hindfoot.

program should be begun. Mann and Inman (13) found a higher incidence of intrinsic muscle activity in flatfoot deformity, which may result in fatigue and pain during prolonged standing. Over-the-counter or custom-molded shoe inserts have been shown to relieve or diminish symptoms (179). Although arch supports do seem to provide relief in a number of cases, Miller et al. (180) were unable to show any change in ground reaction forces relating to the use of orthotic devices. The data were contrary to the current hypothesis about the benefits of the use of an orthotic device.

Whether or not the ground reaction forces can be altered by an orthotic device, it appears that symptoms can be significantly decreased. With an external rotation position of the foot in push-off, stresses over the midfoot are exacerbated. Use of an orthotic device and/or supportive shoe may be of value in such cases. Surgery is rarely indicated in flexible flatfoot deformity. However, in select cases, despite attempts at conservative therapy with an exercise program and proper arch support, surgery should be considered. Alignment of the entire lower extremity emphasizing valgus alignment at the knee and ankle and rotational alignment of the femur and tibia should be considered. When surgery is to be considered, options include soft-tissue reconstruction, osteotomy,

arthroereisis, and arthrodesis. Surgery for flexible flatfoot should be an infrequent procedure, employed in cases of intolerable pain despite maximal conservative management. Weight loss and correction of angular and rotational malalignment of the legs, including ankle valgus, should be considered preoperatively. In an occasional patient with a tight heel cord despite a vigorous stretching program, judicious heel cord lengthening may have a role in the management of flexible flatfoot, as an isolated procedure. Beyond this, soft-tissue reconstruction plays no part in the management of a persistently painful flexible flatfoot deformity. Fusion, including localized midtarsal, subtalar, and triple arthrodesis, has been recommended for the treatment of a flexible flatfoot deformity over the past 70 years. Localized midtarsal arthrodeses are all variants of a Hoke navicular cuneiform type fusion (181–187). Each of these reconstruction arthrodeses may improve alignment of the foot, but long-term results indicate poor outcomes in 49% to 70% of cases. The results were classified as unsatisfactory based on degenerative arthritis primarily involving the talonavicular joint, pain, or recurrence of deformity. In response to unsatisfactory results of limited arthrodeses, some have recommended triple arthrodesis as a procedure of value to prevent midfoot and hindfoot arthritis. Long-term results of triple arthrodeses indicate that this

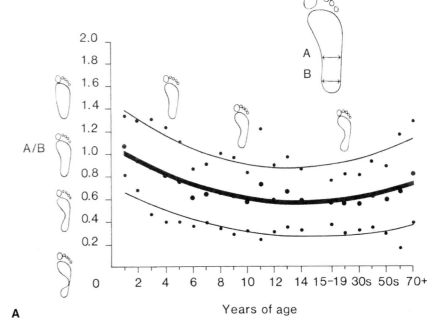

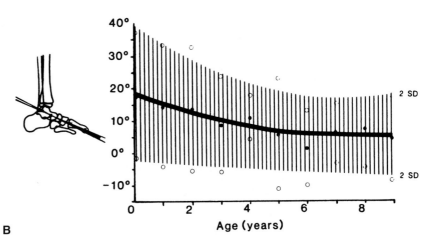

**Figure 30.31** **A:** Footprints from individuals of all ages show that children are more flat-footed than adults, that there is a wide range of healthy arch heights, and that the arch generally elevates spontaneously during the first decade of life. **B:** Radiographs from children of all ages confirm the footprint data. The drawing and graph represent the lateral talus-first-metatarsal angle. (**A** from Staheli LT, Chew DE, Corbett M. The longitudinal arch. A survey of eight hundred and eighty-two feet in normal children and adults. *J Bone Joint Surg Am* 1987;69:426–428, with permission; **B** from Vanderwilde R, Staheli LT, Chew DE, et al. Measurements on radiographs of the foot in normal infants and children. *J Bone Joint Surg Am* 1988;70:407–415, with permission.)

procedure also carries a significant risk of long-term negative consequences based on adjacent degenerative arthritis and pain (188). Therefore, present recommendations primarily include trying to reconstruct the foot while maintaining all normal articulations.

Joint-sparing procedures based upon osteotomy appear to be the option of choice for a flexible flatfoot at this time. Such procedures improve alignment while maintaining mobility. There are two osteotomies that hold promise for long-term relief of symptoms. Both are calcaneal procedures, but one translates the calcaneal tuberosity medially whereas the other lengthens the calcaneus with a positive effect on hindfoot and forefoot alignment.

The calcaneal osteotomy that translates the tuberosity medially (189) will not elevate the plantar-flexed talus, but will realign the weight-bearing axis of the hindfoot. The isolated hindfoot osteotomy may be combined with a closing wedge osteotomy of the medial cuneiform and an opening wedge osteotomy of the cuboid to restore forefoot and midfoot alignment, as described by Rathjen and

Mubarak (190), with good results. In cases in which the talus is not exceedingly plantar-flexed and the navicular is not dorsolaterally translated, this appears to be a valuable procedure, perhaps even the procedure of choice. If there is a tight heel cord, one should consider a fascial lengthening in association with this osteotomy.

The calcaneal lengthening osteotomy first described by Evans (161) and later popularized by Mosca (102,157–159) appears to offer the best opportunity to correct the flexible flatfoot deformity, maintaining joint mobility while reconstructing bony alignment. In this procedure, an opening-wedge osteotomy is performed through the neck of the calcaneus between the anterior and middle facet (Fig. 30.32), inserting a trapezoidal graft (generally allograft) to maintain length. The effect of this osteotomy in lengthening the calcaneus is correction of the eversion of the subtalar joint. The osteotomy improves the valgus alignment of the calcaneus, reduces the dorsolateral translation of the navicular into proper alignment with the long axis of the talus, and improves the talocalcaneal relation.

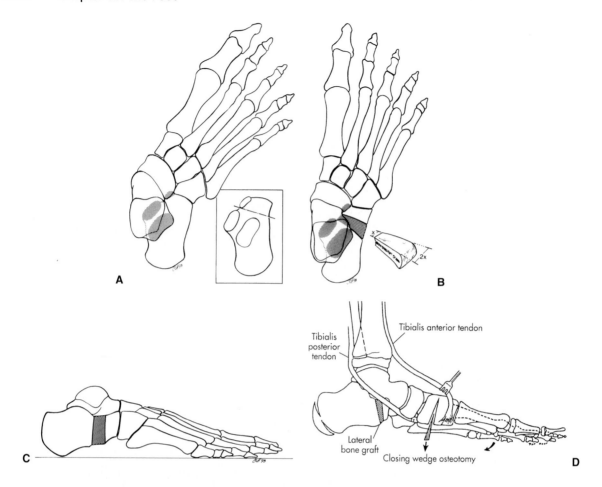

**Figure 30.32  A:** Calcaneal lengthening osteotomy. Dashed line indicates the position of the oblique osteotomy between the anterior and middle facets of the calcaneus. **B,C:** Insertion of the trapezoid-shaped tricortical iliac crest bone graft corrects all components of the valgus deformity of the hindfoot. **D:** A plantar-based closing wedge osteotomy of the medial cuneiform corrects the supination deformity of the forefoot. Lengthening of the gastrocnemius or the Achilles tendon is almost always necessary. (**A, B,** and **C** from Mosca VS. Calcaneal lengthening for valgus deformity of the hindfoot. Results in children who had severe, symptomatic flatfoot and skewfoot. *J Bone Joint Surg Am* 1995;77:500–512; **D** from Anderson AF, Fowler SB. Anterior calcaneal osteotomy for symptomatic juvenile pes planus. *Foot Ankle* 1984;4:274–283, with permission.)

The alignment of the first metatarsal and long axis of the talus as seen on the lateral view (Meary angle) is likewise improved by this procedure (102,161,191–193). Although the effects of this procedure on a flexible flatfoot are primarily positive, it may supinate the forefoot elevating the first ray. If this occurs, a plantar-flexion osteotomy through the first cuneiform is mandatory in order to restore the tripod of the foot and prevent an exacerbation of forefoot supination deformity (Fig. 30.32). The effect of elevating the first ray is counteracted by an intact peroneus longus that should be maintained while doing this lengthening osteotomy. Heel cord lengthening and peroneus brevis lengthening are always done as a part of this procedure.

Finally, "arthroereisis" should be discussed. In this procedure, a block of material is placed in the subtalar joint in order to eliminate motion in the flexible flatfoot (194,195). The block may be sylastic or high-molecular-weight polyethylene, but in either case there is a significant incidence of loosening, displacement, and synovitis related to this

procedure. Black et al. (196) and Verheyden et al. (197) both recommended abandonment of this procedure because of a high rate of negative outcomes. This is in contrast to the work of Grady (198) who reported consistently excellent results in 234 children. Although the author has no experience personally with this procedure, the use of a nonbiologic implant in young children for what is generally a self-limited condition seems illogical. Osteotomies seem to be of benefit in the occasional patient to correct deformity and relieve symptoms. Treating the asymptomatic flatfoot in children with a surgical reconstructive procedure appears to be generally unwise and unnecessary. In the face of neurologic conditions and pathologic degrees of ligamentous laxity, however, some method of management of the flexible flatfoot deformity may include such procedures, as described by Smith and Millar (195).

### Summary

A flexible flatfoot is a variant of the healthy foot that should be treated if it is painful or causing excessive shoe wear. Conservative or surgical management of the commonly associated tight heel cord is mandatory for successful outcome.

## Congenital Vertical Talus

In congenital vertical talus, the navicular is dislocated dorsolaterally on the head of the talus. Associated with this in varying degrees are hindfoot equinus, dorsal cuboid dislocation, and anterior soft-tissue contracture including toe extensors, peroneals, and anterior tibial tendons (199). Taken together, these describe the deformity in congenital vertical talus.

### Epidemiology

Congenital vertical talus is exceedingly rare. Although it occurs as an isolated congenital abnormality in 50% of cases (200–203), it is commonly associated with neuromuscular and genetic disorders including trisomy 13–15 (204) and trisomy 18 (205). Fifty percent of children have bilateral involvement, and there is no sex predilection (202).

### Pathogenesis

Most cases are sporadic or associated with underlying neuromuscular diseases. Case reports have indicated autosomal dominant transmission with incomplete penetrance (203,206) in some cases. Congenital vertical talus is associated with myelomeningocele, sacral agenesis, diastematomyelia, and arthrogryposis. In Sharrard and Grosfield's series of patients with myelomeningocele (207), 10% of patients had vertical talus associated with spinal dysraphism. Given the frequency with which this deformity is associated with neuromuscular disorders, a thorough evaluation of the neuroaxis with MRI is indicated in patients with vertical talus.

### Clinical Features

Congenital vertical talus has a rigid, convex plantar surface, with a hindfoot resting in equinus and a hypoplastic, laterally deviated forefoot (Fig. 30.33). Lloyd-Roberts and

Spence (208) described the appearance as "a prominence in the sole of the foot from which the heel and forefoot rise in a gentle curve." The Achilles tendon is always contracted with a fixed equinovalgus position. The head of the talus is palpable in the medial aspect of the midfoot. Upon plantar-flexing the foot, a gap can be felt anterior and medially to the medial malleolus as a space where the normal neck of the talus should be, when the navicular plantar flexes over the head of the talus. In contrast to a flexible flatfoot or a positional calcaneovalgus foot, the talonavicular joint cannot be reduced by manipulation. Some authors have differentiated a vertical talus from an oblique talus (175,209). An oblique talus is one in which there is dorsal subluxation of the navicular, but some flexibility of the foot exists such that a rigid dislocation of the navicular is not present; however, the foot is significantly more rigid than a common flexible flatfoot. This term may be confusing, but it is helpful if one considers it as describing a foot that appears on physical examination to be nearly like a vertical talus but that nearly reduces fully on a plantar-flexion view radiograph. In such a foot, an oblique talus can be improved by conservative management with casting and arch support, whereas surgery is always required in a true congenital vertical talus.

### Radiographic Features

Anteroposterior and lateral radiographs of the foot should be taken in a neutral position, as in any pediatric foot disorder. Standing radiographs are taken in a child able to stand; however, in the infant, these radiographs are taken in a neutral position. The diagnostic x-ray film of a vertical talus is a forced plantar-flexion view (Fig. 30.30) in which persistent malalignment of the long axis of the talus and the first metatarsal are confirmed. Because the navicular and first cuneiform are not ossified in infancy, the dislocation is implied by virtue of the lack of colinear alignment of the first metatarsal with the long axis of the talus. In a lateral x-ray film of a healthy, unstressed foot, the first metatarsal is aligned with a long axis of the talus. The position of the cuboid relative to the calcaneus should be determined, as this is indicative of the severity of a vertical

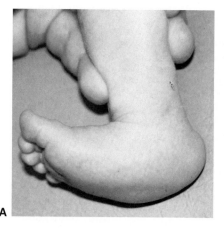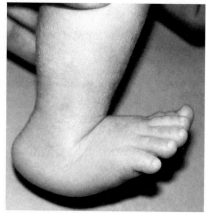

**Figure 30.33** Congenital vertical talus in an infant. **A:** Medial. **B:** Lateral.    **A**    **B**

talus. In the most severe form, there is a dorsal dislocation of the cuboid on the calcaneus.

### Pathoanatomy

Autopsy and surgical findings have confirmed consistent abnormalities in the musculature of the foot in vertical talus (210–213). Most have found contractures of the tibialis anterior, extensor hallucis longus, extensor hallucis brevis, peroneus tertius, peroneus longus, peroneus brevis, and the Achilles tendon. The peroneus longus and peroneus brevis may be anteriorly subluxed over the lateral malleolus, and the posterior tibial tendon may be subluxed anteriorly over the medial malleolus. The head of the talus is generally protruding below the posterior tibial tendon and the calcaneonavicular, or spring ligament, is markedly attenuated. The calcaneus is severely externally rotated and everted, with its posterolateral border in proximity to the fibula. Sustentaculum talae and anterior facet of the subtalar joint are exceedingly hypoplastic or absent in the most severe cases. The dorsal capsule of the talonavicular joint is thickened and contracted.

### Natural History

Untreated, a congenital vertical talus causes significant disability, with poor push-off, difficult shoe fitting, and a gait that is similar to one seen in a patient who has had a Symme amputation. The forefoot becomes atrophic over time, with thick plantar callosity forming over the head of the talus. No weight bearing occurs either on the true heel pad over the calcaneus nor under the forefoot. Eventually, push off becomes impossible.

### Treatment

Where cast treatment of clubfoot using the Ponseti method has markedly decreased the role of surgical management in this deformity, cast treatment of vertical talus has been rather ineffective beyond providing stretching of the dorsolateral soft tissues. In general, the foot is placed in a series of corrective casts in order to stretch the dorsal structures, hoping that surgical treatment will be rendered less complex. Casting is considered important by nearly all who have studied this problem (202,203,212,214). Following a series of corrective casts, an exercise program and, perhaps, a bivalve cast or splint is used until the time of surgery. Surgical options include one-stage or two-stage releases, talectomies, naviculectomy, subtalar arthrodesis, and triple arthrodesis. Consensus has lead to a single-stage procedure in most cases at this point.

Talectomy was recommended by Lamy in 1939 (199) but was soon abandoned. It was destructive and resulted in unacceptable outcome, not addressing the underlying pathology. It also left no options for future reconstruction and has been thoroughly abandoned. The primary choices for operative management of congenital vertical talus in a child younger than 2 years are one-stage versus two-stage reconstruction involving release of tight tendons and ligaments and realignment of osseous structures. If a two-stage procedure is chosen, the first stage consists of lengthening the contracted dorsolateral tendons and release of the contracted dorsolateral joint capsule with reduction of the midfoot on the hindfoot. The second stage consists of a posterolateral release of the contracted Achilles tendon, peroneal tendons, and posterior capsule. Ogata et al. (203) and Mazzocca et al. (215) found increased complications in the two-stage release. Included in the complications described by Ogata was avascular necrosis of the talus.

Most doctors now recommend a one-stage procedure (203,214,216–219) and report results that are comparable to or better than those reported for the two-stage procedures (216,220,221). Mazzocca and Romness compared the dorsal to the posterior approach for one-stage correction of congenital vertical talus. The dorsal approach was found to be associated with shorter operative time and better clinical score with fewer complications than the posterior approach. Several authors have reported the addition of a full or split transfer of the tibialis anterior to the head or neck of the talus (214,216,217,222,223). Although the transfer adds little time to the procedure, it would seem that a dynamic stabilizer of the talus would be unlikely to be particularly effective in maintaining talonavicular alignment, and that this procedure, although brief, may complicate an already somewhat difficult procedure. The author would not recommend the addition of the anterior tibialis transfer. The peroneus longus, is a plantar flexor of the first ray, is particularly strong, and complete transfer of the anterior tibial tendon may lead to an unopposed plantar flexion force, providing another reason not to alter the anterior tibial insertion.

It is not clear what the upper age limit for this reconstructive approach is. There is disproportionate growth between the medial and lateral borders of the foot in an unreduced vertical talus and marked atrophy of forefoot and midfoot. The abnormality of the middle and anterior facet of the subtalar joint become progressively more severe in the unreduced state. Until the age of 2 or 3 years, there may be stimulus toward further growth of cartilage and improvement of the talonavicular joint following reduction. Beyond this, shortening of the medial column and lengthening of the lateral column are approaches to management that may be required. Some authors have recommended naviculectomy (224,225) as a primary salvage procedure in congenital vertical talus. It may be an effective procedure to shorten the medial column and allow improvement of the position of the foot in the older child. Posterolateral release has been combined with naviculectomy for full deformity correction in a group of older children (Fig. 30.34). Coleman (106) has recommended subtalar arthrodesis in children older than 3 years; another alternative for this deformity is lengthening of the lateral column, which may be done in association with peroneal lengthening in select cases. Early diagnosis and treatment should eliminate the need for surgical options in the older child. Nevertheless, occasional cases requiring subtalar (222,223) and triple arthrodesis have been reported. If triple arthrodesis is indicated in this procedure, bone grafting will necessarily be used to supplement

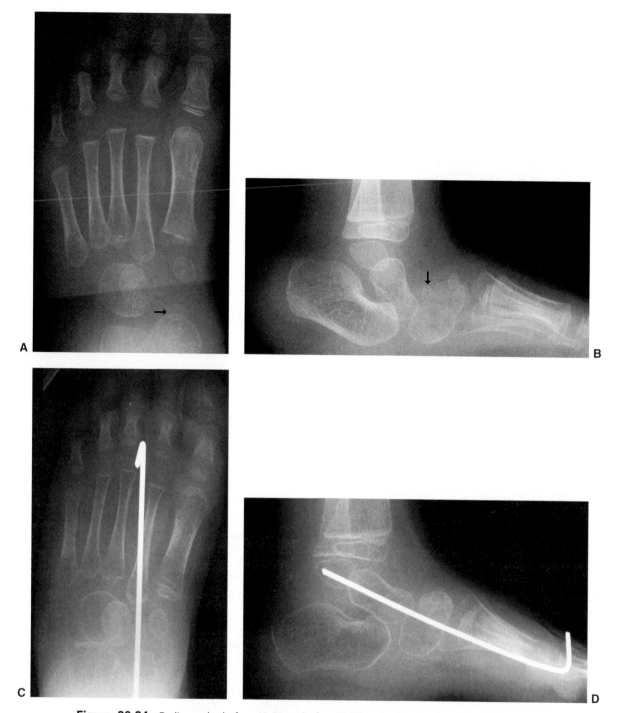

**Figure 30.34** Radiographs before **(A,B)** and after **(C,D)** naviculectomy for congenital vertical talus in an older child. *Arrow* indicates the navicular.

the correction of the foot and restore proper alignment. The literature clearly shows, however, that arthrodesis does result in a significant rate of degenerative arthritis at the ankle and midtarsal joints in the long term (188,226–232). Napiontek (233) reported overcorrection of the valgus foot in half the patients who underwent peritalar reduction combined with subtalar arthrodesis. Arthrodesis of the joints of the hindfoot, therefore, should be reserved for salvage procedures in adolescents and those with recurrent deformity or painful degenerative arthritis.

## Positional Calcaneovalgus Foot

### Definition

Positional calcaneovalgus foot is a foot deformity (Fig. 30.35) in which the foot is hyperdorsiflexed, often with the dorsal surface of the forefoot resting on the anterior surface of the lower leg. It is thought to be primarily a positional deformity.

### Epidemiology

Because flatfoot deformity is very frequent in infancy, the incidence of calcaneovalgus foot depends on how liberally

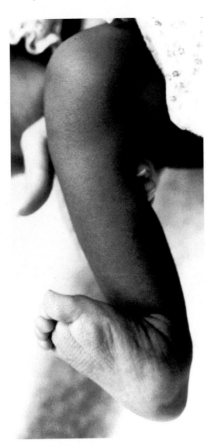

**Figure 30.35**   Positional calcaneovalgus foot deformity.

the term is used. Wynne-Davies et al. (234) reported the incidence to be 1 per 1000 live births, whereas Wetzenstein (235) noted a 30% to 50% incidence in the newborn, as well as a significant correlation to flexible flatfoot in older children. It is more common in girls and firstborn children.

### Pathogenesis

The probable cause of this deformity is intrauterine malpositioning, rather than a truly congenital deformation. Contracture without congenital deformity or dislocation is the hallmark of this condition.

### Clinical Features

Recognition of this generally benign condition, differentiating it from pathologic states requiring orthopaedic intervention, is mandatory. The calcaneovalgus foot deformity should be differentiated from the following conditions:

1. Paralytic calcaneus foot deformity seen in myelodyplasia and other conditions with absent gastrocsoleus.
2. Posteromedial bow of the tibia (Fig. 30.36).
3. Congenital vertical talus (Fig. 30.33).

Posteromedial bow of the tibia is a condition in which a calcaneovalgus foot is always present but is associated with a bowed, shortened tibia. The anterior compartment muscles appear to be somewhat hypoplastic over the concavity of the bow at the distal tibia. The bow (Fig. 30.36C) is benign and

progressive straightening of the tibia occurs, but leg-length discrepancy is always present. A vertical talus has a fixed dislocation of the navicular on the talar head, as described in this chapter. There is far less flexibility in a vertical talus than in a calcaneovalgus foot deformity. A motor exam can differentiate the paralytic calcaneovalgus foot deformity from the true positional abnormality. If the foot is sufficiently flexible for the examiner to be confident of the diagnosis of positional calcaneovalgus foot deformity, no x-ray films are taken. In cases in which there is confusion between a calcaneovalgus foot deformity and a true vertical talus, a plantar-flexion lateral radiograph is indicated (Fig. 30.30). Anteroposterior and lateral x-ray films are taken with which a calcaneovalgus foot can be differentiated from a vertical talus. In most cases, x-ray films are not required.

### Treatment

If the foot cannot be plantar-flexed below neutral, casting is indicated. Exercises to stretch the tightened anterior soft-tissue structures may be beneficial in speeding the resolution of this positional deformity. Larson et al. (8) found no difference between cases managed with exercise versus observation of this deformity at follow-up of 3 to 11 years. Severity of the initial deformity bears no relation to final outcome. Wetzenstein (235) found correlation between a calcaneovalgus foot and flexible flatfoot deformity in the long term. Corrective casting is rarely judged to be of benefit if the foot cannot be plantar-flexed below neutral, and particularly if there are associated tight peroneal muscles and lateral deviation of the forefoot with external tibial torsion.

Surgical treatment of calcaneovalgus foot is not required.

## Tarsal Coalition

### Definition

A tarsal coalition is a fibrous, cartilaginous, or bony connection between two or more bones of the hindfoot and midfoot.

### Epidemiology

The tarsal coalition has been associated with peroneal spastic flatfoot (236) since 1921 when Slomann (237) linked the two conditions. A "peroneal spastic flatfoot" is a rigid flatfoot deformity in which subtalar motion is exceedingly limited. The rigid foot deformity is accompanied by spasm of the extensor digitorum communis and the peroneal muscles in many cases. Harris and Beath (238) further associated the findings of talocalcaneal coalition with peroneal spastic flatfoot. Interestingly, tarsal coalition has also been linked with an infrequently occurring tibialis posterior spastic varus deformity (239,240).

Tarsal coalitions have been noted to occur with a number of other disorders, including fibular hemimelia (241), clubfoot (242), Apert syndrome (243) and Nievegert-Pearlman syndrome. Such coalitions have also been seen in lower-limb congenital abnormalities. Tarsal coalitions have been found in monozygotic twins (244).

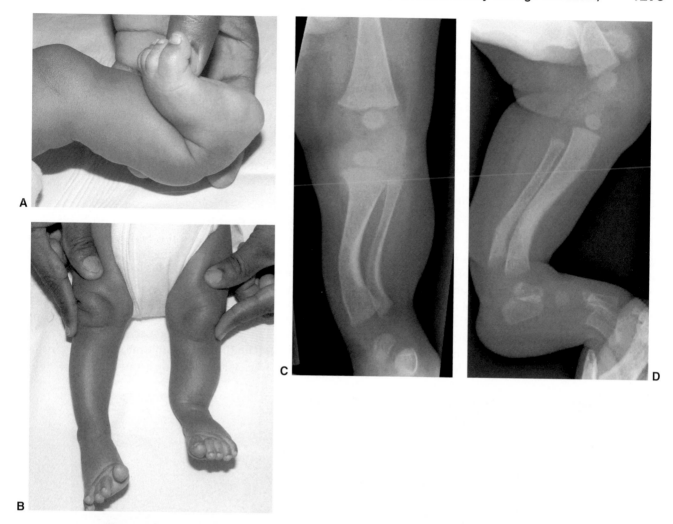

**Figure 30.36  A,B:** This patient has a calcaneovalgus foot but with an apparent bow to the tibia with shortening. **C,D:** A calcaneovalgus foot should be differentiated from that associated with posteromedial bow of the tibia, as seen on radiographs.

The overall incidence of tarsal coalitions was proposed by Harris and Beath in 1948 to be 2%, on the basis of routine physical examination of Canadian Army enlistees (238). On the basis of a cadaveric study by Phitzner in 1896, the rate of calcaneal navicular synostosis was found to be 2.9%, and if talocalcaneal coalitions are included as well, its incidence might reach 6% (245,246). More recently, a study by Lysack and Fenton (247) documented a general prevalence of calcaneal navicular coalition of 5.6% in a radiographic study, which was significantly greater than previously reported. The most common sites of tarsal coalition include the middle facet of the talocalcaneal joint and the calcaneonavicular coalition (238). Together these account for 90% of all coalitions (248). Tarsal coalitions are bilateral in 50% to 60% of cases. Clarke (249) documented multiple coalitions in 6 of 30 patients on review examination of CT scans, raising the question of what the true percentage of feet with multiple coalitions may be. Also reported are talonavicular coalitions, calcaneal cuboid coalitions, and navicular cuneiform coalitions, although all of these are uncommon (248,250) (Fig. 30.37).

Wray and Herndon (251) have suggested autosomal dominant inheritance with variable penetrance based on a single family study. Leonard (252) has confirmed the autosomal dominant pattern of inheritance.

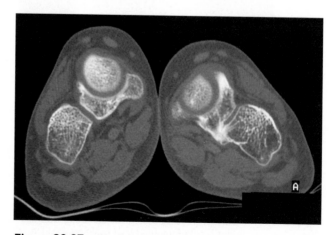

**Figure 30.37**   This computed tomography (CT) scan of the midfoot demonstrates a rare cubonavicular coalition.

### Pathogenesis

The tarsal coalition appears to be a relatively frequent finding in the general population, with symptoms developing in late childhood and adolescence. The possible etiologies of the painful tarsal coalition associated with rigid flatfoot are (i) stress fracture at a time when progressive ossification is occurring or (ii) limited motion with altered hindfoot mobility causing increased stress across involved joints. In either case, bone scan often shows increased uptake in the area of the tarsal coalition. Children with syndromes such as Apert syndrome have multiple coalitions and generally decreased activity to a level where symptoms of the coalitions are limited.

### Clinical Features

Pain associated with valgus hindfoot deformity and limited subtalar motion is the hallmark of tarsal coalition and peroneal spastic flatfoot. Frequently, an insidious onset of aching pain over the medial aspect of the foot in the talocalcaneal coalition, and the sinus tarsi in the calcaneonavicular coalition, is present. Pain is generally aggravated by activity and relieved by rest. Ankle spraining associated with this is common. The flatfoot deformity present is often severe and progressive in a child who has previously had an intact longitudinal arch. Rigidity is because of restriction of subtalar motion, so that the foot cannot be inverted as in the normal physical examination. When the patient rises on tiptoes, the hindfoot does not invert into its normal varus position (253) (Fig. 30.38).

The rigid flatfoot deformity, or peroneal spastic flatfoot, can also be seen with juvenile rheumatoid arthritis, bone lesions of the talus, calcaneus or midfoot, and trauma. Ruling out arthritis and the other causes of rigid flatfoot deformity is mandatory.

### Radiographic Features

A calcaneonavicular coalition is best seen on an oblique radiograph (Fig. 30.39A) of the foot. The failure of segmentation of the tarsal bones in their cartilaginous state results in a cartilaginous bridge, which progressively ossifies forming a synostosis with age. On a standing lateral view, an elongated process of the calcaneus to navicular can be seen as the "anteater's nose" (254) (Fig. 30.39B). Radiographic findings of talocalcaneal coalition include the C-sign (Fig. 30.40) as a line formed from the outline

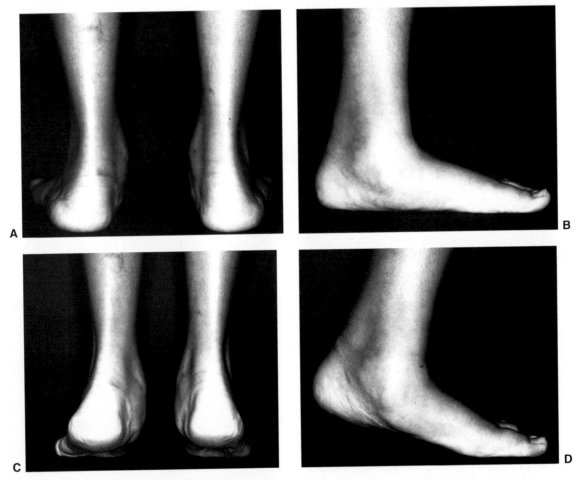

**Figure 30.38** **A,B:** Rigid flatfoot. **C,D:** The arch will not elevate, and the hindfoot valgus will not correct to varus during toe standing, because of immobility of the subtalar joint. (From Mosca VS. Flexible flatfoot and tarsal coalition. In: Richards B, ed. *Orthopaedic knowledge update: pediatrics*, Rosemont, IL: American Academy of Orthopaedic Surgeons, 1996:211, with permission.)

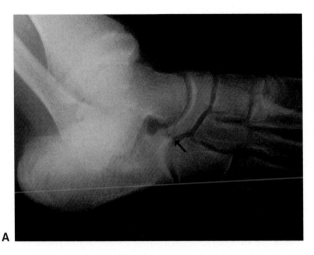 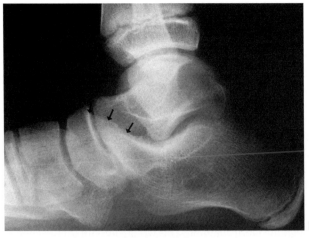

A                                                                              B

**Figure 30.39**  **A:** A calcaneonavicular coalition (*arrow*) is best seen on an oblique radiograph of the foot. **B:** Lateral radiograph demonstrating the anteater nose sign (*arrows*), indicating a calcaneonavicular coalition.

of the talar dome extending around the inferior margin of the sustentaculum tali. This has been thought to be a reliable indicator of talocalcaneal coalition; however, Taniguchi et al. (255) found the C-sign to have low sensitivity, meaning that the diagnosis of tarsal coalition is not negated by the absence of a C-sign. Brown et al. (173) found the C-sign to be specific for a flatfoot deformity but neither sensitive nor specific for the diagnosis of subtalar coalition. Liu et al. (256) found that the absent middle facet was a more accurate sign in the diagnosis of a subtalar coalition than either talar beaking or the C-sign (Fig. 30.40).

In all cases of suspected tarsal coalition, a standing anterior and posterior radiograph of the ankle should be obtained. A ball-and-socket ankle may be seen in cases of long-standing tarsal coalition (257,258).

A talocalcaneal coalition can be seen on an axial or Harris view (238), but the best way to assess a coalition is with CT scan (Fig. 30.41) (259,260). More recently, Emery

et al. (261) showed that MRI was nearly as good as the "gold standard" CT imaging for subtalar coalition. In cases where diagnoses such as bone lesions of the hindfoot or midfoot are considered in the differential diagnosis, an MRI is indicated rather than a CT scan. While MRI should not be the first-line study, it can also identify possible fibrous coalitions (262). Bone scan can also help in identifying the cause of foot pain with an atypical history or pain pattern (260). Because a rigid flatfoot deformity can result from infection or other inflammatory disease as well as bone lesions, a laboratory work-up including a complete blood count (CBC) with differential, sedimentation rate, C-reactive protein, ANA, and rheumatoid factor may be warranted. Rheumatologic evaluation in difficult cases with adjacent joint space narrowing may be helpful as well.

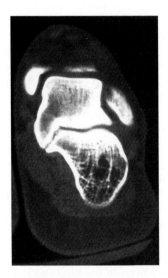

**Figure 30.41**  Talocalcaneal coalitions are best seen on computed tomography (CT) scans taken in the coronal plane. The middle facet is narrow, irregular, and down-sloping. (From Mosca VS. Flexible flatfoot and tarsal coalition. In: Richards B, ed. *Orthopaedic knowledge update: pediatrics*, Rosemont, IL: American Academy of Orthopaedic Surgeons, 1996:211, with permission.)

**Figure 30.40**  A dorsal talar beak (*white arrow*) in a foot with a talocalcaneal coalition. This represents a traction spur, not degenerative arthritis. The C-sign of Lefleur (*black arrows*) is a nonspecific indication of a talocalcaneal coalition.

### Pathoanatomy

The cause of tarsal coalition remains unknown. The bones of the foot are separate in infancy in 99% of individuals. Lack of segmentation of the cartilaginous anlage occurs in some cases, and it is possible that a fibrous connection between bones undergoes metaplasia to cartilage (syndesmosis to synchondrosis) and finally to synostosis (238,263,264). A coalition alters the normal movement of the subtalar complex in gait. When rotation and gliding are eliminated by the tarsal coalition, increased force is concentrated across the talonavicular, calcaneocuboid, and subtalar joints (265). The altered motion may lead to degenerative changes in joints over time as the stresses on cartilage may exceed tolerable limits. Another possible etiology for symptoms is a stress fracture through the tarsal coalition. This would account for the large number of individuals who become symptomatic in adolescence when size and ossification concentrate stress in the coalition. It is possible that this relates to ligament sprain, peroneal muscle spasm, irritation of the sinus tarsi, and irritation of adjacent joints in addition to the arthritis and stress fracture previously mentioned (236). In general, however, the cause of the pain remains unknown (238,248).

### Natural History

According to Leonard (252), only about 25% of individuals with tarsal coalitions become symptomatic. The onset of pain coincides with the progression of the fusion of the coalition. This generally occurs between 8 and 12 years of age for calcaneonavicular coalitions and between 12 and 16 years of age for talocalcaneal coalitions. As the feet become symptomatic, progressive valgus deformity of the hindfoot, flattening of the longitudinal arch, and restriction of subtalar motion occur (251,253,254,257–260,262,263,266).

### Treatment

The goal of treatment is relief of pain and the restoration of motion. The specific goal of reestablishment of the longitudinal arch is less clear. Treatment is indicated only for symptomatic tarsal coalitions (238,257,267). It is not clear that an asymptomatic tarsal coalition with mild restriction would benefit from a surgical excision.

In general, upon presentation with a painful foot and diagnosis of tarsal coalition, attempts should be made to relieve symptoms by nonoperative means including activity modification, nonsteroidal antiinflammatory drugs, shoe inserts, and cast immobilization in a below-knee walking cast. Pain may be eliminated rapidly following cast application, and as many as 30% of patients remain pain-free after cast removal following 6 weeks of immobilization (263). However, Saxena et al. (268) found that patients who underwent tarsal coalition excision reached levels of activity beyond the level reached by a matched group of patients forgoing surgical excision, questioning the wisdom of a nonoperative approach in the marginally symptomatic patient.

Surgical options for patients with recurrent or disabling symptoms include resection of the coalition, osteotomy, and arthrodesis. This chapter will first consider these options applied to the calcaneonavicular coalition first described by Badgley (269) in 1927. In this procedure, the coalition is excised and an interposition material inserted to prevent refusion between the calcaneus and the navicular. The extensor digitorum brevis as an interposition material improved outcome, preventing recurrence of the fusion and providing relief from long-term pain (270–272). The presence of a talar beak is not indicative of degenerative arthrosis and is not by itself a contraindication to resection (273–276). Prior to resection of a calcaneonavicular coalition, one should ensure that a second coalition is not present by analysis of a CT scan of the hindfoot. The absence of degenerative changes in the talonavicular joint and calcaneocuboid joint should be ensured. Significant degenerative arthritis is a contraindication to surgical excision. Cooperman et al. (277) demonstrated significant variation in the extent of the fusion of the anterior aspect of the calcaneus with the navicular. In his analysis of 30 specimens, the anterior facet of the subtalar joint was totally spared in 8. The anterior facet was partially replaced in 7 of 30 specimens and completely replaced in 15. This variation in the anterior portion of the subtalar joint, related to calcaneonavicular coalitions, may result in some variation in outcome and certainly relates to the extent and depth of the resection required to adequately treat this problem. Failure to resolve symptoms with excision is often related to inadequate resection at the time of the primary procedure with respect to depth and breadth of this osseous fusion. A CT scan analysis of the relation of the anterior facet of the subtalar joint to the calcaneal navicular coalition will assist in surgical planning.

Indications for surgical resection of talocalcaneal coalitions are a bit less clear and more complicated. The coalition is located on the medial side, or tension side, of the valgus foot deformity, and resection of a portion of the subtalar joint may lead to further collapse into the valgus. It is stated that resection should not be done if more than 50% of the subtalar joint surface is involved with the coalition (273). Wilde et al. (276) reported unsatisfactory results of resection in feet with a ratio of the surface area of the coalition to the surface area of the posterior facet greater than 50%, on the basis of CT scan evaluation. Luhmann and Schoenecker (278) reported that there were good postoperative results in feet with valgus deformities of less than 21 degrees but with posterior facet involvement of more than 50%. However, valgus abnormality in excess of 21 degrees required postoperative bracing and had compromised results. Many feet with poor outcomes have narrow posterior facet or impingement of the lateral process of the talus on the calcaneus. The resection of the talocalcaneal coalitions therefore remains more controversial, and further study is required for redefining the indications for resection.

Degenerative arthritis in either coalition is considered a contraindication to resection, but this diagnosis may be difficult to make. Talar beaking (Fig. 30.40) is not a sign of degenerative arthritis and not a contraindication to resection (273–276). Successful resection and interposition in talocalcaneal coalition and calcaneonavicular coalitions have been found to occur in up to 90% of cases at 10-year follow-up. Interposition materials in the talocalcaneal coalitions include fat (273,279) or a split portion of the flexor hallucis longus tendon (280). Documented degenerative arthrosis with persistent and recurring pain after coalition, particularly in adults, represents an indication for arthrodesis (236). This may be either a triple arthrodesis or a subtalar arthrodesis (281), depending on the joint and extent of involvement. Osteotomies to improve realignment remain an alternative to arthrodesis, and the medial closing wedge osteotomy of the calcaneus or sliding osteotomy to treat severe valgus deformity should be considered (279,282). Another surgical procedure that should be considered in feet with some mobility is the calcaneal lengthening procedure described by Evans; it can be used following resection of an osseous coalition of the middle facet in select cases. Although long-term studies are not documented for this procedure, recognized problems with long-term outcome of triple arthrodesis are well recognized and alternatives should be sought (188,226,227,232).

## Juvenile Hallux Valgus

### Definition
Juvenile hallus valgus, or bunion deformity, is characterized by lateral deviation of the great toe with prominence of the first metatarsal head medially. The apex of the deformity is at the first metartarsal phalangeal joint and it is often associated with a flatfoot, more commonly in women.

### Epidemiology
The true incidence of hallux valgus deformity is unknown. It is more common in girls than in boys, with girls accounting for more than 80% of cases. Usually there is a strong family history, with most patients inheriting the deformity from their mothers (283–287). Coughlin and Roger (288) found a positive family history of bunion deformity in nearly three fourths of patients reported in his series. No inheritance was present in 70% of cases (288,289). The Mendellian inherence pattern of juvenile hallux valgus has been proposed to be X-linked dominant or autosomal dominant with very variable penetrance (290,292). As in many cases where complex inheritance patterns are present, it has been described as a polygeneic or multifactorial inheritance pattern as well. The cause of hallux valgus deformity is both extrinsic and intrinsic. Studies of hallux valgus in children who wear shoes compared to those who do not show an increased risk with footwear (152,292). However, most evidence leads to the conclusion that juvenile hallux valgus is a deformity negatively influenced by constricting footwear but usually secondary to a structural abnormality of the foot (288,289,293).

Flatfoot deformity has been determined to be a risk factor for the development of hallux valgus, as well as its recurrence following surgical correction, by a number of authors (284,294,295). However, others feel that flatfoot deformity does not predispose to the occurrence of juvenile hallux valgus deformity. Coughlin and Roger (288), Kilmartin and Wallace (296), and Canale et al. (285) found no correlation between pes planus and the rate of success with surgical correction. The relation between the length of the first metatarsal and the development of hallux valgus has been studied as well. Excessively long first metatarsal (284,288,297) and a short metatarsal (298) have been implicated in the incidence and severity of juvenile hallux valgus. However, Coughlin and Roger (288) have shown that the lengths of the first and second metatarsal in children with adolescent bunions are similar to those in a healthy population.

There is an association between metatarsus primus varus, which is defined as an intermetatarsal angle between the first and second rays of greater than 10 degrees, and juvenile hallux valgus. The cause of the varus deformity of the first metatarsal may lie in an abnormal cuneiform–first-metatarsal articulation. The distal articular surface of the first cuneiform is normally transverse; however, an oblique orientation of this joint may predispose to a varus deformity of the first metatarsal (295). The second angle that is important in quantifying the hallux valgus deformity is the hallux valgus angle defined by Hardy and Clapham (289). This angle is measured by the intersections of the longitudinal axis of the proximal phalanx and the first metatarsal (Fig. 30.42). The normal hallux valgus angle is less than 16 degrees (299).

The final important skeletal abnormality to consider in the quantification of the juvenile hallux valgus deformity is the lateral deviation of the articular surface of the first metatarsal. The distal metatarsal articular angle (DMAA) quantifies this alignment (Fig. 30.43) (288,290,300,301). The higher the DMAA, the greater the valgus deformity of the distal metatarsal articulation. Coughlin and Roger (288) reported a 48% incidence of juveniles with hallux valgus having an increased DMAA and a congruous first metatarsal phalangeal joint, significantly greater than in adults (300). He noted that the DMAA was significantly higher in patients with positive family histories and early onset of hallux valgus.

As the deformity of hallux valgus progresses, the flexor tendons and sesamoids sublux laterally; the adductor of the great toe inserting on the proximal phalanx increases the deformity, and finally, once the hallux valgus deformity is present, the abductor hallucis with its plantar insertion on the proximal phalanx has no ability to abduct the great toe.

### Clinical Features
Most adolescents with hallux valgus are asymptomatic, and the mild pressure present over the metatarsal head medially can be relieved by proper shoe fitting. When pain is present, it is generally directly over the medial prominence of the first metatarsal head, as well as overlapping of the second toe over the laterally deviated great toe. Intraarticular pain and arthritis are rare in juvenile hallux valgus. Restriction of motion at the metatarsal phalangeal joint is also rare.

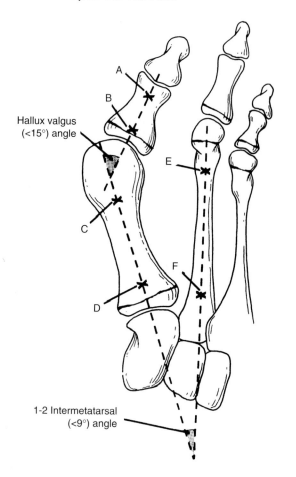

**Figure 30.42** Hallux valgus and first-second intermetatarsal angle. *A-B* axis of proximal phalanx; *C-D* axis of first metatarsal; *E-F* axis of second metatarsal. (From Coughlin M. Juvenile hallux valgus. In: Coughlin M, Mann R, eds. *Surgery of the foot and ankle*, 7th ed. St. Louis, MO: Mosby, 1999:270, with permission.)

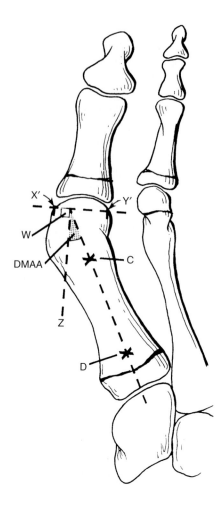

**Figure 30.43** The distal metatarsal articular angle (DMAA) quantifies the angular relation between the articular surface and the shaft of the metatarsal. The DMAA is the angle between the metatarsal shaft (*C-D*) and the line (*W-Z*) that is perpendicular to the articular surface (*X'-Y'*). (From Coughlin M. Juvenile hallux valgus. In: Coughlin M, Mann R, eds. *Surgery of the foot and ankle*, 7th ed. St. Louis, MO: Mosby, 1999:270, with permission.)

In general, juvenile hallux valgus is present bilaterally in women with positive family history. In cases of unilateral deformity in a woman with a negative family history, be aware of other causes of muscle imbalance that might lead to a bunion deformity. Examples of these are central nervous system lesions such as cerebral palsy, spinal dysraphism, or other spinal cord abnormality, and peripheral nerve lesions.

On physical examination, look for associated flatfoot deformity, particularly with tight Achilles tendon. Also look for other causes of pain surrounding the metatarsal phalangeal joint such as arthritis, inflammation, or lesions of local soft tissue or bone.

### Radiographic Features
Standing anteroposterior and lateral radiographs of the foot are necessary in order to evaluate hallux valgus. First, the overall alignment of the foot should be documented on standing views, measuring calcaneal pitch and the first metatarsal to long axis of the talus (Meary angle) on the lateral view. With respect to the bunion deformity, the hallux valgus angle, the intermetatarsal angle and the DMAA should be measured. Look for metatarsal phalangeal joint congruity and relative lengths of the first and second metatarsal. An

abnormality of the proximal phalanx with trapezoidal shape or an abnormal interphalangeal joint may be present with hallux valgus. Cadaver study by Vittetoe et al. showed that the intraobserver reliability of DMAA measurement was high, and interobserver reliability was poor (302).

### Natural History
The natural history of juvenile hallux valgus is not known. Piggott (300) believed that congruous joints with juvenile hallux valgus were stable and less likely to progress than those with subluxations. Congruous, laterally deviated metatarsal phalangeal articulation is much more common in children than in adults. A congruous first metatarsal phalangeal joint is found in 9% of adults (300) but in 47% of juvenile patients with bunions (288).

### Treatment
Patients seeking treatment of hallux valgus either complain of deformity, or pain, or both. There is an assumption on the part of many patients and parents that prompt treatment of

the deformity will resolve and cure this problem. This approach—early correction of the deformity to alleviate the potential for long-term difficulty—has no role in management of hallux valgus deformity. In pediatric orthopaedics, we often try to correct deformities early, in order to keep them from becoming significant problems in the future; not so for bunions. This "hands off" approach is counterintuitive, both to patients and their parents. Pain is the primary indication for treatment of hallux valgus deformity rather than malalignment, because of the significant recurrence rate. Perhaps there is a role for early conservative management with night splinting to prevent progressive bunion deformity. This opinion is based on the work of Groiso (286), who reported a 50% success rate in night splinting, using an orthoplast precut splint, holding the great toe in an abducted position at night. His series included 56 children with 2- to 6-year follow-up. Half the children showed significant improvements in the metatarsal phalangeal angle and the intermetatarsal angle. A contrary view was expressed by Kilmartin et al. (303), who found that hallux valgus deformity increased more in patients who used splints than those who did not. The pillar of conservative management is finding shoes that fit appropriately and have a widened toe box. The upper portion of the shoe should be soft, and an arch support can be used to decrease the tendency for pronation of the foot.

Surgery is indicated when pain cannot be managed with alteration of footwear, and a significant change in activity is required in a child. The age of the patient at the time of surgery is a significant consideration. Poor results with high complication rates have been reported consistently in 30% to 60% of young children who have had hallux valgus surgery (273,304–307). The results have been attributed to a number of factors, including further epiphyseal growth causing progressive deformity (283), growth arrest of the proximal first metatarsal and proximal phalanx, and return of the proximal phalanx to its position of congruent articulation. The return of the great toe to a position of congruent articulation with increasing bunion deformity is a particularly significant problem in patients with an elevated DMAA. Coughlin and Roger (288) and others (307) have, however, performed successful surgical reconstructions with low complication rates in adolescents with open growth plates. The authors stress that if possible, surgery should be delayed until the end of growth.

All surgical procedures have the following components: distal soft tissue realignment (McBride procedure), metatarsal osteotomy (either proximal or distal), and attention to the DMAA.

Also, the excision of the medial eminence in hallux valgus should not be aggressive, because a large protuberant medial eminence is rarely seen in children.

Soft tissue realignment should not be performed in isolation because recurrent deformity will uniformly result. In the face of a subluxed metatarsal phalangeal joint, soft tissue realignment may be valuable. In addressing soft tissue abnormalities, medial soft tissue realignment generally involves a VY reconstruction of the medial capsule, as well

as a lateral release of the adductor tendon. With soft tissue realignment as an isolated procedure without osteotomy, there is a 50% to 75% recurrence rate in adolescents (284,288). Hallux varus has also been reported following this procedure (308,309). Therefore, soft tissue repair alone has been abandoned.

Osteotomies are central to the treatment of juvenile hallux valgus deformity. The osteotomies may be the distal first metatarsal as used in a chevron or Mitchell type osteotomy, the proximal first metatarsal, or the medial cuneiform. In order to make the decision of where to do the procedure, radiologic evaluation is required. For the congruous metatarsal phalangeal joint, a distal osteotomy may be used to correct the DMAA, whereas a proximal metatarsal osteotomy or medial cuneiform osteotomy is used to correct the metatarsus primus varus (290,310) (Fig. 30.44). In some cases, an additional osteotomy at the base of the proximal phalanx is required. If the intermetatarsal angle is less than 15 degrees, a simple distal osteotomy, either Mitchell or chevron, can be used. Standard uniplanar chevron or Mitchell osteotomies do not correct the DMAA. Translating the metatarsal head laterally and correcting the angular deformity can be done with effort, using internal fixation with K-wires to maintain angular correction of the distal fragment and correction of the DMAA (283,285,290,304, 306,311–314). Minimal lateral soft tissue release should be combined with distal metatarsal osteotomy because of the risk of avascular necrosis (315).

Results of the Mitchell osteotomy vary among series. Ball and Sullivan (304) reported a recurrent valgus deformity in 11 of 17 patients, or 61%. Canale et al. (285) reported 31% of patients in their series with a fair or poor outcome; the less than satisfactory results related primarily to poor position of the displaced distal fragment, resulting in recurrent deformity, or plantar angulation resulting in transfer lesions to the second metatarsal head. Such problems can be decreased with appropriate use of internal fixation.

A number of very positive series, using the Mitchell osteotomy, have been reported, with positive outcomes ranging from 81% to 95% (66,283,311,316). Positive outcome from this osteotomy related to preserving the length of the first metatarsal and never dorsiflexing the metatarsal head while stabilizing the osteotomy with a screw or K-wire.

Another distal metatarsal osteotomy that is highly effective in managing a bunion deformity with an intermetatarsal angle of less than 15 degrees is the chevron osteotomy. The chevron (314) osteotomy is a transverse osteotomy through the distal portion of the metatarsal with a chevron shape. The apex of the chevron osteotomy is at the midportion of the metatarsal head, and the angular limbs transverse the cortex of the metatarsal, proximal to the capsular insertion (317). Good results from this osteotomy have been reported by Zimmer et al. (314) in 85% of adolescents despite a recurrence rate of 20%. The intrinsically stable osteotomy avoids the problem of metatarsal shortening. The DMAA can be corrected by angulating the distal articular surface.

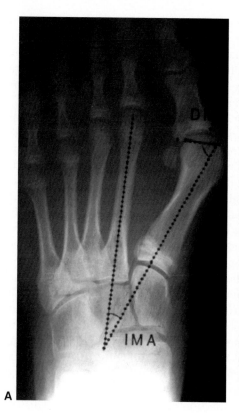

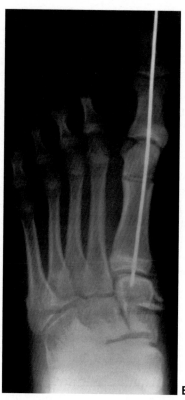

**Figure 30.44 A:** Preoperative radiographs of juvenile hallux valgus. *IMA*, intermetatarsal angle. **B:** Radiograph after medial cuneiform opening wedge osteotomy and distal first metatarsal closing wedge osteotomy. (**A** from Mosca VS. Ankle and foot: pediatric aspects. In: Beaty J, ed. *Orthopaedic knowledge update 6.* Rosemont, IL: American Academy of Orthopaedic Surgeons, 1999:583.)

In cases where the intermetatarsal angle (Fig. 30.44) exceeds 15 degrees, correction of the primary varus deformity of the first ray is necessary (288,290,305). If the medial cuneiform distal surface is angulated, an opening wedge osteotomy through the cuneiform can be done. Peterson and Newman (310) described a two-level osteotomy for adolescent bunions doing a closing distal medially based osteotomy with an opening proximal-based metatarsal osteotomy in which the length of the metatarsal is preserved, the varus deformity corrected, and the DMAA properly aligned.

There is no role for excisional type arthroplasties in the management of bunion deformity in children. Occasionally, an Akin osteotomy, which is a medial closing wedge of the proximal phalanx (318), may be used to improve the alignment of a toe in which the metatarsal alignment is proper and the DMAA appears satisfactory. Hallux valgus, therefore, should be corrected where the deformity lies. In the presence of cerebral palsy, bunion deformities are quite common, both dorsal bunions and hallux valgus. Because of exceedingly high recurrence rates, fusion of the first metatarsal phalangeal joint is the procedure of choice (319–321).

In summary, treatment of adolescent bunions may involve conservative treatment with night splinting and observation. Appropriate footwear should always be encouraged. Surgical treatment should be delayed until the end of growth if possible, and the procedure chosen should treat the deformity present in a given case. There is no indication for isolated soft tissue repair in the juvenile bunion deformity.

## Congenital Overriding Fifth Toe

### Definition
Congenital overriding fifth toe is an abnormality present at birth, in which the fifth toe is adducted, dorsiflexed, and medially deviated, generally lying over the metatarsal phalangeal joint of the fourth toe (Fig. 30.45).

### Epidemiology
The true incidence of this deformity is unknown, because mild forms of the disorder are present in an asymptomatic state, below the threshold for treatment. There is no sex predilection. In 20% to 30% of cases, bilateral involvement is present (322–324).

### Pathogenesis
The cause of a dorsal dislocation or overriding fifth toe is unknown but there is a familial predilection for this deformity (323).

### Clinical Features
In this state, the fifth toe is dorsiflexed and overlies to some degree the fourth toe and fourth metatarsal phalangeal joint. The interphalangeal joints are normal. The skin tends to be contracted a bit dorsally and medially, but there is no stress or abnormality on the skin.

### Radiographic Features
Although difficult to image, x-ray films should be taken to determine whether or not the metatarsal phalangeal joint is subluxed or dislocated prior to surgical treatment.

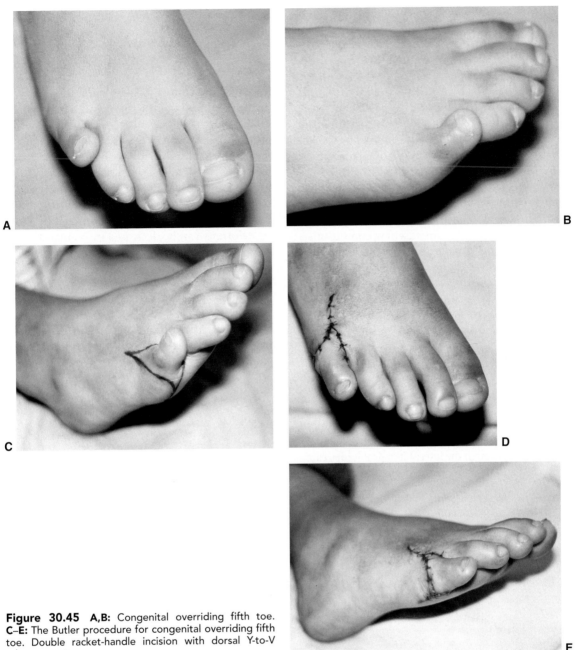

**Figure 30.45 A,B:** Congenital overriding fifth toe. **C–E:** The Butler procedure for congenital overriding fifth toe. Double racket-handle incision with dorsal Y-to-V advancement.

### Pathoanatomy

There is a contracture of the dorsomedial capsule of the fifth metatarsal phalangeal joint, but the toe is not a clawed toe. Flexion deformity of the interphalangeal joint does not occur. Shortening of the extensor tendons of the fifth toe is generally present and must relate to the dorsal position of the toe. The entire toe is translated proximally and medially.

### Natural History

Actual incidence of pain from this condition is uncertain, but it has been stated that approximately half of affected individuals will experience symptoms from this deformity, generally from shoe wear (323).

### Treatment

Although there is no proven efficacy to stretching and taping of the toe, it may be of benefit to patients in whom the deformity is somewhat mild. Education about the reasonably good prognosis of the untreated state is worth pursuing; however, in the case of a committed family with a patient having mild deformity, taping may be of value. In taping, a loop of standard adhesive tape is brought around the toe and it provides a plantar tether to the toe.

Surgery is indicated for roughly 50% of adolescents and adults who experience pain with shoe fitting (323). The toe in its medially deviated and dorsiflexed state will overlie the metatarsal phalangeal joint just at the point where the shoe fold will lie.

Many surgical procedures have been proposed to correct this, including partial or complete excision of the proximal phalanx and syndactylization to the fourth toe (325). Only fair results have been reported with this approach, and secondary deformities persist in many cases (325). Amputation is only a salvage procedure. The Butler procedure (322,324) originally reported by Cockin (323) is a very successful approach for the management of this condition. A racket-handle incision is made to release the contracted soft tissues dorsally and medially, mobilize the neurovascular bundles, and free the toe for translation. The toe is then translated plantarlaterally. Although there is a risk of neurovascular compromise, this is very infrequent. Plantar skin reconstruction with a VY advancement resolves the problem of the soft tissue tether. If the toe spontaneously subluxes, further release of the dorsal capsule and dorsal soft tissues should be done, and the toe can be pinned in position across the metatarsal phalangeal joint at the time of the soft-tissue reconstruction.

## Curly Toe

### Definition

A "curly toe" is a congenital deformity in which one or more of the toes are flexed and have a varus deformity, generally with lateral rotation through the interphalangeal joints, causing the toe to curl and lie under the adjacent or more medial toe (Fig. 30.46).

### Epidemiology

Curly toe is a very common deformity, although the true incidence is not known. It is very frequently bilateral and symmetric, with high familial incidence (326,327).

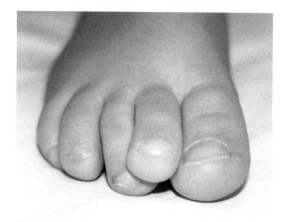

**Figure 30.46** The curly toe deformity generally results from a tight toe flexor as seen in the third toe in this patient. Another possible etiology is an abnormally shaped phalanx that may result in fixed deformity and require osteotomy or fusion for correction of persistent deformity.

### Pathogenesis

The cause is unknown; the condition is often associated with a tight toe flexor, but not always.

### Clinical Features

The third and fourth toes are most frequently involved. The distal phalanx or the distal and middle phalanges are pulled under the adjacent medial toe with flexion, varus, and external rotation of the distal and proximal phalanges. The nail plate of the affected toe often faces laterally. If the deformity is magnified when dorsiflexion of the foot and the MP joint tighten the flexor tendon of the toe, the primary pathologic structure causing the deformity is probably the toe flexor. This can be confirmed by showing that the deformity can be decreased by plantar-flexing the foot and ankle, thereby relaxing the toe flexor.

### Radiographic Features

Radiographs are neither needed nor helpful in the young child.

The flexor digitorum longus and the flexor digitorum brevis tendons may be affected and contracted in curly toe deformity (328). Joint capsules are generally not affected. Occasionally this deformity results from a trapezoidal deformity of the bone, and the curly toe deformity is unrelated to flexor tendon but secondary to structural abnormality of the toe.

### Natural History

Curly toes are generally asymptomatic in young children. Many improve in shape spontaneously (327,328). They may become symptomatic in older children, adolescents, or adults, because of exaggerated pressure on the skin and nails of malaligned toes. The nail of the underlying toe often cuts the plantar surface of the overlying toe, causing symptoms.

### Treatment

Stretching and taping have no proven efficacy in the treatment of curly toes (327) but may work in mild cases. The family may be educated that, in general, symptoms are rare and long-term disability is unlikely. Some patients do experience continued pain and problems from curly toe deformity. If associated with a tight toe flexor, stretching exercises might be of benefit. Prior to embarking on surgical treatment, an attempt at correction of a tight tendon may be of value. Surgery is indicated if there are callosities and cutting of one toe into the other, secondary to this deformity. Another indication is an unacceptable problem with nail deformity.

Tenotomy of the flexor tendon has been successful in 95% to 100% of cases (326,328). A double-blind, randomized prospective study comparing simple tenotomy of the long toe flexor to Girdlestone-Taylor transfer showed no difference in outcome (329). In this study, 19 patients with bilateral deformity involving the third and fourth toes were operated on, using a flexor tenotomy release on one side and a flexor tenotomy with flexon transfer procedure on the other. At 4-year follow-up, it appeared that there was no difference between the two procedures and that simple tenotomy of the flexor tendon is sufficient treatment for the symptomatic curly toe.

## Accessory Navicular

### Definition

"Accessory navicular" is a term applied to a plantar medial enlargement of the tarsal navicular beyond its normal size. A separate bone, either in the posterior tibial tendon (such as sesamoid bone) or with a true articulation with the navicular, is within the breadth of this diagnosis. Other terms that have been used to describe the separate ossicle are the os tibiale externum, the navicular secundum, or the prehallux (Fig. 30.47).

### Epidemiology

The accessory tarsal navicular is the most common accessory bone in the foot, occurring in between 4% and 14% of the population (162,330,331). It is frequently bilateral and occurs more commonly in women. Geist (331) recognized a higher incidence of accessory naviculars in young patients evaluated radiologically than in cadaver studies.

### Pathogenesis

McKusick (332) believed that accessory navicular was inherited as an autosomal dominant trait. Geist (332) suggested that three possible situations accounted for the accessory navicular: (i) bone within the substance of the posterior tibial tendon as a sesamoid bone, (ii) bone with a true articulation (synovial-joint) with the navicular and (iii) a synchondrosis.

### Clinical Features

Accessory navicular tends to produce symptoms in adolescents. There is a firm prominence distal to the talar head on the plantar medial aspect of the midfoot. This may be associated with flexible flatfoot (333–336). The accessory navicular, however, is a primary abnormality in the navicular and posterior tibial tendon relationship and is not related to flexible flatfoot (337). The prominence of the navicular is associated with point tenderness; it can be differentiated from the prominence of the talar head in a flatfoot deformity by inverting and everting through the subtalar joint with a thumb over the bony prominence.

Individuals suspected of having an accessory navicular should have standing anteroposterior and lateral radiographs in order to define the abnormality of the navicular. Bilateral films may be indicated, as there is a high incidence of symmetrical abnormalities.

Accessory navicular may be a pathologic finding leading to foot pain, or perhaps an associated abnormality not related to the clinical disorder with which the patient presents for evaluation. Therefore, careful examination differentiating other causes of foot pain is mandatory. Patients with accessory navicular may present with complex pain patterns requiring very careful examination prior to treatment (338). They may even have a peroneal spastic flat foot.

### Radiographic Features

In general, standing anteroposterior and lateral radiographs of the foot are diagnostic of accessory navicular. There are three types of accessory navicular (339) (Fig. 30.47). In type I accessory navicular, which is rarely symptomatic, a small sesamoid bone is located in the posterior

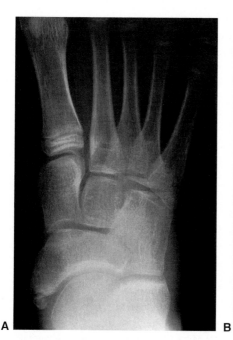
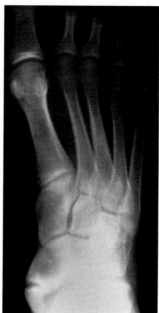
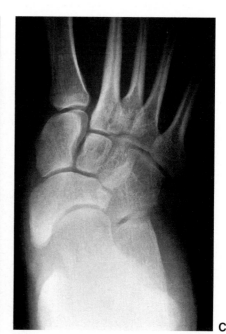

**Figure 30.47** Accessory navicular. **A:** Type I. **B:** Type II. **C:** Type III.

tibialis tendon. Type II accessory navicular is the most frequently symptomatic type, which is a bullet-shaped ossicle joined to the tuberosity of the navicular by a synchondrosis. Type III is a large horn-shaped navicular, which most likely is the result of fusion of a type II accessory navicular with the progress of age.

### Pathoanatomy

There is proliferating vascular and mesenchymal tissue, with growth of fibrocartilage and evidence of bone turnover, in the tissue between the ossicle and the main body of the navicular in the painful type II accessory navicular (339). These histologic findings are consistent with healing microfracture or a chronic stress fracture, substantiating the opinion that repetitive stress leads to this injury. There is a possibility of finding inflammatory cells at some stage in the healing process, but the primary pathology is associated with healing microfracture rather than chronic inflammation.

### Natural History

Accessory naviculars are for the most part asymptomatic. If symptoms do occur, a period of protection from stress and injury generally returns the patient to the asymptomatic state (335).

### Treatment

Nonsurgical treatment of accessory navicular often relieves symptoms. Pain is related to a state similar to that seen in stress fracture or Osgood-Schlatter disease. The decrease in direct pressure over the accessory navicular, as well as decreasing stress from the posterior tibial tendon insertion, may result in relief of symptoms. This can be done with an orthotic device or arch support or a soft shoe and a pad placed around the navicular to decrease direct pressure over it. Finally, the patient can be given a short leg cast to decrease symptoms by decreasing stress from the posterior tibial tendon insertion.

If pain is persistent after a period of observation and immobilization, surgery is indicated. There are two possible operations for treating the accessory navicular. The first is simple excision of the ossicle and the expanded portion of the navicular through a tendon-splitting approach (331–344). In this procedure, the skin incision should be made dorsal to the prominence of the accessory navicular. The bone is removed to a point where the medial foot has no bony prominence over the navicular, between the head of the talus and the first cuneiform. This generally requires removing the accessory navicular as well as a prominent portion of the navicular. Symptoms are relieved in 90% of cases by this procedure.

The second possible procedure is a Kidner procedure (333,334), in which the posterior tibial tendon is advanced along the medial side of the foot with the hope of supporting the longitudinal arch. In this procedure, the ossicle and the prominent medial aspect of the navicular are excised, just as in the simple excision procedure, but the posterior tibial tendon is advanced. There appears to be no benefit to the advancement of the posterior tibial tendon relative to the simple excision procedure (12,340).

## Congenital Hallux Varus

### Definition

Congenital hallux varus is the medial deviation of the great toe on the first metatarsal, present at birth. It occurs as an isolated deformity but is often associated with other malformations of the foot, particularly, short first metatarsal; bracket epiphysis of the first metatarsal, both pre- and postaxial polydactyly; and a fibrous band that acts as a tether along the medial side of the great toe, extending to the base of the first metatarsal (Fig. 30.48) (345,346).

### Epidemiology

This is a rare condition with unknown incidence. Inheritance pattern and other characteristics are not reported.

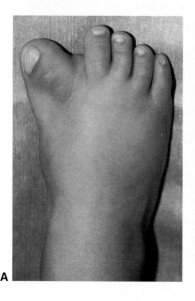 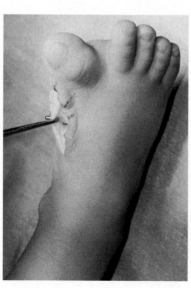

**Figure 30.48   A:** Clinical appearance of congenital hallux varus. **B:** Fibrous band between the hallux and the cartilaginous duplicate tarsal anlage.

### Pathogenesis

The cause of this deformity is not known, but it is associated with a first metatarsal that is short and rounded, leading to a very abnormal metatarsal-phalangeal articulation and medial deviation of the great toe with an enlarged web space between the first and second digit. Healthy growth of the first metatarsal is generally compromised, and the medial tether leads to recurrence.

### Clinical Features

The great toe may be adducted as much as 90 degrees and cannot be aligned by passive manipulation (Fig. 30.48). This should be differentiated from the medial deviation of the great toe, which is a flexible and very common deformity seen in association with metatarsus adductus. The hallmarks of the congenital deformity are the fibrous band along the medial side of the foot, the widened web space between the first and second digit, and the abnormality of the first metatarsal. Duplication of the great toe with preaxial polydactyly is quite common, and this may be associated with a complex syndactyly, as seen in Apert syndrome (243).

### Radiologic Features

A standing anteroposterior and lateral radiograph should be done to assess the varus alignment of the great toe. The deformity of the first metatarsal can be partially delineated on initial x-ray films. However, the longitudinal physeal bracket, which may not be easily seen on initial films, is suggested by a D-shape to the metatarsal, with no cortical differentiation along the convex medial border of the epiphysis (347) (Fig. 30.49A).

### Pathoanatomy

A possible explanation for a single varus toe is that the origin of the deformity is related to preaxial polydactyly or duplication of the great toe. The more medial extra digit degenerates into a fibrous band, rather than fully forming a digit with a corresponding metatarsal. The rudimentary medial structure then forms a fibrous band that acts as a bowstring, pulling the hallux into a varus position (348) (Fig. 30.48B).

In the foot with a longitudinal bracket epiphysis, a growth disorder leading to progressive relative shortening of the first metatarsal occurs, unless addressed.

### Natural History

In the absence of treatment, shoe fitting becomes increasingly difficult or impossible (346). Mild forms of hallux varus with a flexible deformity generally resolve spontaneously, but that condition should be differentiated from congenital hallux varus.

### Treatment

There is no role for conservative management of this deformity. Surgical management is indicated with the specific procedures to be done depending upon the anatomy in the individual case. The issues to be considered are correction of polydactyly if present; correction of the soft tissue tether on the medial side of the foot and the enlarged web space between the great and second toe; correction of metatarsal-phalangeal joint incongruity; and correction of metatarsal or bracket epiphyseal deformity (349).

Soft tissue release and resection procedures have been described by McElvenny (345) and Farmer (350) when the metatarsal is normal. Mills and Menelaus (348) found that soft tissue realignment procedures were often unsatisfactory

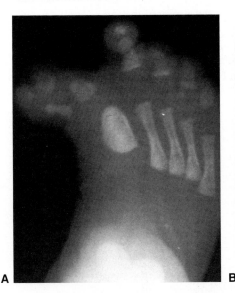
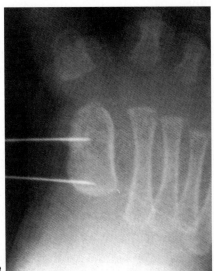
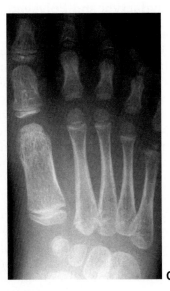

**Figure 30.49**  **A:** Radiographic appearance of congenital hallux varus with a metatarsal longitudinal epiphyseal bracket. **B:** Pins mark the extent of the resection of the longitudinal epiphyseal bracket. **C:** Radiographic appearance 5 years after resection and fat grafting of the longitudinal epiphyseal bracket. The metatarsal has grown normally.

because of shortness of the first metatarsal and growth disorder. In the soft tissue reconstruction of this deformity, which is part of any surgical procedure, lengthening the medial tether is mandatory. This requires resection of the fibrous band as well as Z-plasties in the skin to increase the length along the medial side of the foot. The abductor hallucis must be released and the tether on the capsule must also be released.

The skin of the web space between the first and second toe is resected and the medial reefing of the capsule done if possible. The incongruity of the metatarsal phalangeal joint may need to be dealt with by using a K-wire to hold the great toe in position while remodeling occurs following surgical reconstruction.

The second issue to be dealt with is the bony deformity of the metatarsal. Mubarak et al. (347) demonstrated that resection and interposition grafting of a longitudinal epiphyseal bracket is an effective technique to treat growth disorders resulting from this epiphyseal deformity (Fig. 30.49B and C). When the longitudinal portion of the bracket is excised, interposition material with fat or methylmethacrylate can be used, as with any physeal bridge resection. This procedure is always combined with a soft tissue reconstruction and resection of duplication of the digits. An opening wedge osteotomy may be combined in some cases in which the extra bone from the toe can be used as part of an opening wedge osteotomy.

Late onset of degenerative arthrosis of the first metatarsal phalangeal joint can be managed by arthrodesis (346). Alternative treatments for pain with residual shortening and deformity include metatarsal lengthening and amputation. Amputation is a particularly valuable alternative in the management of severe congenital hallux varus deformity in Apert syndrome (243).

## Polydactyly and Polysyndactyly

### Definition
Polydactyly refers to a congenital abnormality in which extra digits are present, with or without duplication of the corresponding metatarsal. Preaxial polydactyly refers to the medial side of the foot and postaxial polydactyly to the lateral side of the foot. Simple syndactyly refers to a failure of separation of otherwise healthy digits with skin connection only. Complex syndactyly refers to fusion of bone in the digit or metatarsals in adjacent rays.

### Epidemiology
The incidence of polydactyly is 0.3 to 1.3 per 1000 live births in whites and 3.6 to 13.9 per 1000 live births in blacks (351,352). Fifty percent of cases are bilateral, and of the bilateral cases 62% are symmetric (353). Of the patients with polydactyly of the feet, 34% have hand involvement (353). Polydactyly may be inherited as an autosomal dominant trait with variable penetrance (354) but is more likely to occur as an isolated trait.

### Pathogenesis
The cause of polydactyly is unknown. Presumably, there is failure of differentiation in the apical ectodermal ridge (AER) during the first trimester of pregnancy, leading to polydactyly and polysyndactyly (353). Experimentally, polydactyly can be produced by radiation, cytotoxins, and folic acid deprivation.

### Clinical Features
Temtami and McKusick (354) classified polydactyly as preaxial if the great toe is duplicated and postaxial if the duplication involved the lateral side of the foot. The term "central" may be applied to a duplication of the second, third, or fourth toe, if this can be differentiated. Phelps and Grogan (353) in a review of 194 supernumerary toes showed 79% to be postaxial, whereas 15% were preaxial and 6% central. Considerable variation exists and more than one type may be present in a single foot (Fig. 30.50). Syndactyly may accompany the extra digit, and toenails may be fused or separated. Central and postaxial polydactyly tend to be well aligned, whereas the preaxial polydactyly may be associated with congenital hallux varus, short first metatarsal, and longitudinal bracket epiphysis (347,349).

### Radiographic Features
A morphologic classification of the abnormalities of metatarsals and phalanges in the foot was proposed by Venn-Watson (355) (Fig. 30.51). The classification system is based primarily on metatarsal abnormalities. The metatarsals are present on radiographic views at birth, but generally radiographic evaluation is delayed in order to allow full ossification of the phalanges for surgical planning.

### Natural History
Untreated polydactyly may cause problems with shoe fitting and angular deformity of the toe.

### Treatment
The management of a duplicated digit is determined by the family to some degree. A postaxial or central polydactyly

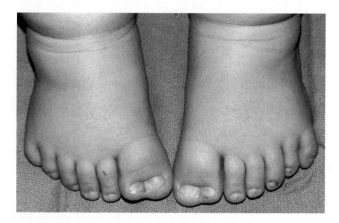

**Figure 30.50** Preaxial and postaxial bilateral polydactyly.

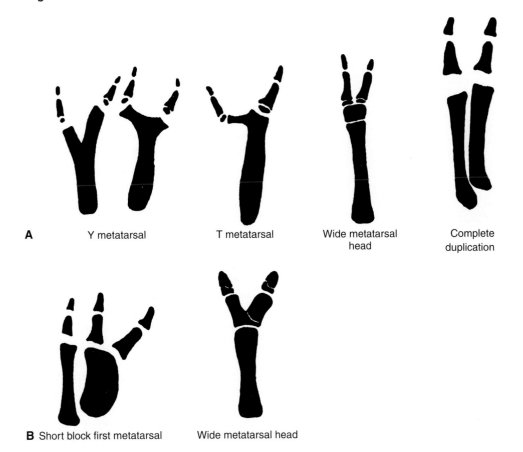

**Figure 30.51**    Venn-Watson classification of polydactyly. **A:** Postaxial. **B:** Preaxial. (From Venn-Watson EA. Problems in polydactyly of the foot. *Orthop Clin North Am* 1976;7:909–927, with permission.)

with proper alignment of the digit may remain in place unless the foot is significantly widened. However, a malaligned toe, particularly preaxial polydactyly, requires surgical treatment. Lateral or postaxial polydactyly is generally treated with excision, with the assumption that this is a relatively simple procedure in infancy and the wide foot will become a problem with shoe fitting in the future.

In general, the most malaligned toe is resected, but effort is made to always remove the border digit of the foot (353,356). Division of a synchondrosis at the base of the proximal phalanx is quite safe, and growth arrest is highly unlikely. Likewise, an enlarged metatarsal head may be reduced in size by performing a transphyseal longitudinal osteotomy (353). In a case with a duplicated metatarsal or Y-shaped metatarsal, the corresponding metatarsal abnormality should always be removed at the time of resection of the extra digit.

In cases of polysyndactyly, the most malaligned phalanges and associated toenail generally are removed through a racket-type incision (353,356). The nail fold should be recreated to prevent problems with chronic ingrown toenail. As polydactyly is often associated with syndactyly, a decision must be made about reconstruction of both the extra digit and the syndactyly. In general, the skin bridge between the toes is left in place and the lateral border digit removed, if surgery is chosen (356).

Postaxial polydactyly generally results in satisfactory outcome with excellent results. Preaxial polydactyly, on the other hand, is more likely to result in residual varus deformity, short metatarsal, and unsatisfactory outcome. Attention to the longitudinal epiphyseal bracket (347) may result in improved length of the first ray and should be considered in cases when this deformity is present with preaxial polydactyly.

## Syndactyly

### Definition

Syndactyly of the toes is a fusion of adjacent digits involving soft tissue (simple syndactyly), or soft tissue and bone (complex syndactyly). The most common fused digits are the second and third, which may be either complete or incomplete (Fig. 30.52).

### Epidemiology

Syndactyly is a common, often inherited trait that is frequently bilateral.

### Pathogenesis

Pathogenesis is unknown, but presumably in early fetal development there is a failure of separation of cells in the AER.

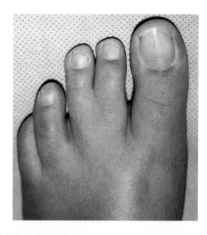

**Figure 30.52**   Clinically benign zygosyndactyly.

### Clinical Features

Webbing of the toes is rarely associated with the angular abnormality of the digit that causes problems. Occasionally, differential length of the toes may result in a flexion deformity of the longer toe and a callus over the proximal interphalangeal (PIP) joint. Rarely, this may become a problem with pain.

### Radiographic Features

Radiographs should be done if deformity is present and surgical management is planned, in order to differentiate simple from complex syndactyly.

### Natural History

In general, syndactyly of adjacent digits is asymptomatic throughout life, and surgical treatment and adaptive shoe wear are generally not needed.

### Treatment

Surgical treatment in general is not warranted for syndactyly as comfort and function are not impaired. Given presently available footwear, which often includes a strap between the first and second toes, a case can be made for surgical management in select cases. Caution must be exercised, as the surgical scars may be less cosmetically pleasing than the condition itself and lead to angular deviation of digits from contracture, where satisfactory alignment was present in the preoperative state. Unlike fingers, discriminatory function of individual digits is not required in the toes, and toe syndactyly is rarely surgically managed. If toe deformity is occurring because of differential growth, a case for surgical reconstruction may be made.

## Macrodactyly

Macrodactyly is a term used to describe enlargement of both hands and feet. It may involve single digits or the entire hand or foot. Macrodactyly may occur as part of a syndrome such as Proteus syndrome (357) or Klippel-Trenaunay-Weber syndrome (venous lymphatic malformation). Some have described the condition of macrodactyly as congenital lipofibromatosis. Another term similarly applied to it is macrodystrophia lipomatosa. Finally, the findings of macrodactyly may be present in a lymphatic malformation or in patients with lymphedema. CT scan, MRI, and physical examination will help to differentiate the above conditions.

Kalen et al. (358) reported a large series of patients with macrodactyly, in which they documented the low incidence of this condition, as well as a male predilection. It was also determined that the second digit is most commonly involved, and multiple digit involvement is present in approximately 50% of cases (Fig. 30.53).

### Pathogenesis

The cause of this condition is unknown and there is no clear inheritance pattern (358). Turra et al. (359) hypothesized a nerve trunk disease as the cause of macrodactyly, but this theory has not been confirmed (358).

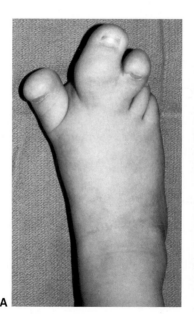
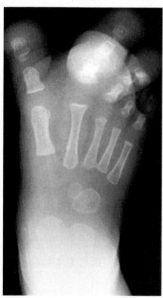

**A**   **B**

**Figure 30.53  A:** Macrodactyly most commonly involves the second ray; in this case, the first and third are involved to some degree. **B:** Radiographic appearance demonstrates enlargement of bone as well as soft tissue.

### Clinical Features

An enlarged digit is present at birth and characterized as "macrodactyly." Features of Klippel-Trenaunay-Webber and neurofibromatosis should be checked for. In neurofibromatosis, café au lait spots are frequently apparent. In Proteus syndrome, a cerebriform skin pattern on the plantar surface of the foot as well as asymmetries of growth and nevi are present. Surprisingly, in Klippel-Trenaunay-Webber, a syndrome of venous lymphatic malformation, ipsilateral macrodactyly is frequently present with a vascular component, and contralateral macrodactyly is present as a fibrofatty disorder. Fifty percent of patients with foot involvement in macrodactyly have a dorsally angled digit with weak toe flexors (360).

### Radiographic Features

Standing anteroposterior and lateral radiographs of the foot are useful for monitoring growth rates of digits and for surgical planning. MRI (361) is of value in macrodactyly in order to differentiate cases of vascular malformation in association with macrodactyly from true fibro-fatty disorders or lymphedema.

### Pathoanatomy

There is enlargement of both soft tissue and bony tissues in the foot. In general, there is an overabundance of fibrofatty tissue, often in a neural distribution. The cause of the overgrowth remains unknown.

### Natural History

Macrodactyly may be progressive, with proportional growth throughout the life of the child. It may, however, be progressive with disproportionate overgrowth compared to healthy digits (362). The type with progressive overgrowth is more likely (358). It may be disabling, with respect to shoe fitting and the possibility of wearing commercially available shoes.

### Treatment

In cases of macrodactyly, the treatment of a child needs to be individualized and must be recognized to be a long-term commitment to that child and family. Treatment involves several options including soft tissue debulking, amputation, and epiphyseodesis. In general, ray resection of the toe and corresponding metatarsal are the most satisfactory procedures to use in dealing with this condition of the foot (363). Toe amputation alone has not been cosmetically satisfactory, nor has it resulted in significant improvement of the foot deformity. In mild cases, epiphyseodesis of the proximal phalanx (364) and of the distal metatarsal, as well as surgical debulking, may be of some value (358,359,364–367). Ray resection combined with debulking of soft tissue has the best outcome and lowest risk of recurrent deformity, achieving the goal of shoe fitting with commercially available footwear in some cases (358,359,367) (Fig. 30.54). In selecting the timing for epiphyseodesis of the foot, the author generally uses an x-ray film of the affected child's parent's foot in order to predict the approximate rate of growth of the healthy foot and therefore timing of epiphyseodesis. Growth charts for the size of the foot were developed by Green (Fig. 30.1); however, it is preferable to use the size of the parent's foot and the size of the contralateral foot for timing of epiphyseodesis. A successful ray resection should remove the entire metatarsal. If the proximal metatarsal is left in place, the space between the first and second metatarsal remains wide and an unsatisfactory outcome will result.

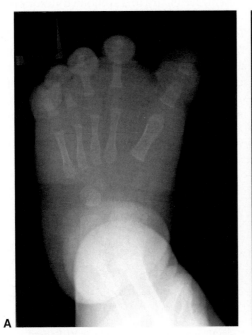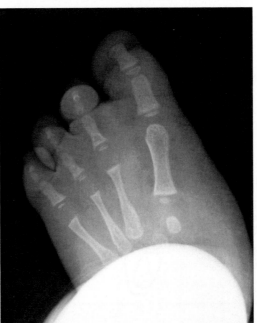

A B

**Figure 30.54** Macrodactyly of the foot is most effectively managed by a second ray resection in general. The width of the foot can be reduced by resecting the entire second metatarsal.

One should expect multiple debulking procedures to be necessary in the management of macrodactyly, and the parents should understand this at the outset of the procedure. The author has found that debulking procedures in the presence of lymphedema are less successful than in cases of fibro-fatty type macrodactyly or vascular malformation.

## Cleft Foot (Ectrodactyly)

### Definition

A cleft foot is characterized by a central deficiency involving soft tissue and bone (368). The term "lobster claw foot" used by Cruveilhier (368) in 1829 is no longer appropriate as a description of this clinical condition.

### Epidemiology

The cleft foot is a rare condition with an overall occurrence rate of 1 per 90,000 live births (369). The most common form of this condition is inherited as an autosomal dominant condition with variable penetrance (369–371). The much less common form of this condition has an incidence of approximately 1 per 150,000 live births, in which there is a spontaneous mutation and no evidence of a familial condition. Approximately 10% of cleft feet are of this pattern (372). Boys are affected more frequently than girls.

### Pathogenesis

This condition results from an abnormality in tissue differentiation at the AER (373); such a defect might be caused by genetic or toxic influence, leading to an error in differentiation. Such irregularities may lead to polydactyly or syndactyly or the much more rare central defect of cleft foot. Watson and Bonde (374) proposed that a specific region in the AER localized to the second or third ray, which is the typical area for deficiency in a cleft foot. They further proposed that the extent of damage to the AER would relate to both the width and depth of the cleft defect of the foot.

### Clinical Features

The range of cleft foot is from a simple deepening of an interdigital space to a central ray deficiency or even a monodactylous foot (375). Associated abnormalities include cleft hand, cleft lip and palate, deafness, urinary tract abnormalities, triphalangeal thumbs, and tibial hemimelia.

### Radiographic Features

The classification of the cleft foot into six types (Fig. 30.55) was done by Blauth and Borisch (375). The classification system is based on the extent of bony deficiency of the central rays, culminating in a foot with a nearly absent medial ray.

Beyond this classification system are two forms of cleft foot: the monodactylous foot with a single ray, and a tibial diastasis with central ray deficiency of the foot. Other variations include cross bones and synostosis (Fig. 30.56). Radiographs of the foot should be taken at presentation in order to classify the deformity appropriately. Other diagnostic studies include renal ultrasonography as indicated to rule out renal abnormalities as they are frequently associated with cleft foot.

### Pathoanatomy

Synostosis and significant abnormalities of the tarsal bones may coexist with cleft foot and should be considered (375). Often a hallux valgus results from the pull of a conjoined flexor and extensor, resulting in an abductor as a component of this deformity.

### Natural History

Many patients with cleft foot function well and can wear regular shoes without pain or compromise of function. For such individuals, no surgical treatment may be required. However, in many cases of cleft feet there is a marked increase in width (Fig. 30.57), which prevents normal shoe fitting. Painful callosities develop over the medial and lateral metatarsal heads. A severe hallux valgus is frequently present, secondary to a conjoined flexor extensor tendon.

### Treatment

Treatment of the cleft foot should focus on the goal of the ability to wear a standard shoe without pain and with good function. A secondary goal is reconstructing the foot to a socially acceptable appearance. Surgical repair is recommended for feet in which a significant improvement can be

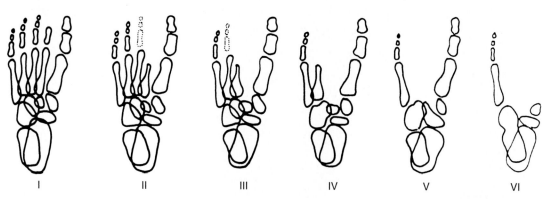

**Figure 30.55**   Cleft foot classification according to Blauth and Borisch. (From Blauth W, Borisch NC. Cleft feet. Proposals for a new classification based on roentgenographic morphology. *Clin Orthop* 1990; 258:41–48, with permission.)

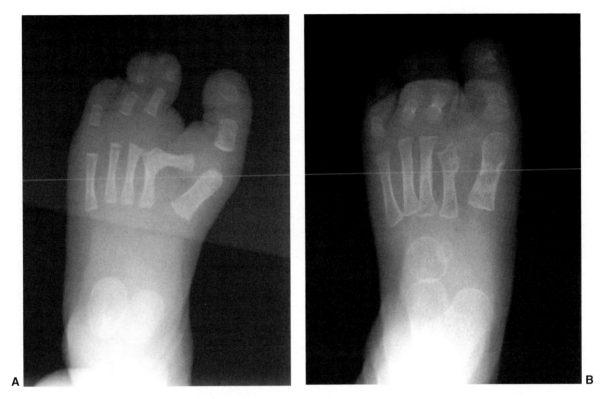

**Figure 30.56    A:** This patient had a mild cleft foot with a transverse metatarsal bridging the cleft and widening the foot. **B:** With repair of the cleft and removal of the transverse metatarsal, a healthy foot resulted.

made in the shape of the foot, facilitating shoe wear and improving function. In recommending surgical repair, it should be remembered that most cleft feet can function quite well without repair. Bony prominences, medially and laterally, cause pain because of direct pressure from footwear, rather than pain from walking. Wood et al. (376) recommended surgical therapy for closure of a cleft foot, in which soft tissue is reconstructed by a series of rectangular flaps. The flaps are approximated and metatarsal osteotomies performed. Their reported experience was of 42 operations in 15 affected feet that were felt to warrant surgical repair, and their recommended age of patients was between 6 and 12 months. The author has resorted to

reconstruction, creating a web space using a Barsky flap from one of the border digits to define the depth of the new web space, and closure of the cleft using a zigzag skin repair. In addition to the skin repair, the underlying tendon reconstruction and metatarsal osteotomies are important in this reconstruction (Fig. 30.58). There frequently is a conjoined flexor and extensor tendon to the great toe functioning as an adductor and causing a severe hallux valgus. The recognition of this with centralization of both the extensor and flexor tendon and division of the conjoined tendon as an adductor is important. Metatarsal osteotomies and midtarsal osteotomies are used to narrow the foot and reconstruct the cleft, in addition to soft tissue repair. Complex plastic surgical procedures to create the appearance of toes have been described, but they do not produce functional benefit (377).

## ACQUIRED CONDITIONS

### Cavus Foot Deformity

#### Definition

The cavus foot is one with an elevated longitudinal arch. The high arch may be secondary to plantar-flexion deformity of the forefoot (forefoot equinus) or dorsiflexion of the calcaneus (378). The hindfoot is generally in varus, but may be laterally oriented or in valgus at times. The forefoot is generally pronated with a plantar-flexed first ray.

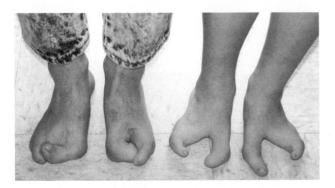

**Figure 30.57**    Father and son with cleft feet.

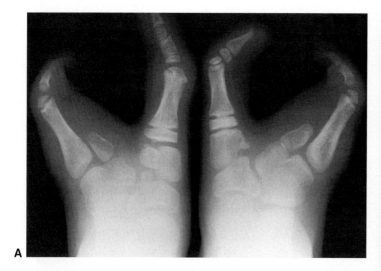

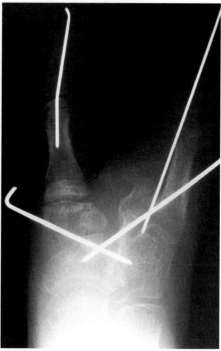

**Figure 30.58** Preoperative **(A)** and postoperative **(B)** radiographs of symptomatic cleft foot treated with osteotomies.

### Pathogenesis

A cavus foot results from muscle imbalance between opposing extrinsic or intrinsic muscle groups. A very high proportion, greater than two thirds, of patients with a cavus foot have an underlying neurologic disorder (379). The number of cases termed "idiopathic" cavus foot continues to decrease as diagnostic methods improve. The diagnosis of hereditary sensory motor neuropathy (HSMN), which includes the types I and II Charcot-Marie-Tooth (CMT) (380), is the most common neurologic disorder resulting in this deformity. On physical examination, in addition to considering the array of systemic diseases resulting in cavus foot, one should also explore the structural abnormality and muscle imbalance that leads to this

disorder. Forefoot plantar flexion involving primarily the first ray is the most common structural problem leading to a cavus foot. In this state, the first ray plantar flexion compromises the normal tripod structure of the foot, shifting weight bearing laterally and driving the hindfoot into varus. This may result from weak anterior tibial muscle relative to peroneus longus muscle (7), overpull of the extensor hallucis longus compensating for a weak anterior tibial muscle (68), or intrinsic muscle contracture of the foot with weakness (2). With time, the plantar fascia contracts and the varus hindfoot deformity becomes fixed. The second major group of cavus feet are those with a dorsiflexion deformity of the calcaneus; this generally is the result of weakness in the gastrocsoleus complex (Fig. 30.59) and a

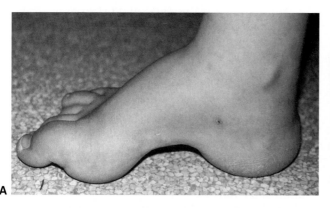

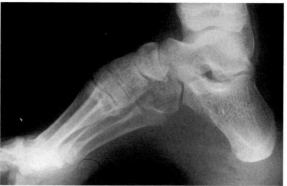

**Figure 30.59** Calcaneocavus deformity in a child with myelomeningocele. **A:** Transtarsal cavus with thick callosities under the calcaneus and the metatarsal heads. **B:** Radiograph of the calcaneocavus "pistol-grip" deformity.

compensatory push-off augmented by toe flexors. Any abnormality in the neuromuscular axis may affect muscle balance in the foot, contributing to a cavus deformity. Bilateral involvement suggests a systemic condition, whereas unilateral cavus deformities suggest a more localized differential diagnosis (Table 30.2).

## Epidemiology

The cavus foot occurs at the frequency of the underlying neurologic condition. That is, the frequency of CMT or Freidrich ataxia in a given population will define the frequency of the cavus foot that is secondary to these deformities.

## Clinical Features and Presentation

Presenting symptoms of a patient with cavus foot are generally related to either instability or pain. Instability may be secondary to muscle weakness, sensory loss, or deformity (381). The pain is generally related to prominence of the metatarsal heads, callosities over the toes, or malalignment increasing the stresses of weight bearing. Muscle contraction is not required to maintain erect posture with a healthy, balanced foot. With excessive plantar flexion of the first ray, the normal tripod (first metatarsal, fifth

## TABLE 30.2
### CAUSES OF CAVUS FOOT DEFORMITY

**Bilateral**
Charcot-Marie-Tooth disease
Friedreich ataxia
Dejerine-Sottas interstitial hypertrophic neuritis
Polyneuritis
Roussy-Lévy syndrome
Spinal muscular atrophy
Myelomeningocele
Syringomyelia
Spinal cord tumor
Diastematomyelia
Spinal dysraphism (tethered cord)
Muscular dystrophy
Cerebral palsy—paraparesis or quadriparesis (although usually planus deformities)
Familial (consider Charcot-Marie-Tooth disease)
Clubfoot/recurrent clubfoot
Idiopathic cause (diagnosis of exclusion)

**Unilateral**
Traumatic injury of a peripheral nerve or spinal root nerve
Poliomyelitis
Syringomyelia
Lipomeningocele
Spinal cord tumor
Diastematomyelia
Spinal dysraphism (tethered cord)
Tendon laceration
Overlengthened Achilles tendon
Cerebral palsy—hemiparesis
Clubfoot/recurrent clubfoot
Compartment syndrome of the leg
Severe burn of the leg
Crush injury of the leg

metatarsal, and calcaneus) is lost, leading to an abnormal force distribution. In the malaligned state, not only are stresses increased across joints and pressures increased on bony prominences, but also muscle strength is required to maintain posture. The combination of these leads to pain, fatigue, and instability.

Clinical presentation varies from patient to patient. A frequently reported symptom is a recurrent spraining of the ankle with a feeling of giving out. Ligament injuries as well as the malalignment lead to pain. Blistering and calluses result over bony prominences. This is particularly true over the dorsal aspects of the interphalangeal (IP) and PIP joints, as well as the plantar aspect under the metatarsal head and lateral border of the fifth metatarsal. Muscle weakness related to the underlying condition leads to giving out with loss of the dynamic stabilizers of the ankle, particularly the peroneal muscles. Finally, sensory loss, particularly position and vibratory, disrupts the normal feedback loop that provides dynamic stabilization of the ankle.

As a cavus foot is generally secondary to an underlying neuromuscular abnormality, symptoms at presentation may reflect the underlying condition. A history of change in foot shape or change in foot size is important. Family history is critical; if possible, examination of other members of the family, rather than simply asking for history of underlying medical conditions, can often be revealing because a subtle cavus foot may be present. Further medical, birth, and developmental histories, as well as a review of systems, are mandatory in searching for underlying causes of cavus foot.

The clinical examination should be done, observing a patient's stance (Fig. 30.60) and gait first. In a sitting position, the foot can appear to have a high arch but be completely flat in stance. In the swing phase of gait, the foot dorsiflexion may be the result of isolated extensor hallucis longus (EHL) contraction, rather than a coordinated activity of anterior tibial as well as EHL and toe extensors. Look at foot position at heel strike, as weight may immediately shift to the lateral border of the foot. Does heel strike occur or is forefoot equinus preventing heel strike and there is no contact of the calcaneus with the ground? Are there any compensatory features of gait present such as knee hyperextension or Trendelenburg compensation at the hip? The spine should be evaluated for evidence of scoliosis, cutaneous defects over the spine typical in diastomatomyelia, or fatty deposits seen in lipomeningoceles.

A detailed muscle examination including strength testing and reflexes must be done in all cases. Sensory examination should include light touch, pain, and vibratory sense. Stocking and glove sensory loss may be reflective of underlying peripheral neuropathy. Despite varied patterns of muscle imbalance, the cavus deformity with a plantar-flexed first ray is rather constant (382–384).

The foot should be observed for flexibility with localization of the deformity to the forefoot or hindfoot. A tight plantar fascia is palpable as a subcutaneous band along the longitudinal arch with stretching of the forefoot. The

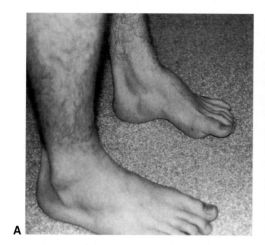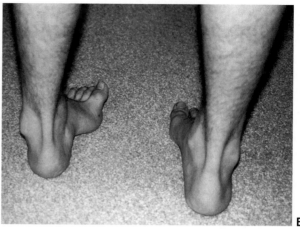

**A**

**B**

**Figure 30.60**  Cavovarus deformity in this individual with Charcot-Marie-Tooth disease. **A:** The arch is elevated only along the medial border of the foot. **B:** Varus and adduction can be appreciated.

hindfoot is evaluated using the Coleman block test (Fig. 30.15) (385). In this test, a 1-inch block is placed under the lateral border of the foot allowing the first ray to plantar-flex without driving the hindfoot into varus. In the common case where the plantar-flexed first ray is the primary problem in cavus foot, the hindfoot will shift beyond neutral into a position of slight valgus, as stance is assumed (Fig. 30.61). The hindfoot should also be examined with the patient in prone position or kneeling in order to evaluate the isolated position of the hindfoot and eliminate forefoot deformity. The degree of hindfoot flexibility is vital for surgical planning.

Hindfoot equinus is very uncommon in the cavus foot, whereas varus and calcaneus deformity are seen quite frequently. Flexibility or rigidity must be determined, as treatment implications are critical. With the flexible state, tendon-balancing procedures are effective, whereas rigidity of deformity requires osteotomy and at times arthrodesis. Toe deformity with MP hyperextension and PIP flexion are important to identify and treat. With the foot dorsiflexed, the toe flexion deformity is accentuated by tightening the

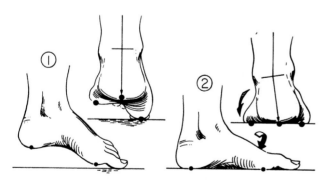

**Figure 30.61**  The tripod effect. The hindfoot must assume a varus position when weight bearing if the first metatarsal is fixed in plantar flexion (*1*). Initial contact of plantar-flexed first metatarsal (*2*). Fifth metatarsal makes contact through supination of the forefoot (*arrow*), which also drives the hindfoot into varus. (From Paulos L, Coleman SS, Samuelson KM. Pes cavovarus. Review of a surgical approach using selective soft-tissue procedures. *J Bone Joint Surg Am* 1980;62:942–953, with permission.)

flexor hallucis longus and the flexor digitorum communis. With plantar flexion, the extrinsic toe flexors are relaxed and the deformity of the PIP and MP joints can be determined. Tender callosities over joints must be documented.

### Radiologic Features

Standing anteroposterior and lateral radiographs of the foot are obtained in all cases as part of the initial evaluation. Even in mild cases, knowing the radiologic appearance of the foot establishes a baseline on which future evaluation of progression can be judged. The standing lateral film is most important for evaluation. The long axis of the talus should be collinear with the long axis of the first metatarsal. Deviation from this with the dorsal apex is seen in cavus foot deformity. This has been termed the *Meary angle*. The angle between the first metatarsal and the long axis of the calcaneus is the Hibb angle, and this is a gauge of the elevation of the longitudinal arch. In the normal state it is greater than 150 degrees but it steadily decreases as cavus foot worsens (Fig. 30.62). Finally, the calcaneal pitch is the angle between the calcaneus and the horizontal and is a measure of hindfoot sagittal plane deformity. Cock-up toe deformity and MP dorsal subluxations should be observed as well. In the anteroposterior view, there is normally an angle of approximately 30 degrees between the talus and calcaneus. With increased varus deformity of the hindfoot, this angle lessens and the talus and calcaneus become increasingly parallel. Further diagnostic studies generally involve anteroposterior and lateral views of the spine and sacrum, looking for underlying deformity that may relate to etiology. Beyond this, MRI of the neuroaxis may be indicated, as well as complete neurologic evaluation, electromyography (EMG), and nerve conduction velocities in order to complete the search for etiology.

### Treatment

Although some have said that there is little role for nonoperative treatment of the cavus foot, the author believes this should be reconsidered. This is a frequently progressive

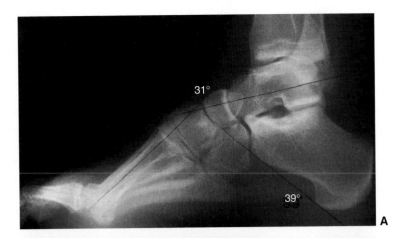

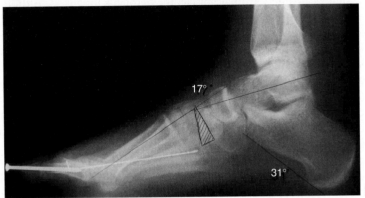

**Figure 30.62** Lateral radiograph of a cavovarus foot deformity before (**A**) and after (**B**) a medial cuneiform plantar-based opening wedge osteotomy. The axis lines of the first metatarsal and the talus cross each other in the body of the medial cuneiform, indicating that as the site of deformity. (From Mosca VS. Ankle and foot: pediatric aspects. In: Beaty J, ed. *Orthopaedic knowledge update 6.* Rosemont, IL: American Academy of Orthopaedic Surgeons, 1999:583.)

deformity that must be monitored. Tightness in the heel cord should be managed with a stretching program, and weakness in dorsiflexion and peroneals may be countered by an exercise program to improve strength and a lightweight brace or angle foot orthoses (AFO) to prevent recurrent spraining or injury. Although a specific program to stretch the longitudinal arch or plantar fascia may not be effective in altering the natural history of this condition, preventing equinus deformity is valuable, and attempts to improve or maintain muscle balance should be pursued. Plantar callosities are often bothersome and painful to patients. These symptoms may be ameliorated with an appropriate arch support with metatarsal pad. A properly made orthotic may significantly improve symptoms and delay or prevent the need for surgical reconstruction (386). Management rather than cure of the cavus foot is the concept to remember. As cavus deformity is usually secondary to neuromuscular disease, continued problems and further treatment should be anticipated (188,226,227,378,386,387).

Surgical correction is dependent upon the definition of the deformity present, determined by physical exam and radiographic evaluation. The elevation of the longitudinal arch (Hibb angle) universally requires a plantar fascia release. A plantar-flexed first ray that is flexible may be balanced by tendon transfer, whereas a rigid deformity requires an osteotomy in order to correct the plantar-flexion deformity. The hindfoot may have fixed varus deformity (Coleman block test) (385) and require an osteotomy for

correction, or it may be flexible and assume normal posture simply with correction of the first ray or forefoot deformity. On the other hand, the entire forefoot may be involved in such a way that midfoot osteotomy is required in order to achieve correction. Finally, toe deformity must be corrected. No single prescription for surgical correction of cavus foot can be found, but a group of operations applied to specific deformities for individual patients allow satisfactory management of the cavus foot deformity.

Plantar fascia release is a standard in all cavus foot procedures (383,386). In this procedure, the plantar fascia and the origin of the abductor hallucis is released. The neurovascular bundle is identified under the fascia of the abductor hallucis and followed distally into the plantar aspect of the foot. In doing this, the plantar fascia can be safely released. Open rather than percutaneous release should be done, as tight plantar structures need to be released in addition to simply dividing the superficial fascia. Steindler (388) described a procedure in which the intrinsic muscles of the foot were released extraperiosteally with correction of the deformity. Release of the calcaneonavicular ligament may facilitate correction of a severe elevation of the longitudinal arch when combined with corrective casting. Plantar midfoot and hindfoot release when combined with corrective casting has been shown to be of some value by Paulos, Coleman, and Samuelson (383) as well as by Sherman and Westin, who (389) noted that in up to 85% of patients, significant correction of residual cavus deformity in clubfoot could be treated with extensive plantar release and corrective casting. Corrective casting has no role in a calcaneal cavus foot with increased calcaneal pitch. Further stretching of the hindfoot and weakening of the gastrocsoleus will result without significant correction of the longitudinal arch. In poliomyelitis, or conditions in which the deformity is secondary to weak gastrocsoleus and a pistol-grip calcaneus deformity is present, there is no role for corrective casting.

The concept of muscle-balancing procedures affecting first ray deformity should be considered next. Figure 30.63 shows the effect of two pairs of opposing muscle forces on the first ray. These opposing force couples are the anterior tibial muscle versus the peroneus longus, and the extensor hallucis longus versus the flexor hallucis longus and intrinsics. In the face of a weak anterior tibial muscle, the peroneus longus plantar flexes the first ray. The EHL overpulls with dorsiflexion of the great toe, plantar flexing the metatarsal head as the toe flexor produces an IP flexion deformity as well. Two muscle-balancing procedures providing benefit to the first ray in a cavus foot are the peroneus longus to brevis transfer and the Jones transfer, or EHL, to first metatarsal head, accompanied by IP fusion. In the peroneus longus to brevis transfer, the two tendons are sewn together just distal to the fibula, and the distal portion of the peroneus longus tendon is divided. In the EHL transfer (Jones procedure), the tendon is divided at the MP joint and the proximal tendon is placed through the metatarsal. The distal stump of the EHL tendon is transferred to the extensor brevis, and an IP fusion of the great toe is done to prevent subsequent flexion deformity of the great toe. Tynan and Klenerman (390) showed that this transfer was highly effective in treating clawing of the hallux and plantar-flexion deformity of the first ray in 90% of cases; it was, however, unreliable in curing pain under the first metatarsal head, helping only in 43% of patients at follow-up. Breusch et al. (391) showed that the overall rate of patient satisfaction was 86%, but that the problems of catching of the big toe when walking barefoot and transfer lesion to the second metatarsal head occurred. They also noted that transfer of the peroneus longus to peroneus brevis was a significant risk factor for elevation of the first metatarsal. In cases with significant peroneal weakness it should not routinely be used as in many cases of cavus foot, the lesser toes are involved with clawing, with plantar flexion of the lesser metatarsal heads as well, resulting in pain and deformity. The balancing procedures for the lesser toes involve transfer of the extensors to the metatarsal heads with IP fusion, with or without flexor tenotomy. Another alternative in a case with a weak anterior tibial tendon is transfer of the entire group of extensor tendons to the cuneiforms in an effort to augment weak dorsiflexion, as described by Cole (392). Mulier, Dereymaeker, and Fabry (393) found an association between metatarsalgia and long, clawed toes. With transfer of the extensor digitorum longus tendons to the metatarsal necks, symptoms were relieved in 25 of 33 affected feet. Although symptoms were improved in the remainder, residual deformity remained. Fabry believed that the transfer of the long extensor tendons to their respective metatarsal necks with IP joint fusion was an excellent procedure for patients with metatarsalgia and pes cavus deformity.

A rigid deformity of the first ray requires corrective osteotomy prior to or in association with tendon transfer. Following plantar fascia release, one must make a decision about the correctibility of the first ray deformity or flexibility of the foot. If one has any question about the persistence of a plantar-flexion first ray deformity, osteotomy is required. The osteotomy may be a plantar opening wedge of the first cuneiform (Fig. 30.62); this is a stable osteotomy in which bone graft can be used to maintain the corrected position of the osteotomy. Cuneiform osteotomy avoids the risk of growth arrest in the proximal first metatarsal in a growing child. Frequently, the center of rotation in a cavus foot is in the midfoot or cuneiform, making this osteotomy preferable to metatarsal procedures. For more severe deformities of the midfoot, a first cuneiform osteotomy will not be sufficient. Midfoot osteotomies, as described by Cole (392), Japas (394), Jahss (395), and Wilcox and Weiner (396) may be used to correct the forefoot and midfoot component of the cavus deformity. These procedures sacrifice midfoot joints and mobility but correct forefoot deformity. The talonavicular joint and calcaneal cuboid joints are preserved in midfoot

Medial view

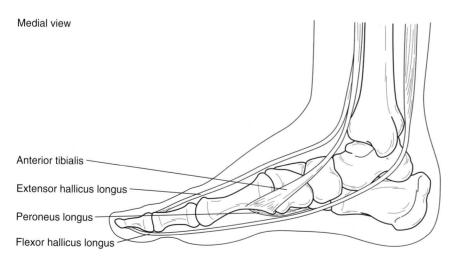

Anterior tibialis

Extensor hallicus longus

Peroneus longus

Flexor hallicus longus

**Figure 30.63** Opposing muscles, anterior tibial versus peroneus longus and extensor hallucis longus versus flexor hallucis longus and intrinsics, create deformity if unbalanced.

osteotomies. The amount of correction achievable with midfoot osteotomy is dependent upon the shortening of the foot and the size of the wedge that is removed. They are accompanied by plantar release. Maximal correction for midfoot osteotomies is in the range of 20 to 25 degrees. Excessive correction through the midfoot may lead to a rocker-bottom deformity of the foot and should be avoided. In select cases, metatarsal osteotomies may be of value in correction of forefoot deformity. This is particularly true if residual medial deviation of the forefoot remains after soft tissue release. A greenstick dorsal closing wedge of the metatarsals has been described by Swanson et al. (397) and Gould (398). Watanabe (399) found 84% good or excellent results in individuals treated in this manner.

With respect to the hindfoot, ignored so far in this discussion of cavus foot, one must ensure that varus deformity is corrected. Rarely is calcaneal pitch decreased with equinus coming primarily from the hindfoot in cavus foot deformity. In reviewing a large number of patients with CMT, Atkas and Sussman (400) found the hindfoot always to be in slight dorsiflexion, with equinus deformity resulting primarily from forefoot and midfoot alteration in anatomy. Rigid hindfoot varus is best addressed by a modified Dwyer osteotomy. In this osteotomy, closing lateral wedge of the calcaneus is combined with a slide or translation of the calcaneal tuberosity to achieve improved correction. Sammarco and Taylor (401) reported on a series of combined calcaneus and metatarsal osteotomies for cavus foot in 15 patients with excellent results, both clinically and radiologically. Symptoms of metatarsalgia as well as instability were corrected by this procedure. A pain-free, plantigrade foot was achieved without sacrificing motion as would be required with arthrodesis. Occasionally, deformity is sufficiently severe and rigid that there is no alternative to triple arthrodesis. Although it was generally thought that a triple arthrodesis would provide long-term plantigrade foot, Schwend and Drennan (402) have shown that progressive deterioration over time, secondary to muscle imbalance, occurs even after triple arthrodesis. Balancing procedures, therefore, are recommended in association with this hindfoot fusion. The two types of triple arthrodeses that are indicated in severe deformities are the Beak triple arthrodesis as described by Siffert et al. (115) and the Lambrinudi triple arthrodesis as modified by Hall and Calvert (116). In these operations, the wedges of bone removed allow correction to a plantigrade foot. In the Beak triple arthrodesis, a portion of the talus and navicular is removed to achieve satisfactory alignment of the foot. In the Lambrinudi procedure, a wedge of talus is removed with a cut perpendicular to the long axis of the tibia, allowing correction of equinus deformity through bony cuts of the triple arthrodesis. Similarly, varus deformity is corrected in this manner and internal fixation achieved with staples or screws.

Complications of triple arthrodesis include pseudarthrosis, primarily of the talonavicular joint. Adelaar et al. (188) described a long-term follow-up with a 61% success rate, compared to Schwend and Drennan's series (402), which had a very low long-term success rate after triple arthrodesis.

Patients in Adelaar's group were primarily affected with poliomyelitis, whereas patients in Schwend and Drennan's group had neuromuscular disease with progressive muscle weakness and therefore progressive imbalance. Triple arthrodesis should be reserved for patients where other procedures will not provide sufficient correction of deformity to achieve a plantigrade foot. In equivocal cases, patients should be aware of the need to attempt correction through osteotomies and soft tissue releases, withholding arthrodesis for severe, recurrent, or residual deformities in which no alternative is present. Finally, Ilizarov management has been used in a number of cases of severe foot deformity with reasonable improvement. A combination of distraction osteotomy and joint correction is used in order to achieve satisfactory alignment. This may represent a valuable alternative to triple arthrodesis, but more data is required in this area. Kucukkaya et al. (403) have recommended a V osteotomy using the Ilizarov frame and method for management of foot deformity in poliomyelitis and CMT. In a series of patients treated in this manner, they documented nearly uniform achievement of a painless plantigrade foot. It appears that there is a role for a combination of soft tissue stretching and osteotomy in the correction of severe deformity using an Ilizarov frame (403).

## Kohler Disease

### Definition
In 1908, Kohler described a condition causing foot pain in young children in whom radiographic findings of the foot showed characteristic flattening, sclerosis, and irregular ossification pattern (404). This is a self-limiting condition, with restitution of healthy bony architecture in all cases.

### Epidemiology
Kohler disease is more common in boys than in girls, with a ratio of 4:1 (405,406) and is frequently bilateral (406,407). Tsirikos et al. have reported bilateral Kohler disease in identical twins, suggesting a genetic predilection for this relatively rare condition (408).

### Pathogenesis
The etiology of Kohler disease remains unknown, but the condition is characterized by disordered enchondral ossification including both osteogenesis and chondrogenesis, presumably related to mechanical stress at the time of early ossification. Karp (409) found that ossification of the navicular occurs earlier in girls than in boys. Half of the girls studied had a navicular that was ossified by the age of 2 years, and one third of the boys were more than $3\frac{1}{2}$ years of age by the time ossification occurred. Karp's feeling was that the delay in ossification predisposed boys to mechanical injury at the time of early ossification of the cartilaginous navicular.

In addition to the effects of mechanical stress at the time of ossification, avascular necrosis appears to play a role in the development of Kohler disease. The blood supply to the navicular bone is significant, with a network of perichondral vessels. However, at the time of early ossification, arteries penetrate the cartilaginous navicular without their mature anastomotic network, predisposing them to vascular injury. Vascular theories are supported by biopsy studies showing areas of necrosis in the navicular (404).

### Clinical Features

The typical child with Kohler disease is a young boy, presenting with an antalgic gait, tending to walk on the lateral border of the foot. There is often dorsal medial swelling and tenderness, at times with redness and warmth, which might suggest infection or arthritis. Range of motion is generally intact.

### Radiographic Features

Standing anteroposterior and lateral x-ray films of the foot demonstrate characteristic findings of sclerosis, fragmentation, and flattening of the navicular bone (Fig. 30.64). The navicular is the last bone in the foot to ossify. The ossific nucleus is first seen in girls between 18 and 24 months of age and in boys 30 to 36 months of age (409). Irregularity in ossification is common, with coalescence of early ossification centers (409). Kohler disease is a clinical diagnosis, rather than a radiologic one; that is, a patient with irregular ossification pattern does not have Kohler disease in the absence of symptoms.

### Other Imaging Studies

Occasional cases are relatively severe, mimicking infection, and an evaluation including CBC, sedimentation rate, and C-reactive protein is beneficial. Occasionally an MRI is helpful in differentiating these conditions. Stress fractures to the tarsal navicular exist, generally in adults, and avascular necrosis of the tarsal navicular has been associated with diabetes, but again in adults, not in young children.

### Pathoanatomy

Waugh (410) found two patterns of blood supply to the navicular. The most common pattern was a diffuse network of five or six perichondrial vessels. The most common pattern was a single dorsal or plantar artery. The single vessels at the time of ossification predispose to mechanical injury and secondary avascular necrosis. Histologic examination of affected bones demonstrates necrosis, resorption of dead bone, and formation of new bone consistent with remodeling after vascular injury.

### Natural History

This is a self-limiting condition with onset in early childhood. The navicular reconstitutes itself somewhere between 4 months and 4 years of age and is normal at skeletal maturity (405–407). There is no residual deformity or disability in adults.

### Treatment

Treatment is symptomatic. An over-the-counter arch support may relieve mild symptoms. For persistent or intense pain, a short leg cast has been shown to be beneficial. Borges et al. (407), Ippolito et al. (405), and Williams et al. (406) found that treatment with a below-knee cast for a minimum of 8 weeks reduced the duration of symptoms. Use of a walking cast was found to be as effective as use of

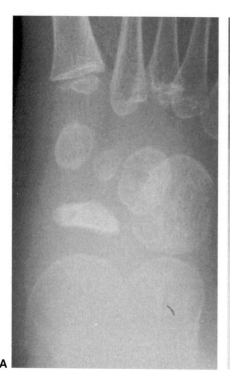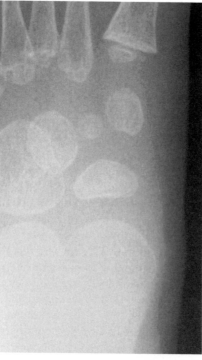

**Figure 30.64** **A:** Kohler disease manifested as sclerotic and flattened right tarsal navicular. **B:** Healthy left navicular.

a nonwalking cast. As symptoms were routinely relieved by a short leg cast in this self-limiting condition, failure to follow the expected course might be an indication for biopsy. There is, however, no role for biopsy or surgery in typical cases of Kohler disease.

## Sever Apophysitis

### Definition

Sever (411) described a disorder of the os calcis leading to heel pain in a growing child, which he thought was an inflammatory disorder. The advent of radiologic imaging in the early 20th century led Kohler, Freiberg, and many others to the identification of clinical conditions characterized by similar radiographic findings called "osteochondroses."

### Epidemiology

Sever calcaneal apophysitis is a very common cause of heel pain in immature athletes (412). The average age at presentation is 11.5 years; it is two to three times more common in boys than in girls, and 60% of patients have bilateral involvement (412). As girls become more athletically active, the author suspects that there will be no sexual predilection for this condition.

### Pathogenesis

The cause of Sever apophysitis is unknown. It is considered to be a nonarticular osteochondrosis (413). Repetitive microtrauma and overuse lead to this "apophysitis" in constitutionally susceptible children (412). It appears much like a stress fracture encountered in Osgood-Schlatter disease.

### Clinical Features

The typical child with Sever apophysitis is a 10- to 12-year-old athletically inclined boy. The patient has pain secondary to impact as well as repetitive pull of the gastrocsoleus on the apophysis. The pain is limited to the heel. It may be associated with warmth, swelling, and even redness. The characteristic finding is pain with medial lateral compression over the tuberosity of the calcaneus.

It must be differentiated from other causes of heel pain, which include cystic lesions of the calcaneus and osteomyelitis. Frequently, children with calcaneal apophysitis have a tight Achilles tendon.

### Radiologic Features

The diagnosis of Sever apophysitis is a clinical one because there is no diagnostic radiographic finding. In a review of radiographs of children with and without Sever apophysitis, sclerosis appears with equal frequency in the healthy and diseased state. Fragmentation of the apophysis (414), however, is the radiologic finding seen with increasing frequency in Sever disease (Fig. 30.65).

Other imaging studies: A bone scan may be helpful in localizing pathology but is generally not needed. An MRI will be helpful in making the differentiation between disease states involving the body of the calcaneus and apophysis.

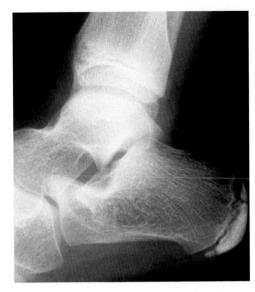

**Figure 30.65** Lateral radiograph showing the normal irregularities of ossification of the apophysis of the os calcis in the growing child.

Such conditions include stress fracture, lytic lesion, or osteomyelitis.

### Pathoanatomy

The apophysis of the os calcis is subjected to opposing forces from the plantar fascia and the Achilles tendon during weight bearing (413,415,416). It is also subjected to impact with heel strike in gait. The combination of direct impact and tension forces from the plantar fascia and the pull of the gastrocsoleus complex lead to a stress fracture from repeated microtrauma. Liberson et al. (415) reviewed the pathology of the apophysis of the os calcis in children. Their data supported the hypothesis of a stress fracture as a cause of this injury.

### Natural History

Sever apophysitis is a self-limiting condition that resolves with maturation and the closure of the apophysis of the os calcis.

### Treatment

Treatment of Sever apophysitis is symptomatic. In general, patients respond to activity restriction and use of a heel pad in the shoe, making them comfortable. Stretching exercises of the Achilles tendon may be helpful in decreasing symptoms, and certainly in decreasing recurrent episodes of Sever apophysitis. Nonsteroidal antiinflammatory medicines may be of some value. For persistent symptoms, a short leg cast will relieve pain. With the use of a short leg cast for patients with symptoms, the average time for relief and return to activity is 2 months, with the range of time being from 1 to 6 months (412). The recurrence of symptoms is relatively common in adolescents. There may be some benefit in the long-term use of heel pads and a heel cord stretching program in the prevention of recurrence of this condition.

In general, there is no role for surgery in the treatment of Sever apophysitis.

## Freiberg Infraction

### Definition

Freiberg (417) described a painful condition of the second metatarsal head, characterized by flattening of the articular surface of bone with both lucency and sclerosis in the metatarsal head. The term "infraction" implied a traumatic origin, whereas "infarction" would imply an ischemic origin.

### Epidemiology

The incidence of this condition is unknown, but it occurs most commonly in adolescent girls and is, surprisingly, the only "osteochondrosis" with a predilection for the female sex. The second metatarsal head is most commonly affected, followed by the third. Less commonly, the first, fourth, and fifth metatarsals are involved. Less than 10% of individuals have bilateral involvement.

### Pathogenesis

The cause of this disease is unknown, but it is classified under an osteochondrosis that is characterized by disordered enchondral ossification. It has been classified by Siffert (413) as primarily an articular osteochondrosis that may or may not disrupt the associated epiphysis. Proposed theories for etiology include trauma, repetitive stress, vascular abnormalities, or high heeled shoes (418,419).

### Clinical Features

Typically, girls present with foot pain, exacerbated by weight-bearing activities or athletics. There is soft tissue swelling about the metatarsal head and tenderness with restriction of motion on examination. The differential diagnosis includes arthritis as well as a metatarsal stress fracture.

### Radiologic Features

The appearance of Freiberg infraction (Fig. 30.66) is one of increased sclerosis, flattening of the articular surface, and lucency. It has an appearance somewhat like Perthes disease of the metatarsal head. The prognosis cannot be accurately determined by the extent of involvement seen radiographically. Classification systems for this disease based on radiographic appearance exist (419–421) but have not been particularly useful in clinical management.

### Pathoanatomy

There are three stages of pathologic changes in this condition (422). Stage 1 is associated with swelling and pain in the absence of radiologic changes. In stage 2, the cells of the chondrocytes in the epiphysis die secondary to loss of nutrition by diffusion from joint fluid or loss of oxygen from blood flow. In stage 3, repair takes place with gradual replacement of necrotic bone and healing. Intraarticular loose bodies may complicate the clinical course of Freiberg infraction.

### Natural History

The disease generally progresses through the three stages as listed in the preceding text, with reconstitution of a satisfactory articular surface and relief of pain. The long-term results depend on the severity of the damage to the articular surface and whether loose bodies result.

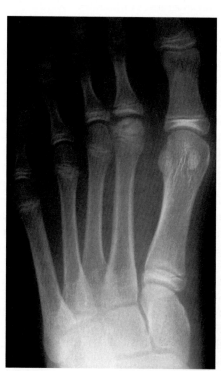 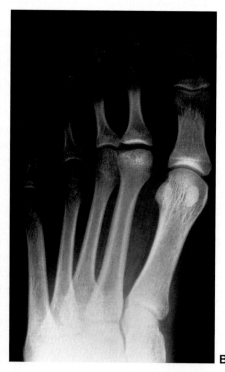

A   B

**Figure 30.66   A:** Freiberg infraction of the second metatarsal head. Early stage with crescent sign. **B:** Later stage with collapse of the metatarsal head. The patient, a young woman, was asymptomatic.

## Treatment

Nonoperative treatment is indicated to relieve symptoms and allow healing of this condition in most cases. Treatments include avoidance of activity, use of shoe inserts with a metatarsal pad, and the use of well-padded shoes. Avoiding high-heeled shoes that place more pressure on the metatarsal heads is advised. Surgery for this condition generally includes joint debridement and removal of loose bodies (417,420,423), elevation of a collapsed articular surface with bone grafting (421), excision of a metatarsal head and shortening of a metatarsal (424), and metatarsal dorsiflexion osteotomy (419,420,423). Debridement of periarticular osteophytes or prominent bone impinging on metatarsal phalangeal joint motion is a procedure that usually gives satisfactory symptomatic relief (417,420,423) if required. The distal metatarsal dorsiflexion osteotomy has been reported to relieve symptoms (419,420,425). In any procedure, it is important to avoid damage to the blood supply of the metatarsal head at the time of surgery, limiting soft tissue dissection (419).

## REFERENCES

1. Staheli LT, Chew DE, Corbett M. The longitudinal arch. A survey of eight hundred and eighty-two feet in normal children and adults. *J Bone Joint Surg Am* 1987;69:426–428.
2. Farsetti P, Weinstein SL, Ponseti IV. The long-term functional and radiographic outcomes of untreated and non-operatively treated metatarsus adductus. *J Bone Joint Surg Am* 1994;76:257–265.
3. Ponseti IV, Becker JR. Congenital metatarsus adductus: the results of treatment. *J Bone Joint Surg Am* 1966;48:702.
4. Rushforth GF. The natural history of hooked forefoot. *J Bone Joint Surg Br* 1978;60-B:530–532.
5. Sim-Fook L, Hodgson AR. A comparison of foot forms among the non-shoe and shoe-wearing Chinese population. *J Bone Joint Surg Am* 1958;40-A:1058–1062.
6. Rao UB, Joseph B. The influence of footwear on the prevalence of flat foot. A survey of 2300 children. *J Bone Joint Surg Br* 1992;74:525–527.
7. Salenius P, Vankka E. The development of the tibiofemoral angle in children. *J Bone Joint Surg Am* 1975;57:259–261.
8. Larsen B, Reimann I, Becker-Andersen H. Congenital calcaneovalgus. With special reference to treatment and its relation to other congenital foot deformities. *Acta Orthop Scand* 1974;45:145–151.
9. Anderson M, Blais MM, Green WT. Lengths of the growing foot. *J Bone Joint Surg Am* 1956;38-A:998–1000.

### Anatomy

10. Wulker N, Stukenborg C, Savory KM, et al. Hindfoot motion after isolated and combined arthrodeses: measurements in anatomic specimens. *Foot Ankle Int* 2000;21:921–927.
11. Gray H. Skeletal system: ankle and foot. In: Gray H, Williams PL, Bannister LH, eds. *Gray's anatomy: the anatomical basis of medicine and surgery*, New York: Churchill Livingstone, 1995:712.
12. Basmajian JV, Stecko G. The role of muscles in arch support of the foot. *J Bone Joint Surg Am* 1963;45:1184–1190.
13. Mann R, Inman VT. Phasic activity of intrinsic muscles of the foot. *J Bone Joint Surg Am* 1964;46:469–481.

### Congenital Deformities And Malformations Of The Foot (Natural History Through Treatment)

14. Irani RN, Sherman MS. The pathological anatomy of idiopathic clubfoot. *Clin Orthop* 1972;84:14–20.
15. Gilbert JA, Roach HI, Clarke NM. Histological abnormalities of the calcaneum in congenital talipes equinovarus. *J Orthop Sci* 2001;6:519–526.
16. Danielsson LG. Incidence of congenital clubfoot in Sweden. 128 cases in 138,000 infants 1946–1990 in Malmo. *Acta Orthop Scand* 1992;63:424–426.
17. Wynne-Davies R. Family studies and the cause of congenital club foot. Talipes equinovarus, talipes calcaneo-valgus and metatarsus varus. *J Bone Joint Surg Br* 1964;46:445–463.
18. Wynne-Davies R. Genetic and environmental factors in the etiology of talipes equinovarus. *Clin Orthop* 1972;84:9–13.
19. Carey M, Bower C, Mylvaganam A, et al. Talipes equinovarus in Western Australia. *Paediatr Perinat Epidemiol* 2003;17:187–194.
20. Gourineni V, Carroll N. Clubfoot. *Foot Ankle Clin* 1998;3:633.
21. Cowell HR, Wein BK. Genetic aspects of club foot. *J Bone Joint Surg Am* 1980;62:1381–1384.
22. Skelly AC, Holt VL, Mosca VS, et al. Talipes equinovarus and maternal smoking: a population-based case-control study in Washington state. *Teratology* 2002;66:91–100.
23. Honein MA, Paulozzi LJ, Moore CA. Family history, maternal smoking, and clubfoot: an indication of a gene-environment interaction. *Am J Epidemiol* 2000;152:658–665.
24. Rebbeck TR, Dietz FR, Murray JC, et al. A single-gene explanation for the probability of having idiopathic talipes equinovarus. *Am J Hum Genet* 1993;53:1051–1063.
25. Isaacs H, Handelsman JE, Badenhorst M, et al. The muscles in club foot—a histological, histochemical and electron microscopic study. *J Bone Joint Surg Br* 1977;59-B:465–472.
26. Bechtol CO, Mossman HW. Clubfoot: an embryological study of associated muscle abnormalities. *J Bone Joint Surg Am* 1950;32:827–838.
27. Feldbrin Z, Gilai AN, Ezra E, et al. Muscle imbalance in the aetiology of idiopathic club foot. An electromyographic study. *J Bone Joint Surg Br* 1995;77:596–601.
28. Ippolito E, Ponseti IV. Congenital club foot in the human fetus. A histological study. *J Bone Joint Surg Am* 1980;62:8–22.
29. Zimny ML, Willig SJ, Roberts JM, et al. An electron microscopic study of the fascia from the medial and lateral sides of clubfoot. *J Pediatr Orthop* 1985;5:577–581.
30. Fukuhara K, Schollmeier G, Uhthoff HK. The pathogenesis of club foot. A histomorphometric and immunohistochemical study of fetuses. *J Bone Joint Surg Br* 1994;76:450–457.
31. Sano H, Uhthoff HK, Jarvis JG, et al. Pathogenesis of soft-tissue contracture in club foot. *J Bone Joint Surg Br* 1998;80:641–644.
32. Khan AM, Ryan MG, Gruber MM, et al. Connective tissue structures in clubfoot: a morphologic study. *J Pediatr Orthop* 2001;21:708–712.
33. van der Sluijs JA, Pruys JE. Normal collagen structure in the posterior ankle capsule in different types of clubfeet. *J Pediatr Orthop B* 1999;8:261–263.
34. Muir L, Laliotis N, Kutty S, et al. Absence of the dorsalis pedis pulse in the parents of children with club foot. *J Bone Joint Surg Br* 1995;77:114–116.
35. Katz DA, Albanese EL, Levinsohn EM, et al. Pulsed color-flow Doppler analysis of arterial deficiency in idiopathic clubfoot. *J Pediatr Orthop* 2003;23:84–87.
36. Laaveg SJ, Ponseti IV. Long-term results of treatment of congenital club foot. *J Bone Joint Surg Am* 1980;62:23–31.
37. Simons GW. A standardized method for the radiographic evaluation of clubfeet. *Clin Orthop* 1978;135:107–118.
38. Miyagi N, Iisaka H, Yasuda K, et al. Onset of ossification of the tarsal bones in congenital clubfoot. *J Pediatr Orthop* 1997;17:36–40.
39. Cahuzac JP, Baunin C, Luu S, et al. Assessment of hindfoot deformity by three-dimensional MRI in infant club foot. *J Bone Joint Surg Br* 1999;81:97–101.
40. Howard CB, Benson MK. The ossific nuclei and the cartilage anlage of the talus and calcaneum. *J Bone Joint Surg Br* 1992;74:620–623.
41. Brennan R, Davidson R, Dormans J, et al. Radiographs of the infant foot: a study of reproducibility of measurement and positioning. *Orthop Trans* 1994;18:996.
42. Dimeglio A, Bonnet F, Mazeau P, et al. Orthopaedic treatment and passive motion machine: consequences for the surgical treatment of clubfoot. *J Pediatr Orthop B* 1996;5:173–180.
43. Hudson I, Catterall A. Posterolateral release for resistant club foot. *J Bone Joint Surg Br* 1994;76:281–284.
44. Bensahel H, Csukonyi Z, Desgrippes Y, et al. Surgery in residual clubfoot: one-stage medioposterior release "a la carte." *J Pediatr Orthop* 1987;7:145–148.
45. Beatson TR, Pearson JR. A method of assessing correction in club feet. *J Bone Joint Surg Br* 1966;48:40–50.

46. Vanderwilde R, Staheli LT, Chew DE, et al. Measurements on radiographs of the foot in normal infants and children. *J Bone Joint Surg Am* 1988;70:407–415.

47. Spiegel DA, Loder RT. Leg-length discrepancy and bone age in unilateral idiopathic talipes equinovarus. *J Pediatr Orthop* 2003;23:246–250.

48. Dimeglio A, Bensahel H, Souchet P, et al. Classification of clubfoot. *J Pediatr Orthop B* 1995;4:129–136.

49. Pirani S. *A reliable and valid method of assessing the amount of deformity in the congenital clubfoot.* St. Louis, MO: Pediatric Orthopaedic Society of North America, 2004.

50. Flynn JM, Donohoe M, Mackenzie WG. An independent assessment of two clubfoot-classification systems. *J Pediatr Orthop* 1998;18:323–327.

51. Wainwright AM, Auld T, Benson MK, et al. The classification of congenital talipes equinovarus. *J Bone Joint Surg Br* 2002;84:1020–1024.

52. Keret D, Ezra E, Lokiec F, et al. Efficacy of prenatal ultrasonography in confirmed club foot. *J Bone Joint Surg Br* 2002;84:1015–1019.

53. Ryu JK, Cho JY, Choi JS. Prenatal sonographic diagnosis of focal musculoskeletal anomalies. *Korean J Radiol* 2003;4:243–251.

54. Bakalis S, Sairam S, Homfray T, et al. Outcome of antenatally diagnosed talipes equinovarus in an unselected obstetric population. *Ultrasound Obstet Gynecol* 2002;20:226–229.

55. Rijhsinghani A, Yankowitz J, Kanis AB, et al. Antenatal sonographic diagnosis of club foot with particular attention to the implications and outcomes of isolated club foot. *Ultrasound Obstet Gynecol* 1998;12:103–106.

56. Tillett RL, Fisk NM, Murphy K, et al. Clinical outcome of congenital talipes equinovarus diagnosed antenatally by ultrasound. *J Bone Joint Surg Br* 2000;82:876–880.

57. Treadwell MC, Stanitski CL, King M. Prenatal sonographic diagnosis of clubfoot: implications for patient counseling. *J Pediatr Orthop* 1999;19:8–10.

58. Woodrow N, Tran T, Umstad M, et al. Mid-trimester ultrasound diagnosis of isolated talipes equinovarus: accuracy and outcome for infants. *Aust N Z J Obstet Gynaecol* 1998;38:301–305.

59. Ramin KD, Raffel C, Breckle RJ, et al. Chronology of neurological manifestations of prenatally diagnosed open neural tube defects. *J Matern Fetal Neonatal Med* 2002;11:89–92.

60. Shipp TD, Benacerraf BR. The significance of prenatally identified isolated clubfoot: is amniocentesis indicated? *Am J Obstet Gynecol* 1998;178:600–602.

61. Malone FD, Marino T, Bianchi DW, et al. Isolated clubfoot diagnosed prenatally: is karyotyping indicated? *Obstet Gynecol* 2000;95:437–440.

62. Kite JH. Principles involved in the treatment of congenital clubfoot. 1939. *J Bone Joint Surg Am*, 2003;85-A:1847; discussion 1847.

63. Kite J. *The clubfoot.* New York: Grune & Stratton, 1964.

64. Lovell WW, Bailey T, Price CT, et al. The nonoperative management of the congenital clubfoot. *Orthop Rev* 1979;8:113–115.

65. Ponseti IV. *Congenital clubfoot: fundamentals of treatment.* Oxford: Oxford University Press, 1996.

66. Morcuende JA, Weinstein S, Dietz F, et al. Plaster cast treatment of clubfoot: the Ponseti method of manipulation and casting. *J Pediatr Orthop B* 1994;3:161.

67. Ponseti IV. Treatment of congenital club foot. *J Bone Joint Surg Am* 1992;74:448–454.

68. Staheli LT, Corbett M, Wyss C, et al. Lower-extremity rotational problems in children. Normal values to guide management. *J Bone Joint Surg Am* 1985;67:39–47.

69. Carroll NC, McMurtry R, Leete SF. The pathoanatomy of congenital clubfoot. *Orthop Clin North Am* 1978;9:225–232.

70. Carroll NC. Pathoanatomy and surgical treatment of the resistant clubfoot. *Instr Course Lect* 1988;37:93–106.

71. Coss HS, Hennrikus WL. Parent satisfaction comparing two bandage materials used during serial casting in infants. *Foot Ankle Int* 1996;17:483–486.

72. Cooper DM, Dietz FR. Treatment of idiopathic clubfoot. A thirty-year follow-up note. *J Bone Joint Surg Am* 1995;77:1477–1489.

73. Herzenberg JE, Radler C, Bor N. Ponseti versus traditional methods of casting for idiopathic clubfoot. *J Pediatr Orthop* 2002; 22:517–521.

74. Lehman WB, Mohaideen A, Madan S, et al. A method for the early evaluation of the Ponseti (Iowa) technique for the treatment of idiopathic clubfoot. *J Pediatr Orthop B* 2003; 12:133–140.

75. Hattori T, Ono Y, Kitakoji T, et al. Effect of the Denis Browne splint in conservative treatment of congenital club foot. *J Pediatr Orthop B* 2003;12:59–62.

76. Kuhns LR, Koujok K, Hall JM, et al. Ultrasound of the navicular during the simulated Ponseti maneuver. *J Pediatr Orthop* 2003; 23:243–245.

77. Pirani S, Zeznik L, Hodges D. Magnetic resonance imaging study of the congenital clubfoot treated with the Ponseti method. *J Pediatr Orthop* 2001;21:719–726.

78. Dobbs MB, Corley CL, Morcuende JA, et al. Late recurrence of clubfoot deformity: a 45-year followup. *Clin Orthop* 2003;411:188–192.

79. Masse P. Le traitement du pied bot par la methode "fonctionnelle." *Cahier d'enseignement de la SOFCOT*, Vol. 3. Paris: Expansion Scientific, 1977:51–56.

80. Bensahel H, Guillaume A, Czukonyi Z, et al. Results of physical therapy for idiopathic clubfoot: a long-term follow-up study. *J Pediatr Orthop* 1990;10:189–192.

81. Dimeglio A. Orthopaedic treatment and passive motion machine in clubfoot. *Pediatric Orthopaedic Society of North America 2000 annual meeting.* Rosemont, IL: Pediatric Orthopaedic Society of North America, 2000:47.

82. Noonan KJ, Richards BS. Nonsurgical management of idiopathic clubfoot. *J Am Acad Orthop Surg* 2003;11:392–402.

83. Richards BS, Wilson H, Johnston CE, et al. Nonoperative clubfoot treatment using the French method: comparing clinical outcome with radiographs. *Pediatric Orthopaedic Society of North America 2001 annual meeting.* Rosemont, IL: Pediatric Orthopaedic Society of North America, 2001:142.

84. Van Campenhout A, Molenaers G, Moens P, et al. Does functional treatment of idiopathic clubfoot reduce the indication for surgery? Call for a widely accepted rating system. *J Pediatr Orthop B* 2001;10:315–318.

85. Cohen-Sobel E, Caselli M, Giorgini R, et al. Long-term followup of clubfoot surgery: analysis of 44 patients. *J Foot Ankle Surg* 1993;32:411–423.

86. Ryoppy S, Sairanen H. Neonatal operative treatment of club foot. A preliminary report. *J Bone Joint Surg Br* 1983;65: 320–325.

87. Pous JG, Dimeglio A. Neonatal surgery in clubfoot. *Orthop Clin North Am* 1978;9:233–240.

88. Turco VJ. Surgical correction of the resistant club foot. One-stage posteromedial release with internal fixation: a preliminary report. *J Bone Joint Surg Am* 1971;53:477–497.

89. Turco VJ. Resistant congenital club foot—one-stage posteromedial release with internal fixation. A follow-up report of a fifteen-year experience. *J Bone Joint Surg Am* 1979;61:805–814.

90. Simons GW. Complete subtalar release in club feet. Part I—A preliminary report. *J Bone Joint Surg Am* 1985;67:1044–1055.

91. McKay DW. New concept of and approach to clubfoot treatment: section I—principles and morbid anatomy. *J Pediatr Orthop* 1982;2:347–356.

92. McKay DW. New concept of and approach to clubfoot treatment: section II—correction of the clubfoot. *J Pediatr Orthop* 1983;3:10–21.

93. Goldner J, Fitch R. Idiopathic congenital talipes equinovarus (clubfoot). In: Jahss M, ed. *Disorders of the foot and ankle: medical and surgical management,* 2nd ed. Philadelphia, PA: WB Saunders, 1991:771.

94. Goldner JL. Congenital talipes equinovarus—fifteen years of surgical treatment. *Curr Pract Orthop Surg* 1969;4:61–123.

95. Carroll N. Surgical technique for talipes equinovarus. *Oper Tech Orthop* 1993;3:115.

96. Simons GW. Complete subtalar release in club feet. Part II—Comparison with less extensive procedures. *J Bone Joint Surg Am* 1985;67:1056–1065.

97. Simons GW. Calcaneocuboid joint deformity in talipes equinovarus: an overview and update. *J Pediatr Orthop B* 1995;4:25–35.

98. Crawford AH, Marxen JL, Osterfeld DL. The Cincinnati incision: a comprehensive approach for surgical procedures of the foot and ankle in childhood. *J Bone Joint Surg Am* 1982;64: 1355–1358.

99. Ferlic RJ, Breed AL, Mann DC, et al. Partial wound closure after surgical correction of equinovarus foot deformity. *J Pediatr Orthop* 1997;17:486–489.

100. Karol LA, Concha MC, Johnston CE II. Gait analysis and muscle strength in children with surgically treated clubfeet. *J Pediatr Orthop* 1997;17:790–795.

101. Napiontek M. Muscular strength after extensive operative treatment of congenital talipes equinovarus. *J Pediatr Orthop B* 2000; 9:128–136.

102. Mosca VS. Calcaneal lengthening for valgus deformity of the hindfoot. Results in children who had severe, symptomatic flatfoot and skewfoot. *J Bone Joint Surg Am* 1995;77:500–512.

103. Davids JR, Valadie AL, Ferguson RL, et al. Surgical management of ankle valgus in children: use of a transphyseal medial malleolar screw. *J Pediatr Orthop* 1997;17:3–8.

104. Stevens PM, Belle RM. Screw epiphysiodesis for ankle valgus. *J Pediatr Orthop* 1997;17:9–12.

105. Evans D. Relapsed club foot. *J Bone Joint Surg Br* 1961;43:722.

106. Coleman SS. *Complex foot deformities in children.* Philadelphia, PA: Lea & Febiger, 1983.

107. Kuo KN, Jansen LD. Rotatory dorsal subluxation of the navicular: a complication of clubfoot surgery. *J Pediatr Orthop* 1998; 18:770–774.

108. Wei SY, Sullivan RJ, Davidson RS. Talo-navicular arthrodesis for residual midfoot deformities of a previously corrected clubfoot. *Foot Ankle Int* 2000;21:482–485.

109. Kuo KN, Hennigan SP, Hastings ME. Anterior tibial tendon transfer in residual dynamic clubfoot deformity. *J Pediatr Orthop* 2001;21:35–41.

110. Garceau GJ. Anterior tibial tendon transfer for recurrent clubfoot. *Clin Orthop* 1972;84:61–65.

111. Lichtblau S. A medial and lateral release operation for club foot. A preliminary report. *J Bone Joint Surg Am* 1973;55:1377–1384.

112. McKay DW. Dorsal bunions in children. *J Bone Joint Surg Am* 1983;65:975–980.

113. Ezra E, Hayek S, Gilai AN, et al. Tibialis anterior tendon transfer for residual dynamic supination deformity in treated club feet. *J Pediatr Orthop B* 2000;9:207–211.

114. Huber H, Dutoit M. Dynamic foot-pressure measurement in the assessment of operatively treated clubfeet. *J Bone Joint Surg Am* 2004;86-A:1203–1210.

115. Siffert RS, Forster RI, Nachamie B. "Beak" triple arthrodesis for correction of severe cavus deformity. *Clin Orthop* 1966;45: 101–106.

116. Hall JE, Calvert PT. Lambrinudi triple arthrodesis: a review with particular reference to the technique of operation. *J Pediatr Orthop* 1987;7:19–24.

117. Bennett GL, Graham CE, Mauldin DM. Triple arthrodesis in adults. *Foot Ankle* 1991;12:138–143.

118. Grill F, Franke J. The Ilizarov distractor for the correction of relapsed or neglected clubfoot. *J Bone Joint Surg Br* 1987;69: 593–597.

119. Wallander H, Hansson G, Tjernstrom B. Correction of persistent clubfoot deformities with the Ilizarov external fixator. Experience in 10 previously operated feet followed for 2-5 years. *Acta Orthop Scand* 1996;67:283–287.

120. Choi IH, Yang MS, Chung CY, et al. The treatment of recurrent arthrogrypotic club foot in children by the Ilizarov method. A preliminary report. *J Bone Joint Surg Br* 2001;83:731–737.

121. Bradish CF, Noor S. The Ilizarov method in the management of relapsed club feet. *J Bone Joint Surg Br* 2000;82:387–391.

122. Steinwender G, Saraph V, Zwick EB, et al. Complex foot deformities associated with soft-tissue scarring in children. *J Foot Ankle Surg* 2001;40:42–49.

123. Goldner JL, Fitch RD. Classification and evaluation of congenital talipes equinovarus. In: Simons GW, ed. *The clubfoot.* New York: Springer-Verlag, 1993.

124. Hunziker UA, Largo RH, Duc G. Neonatal metatarsus adductus, joint mobility, axis, and rotation of the lower extremity in preterm and term children 0-5 years of age. *Eur J Pediatr* 1988; 148:19–23.

125. Kite JH. Congenital metatarsus varus; report of 300 cases. *J Bone Joint Surg Am* 1950;32-A:500–506.

126. Kite JH. Congenital metatarsus varus. *J Bone Joint Surg Am* 1967; 49:388–397.

127. McCormick DW, Blount WP. Metatarsus adductovarus: "skewfoot." *JAMA* 1949;141:449.

128. Jacobs JE. Metatarsus varus and hip dysplasia. *Clin Orthop* 1960;16:203–213.

129. Kumar SJ, MacEwen GD. The incidence of hip dysplasia with metatarsus adductus. *Clin Orthop* 1982;164:234–235.

130. Gruber MA, Lozano JA. Metatarsus varus and developmental dysplasia of the hip: is there a relationship? *Orthop Trans* 1991;15:336.

131. Kollmer CE, Betz RR, Clancy M, et al. Relationship of congenital hip and foot deformities: a national Shriner's Hospital survey. *Orthop Trans* 1991:96.

132. Morcuende JA, Ponseti IV. Congenital metatarsus adductus in early human fetal development: a histologic study. *Clin Orthop* 1996;333:261–266.

133. Reimann I, Werner HH. The pathology of congenital metatarsus varus: a post-mortem study of a newborn infant. *Acta Orthop Scand* 1983;54:847.

134. Ghali NN, Abberton MJ, Silk FF. The management of metatarsus adductus et supinatus. *J Bone Joint Surg Br* 1984;66:376–380.

135. Browne RS, Paton DF. Anomalous insertion of the tibialis posterior tendon in congenital metatarsus varus. *J Bone Joint Surg Br* 1979;61:74–76.

136. Peabody CW, Muro F. Congenital metatarsus varus. *J Bone Joint Surg Am* 1933;15A:171.

137. Cappello T, Mosca VS. Metatarsus adductus and skewfoot. *Foot Ankle Clin* 1998:683.

138. Bleck EE. Metatarsus adductus: classification and relationship to outcomes of treatment. *J Pediatr Orthop* 1983;3:2–9.

139. Smith JT, Bleck EE, Gamble JG, et al. Simple method of documenting metatarsus adductus. *J Pediatr Orthop* 1991;11: 679–680.

140. Berg EE. A reappraisal of metatarsus adductus and skewfoot. *J Bone Joint Surg Am* 1986;68:1185–1196.

141. Cook DA, Breed AL, Cook T, et al. Observer variability in the radiographic measurement and classification of metatarsus adductus. *J Pediatr Orthop* 1992;12:86–89.

142. McCauley J Jr., Lusskin R, Bromley J. Recurrence in congenital metatarsus varus. *J Bone Joint Surg Am* 1964;46:525–532.

143. Thompson SA. Hallux varus and metatarsus varus. *Clin Orthop* 1960;16:109.

144. Asirvatham R, Stevens PM. Idiopathic forefoot-adduction deformity: medial capsulotomy and abductor hallucis lengthening for resistant and severe deformities. *J Pediatr Orthop* 1997;17: 496–500.

145. Heyman CH, Herndon CH, Strong JM. Mobilization of the tarsometatarsal and intermetatarsal joints for the correction of resistant adduction of the fore part of the foot in congenital club-foot or congenital metatarsus varus. *J Bone Joint Surg Am* 1958;40-A:299–309; discussion 291–309.

146. Stark JG, Johanson JE, Winter RB. The Heyman-Herndon tarsometatarsal capsulotomy for metatarsus adductus: results in 48 feet. *J Pediatr Orthop* 1987;7:305–310.

147. Kendrick RE, Sharma NK, Hassler WL, et al. Tarsometatarsal mobilization for resistant adduction of the fore part of the foot. A follow-up study. *J Bone Joint Surg Am* 1970;52:61–70.

148. Berman A, Gartland JJ. Metatarsal osteotomy for the correction of adduction of the fore part of the foot in children. *J Bone Joint Surg Am* 1971;53:498–506.

149. Steytler JC, Van der Walt ID. Correction of resistant adduction of the forefoot in congenital club-foot and congenital metatarsus varus by metatarsal osteotomy. *Br J Surg* 1966;53:558–560.

150. Gamble JG, Decker S, Abrams RC. Short first ray as a complication of multiple metatarsal osteotomies. *Clin Orthop* 1982: 241–244.

151. Holden D, Siff S, Butler J, et al. Shortening of the first metatarsal as a complication of metatarsal osteotomies. *J Bone Joint Surg Am* 1984;66:582–587.

152. Fowler SB, Brooks AL, Parrish TF. The cavo-varus foot. *J Bone Joint Surg Am* 1959;41:757.

153. Anderson DA, Schoenecker PL, Blair VPI. Combined lateral column shortening and medial column lengthening in the treatment of severe forefoot adductus. *Orthop Trans* 1991;15:768.

154. Conklin MJ, Kling TF. Open-wedge osteotomies of the first cuneiform for metatarsus adductus. *Orthop Trans* 1991:106.

155. Lincoln CR, Wood KE, Bugg EI Jr. Metatarsus varus corrected by open wedge osteotomy of the first cuneiform bone. *Orthop Clin North Am* 1976;7:795–798.

156. McHale KA, Lenhart MK. Treatment of residual clubfoot deformity—the "bean-shaped" foot—by opening wedge medial cuneiform osteotomy and closing wedge cuboid osteotomy. Clinical review and cadaver correlations. *J Pediatr Orthop* 1991; 11:374–381.

157. Mosca VS. Skewfoot deformity in children: correction by calcaneal neck lengthening and medial cuneiform opening wedge
osteotomies. *J Pediatr Orthop* 1993;13:807.

158. Mosca VS. Flexible flatfoot and skewfoot. *Instr Course Lect*
1996;45:347–354.

159. Mosca VS. Flexible flatfoot and skewfoot. In: Drennan JC, ed.
*The child's foot and ankle*. New York: Raven Press, 1992:355.

160. Peterson HA. Skewfoot (forefoot adduction with heel valgus).
*J Pediatr Orthop* 1986;6:24–30.

161. Evans D. Calcaneo-valgus deformity. *J Bone Joint Surg Br* 1975;
57:270–278.

162. Harris RI. *Army foot survey: an investigation of foot ailments in
Canadian soldiers*. National Research Council of Canada, 1947.

163. Harris R, Beath T. Hypermobile flatfoot with the short tendo
Achillis. *J Bone Joint Surg Am* 1948;30:116.

164. Reimers J, Pedersen B, Brodersen A. Foot deformity and the
length of the triceps surae in Danish children between 3 and 17
years old. *J Pediatr Orthop B* 1995;4:71–73.

165. Echarri JJ, Forriol F. The development in footprint morphology
in 1851 Congolese children from urban and rural areas, and the
relationship between this and wearing shoes. *J Pediatr Orthop B*
2003;12:141–146.

166. Hicks JH. The mechanics of the foot. II. The plantar aponeurosis
and the arch. *J Anat* 1954;88:25–30.

167. Kanatli U, Yetkin H, Cila E. Footprint and radiographic analysis
of the feet. *J Pediatr Orthop* 2001;21:225–228.

168. Lin CJ, Lai KA, Kuan TS, et al. Correlating factors and clinical
significance of flexible flatfoot in preschool children. *J Pediatr
Orthop* 2001;21:378–382.

169. Cowan DN, Jones BH, Robinson JR. Foot morphologic characteristics and risk of exercise-related injury. *Arch Fam Med* 1993;
2:773–777.

170. Kaufman KR, Brodine SK, Shaffer RA, et al. The effect of foot
structure and range of motion on musculoskeletal overuse
injuries. *Am J Sports Med* 1999;27:585–593.

171. Steel MW, III, Johnson KA, DeWitz MA, et al. Radiographic measurements of the normal adult foot. *Foot Ankle* 1980;1: 151–158.

172. Meary R. On the measurement of the angle between the talus
and the first metatarsal. Symposium: Le Pied Creux Essential.
*Rev Chir Orthop* 1967;53:389.

173. Brown RR, Rosenberg ZS, Thornhill BA. The C sign: more specific for flatfoot deformity than subtalar coalition. *Skeletal
Radiol* 2001;30:84–87.

174. Bleck EE, Berzins UJ. Conservative management of pes valgus
with plantar flexed talus, flexible. *Clin Orthop* 1977;122:85–94.

175. Gould N, Moreland M, Alvarez R, et al. Development of the
child's arch. *Foot Ankle* 1989;9:241–245.

176. Wenger DR, Mauldin D, Speck G, et al. Corrective shoes and
inserts as treatment for flexible flatfoot in infants and children.
*J Bone Joint Surg Am* 1989;71:800–810.

177. Penneau K, Lutter LD, Winter RD. Pes planus: radiographic
changes with foot orthoses and shoes. *Foot Ankle* 1982;2:
299–303.

178. Garcia-Rodriguez A, Martin-Jimenez F, Carnero-Varo M, et al.
Flexible flat feet in children: a real problem? *Pediatrics* 1999;
103:e84.

179. Theologis TN, Gordon C, Benson MK. Heel seats and shoe wear.
*J Pediatr Orthop* 1994;14:760–762.

180. Miller CD, Laskowski ER, Suman VJ. Effect of corrective rearfoot
orthotic devices on ground reaction forces during ambulation.
*Mayo Clin Proc* 1996;71:757–762.

181. Duncan JW, Lovell WW. Modified Hoke-Miller flatfoot procedure. *Clin Orthop* 1983;181:24–27.

182. Hoke M. An operation for the correction of extremely relaxed
flatfeet. *J Bone Joint Surg Am* 1931;13:773.

183. Miller O. A plastic flat-foot operation. *J Bone Joint Surg Am*
1927; 9:84.

184. Jack EA. Naviculo-cuneiform fusion in the treatment of flat foot.
*J Bone Joint Surg Br* 1953;35-B:75–82.

185. Seymour N. The late results of naviculo-cuneiform fusion.
*J Bone Joint Surg Br* 1967;49:558–559.

186. Butte F. Navicular-cuneiform arthrodesis for flatfoot: an end-
result study. *J Bone Joint Surg Am* 1937;19:496.

187. Crego CH Jr, Ford LT. An end-result of various operative procedures for correcting flat feet in children. *J Bone Joint Surg Am*
1952;34-A:183–195.

188. Adelaar RS, Dannelly EA, Meunier PA, et al. A long-term study
of triple arthrodesis in children. *Orthop Clin North Am* 1976; 7:
895–908.

189. Koutsogiannis E. Treatment of mobile flat foot by displacement
osteotomy of the calcaneus. *J Bone Joint Surg Br* 1971;53: 96–100.

190. Rathjen KE, Mubarak SJ. Calcaneal-cuboid-cuneiform osteotomy
for the correction of valgus foot deformities in children. *J Pediatr
Orthop* 1998;18:775–782.

191. Anderson AF, Fowler SB. Anterior calcaneal osteotomy for symptomatic juvenile pes planus. *Foot Ankle* 1984;4:274–283.

192. Armstrong G, Carruthers C. Evans elongation of lateral column of
the foot for valgus deformity. *J Bone Joint Surg Am* 1975; 57:530.

193. Phillips GE. A review of elongation of os calcis for flat feet.
*J Bone Joint Surg Br* 1983;65:15–18.

194. Miller GR. The operative treatment of hypermobile flatfeet in
the young child. *Clin Orthop* 1977;122:95–101.

195. Smith SD, Millar EA. Arthrorisis by means of a subtalar polyethylene peg implant for correction of hindfoot pronation in
children. *Clin Orthop* 1983;15–23.

196. Black PR, Betts RP, Duckworth T, et al. The Viladot implant in
flatfooted children. *Foot Ankle Int* 2000;21:478–481.

197. Verheyden F, Vanlommel E, Van Der Bauwhede J, et al. The sinus
tarsi spacer in the operative treatment of flexible flat feet. *Acta
Orthop Belg* 1997;63:305–309.

198. Grady JF, Dinnon MW. Subtalar arthroereisis in the neurologically normal child. *Clin Podiatr Med Surg* 2000;17:443–457, vi.

199. Lamy L. Congenital convex pes valgus. *J Bone Joint Surg Am*
1939:79.

200. Dodge LD, Ashley RK, Gilbert RJ. Treatment of the congenital
vertical talus: a retrospective review of 36 feet with long-term
follow-up. *Foot Ankle* 1987;7:326–332.

201. Hamanishi C. Congenital vertical talus: classification with 69
cases and new measurement system. *J Pediatr Orthop* 1984;4:
318–326.

202. Jacobsen ST, Crawford AH. Congenital vertical talus. *J Pediatr
Orthop* 1983;3:306–310.

203. Ogata K, Schoenecker PL, Sheridan J. Congenital vertical talus
and its familial occurrence: an analysis of 36 patients. *Clin
Orthop* 1979;139:128–132.

204. Townes PL, Dehart GK Jr, Hecht F, et al. Trisomy 13-15 in a male
infant. *J Pediatr* 1962;60:528–532.

205. Uchida IA, Lewis AJ, Bowman JM, et al. A case of double trisomy: trisomy No. 18 and triplo-X. *J Pediatr* 1962;60:498–502.

206. Stern HJ, Clark RD, Stroberg AJ, et al. Autosomal dominant
transmission of isolated congenital vertical talus. *Clin Genet*
1989;36:427–430.

207. Sharrard WJ, Grosfield I. The management of deformity and
paralysis of the foot in myelomeningocele. *J Bone Joint Surg Br*
1968;50:456–465.

208. Lloyd-Roberts GC, Spence AJ. Congenital vertical talus. *J Bone
Joint Surg Br* 1958;40-B:33–41.

209. Kumar SJ, Cowell HR, Ramsey PL. Vertical and oblique talus.
*Instr Course Lect* 1982;31:235–251.

210. Patterson WR, Fitz DA, Smith WS. The pathologic anatomy of
congenital convex pes valgus. Post mortem study of a newborn
infant with bilateral involvement. *J Bone Joint Surg Am* 1968; 50:
458–466.

211. Drennan JC, Sharrard WJ. The pathological anatomy of convex
pes valgus. *J Bone Joint Surg Br* 1971;53:455–461.

212. Seimon LP. Surgical correction of congenital vertical talus under
the age of 2 years. *J Pediatr Orthop* 1987;7:405–411.

213. Specht EE. Congenital paralytic vertical talus. An anatomical
study. *J Bone Joint Surg Am* 1975;57:842–847.

214. Drennan JC. Congenital vertical talus. *Instr Course Lect* 1996; 45:
315–322.

215. Mazzocca AD, Thomson JD, Deluca PA, et al. Comparison of the
posterior approach versus the dorsal approach in the treatment of
congenital vertical talus. *J Pediatr Orthop* 2001;21: 212–217.

216. Duncan RD, Fixsen JA. Congenital convex pes valgus. *J Bone
Joint Surg Br* 1999;81:250–254.

217. Kodros SA, Dias LS. Single-stage surgical correction of congenital vertical talus. *J Pediatr Orthop* 1999;19:42–48.

218. Oppenheim W, Smith C, Christie W. Congenital vertical talus.
*Foot Ankle* 1985;5:198–204.

219. Stricker SJ, Rosen E. Early one-stage reconstruction of congenital
vertical talus. *Foot Ankle Int* 1997;18:535–543.

220. Coleman SS, Stelling FH III, Jarrett J. Pathomechanics and treatment of congenital vertical talus. *Clin Orthop* 1970;70:62–72.

221. Walker AP, Ghali NN, Silk FF. Congenital vertical talus. The results of staged operative reduction. *J Bone Joint Surg Br* 1985;67:117–121.

222. Grice DS. An extra-articular arthrodesis of the subastragalar joint for correction of paralytic flat feet in children. *J Bone Joint Surg Am* 1952;34A:927–940; passim.

223. Grice DS. Further experience with extra-articular arthrodesis of the subtalar joint. *J Bone Joint Surg Am* 1955;37-A:246–259; passim.

224. Colton CL. The surgical management of congenital vertical talus. *J Bone Joint Surg Br* 1973;55:566–574.

225. Clark MW, D'Ambrosia RD, Ferguson AB. Congenital vertical talus: treatment by open reduction and navicular excision. *J Bone Joint Surg Am* 1977;59:816–824.

226. Angus PD, Cowell HR. Triple arthrodesis. A critical long-term review. *J Bone Joint Surg Br* 1986;68:260–265.

227. Drew AJ. The late results of arthrodesis of the foot. *J Bone Joint Surg Br* 1951;33-B:496–502.

228. McCall RE, Lillich JS, Harris JR, et al. The Grice extraarticular subtalar arthrodesis: a clinical review. *J Pediatr Orthop* 1985;5:442–445.

229. Ross PM, Lyne ED. The Grice procedure: indications and evaluation of long-term results. *Clin Orthop* 1980;153:194–200.

230. Scott SM, Janes PC, Stevens PM. Grice subtalar arthrodesis followed to skeletal maturity. *J Pediatr Orthop* 1988;8:176–183.

231. Smith JB, Westin GW. Subtalar extra-articular arthrodesis. *J Bone Joint Surg Am* 1968;50:1027–1035.

232. Southwell RB, Sherman FC. Triple arthrodesis: a long-term study with force plate analysis. *Foot Ankle* 1981;2:15–24.

233. Napiontek M. Congenital vertical talus: a retrospective and critical review of 32 feet operated on by peritalar reduction. *J Pediatr Orthop B* 1995;4:179–187.

234. Wynne-Davies R, Littlejohn A, Gormley J. Aetiology and interrelationship of some common skeletal deformities. (Talipes equinovarus and calcaneovalgus, metatarsus varus, congenital dislocation of the hip, and infantile idiopathic scoliosis). *J Med Genet* 1982;19:321–328.

235. Wetzenstein H. The significance of congenital pes calcaneo-valgus in the origin of pes plano-valgus in childhood. Preliminary report. *Acta Orthop Scand* 1960;30:64–72.

236. Mosier KM, Asher M. Tarsal coalitions and peroneal spastic flat foot. A review. *J Bone Joint Surg Am* 1984;66:976–984.

237. Slomann W. On coalitio calcaneo-navicularis. *J Orthop Surg* 1921;3:586.

238. Harris R, Beath T. Etiology of peroneal spastic flatfoot. *J Bone Joint Surg Br* 1948;30:624.

239. Simmons EH. Tibialis spastic varus foot with tarsal coalition. *J Bone Joint Surg Br* 1965;47:533–536.

240. Stuecker RD, Bennett JT. Tarsal coalition presenting as a pes cavo-varus deformity: report of three cases and review of the literature. *Foot Ankle* 1993;14:540–544.

241. Grogan DP, Holt GR, Ogden JA. Talocalcaneal coalition in patients who have fibular hemimelia or proximal femoral focal deficiency. A comparison of the radiographic and pathological findings. *J Bone Joint Surg Am* 1994;76:1363–1370.

242. Spero CR, Simon GS, Tornetta P III. Clubfeet and tarsal coalition. *J Pediatr Orthop* 1994;14:372–376.

243. Mah J, Kasser J, Upton J. The foot in Apert syndrome. *Clin Plast Surg* 1991;18:391–397.

244. Glessner JR Jr, Davis GL. Bilateral calcaneonavicular coalition occurring in twin boys. A case report. *Clin Orthop* 1966;47:173–176.

245. Heiple KG, Lovejoy CO. The antiquity of tarsal coalition. Bilateral deformity in a Pre-Columbian Indian skeleton. *J Bone Joint Surg Am* 1969;51:979–983.

246. Herschel H, Von Ronnen JR. The occurrence of calcaneonavicular synosteosis in pes valgus contractus. *J Bone Joint Surg Am* 1950;32A:280–282.

247. Lysack JT, Fenton PV. Variations in calcaneonavicular morphology demonstrated with radiography. *Radiology* 2004; 230: 493–497.

248. Stormont DM, Peterson HA. The relative incidence of tarsal coalition. *Clin Orthop* 1983;181:28–36.

249. Clarke DM. Multiple tarsal coalitions in the same foot. *J Pediatr Orthop* 1997;17:777–780.

250. Piqueres X, de Zabala S, Torrens C, et al. Cubonavicular coalition: a case report and literature review. *Clin Orthop* 2002;396: 112–114.

251. Wray J, Herndon C. Hereditary transmission of congenital coalition of the calcaneus to the navicular. *J Bone Joint Surg Am* 1963; 45:365.

252. Leonard MA. The inheritance of tarsal coalition and its relationship to spastic flat foot. *J Bone Joint Surg Br* 1974;56B:520–526.

253. Mosca VS. Flexible flatfoot and tarsal coalition. In: Richards B, ed. *Orthopaedic knowledge update: pediatrics*. Rosemont, IL: American Academy of Orthopaedic Surgeons, 1996:211.

254. Oestreich AE, Mize WA, Crawford AH, et al. The "anteater nose": a direct sign of calcaneonavicular coalition on the lateral radiograph. *J Pediatr Orthop* 1987;7:709–711.

255. Taniguchi A, Tanaka Y, Kadono K, et al. C sign for diagnosis of talocalcaneal coalition. *Radiology* 2003;228:501–505.

256. Liu PT, Roberts CC, Chivers FS, et al. "Absent middle facet": a sign on unenhanced radiography of subtalar joint coalition. *AJR Am J Roentgenol* 2003;181:1565–1572.

257. Drennan JC. Tarsal coalitions. *Instr Course Lect* 1996;45: 323–329.

258. Conway JJ, Cowell HR. Tarsal coalition: clinical significance and roentgenographic demonstration. *Radiology* 1969;92:799–811.

259. Herzenberg JE, Goldner JL, Martinez S, et al. Computerized tomography of talocalcaneal tarsal coalition: a clinical and anatomic study. *Foot Ankle* 1986;6:273–288.

260. Deutsch AL, Resnick D, Campbell G. Computed tomography and bone scintigraphy in the evaluation of tarsal coalition. *Radiology* 1982;144:137–140.

261. Emery KH, Bisset GS, 3rd, Johnson ND, et al. Tarsal coalition: a blinded comparison of MRI and CT. *Pediatr Radiol*, 1998; 28: 612–616.

262. Wechsler RJ, Schweitzer ME, Deely DM, et al. Tarsal coalition: depiction and characterization with CT and MR imaging. *Radiology* 1994;193:447–452.

263. Jayakumar S, Cowell HR. Rigid flatfoot. *Clin Orthop* 1977;122: 77–84.

264. Kumai T, Takakura Y, Akiyama K, et al. Histopathologic study of nonosseous tarsal coalition. *Foot Ankle Int* 1998;525.

265. Outland T, Murphy ID. The pathomechanics of peroneal spastic flat foot. *Clin Orthop* 1960;16:64–73.

266. Lateur LM, Van Hoe LR, Van Ghillewe KV, et al. Subtalar coalition: diagnosis with the C sign on lateral radiographs of the ankle. *Radiology* 1994;193:847–851.

267. Cowell HR. Tarsal coalition—review and update. *Instr Course Lect* 1982;31:264–271.

268. Saxena A, Erickson S. Tarsal coalitions. Activity levels with and without surgery. *J Am Podiatr Med Assoc* 2003;93:259–263.

269. Badgley C. Coalition of the calcaneus and the navicular. *Arch Surg* 1927;15:75.

270. Cowell H. Extensor brevis arthroplasty. *J Bone Joint Surg Am* 1970;82:820.

271. Gonzalez P, Kumar SJ. Calcaneonavicular coalition treated by resection and interposition of the extensor digitorum brevis muscle. *J Bone Joint Surg Am* 1990;72:71–77.

272. Moyes ST, Crawfurd EJ, Aichroth PM. The interposition of extensor digitorum brevis in the resection of calcaneonavicular bars. *J Pediatr Orthop* 1994;14:387–388.

273. Scranton PE Jr. Treatment of symptomatic talocalcaneal coalition. *J Bone Joint Surg Am* 1987;69:533–539.

274. Swiontkowski MF, Scranton PE, Hansen S. Tarsal coalitions: long-term results of surgical treatment. *J Pediatr Orthop* 1983;3: 287–292.

275. Takakura Y, Sugimoto K, Tanaka Y, et al. Symptomatic talocalcaneal coalition. Its clinical significance and treatment. *Clin Orthop* 1991;249–256.

276. Wilde PH, Torode IP, Dickens DR, et al. Resection for symptomatic talocalcaneal coalition. *J Bone Joint Surg Br* 1994;76: 797–801.

277. Cooperman DR, Janke BE, Gilmore A, et al. A three-dimensional study of calcaneonavicular tarsal coalitions. *J Pediatr Orthop* 2001;21:648–651.

278. Luhmann SJ, Schoenecker PL. Symptomatic talocalcaneal coalition resection: indications and results. *J Pediatr Orthop* 1998; 18:748–754.

279. Olney BW, Asher MA. Excision of symptomatic coalition of the middle facet of the talocalcaneal joint. *J Bone Joint Surg Am* 1987;69:539–544.

280. Kumar SJ, Guille JT, Lee MS, et al. Osseous and non-osseous coalition of the middle facet of the talocalcaneal joint. *J Bone Joint Surg Am* 1992;74:529–535.

281. Mann RA, Beaman DN, Horton GA. Isolated subtalar arthrodesis. *Foot Ankle Int* 1998;19:511–519.

282. Cain TJ, Hyman S. Peroneal spastic flat foot. Its treatment by osteotomy of the os calcis. *J Bone Joint Surg Br* 1978;60-B:527–529.

283. Luba R, Rosman M. Bunions in children: treatment with a modified Mitchell osteotomy. *J Pediatr Orthop* 1984;4:44–47.

284. Scranton PE Jr., Zuckerman JD. Bunion surgery in adolescents: results of surgical treatment. *J Pediatr Orthop* 1984;4:39–43.

285. Canale PB, Aronsson DD, Lamont RL, et al. The Mitchell procedure for the treatment of adolescent hallux valgus. A long-term study. *J Bone Joint Surg Am* 1993;75:1610–1618.

286. Groiso JA. Juvenile hallux valgus. A conservative approach to treatment. *J Bone Joint Surg Am* 1992;74:1367–1374.

287. Glynn MK, Dunlop JB, Fitzpatrick D. The Mitchell distal metatarsal osteotomy for hallux valgus. *J Bone Joint Surg Br* 1980;62-B:188–191.

288. Coughlin MJ, Roger A. Mann award. Juvenile hallux valgus: etiology and treatment. *Foot Ankle Int* 1995;16:682–697.

289. Hardy RH, Clapham JC. Observations on hallux valgus; based on a controlled series. *J Bone Joint Surg Br* 1951;33-B:376–391.

290. Coughlin M. Juvenile hallux valgus. In: Coughlin M, Mann R, eds. *Surgery of the foot and ankle*, 7th ed. St. Louis, MO: Mosby, 1999:270.

291. Johnston O. Further studies of the inheritance of hand and foot anomalies. *Clin Orthop* 1954;146.

292. Shine IB. Incidence of hallux valgus in a partially shoe-wearing community. *Br Med J* 1965;5451:1648–1650.

293. Jones A. Hallux valgus in the adolescent. *Proc R Soc Med* 1948:392.

294. Inman VT. Hallux valgus: a review of etiologic factors. *Orthop Clin North Am* 1974;5:59–66.

295. Kalen V, Brecher A. Relationship between adolescent bunions and flatfeet. *Foot Ankle* 1988;8:331.

296. Kilmartin TE, Wallace WA. The significance of pes planus in juvenile hallux valgus. *Foot Ankle* 1992;13:53–56.

297. Price GF. Metatarsus primus varus: including various clinicoradiologic feautres of the female foot. *Clin Orthop* 1979; 145: 217–223.

298. Goldner JL, Gaines RW. Adult and juvenile hallux valgus: analysis and treatment. *Orthop Clin North Am* 1976;7:863–887.

299. Thompson GH. Bunions and deformities of the toes in children and adolescents. *Instr Course Lect* 1996;45:355–367.

300. Piggott H. The natural history of scoliosis in myelodysplasia. *J Bone Joint Surg Br* 1980;62-B:54–58.

301. Richardson EG, Graves SC, McClure JT, et al. First metatarsal head-shaft angle: a method of determination. *Foot Ankle* 1993; 14:181–185.

302. Vittetoe DA, Saltzman CL, Krieg JC, et al. Validity and reliability of the first distal metatarsal articular angle. *Foot Ankle Int* 1994; 15:541–547.

303. Kilmartin TE, Barrington RL, Wallace WA. A controlled prospective trial of a foot orthosis for juvenile hallux valgus. *J Bone Joint Surg Br* 1994;76:210–214.

304. Ball J, Sullivan JA. Treatment of the juvenile bunion by Mitchell osteotomy. *Orthopedics* 1985;8:1249–1252.

305. Bonney G, Macnab I. Hallux valgus and hallux rigidus; a critical survey of operative results. *J Bone Joint Surg Br* 1952;34-B:366–385.

306. Helal B, Gupta SK, Gojaseni P. Surgery for adolescent hallux valgus. *Acta Orthop Scand* 1974;45:271–295.

307. Simmonds FM, Menelaux MB. Hallux valgus in adolescents. *J Bone Joint Surg Br* 1960;42:761.

308. Mann RA, Pfeffinger L. Hallux valgus repair. DuVries modified McBride procedure. *Clin Orthop* 1991;272:213–218.

309. McGrory BJ, Amadio PC, Dobyns JH, et al. Anomalies of the fingers and toes associated with Klippel-Trenaunay syndrome. *J Bone Joint Surg Am* 1991;73:1537–1546.

310. Peterson HA, Newman SR. Adolescent bunion deformity treated with double osteotomy and longitudinal pin fixation of the first ray. *J Pediatr Orthop* 1993;13:80–84.

311. Geissele AE, Stanton RP. Surgical treatment of adolescent hallux valgus. *J Pediatr Orthop* 1990;10:642–648.

312. Helal B. Surgery for adolescent hallux valgus. *Clin Orthop* 1981; 157:50–63.

313. Wilson JN. Oblique displacement osteotomy for hallux valgus. *J Bone Joint Surg Br* 1963;45:552–556.

314. Zimmer TJ, Johnson KA, Klassen RA. Treatment of hallux valgus in adolescents by the chevron osteotomy. *Foot Ankle* 1989; 9: 190–193.

315. Jones KJ, Feiwell LA, Freedman EL, et al. The effect of chevron osteotomy with lateral capsular release on the blood supply to the first metatarsal head. *J Bone Joint Surg Am* 1995;77:197–204.

316. Barnett RS. Medial/lateral column separation (Third Street operation) for dorsal talonavicular subluxation. In: Simons G, ed. *The clubfoot: the present and a view of the future*. New York: Springer-Verlag, 1994:268.

317. Austin DW, Leventen EO. A new osteotomy for hallux valgus: a horizontally directed "V" displacement osteotomy of the metatarsal head for hallux valgus and primus varus. *Clin Orthop* 1981;157:25–30.

318. Akin O. The treatment of hallux valgus: a new operative procedure and its results. *Med Sentinel* 1925;33:678.

319. Fulford GE. Surgical management of ankle and foot deformities in cerebral palsy. *Clin Orthop* 1990;253:55–61.

320. Goldner JL. Hallux valgus and hallux flexus associated with cerebral palsy: analysis and treatment. *Clin Orthop* 1981;157:98–104.

321. Holstein A. Hallux valgus—an acquired deformity of the foot in cerebral palsy. *Foot Ankle* 1980;1:33–38.

322. Black GB, Grogan DP, Bobechko WP. Butler arthroplasty for correction of the adducted fifth toe: a retrospective study of 36 operations between 1968 and 1982. *J Pediatr Orthop* 1985;5:439–441.

323. Cockin J. Butler's operation for an over-riding fifth toe. *J Bone Joint Surg Br* 1968;50:78–81.

324. DeBoeck H. Butler's operation for congenital overriding of the fifth toe: retrospective 1-7-year study of 23 cases. *Acta Orthop Scand* 1993;64:343.

325. Janecki CJ, Wilde AH. Results of phalangectomy of the fifth toe for hammertoe. The Ruiz-Mora procedure. *J Bone Joint Surg Am* 1976;58:1005–1007.

326. Pollard JP, Morrison PJ. Flexor tenotomy in the treatment of curly toes. *Proc R Soc Med* 1975;68:480–481.

327. Sweetnam R. Congenital curly toes; an investigation into the value of treatment. *Lancet* 1958;2:398–400.

328. Ross ER, Menelaus MB. Open flexor tenotomy for hammer toes and curly toes in childhood. *J Bone Joint Surg Br* 1984; 66: 770–771.

329. Hamer AJ, Stanley D, Smith TW. Surgery for curly toe deformity: a double-blind, randomised, prospective trial. *J Bone Joint Surg Br* 1993;75:662–663.

330. Shands AR Jr, Wentz IJ. Congenital anomalies, accessory bones, and osteochondritis in the feet of 850 children. *Surg Clin North Am* 1953;97:1643–1666.

331. Geist ES. The accessory scaphoid bone. *J Bone Joint Surg Am* 1925;7:570.

332. McKusick VA. *Mendelian inheritance in man: catalogs of autosomal dominant, autosomal recessive and X-linked phenotypes*, 2nd ed. Baltimore, MD: The Johns Hopkins University Press, 1968.

333. Kidner F. The pre-hallux (accessory scaphoid) in its relation to flat-foot. *J Bone Joint Surg Am* 1929;11:831.

334. Kidner F. The pre-hallux in relation to flatfoot. *JAMA* 1933; 101:1539.

335. Leonard MH, Gonzalez S, Breck LW, et al. Lateral transfer of the posterior tibial tendon in certain selected cases of pes plano valgus (kidner operation). *Clin Orthop* 1965;40:139–144.

336. Zadek I, Gold A. The accessory tarsal scaphoid. *J Bone Joint Surg Am* 1948;30A:957.

337. Sullivan JA, Miller WA. The relationship of the accessory navicular to the development of the flat foot. *Clin Orthop* 1979; 144: 233–237.

338. Ray S, Goldberg VM. Surgical treatment of the accessory navicular. *Clin Orthop* 1983;177:61–66.

339. Grogan DP, Gasser SI, Ogden JA. The painful accessory navicular: a clinical and histopathological study. *Foot Ankle* 1989;10:164–169.

340. Jones RL. The human foot: an experimental study of its muscles and ligaments in the support of the arch. *Am J Anat* 1941;68:1.

341. Bennett GL, Weiner DS, Leighley B. Surgical treatment of symptomatic accessory tarsal navicular. *J Pediatr Orthop* 1990;10:445–449.

342. Macnicol MF, Voutsinas S. Surgical treatment of the symptomatic accessory navicular. *J Bone Joint Surg Br* 1984;66:218–226.

343. Veitch JM. Evaluation of the Kidner procedure in treatment of symptomatic accessory tarsal scaphoid. *Clin Orthop* 1978;131:210–213.

344. Giannestrus NJ. *Foot disorders: medical and surgical management*. Philadelphia, PA: Lea & Febiger, 1973.

345. McElvenny R. Hallux varus. *Q Bull Northwest Univ Med Sch* 1941;15:277.

346. Mills JA, Menelaus MB. Hallux varus. *J Bone Joint Surg Br* 1989; 71:437–440.

347. Mubarak SJ, O'Brien TJ, Davids JR. Metatarsal epiphyseal bracket: treatment by central physiolysis. *J Pediatr Orthop* 1993;13:5–8.

348. Beaty J. Congenital foot deformities. In: Coughlin M, Mann R, eds. *Surgery of the foot and ankle*, 7th ed. St. Louis, MO: Mosby, 1999:1320.

349. Light TR, Ogden JA. The longitudinal epiphyseal bracket: implications for surgical correction. *J Pediatr Orthop* 1981;1:299–305.

350. Farmer AW. Congenital hallux varus. *Am J Surg* 1958; 95: 274–278.

351. Frazier TM. A note on race-specific congenital malformation rates. *Am J Obstet Gynecol* 1960;80:184–185.

352. Woolf C, Myrianthopoulos N. Polydactyly in American negroes and whites. *Am J Hum Genet* 1973;25:397.

353. Phelps DA, Grogan DP. Polydactyly of the foot. *J Pediatr Orthop* 1985;5:446–451.

354. Temtamy S, McKusick V. Synopsis of hand malformations with particular emphasis on genetic factors. *Birth Defects* 1969;5:125.

355. Venn-Watson EA. Problems in polydactyly of the foot. *Orthop Clin North Am* 1976;7:909–927.

356. Nogami H. Polydactyly and polysyndactyly of the fifth toe. *Clin Orthop* 1986;204:261–265.

357. Biesecker LG, Happle R, Mulliken JB, et al. Proteus syndrome: diagnostic criteria, differential diagnosis, and patient evaluation. *Am J Med Genet* 1999;84:389–395.

358. Kalen V, Burwell DS, Omer GE. Macrodactyly of the hands and feet. *J Pediatr Orthop* 1988;8:311–315.

359. Turra S, Santini S, Cagnoni G, et al. Gigantism of the foot: our experience in seven cases. *J Pediatr Orthop* 1998;18:337–345.

360. Chen SH, Huang SC, Wang JH, et al. Macrodactyly of the feet and hands. *J Formos Med Assoc* 1997;96:901–907.

361. DeCosta H, Hunter D. Magnetic resonance imaging in macrodactyly. *Br J Radiol* 1996;69:1189–1194.

362. Barsky A. Macrodactyly. *J Bone Joint Surg Am* 1967;49:1255.

363. Chang CH, Kumar SJ, Riddle EC, et al. Macrodactyly of the foot. *J Bone Joint Surg Am* 2002;84-A:1189–1194.

364. Topoleski TA, Ganel A, Grogan DP. Effect of proximal phalangeal epiphysiodesis in the treatment of macrodactyly. *Foot Ankle Int* 1997;18:500–503.

365. Dedrick D, Kling D. Ray resection in the treatment of macrodactyly of the foot in children. *Orthop Trans* 1985:145.

366. Dennyson WG, Bear JN, Bhoola KD. Macrodactyly in the foot. *J Bone Joint Surg Br* 1977;59:355–359.

367. Grogan DP, Bernstein RM, Habal MB, et al. Congenital lipofibromatosis associated with macrodactyly of the foot. *Foot Ankle* 1991;12:40–46.

368. Cruveilhier J. *Anatomie pathologique de corps humaine*. Paris: S. Balliere, 1829.

369. Birch-Jensen A. *Congenital deformities of the upper extremities*. Copenhagen: Ejnar Munksgaard, 1949.

370. McMullen G, Pearson K. One the inheritance of the deformity known as split foot or lobster claw. *Biometrika* 1913;9:381.

371. Stiles K, Pickard JS. Hereditary malformations of the hands and feet. *Plast Reconstr Surg* 1943:627.

372. Walker JC, Clodius L. The syndromes of cleft lip, cleft palate, and lobster-claw deformities of hands and feet. *Plast Reconstr Surg* 1963;32:627–636.

373. O'Rahilly R, Gardner E, Gray DJ. The ectodermal thickening and ridge in the limbs of staged human embryos. *J Embryol Exp Morphol* 1956;4:254.

374. Watson AG, Bonde RK. Congenital malformations of the flipper in three West Indian manatees, Trichechus manatus, and a proposed mechanism for development of ectrodactyly and cleft hand in mammals. *Clin Orthop* 1986;202:294–301.

375. Blauth W, Borisch NC. Cleft feet. Proposals for a new classification based on roentgenographic morphology. *Clin Orthop* 1990; 258:41–48.

376. Wood VE, Peppers TA, Shook J. Cleft-foot closure: a simplified technique and review of the literature. *J Pediatr Orthop* 1997;17:501–504.

377. Sumiya N, Onizuka T. Seven years' survey of our new cleft foot repair. *Plast Reconstr Surg* 1980;65:447–459.

## Acquired Conditions

378. Samilson RL, Dillin W. Cavus, cavovarus, and calcaneocavus. An update. *Clin Orthop* 1983;177:125–132.

379. Brewerton DA, Sandifer PH, Sweetnam DR. "Idiopathic" Pes Cavus: an investigation into its aetiology. *Br Med J* 1963;5358:659–661.

380. Holmes JR, Hansen ST Jr. Foot and ankle manifestations of Charcot-Marie-Tooth disease. *Foot Ankle* 1993;14:476–486.

381. Olney B. Treatment of the cavus foot. Deformity in the pediatric patient with Charcot-Marie-Tooth. *Foot Ankle Clin* 2000;5:305–315.

382. Mann RA, Missirian J. Pathophysiology of Charcot-Marie-Tooth disease. *Clin Orthop* 1988;234:221–228.

383. Paulos L, Coleman SS, Samuelson KM. Pes cavovarus. Review of a surgical approach using selective soft-tissue procedures. *J Bone Joint Surg Am* 1980;62:942–953.

384. Sabir M, Lyttle D. Pathogenesis of pes cavus in Charcot-Marie-Tooth disease. *Clin Orthop* 1983;175:173–178.

385. Coleman SS, Chesnut WJ. A simple test for hindfoot flexibility in the cavovarus foot. *Clin Orthop* 1977;123:60–62.

386. Alexander IJ, Johnson KA. Assessment and management of pes cavus in Charcot-Marie-Tooth disease. *Clin Orthop* 1989; 246:273–281.

387. Levitt RL, Canale ST, Cooke AJ Jr, et al. The role of foot surgery in progressive neuromuscular disorders in children. *J Bone Joint Surg Am* 1973;55:1396–1410.

388. Steindler A. Stripping of the os calcis. *Am J Orthop Surg* 1920; 2:8.

389. Sherman FC, Westin GW. Plantar release in the correction of deformities of the foot in childhood. *J Bone Joint Surg Am* 1981;63:1382–1389.

390. Tynan MC, Klenerman L. The modified Robert Jones tendon transfer in cases of pes cavus and clawed hallux. *Foot Ankle Int* 1994;15:68–71.

391. Breusch SJ, Wenz W, Doderlein L. Function after correction of a clawed great toe by a modified Robert Jones transfer. *J Bone Joint Surg Br* 2000;82:250–254.

392. Cole WH. The classic. The treatment of claw-foot. By Wallace H. Cole. 1940. *Clin Orthop*, 1983:3–6.

393. Mulier T, Dereymaeker G, Fabry G. Jones transfer to the lesser rays in metatarsalgia: technique and long-term follow-up. *Foot Ankle Int* 1994;15:523–530.

394. Japas LM. Surgical treatment of pes cavus by tarsal V-osteotomy. Preliminary report. *J Bone Joint Surg Am* 1968;50:927–944.

395. Jahss MH. Tarsometatarsal truncated-wedge arthrodesis for pes cavus and equinovarus deformity of the fore part of the foot. *J Bone Joint Surg Am* 1980;62:713–722.

396. Wilcox PG, Weiner DS. The Akron midtarsal dome osteotomy in the treatment of rigid pes cavus: a preliminary review. *J Pediatr Orthop* 1985;5:333–338.

397. Swanson AB, Braune HS, Coleman JA. The cavus foot concept of production and treatment by metatarsal osteotomy. *J Bone Joint Surg Am* 1966;48-A:1019.

398. Gould N. Surgery in advanced Charcot-Marie-Tooth disease. *Foot Ankle* 1984;4:267–273.

399. Watanabe RS. Metatarsal osteotomy for the cavus foot. *Clin Orthop* 1990;252:217–230.

400. Aktas S, Sussman MD. The radiological analysis of pes cavus deformity in Charcot Marie Tooth disease. *J Pediatr Orthop B* 2000;9:137–140.

401. Sammarco GJ, Taylor R. Cavovarus foot treated with combined calcaneus and metatarsal osteotomies. *Foot Ankle Int* 2001; 22:19–30.

402. Schwend RM, Drennan JC. Cavus foot deformity in children. *J Am Acad Orthop Surg* 2003;11:201–211.

403. Kucukkaya M, Kabukcuoglu Y, Kuzgun U. Management of the neuromuscular foot deformities with the Ilizarov method. *Foot Ankle Int* 2002;23:135–141.

404. Kidner F. Kohler's disease of the tarsal scaphoid or os navicular. *JAMA* 1924:650.

405. Ippolito E, Ricciardi Pollini PT, Falez F. Kohler's disease of the tarsal navicular: long-term follow-up of 12 cases. *J Pediatr Orthop* 1984;4:416–417.

406. Williams GA, Cowell HR. Kohler's disease of the tarsal navicular. *Clin Orthop* 1981:53–58.

407. Borges JL, Guille JT, Bowen JR. Kohler's bone disease of the tarsal navicular. *J Pediatr Orthop* 1995;15:596–598.

408. Tsirikos AI, Riddle EC, Kruse R. Bilateral Kohler's disease in identical twins. *Clin Orthop* 2003:195–198.

409. Karp M. Kohler's disease of the tarsal scaphoid. *J Bone Joint Surg Br* 1937:84.

410. Waugh W. The ossification and vascularisation of the tarsal navicular and their relation to Kohler's disease. *J Bone Joint Surg Br* 1958;40-B:765–777.

411. Sever J. Apophysitis of the os calcis. *NY State J Med* 1912; 95:1025.

412. Micheli LJ, Ireland ML. Prevention and management of calcaneal apophysitis in children: an overuse syndrome. *J Pediatr Orthop* 1987;7:34–38.

413. Siffert RS. Classification of the osteochondroses. *Clin Orthop* 1981;158:10–18.

414. Ferguson AB Jr, Gingrich RM. The normal and the abnormal calcaneal apophysis and tarsal navicular. *Clin Orthop* 1957;4: 87–95.

415. Liberson A, Lieberson S, Mendes DG, et al. Remodeling of the calcaneus apophysis in the growing child. *J Pediatr Orthop B* 1995;4:74–79.

416. Katz JF. Nonarticular osteochondroses. *Clin Orthop* 1981;158: 70–76.

417. Freiberg A. Infraction of the second metatarsal bone: a typical injury. *Surg Gynecol Obstet* 1914;19:191.

418. Duthie RB, Houghton GR. Constitutional aspects of the osteochondroses. *Clin Orthop* 1981;158:19–27.

419. Katcherian D. Treatment of Freiberg's disease. *Orthop Clin North Am* 1994;25:69.

420. Gauthier G, Elbaz R. Freiberg's infraction: a subchondral bone fatigue fracture. A new surgical treatment. *Clin Orthop* 1979:93–95.

421. Smillie I. Freiberg's infraction (Kohler's second disease). *J Bone Joint Surg Br* 1957;39B:580.

422. Omer GE Jr. Primary articular osteochondroses. *Clin Orthop* 1981;158:33–40.

423. Sproul J, Klaaren H, Mannarino F. Surgical treatment of Freiberg's infraction in athletes. *Am J Sports Med* 1993; 21: 381–384.

424. Smith TW, Stanley D, Rowley DI. Treatment of Freiberg's disease. A new operative technique. *J Bone Joint Surg Br* 1991;73:129–130.

425. Kinnard P, Lirette R. Freiberg's disease and dorsiflexion osteotomy. *J Bone Joint Surg Br* 1991;73:864–865.

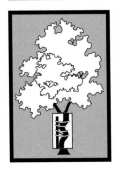

# 31

# The Child with a Limb Deficiency

*Raymond T. Morrissy*  *Brian J. Giavedoni*  *Colleen Coulter-O'Berry*

There is little information on the incidence of congenital limb deficiency in the population, and what is reported varies widely, from 1 per 4264 in Canada (1) to 5 per 10,000 in Australia (2) to 310 per 10,000 in Tayside, Scotland (3). This fact illustrates that this information should be interpreted with caution because the methods of gathering it vary.

Although such figures, if available, would be of use to health planning agencies, the fact is that to the orthopaedic surgeon, a child with a limb deficiency is not a common problem. Most limb deficiencies seen in childhood are congenital in origin. This is followed at a distant second by those caused by trauma and lastly by those caused by tumors. This infrequency creates a lack of experience for the practioner in a complex problem, creating a need for these patients to be seen in an organized program in which knowledge and experience are available.

Fibular deficiency is the most common long-bone deficiency. The incidence is between 7.4 and 20 per million live births (4,5). The prevalence of tibial deficiencies is far less, and is reported to be approximately one per million live births. The incidence of proximal femoral focal deficiency (PFFD) ranges from 1 in 50,000 to 1 in 200,000 live births. Although this is a more common anomaly than fibular deficiency, the explanation lies in the difficulty in separating congenital short femur from true PFFD.

The incidence of upper-extremity amputations is not precisely known. However, two general facts are easily accepted. Although upper-extremity amputations of all types are unusual, in children congenital amputations are far more common than acquired amputations. In one multicenter review, 85% of bilateral deficiencies were congenital (6). In addition, one congenital upper-extremity deficiency, below-elbow transverse deficiency, is more common than all others, combined. Few physicians, other than those working in a limb-deficiency program, will have much experience with these amputations.

## CLASSIFICATION

The attempt to classify congenital anomalies has taken many paths, and most clinics choose to use some combination of these classification systems to best categorize the child's deficiency. These different classifications are an attempt to convey the particular anomaly more precisely.

The first attempt to devise a classification system for congenital anomalies was that of Frantz and O'Rahilly (7) (Fig. 31.1). This system was widely adopted in the United States, and is still widely used by clinicians today to describe longitudinal deficiencies. However, it was not acceptable to European physicians because of problems created in translating terms such as "hemimelia." This led to the classification system devised by the International Standards Organization (ISO) and the International Society for Prosthetics and Orthotics (ISPO) (8).

The classification of Frantz and O'Rahilly begins with seven descriptive terms derived from Greek root words. Three of the terms are from the root word *melos*, meaning limb:

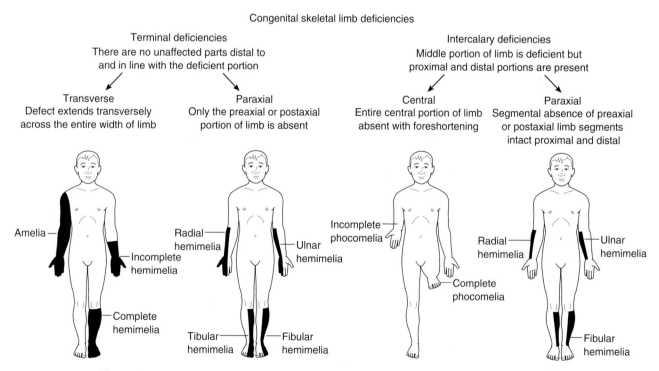

**Figure 31.1** Diagrammatic representation of the Frantz and O'Rahilly classification of congenital limb deficiencies. (From Frantz C, O'Rahilly R. Congenital skeletal limb deficiencies. *J Bone Joint Surg Am* 1961;43:1202, with permission)

amelia, absence of a limb; hemimelia, absence of a large part or half of a limb; and phocomelia, or a flipperlike limb (*phoke;* seal). The hemimelias can be divided into complete, partial, and paraxial hemimelias. The remaining four terms refer to the hands (*cheir*), feet (*pous, podos*), metacarpals (*daktylos*), and phalanges (*phalanx*) (Table 31.1).

The hemimelias can have three additional descriptions: complete, when the entire distal half of the limb is missing; partial, when only a portion of the distal half is missing; and paraxial, when either the preaxial or postaxial side of the distal portion of the limb is missing. The hemimelia is named after the missing portion of the limb. Therefore, a complete absence of the fibula is a fibular hemimelia.

Next, the deficiencies are either terminal, in which all of the parts of the limb distal to and in line with the defect are affected; or intercalary, in which the parts of the limb proximal and distal to the defect are present. Finally, the terminal and intercalary deficiencies are further divided into transverse deficiencies, in which the defect extends across the entire limb, and longitudinal deficiencies, in which only the pre- or postaxial portion is affected.

The ISO/ISPO system of classification of deficiencies present at birth (ISO 8548-1 Method of Describing Limb Deficiencies Present at Birth) was adopted by the ISO and the ISPO (8,9). In this system, the deficiency is first described as transverse, in which the entire limb is missing; or as longitudinal, in which all or part of one or more bones in a limb are missing. In a longitudinal deficiency ("paraxial" in the Franz and O'Rahilly classification), there may be parts of the limb present distal to the deficiency. In

## TABLE 31.1
### CLASSIFICATION OF CONGENITAL SKELETAL LIMB DEFICIENCIES

#### Terminal (T)

| Transverse (-) | Longitudinal (/) |
|---|---|
| 1. Amelia (absence of limb) | 1. Complete paraxial hemimelia (complete absence of one of the forearm or leg elements, and of the corresponding portion of the hand or foot)—R, U, TI, or FI[a] |
| 2. Hemimelia (absence of forearm and hand or leg and foot) | 2. Incomplete paraxial hemimelia (similar to the above, but part of the defective element is present)—r, u, ti, or fi[a] |
| 3. Partial hemimelia (part of forearm or leg is present) | 3. Partial adactylia (absence of one to four digits and their metacarpals or metatarsals): 1, 2, 3, 4, or 5 |
| 4. Acheiria or apodia (absence of hand or foot) | 4. Partial aphalangia (absence of one or more phalanges from one to four digits): 1, 2, 3, 4, or 5 |
| 5. Complete adactylia (absence of all five digits and their metacarpals or metatarsals) | |
| 6. Complete aphalangia (absence of one or more phalanges from all five digits) | |

#### Intercalary (I)

| Transverse (-) | Longitudinal (/) |
|---|---|
| 1. Complete phocomelia (hand or foot attached directly to trunk) | 1. Complete paraxial hemimelia (similar to corresponding terminal defect but hand or foot is more or less complete)—R, U, TI, or FI[a] |
| 2. Proximal phocomelia (hand and forearm, or foot and leg, attached directly to trunk) | 2. Incomplete paraxial hemimelia (similar to corresponding terminal defect but hand or foot is more or less complete)—r, u, ti, or fi[a] |
| 3. Distal phocomelia (hand or foot attached directly to arm or thigh) | 3. Partial adactylia (absence of all or part of a metacarpal or metatarsal): 1 or 5 |
| | 4. Partial aphalangia (absence of proximal or middle phalanx, or both, from one or more digits):1, 2, 3, 4, or 5 |

-, transverse; /, longitudinal; 1, 2, 3, 4, or 5 denotes the digital ray involved; FI or fi, fibular; I, intercalary; R or r, radial; T, terminal; TI or ti, tibial; U or u, ulnar.
A line below a numeral denotes upper limb involvement; for example, T-2 represents terminal transverse hemimelia of the upper limb. A line above a numeral denotes lower limb involvement, for example, I-1 represents intercalary transverse complete phocomelia of the lower limb.
[a]In capital letters when the paraxial hemimelia is complete, in small letters when the defect is incomplete.
From Frantz C, O'Rahilly R. Congenital skeletal limb deficiencies. *J Bone Joint Surg Am* 1961;43:1202, with permission.

the transverse deficiencies, the part of the segment in which the limb ends is named, and extent may be stated. A complete loss of the limb distal to the tibial tubercle would be "transverse leg upper third." In a longitudinal deficiency, the bone or bones missing are named and described as "partial" or "total." Therefore, a fibular deficiency with part of the distal fibula present would be described as "longitudinal fibula partial." Because this system does not characterize deficiencies (e.g., PFFD, phocomelia, and amelia), these terms may still be used.

A second system for describing acquired (traumatic or surgical) amputations (ISO 8549-2.1) uses three adjectives: trans, disarticulation, and partial. The term trans is used to describe any amputation across the axis of a long bone. A child who has an amputation performed through the upper third of the tibia is not a case of below-knee (B-K) amputation in this classification but one of "transtibial, upper third." "Disarticulation" refers to any amputation through a joint. Therefore, a Syme amputation is an ankle disarticulation. "Partial" refers to any amputation distal to the wrist or ankle joint. Therefore, a Boyd amputation is a partial foot amputation, with qualifiers added to distinguish it from a Chopart amputation.

## ETIOLOGY

There are at least three ways in which limb deficiencies can be caused: errors in the genetic control of limb development; disruption of the developing arterial supply, such as "the subclavian artery supply disruption sequence;" (10) and intrauterine amputation from amniotic bands.

The oldest and most commonly held etiology for congenital amputation in the past was the mechanical amputation of limbs by amniotic bands. Streeter, whose name is associated with this concept of limb deficiency, actually felt that the bands and constrictions were due to an intrinsic defect in the growth of the fetal limb (11). There is, however, evidence that amniotic bands can form a constriction around the developing limb that interferes with the growth of the limb. The resulting constriction can lead to any degree of damage, from a constriction band around a limb that is otherwise normal to a complete transverse amputation. The previously developed limb has actually been recovered at the time of birth, indicating the mechanism (12). Most children with amniotic band syndrome have either craniofacial abnormalities or other evidence of band formation.

Modern genetics has shown that the development of the limb is a complex phenomenon that requires the precise interaction of a large number of genes and their effects, which are described in Chapter 1 and other review articles (13,14). The opportunity for errors in this system is great, and animal experimentation has identified the probable mechanism in several limb anomalies.

The disruption of the subclavian artery and its blood supply to the tissues explains the overlap of many of the

common orthopaedic conditions seen, for example, Poland syndrome, Klippel-Feil syndrome, Mobius syndrome, Sprengle deformity, and transverse limb deficiencies. There are several possible mechanisms by which this disruption may occur. For more details, the reader is referred to an excellent review article (15).

This understanding of the various etiologies is of importance to the clinician. With genetic control and vascular disruptions playing a large role in the development of the limb and having consequences in other organs and systems, the association of limb deficiencies with other abnormalities creating syndromes is likely. There are two implications when children present with limb deficiencies; a thorough examination for other abnormalities is necessary and any heritable genetic defect should be identified. The possibility of a teratogen always arises in the parent's mind. Although there may be many suspected agents, to date, thalidomide remains the only drug proven to have caused many congenital limb deficiencies, and other teratogens do not appear to play a role in the congenital limb deficiencies of today. The role of retinoic acid and low cholesterol on gene expression is discussed in Chapter 1.

Although most congenital limb deficiencies are sporadic and not transmissible (transverse below-elbow), a few are (tibial deficiency and cleft hand and foot). This is often something parents desire to know. Understanding the cause of the deficiency is important to the resolving of the guilt that parents will initially feel. The possibility of a transmissible defect is certainly something their affected offspring will also need to know. A recent study from the Medical Birth Registry of Norway showed that children born to a mother with a limb deficiency had a relative risk of 5.6% of having the same defect as the mother (16). This is similar to the relative risk of clubfoot. For the physician, knowing the existence of other problems and the natural history of the syndrome is necessary for the care of the child.

## THE CHILD WITH AN AMPUTATION

### Psychosocial Development

The child with an amputation is essentially different—something that no child wants to be. However, almost all children are different in various ways. Some differ in physical appearance, some in physical ways that are not immediately visible, and some in personality and intellectual development. The more children perceive themselves to be different from peers, the more they understand their disability. Children's understanding of their disability is general and incomplete at 6 years of age, but within a few years, around the age of 8 or 9 years, they come to a much more complete understanding of their handicap (17). Therefore, if parents have not discussed this with the child, they can expect the more difficult questions from their child to begin at around this age.

All children with disabilities are vulnerable to social isolation. This, in turn, can have negative effects on the development of self-esteem, body image, and the child's identity, which are developed through the interaction with parents, teachers, friends, classmates, and others. As children develop these interactions, the issue of "first appearance" becomes important because it serves as a clue to perceived personal characteristics, and can be an obstacle to further healthy interaction. Children in peer groups tend to devalue those with handicaps, a factor that may greatly interfere with these relationships (18). Parents especially understand this and fear for their child in this regard.

There has been a great deal of study on the nonhandicapped child's reaction to various handicaps, showing that children prefer other children without handicaps, and that they dislike some handicaps more than they dislike others (19–21). In addition, it is known that young adults show signs of anxiety when face-to-face with a handicapped person. However, there is some evidence that young children do not share their parents' values toward various handicaps when young, but between the ages of 6 and 18 years, they gradually develop values almost identical to those of their parents (20). This would suggest that these values may be subjected to modification among young children and emphasizes that organized discussions with classmates in school about the child's handicap may be of great value.

Despite the negative "first impression" that physical differences hold for children, there is evidence demonstrating that the age of the patient, the gender, the degree of limb loss, or socioeconomic status are not predictors of low self-esteem or of depressive symptoms. Rather, social factors, for example, stress and hassle, parental discord, and social support from classmates, parents, and teachers, along with the child's own perceptions of competency and adequacy, gained through peer acceptance, scholastic achievement, and athletic accomplishments, play the largest role in the development of self-esteem (22–24).

The importance of this information for parents, physicians, therapists, prosthetists, and teachers is that although limb deficiency is the visible problem and is subject to little modification, the important factors in the development of self-esteem are independent of the deficiency and can be positively affected.

## Differences in Amputees

The difference between the juvenile amputee and the adult amputee are as different as are the child and the adult. Acquired amputation in the adult is usually of the lower extremity and involves only one limb. In the child, it is most often congenital and more frequently has upper- and multiple-limb involvement.

The more important difference, however, lies in the fact that children are born dependent and are naturally in the process of becoming independent, whereas adults and older children are independent and far less changeable. The child with a congenital amputation or congenital deformity requiring an amputation will adapt far better to a missing limb than will an older child or adult who suddenly loses a limb. In addition to their adaptability in the physical arena, they will have far more adaptability in the psychosocial arena.

Similar differences apply to congenital and acquired juvenile amputees. The congenital amputee has a difference; the acquired amputee must adjust to a loss. The difference is dependent on the age and the deficiency. A child born with bilateral amelia will learn to use the feet for all activities of daily living, as will a child with traumatic loss of both upper limbs at an early age. However, bilateral upper-extremity loss in the older child who has functioned with both hands for years will not be so well compensated for by use of the feet.

## THE PARENTS

When a child with a congenital deformity or congenital amputation first presents, one of the first concerns has to be the parents. The child does not need a doctor yet, but the parents do. The issues around the child's deficiency, especially if amputation or surgery is required, are not urgent. However, the mental turmoil in the parents' lives is urgent. They did not expect to give birth to anything but a healthy, normal child, unless forewarned by ultrasonography. They are now there to see a doctor, with the certainty that their child is anything but healthy and with the unrealistic desire for an expert to make the deficient limb normal.

One of the earliest emotions the parents will have is guilt. What did I take or do during my pregnancy to cause this? Even worse, they may be wondering from which side of the family did this affliction come. It is a time of anticipated joy that has turned into a period of great stress for both the individuals and, often, for the marriage. Taking time at the first visit and again looking for the opportunity later to explain what is known about the cause of these problems is essential. Obtaining a genetic consultation, even when the deficiency is not known to be hereditary or caused by teratogens, can be therapeutic in this regard. It is usually much more thorough than what the orthopaedic surgeon can do and is done by an expert in that particular area, giving the parents additional reassurance.

Soon, the feeling of guilt will be mixed with anxiety about the child's future. Will he walk? Can he play sports? Will she have children of her own? The parents probably have never known a child or an adult with an amputation and have no frame of reference to answer these questions. Although one may try to anticipate and answer many of their questions, it is not possible to alleviate their fears through conversation. The best one can do during the first visit of the parents is to gain their confidence and give them realistic hope. Fortunately, there are usually no emergent decisions to be made, and there is time to help the parents answer these questions for themselves.

Because "seeing is believing," the next several months are a good time for the parents to meet children with similar deficiencies and to see what their child might actually be like in the future. This makes known the previously unknown, and the problems become easier to deal with. In addition, the parents can see the various surgical options that might be recommended for their child. Because there is no need for intervention in the congenital deficiency for a few months to a few years, the parents have time to learn about their child's problem. Introducing the family to other families who have children with similar limitations is one of the most important interventions. A recent study has demonstrated that although parents benefit from the support of friends and health professionals, they do not receive the level of support they need (25). This support is found by contact with other parents whose children have similar disabilities.

With information from the lay press or the Internet, and encouraged by well-meaning friends, many parents will ask about a miracle cure—whether the doctor can sew on a new arm, for example. The Internet can be both helpful and harmful and is used by virtually all parents with a child with a limb deficiency. What the parents often find may be more advertisement than information, and they usually have difficulty placing their child in the correct context of the information they read. Carefully listening to and explaining what they have read or heard will usually suffice for most. Seeing other patients and talking to their parents is also of great help because they are parents who went through the same thing, and they likely asked the same questions.

During this initial period, physicians also need to be careful about what they tell the parents. In an effort to help the parents feel better, although not knowing how to deal with this difficult role, physicians may offer false hope and mention treatments that are totally unrealistic. Physicians who do not know, or who do not wish to take on this role, should assure the parents that they are referring them to the best possible care rather than tell them not to worry and that medical science has amazing cures today.

The relationship between the parents and the physician (as well as all members of the team) is important. In this regard, the first thing the parents must be made to understand is that all the decisions will be theirs. No one will make them do anything they do not wish to do. In this regard, it becomes the role of the physician to educate the parents through repetitive explanation and answering parents' questions. It is helpful if this process occurs not only with the physician but also with the therapist and prosthetist, all of whom should be working together. In fact, the parents will usually hear and retain more information from a knowledgeable therapist or prosthetist than from the physician. Again, nothing helps like seeing other patients and parents.

Parents will often refuse a recommendation such as an amputation (26). It is important for the treating physician to recognize the factors that affect their decision and to do his or her best to educate the parents. Frequently, the child will have a near-normal appearing foot, and all the parents see is a small amount of shortening. The child may be able to walk in the first few years of life, and the parents may not understand the progressive shortening that will develop. Along with these observations, they share the popular public belief that modern science can cure everything—next year, if not now. They have all heard of miraculous lengthening of limbs in the popular press, and more recently, the "successful" transfer of limbs. It can be difficult to align the parents' expectations with reality.

Finally, it may need to be constantly reinforced that the child with a limb deficiency is more normal than abnormal. During this first year, the parents need to resolve their disappointment and loss, accept the child, and see the potential for the future. They need to bond to the child and begin to think of the child as an independent person. Most parents will begin to see their children this way as they grow and develop. Again, this process can be accelerated by seeing other children with similar problems. One recommendation that often needs repeating to the parents is that children tend to acquire the fears of their parents and that supporting any activity the child expresses interest in will allow the child to develop his or her natural abilities to the fullest.

## ORGANIZATION OF CARE

The management of pediatric limb deficiency is considered a specialized area of practice. There are several reasons for this. First, these anomalies are rare to any one practitioner outside a limb-deficiency center. The experience of an orthopaedic surgeon, therapist, or prosthetist who has treated several of these different anomalies can be important. Second, all patients and parents benefit by knowing they are not alone. In particular new parents, and later their children, will benefit immensely by seeing other parents and children like themselves. No amount of explanation, pictures, or movies can educate parents so well as talking to other parents like themselves and seeing children like their own.

The team should be made up of a physician and surgeon, a prosthetist, a physical and occupational therapist, and a social worker or child psychologist, all of whom are knowledgeable in normal childhood development and who can anticipate the deviations that will occur in development. The adult acquired amputees know what they had and what they want. The child and parents of a congenital amputee know little, and need education and guidance that usually cannot be provided by an orthopaedic surgeon referring the patient to a prosthetist. The parents will be making decisions for their child that the child will live with for the remainder of his or her life, and they are acutely aware of this responsibility. The professionals caring for the family must provide the necessary education and framework in which the parents can make these decisions.

Family involvement is the essential setting for the treatment program (27). The child has a condition he or she will adapt to. This is not a disease that will be cured. Hence, the condition should not be "medicalized," but rather treated within the context of family, home, school, and play, not through clinic visits.

## GENERAL CONSIDERATIONS

### Growth

It has been observed that the percentage of shortening in a congenital limb deficiency remains relatively constant. This principle has been established for congenital short femur (28–30), and fibular hemimelia (31,32). Clinical experience indicates this to be true for the tibial hemimelias also. It is important for the clinician and the parents to be aware that this percentage difference will translate into significant differences as the limb grows. Therefore, in discussing centimeters of shortening and planning treatment, it is important to calculate what the discrepancy will be at maturity.

Because the percentage of shortening remains relatively constant, it is possible to calculate the ultimate discrepancy in centimeters at an early age. Knowing the percentile height of the child, the length of the femoral and tibial segments of the normal limb can be estimated from the Green and Anderson growth charts (33) (Tables 31.2 and 31.3). Then, knowing the length of the normal segments and the percentage by which the affected segments are short, the length of the affected segments at maturity can be estimated.

Although the preceding method of calculating the eventual discrepancy at maturity is clinically valid, the clinician should be aware of the effect that surgical procedures could have on the growth of the limb. Following amputation, the epiphysis of the bone may not grow at the normal rate. Christi et al. showed that in 20 B-K amputations in children, only three tibias grew at the expected rate (34). The congenital group of tibias grew to 36% of what would have been expected, and the acquired group grew to 53% of the expected level. Various reasons for this may be the lack of stress across the growth plate, the decreased blood flow to the bone, or the result of the congenital insult that produced the limb deficiency.

### Timing of Amputation

The timing of an amputation in a congenital limb-deficient child is best understood in the context of the purpose of the amputation in an already limb-deficient child and the development of the child. The amputation is done for two reasons: to correct a severe discrepancy in length or to enhance prosthetic fitting.

In general, elective lower-extremity amputations, designed to aid prosthetic fitting of congenital deficiencies, are performed at the time the children are ready to walk, as indicated by their pulling to stand. For children with tibial and fibular deficiencies who will be treated with amputation, pulling to stand and cruising are the signals that the child is ready to begin walking. This would be the time for an amputation and prosthetic fitting, so that the child can maintain a normal developmental sequence. In some unusual cases in which the deformed extremity is interfering with crawling and other prewalking activities, amputation may be performed earlier. However, prosthetic fitting should wait until it will be of some value. It is very difficult to keep a prosthesis on a crawling child.

In other cases (e.g., PFFD), prosthetic fitting will usually be done when the child is ready to walk, but definitive surgical treatment to permit a more functional prosthesis will be done later for technical reasons.

Finally, there will be cases in which leg lengthening is the treatment of choice, but the difference in length must be compensated for before lengthening at a later age. Occasionally, it will be necessary to fit such patients with nonconventional prostheses, when shoe lifts are not sufficient.

Although it is poorly documented, there is the impression among both parents and surgeons that with early amputation the child does not experience the loss in body image that accompanies amputation at a later stage. Also important is that as a general rule, the earlier the amputation, the better the adaptation of the child's neurologic plasticity to the alteration.

## COMPLICATIONS

### Overgrowth

Bony overgrowth at the end of the residual limb is the most common problem in juvenile amputees. Its occurrence is reported to be between 4% and 35%, and depends on the cause of the amputation, the age of the patient at the time of amputation, and the bone involved (35–37). It occurs most commonly following traumatic amputation or elective amputation through a bone. It is seen in congenital amputations because of amniotic band syndrome but not in those due to failure of limb development. It is not seen in amputations through joints (38). Overgrowth occurs most often in below-knee amputations, with the problem being present in the fibula more often than in the tibia, and in transhumeral amputations. Recurrence is common and is felt by some to be more common during periods of rapid growth when bone turnover is high (e.g., adolescence).

Contraction of the soft tissue and growth of the bone, pushing it through the skin, were originally thought to be

**TABLE 31.2**

**GIRLS: LENGTHS OF THE LONG BONES INCLUDING EPIPHYSES**[a]

**Femur**

| No. | Age (yr) | Mean | $\sigma_d$ | $\sigma_m$ | Distribution | | | |
|---|---|---|---|---|---|---|---|---|
| | | | | | $+2\sigma_d$ | $+1\sigma_d$ | $-1\sigma_d$ | $-2\sigma_d$ |
| 30 | 1 | 14.81 | 0.673 | 0.082 | 16.16 | 15.48 | 14.14 | 13.46 |
| 52 | 2 | 18.23 | 0.888 | 0.109 | 20.01 | 19.12 | 17.34 | 16.45 |
| 63 | 3 | 21.29 | 1.100 | 0.134 | 23.49 | 22.39 | 20.19 | 19.09 |
| 66 | 4 | 23.92 | 1.339 | 0.164 | 26.60 | 25.26 | 22.58 | 21.24 |
| 66 | 5 | 26.32 | 1.437 | 0.176 | 29.19 | 27.76 | 24.88 | 23.45 |
| 66 | 6 | 28.52 | 1.616 | 0.197 | 31.75 | 30.14 | 26.90 | 25.29 |
| 67 | 7 | 30.60 | 1.827 | 0.223 | 34.25 | 32.43 | 28.77 | 26.95 |
| 67 | 8 | 32.72 | 1.930 | 0.236 | 36.59 | 34.66 | 30.78 | 28.85 |
| 67 | 9 | 34.71 | 2.117 | 0.259 | 38.94 | 36.83 | 32.59 | 30.48 |
| 67 | 10 | 36.72 | 2.300 | 0.281 | 41.32 | 39.02 | 34.42 | 32.12 |
| 67 | 11 | 38.81 | 2.468 | 0.302 | 43.75 | 41.28 | 36.34 | 33.87 |
| 67 | 12 | 40.74 | 2.507 | 0.306 | 45.75 | 43.25 | 38.23 | 35.73 |
| 67 | 13 | 42.31 | 2.428 | 0.310 | 47.17 | 44.74 | 39.88 | 37.45 |
| 67 | 14 | 43.14 | 2.269 | 0.277 | 47.68 | 45.41 | 40.87 | 38.60 |
| 67 | 15 | 43.47 | 2.197 | 0.277 | 47.86 | 45.67 | 41.27 | 39.08 |
| 67 | 16 | 43.58 | 2.193 | 0.268 | 47.97 | 45.77 | 41.39 | 39.19 |
| 67 | 17 | 43.60 | 2.192 | 0.268 | 47.98 | 45.79 | 41.41 | 39.22 |
| 67 | 18 | 43.63 | 2.195 | 0.269 | 48.02 | 45.82 | 41.44 | 39.24 |

**Tibia**

| No. | Age (yr) | Mean | $\sigma_d$ | $\sigma_m$ | Distribution | | | |
|---|---|---|---|---|---|---|---|---|
| | | | | | $+2\sigma_d$ | $+1\sigma_d$ | $-1\sigma_d$ | $-2\sigma_d$ |
| 61 | 1 | 11.57 | 0.646 | 0.082 | 12.86 | 12.22 | 10.92 | 10.28 |
| 67 | 2 | 14.51 | 0.739 | 0.090 | 15.99 | 15.25 | 13.77 | 13.03 |
| 67 | 3 | 16.81 | 0.893 | 0.109 | 18.00 | 17.70 | 15.92 | 15.02 |
| 67 | 4 | 18.86 | 1.144 | 0.140 | 21.15 | 20.00 | 17.72 | 16.57 |
| 67 | 5 | 20.77 | 1.300 | 0.159 | 23.37 | 22.07 | 19.47 | 18.17 |
| 67 | 6 | 22.53 | 1.458 | 0.178 | 25.45 | 23.99 | 21.07 | 19.61 |
| 67 | 7 | 24.22 | 1.640 | 0.200 | 27.50 | 25.86 | 22.58 | 20.94 |
| 67 | 8 | 25.89 | 1.786 | 0.218 | 29.46 | 27.68 | 24.10 | 22.32 |
| 67 | 9 | 27.56 | 1.993 | 0.243 | 31.55 | 29.55 | 25.57 | 23.57 |
| 67 | 10 | 29.28 | 2.193 | 0.259 | 33.67 | 31.47 | 27.09 | 24.89 |
| 67 | 11 | 31.00 | 2.384 | 0.291 | 35.77 | 33.38 | 28.62 | 26.23 |
| 67 | 12 | 32.61 | 2.424 | 0.296 | 37.46 | 35.03 | 30.19 | 27.76 |
| 67 | 13 | 33.83 | 2.374 | 0.290 | 38.58 | 36.20 | 31.46 | 29.08 |
| 67 | 14 | 34.43 | 2.228 | 0.272 | 38.89 | 36.66 | 32.20 | 29.97 |
| 67 | 15 | 34.59 | 2.173 | 0.265 | 38.94 | 36.76 | 32.42 | 30.24 |
| 67 | 16 | 34.63 | 2.151 | 0.263 | 38.93 | 36.78 | 32.48 | 30.33 |
| 67 | 17 | 34.65 | 2.158 | 0.264 | 38.97 | 36.81 | 32.49 | 30.33 |
| 67 | 18 | 34.65 | 2.161 | 0.264 | 38.97 | 36.81 | 32.49 | 30.33 |

[a]Orthoradiographic measurements from longitudinal series of 67 children.
From Anderson M, Messner MB, Green WT. Distribution of lengths of the normal femur and tibia in children from one to eighteen years of age. *J Bone Joint Surg Am* 1964;46:1197, with permission.

responsible for bone overgrowth. Aitken disproved these theories when he demonstrated by implanting metallic markers that the overgrowth took place distal to the end of the bone (35,39). The new bone is formed by periosteal and endosteal bone. Overgrowth results from the typical process of wound contracture as has been demonstrated by Speer (40). Following amputation through a bone, the periosteum continues to grow. As it grows over the end of the bone, it grows over the open medullary canal, where it contracts and is drawn into the canal from which it can continue to grow, producing the overgrowth at the end of the bone.

The patient will often notice pain on weight bearing or prosthetic use. An antalgic gait with decreased stance time may be noticed. Decreased range of motion, to limit pulling

### TABLE 31.3
## BOYS: LENGTHS OF THE LONG BONES INCLUDING EPIPHYSES[a]

### Femur

| No. | Age (yr) | Mean | $\sigma_d$ | $\sigma_m$ | Distribution | | | |
|---|---|---|---|---|---|---|---|---|
| | | | | | $+2\sigma_d$ | $+1\sigma_d$ | $-1\sigma_d$ | $-2\sigma_d$ |
| 21 | 1 | 14.48 | 0.628 | 0.077 | 15.74 | 15.11 | 13.85 | 13.22 |
| 57 | 2 | 18.15 | 0.874 | 0.107 | 19.90 | 19.02 | 17.28 | 16.40 |
| 65 | 3 | 21.09 | 1.031 | 0.126 | 23.15 | 22.12 | 20.06 | 19.03 |
| 66 | 4 | 23.65 | 1.197 | 0.146 | 26.04 | 24.85 | 22.45 | 21.26 |
| 66 | 5 | 25.92 | 1.342 | 0.164 | 28.60 | 27.26 | 24.58 | 23.24 |
| 67 | 6 | 28.09 | 1.506 | 0.184 | 31.10 | 29.60 | 25.58 | 25.08 |
| 67 | 7 | 30.25 | 1.682 | 0.205 | 33.61 | 31.93 | 28.57 | 26.89 |
| 67 | 8 | 32.28 | 1.807 | 0.221 | 35.89 | 34.09 | 30.47 | 28.67 |
| 67 | 9 | 34.36 | 1.933 | 0.236 | 38.23 | 36.29 | 32.43 | 30.49 |
| 67 | 10 | 36.29 | 2.057 | 0.251 | 40.40 | 38.35 | 34.23 | 32.18 |
| 67 | 11 | 38.16 | 2.237 | 0.276 | 42.63 | 40.40 | 35.92 | 33.69 |
| 67 | 12 | 40.12 | 2.447 | 0.299 | 45.01 | 42.57 | 37.67 | 35.23 |
| 67 | 13 | 42.17 | 2.765 | 0.338 | 47.70 | 44.95 | 39.40 | 36.64 |
| 67 | 14 | 44.18 | 2.809 | 0.343 | 49.80 | 46.99 | 41.37 | 38.56 |
| 67 | 15 | 45.69 | 2.512 | 0.307 | 50.71 | 48.20 | 43.19 | 40.67 |
| 67 | 16 | 46.66 | 2.244 | 0.274 | 51.15 | 48.90 | 44.42 | 42.17 |
| 67 | 17 | 47.07 | 2.051 | 0.251 | 51.17 | 49.12 | 45.02 | 42.97 |
| 67 | 18 | 47.23 | 1.958 | 0.239 | 51.15 | 49.19 | 45.27 | 48.31 |

### Tibia

| No. | Age (yr) | Mean | $\sigma_d$ | $\sigma_m$ | Distribution | | | |
|---|---|---|---|---|---|---|---|---|
| | | | | | $+2\sigma_d$ | $+1\sigma_d$ | $-1\sigma_d$ | $-2\sigma_d$ |
| 61 | 1 | 11.60 | 0.620 | 0.074 | 12.84 | 12.22 | 10.98 | 10.36 |
| 67 | 2 | 14.54 | 0.809 | 0.099 | 16.16 | 15.35 | 13.73 | 12.92 |
| 67 | 3 | 16.79 | 0.935 | 0.114 | 18.66 | 17.72 | 15.86 | 14.92 |
| 67 | 4 | 18.67 | 1.091 | 0.133 | 20.85 | 19.76 | 17.58 | 16.49 |
| 67 | 5 | 20.46 | 1.247 | 0.152 | 22.95 | 21.71 | 19.21 | 17.97 |
| 67 | 6 | 22.12 | 1.418 | 0.173 | 24.96 | 23.54 | 20.87 | 19.46 |
| 67 | 7 | 23.76 | 1.632 | 0.199 | 27.02 | 25.39 | 22.13 | 20.50 |
| 67 | 8 | 25.38 | 1.778 | 0.217 | 28.94 | 27.16 | 23.60 | 21.82 |
| 67 | 9 | 26.99 | 1.961 | 0.240 | 30.91 | 28.95 | 25.02 | 23.06 |
| 67 | 10 | 28.53 | 2.113 | 0.258 | 32.76 | 30.64 | 26.42 | 24.30 |
| 67 | 11 | 30.10 | 2.301 | 0.281 | 34.70 | 32.40 | 27.80 | 25.50 |
| 67 | 12 | 31.75 | 2.536 | 0.310 | 36.82 | 34.29 | 29.21 | 26.68 |
| 67 | 13 | 33.49 | 2.833 | 0.345 | 39.16 | 36.32 | 30.66 | 27.82 |
| 67 | 14 | 35.18 | 2.865 | 0.350 | 40.91 | 38.04 | 32.32 | 29.45 |
| 67 | 15 | 36.38 | 2.616 | 0.320 | 41.61 | 39.00 | 33.76 | 31.15 |
| 67 | 16 | 37.04 | 2.412 | 0.295 | 41.86 | 39.45 | 34.63 | 32.22 |
| 67 | 17 | 37.22 | 2.316 | 0.283 | 41.85 | 39.54 | 34.00 | 32.59 |
| 67 | 18 | 37.29 | 2.254 | 0.275 | 41.80 | 39.54 | 35.04 | 32.78 |

[a]Orthoradiographic measurements from longitudinal series of 67 children.
From Anderson M, Messner MB, Green WT. Distribution of lengths of the normal femur and tibia in children from one to eighteen years of age. *J Bone Joint Surg Am* 1964;46:1197, with permission.

of the skin at the end of the limb, is an additional symptom. Clinically, the patient presents with tenderness and pain at the end of the residual limb. There may be inflammation, bursal formation, or the bone end may be protruding through the skin. Commonly, the bony spike can be palpated within a small, tender bursa. Careful medical supervision can often anticipate the problem, which in turn allows the patient to plan for surgical correction. Prosthetic

adjustments may help delay surgical revision, but will seldom be sufficient with significant overgrowth.

In an effort to disrupt the pathologic sequence of overgrowth, various plastic and metallic devices have been used to cap or plug the end of the bone. However, these techniques have been abandoned because the results were not as good as with the use of biologic material (41,42). Marquardt reported in the mid-1970s, in the German literature, on the capping of the bone end with a cartilage-bone graft. More recently, Tenholder et al. reported comparable results with the use of a polytetrafluoroethylene felt pad (43). Various reports for both acquired and congenital amputees indicate generally favorable results, with most revisions being for technical reasons (41,42,44,45).

When a patient presents with pain and bursa formation, prosthetic modification and other conservative measures should be used first unless a bony spike is felt. If revision surgery is necessary, a capping procedure should be considered. In the case of a primary amputation, it is advisable to use available parts from the amputated portion of the limb to cap the end of the bone, if conditions permit. The most common procedure is the use of the proximal fibula to cap the tibia. As in any revision, adequate resection of the bone is essential to provide a healthy soft-tissue envelope. (Fig. 31.2).

Following surgery, the therapist should supervise and educate the child and parents in edema control to hasten return to prosthetic use. In addition, range of motion and strengthening exercises hasten, and may even be necessary to regain, full function of the prosthesis. Users of myoelectric prostheses may need readjustment of their electrodes and, for a while, may have difficulty activating the prosthesis. This is because of swelling and reshaping of the limb, which may alter the optimal sites for electrode placement.

## Short Residual Limb

In some patients with either congenital or acquired amputation, the residual limb will be too short for satisfactory or comfortable prosthetic fitting. In such cases it may be possible to lengthen the residual limb. Watts has written an excellent review of this subject and reports his experience with 32 limbs in 27 patients (46). Alekberov et al. report on six patients who had successful lengthening of 3.4 to 8.4 cm in congenital below-elbow segments (47). The remainder of the literature to date is largely case reports.

The lengthening of residual limbs is fraught with complications, and careful consideration needs to be given to the potential benefits versus the possible complications. Skin problems are frequent and often limit the length to be gained. Tissue expanders generally do not provide the solution. Free tissue flaps may be used when skin coverage is

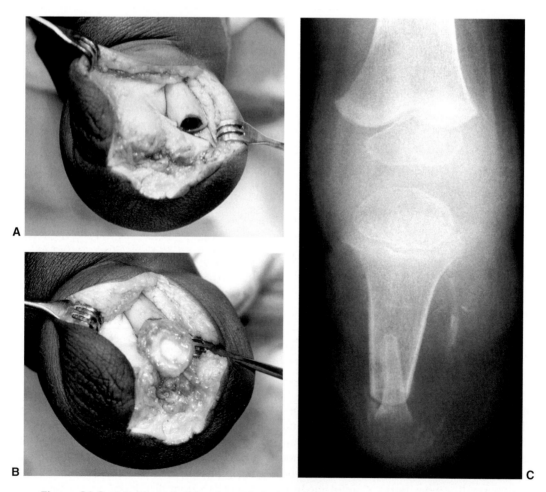

**Figure 31.2 A,B:** The end of the tibia with the bony overgrowth removed and the head of the fibula inserted into the medullary canal of the tibia (Marquardt procedure). **C:** The anteroposterior view of the tibia 6 weeks after the procedure.

inadequate. Free flaps often remove sensation from the end of the residual limb, and especially in the upper limb this can affect the function of the limb both with and without the prosthesis. The child will be without the use of the prosthesis for a prolonged period, an especially difficult problem when the lower extremity is involved.

## Phantom Sensation/Pain

The term "phantom limb" was coined by the neurologist Silas Weir Mitchell in the middle of the 19th century. He described these sensations as replicas of the lost limb, some being painful and some not. Phantom sensation of the limb is often described by patients as the feeling that they can move the part, tell how the part is positioned, or feel it itching or tingling. Phantom pain, however, is perceived by the patient as just that—painful. It often is the same as the pain before an amputation or may be cramping, shooting, burning, or of any other characterization.

It has been a general idea that children born without limbs do not have sensations of them; nor do these children experience the phantom pain or phantom sensation seen in the acquired amputee (48). Recent reports call this commonly accepted truism into question (49,50). Whatever this pain is, those who care for children with limb deficiencies will recognize that these children do not have the same problem as the true chronic phantom pain seen in adult amputees.

Melzack et al. reported that phantom limb was present in at least 20% of children with congenital limb deficiency and in 50% of those who underwent amputation before age 6 (50). In addition, 20% of the congenitally deficient group described the sensations as painful, whereas 42% of the acquired amputees described them as painful. To explain the phenomenon of phantom limb in a child who has never had a limb, Melzack et al. have proposed that there is a genetically or innately determined neural network that is distributed in the cortex (not focal), which is responsible for the representation of the limb, even though the limb bud development was not normal.

Phantom pain and distal residual limb pain are also associated, and in general seen to be associated with, other pains; such as, headache, bone, or joint pain (49,51). The phantom sensations may occur frequently or rarely. They are often triggered by a wide variety of stimuli. Feeling nervous or happy, not wearing a prosthesis, being cold, or being ill are frequent triggers. Fortunately, these sensations do not interfere with the child's usual activity, and most say they just try to ignore the sensations (52).

There is no single highly successful treatment for phantom limb pain, most likely because there is usually not one single cause. Because many of these problems resolve with prosthetic alterations or physical therapy modalities, a multidisciplinary approach has proven to be the best intervention in evaluating and properly treating the phantom limb phenomenon when it becomes a problem.

A properly fitting socket, with appropriate suspension and sock thickness, is the best and first treatment of choice (52,53). A heavy, tight shrinker, either worn inside the prosthesis or when the prosthesis is off, may provide relief. Physical therapy interventions, including weight bearing and graduating pressures such as tapping, rubbing, and massage to the residual limb, have been reported to give temporary or permanent relief. Rubbing and massaging the uninvolved limb at similar points to those in which they are experiencing the phantom limb sensation may provide relief. Various physical modalities have been utilized in the treatment of phantom sensations in children, including transcutaneous electrical nerve stimulation (TENS), biofeedback, ultrasound, and the physical agents of heat and cold (54).

For the occasional adolescent amputee who has problems with phantom pain following an amputation, gabapentin (Neurontin, Park-Davis) has proven a useful medication for some patients.

# CONGENITAL DEFICIENCIES OF THE LOWER EXTREMITY

## Fibular Deficiency

### Classification

According to the ISO terminology, fibular deficiency is longitudinal deficiency that is either partial or complete. But this does little to accurately portray the spectrum of deficiency that is seen.

Numerous classifications specific for fibular deficiency have been proposed (26,31,55–57). To be useful, a classification should guide treatment or aid in prognosis. As treatment changes, it may be reasonable to expect that classifications change.

Most classifications are anatomic and are based on the radiographic appearance. Maffulli and Fixsen describe total aplasia of the fibula and a *forme fruste* of the same condition in which the fibula and tibia are short to varying degrees (58,59). A more specific classification, which is probably the most widely used today, was proposed by Achterman and Kalamchi (31) (Figs. 31.3 to 31.5). They correlated the classification with the discrepancy in length, and recommended treatment on the basis of the classification.

Recently, Birch et al. have proposed a functional classification on the basis of the functionality of the foot and the limb-length discrepancy as a percentage of the opposite side (60). As they point out, however, the problem is picking the correct treatment for the individual patient.

Given the large variation in the different aspects of fibular deficiency, including the parents' desire, it remains unlikely that classifications will provide anything more than a rough guide and a method of comparing patients in different reports. In addition, the protean effects on the femur, tibia, knee, ankle, and foot demonstrate the difficulty of classifying this deficiency accurately by the radiographic appearance of the fibula.

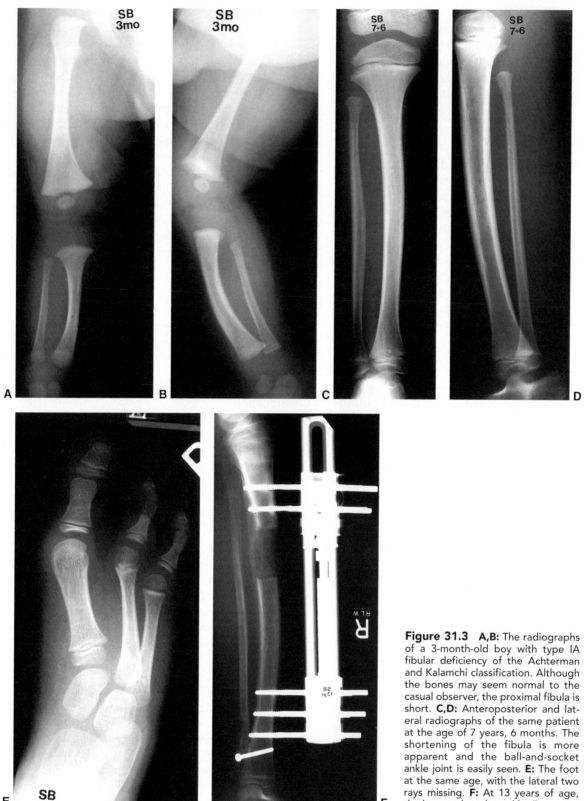

**Figure 31.3  A,B:** The radiographs of a 3-month-old boy with type IA fibular deficiency of the Achterman and Kalamchi classification. Although the bones may seem normal to the casual observer, the proximal fibula is short. **C,D:** Anteroposterior and lateral radiographs of the same patient at the age of 7 years, 6 months. The shortening of the fibula is more apparent and the ball-and-socket ankle joint is easily seen. **E:** The foot at the same age, with the lateral two rays missing. **F:** At 13 years of age, the leg was lengthened by 7 cm.

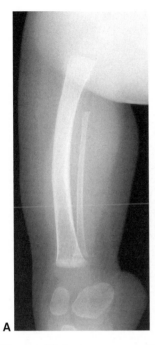
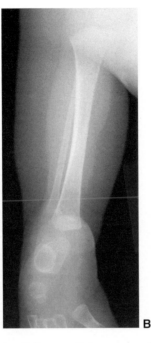

**Figure 31.4  A,B:** Type IB fibular deficiency (Achterman and Kalamchi), in which the proximal fibula is missing. This type is often associated with proximal focal deficiency, as in this child.

### Clinical Appearance

The appearance and physical findings of the leg are indicative of the widespread abnormality that may be present, along with hypoplasia or absence of the fibula, which gives the deficiency its name.

The appearance of a limb with fibular deficiency, especially in the first year of life, can vary from practically normal to severely deformed. However, the typical limb is characterized by a rigid valgus foot, often with one or two lateral (postaxial) rays missing, a shortened leg and (often) thigh, a valgus knee, and variable anterior bowing of the tibia with a dimple over the apex (Fig. 31.5E,F). Further examination will demonstrate an anteroposterior instability of the knee along with a small patella.

Radiographically, the fibula will usually be seen to be shortened in relation to the tibia. This may occur either proximally or distally or both (Fig. 31.3). Often a portion of the fibula is absent in part (Fig. 31.4) or in its entirety (Fig. 31.5). In those cases in which the fibula is of normal or near-normal length, the diagnosis can be difficult during the first year of life. Radiographically, the condylar notch of the femur is shallow and the tibial spines are small.

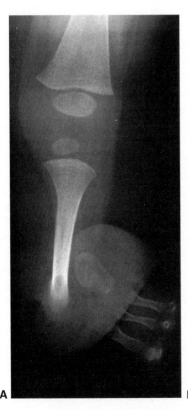
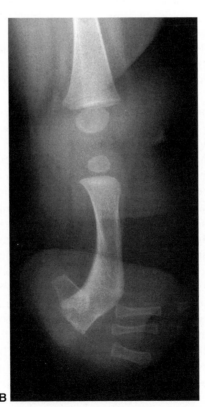
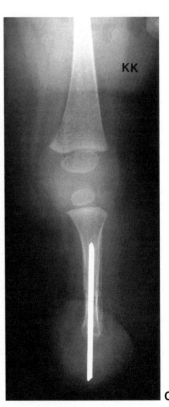

**Figure 31.5  A,B:** Anteroposterior and lateral radiographs of a type II fibular deficiency (Achterman and Kalamchi), in which the entire fibula is missing. Note the missing lateral rays of the foot and the severe angulation of the tibia. **C,D:** The limb, 6 weeks after Syme amputation and an anterior closing-wedge osteotomy of the tibia. Placing the pin through the anterior cortex of the proximal fragment provides rigid fixation, which is not obtained if the pin is simply passed up the medullary canal. The pin was removed in the office at the time of cast removal. **E,F:** The clinical appearance of the same deficiency at the time of surgery in another patient. Note the short tibial segment, the valgus knee and foot, and the dimple over the tibia.

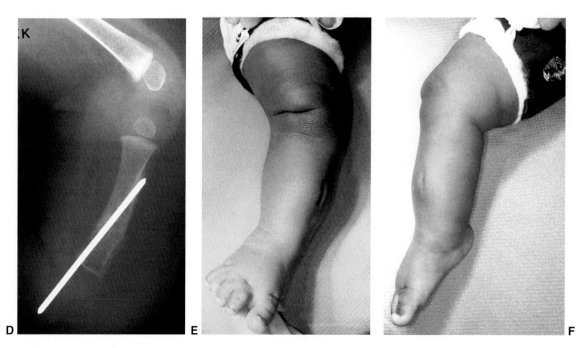

**Figure 31.5** *(continued)*

The femoral shortening may be slight to severe, varying from a few centimeters of shortening to a true PFFD. Amstutz (29) reported femoral deficiency in 15% of those with fibular deficiency, whereas Bohne and Root (61) reported femoral deficiencies in almost two-thirds of their patients. Kalamchi noted that 70% of type I and 50% of type II deficiencies were associated with shortening or deformity of the femur (62).

The valgus deformity of the knee, which is not associated with varus/valgus instability (63), results at least in part from a small hypoplastic lateral femoral condyle (64). The natural history of this deformity is that it usually worsens with growth (32,61,65,66). In some cases, the degree of valgus is more severe than can be explained by the smaller lateral femoral condyle alone, and its recurrence after correction speaks of a more dynamic cause.

The ankle may appear normal in some patients with mild deficiencies, but by skeletal maturity there is usually a valgus deformity. The classic appearance of the ball-and-socket ankle joint in these deficiencies is seen in Figs. 31.3C,D. There is disagreement about the origin of this abnormality. Some authors feel that it is congenital (67), whereas others feel that it develops secondary to the tarsal coalitions (68). If it is caused by the tarsal coalition, it is difficult to explain its absence in tarsal coalitions without fibular deficiency. In slightly more severe cases, if the fibula is present it is short and may not reach the level of the ankle joint. The distal tibial epiphysis shows a triangular appearance.

Although not seen on radiographs at birth, tarsal coalitions are present in most of the feet associated with fibular deficiency. Grogan et al. noted such coalitions in 54% of anatomic specimens, although the abnormality could be seen radiographically on only 15% of the specimens because of the cartilaginous nature of the coalition (69). The missing lateral rays are easily seen without radiographs.

### Treatment Options

The main problems in the treatment of fibular deficiency are the limb-length discrepancy and the deformity and instability of the foot and ankle. It is very important to realize that the discrepancy will become worse with growth, and it is the ultimate discrepancy at maturity that is important.

***Amputation and Lengthening.*** Until the 1960s, amputation for fibular deficiency was recommended only as a last resort (70). In reaction to the results of these early attempts to save the limbs, several reports emphasized the advantages of amputation for severe cases (32,71–73). The indications are based primarily on the difference in length and the functionality of the foot. Wood et al. recommended amputation for: a discrepancy of 3 inches or more at the time of decision, or if predicted at maturity; for a nonfunctional foot; for a limb that would have severe cosmetic or functional problems; or for children who cannot endure the psychologic trauma of repeated hospitalizations and surgery (73). These recommendations were reaffirmed in a later publication from the same institution, following up many of the same patients (32).

More recent recommendations begin to stretch the extent to which length can be restored, reflecting improvements in limb lengthening. Westin et al. suggested amputation for any discrepancy that would be greater than 7.5 cm at maturity (32). For Letts and Vincent, the number was greater than 10 cm (26), and for Hootnick et al. it was between 8.7 cm and 15 cm (74).

Although modern prosthetics have made amputation a somewhat more acceptable alternative, the improved ability to lengthen limbs has also made limb salvage a more feasible option. The recommendations of Birch et al. are an effort to account for these changes (60). They would recommend amputation for those with a nonfunctional foot, regardless of leg length, unless the upper extremities were nonfunctional. For those with a functional foot, but a leg-length discrepancy of 30% or more, amputation would be recommended. For those with a functional foot and a discrepancy of less than 10%, epiphysiodesis or lengthening is reasonable. There is little disagreement about these indications today.

It is between those two groups that the controversy regarding treatment lies, and the greater the discrepancy in length, the greater the controversy. According to Birch et al., those patients with a functional foot and a discrepancy between 10% and 30% are candidates for either amputation or lengthening (60). The parents, who are the decision-makers, are weighing the hope for their child to retain the limb against what that will entail. They most likely have never seen a child or adult with an amputation; they visualize something horrible. At the same time they cannot really know what a lengthened limb will be like at the end of treatment; they imagine the limb will be normal. Although they may understand that they will need two or three lengthening procedures, they cannot know what the impact will be on their child or their family, what complications they will encounter on the way, or how their child will look or function at the end of the treatment.

As yet, there are but a few preliminary reports of lengthening in fibular deficiencies with discrepancies greater than 10 cm. These preliminary reports, using the Ilizarov methods, deal mainly with the extent of length achieved, often before maturity, but with little information on cosmetic and functional result (75–79).

One way to begin to assess the problem is to look at what amount of length is required. The combined femoral and tibial length for a girl of average height at maturity will be approximately 80 cm (33) (Table 31.2). A 10% discrepancy would be approximately 8 cm, a 20% discrepancy would be 16 cm, and a 30% discrepancy would be 24 cm. To achieve greater than 10 cm of length in a congenital limb deficiency with anteroposterior knee instability, ankle instability, foot deformity, and congenitally short soft tissues is a significant undertaking (79–81).

Reports comparing Syme amputation with lengthening are few and incomplete, but begin to give an appreciation of the problems associated with lengthening severe deficiencies (55,82–84). These reports conclude that lengthening should be reserved for those with more normal feet and less discrepancy in length, although early Syme amputation is the best treatment for the more severe problems. Herring gives a philosophical perspective on the dilemma (85). Birch et al. reviewed a series of adults who were treated with Syme amputation in childhood. These authors conducted physical examination, prosthetic assessment, psychologic testing, and physical performance testing, and commented that the results of multistaged lengthenings for this condition would have to match these results to be justified (86). They currently offer lengthening to patients whose limb-length discrepancy is 20% or less.

***Bilateral.*** In patients with bilateral fibular deficiency, the three problems are the foot deformity, the discrepancy in length between the two limbs, and the overall shortening in height because of two short limbs. Without extenuating circumstances (e.g., nonfunctional upper extremities), disarticulation of the foot and prosthetic fitting is the best solution. For those children with nonfunctional upper extremities who will use their feet for many of the activities of daily living, amputation of the feet is not an option.

In children with bilateral fibular deficiency, there is usually little discrepancy between the two limbs, but rather a discrepancy between their height and what their normal height should be. As they enter into their peer group this becomes an increasing problem. This problem is most easily solved by the prosthetist. If there is a significant difference between the length of the two limbs that cannot be solved by prosthetic adjustment, lengthening of the short limb becomes an attractive option.

It is easy to miss a case of bilateral deficiency when the deficiency on one side is mild. The focus on the severe deficiency distracts the examiner. The lesser deficiency will become apparent with time, however, causing disappointment and loss of confidence.

***Syme and Boyd Amputation.*** The amputation described by Syme (87) seems to have been accepted for adults before it was accepted for children, and its use in boys was advocated before its use in girls because it was said that the Syme amputation produced an unsightly bulkiness around the ankle. This resulted in many children receiving a transtibial amputation rather than a Syme amputation. It was subsequently learned, however, that the ankle does not enlarge following amputation in a young child, and the cosmetic appearance is excellent as the child grows.

Thompson et al. were the first to recommend the Syme amputation, rather than transtibial amputation, although only as a last resort (70). Subsequent reports by Kruger and Talbott (72) and Westin et al. (32) not only confirmed the advantages of the Syme amputation in both boys and girls but also advocated its early use for severe deficiencies. Several studies now confirm the value of Syme amputation (66,72,85,88–92).

One of the major advantages of the Syme amputation is the ability to bear weight on the end of the residual limb. One of the major complications of the Syme amputation is migration of the heel pad off the end of the residual limb. This is particularly true in congenital limb deficiencies, in which the heel may be on the back of the tibia, making repositioning of the heel pad on the end of the limb difficult or impossible. Although suggestions to remove a piece of the Achilles tendon, suture the extensor tendons into the anterior portion of the heel pad, or fix the heel pad with a Kirschner wire may each have their place, most authors agree that migration of the heel pad does not produce any insurmountable problem for the patient or the prosthetist (65,88). Most other problems in patients with Syme amputation are caused by other effects of the underlying disorder (65,66,88,90).

In the most complete study to date on the outcome of Syme amputation in children, Herring et al. examined the functional and psychologic status of 21 patients with a Syme amputation (65). They noted that family stress was the factor that had the greatest influence on the patients' psychologic functioning, and that children who had the amputation after several failed attempts at salvage were at considerable risk for emotional disturbance. Green and Cary found that patients were able to function at the average levels for their age group, and the authors did not find that adolescents were less likely to participate in athletics (93). In summary, these studies indicate that Syme amputation may be compatible with the athletic and psychologic function of a nonhandicapped child.

A variation of Syme amputation was described by Boyd (94). In the Boyd amputation, the talus is excised and the retained calcaneus with the heel pad is arthrodesed to the tibia. The surgery was initially devised to avoid the complication of posterior migration of the heel pad seen in some children with Syme amputation. However, the main complication of the Boyd amputation is the migration of the calcaneus if arthrodesis is not achieved. This requires an additional surgery, which is often conversion to a Syme amputation. An advantage of the Boyd amputation is that with the retained calcaneus, the heel pad tends to grow with the child, rather than remaining small as in the Syme amputation. The Boyd amputation also adds length. This can be a problem when children who do not have significant shortening of the limb are fitted for various prosthetic feet and may require a shoe lift on the normal side.

Eilert and Jayakumar (89) compared the two surgeries, and found the migration of the heel pad to be the only complication in the Syme amputation, whereas the Boyd amputation had more perioperative wound problems and migration or improper alignment of the calcaneus. In the authors' clinic, all of the children, even bilateral amputees, can and do walk on the ends of their residual limbs, either with or without the heel pad in place. If the heel pad migrates posteriorly, it may alter the weight-bearing aspects of prosthetic fitting, especially as the child gets older.

In fitting a Syme amputation, there are two prosthetic advantages to having the deficient limb shorter. The first is the ability to make a narrower and more cosmetic ankle in the prosthesis. The second is that some shortening, rather than additional lengthening, makes it easier to fit more durable, energy-storing feet. In fibular deficiencies, length is never a problem, because these limbs are always short.

*Correction of Tibial Bow.* The anterior bow in the diaphysis of the tibia varies from nonexistent to severe. Severe bowing is usually seen in the more severe deficiencies with complete absence of the fibula. Westin et al. reported this to be of little consequence (32). However, observations in the authors' center have shown this to be a frequent prosthetic problem, requiring osteotomy during the first decade.

With the tibial bow, the foot is displaced posterior to the weight-bearing axis that passes through the knee. If the foot is placed at the distal end of the tibia (which the parents want for cosmetic reasons), the ground reaction force places a large moment through the toe-break area, leading to premature failure of the foot component and skin problems caused by abnormal pressure. The problem is then blamed on the foot component or the prosthetist.

A reasonable recommendation would be to correct any significant bow at the time of Syme amputation. A small anterior incision, removal of an anterior-based wedge of the tibia, and fixation with a temporary Steinmann pin placed up through the heel pad solves the problem and does not result in any delay in prosthetic fitting (Fig. 31.5). When correction of the bow is necessary in older children who are already in their prosthesis, the authors have preferred the Williams rod technique, because this speeds resumption of prosthetic wearing.

*Correction of Genu Valgum.* Development of progressive genu valgum has long been known as a complication of fibular deficiency. It is one of the major problems seen in the gait of children with this problem. At first, it is merely cosmetic and can be accommodated with prosthetic alterations. However, if it becomes more severe, it will increase the forces on the lateral compartment and make good alignment impossible.

The cause of the deformity has been controversial. Initially, it was thought to result from tethering by the fibular anlage; however, release of this lateral band does not prevent or lessen the deformity (29).

Westin et al. noted that the tibia often developed an anterior flexion along with the valgus, and attributed the problem to an abnormality in growth in the lateral and posterior portions of the proximal tibial physis (32). This problem is different from anterior bow in the diaphysis of the tibia.

Most recently, Boakes et al. documented a decrease in the height of the lateral femoral condyle that was not present prior to walking (64). There was a suggested relation between the extent of anteromedial bowing of the tibia and subsequent decrease in height of the lateral femoral condyle. They suggested that tibial osteotomy might prevent the changes in the lateral femoral condyle and correct the anteromedial bowing. If the deformity was present in the lateral femoral condyle, they suggested temporary stapling of the medial femoral condyle, since osteotomy has a very high recurrence rate unless performed near the end of growth. The authors' experience indicates that it is not as simple as this and that the recurring nature of the valgus following good correction of alignment suggests other causes of this problem.

*Ankle Reconstruction.* Any attempt to save the limb of a child with significant fibular deficiency will require efforts to realign and stabilize the ankle. There is renewed interest in this subject with attempts to lengthen the leg.

The Gruca procedure is designed to provide lateral stability to the foot in the absence of the fibula. Serafin gives the first report of the technique in the English literature, and recounts the various attempts at bone grafting and other procedures that were described before Gruca developed his technique (95).

In the Gruca procedure the tibia is split longitudinally. The medial segment is displaced proximally with the talus, leaving the lateral fragment as a lateral buttress. Thomas and Williams describe the early results in nine patients treated with this procedure. The follow-up is short and the evaluation of function incomplete (96). The surgery has not been widely used and would seem to have little to recommend it.

Arthrodesis of the talus to the distal tibia is a logical plan in conjunction with leg lengthening, but there are no reports on its outcome. It is likely that this would also require release of all of the tendons crossing the ankle joint to prevent foot deformity. Drift of the foot through the physis or the fusion itself with lengthening and over time seems a possibility.

The ball-and-socket ankle joint, seen in the Kalamchi type IA deficiencies, usually require no treatment. The authors have, however, seen several children with increasing valgus during adolescence or following leg lengthening who become symptomatic with normal athletic activity. They have been successfully treated by a Wiltse osteotomy of the distal tibia.

*Prosthetic Management.* Prosthetic management of the fibular-deficient limb is treated differently than management of a comparable Syme disarticulation in an adult after trauma. In the child, the prosthesis is designed to accommodate growth and to help stabilize knee laxity and hyperextension through socket design and alignment. Emphasis is placed on socket alignment and minimizing rotational forces acting on the knee.

The socket fitting for a Syme amputation may be designed to take all of the weight on the end of the residual limb, as intended, all of the weight on the patellar tendon and flare of the proximal tibial condyles, as in a transtibial amputation, or both. As the child grows, it is a good idea to begin to shift some of the weight bearing to the proximal structures to prepare the child for the time when full weight bearing on the end may not be possible. Failure to shift weight bearing proximally with age usually leads to problems with fittings resulting from tolerance issues. This discomfort probably arises from the small distal weight-bearing surface seen in many of the congenitally deformed limbs. This is an important consideration in the bilateral amputee, in whom disproportionate weight shifting to the sound side is not possible for comfort.

As with most amputations done at a young age, the condyles will be small at the time of amputation, will not grow to normal size, and therefore, do not need to be trimmed as in the adult. The brim of the socket is designed with supracondylar medial and lateral trim lines, in an effort to control any knee valgus instability and/or patellar instability. The type of suspension will depend on the size of the distal end of the residual limb. If it is very large, an obturator or window may be necessary. With further growth, the distal end may not be sufficient for suspension, and a different design will be necessary. These are discussed later.

To best utilize current prosthetic feet in children who are older and large enough to take advantage of them, it is necessary that at least 4 cm of space be available at the distal end. If the prosthetist is to offer the latest in technologic advances in components, greater residual limb-length differences will be required. This need can be anticipated, and an arrest of the distal or proximal tibial and fibular physes performed at the appropriate time. This length differential is usually not a problem in children with congenital limb deficiency, because the deficient limb will usually be shorter than the other limb. It is relevant in children with acquired deficiency treated by Syme or, more often, Boyd amputations. Although the longer lever arm of the Syme amputee tends to compensate for the lack of more elaborate prosthesis components, when fit is possible, they can be an advantage.

## Tibial Deficiency

### Classification
There are two classifications specific for tibial deficiencies, both based on the radiographic findings. Anatomic studies of available specimens have not proven helpful in classification (97,98).

The simplest classification is that of Kalamchi and Dawe (99). Type I is the complete absence of the tibia (Fig. 31.6). Type II is the absence of the distal tibia, with a proximal portion that forms a relatively normal articulation with the femur (Fig. 31.7). Type III is distal tibiofibular diastasis (Fig. 31.8).

The classification of Jones et al. divides the type I tibial deficiency of Kalamchi and Dawe into 1a and 1b. In neither is the proximal tibia visible radiographically at birth. In type 1a it is actually absent and without an extensor mechanism, whereas in type 1b it is present as a cartilaginous remnant that will later ossify, suggesting that the extensor mechanism is intact.

The Jones classification adds an additional type, a very unusual variant with a diaphyseal and distal remnant of tibia but no proximal tibia, as type 3. The diastasis of the distal tibiofibular joint is type 4 in this classification.

The most important point in deciding on the treatment is the presence of active knee extension, which implies an adequate active quadriceps muscle and insertion on the tibia. This usually depends on the presence of a proximal tibial segment. Because this proximal portion of the tibia may be present, but not be visible, in the Jones type 1b

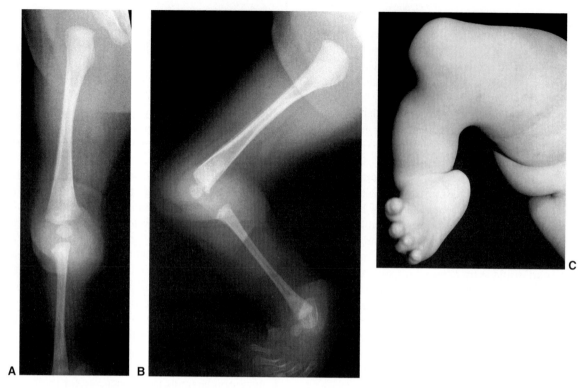

**Figure 31.6   A,B:** Radiographs of an infant with a type I tibial deficiency of Kalamchi and Dawe (99) (type 1a of Jones et al.) (120), in which the entire tibia is absent. There was no extensor mechanism and no proximal tibia. If there were a proximal remnant of tibia that would later ossify, this would be a type 1b deficiency of Jones et al. **C:** The clinical appearance, with the medial deviation and severe equinus of the foot and the absence of any tibial structure below the distal femur.

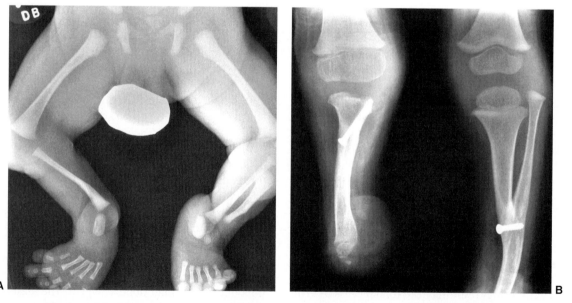

**Figure 31.7   A:** Anteroposterior radiographs of a 4-month-old child with type I tibial deficiency of the right leg and type II deficiency of the left leg. **B:** On the right leg, he underwent a Brown procedure. Despite the favorable radiographic appearance 4 years after surgery, he developed a severe valgus/flexion deformity, and subsequently had a knee disarticulation on this side. On the left leg, he underwent a synostosis of the fibula to the tibia and a Syme amputation. It is best to excise the proximal remnant of the fibula when performing this procedure, because the continued growth of the proximal fibula produces a large prominence that will interfere with prosthetic fitting. This was resected at the time of his right knee disarticulation.

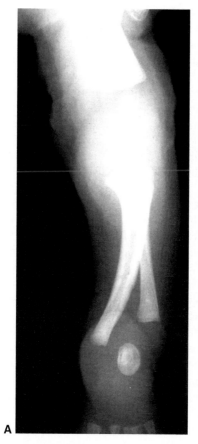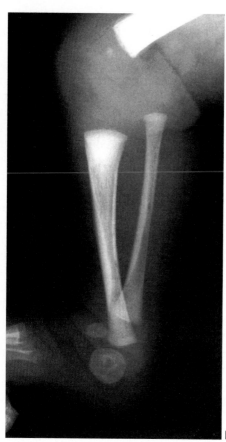

**Figure 31.8 A,B:** Anteroposterior and lateral views of tibial deficiency of type III of Kalamchi and Dawe, or type 4 of Jones et al. This is sometimes referred to as a diastasis of the ankle mortise. Notice the shortened tibia and the disruption of the normal relation between the tibia and the fibula.

A

B

deficiencies, some authors have recommended direct surgical exploration, sonography (100), or magnetic resonance imaging to detect its presence. This should seldom be necessary because it is the extension power to the tibial segment that is important, and not the presence of a tibial segment. A good radiographic clue is that in patients who have a proximal portion of the tibia, the distal femoral condyle is wider and the ossification of the epiphysis is better than if it is not present.

An unusual type of tibial deficiency is that seen in association with fibular dimelia. Kumar and Kruger summarized the sporadic reports until 1993 and presented the findings, associated anomalies, and treatments in six patients (101). In this deficiency, the tibia is absent and there is a duplication of the fibula. There is a high incidence of other anomalies, including visceral anomalies, in these patients. These authors recommended knee disarticulation if the femur is of normal length, and fusion of the fibula to create a sufficient lever arm if there is associated PFFD.

### Clinical Appearance

The characteristic appearance of an infant with tibial deficiency is a markedly shortened tibia with a rigid equinovarus-supinated foot pointing toward the perineum (Fig. 31.6C). Preaxial polydactyly is characteristic of tibial deficiencies, although absence of the preaxial rays can also be seen. The fibula is relatively long. Other congenital

limb anomalies will frequently be seen in association with tibial deficiency.

Children with congenital tibial deficiencies, regardless of type, frequently have other associated abnormalities, frequently musculoskeletal (102,103). The incidence of associated anomalies is reported to be between 60% and 75% (99,104,105). Although most of these anomalies are in the musculoskeletal system, there may occasionally be problems in other organ systems (106).

In addition, many of the children with tibial deficiency and other anomalies will represent an inherited syndrome (102,103,107,108). Although it is not necessary for the orthopaedic surgeon to know all of these syndromes, he or she must be aware of the need for a thorough examination of the affected children, and of the high potential for genetic transmission of the disorder (108,109). These patients should probably have formal genetic counseling.

### Treatment

The treatment of the type I of Kalamchi and Dawe or the 1a of Jones is knee disarticulation. Without the presence of active knee extension, there is no possibility for reconstruction of the leg. Notwithstanding this common orthopaedic principle, there have been attempts to centralize the fibula under the femoral condyle.

Adopted from others (110,111) and popularized in the United States by Brown (112), the Brown procedure, as it is commonly known in the United States, is the centralization of the fibula under the femur. It was Brown's recommendation that fibular centralization be done only with active extension. Apparently, there are occasional deficiencies in which some part of the extensor mechanism inserts into the fibula. On reviewing the literature on the results of Brown's procedure, it is not apparent that this is always present before surgery. The surgery has now been evaluated in several clinical trials (102,103,113–117). This procedure is distinct from synostosis of the fibula to a tibial remnant, a point that may not always be clear in reports on the subject.

Most of those reporting on the procedure recommend against it, preferring the early function obtained with knee disarticulation (102,103,114). Loder (118) examined 87 cases from the literature using the minimal requirements for a good result, as suggested by Jayakumar and Eilert, of acceptable gait, active knee motion of 10 degrees to 80 degrees of flexion, varus/valgus instability less than 5 degrees, and no flexion contracture (119). He found that 53 of the 55 cases of Jones type 1a deficiency treated by Brown's procedure had a poor result because of flexion contracture. This echoes the reported experience of most others, and emphasizes the need for strong, active knee extension, which is usually not present without a remnant of the proximal tibia (102,113,114,116,117). Simmons et al. were satisfied with the results from their evaluation of Brown's procedure (115). Their satisfaction was based more on the patients' feelings than objective assessment.

It has been said that it is difficult to assess active quadriceps function clinically, prior to surgery (102). However, it might be a wise clinical decision to consider quadriceps function to be at least inadequate, if not absent, if it cannot be observed during the first year of the patient's life by an experienced physician and therapist.

In patients with Jones type 1b deficiency, in which a radiographically invisible cartilaginous remnant of the tibia is present, it is important to assess it over time for ossification and development, as well as to verify good active extension. It is possible that this remnant will be present, but good active extension will be absent or the remnant will not ossify. If there is active extension in a child, but the remnant is not sufficiently ossified by 1 year of age, the surgeon may choose to attempt to transfer the fibula to the unossified segment or perform a Syme amputation, fit with a prosthesis, and wait for ossification before performing the transfer.

In patients with type I deformities and proximal femoral deficiency with a very short limb, the best option may be to arthrodese the fibula to the distal end of the femur. The goal of this procedure is to increase the lever arm of the femoral segment, for the same reasons that a knee fusion is performed in children with PFFD.

In type II deficiencies in either classification, the tibial remnant will ossify and form a satisfactory joint. In these cases, it is usually best to create a synostosis between the existing fibula and the tibial remnant to increase the length of the lever arm. A Syme amputation is performed at the same time, and the patient is fit with a below-knee prosthesis. When performing the synostosis, it is important to achieve good alignment of the fibula in relation to the knee joint. The residual proximal fibula should be removed to avoid problems later with prosthetic fit.

Type 3 deficiencies of Jones (not classified by Kalamchi and Dawe) are very unusual, and there is not much published experience. Jones et al. reported one case that was bilateral (120). They described a cartilaginous portion of the tibia, proximal to the ossified portion, which was "under voluntary muscle control." Their patient was treated with excision of the proximal fibula and Syme amputation. Fernandez-Palazzi et al. had two cases in their report. Both were treated with Syme amputation, implying that there was an active quadriceps mechanism (121).

Type III deficiency of Kalamchi (type 4 in the Jones classification) presents a unique problem. At birth, the foot is deformed, often appearing like a clubfoot to the inexperienced. In addition, the amount of tibial shortening that will result is not apparent. All of this makes it difficult for the parents to accept amputation. The difficulty for the surgeon is that this deformity is a spectrum of deformity. Garbarino et al. have emphasized the distinction between a short tibia with a varus foot and a true congenital diastasis of the ankle joint (122). The former is usually amenable to reconstruction according to Schoenecker (105), whereas the true type 4 deficiency with diastasis of the ankle joint usually is treated with amputation (120,123).

There are reports of reconstruction for the type 4 deficiencies, but in general the follow-up is short and the problems of a plantigrade foot and limb-length discrepancy are just beginning in these patients (122,124–126). One patient followed up to the age of 15 years is described as having satisfactory ankle function and 6.5 cm of shortening (127), while another followed up to the age of 10 years (6 years after reconstructive surgery) is reported as having a stable ankle and plantigrade foot, but projected limb-length discrepancy is not mentioned (128).

In their review of tibial deficiencies, Schoenecker et al. reported on ten patients with Jones type 4 deficiencies, of which nine had initial reconstruction of the foot. A Syme amputation was subsequently done in six of them, usually at the parents' request. Of the four who retained the foot, two had contralateral deficiencies in which the prosthesis accommodated the length discrepancy. One had a lengthening of 4.6 cm and one remained 4.8 cm short.

From the available information it would seem reasonable to attempt to retain the foot, if the deformity is at the less severe end of the spectrum, or if there is a significant contralateral deficiency. In most other cases, Syme amputation seems most reasonable.

***Prosthetic Management.*** With the various surgical interventions dependent on the severity of the anomaly, there are several prosthetic approaches to management. In children with type I tibial deficiency who have been treated with knee disarticulation and have a flare at the condyles, the prosthetic socket consists of a nonischial weight-bearing design with rotational control achieved through the intimate fit of the distal end of the socket over the femoral condyles and a well-formed gluteal impression. Suspension is usually achieved with the use of a segmented liner or bladder design that allows the wider condyles to pass through, while maintaining pressure over the femur just proximal to the condyles.

In cases in which the condyles are absent or there is the need to fit with a transfemoral socket, rotational control is achieved through proper contouring of the socket relative to the femur—the musculature surrounding the femur has a slight triangular shape in a cross-sectional view, with a flatter contour on the lateral surface, especially proximally. This allows a locking of the musculature which, with proper socket fit, decreases rotation. In addition, a silicone sleeve suspension may be used in conjunction with a pull-through strap to secure the liner. If all other procedures fail, a standard Silesian belt (around the pelvis) may be utilized. The total elastic suspension (TES) belt offers excellent suspension and flexibility of form, and it aids in control of the prosthesis. However, the Silesian belt and TES will interfere with grooming and toilet training.

In the knee disarticulation (or transfemoral) prosthesis for children, there are differences of opinion as to when young children are able to handle an articulated knee. Traditional established practice is to first fit the child with a locked knee, and allow an articulating knee at approximately 3 to 5 years of age. In contrast, Wilk et al. (129) advocate the use of articulating knees in children as young as 17 months. Children as young as 11 months can be appropriate candidates for articulated knees (128). The children learn how to handle the knee very quickly, and there is very little need for any type of device to temporarily stabilize the knee. The use of a knee joint at this stage permits more normal development, allowing bent-knee sitting, side sitting, crawling and kneeling on hands and knees, and easier pull to a stand. With a pediatric knee, children can reduce or eliminate a circumducted gait pattern.

In type II cases, in which a tibial segment has been preserved or the fibula has been joined to the tibial remnant, a modified transtibial prosthesis or a Syme prosthesis is utilized. Unlike the standard transtibial design, the socket will incorporate supracondylar and suprapatellar proximal brim lines that will aid in the control and stability of the knee and prevention of a hyperextension moment, respectively. In some instances in which knee stability is less than optimal, outside joints and a thigh cuff or lacer may be required. These are used as a last resort and often contribute to increased weakening of the musculature as a trade-off for increased control and alignment.

## Femoral Deficiency

### Classification

There have been numerous classifications of PFFD (28,30,57,130–134). These classifications range from attempts to unify all radiographic defects of femoral development to a simple two-part classification based on limb-length inequality. Some classifications are radiologic, some functional, and some are designed to suit the authors' preferred treatment. In addition, no classification is able to account for the length, radiographic, and muscle abnormalities, all of which are important in the treatment and outcome.

The most widely used classification is that proposed by Aitken (130). It divides the true PFFD cases into four categories on the basis of the radiographic findings. It is important to keep in mind that in PFFD, as in other congenital deficiencies, the bone may be late in ossifying and therefore may be present but unseen on radiographs. Also, these different groups are not distinct, but rather form a continuous spectrum.

In class A, the femur is short, with its proximal end at or slightly above the acetabulum (Fig. 31.9). There is a defect in the subtrochanteric region. The femoral head may be

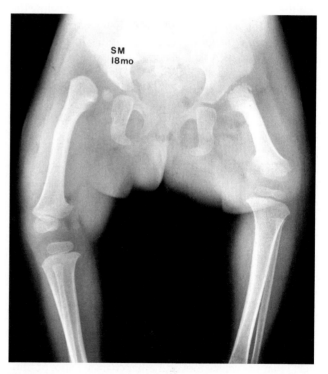

**Figure 31.9** Anteroposterior pelvis of an 18-month-old child with bilateral proximal femoral focal deficiency (PFFD). The right hip is an Aitken class A and demonstrates the presence of the ossific nucleus and a good acetabulum. The femoral metaphysis lies above the level of the ossific nucleus. There is a cartilaginous connection between the metaphysis and the femoral head, which will usually ossify by skeletal maturity, but often with a significant varus deformity. The opposite hip is an Aitken class C PFFD. This patient demonstrates the difficulty with limb-length difference in some patients with bilateral PFFD.

absent, but will later ossify, and its presence is indicated by a well-developed acetabulum. The subtrochanteric defect will eventually ossify, establishing bony continuity, although usually with considerable varus deformity. The location of this varus deformity in the subtrochanteric region, rather than the femoral neck, is what distinguishes PFFD from congenital coxa vara.

In class B, there is a more extensive defect or absence of the proximal femur (Fig. 31.10). The femoral head is present, although its ossification may be delayed. There is usually a bony tuft on the proximal end of the femoral shaft. The defect will not heal spontaneously, and the proximal end of the femur will be above the acetabulum.

In Aitken class C, the femoral head is absent, and the acetabulum is severely dysplastic (Fig. 31.11). The femoral shaft is shorter than in class B, and the entire proximal portion of the femur, including the trochanters, will not appear.

In Aitken class D, the femoral shaft is extremely short, often with only a tuft of irregularly ossified bone proximal to the distal femoral epiphysis (Fig. 31.12). The lateral pelvic wall is flat, without hint of an acetabulum.

Gillespie (132) proposed classifying femoral deficiencies into three groups for purposes of treatment. Group A are those with congenital short femur indicated by clinical hip stability, lack of significant knee flexion contracture, and the foot of the affected extremity lying at or below the midpoint of the opposite tibia. These patients may be candidates for limb lengthening. His group B patients include those classified as Aitken classes A, B, and C, whereas his group C represents the Aitken class D patients. He recommends lengthening for his group A patients, and prosthetic treatment for his group B and C patients.

An unusual variant of PFFD is that seen with a bifurcated (not duplicated) femur. In this condition, the femur has two distal ends, which form a "Y" (135). There is always an associated Kalamchi and Dawe type I tibial deficiency without active extension, and treatment is by knee disarticulation and removal of the segment of femur in poorest alignment.

### Clinical Appearance

The appearance is classic and should be easily recognized. It will be bilateral in 15% of the cases. The femoral segment is short, flexed, abducted, and externally rotated. The hip and knee joints exhibit flexion contractures. The proximal thigh is bulbous and rapidly tapers to the knee joint. Fibular deficiencies are so common in association with PFFD that the valgus foot and other characteristics of fibular deficiency are almost a part of PFFD (Fig. 31.13). PFFD is associated with fibular deficiency in 70% to 80% of cases (136). In addition, approximately 50% of the patients will have anomalies involving other limbs (130,136).

Examination of the hip joint is difficult because of the bulbous thigh and short femoral segment. Pistoning may be apparent because of associated hip instability. The knee is always unstable in the anteroposterior direction.

### Treatment

The treatment aims to compensate for the functional problems the patient experiences. The most obvious of these is the shortening of the limb. Less obvious is the problem with hip function and its relation to alignment of the limb. Because of the flexed and externally rotated femoral segment, the knee remains flexed, and the leg and foot are anterior to the axis of the body (Figs. 31.13 and 31.14D). With or without skeletal hip stability, there is a deficiency of the muscles around the hip, resulting in a significant lurch to shift the center of gravity in single-leg stance. The knee will have varying degrees of instability. The function of the foot will depend on the severity of any associated deficiencies of the leg, for example, fibular deficiency.

There are more options and variations in the treatment of PFFD than in that of almost any other congenital limb deficiency. Fortunately, most of these decisions can be postponed until $2\frac{1}{2}$ to 3 years of age, because this is the best age to perform these surgical options. Before this age, several important decisions need to be made. The first is whether the child is a suitable candidate for limb lengthening.

According to most literature on this subject, the limb may be judged to be suitable for lengthening if the predicted discrepancy at maturity is not greater than 20 cm, the hip is, or can be, made stable, and there is a good knee, ankle, and foot. In such cases, multiple staged lengthenings can be planned. The timing and staging of these procedures depends on the choice of the physician, but will usually not start before the age of 3 years. Although it is possible to obtain 20 cm length, there are as yet no good reports on the functional outcome of such lengthenings in patients followed up to maturity and into adulthood.

If the discrepancy is predicted to be greater than 20 cm at maturity, or for any other reason lengthening is not chosen as a treatment, a decision should be reached about the best approach to prosthetic fitting.

The aim of the initial treatment of children with unilateral PFFD is, as in other congenital deficiencies, to parallel normal development. Therefore, when the child is ready to stand, regardless of the treatment planned for the future, he or she is fitted with a prosthesis to equalize the leg lengths and permit standing and walking. The prosthesis is often called a *nonconventional* or *extension* prosthesis. It is designed to fit the extremity without any surgical modification to it (Fig. 31.14). The flexion, abduction, and external rotation of the proximal segment (the femur) are accommodated in the alignment. Although it is customary to omit a knee joint, all efforts should be made to incorporate an articulated prosthetic knee or outside knee joints. The level of the prosthetic knee as compared to the contralateral side is of no consequence. The benefit is to allow flexion and ground clearance and thereby reduce compensatory patterns (128).

This allows the infant knee flexion during all developmental functions: one-half kneel, squat, pull-to-stand, and climb on toys and furniture. The authors have found that

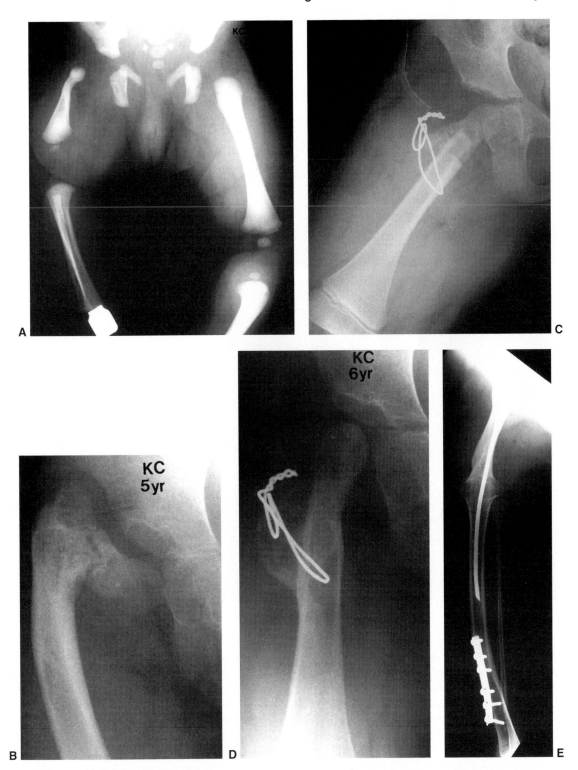

**Figure 31.10** **A:** Anteroposterior radiograph of the pelvis and limbs of a newborn girl with Aitken class B proximal femoral focal deficiency. Note the short femoral segment and the well-developed acetabulum, although the femoral head is not visible. **B:** By 5 years of age, the femoral head is ossified and the cartilaginous connection between the femoral head and the subtrochanteric region of the femur has undergone considerable ossification. However, a pseudarthrosis persists and a significant varus deformity has developed. **C:** The femur after correction of the varus with a spike type of osteotomy. **D:** The result 1 year later. Now faced with a projected discrepancy of 20 cm, the parents elect a van Nes rotationplasty. This was done with part of the rotation through the knee arthrodesis, and the remainder through the tibia. **E:** The radiographic result. The patient had one additional derotation performed through the midtibia at the age of 10 years.

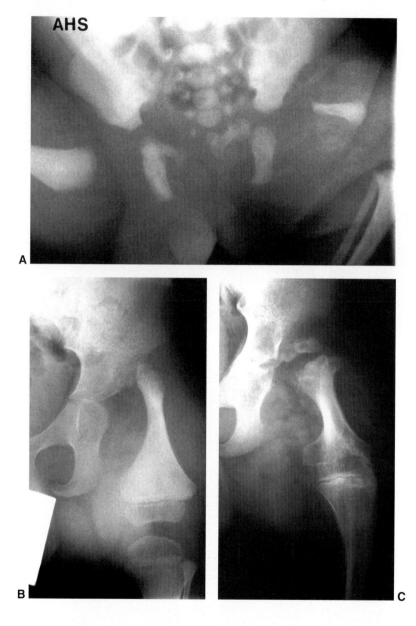

**Figure 31.11** The anteroposterior pelvis and limbs of a newborn boy **(A)** and at 3 years of age, just before surgery **(B)**, with Aitken class C proximal femoral focal deficiency. Note the very short femoral segment and the lack of acetabular development. The same patient is seen in **(C)** at the age of 12, following a Syme amputation and knee arthrodesis with preservation of the proximal tibial physis. There is still no appearance of a proximal femoral ossific nucleus.

infants who are fitted with knees learn very rapidly to extend their hips to control knee extension throughout all their movements. Less vaulting and fewer deviations on the nonprosthetic side are also noted if a knee joint is placed within the prosthesis. There is no knee joint in the prosthesis if the length of the limb is too long to fit a prosthetic foot that includes a knee.

This nonconventional prosthesis will permit ambulation for the young child. However, as the child grows older, the limitations of this prosthesis soon become apparent (Fig. 31.14D). The continued flexion, abduction, and external rotation of the femoral segment result in limb alignment anterior to the body's axis, along with the hip instability and the flexed knee, which is difficult to contain within the prosthesis; all these are factors that make a very poor lever arm to move the prosthesis. The

foot frequently lies at the level of the midcalf of the opposite limb, making the placement of the knee joint less than ideal. The primary goal of surgical correction of these problems is to make the limb a more efficient lever arm for the prosthesis. The secondary goal is to provide a more cosmetic prosthesis. Among the usual surgical choices are knee arthrodesis, amputation of the foot, rotationplasty of the limb, and reconstruction of the hip. Additional possibilities are iliofemoral arthrodesis, with or without rotation, and prosthetic fitting without modification to the limb. Thigh reduction by surgical resection and liposuction are of great value in prosthetic fitting as the patient grows older.

The treatment of children with bilateral PFFD is very different. In these children, the feet should be preserved and knee fusion is not indicated. This is because these

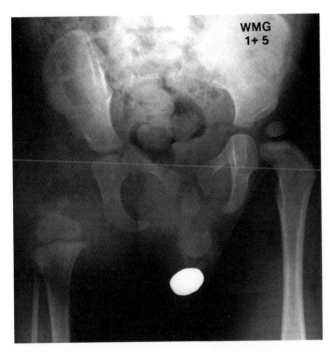

**Figure 31.12** Anteroposterior radiograph of the pelvis and femur of a boy aged 1 year and 5 months with Aitken class D proximal focal deficiency. There is little femur present, and no sign of acetabular development. He underwent knee arthrodesis and Syme amputation at 2½ years of age.

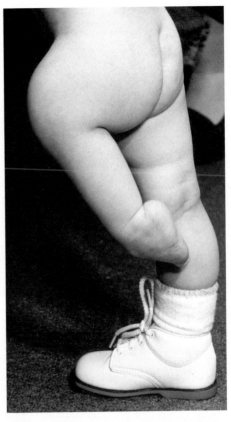

**Figure 31.13** This photo of a 12-month-old girl who is pulling to the standing position demonstrates the clinical features of proximal femoral focal deficiency: a very short and bulbous femoral segment, which is flexed, abducted, and externally rotated.

children will spend most of their lives walking without prostheses. The two biggest problems in these children are foot deformities and unequal limb lengths. Surgical release of the foot and long-term orthotic use can usually provide for a useful foot. Limb-length discrepancy, when significant, is more difficult because of the problem of shortening the child more, on the one hand, and the difficulty of lengthening these limbs, on the other. No firm recommendation can be made regarding this, and each case should be decided on its own merits.

*Knee Arthrodesis.* Arthrodesis of the knee joint is a standard procedure in children with PFFD. It creates a single, longer, and more efficient lever arm, which is easier to contain within the prosthesis. This will greatly enhance prosthetic function and reduce energy consumption. Within 6 months of knee fusion and prosthetic fitting, the abduction and flexion deformity at the hip joint will correct, thereby aligning the limb under the axis of the body.

Depending on the length of the femoral segment and the limb as a whole, it is usually desirable to remove at least one of the growth plates at the knee at the time of fusion. This is usually the case in Aitken class A, B, and C deformities. If this is not done, the limb will remain too long for fitting of a suitable knee joint at maturity. In some cases, depending on the length, it may be advisable to remove both or neither growth plates (137). Calculation of

the anticipated length of both limbs at maturity by means of the Green-Anderson growth charts (Tables 31.2 and 31.3), as described earlier, will help with the answer.

The fusion is usually performed for children between 2 and 3 years of age. After excision of the epiphysis and physis from one side, usually the femur, and the joint surface from the other, the femur and tibia are fixed with a rigid rod, for example, a Rush rod placed from proximal to distal. This is supplemented with a spica cast. The patient is usually ready for prosthetic fitting in 6 weeks and for ambulation as soon as the prosthesis is ready.

*Amputation of the Foot.* With the knee fused, ablation of the foot is desirable in most situations. One reason is length—the new lever arm, consisting of the femur and the tibia, needs to be short enough to accommodate an internal knee joint when the child is older. The foot adds unnecessary length. In addition, as the foot grows, it becomes increasingly difficult to accommodate in a cosmetically acceptable socket. The advantages and disadvantages of the Syme and Boyd amputations have been discussed. Amputation is best performed at the time of knee fusion.

*van Nes Rotationplasty.* In the van Nes rotationplasty, the limb is rotated 180 degrees, through the knee arthrodesis,

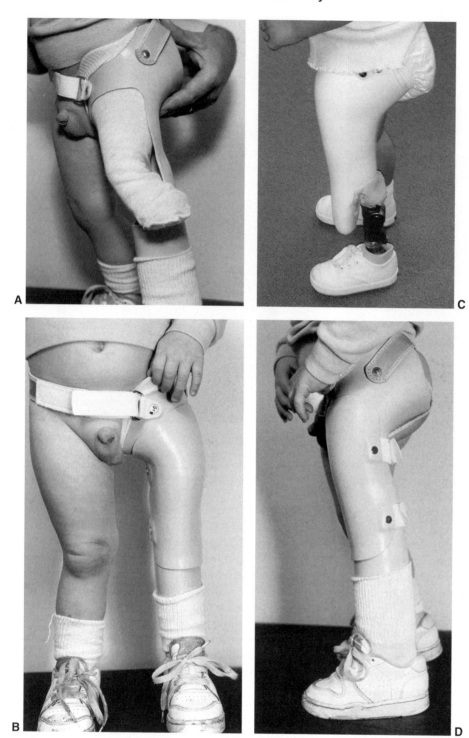

**Figure 31.14** The nonconventional or extension prosthesis allows the child to "stand" on the prosthesis, extending his limb to the floor and accommodating the deformity. **A,B:** The nonconventional or extension prosthesis without a knee joint, which is usual. It is possible to add a knee joint to the prosthesis. **C:** The children rapidly learn to control the knee joint. **D:** Lateral view of the patient with the prosthesis, demonstrating why this prosthesis is not a good long-term solution. The knee is at the brim of the socket, is poorly contained, and provides a very poor lever arm. The weight-bearing line of the leg remains anterior to the axis of the body; the flexion and external rotation of the hip persist.

the tibia, or a combination of both. The goal is to have the ankle of the short limb at the level of the knee on the long limb at maturity. The foot now functions like the residual tibia in a below-knee amputation, thereby allowing the patient to function more like a B-K amputee than one with a knee disarticulation (Fig. 31.15). An obvious prerequisite is reasonable function of the foot and ankle. Because this procedure is also used in the treatment of both malignant skeletal tumors around the knee and traumatic loss of the

knee with its corresponding growth plates, it is important to keep in mind that these patients are very different from those with PFFD. Although some lessons from one group are applicable to the other, care must be taken.

The rotationplasty was first described in 1930 by Borggreve (138), for an acquired limb-length discrepancy, and later by van Nes (139) for three cases of congenital deficiency of the femur. Initial reports of rotationplasty for treatment of PFFD by Kostuik et al. (140) and Torode and

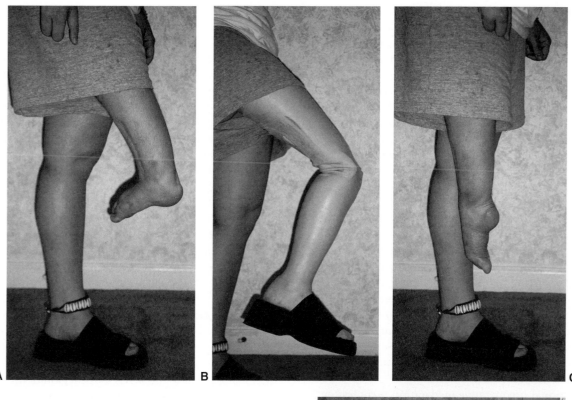

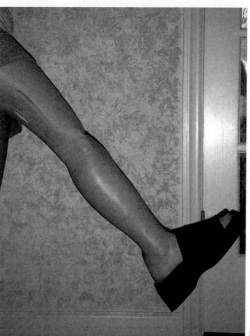

**Figure 31.15** The results of a van Nes rotationplasty are seen in this 17-year-old girl with proximal femoral focal deficiency (PFFD) (same patient as in Fig. 31.10). With the ankle rotated 180 degrees, dorsiflexion of the ankle **(A)** results in flexion of the prosthetic knee **(B)**, and plantar flexion **(C)** results in extension of the prosthetic knee **(D)**.

Gillespie (141) have been followed by more recent reports by Friscia et al. (142) and Alman et al. (143).

The main complication of the procedure is either failure to achieve sufficient rotation at surgery or subsequent derotation with growth. Kostuik et al. (140), in one of the earliest reports on this procedure, recommended waiting to perform the surgery until the child was older. However, this delays the procedure many years beyond when the patient can learn to use the prosthesis and benefit from the procedure. Because the complication is easily treated, there seems to be little reason to wait. Subsequent reports have not found this to be so great a problem.

When this procedure is considered, a potential problem of concern to patients, parents, physicians, and prosthetists is the cosmetic appearance. It appears, however, that this problem is overrated by medical staff, compared to the patients themselves. The procedure has been more widely used and accepted in Canada than in the United States, except in large limb-deficiency centers. Alman et al. found no difference in the perceived physical appearance of children treated with rotationplasty, compared to knee arthrodesis and Syme amputation (143). In the report of Friscia et al. (142), one patient subsequently had a Syme amputation at the parents' request. Two recent studies evaluating the quality of life in patients who had rotationplasty for sarcoma treatment demonstrated that although physical function was less than that in healthy peers, psychosocial adaptation and life contentment were about the same (144,145). This emphasizes the importance of proper preparation of the parents and of the patient, if she or he is old enough. This is best accomplished by seeing other patients with a rotationplasty, along with the use of videos of patients, teaching dolls, and so on.

It needs to be emphasized that the ankle must be sufficiently normal to serve as a knee. This is particularly important, because up to 70% of children with PFFD will also have a fibular deficiency on the same side. Although some valgus alignment of the foot and ankle can be compensated for in the prosthetic alignment, the deformity may tend to become greater with age. Severe valgus and equinus deformities, with a deficient foot, are contraindications to the procedure.

Additional preoperative preparation includes toe and ankle strengthening, in particular, because these are the structures that will power the new knee joint. Equinus position should be emphasized, because this will place the foot in the best mechanical position. Children who have mild equinus contractures of 30 degrees or less will usually stretch these out with prosthetic use, and do not need special attention preoperatively. Crutch training should be done preoperatively, as in all elective surgery that will require crutch use postoperatively.

The improvement in function with the rotationplasty, compared to other procedures, has been documented both for patients with tumor (146–148) and for those with PFFD (143,149). These studies demonstrate that those with rotationplasty function better than those with knee arthrodesis and Syme amputation, not quite so well as those with a below-knee amputation, and not as well as those who have rotationplasty for noncongenital conditions, for example, tumor. Those with rotationplasty for noncongenital conditions probably do better because of the normal hip function that remains one of the major problems in those with PFFD.

### Stabilization of the Hip

Most patients with PFFD who are to be managed with prosthetic fitting will have hip instability. This is not only because of the deficient bony anatomy, but also the deficient musculature. This has resulted in some controversy about the value of surgical procedures to stabilize the hip. Some feel that nothing of functional value is gained and surgical intervention is not warranted (136,137,150), whereas others feel that surgical correction can be of value

(28,151–153). It is the authors' opinion that in Aitken class A and B patients who have a femoral head within the acetabulum, surgical correction of the pseudarthrosis with correction of the varus deformity is beneficial (Fig. 31.10B to D).

There are two problems to consider: the pseudarthrosis and consequent malalignment, and the bony stability of the femoral-pelvic articulation. In those patients for whom lengthening is planned, it is necessary to obtain good containment of the femoral head, which may require an acetabular procedure. In these patients, retroversion and varus are usually present, and should be corrected prior to lengthening.

In patients with Aitken class B PFFD, there will be a pseudarthrosis of the femoral neck. This can be repaired while, at the same time, restoring more normal alignment. It may not be necessary to wait until complete ossification of the femoral neck to perform this procedure (154). Ossification may accelerate after realignment.

***Iliofemoral Arthrodesis.*** There are two types of iliofemoral arthrodeses described. These procedures are an attempt to address the problem of hip instability.

In 1987, Steel (155) described arthrodesis of the distal femoral segment to the pelvis in the region of the acetabulum in four patients. The femur was flexed 90 degrees so that it was perpendicular to the axis of the body. This results in knee extension being equivalent to hip flexion, and knee flexion being equivalent to hip extension.

More recently, Brown (156) has described a rotationplasty in conjunction with iliofemoral arthrodesis. In this procedure, the distal end of the femur is rotated 180 degrees before it is joined to the ilium with its axis in line with that of the body. The knee now functions as the hip joint, and the ankle now functions as the knee joint, as in a van Nes rotationplasty.

Both of these procedures have had limited use. There are significant problems in achieving an arthrodesis, and the distal femoral segment cannot be allowed to grow too long. Additional surgical procedures are to be expected. As yet, there are only very limited reports on the functional advantages (155,156).

***Thigh Reduction.*** The bulbous proximal portion of the thigh makes prosthetic fitting difficult in some patients and results in discomfort for others. This problem usually manifests itself during adolescence and can be resolved by thigh reduction with a combination of surgical excision and liposuction.

***Prosthetic Management.*** Initial prosthetic management of the child presenting with PFFD begins with the extension or nonstandard prosthesis, with or without an activated knee joint (Fig. 31.14). With the foot positioned in plantar flexion, the limb is cast proximal to the hip joint, and the prosthesis fabricated with a prosthetic foot positioned under the shortened limb. The socket, with ischial containment, has been called a "ship's funnel" design because of the resemblance to the engine air intake funnels of ocean vessels. This drastic socket design is necessary because of the flexed hip and knee that must be contained within the socket while attempting to gain ischial support.

The purpose of the extension-type prosthesis is to equalize the length between the prosthetic and the sound limb, in preparation for early ambulation, while affording time for surgical decisions. There are four indications that have been identified relating to the fitting of nonstandard prostheses (157):

1. When the patient is still too young for surgical conversion.
2. When the patient or parent refuses surgical intervention, and a prosthesis is necessary for ambulation.
3. In bilateral cases, when extra height or better balance is the goal.
4. When there is lower-extremity involvement, combined with bilateral upper-extremity absence, requiring the feet for activities for daily living (ADL).

When a Syme amputation with knee fusion option is chosen, the prosthesis resembles a knee disarticulation prosthesis, except for the need for ischial weight bearing and high lateral brim containment to aid in hip stability. Weight bearing is divided between the ischium and the distal heel pad. Full distal weight bearing would severely compromise hip function over a period of time, because of the inherent instability of the hip with possible proximal migration of the femur. Prosthetically, fusion of the knee with correction of the angular deformities results in improved gait and ease of fitting because of the single skeletal lever arm (158). During growth, the child should be evaluated periodically for the relative length of the two limbs so that, if needed, distal femoral epiphysiodesis can be performed. This will allow fitting of an optimal knee joint when the patient is fully grown, while maintaining the knees at the same level.

In the small child, and when the residual limb is longer than the opposite femoral segment, external knee joints may be used. As the child grows, an internal four-bar knee can be used. More about the indications and selection of knee joints is discussed later in this chapter.

A Syme amputation without knee fusion results in difficulty with prosthetic management. Movement within the prosthesis, at the level of the anatomic knee, and the increased need for an intimately fitted socket, foster a decreased stride length and increased pelvic movement. However, in the child with an Aitken class D PFFD and only a remnant of distal femoral epiphysis in which knee fusion will have little to offer, this may be a suitable choice.

The van Nes rotationplasty requires a nonconventional prosthesis with the ankle functioning as the new knee. This is a very difficult prosthesis to align and fit, although it gives excellent function (142,159). The prosthesis has a lower padded foot socket that contains the rotated foot in full plantar flexion. Lateral and medial external joints are attached to the upper thigh section to increase stability and to prevent hyperextension of the lower shank (159). The original design incorporated a laminated thigh section with ischial weight bearing. For patients with good hip stability, for example, in those who had a tumor and trauma, the laminated section is often replaced with a leather thigh lacer and no ischial weight bearing. It is imperative for proper function that the external joints be aligned with the axis of rotation of the ankle/subtalar complex, while maintaining the line of progression. Failure to ensure this alignment, regardless of the anatomic joint, will result in a poor gait pattern and skin breakdown. The prosthetist should incorporate mechanical joint placement with slight external rotation on a new prosthesis, in anticipation of the mild internal derotation inevitable during growth.

# CONGENITAL DEFICIENCIES OF THE UPPER EXTREMITY

Some of the differences between upper- and lower-extremity amputations have been discussed previously. One additional difference requires emphasis here: Upper-extremity amputations are very visible. The hand is one of the most noticed parts of the human body. Therefore, unlike the child with a below-knee amputation who walks without a limp and can often match his or her peers in physical activity, the child with an upper-extremity amputation is more easily seen as different.

This section deals with those congenital deficiencies of the upper extremity that are transverse in nature. The longitudinal deficiencies, for example, radial club hand and the other classic anomalies that are confined to the hand, are discussed in Chapter 23.

Most transverse deficiencies of the upper extremity will be treated with prosthetic fitting, if they are treated at all. An upper-extremity prosthesis is a way to improve the ability of the deficient limb to assist the intact limb in its activities; it does not replace the function of the missing part as adequately as it does in the lower limb.

The main purpose of the upper extremity, or a prosthetic substitute, lies in the function of the hand, with the rest of the limb used to position the hand. In addition, the upper limb, or a prosthesis, also plays a role in support, balance, and trunk stability. In these latter functions, the prosthesis can do well, but in the main function of prehension, it functions poorly when compared to the normal hand. A prosthesis has no sensory feedback, which requires that the child watch the prosthetic hand in use. This, plus the thought and mental practice that goes into making a mechanical device work, makes the upper-extremity prosthesis a far less efficient tool than the lower-extremity prosthesis.

It is important to recognize that many transverse upper-extremity deficiencies will not be well served by prosthetic prescription. If the prosthesis does not afford the child a functional gain or cosmetic benefit, he or she will be quick to reject it. The prosthesis must aid the child in some function he or she wishes to do, that is, an age-appropriate function that requires the use of two hands. The reasons for some children becoming good users of a prosthesis, whereas others with the same characteristics reject it, are not well understood. Although the parents' acceptance and compliance are important, this is not the whole answer. The inability of the prosthesis to substitute for a normal limb, and the hand in particular, is also a partial explanation. These facts, coupled with the incredible ability of the young child to learn to use one hand assisted by the residual limb with minimal concession to activities that are assumed to require two hands, must also be a significant factor.

Judging the success of an upper-extremity prosthesis is very specific to the particular patient, and difficult to quantify. The hours of use alone is not a good criterion. Many children will use the prosthesis for specific tasks (riding a bike), and prefer to remove it for others (swimming). Some children will wear it very little during the summer while playing, but will wear and use it every day in school, when different bimanual motor tasks are a significant part of the activity.

What the child can do with the prosthesis when asked and what he or she actually does with it in normal activities can be very different. Although some children develop an amazing facility with the prosthesis in their everyday activities, many will demonstrate their skill with the prosthesis only in the medical setting while they continue to use the prosthesis much as they would their residual limb, and not as a prehensile tool, during daily activities. Standardized tests have been developed to measure spontaneous use versus voluntary control as it relates to age-appropriate activities. The University of New Brunswick test of myoelectric control is used by therapists to assess the child's ability to use the prosthesis in a controlled situation. The Prosthetic Upper Extremity Functional Index is a self-reported measure of the child's functional abilities during daily activities.

Although children often will not use a hand for functional purposes, the importance of the hand in appearance must be remembered. Besides the face, the hand (or its absence) is the most readily noted feature of the body. Good cosmetic hands can be of great help to children, especially adolescents, who desire them, and their benefit to the child should not be minimized because of their nonfunctional nature.

The higher the deficiency, the more the disability, the harder it is to replace the function with a prosthesis, and the less will be the patient's acceptance of it. Lack of heat dissipation, weight, energy expenditure, concentration necessary to work it, and lack of functionality are all reasons for children with more proximal deficiencies to be less likely to use a prosthesis.

The main purpose of the upper extremities is the grasp and manipulation of objects. Early in infancy, the upper extremity reaches and touches objects within the visual fields and provides a rich sensory feedback to the child. This sensory feedback is an essential element of upper-extremity function. For the child with a limb deficiency or high-level amputation, especially if bilateral, sensation seems to be the single most desirable attribute of the extremities. Therefore, if the upper extremities meet in the midline, the child will usually reject a prosthesis. If the extremities will not meet, or sometimes, when they meet where they cannot be seen, the patient may prefer a prosthesis for the function it affords.

The fitting of an upper-extremity prosthesis is much more individualized than a lower-extremity prosthesis. For those with a unilateral below-elbow amputation, fitting with a passive hand at approximately 4 to 6 months of age is an easy decision because it is relatively inexpensive, well tolerated by the patient, and helpful in deciding on fitting with a more complex prosthesis later. However, in cases of high-level amputations, especially if they are bilateral, such a program of routine fitting will frequently result in failure (6).

The age for fitting is based on the normal development of the child. By 4 months of age, the child brings the hands to the midline while supine, and props on the elbows while prone. Eye–hand coordination develops as the hands are brought into the visual fields. By 6 months, the child is beginning to prop on the extended arms when sitting, and is rolling in all directions. Early prosthetic fitting between 4 and 6 months allows the infant to incorporate the prosthesis in all gross and fine motor functions that are developing.

Children with bilateral high-level amputations will primarily use adaptive performance techniques with their mouth, chin, neck, shoulder, and feet. Therapeutic interventions should first focus on promoting these techniques, and secondarily on adapting the environment to assist the child in age-appropriate activities. Attempts should not be made at this point to modify the child with prosthetics. Children with high levels or complete absence of the upper limbs will use their feet to accomplish everyday two-handed activities. The use of the foot in play, and in ADL appropriate for the child's stage of development should be incorporated in all therapy home programs. It may take considerable persuasion to win the parents to this view.

Nonetheless, children with bilateral high-level amputations should probably be given an opportunity for prosthetic use. In addition to possible functional gains, the families experience a significant benefit in knowing that all has been tried, and the patients gain a valuable experience in having tried prostheses. A multicenter review of bilateral upper-limb deficiencies showed that 50% of patients were still wearing a prosthesis at age 17 years or more (6). Fitting in such children should rarely be attempted before 1 year of age, despite the parents' anxieties. Fitting should be done to help the child perform appropriate tasks for his or her stage of development, or to aid in certain specific activities. It is usually best to fit a child with only one prosthesis at a time because the problems with two may lead to early rejection.

## Amelia

The child with unilateral absence of the arm will be less likely to fully accept a functional prosthesis than those with lower levels of amputation. If body-powered components are used, the patient has difficulty in controlling the devices because there is no lever arm. Externally powered prostheses are heavy. The weight and increased body heat due to the necessary suspension make this a difficult prosthesis to wear. When coupled with the problems of function in using an artificial shoulder, elbow joint, and hand, the child will usually choose to function without the prosthesis.

Many children with amelia of the upper extremity are affected bilaterally. The choices for these children are to help them develop their lower extremities to substitute for the upper extremities, to fit them with prostheses, or to attempt a combination of both. There is universal agreement that there is no place for attempting to limit the child's use of the feet or attempting to provide all of the child's upper-extremity function with prostheses. The feet are the best substitute for the hands. Children with bilateral amelia and relatively normal lower extremities can usually master all ADL, while leading full lives with family, children, and employment. Until the physician becomes acquainted with a child or, preferably an adult, with bilateral amelia, she or he cannot understand the extent to which the legs and feet can substitute for the arms and hands. Most of these children will reject prostheses.

The question of prosthetic fitting most often arises in the child with bilateral amelia and significant lower-extremity anomalies that limit their substitution for upper-extremity function. In such cases, unilateral fitting may be indicated, but is likely to gain limited acceptance, and then only after many years of struggle.

Children with bilateral amelia will often walk late. They will need help in pushing to stand. In addition, the fear of falling, because they cannot protect themselves, comes early. Helmets or some protective headgear are needed until the child is independent in gait. Therapy is directed at trunk control and strength, along with training in the use of their feet for all activities. These children are also prone to develop a progressive scoliosis, often before adolescence. This presents a difficult problem. Bracing restricts the use of their feet in activities of daily living. Surgical fusion does the same. However, often these curves will require fusion, and in such cases, as short a fusion as possible should be done.

## Phocomelia

In phocomelia, the distal portion of the extremities appear to attach directly to the body. There are wide variations in this deficiency. In some, the hands may be close to normal, with some remnants of the arm bones, whereas in others the hand may be no more than a single functionless digit with little residue of the arm. Patients with phocomelia usually have some mobility in their residual limbs, and therefore differ in one significant way from the child with bilateral amelia—they have a sensate limb often capable of some grasping function. The function of these limbs depends on the function of the hand, the length and function of the arm itself, and the ability to bring the hands together at the midline or to the face.

Those children who cannot bring their hands to the midline or to the mouth will use their feet to substitute in the ADL (Fig. 31.16A–D). They should be encouraged from an early age to develop their foot skills and the body strength that is necessary to use the feet. In those children with better function and length, little else than adaptive equipment to aid in dressing and so on may be necessary (Fig. 31.16E).

Therapy to increase the range of motion of the scapula and limbs and to strengthen any muscle power in the residual digits may prove of benefit. Adaptive equipment to aid in the use of the residual limbs can be very useful for some activities such as feeding, dressing, and so on. The residual limbs can manipulate switches for powered prostheses, and therefore, the temptation to find for a prosthetic solution to their problem arises. However, like the child with bilateral amelia, these children will function in most activities by substituting foot function for what they cannot do with their upper extremities. Fitting the older child with a unilateral prosthesis for a specific function may be indicated, but routine wear is not common.

## Transverse Complete Humeral Deficiency

There is little published experience in this deficiency. Although some children with unilateral above-elbow amputation will develop surprising facility with a prosthesis, they will often wear it only for specific activities, such as sports, or for cosmetic reasons. If there is a humeral segment of any reasonable length, the humeral-thoracic pinch provides useful assistance for the normal opposite extremity. Prosthetic use will be in accord with the patient's functional needs, and will generally relate to specific tasks. These may be as limited as riding a bicycle or full-time use at school. These patients should be offered the opportunity for prosthetic fitting.

Patients with bilateral congenital transhumeral deficiencies are more inclined to use their own body, rather than a prosthesis. These children may benefit more from assistive devices than from prostheses. Such patients will often prefer prosthetic fitting on one side, where they use the humeral-thoracic pinch, with intact sensory feedback on the other side and in their feet. Again, it is important to make the distinction between the congenital and acquired amputee. The congenital amputee will be less inclined to

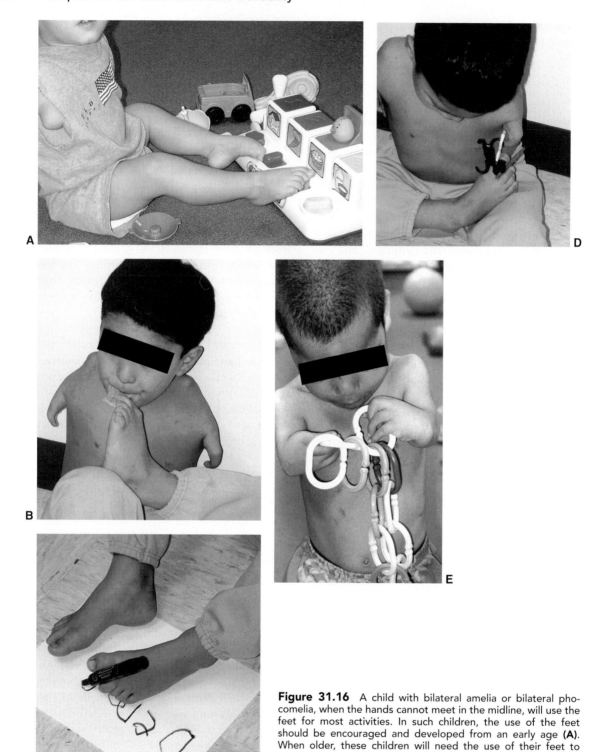

**Figure 31.16** A child with bilateral amelia or bilateral pho-comelia, when the hands cannot meet in the midline, will use the feet for most activities. In such children, the use of the feet should be encouraged and developed from an early age **(A)**. When older, these children will need the use of their feet to accomplish the activities of daily living **(B,C)**. If there is any motor power in the extremities, they may be capable of useful function and assist the feet **(D)**. When the hands can meet in the midline and have good motor power, excellent function is possible **(E)**.

use prostheses, and the traumatic amputee will be more inclined.

For the patient with bilateral above-elbow transhumeral deficiencies, Marquardt has recommended an angulation osteotomy of the humerus (160). The osteotomy angles the distal 3 to 5 cm of the humerus anteriorly by 70 to 90 degrees. This allows for suspension of the prosthesis without the usual shoulder cap, makes it easier to put on, permits better shoulder motion, and gives better control of rotation. This procedure should only be performed if the humeral length is sufficient and there is a need for a unilateral prosthesis.

## Transverse Complete Forearm Deficiency (Congenital Below-Elbow Amputation)

The congenital below-elbow amputation is the most common of all of the upper-extremity deficiencies. It is more often the left arm (Fig. 31.17). It is sporadic and without known cause. Children with this deficiency present the most ideal upper-extremity deficiencies for prosthetic fitting. Children with this deficiency are unlike those with a transverse amputation through the carpal bones, which usually have partial grasping function with sensation. They are also unlike the above-elbow deficiencies in that they have a normal shoulder and elbow that allow accurate placement of a relatively light prosthetic terminal device.

Despite the fact that congenital below-elbow amputees are ideal candidates for prosthetic use, not all children will remain good prosthetic users during their childhood. Scotland and Galway reviewed the experience at the Ontario Crippled Children's Center, and found that 32% had stopped using their prosthesis, upon follow-up of 7 to 17 years (161). How many of these may resume use of the prosthesis in the work environment is unknown. They, like

Brooks and Shaperman (162), noted greater acceptance of the prosthesis if fitting was done before the age of 2 years.

In the congenital group of Brooks and Shaperman (162), 22% of those fitted before 2 years of age, and 58% of those fitted after, had stopped using their prosthesis. However, of those who continued to use their prosthesis, there was no difference in the extent of use between the two groups. The most common age at which patients discontinued use of their prosthesis was at 13 years, and the most common reasons they gave were that the prosthesis was cosmetically unacceptable and that they could do everything without it. Sorbye (163) reported that, of the patients in their clinic who were younger than 24 years, 87% were using their myoelectric prosthesis, and 65% of these used it all day and for all activities. Hubbard et al. (164), reporting on the Toronto experience, found that 70% of the below-elbow amputees were using their prosthesis, whereas 30% had rejected it.

With this and other evidence, it is now the usual practice to recommend fitting around the age of 4 to 6 months with a passive hand to aid in normal development. It is in this age range that the child brings his or her hands to midline

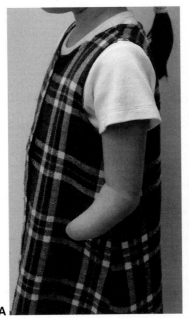
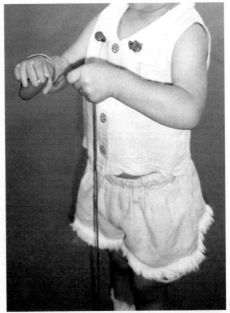
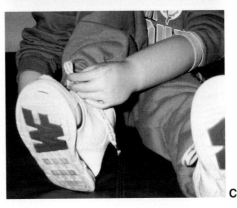

**Figure 31.17** **A:** A typical patient with a congenital below-elbow amputation. There is usually enough length to fit a prosthetic arm and still permit good active elbow motion. **B,C:** Two different children with transverse incomplete forearm deficiency fitted with a myoelectric-powered hand performing common functions of childhood. Many of the children who use the prosthesis develop amazing skills in its use.

while supine, props on the elbows while prone, and then props on extended arms while sitting and rolling over. This lightweight prosthesis is used to have the child become comfortable with a prosthesis, and to acquaint the child with the two-handed activities that a normal child would perform, in an effort to develop the central cortical pathways for bimanual dexterity.

Depending on the child's acceptance and use of this passive prosthesis and the choice of a terminal device, a more functional terminal device is fit between 15 and 18 months (27,165). Today, there are a number of terminal devices available (166). There are two choices to power the device: battery (myoelectric) and body (cables). Although there will be many factors to consider in the selection (cost and funding, clinic philosophy, and parent choice), virtually all centers today in North America are fitting most children with myoelectric-powered terminal devices (Fig. 31.17). Table 31.4 compares the advantages and disadvantages of myoelectric and body-powered terminal devices for the child with a congenital below-elbow amputation.

## Terminal Transverse Transcarpal Deficiency

The congenital transcarpal amputation is the second most common deficiency of the upper limb and occurs in a characteristic pattern, with some or all of the proximal row of carpal bones preserved. The existing flexion of the carpals on the radius allows for limited grasping function, which along with normal sensation, makes this an assistive hand for which no prosthesis can substitute (Fig. 31.18). Occasionally, children will benefit from a volar opposition post for certain activities. They will usually wear it only for certain tasks, for example, as a guitar pick adapter or to grasp the handle bars on a bicycle.

The authors' experience with such children is that they have much more difficulty with the cosmetic aspect of their deficiency than do those children with transverse amputations at higher levels. In the older child and adolescent, it may be wise to explore the desire for a cosmetic hand that would be used in certain circumstances or would provide a psychosocial benefit. Some cosmetic hands have a passive spring grasp to provide limited function.

## Prosthetic Management

Generally, upper-extremity prostheses and their control systems can be subdivided into three categories: *passive, externally powered,* or *body-powered devices.* The Ballif arm (circa 1400) was the first body-powered prosthesis to introduce the use of prosthetic hand operation by transferring

## TABLE 31.4

### COMPARISON OF MYOELECTRIC WITH BODY-POWERED PROSTHESES

| Myoelectric | Body-powered |
| --- | --- |
| **Weight** Heavier; passive prostheses are weighted to prepare patient for the myoelectric system | Weight spread across the shoulders |
| **Grip Strength** Stronger than a body-powered prosthesis; strength built into the system; less work for the child | Strength is provided by rubber bands that increase or decrease the tension and force needed to open the hand; more work needed through scapular control |
| **Cosmesis** More accepted; resembles the hand; more self-esteem for the child; greater parental acceptance | Hooklike or clawlike in appearance; usually rejected by the child or parent; object of ridicule by other children |
| **Maintenance** Requires gloves; requires maintenance and electronics; electrodes lose contact and require occasional adjustment; adjustments required for growth | Requires gloves if mechanical hand is used; frequently requires repair for broken cables caused by friction; requires adjustments for growth on a regular basis |
| **Harness** No harness or straps on body; suspension through socket | Harness is bulky on a toddler, difficult to keep on without pinning to undergarment; children dislike harness especially in summer months |
| **Muscle Control** Uses muscles in limb to control terminal device; with prosthetic hand child can experience direct "cause and effect" | Uses muscles distant from the terminal device, biscapular abduction to control hand or hook; very confusing for toddler whose control and balance is developing; easier for older children |
| **Grip Control** Maintains grip more easily through muscle contraction at the end of the residual limb; is the most successful type of control | Toddlers loose grip very easily, overall gross movements allow the object being grasped to release and fall involuntarily; tension on the cable to the harness does not remain constant; becomes very frustrating for the child |

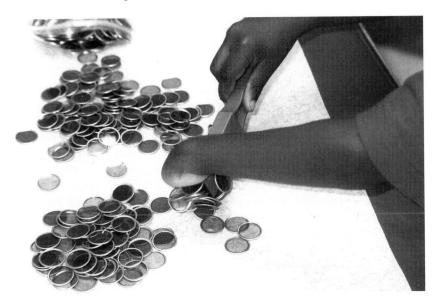

**Figure 31.18** This young boy with a transverse transcarpal deficiency demonstrates the partial grasp at the flexor crease that, when combined with sensation, usually proves superior in function to a prosthesis.

shoulder movement to activate the terminal device (167). A harness over the contralateral shoulder is connected with a thin cable and housing to a terminal device. Through the use of scapular abduction, the fixed cable is stretched over a greater distance and causes the prosthetic hook or hand to open or close, depending on the configuration of the terminal device. A good analogy is the braking system on most bicycles. Most parents prefer the cable-operated prosthetic hand over the cantered hook for cosmetic reasons. Unfortunately, the hook is far superior in function, but has fallen from favor because of the desire to have the prosthesis look as natural as possible, even at the sacrifice of function. Most hooks are canted in design, and this allows a full field of view of the device while using it, compared to the mechanical hand that obstructs the view and results in awkward arm positions to grasp objects.

The externally powered prosthesis can be further subdivided into *switch control* or *myoelectric control*. In both systems, a battery, relay switch, electric hand, and electronic control system are present. It should be noted that the myoelectric hand is the only terminal device available for children using the externally powered prosthesis. In the myoelectric prosthesis (Fig. 31.19), an electrode placed on the surface of the skin acts to pick up the electromyographic (EMG) signal, which in turn is amplified with the help of an electronic relay switch, and this, in turn, operates the electric hand (168). The entire system is generally referred to as a one-site or two-site system. This denotes the number of electrodes that are used for signal recognition.

The one-site system can be further categorized as voluntary opening–automatic closing, rate-sensitive, and level-sensitive. The first fitting of a myoelectric arm occurs at younger than 2 years and utilizes a voluntary opening–automatic closing (cookie-cruncher) configuration. The muscle signal opens the electric hand, and relaxing of the signal causes the hand to close automatically. This system is used for children under 4 years of age. The rate-sensitive and level-sensitive control systems use one muscle to control two functions, and are generally fitted to children over 4 years of age, when two sites are not available. The choice of a system depends on the muscle signal strength, muscle control, and prosthetic design factors (27).

In the two-site system, each electrode operates a specific task. Children can often operate this more complex system

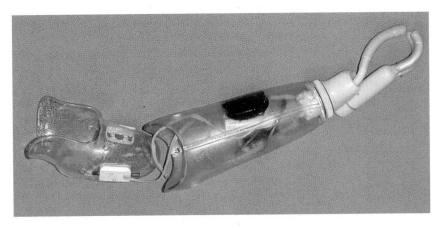

**Figure 31.19** This example of a myoelectric prosthesis, called the Otto Bock Electrohand, was made with a clear socket for teaching purposes. The proximal portion of the socket, which fits on the residual limb, contains the electrodes that pick up the signals from the muscles. This fits into the prosthesis, which contains the electrical and mechanical working parts of the hand.

by 3 to 3 ½ years of age. The EMG signal of the flexors is used to close the hand, whereas the EMG signal of the extensors is used to open the hand. This system is used when children have established good control and good use of their myoelectric prosthesis and have demonstrated the ability to control both the flexors and extensors independently of each other.

Patients with a higher level of upper-extremity amputation are generally good candidates for switch-controlled externally powered prostheses. The electrode is replaced with a miniature switch that can be of a push-pull configuration, a force-sensing resistor, or of a simple on-off design. The incorporation of these switches into the prosthesis depends primarily on the level of amputation and the design of the prosthetic socket or frame.

## Multiple-Limb Deficiencies

Management of the patient with multiple-limb deficiencies, involving both the upper and lower limbs, is a challenge that requires a team with experience to achieve the maximum function for the patient. The problem of bilateral upper-extremity amputation has been covered earlier. Children with one upper and one lower extremity pose no problems beyond the management of each individual limb. Children with bilateral knee disarticulation or transtibial amputations will walk without support, and therefore a unilateral upper-extremity amputation in association poses no special problem, other than donning and doffing the prostheses. With bilateral amputations above the knee disarticulation level, however, walking without support is problematic; upper-extremity function is needed, and a wheelchair may be required for long distances and to conserve energy.

A special caution needs to be given in regard to those children with bilateral upper-extremity amputation and lower-extremity anomalies that might ordinarily be treated with amputation and prosthetic fitting. No amputations of the lower extremity should be performed until it is certain that the child will not require the use of the feet for grasping activities.

One of the most common types of patients seen in the pediatric age-group with this problem is the quadrimembral amputee resulting from meningococcemia. In these patients, it is often necessary to cover the residual extremities with split-thickness skin grafts to maintain length. These grafts, if not adherent to bone, do very well in the prosthesis, and are not a hindrance to fitting. Treatment must be individualized for each patient with certain general guidelines. The first is to help the patient maximize function with his or her residual limbs. This is especially true with the upper extremities, in which sensation is so important to function. Although these children will become proficient in the use of bilateral upper-extremity prostheses, if their residual limbs are long enough, they will usually perform many of their daily activities, especially at home, without their prostheses.

A common mistake is to attempt to fit all four extremities of these children with quadrimembral loss at the same time. Although the pressure to do so is enormous, it may result in actual delay in functional recovery and rejection of the prostheses. In most situations, it is best to first fit the lower extremities and achieve ambulation. After this is accomplished, the upper extremity is fit.

In the child with a congenital quadrimembral deficiency, there will usually come a time when the parents, and perhaps the child, desire prosthetic fitting. Again, it is best to avoid fitting all four extremities at once, but rather focus on meeting specific needs. Although experience shows that most of these children will use their prosthetic devices in a limited fashion, if at all, they and their parents need and are entitled to this experience at least once (Fig. 31.20).

# ACQUIRED DEFICIENCIES

## Causes

Children may undergo an amputation for a variety of reasons. Although there are no good statistics, trauma is the major cause of amputation in childhood (169). In this group, power lawnmowers lead the list of causes, and most commonly, it is a child riding with a family member. Motor vehicle accidents, farm injuries, and gunshot wounds follow in that order (170). In war-torn countries, land mines may be the leading cause of amputation. Because amputation of the digits is most often caused by machinery, upper-extremity amputations are more common than those of the lower extremity. Boys are affected about twice as often as girls.

Tumors, vascular occlusion caused by meningitis or vascular catheterization, and burns are additional causes, and each has its own unique set of circumstances. Indeed, the differences in acquired amputation defy a detailed analysis. Some are semielective and allow for some preparation of the patient and the parents, whereas traumatic amputations do not. It is possible, however, to discuss the common principles that are applicable to acquired amputations in children.

## Principles

When the surgeon is faced with an acutely mangled extremity, it can be difficult to decide on amputation versus limb salvage. The usual criteria and classifications that are applied to adults are not easily transferred to children. It is often necessary to gain the input of a vascular surgeon and others to make the best assessment, while always remembering the tremendous healing and adaptive capacity of the child, compared with the adult.

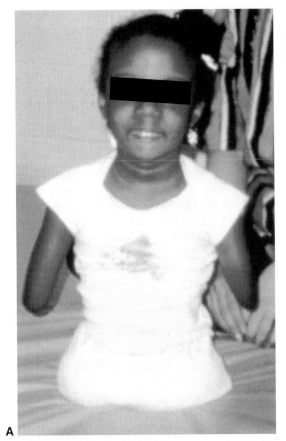

A

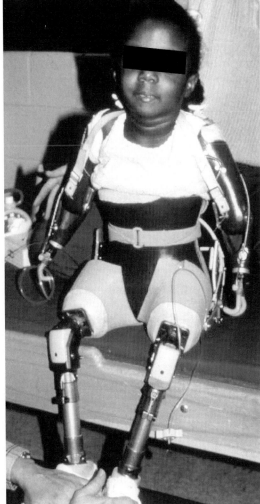

B

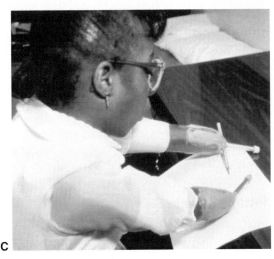

C

**Figure 31.20** This child with congenital bilateral hip disarticulation and transhumeral amputations **(A)** was fitted with four prostheses **(B)**, which she quickly abandoned in favor of her power chair and simple assistive devices **(C)**.

When dealing with feet mangled in a power lawnmower, it is often wise to attempt salvage at the first surgery. However, in the case of a mangled leg that will require vascular and nerve repair, along with bone reconstruction and free tissue transfer, the decision needs to be made more realistically. The more energy expended in saving the limb, the higher the parents' expectations of the result.

The surgeon rarely will have options regarding the level of amputation in trauma. The lack of preparation, coupled with the parents' expectations, usually dictates saving as

much of the limb as possible. This often results in a less functional level of amputation than one that is more proximal. The most obvious example is preservation of the talus and calcaneus, which the parents and child may see as saving at least part of the foot, whereas the result may be a worse gait, worse cosmesis, and more prosthetic problems than with a Syme amputation.

In the child, it is usually advisable to save as much length as possible in amputations of the long bones. This is especially true in the femur, in which 70% of the growth of the bone occurs from the distal physis. A 5-year-old child with a midthigh amputation will have less than ideal length as an adult. In the leg, however, little is lost, so long as an adequate portion of proximal tibia, in which most of the growth occurs, is preserved, and in fact, shortening the bone to achieve good soft-tissue coverage may be the best course.

The common teaching, that skin grafts do not make suitable coverage for a residual limb that will bear weight in a prosthesis, is not applicable to children, especially very young ones. In children, skin grafts do make good coverage so long as they are not adherent to the bone. Split-thickness skin grafts are frequently needed to preserve length in meningococcemia, burns, and some cases of trauma. In older children with traumatic amputations, free vascularized flaps can provide excellent coverage.

Where possible, disarticulations will prevent the problem of bony overgrowth. It is not necessary, or perhaps even advisable, to remove the cartilage from the bone end. Tapering of the bone ends, at the distal tibia, for example, is not necessary unless the child is approaching adulthood. The bony prominences will not develop to adult proportions, and therefore do not present a prosthetic fitting problem. If a young child has a through-bone amputation, it may be possible to salvage a portion of bone and cartilage from the amputated part for capping the bone. This is similar to performing a Marquardt procedure, and has the potential to substantially reduce problems of overgrowth.

It is important not to forget the child during the acute phase of the amputation. Often the surgeon has enough problems dealing with the parents' emotions, and can easily forget that the child also needs emotional as well as physical attention.

In many circumstances, the amputation will be elective. Such is the case with children who have posttraumatic injuries, and are electing surgical modification for better function and prosthetic fitting. Children with gigantism, Klippel-Trenauney-Weber syndrome, and malignant tumors not suitable for limb salvage also are in this category. In many cases the need is obvious, and the child and parents have come to their decision after careful consideration.

In the case of tumors, however, it is usually not so easy, and generally there is not complete acceptance of what is in fact a life-saving procedure. In all cases, the more preparation by the professionals and opportunities for the parents and patient to talk with other patients, the better. It needs to be emphasized that the challenge is to live, and that the surgery is necessary for that. The options revolve around the functional and cosmetic aspects of the different procedures.

There remains a difference of opinion as to whether it is worthwhile to fit the acquired juvenile amputee in the immediate postoperative period. In the young child with a congenital deficiency, there seems little to be gained. However, in the older child, especially when the amputation is caused by trauma, there can be large psychologic benefits from placing the child immediately in a postoperative prosthesis. This also aids in the control of edema and phantom pain.

## PROSTHETICS

In the prosthetic fitting of the pediatric amputee, the single most important guiding principle is that function should never be sacrificed for cosmesis. When dealing with the adult population, overall biomechanical forces resulting from prosthetic alignment can do relatively little damage to skeletal integrity. This is not the case for the pediatric patient, in whom skeletal development is ongoing. Incorrect alignment can have far-reaching and often pronounced negative results.

### Role of the Prosthetist

The role of the prosthetist is to ensure that the highest level of functional need of the patient is met through prosthetic intervention, or through no intervention at all if appropriate. The skilled prosthetist is able to assess anatomic and functional deficiencies and recommend socket design and component selection. In recent years, there has been a tremendous increase in the prosthetic innovations and components available for the pediatric amputee. Current knowledge of these components and their appropriate use will generally be the responsibility of a prosthetist with special interest and experience with children. In addition, he or she must possess the clinical skills, medical knowledge, and the ability to communicate that will enable timely and appropriate flow of knowledge to the other team members and parents, so that realistic expectations can be identified and achieved. Routine servicing of the prosthesis is extremely important so that extensive repairs will be minimized and the need for a new prosthesis recognized. Children are generally not happy to be without their prosthesis.

### Fitting Techniques

The technique will vary, on the basis of the experience of the prosthetist, team approach, integration of ever-changing technology, and the severity of the deficiency. Physiologically, the child is in a constant state of growth and the prosthetic device must be designed to permit weight bearing and allow for the greatest amount of growth without compromising fit and function. Most congenital lower-extremity amputees are able to bear some weight on the distal end of the residual limb, and the prosthetist is able to allow for a slightly less intimate fit of the prosthetic socket than might be the case for the acquired amputee. Unlike the adult, the child's skin has greater tolerance to skin breakdown. The increased activity levels of the child amputee place tremendous expectations on the prosthetic devices and the components. All of these factors are constant challenges to the prosthetic prescription, and emphasize the need for a nonstructured approach to fitting. What may be suitable for one child may be unsuitable for a different child with the same anomaly. Rigid time schedules are discouraged, and developmental levels should be used only as a rough guideline to aid the practitioner.

Fitting the pediatric amputee leads to unique issues not normally seen in the adult population. Disarticulations lead to long residual limbs with knee centers lower than on the sound side. Ischial containment sockets are not normally recommended (unless needed because of hip instability or nondistal weight bearing) because of problems with soft-tissue containment and diapers in infants. Location of bony landmarks is obscured by fatty baby tissue, and casting is difficult and nonexact.

The various stages involved prior to fitting a prosthesis are generally standard within the profession. Upon referral to a clinic, the child is assessed by the team, and a treatment protocol is established. The stages involved in prosthetic fitting include:

1. *CASTING* of the residual limb.
2. *TEST FITTING* of the modified interfacing socket.
3. *DYNAMIC ALIGNMENT AND GAIT TRAINING.*
4. *DELIVERY* of the completed prosthesis.

## Socket Design and Suspension Systems

The cast or impression forms the foundation for the prosthetic design (171). It is only after a well-fitting and comfortable socket-skin interface is achieved that the additional components can be added and expected to function as designed. Casting usually involves the placing of a casting sock on the residual limb, marking all landmarks and wrapping circumferentially with plaster or synthetic bandage. This becomes the negative impression. It is then filled with molding plaster and stripped, forming the positive cast ready for modification. This positive cast is then modified to distribute forces and relieve pressure in the socket for proper hydrostatic control of the residual limb.

Through the use of a clear test or diagnostic socket fabricated over the positive mold, the practitioner is able to ascertain the areas of high and low pressure and to ensure that they are directed over the appropriate areas. Common fitting problems can be flagged and corrected before final socket design.

Computer-aided design/computer-aided manufacture (CAD/CAM) has been used as an alternative tool to plaster casting and modification of the prosthetic socket. In its most simplified form, a residual limb is scanned with an optical laser. The information is relayed to a computer, with which modifications can be made to the scanned shape to allow for increased or decreased weight-bearing areas. The finished design is transferred to a computerized milling machine to form a positive model. This, in turn, is used to fabricate the finished device. Slowly, CAD/CAM

is becoming more widely used within the profession, because of advantages of design reproducibility, record keeping, and flexibility in remote locations (172). Its advantages in the pediatric setting have yet to be proven. All current CAD/CAM systems rely on surface topography of the residual limb, and therefore disregard crucial data such as tissue density, tissue mobility, and underlying skeletal structures (173).

During dynamic alignment in the crawling infant, the prosthetist initially focuses on creating a prosthesis that will aid the infant in preparation for ambulation, transitioning from crawling to standing, with little consideration of gait at this point. Sutherland concluded that mature gait patterns were established by 3 years of age (174), whereas others place the time frame closer to 6 years of age. Early infant gait patterns are, in fact, the processes of suppression of primitive reflexes and the acquisition of postural responses (175). Dynamic alignment is the manipulation of relative position of the socket to the foot and knee while the prosthesis is moving through the various stages of gait. Through the use of alignment mechanisms in the components, the prosthetist is able to shift, tilt, and rotate the knee and foot in relation to the socket. Once independent gait is established in the infant, refinement to gait can be achieved through further prosthetic alignment.

## Lower-extremity Socket Design

The design and fitting of lower-extremity prostheses encompasses numerous biomechanical principles and their application to the residual limb-socket interface, and it is the successful manipulation of these forces that ensures a patient's comfort and function. The accommodation for differences in tissue compressibility, pressure tolerance, underlying bony structures, and vascular integrity are factors taken into account prior to socket design. Dynamic forces exerted through ground reaction forces and resulting moments, including torque and shear forces, increase the vulnerability of the skin-socket interface.

### Hip Disarticulation

Amputees at the hip disarticulation level require extensive prosthetic intervention. The socket encompasses the amputated pelvic remnant, and encloses the contralateral side for suspension. The traditional socket design rises proximally to the waist, and fits similarly to a Boston spinal orthosis. The diagonal socket is a modified version of the standard design, and it affords a more comfortable fit and increased flexibility. Prosthetic hips arc on a single axis, and are mounted on the outside anterior distal aspect of the affected side. Hip and knee flexion are easy to activate through pelvic tilt, if the prosthesis is perfectly aligned. The hip is anterior to the weight line and the knee is posterior. This allows for a stable stance and a smooth gait. The endoskeletal system is used exclusively for this level of amputation because of an increased level of cosmesis and decreased weight. Children with amputations at this level can achieve remarkable gains when fitting begins while the child is pulling to stand and when therapeutic intervention and parental training are incorporated. It is recommended that the knee be locked, initially, so that hip control can first be learned. Once the child is walking independently, the knee can be activated.

### Transfemoral Prosthesis

Transfemoral socket design has evolved significantly over the last 10 years. The quadrilateral socket was the socket design of choice until 1987, when the ISPO formulated recommendations on the narrow medial lateral (ML) socket design (176). Variants of this design (ischial containment socket) continue, including the contoured adducted trochanteric–controlled alignment method (CAT-CAM), the normal shape, normal alignment (NSNA), and the modified quad designs, to name a few (Fig. 31.21). The underlying principle is to adduct the femur while locking the ischial tuberosity within the socket, thereby providing a more anatomically correct alignment during all phases of gait (177). The controversy over these designs has been increasingly dispelled, with further clinical experience.

There are various suspension mechanisms that may be utilized for the secure attachment of the socket to the residual limb. These devices may provide auxiliary suspension which is attached to the socket to suspend or enhance suspension. The suspension may be incorporated in the socket itself, as in suction sockets, supracondylar sockets, and so on.

Pediatric amputees are usually fitted with a *Silesian belt* system of suspension (Fig. 31.14A and B; Fig. 31.22A), until adequate development of the residual limb allows for silicone suspension, at approximately 2 to 3 years of age. The Silesian belt attaches to the anterior/medial aspect and the lateral aspect of the transfemoral socket, and lies across the pelvis at the waist. Tightening the Silesian belt prevents the socket from slipping distally. The TES belt may be used instead of the Silesian belt. The TES belt is a neoprene suspension system that is applied over the proximal portion of the transfemoral socket and is then secured around the waist, and it has become the suspension of choice for the first-time prosthetic user.

Suction sockets are not typically used for the pediatric population because of tight tolerances in fitting that cannot be maintained by a growing child. With the suction socket, the residual limb is pulled into a socket that incorporates a one-way valve in its design (Fig. 31.22B). Once the valve is in place, the amputee expels air every time the prosthesis is in contact with the ground. During swing phase, the negative pressure within the socket holds the prosthesis in place. Air that leaks into the socket is quickly expelled through the one-way valve, and a constant negative pressure is maintained. Total contact suction sockets are generally used for the transfemoral amputee with a mature residual limb, and at the completion of skeletal growth. Short limbs, volumetric changes, and severe scarring are contraindications for the suction-suspended socket.

### Transtibial Prosthesis

The transtibial prosthesis is used the least in the pediatric population. Although most amputations in children are disarticulations, growth changes in the fibular deficiency often result in a transtibial-level residual limb that is a distal-end weight-bearing limb. The true transtibial socket is most often required for the traumatic amputee. Total contact design allows for increased pressure bearing over the patellar tendon, medial flare of the tibia, medial shaft of the tibia, and lateral shaft of the fibula, and the anterior and posterior compartments. Similarly, the weight-sensitive areas most affected include the tibial crest, fibular head, distal tibia and fibula, peroneal nerve, and the patella. The socket design is composed of an outer shell, inner soft liner, and a cosmetic cover.

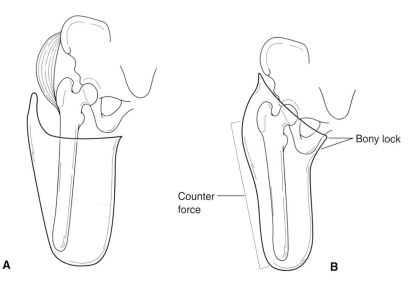

**A**

**B**

**Figure 31.21  A:** The quadrilateral socket is useful for the young child, especially if end bearing is possible. However, it fails to stabilize the femoral segment in a transfemoral amputation. **B:** This has led to the popularity of the narrow medial lateral socket design, such as the ischial containment socket shown here. This design can prove impossible in small infants, because of the fatty thigh and buttocks as well as the diapers.

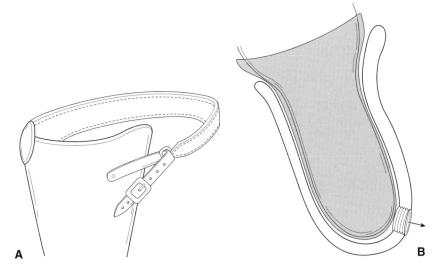

**Figure 31.22** Methods of suspension for transfemoral prostheses. **A:** The Silesian belt is almost universally used in the young pediatric patient to suspend a transfemoral prosthesis or occasionally a knee disarticulation or transtibial prosthesis (Fig. 31.15B). **B:** The suction socket is a tight-fitting socket design with a one-way valve that allows air to be expelled with weight bearing to maintain a suction fit on the residual limb. It is best suited for the older child or adolescent, who has a mature limb that is not changing in size.

The patellar-tendon-bearing (PTB) socket is the standard socket (Fig. 31.23A). It provides the least suspension, and for that reason, is not often suitable for young children. The supracondylar/suprapatellar (SCSP) transtibial socket design (Fig. 31.23B) allows for suspension without the need for belts or cuffs. The medial, lateral, and anterior walls extend proximally, to fully enclose the patella and femoral condyles. The supracondylar (SC) transtibial socket (Fig. 31.23C) is almost identical to the SCSP design, except the anterior proximal brim does not enclose the patella, and therefore allows greater freedom and range of motion. Contraindications for both the SCSP and SC design include obese or muscular limbs and patients with heavy scarring around the knee.

Supracondylar cuff suspension is a common form of suspension for the pediatric transtibial amputee (Fig. 31.23D). The cuff is fabricated from leather and encompasses the femoral condyles and patella. It is attached to the medial and lateral aspects of the socket. The neoprene sleeve suspension is another useful suspension in the pediatric prosthesis (Fig. 31.23E). For the very active child, it provides a great level of security in that the prosthesis will not come off. Recent advances in silicone and urethane technology have increased comfort, flexibility, and cosmesis of the sleeve suspension systems.

Silicone suspension liners have become increasingly popular as a method of suspension without the need for belts or cuffs (Fig. 31.24). The liner is rolled onto the residual limb. At the distal end of the liner is a serrated pin. Inside the distal end of the socket is a shuttle or receptacle mechanism. Once the liner is donned, the amputee places the limb in the socket, and the pin and shuttle engage and lock into place. Pressing of a button hidden on the medial distal aspect of the prosthesis releases the pin, and the residual limb can be removed from the socket. Because of the physical characteristics of the liner, the greater the distracting forces placed on the prosthesis, the tighter the liner grips the residual limb. This system is used extensively in young children. Where space is at a premium, a cushioned silicone liner used in conjunction with a socket expulsion valve, and a silicone sleeve allows the amputee to achieve a remarkable level of suspension using a modified suction technique.

### Ankle Disarticulation Prosthesis (Syme)

The obturator (medial opening) design is most often used when the distal bulbous end is large and the medial malleolus is prominent (Fig. 31.25A). The removable or segmented liner socket incorporates a full foam liner that has been built up to the same circumference as the distal bulbous end. A laminated shell is then formed over this insert. The patient dons the liner first, then slips this into the laminated receptacle (Fig. 31.25B). An atrophied residual limb with a small heel pad is best suited for this design, and the degree of cosmetic restoration will be very good. The silicone or bladder prosthesis utilizes an inner elastic area that stretches to permit passage of the bulbous end of the residuum through the narrower circumference of the tibia and fibula, then constricts once the distal end has passed through (Fig. 31.25C). All of the above designs maintain total contact, and the proximal brim is at the level of the patellar tendon. This ensures that the biomechanical forces are adequately spread up to a load-bearing landmark to increase comfort and function.

## Prosthetic Knees

It has been estimated that more than 100 prosthetic knees are commercially available, and the number is growing each year (178). Although most are for adults, recently there are a number of new knees available for children. The prosthetic knee is composed of the knee mechanism or frame, and may contain a control unit. The control unit consists of a pneumatic, hydraulic, or mechanical system, or some combination of these three. The control unit responds to changes in cadence and dampens sudden, abrupt changes.

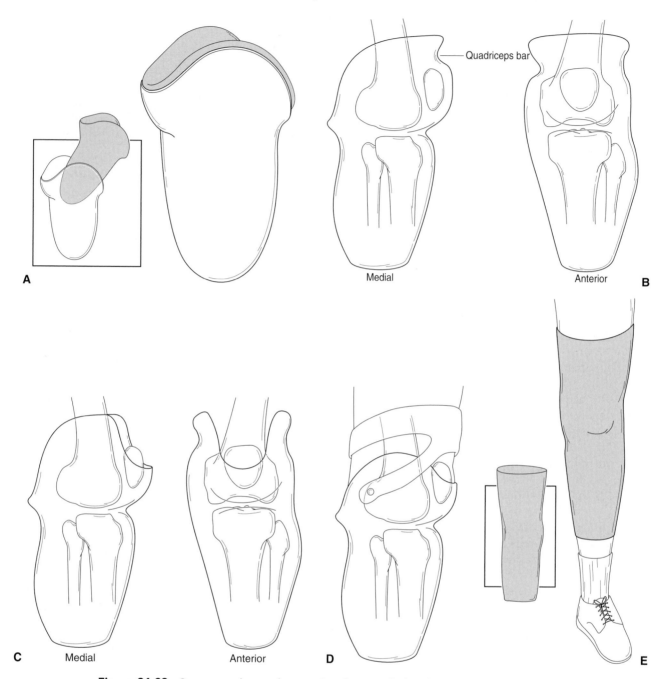

Quadriceps bar

A

Medial                Anterior                                                        B

C        Medial                Anterior                D                                    E

**Figure 31.23** Common sockets and suspensions for transtibial pediatric amputees. **A:** Patellar-tendon-bearing (PTB) socket is most useful for the mature patient. It gives the most freedom of motion, but the least secure suspension. **B:** The supracondylar suprapatellar (PTB-SCSP) design gives the most secure suspension and best knee control of any of the sockets that incorporate the suspension in the socket. **C:** The supracondylar (PTB-SC) socket eliminates the suprapatellar portion of the socket anteriorly, providing better range of motion but less control of hyperextension. **D:** The supracondylar cuff suspension is a common suspension used in the pediatric age range. **E:** The neoprene sleeve suspension provides very secure suspension for the very active amputee. This can also be used for the transfemoral amputee.

The faster a hydraulic or pneumatic unit is compressed, the faster the energy is released, and this helps to regulate the lower shank of the prosthesis. The prosthetic knee unit can be further subdivided into single axis and polycentric types.

The maturation of gait from infant to adult carries with it the need for sound practice in selecting the appropriate knee, on the basis of amputation level, functional level,

and body size. In general, the single-axis internal knee without any control unit is the first knee to be used on the child, because of its light weight, short lever arm, and simplicity. In the single-axis knee joint, the lower shank rotates around a single point in relation to the socket.

A polycentric knee was introduced in 1998 for the infant and toddler, and it may be used if space permits.

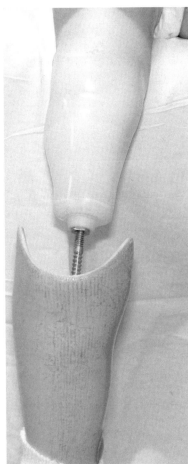

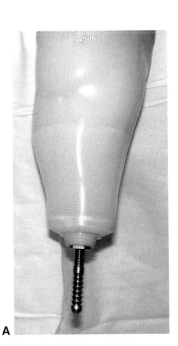

**Figure 31.24** Silicone suspension liners (Triple S socket) have become very popular. The soft silicone liner has a serrated pin incorporated into the bottom of the liner. The patient rolls the liner on the residual limb **(A)**, then inserts the limb into the prosthesis **(B)**. At the bottom of the prosthesis is a socket in which the pin locks. It is released by pushing the button on the medial side of the prosthesis.

Internal polycentric knees move around a center of rotation that varies with the flexion angle of the lower shank (168). The four-bar linkage knee is the most common polycentric knee and the most widely used by prosthetists (179) (Fig. 31.26). The inherent stability during stance, the fluid knee-flexion movement, and the mechanical design to give more ground clearance during flexion increase patient and practitioner confidence in the unit (180).

Changes in design and technology have now widened the boundaries and age distinctions for the prescribing of specific knees. Traditionally, an articulating knee would be introduced in a congenital amputee at approximately 3 to 4 years of age. This age was determined, in part, by the limitations in the size and function of the components. In the experience at the authors' center, as well as others, introduction of a prosthetic knee without a locking feature can be used as the first prosthesis when the child first pulls to stand. A recent report demonstrated the benefits of early fitting with articulated knees in children as young as 17 months. All children learned to walk with an articulated knee, despite their age differences (129).

As the child develops and grows, more sophisticated control systems (e.g., hydraulic knees) can be incorporated into the prosthesis. Most components carry specific weight guidelines, and many children reach these ranges well before adulthood. For example, an adult hydraulic polycentric knee is routinely used on 8-year-old boys whose weight has surpassed 100 lb. This does not mean that every child of a certain age and weight should have a particular knee. Placing a sophisticated knee and control system on an individual who has neither the hip range, muscle strength, nor residual limb length to activate the knee often results in contralateral hip and lower back pain as well as patient frustration.

## Prosthetic Feet

Variations in the materials, design, and alignment of the foot can have profound effects on the performance of the prosthesis. Functionally, prosthetic feet can be categorized into five main groups (181):

- Solid ankle cushion heel
- Single axis
- Multiaxis
- Elastic keel
- Dynamic response

The solid ankle cushion heel (SACH) foot [Therapeutic Recreation Systems, Inc. (TRS)] contains no articulating parts, and foot motion depends on the various compressive properties of the materials used between heel-strike and

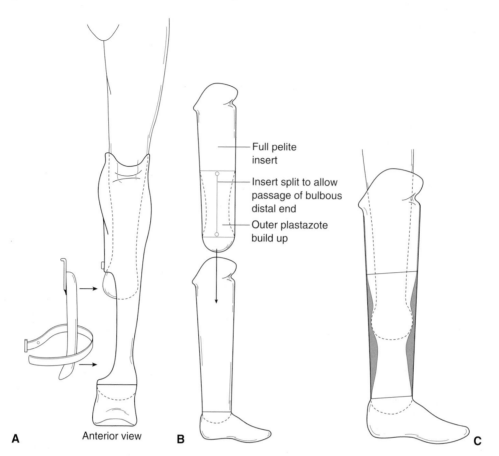

**Figure 31.25**   Common socket designs for Syme amputation prosthesis. **A:** Obturator design is often needed if the distal end of the residual limb is large and bulbous or the medial malleolus is prominent. It is the least cosmetic. **B:** The removable or segmented liner consists of a complete separate foam liner, which has a split in the side to allow the distal end of the limb to pass. Once the patient applies the liner, he or she slides the limb covered by the liner into the prosthesis. The patient must have the manual dexterity and strength to use this suspension, which will eliminate some patients with hand anomalies from using it. Limbs with a small heel do best with this system. **C:** The bladder design has a built-up silicone sleeve, which the patient slides the limb past. This socket fits more loosely, and does not stabilize the heel pad as well as the other designs.

toe-off (Fig. 31.27A). It is generally considered when amputees require maximum late-stance stability because of weak knee extensors, knee-flexion contractures, or poor mid- to late-stance balance (182). The SACH foot is used in pediatrics when the foot size is below 12 cm. The Little Feet is a bolt on type SACH foot designed with unique energy dynamics (Fig. 31.27B). The toes are very flexible because of the use of an elastomer that more closely mimics the child's foot. A special removable heel core allows the foot to be used "barefoot."

The single-axis foot usually contains rubber bumpers that allow passive dorsi- and plantar flexion. By changing the hardness of the bumper, the prosthetist is able to effectively change the properties of the foot. The single-axis foot does not come in a size suitable for the child amputee. This foot is best suited for the transfemoral amputee, in whom full-foot contact with the ground is necessary to increase stability. The multiaxis foot allows passive dorsi- and plantar flexion, inversion, and eversion. The multiaxis foot was once thought best suited for the amputee who because of

uneven terrain or a lifestyle that includes golfing or various sports requires flexibility and some rotational control: It has now found its way into the pediatric population. The multiaxial foot (College Park Truper foot) (Fig. 31.27C) allows controlled resistance in all planes—inversion/eversion, dorsiflexion and plantar flexion, and transverse rotation about the ankle joint. This class of foot has gained wide acceptance within the pediatric arena, in part because of its ability to absorb forces at the ankle and reduce transmission of these forces to the socket. This is particularly useful when fitting a very short residual limb.

Once the child's activity level warrants a higher-functioning foot, the prosthetist can move the child into a dynamic-response foot. This group of feet is distinguished by a spring mechanism in the keel that deflects during gait (Fig. 31.27D). The dynamic-response foot has found its way into competitive-level sports as well as day-to-day activities. Although the variety of componentry for children is still much less than for adults, there is a wide variety of feet with different performance characteristics available. It is important to use

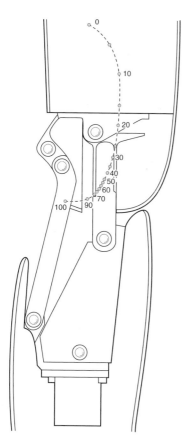

**Figure 31.26** Four-bar linkage is an internal polycentric knee that provides many advantages to the patient, including increased stability and better ground clearance during swing phase. As indicated in this illustration, the point of rotation varies with the degree of flexion. With the knee flexed, the leg folds under the thigh segment, and therefore is very useful for longer residual limbs. There is also a hydraulic version of the four-bar-linkage for children.

components that will maximize performance, and at the same time be appropriate for the patient (183).

At slower walking velocities, there is little difference between the dynamic-response foot and the SACH foot (184). Generally, children are not fitted with the highest-performance dynamic-response feet, because of constant growth and weight changes and the high costs associated with foot replacement. The involvement in competitive sports is usually a good benchmark to initiate fitting adolescents with the highest-performance dynamic-response feet.

In the transfemoral amputee, it is crucial to properly choose a foot that will enhance gait, but also to choose the complementary knee that will aid in controlling the foot during all aspects of the gait cycle. A common mistake is to prescribe a dynamic-response foot with a simple, friction-controlled knee that is incapable of preventing uncontrolled heel rise. The same is true of the transtibial amputee, who lacks the muscle strength to control the foot, often resulting in premature muscle fatigue. In the selection of multiple components, the prosthetist must marry the characteristics of all components, so that maximum benefit can be available to the amputee.

## Partial-Foot Prosthesis

The most important consideration in the fitting of the partial-foot amputee is to ensure that adequate load-bearing is designed into the prosthesis of choice. As a general rule, the more proximal the level of amputation, the higher the prosthesis must fit over the ankle complex and the more proximally it must fit on the tibia and fibula. Tissue condition, function of the remaining foot complex, and activity of the child all play a role in determining the prescription and design of the prosthesis.

Complete or partial absence of the toes usually requires little more than a shoe filler. A carbon fiber insert to better control forces from heel to toe-off may be incorporated in the shoe filler. In the case of the very young child, no intervention may be required until a need has been demonstrated, for example, the inability to keep the shoe on, especially when the child becomes more active in sports.

The prosthesis most commonly used for the moderate/short partial-foot amputee is the Lange silicone partial-foot prosthesis (Fig. 31.28). This incorporates a cosmetic foot shell, silicone-laminated socket with modified foot sole, and a posterior zipper for ease of donning and doffing. The prosthesis is fabricated over a modified model of the patient's partial foot. The socket trim line is proximal to the malleoli, and is fitted intimately to ensure adequate control. The design of a partial-foot prosthesis may also include a removable insert, to accommodate the need for corrective alignment of the residual foot. The prosthesis is then cosmetically finished to resemble the contralateral limb. Overall, this type of prosthesis is perfectly suited for the child amputee, and resists premature wear and tear. If needed, a partial-foot prosthesis should be prescribed once the child is pulling to furniture, so that foot control will begin at an early age. It should be noted that a low-profile insert (distal to the malleoli), used in conjunction with a high-top boot, will offer adequate function and cosmesis until a lower-cut shoe is requested by the parent.

The Chopart, or midtarsal, amputation is rarely used except in special instances (185). In the Chopart partial-foot amputation level, the prosthesis is modified to encompass the calcaneus and talus, and this results in a prosthesis that is often longer than the contralateral limb. The prosthesis must encompass the ankle joint, and it often rises proximally to the patellar tendon in an effort to reduce forces on the tibial crest-socket interface. Selection of prosthetic feet is compromised because of the lack of space distally, and commercially available carbon foot plates require permanent attachment with vulcanizing rubber cement. This negates any changes caused by growth, and realignment to compensate for gait changes is virtually impossible.

## Terminal Devices for the Upper Extremity

The choices left open to the prosthetist are numerous and, at times, controversial. Where some clinics maintain rigid protocols for terminal device selection, other clinics rely more on patient and parent input, combined with historic

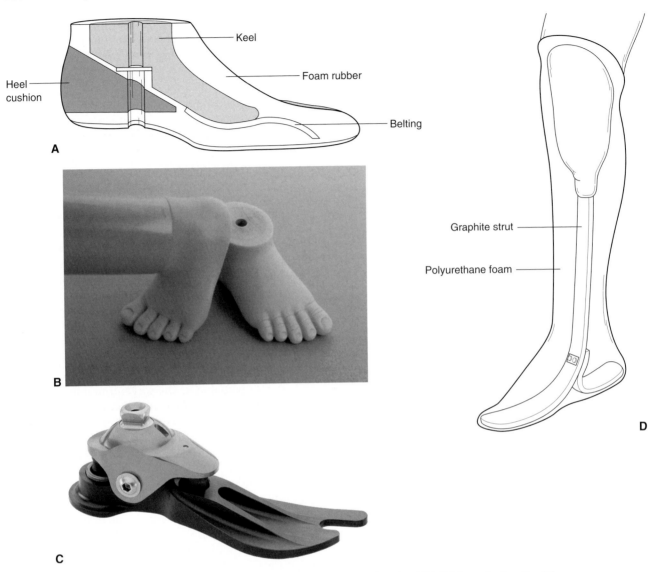

**Figure 31.27** **A:** In the conventional style solid ankle cushion heel (SACH) foot, the length of the keel controls the toe lever arm, and therefore the hyperextension moment at the knee, while the compression of the material at the heel absorbs the forces at heel strike. **B:** The Little Feet type design incorporates unique energy dynamics with flexible toes all in sizes beginning at 10 cm length. The length of the keel controls the toe lever arm and thus the hyperextension moment at the knee, and the compression of the elastomer heel absorbs and deflects the forces at heel strike. **C:** The dynamic multiaxial TruPer foot allows rotation, inversion and eversion, flexion, and extension movements. The outer cosmetic shell can be exchanged for larger shells as the child grows. **D:** The Flex-foot is a dynamic-response foot with much different performance characteristics than the SACH foot or multiaxial foot. It is used for the older, stronger, and physically active child who has the physical ability to use such a foot.

success rates for device types. Clinics that maintain very high caseloads for myoelectric devices, for example, will most likely have far more experience in fitting externally powered prostheses, compared to a clinic that may only see a handful of potential myoelectric candidates.

In simple terms, the terminal devices can be divided into hands and hooks, and they can be body-powered (cable and harness) or externally powered (electric). Hands and hooks can be either voluntary opening or voluntary closing. Patton lists the functional and prescription criteria for the various terminal devices (166).

The initial fitting of a child with upper-extremity limb deficiency begins at 4 months of age in a passive prosthesis with a stylized passive hand. There are several hands manufactured for this age range (Fig. 31.29A). This allows for equal arm lengths for the development of propping up on the amputated side and greater acceptance by the parents. Following initial sitting balance, the clenched-fist terminal device is exchanged for a small infant passive hand. When the infant begins to reach out (at approximately 15 to 18 months of age), the clinic team begins to assess the need for either body-powered or externally powered prostheses. If

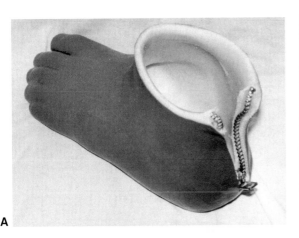
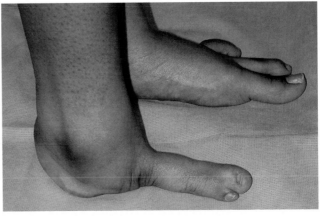

**Figure 31.28** **A:** The Lange silicone partial-foot prosthesis is a custom-made prosthesis that can incorporate a keel to aid in foot stability and push-off in gait. **B:** It is useful for children with partial amputations of the foot or congenital longitudinal deficiencies of the foot, shown here. It is not useful in feet with insufficient length, for example, those with the Chopart amputation.

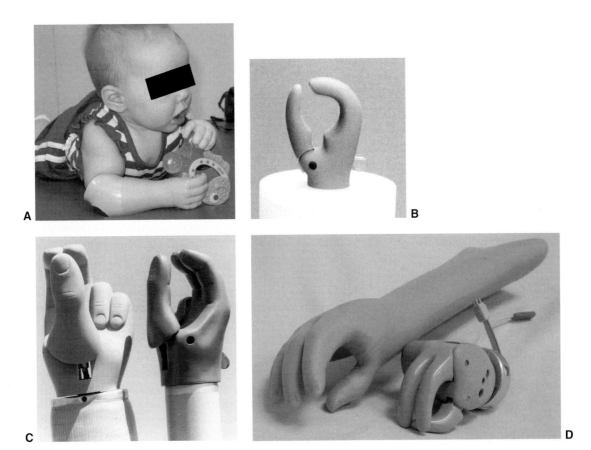

**Figure 31.29** **A:** The TRS ALPHA Infant Hand is an option for the first prosthetic hand offering age-appropriate fine motor activities. This would commonly be fitted between 4 and 6 months of age. The hand incorporates a flexible thumb that allows objects to be placed for simple grasp and release functions. **B:** The ADEPT is a voluntary closing body-powered hook that is fitted at approximately 15 months of age, if the child is ready and a body-powered device is desired. **C:** The Lite-Touch is a voluntary closing hand that would find the same indications as the ADEPT hook. It looks a bit more like a hand, which often makes this option popular with parents. **D:** The Variety Village hand is one of the most commonly used myoelectric hands in the pediatric age group. The Otto Bock Electrohand is shown in Figure 31.19. Both of these electric hands are covered with a cosmetic glove.

body-powered prosthesis is recommended, a cable-operated Hosmer 12P plastic-covered hook (Fig. 31.29B) or an ADEPT infant hand (Fig. 31.29C) will be prescribed. The canted design of the 12P hook allows for greater visual feedback to the wearer. In the event that a myoelectric device is warranted, the Variety Village 0-3 (VV 0-3) electric hand (Fig. 31.29D) or the Otto Bock Electrohand (Fig. 31.19) is used. In the pediatric VV 0-3 hand, the thumb and opposing two fingers operate to form a three-point chuck grip. In the Otto Bock 2000 hand, the same principle is applied, except that from the open to closed position, the thumb sweeps from a lateral position to meet the two opposing fingers upon close.

Progression from this starting point through the various component sizes and versions allows for a relatively smooth transition into adulthood. Prescription criteria are reviewed during each clinic visit, and changes are made on the basis of the child's changing needs. In today's environment of active children and sports activities, the use of sports or other adaptive terminal devices is essential for the amputee. TRS has developed numerous devices for use in sports and recreational activities. These can be interchanged on the prosthesis, so that only one socket is required.

## Endoskeletal versus Exoskeletal Construction

The structure or construction of a prosthesis is referred to as an endoskeletal (internal structure) or exoskeletal (external structure) prosthesis. Generally, transtibial, partial foot, and transradial prostheses are constructed exoskeletally, and transfemoral, knee disarticulation, hip disarticulation, transhumeral, and shoulder disarticulation levels of prostheses are constructed endoskeletally.

Exoskeletally finished prostheses are more durable and better suited to the growing child. There are various techniques and materials used in the construction of the exoskeletal prosthesis. Generally, following the completion of dynamic alignment, the ready-to-be-finished prosthesis is placed within a transfer jig that allows the socket to be separated from the foot, while maintaining alignment. A rigid polyurethane foam is added, and the prosthesis is cosmetically shaped to equal the sound limb. The structure is then laminated with acrylic resin forming the outer "shell." The advantages of this construction are its increased durability, and that it is easy to clean and structurally strong. The major disadvantages are the lack of further alignment capabilities, and that they are less cosmetically acceptable than some other types.

Endoskeletal design was initially used in the immediate postoperative period as a temporary method to initiate ambulation, while maintaining the ability to alter the alignment. This quickly became the norm for fitting in the adult population, and has been used primarily for knee disarticulation or transfemoral prosthesis. The prosthesis is modular and composed of a pylon (tube) and connecting

hardware, and it allows for quick changing of damaged components. In the event that realignment is necessary, the endoskeletal design incorporates alignment jigs within the attachment couplings, and only the cosmetic soft cover needs to be removed for adjustment. For these reasons, advanced components for use by children tend to be engineered for use in this system. The disadvantages of the endoskeletal system are lack of durability of the cosmetic cover, increased maintenance, and increased costs. This is outweighed by the increase in function and ease of adjusting length.

## ROLE OF THE PHYSICAL/ OCCUPATIONAL THERAPIST

The role of the physical/occupational therapist in the care of the limb-deficient child is mostly nontraditional. In addition to the traditional role, the physical/occupational therapist fills the roles of teacher, advocate, friend, and liaison (186). In some situations, all but the traditional role of therapist may be filled by a nurse. In some cases, the role may be shared. What is important is to recognize the need for all of these activities.

The first role of the therapist will usually be that of the educator. In this role, it is important that the therapist, physician, and prosthetist all be of one mind regarding the patient's treatment. First is the education of the parents. Like nurse-practitioners, the therapists will usually have more time and be better heard than the doctor when relaying information to the parents about their child. The therapist will be able to reinforce to the parents the options that have been discussed at the initial meeting with the physician. Most importantly, they can arrange for the family and child to meet others with similar deficiencies during routine sessions. Throughout the child's life, the experienced therapist can be of immense value to the child and young adult in anticipating problems and helping with solutions.

The therapist's first role as advocate will start with the first meeting with the parents. The importance in this role is to bring the parents to see the normal, as well as the abnormal, and to ensure that the initial bonding to the parents occurs. The therapist will frequently need to advocate for the patient to insurance companies and other agencies to help provide for the patient's needs. When the child starts into day care and then school, the therapist will assist in the child's transition into a new world by educating the teachers and the child's peers about the child's differences. This can be extremely important for the child's acceptance and socialization. Later, the same role may be necessary with physical education teachers and coaches to ensure that the child can participate in all the activities he or she is able to.

The therapist (or nurse) with these roles is the ideal liaison among the team members. This close teamwork can spare the child and parents countless visits to clinics and delays in treatment: a very important goal in avoiding the medicalization of a condition for which there is no cure, but only good management.

The traditional role of the therapist will be far more home/community based than hospital/office based, for many reasons. First, the child's condition will be permanent. This means adapting to the environment in which the child exists. None of the child's activities (toileting, eating, dressing, play, sports) will take place in the hospital or an office. Therefore, they should be learned in the normal environment. Second, the parents will be with the child, and are responsible for the child's development and learning. They will have unlimited access to the child for this "therapy." Finally, the child should not come to think of him- or herself as a medical problem, but rather as a child with a difference that can be successfully adapted to. Unnecessary hospital, clinic, or office visits are not a good way in which to communicate this goal of independence.

The traditional medical model does have a role in acute situations, as it does in many diseases or postsurgical situations. These are times when specific therapeutic exercises or the use of new prostheses must be performed, supervised, and taught. During the first months of life of a congenital amputee, the parents are seen by the therapist every 6 to 8 weeks. The child's development is monitored, and the parents are taught activities appropriate for the stage of development, for example, rolling over and coming to stand from sitting. These visits are used to monitor the parents' coping, to listen and answer questions, review treatment options, and arrange for the meeting with other parents and children.

Following surgical intervention and prosthetic fitting, the medical model is more appropriate, and the frequency of the visits increases briefly, while the child and parent are taught the use of the prosthesis. In addition to the usual goals of increasing or maintaining motion and strength following surgery, the therapist plays a critical role in edema control. This is very important if the patient is to resume prosthetic wear quickly. Teaching and supervising elastic wrapping and obtaining shrinkers are important postsurgical issues.

Older children need to be taught ways to become independent in donning and doffing the prosthesis, toileting, and other activities with the prosthesis. Fitting of a new prosthetic component, for example, a hydraulic knee joint, will usually require specific training to maximize the benefits of the new components.

As the child grows out of infancy, the therapist can be helpful in designing and modifying age-appropriate play activities, With the approach of school age, emphasis switches to independence in the activities of daily living, and later, to fine motor skills that may be needed for classroom activities. Adaptations for sports, for example, special terminal devices, if desired, or a swimming leg, are important, as is the advocacy role to allow the children to participate in all possible activities.

In adolescence the need for specific therapeutic interventions is usually minimal. The child has now become fully aware of his or her differences and their significance. The child will usually dictate the needs. Appearance being important, more cosmetic prostheses and improved gait become important issues.

At this time, driving becomes one of the major issues defining independence. The therapist can play a critical role in directing the child and parents to the appropriate agency for the rules of the state, and to a source for evaluation and modifications to the vehicle. As with any adolescent, the amputee should attend driver education training, using modifications if needed. Modifications can range from simple to complex. Switching the brake and gas pedals to accommodate unilateral lower-limb loss is one of the most common examples. Many amputees, even with bilateral lower-extremity loss, drive without adaptations. This must be closely monitored and evaluated by the state's examiners. Hand controls are used most commonly in bilateral lower-extremity loss. A ring adaptation can be used to modify the steering wheel for upper-extremity amputees. A handicap license is appropriate for individuals whose mobility is limited. The higher-level amputee, and those with multilevel limb loss, may benefit from a handicap parking license. All modifications are listed on the amputee's driver's license.

College is often the patient's first test of complete independence, and the needs may be greater than what the child anticipates. The therapist can be of great value in assessing the situation, counseling the patient, and helping with the transition. The Internet can prove to be a great resource in assisting college-bound students and their families.

## ADAPTATIONS FOR ACTIVITIES AND SPORTS

Children of all ages with limb deficiencies or amputations should be encouraged to participate in sports and recreational activities with their peers. The psychologic impact of sports cannot be underestimated. Improving self-esteem and confidence, gaining independence, learning to win and lose, developing decision-making and problem-solving skills, and cooperating as a team member are a few of the benefits that a child carries throughout his or her life. Improving physical fitness, developing balance, strength, coordination and motor skills, increasing endurance, and weight control are benefits of physical activity.

Over the years, there has been an increased awareness of adapted sports and recreation for individuals with physical and mental impairments. The Paralympic and Special Olympics initiatives have been the most obvious and have sparked an increase in availability of programs for special-needs children. Laws also have been passed for children to receive education in the least restrictive environments. PL 94-142 provides free and appropriate education for all children with disabilities (186). Physical therapy and recreation are related services included in this legislation. This allows for adapted physical education to be included in a child's everyday school activities. Physical therapists need to be aware of the resources and adaptations that provide accessibility of a sport to a child within limits of his/her physical abilities in the school and community settings. Gross motor achievements are a measure of a child's development. Learning to toss a ball, jump, run, hop, and ride a bicycle are activities included on standardized developmental screenings and tests. It is important that these activities be included in the child's plan of treatment, so that a child can be offered the same age-appropriate physical challenges as his or her peers.

Special adaptations and specific sports-related prostheses are available, depending on the degree and level of the disability. These adaptations are too numerous to mention. Recreational and sports-related terminal devices are available for the upper-extremity amputee (187,188). Adaptations can be as simple as raising the handlebars on a bicycle and adding a toe strap to highly sophisticated prosthetic components specific to each sport (189). Information and resources for sports and adaptive recreation for the amputee can be obtained through the Amputee Coalition of America (www.amputee-coalition.org; telephone 1-888-267-5669). The Association of Children's Prosthetic and Orthotics Clinics is an excellent resource for services in geographical regions (www.acpoc.org; telephone 847-698-1637).

# REFERENCES

1. McDonnell P. Developmental response to limb deficiency and limb replacement. *Can J Psychol* 1988;42:120.
2. Jones L, Lipson A. The care of the limb deficient child in Australia. *Prosthet Orthot Int* 1991;15:140.
3. Stewart CP, Jain AS. Congenital limb anomalies and amputees Tayside, Scotland 1965-1994. *Prosthet Orthot Int* 1995;19:148.
4. Rogala EJ, Wynne-Davies R, Littlejohn A, et al. Congenital limb anomalies: frequency and aetiological factors. *J Med Genet* 1974;11:221.
5. Froster UG, Baird PA. Congenital defects of lower limbs and associated malformations: a population base study. *Am J Med Genet* 1993;45:60.
6. Clark M, Atkins D, Hubbard S, et al. Prosthetic devices for children with bilateral upper limb deficiencies: when and if, pros and cons. In: Herring JA, Birch JG, eds. *The child with a limb deficiency*, Rosemont, IL: American Academy of Orthopaedic Surgeons, 1998:397.

## Classification

7. Frantz C, O'Rahilly R. Congenital skeletal limb deficiencies. *J Bone Joint Surg Am* 1961;43:1202.
8. Schuch CM. International standards organization terminology: application to prosthetics and orthotics. *J Prosthet Orthot* 1993;6:29.
9. Day HJB. The ISO/ISPO classification of congenital limb deficiency. In: Bowker JH, Michael JW, eds. *Atlas of limb prosthetics: surgical, prosthetic, and rehabilitation principles*, 2nd ed. St. Louis, MO: Mosby, 1992:743.

## Etiology

10. Bavinck JN, Weaver DD. Subclavian artery supply disruption sequence: hypothesis of a vascular etiology for Poland, Klippel-Feil, and Mobius anomalies. *Am J Med Genet* 1986;23:903.

11. Streeter GL. Focal deficiencies in fetal tissues and their relation to intrauterine amputation. *Contrib Embryol* 1930;22:1.
12. Glessner JR. Spontaneous intrauterine amputation. *J Bone Joint Surg Am* 1963;45:351.
13. Sadler TW. Embryology and gene regulation of limb development. In: Herring JA, Birch JG, eds. *The child with a limb deficiency*. Rosemont, IL: American Academy of Orthopaedic Surgeons, 1998:3.
14. Lovett M, Clines G, Wise CA. Genetic control of limb development. In: Herring JA, Birch JG, eds. *The child with a limb deficiency*. Rosemont, IL: American Academy of Orthopaedic Surgeons, 1998:13.
15. Weaver DD. Vascular etiology of limb defects: the subclavian artery supply disruption sequence. In: Herring JA, Birch JG, eds. *The child with a limb deficiency*. Rosemont, IL: American Academy of Orthopaedic Surgeons, 1998:25.
16. Skjaerven R, Wilcos AJ, Lie TR. A population-based study of survival and childbearing among female subjects with birth defects and the risk of recurrence in their children. *N Engl J Med* 1999;340:1057.

## The Child with an Amputation

17. Dunn NL, McCartan KW, Fuqua RW. Young children with orthopedic handicaps: self-knowledge about their disability. *Except Child* 1998;55:249.
18. Vaughn BE, Langolis JH. Physical attractiveness as a correlate of peer status and social competence in preschool children. *Dev Psychol* 1983;19:561.
19. Harper D, Wacker D, Cobb L. Children's social preferences toward peers with visible physical differences. *J Pediatr Psychol* 1986;11:323.
20. Richardson S. Age and sex differences in values toward physical handicaps. *J Health Soc Behav* 1970;11:207.
21. Richardson S. Handicap, appearance and stigma. *Soc Sci Med* 1971;5:621.
22. Varni J, Setoguchi Y, Rappaport L, et al. Effects of stress, social support, and self-esteem on depression in children with limb deficiencies. *Arch Phys Med Rehabil* 1991;72:1053.
23. Varni J, Setoguchi Y. Correlates of perceived physical appearance in children with congenital/acquired limb deficiencies. *J Dev Behav Pediatr* 1991;12:171.
24. Varni JW, Setoguchi Y. Effects of parental adjustment on the adaptation of children with congenital or acquired limb deficiencies. *J Dev Behav Pediatr* 1993;14:13.

## The Parents

25. Kerr SM, McIntosh JB. Coing whe a child has a disability: exploring the imnpact of parent-to parent support. *Child Care Health Dev* 2000;26:309.
26. Letts M, Vincent N. Congenital longitudinal deficiency of the fibula (fibular hemimelia). Parental refusal of amputation. *Clin Orthop* 1993;287:160.

## Organization of Care

27. Hubbard S, Heim W, Giavedoni B. Paediatric prosthetic management. *Curr Orthop* 1997;11:114.

## General Considerations

28. Amstutz HC The morphology, natural history, and treatment of proximal femoral focal deficiency. *A symposium on proximal femoral focal deficiency—a congenital anomaly*. Washington, DC: National Academy of Sciences, 1969:50.
29. Amstutz HC. Natural history and treatment of congenital absence of the fibula. *J Bone Joint Surg Am* 1972;54:1349.
30. Hamanishi C. Congenital short femur: clinical, genetic and epidemiological comparison of the naturally occurring condition with that caused by thalidomide. *J Bone Joint Surg Br* 1980;62:307.
31. Achterman C, Kalamchi A. Congenital deficiency of the fibula. *J Bone Joint Surg Br* 1979;61:133.
32. Westin GW, Sakai DN, Wood WL. Congenital longitudinal deficiency of the fibula: follow-up of treatment by Syme amputation. *J Bone Joint Surg Am* 1976;58:492.
33. Anderson M, Messner MB, Green WT. Distribution of lengths of the normal femur and tibia in children from one to eighteen years of age. *J Bone Joint Surg Am* 1964;46:1197.

34. Christie J, Lamb DW, McDonald JM, et al. A study of stump growth in children with below-knee amputations. *J Bone Joint Surg Br* 1979;61:464.

## Complications

35. Aitken GT. Overgrowth of the amputation stump. *Interclin Inform Bull* 1962;1:1.

36. Jorring K. Amputation in children: a follow-up of 74 children whose lower extremities were amputated. *Acta Orthop Scand* 1971;42:178.

37. Pellicore RJ, Lambert CN, Hamilton RC. Incidence of bone overgrowth in the juvenile amputee population. *Interclin Inform Bull* 1974;8:1.

38. Oneal ML, Bahner R, Ganey TM, et al. Osseous overgrowth after amputation in adoldescnets and children. *J Pediatr Orthop* 1996;16:78.

39. Aitken GT. Surgical amputation in children. *J Bone Joint Surg Am* 1963;45:1735.

40. Speer DP. The pathogenesis of amputation stump overgrowth. *Clin Orthop* 1981;159:294.

41. Abraham E. Operative treatment of bone overgrowth in children who have an acquired or congenital amputation [letter; comment]. *J Bone Joint Surg Am* 1996;78:1287.

42. Davids JR, Meyer LC, Blackhurst DW. Operative treatment of bone overgrowth in children who have an acquired or congenital amputation [see comments]. *J Bone Joint Surg Am* 1995;77:1490.

43. Tenholder M, Davids JR, Gruber HE, et al. Surgical management of juvenile amputation overgrowth with a synthetic cap. *J Pediatr Orthop B* 2004;24:218.

44. Benevina J, Makley JT, Leeson MC, et al. Primary epiphyseal transplants and bone overgrowth in childhood amputations. *J Pediatr Orthop* 1992;12:467.

45. Bernd L, Blasius K, Lukoschek M, et al. The autologous stump plasty: treatment for bony overgrowth in the juvenile amputees. *J Bone Joint Surg Br* 1991;73:203.

46. Watts HG. Lengthening of short residual limbs in children. In: Herring JA, Birch JG, eds. *The child with a limb deficiency*. Rosemont, IL: American Academy of Orthopaedic Surgeons, 1998:397.

47. Alekberov C, Karatosun V, Baran O, et al. Lenghtening of congenital below-elbow amputation stumps by the Ilizarov technique. *J Bone Joint Surg Br* 2000;82:239.

48. Tooms R. Acquired amputations in children. In: Bowker J, Michael J, eds. *Atlas of limb prosthetics: surgical, prosthetic, and rehabilitation principles*, St. Louis, MO: Mosby, 1992:738.

49. Wilkins K, McGrath P, Finley G, et al. Phantom limb sensations and phantom limb pain in child and adolescent amputees. *Pain* 1998;78:7.

50. Melzack R, Israel R, Lacroix R, et al. Phantom limbs in people with congenital limb deficiency or amputation in early childhood. *Brain* 1997;120:1603.

51. Lindesay J. Multiple pain complaints in amputees. *J R Soc Med* 1985;78:452.

52. Davis RW. Phantom sensation, phantom pain and stump pain. *Arch Phys Med Rehabil* 1993;74:79.

53. Sherman RA. A survey of current phantom limb treatments in the United States. *Pain* 1980;8:85.

54. Carabelli R, Kellerman WC. Phantom pain: relief by application of TENS to the contralateral extremity. *Arch Phys Med Rehabil* 1985;66:466.

## Congenital Deficiencies of the Lower Extremity

55. Choi IH, Kumar SJ, Bowen JR. Amputation or limb-lengthening for partial or total absence of the fibula. *J Bone Joint Surg Am* 1990;72:1391.

56. Coventry MB, Johnson EWJ. Congenital absence of the fibula. *J Bone Joint Surg Am* 1952;34:941.

57. Pappas AM. Congenital abnormalities of the femur and related lower extremity malformations: classification and treatment. *J Pediatr Orthop* 1983;3:45.

58. Maffulli N, Fixsen JA. Fibular hypoplasia with absent lateral rays of the foot. *J Bone Joint Surg Br* 1991;73:1002.

59. Maffulli N, Fixsen JA. Management of forme fruste fibular hemimelia. *J Pediatr Orthop B* 1996;5:17.

60. Birch JG, Lincoln TL, Mack PW. Functional classification of fibular deficiency. In: Herring JA, Birch JG, eds. *The child with a limb deficiency*. Rosemont, IL: American Academy of Orthopaedic Surgeons, 1998:161.

61. Bohne WH, Root L. Hypoplasia of the fibula. *Clin Orthop* 1977;125:107.

62. Kalamchi A. *Congenital lower limb deficiencies*. New York: Springer-Verlag, 1989.

63. Torode IP, Gillespie R. Anteroposterior instability of the knee: a sign of congenital limb deficiency. *J Pediatr Orthop* 1983;3:467.

64. Boakes JL, Stevens PM, Moseley RF. Treatment of genu valgus deformity in congenital absence of the fibula. *J Pediatr Orthop* 1991;11:721.

65. Herring JA, Barnhill B, Gaffney C. Symes amputation; an evaluation of the physical and psychological function in young patients. *J Bone Joint Surg Am* 1986;68:573.

66. Davidson WH, Bohne WH. The Syme amputation in children. *J Bone Joint Surg Am* 1975;57:905.

67. Pappas AM, Miller JT. Congenital ball-and-socket ankle joints and related lower-extremity malformations. *J Bone Joint Surg Am* 1982;64:672.

68. Takakura Y, Tamai S, Masuhara K. Genesis of the ball-and-socket ankle. *J Bone Joint Surg Br* 1986;68:834.

69. Grogan DP, Holt GR, Ogden JA. Talocalcaneal coalition in patients who have fibular hemimelia or proximal femoral focal deficiency. A comparison of the radiographic and pathological findings. *J Bone Joint Surg Am* 1994;76:1363.

70. Thompson TC, Straub LR, Arnold WD. Congenital absence of the fibula. *J Bone Joint Surg Am* 1957;39:1229.

71. Farmer AW, Laurin CA. Congenital absence of the fibula. *J Bone Joint Surg Am* 1960;42:1.

72. Kruger LM, Talbot RD. Amputation and prosthesis as definitive treatment in congenital absence of the fibular. *J Bone Joint Surg Am* 1961;43:625.

73. Wood WL, Zlotsky N, Westin GW. Congenital absence of the fibula: treatment by Syme amputation—indications and technique. *J Bone Joint Surg Am* 1965;47:1159.

74. Hootnick D, Boyd NA, Fixsen JA, et al. The natural history and management of congenital short tibia with dysplasia or absence of the fibula. *J Bone Joint Surg Br* 1977;59:267.

75. Miller LS, Bell DF. Management of congenital fibular deficiency by Ilizarov technique. *J Pediatr Orthop* 1992;12:651.

76. Stanitski DF, Shahcheraghi H, Nicker DA, et al. Results of tibial lengthening with the Ilizarov technique. *J Pediatr Orthop* 1996;16:168.

77. Catagni MA, Guerreschi F. Management of fibular hemimelia using the Ilizarov method. In: Herring JA, Birch JG, eds. *The child with a limb deficiency*. Rosemont, IL: American Academy of Orthopaedic Surgeons, 1998:179.

78. Catagni MA. Management of fibular hemimelia using the Ilizarov method. *Instr Course Lect* 1992;41:431.

79. Gibbons PJ, Bradish CF. Fibular hemimelia: a preliminary report on management of the severe abnormality. *J Pediatr Orthop B* 1996;5:20.

80. Ghoneem HG, Wright JG, Cole WG, et al. The Ilizarov method for correction of complex deformities: psychological and functional outcomes. *J Bone Joint Surg Am* 1996;78:1480.

81. Price CT. Editorial: are we there yet? Management of limb-length inequality. *J Pediatr Orthop* 1996;16:141.

82. Naudie D, Hamdy RC, Fassier F, et al. Management of fibular hemimelia: amputation or limb lengthening [see comments]. *J Bone Joint Surg Br* 1997;79:58.

83. Correll J. Management of fibular hemimelia [letter; comment]. *J Bone Joint Surg Br* 1997;79:1040.

84. McCarthy JJ, Glancy GL, Chang FM, et al. Fibular hemimelia; comarison of outcome measurements after amputation and lengthening. *J Bone Joint Surg Am* 2000;82:1732.

85. Herring JA. Symes amputation for fibular hemimelia: a second look in the Ilizarov era. *Instr Course Lect* 1992;41:435.

86. Birch JG, Walsh SJ, Small JM, et al. Syme amputation for the treatment of fibular deficiency. *J Bone Joint Surg Am* 1999;81:1511.

87. Syme J. Amputation at the ankle joint. *Lond Edinb Monthly J Med Sci* 1843;3:93.

88. Anderson L, Westin GW, Oppenheim WL. Syme amputation in children: indications, results, and long-term follow-up. *J Pediatr Orthop* 1984;4:550.

89. Eilert RE, Jayakumar SS. Boyd and Syme ankle amputations in children. *J Bone Joint Surg Am* 1976;58:1139.

90. Fergusson CM, Morrison JD, Kenwright J. Leg-length inequality in children treated by Syme's amputation. *J Bone Joint Surg Br* 1987;69:433.

91. Mazet R Jr. Syme's amputation. A follow-up study of fifty-one adults and thirty-two children. *J Bone Joint Surg Am* 1968;50:1549.

92. Gaine WJ, McCreath SW. Syme's amputation revisited: a review of 46 cases. *J Bone Joint Surg Br* 1996;78:461.

93. Green WB, Cary JM. Partial foot amputations in children. *J Bone Joint Surg Am* 1982;64:438.

94. Boyd HB. Amputation of the foot with calcaneotibial arthrodesis. *J Bone Joint Surg* 1939;21:997.

95. Serafin J. A new operation for congenital absence of the fibula: preliminary report. *J Bone Joint Surg Br* 1967;49:59.

96. Thomas IH, Williams PF. The Gruca operation for congenital absence of the fibula. *J Bone Joint Surg Br* 1987;69:587.

97. Turker R, Mendelson S, Ackman J, et al. Anatomic considerations of the foot and leg in tibial hemimelia. *J Pediatr Orthop* 1996;16:445.

98. Williams L, Wientroub S, Getty CJM, et al. Tibial dysplasia. A study of the anatomy. *J Bone Joint Surg Br* 1983;65:157.

99. Kalamchi A, Dawe RV. Congenital deficiency of the tibia. *J Bone Joint Surg Br* 1985;67:581.

100. Grissom LE, Harcke HT, Kumar SJ. Sonography in the management of tibial hemimelia. *Clin Orthop* 1990;251:266.

101. Kumar A, Kruger LM. Fibular dimelia with deficiency of the tibia. *J Pediatr Orthop* 1993;13:203.

102. Loder RT, Herring JA. Fibular transfer for congenital absence of the tibia: a reassessment. *J Pediatr Orthop* 1987;7:8.

103. Schoenecker PL, Capelli AM, Millar EA, et al. Congenital longitudinal deficiency of the tibia. *J Bone Joint Surg Am* 1989;71:278.

104. Aitken GW. Tibial hemimelia. In: Aitken GW, ed. *Selected lower limb anomalies: surgical and prosthetic management.* Washington, DC: National Academy of Sciences, 1971:1.

105. Schoenecker PL. Tibial deficiency. In: Herring JA, Birch JG, eds. *The child with a limb deficiency.* Rosemont, IL: American Academy of Orthopaedic Surgeons, 1998:209.

106. Setoguchi Y. Medical conditions associated with congenital limb deficiencies. In: Herring JA, Birch JG, eds. *The child with a limb deficiency.* Rosemont, IL: American Academy of Orthopaedic Surgeons, 1998:51.

107. Clark MW. Autosomal dominant inheritance of tibial meromelia. Report of a kindred. *J Bone Joint Surg Am* 1975;57:262.

108. Wilson GN. Heritable limb deficiencies. In: Herring JA, Birch JG, eds. *The child with a limb deficiency.* Rosemont, IL: American Academy of Orthopaedic Surgeons, 1998:39.

109. Goldberg MJ. *The dysmorphic child: an orthopaedic perspective.* New York: Raven Press, 1987.

110. Meyers TH. Congenital absence of the tibia: transplantation of head of fibula: arthrodesis at the ankle joint. *Am J Orthop Surg* 1910;3:72.

111. Sulamaa M, Ryoppy S. Congenital absence of the tibia. *Acta Orthop Scand* 1963;33:262.

112. Brown FW. Construction of a knee joint in congenital total absence of the tibia (paraxial hemimelia tibia). *J Bone Joint Surg Am* 1965;47:695.

113. Christini D, Levy EJ, Facanha FA, et al. Fibular transfer for congenital absence of the tibia. *J Pediatr Orthop* 1993;13:378.

114. Epps CH Jr, Tooms RE, Edholm CD, et al. Failure of centralization of the fibula for congenital longitudinal deficiency of the tibia. *J Bone Joint Surg Am* 1991;73:858.

115. Simmons ED Jr, Ginsburg GM, Hall JE. Brown's procedure for congenital absence of the tibia revisited. *J Pediatr Orthop* 1996;16:85.

116. Wehbe MA, Weinstein SL, Ponseti IV. Tibial agenesis. *J Pediatr Orthop* 1981;1:395.

117. Jayakumar SS, Eilert RE. Fibular transfer for congenital absence of the tibia. *Clin Orthop Relat Res* 1979;139:97.

118. Loder RT. Fibular transfer for congenital absence of the tibia (Brown procedure). In: Herring JA, Birch JG, eds. *The child with a limb deficiency.* Rosemont, IL: American Academy of Orthopaedic Surgeons, 1998:223.

119. Jayakumar SS, Eilert RE. Fibular transfer for congenital absence of the tibia. *Clin Orthop* 1979;139:97.

120. Jones D, Barnes J, Lloyd-Roberts GC. Congenital aplasia and dysplasia of the tibia with intact fibula. Classification and management. *J Bone Joint Surg Br* 1978;60:31.

121. Fernandez-Palazzi F, Bendahan J, Rivas S. Congenital deficiency of the tibia: a report on 22 cases [in process citation]. *J Pediatr Orthop B* 1998;7:298.

122. Garbarino JL, Clancy M, Harcke HT, et al. Congenital diastasis of the inferior tibiofibular joint: a review of the literature and report of two cases. *J Pediatr Orthop* 1985;5:225.

123. Pattinson RC, Fixsen JA. Management and outcome in tibial dysplasia [see comments]. *J Bone Joint Surg Br* 1992;74:893.

124. Bose K. Congenital diastasis of the inferior tibiofibular joint. *J Bone Joint Surg Am* 1976;58:886.

125. Tuli SM, Varma BP. Congenital diastasis of the tibiofibular mortise. *J Bone Joint Surg Br* 1972;54:346.

126. Tokmakova K, Riddle EC, Jay Kumar S. Type IV congenital deficiency of the tibia. *J Pediatr Orthop* 2003;23:649.

127. Sedgwick WG, Schoenecker PL. Congenital diastasis of the ankle joint. *J Bone Joint Surg Am* 1982;64:450.

128. Giavedoni B, O'Berry C. An early leg up. *Orthokinetic Rev* 2003;3:32.

129. Wilk B, Karol L, Halliday S. Characterizing gait in young children with a prosthetic knee joint. *Phys Ther Products* 1999;10:20.

130. Aitken GT. Proximal femoral deficiency. *A symposium on proximal femoral focal deficiency—a congenital anomaly.* Washington, DC: National Academy of Sciences, 1969:1.

131. Gillespie R, Torode IP. Classification and management of congenital abnormalities of the femur. *J Bone Joint Surg Br* 1983;65:557.

132. Gillespie R. Classification of congenital abnormalities of the femur. In: Herring JA, Birch JG, eds. *The child with a limb deficiency.* Rosemont, IL: American Academy of Orthopaedic Surgeons, 1998:63.

133. Kalamchi A, Cowell HR, Kim KI. Congenital deficiency of the femur. *J Pediatr Orthop* 1985;5:129.

134. Fixsen JA, Lloyd-Roberts GC. The natural history and early treatment of proximal femoral focal dysplasia. *J Bone Joint Surg Br* 1974;56:86.

135. Wolfgang GL. Complex congenital anomalies of the lower extremities: femoral bifurcation, tibial hemimelia, and diastasis of the ankle. Case report and review of the literature. *J Bone Joint Surg Am* 1984;66:453.

136. Bevan-Thomas WH, Millar EA. A review of proximal focal deficiencies. *J Bone Joint Surg Am* 1967;49:1376–1388.

137. Epps CH Jr. Proximal femoral focal deficiency. *J Bone Joint Surg Am* 1983;65:867.

138. Borggreve J. Kniegelenksersatz durch das in der Beinlangsachse urn 1800 gedrehtd Fussgelenk. *Arch Orthop Unfall Chir* 1930;28:175.

139. van Nes CP. Rotation-plasty for congenital defects of the femur: making use of the ankle of the shortened limb to control the knee joint of a prosthesis. *J Bone Joint Surg Br* 1950;32:12.

140. Kostuik JP, Gillespie R, Hall JE, et al. Van Nes rotational osteotomy for treatment of proximal femoral focal deficiency and congenital short femur. *J Bone Joint Surg Am* 1975;57:1039.

141. Torode IP, Gillespie R. Rotationplasty of the lower limb for congenital defect of the femur. *J Bone Joint Surg Br* 1983;65:569.

142. Friscia DA, Moseley CF, Oppenheim WL. Rotational osteotomy for proximal femoral focal deficiency. *J Bone Joint Surg Am* 1989;71:1386.

143. Alman BA, Krajbich JI, Hubbard S. Proximal femoral focal deficiency: results of rotationplasy and Syme amputation. *J Bone Joint Surg Am* 1995;77:1876.

144. Veenstra KM, Sprangers MAG, van der Eyen JW, et al. Quality of life in survivors with a van Ness-Borggreve rotationplasty after bone tumour resection. *J Surg Oncol* 2000;73:192.

145. Rodl RW, Pohlmann U, Gosheer G, et al. Rotationplasty: quality of life after 10 years in 22 patients. *Acta Orthop Scand* 2002;73:85.

146. Hillmann A, Hoffmann C, Gosheger G, et al. Malignant tumor of the distal part of the femur of the proximal part of the tibia: endoprosthetic replacement of rotationplasry. *J Bone Joint Surg Am* 1999;81:462.

147. Murray PM, Jacobs PA, Gore DR, et al. Functional performance after tibial rotationplasry. *J Bone Joint Surg Am* 1985;67:392.

148. Steenhoff RM, Daanen HAM, Taminiau HM. Functional analysis of patients who have had a modified van Nes Rotationplasry. *J Bone Joint Surg Am* 1993;75:1451.

149. Fowler E, Zernicke R, Setoguchi Y, et at. Energy expenditure during walking by children who have proximal femoral focal deficiency. *J Bone Joint Surg Am* 1996;78:1857.

150. Westin GW, Gunderson FO. Proximal femoral focal deficiency—a review of treatment experiences. In: Aitken GT, ed. *Proximal femoral focal deficiency. A congenital anomaly.* Washington, DC: American Academy of Sciences, 1969:100.

151. Koman LA, Meyer LC, Warren FH. Proximal femoral focal deficiency: a 50-year experience. *Dev Med Child Neurol* 1982;24:344.

152. Goddard NJ, Hashemi-Nejad A, Fixsen JA. Natural history and treatment of instability of the hip in proximal femoral focal deficiency. *J Pediatr Orthop B* 1995;4:145.

153. Panting AL, Williams PF. Proximal femoral focal deficiency. *J Bone Joint Surg Br* 1978;60:46.

154. Tonnis D, Stanitski DF. Early conservative and operative treatment to gain early normal growth in proximal femoral focal deficiency. *J Pediatr Orthop B* 1997;6:59.

155. Steel HH. Iliofemoral fusion for proximal femoral focal deficiency. In: Herring JA, Birch JG, eds. *The child with a limb deficiency.* Rosemont, IL: American Academy of Orthopaedic Surgeons,1998:99.

156. Brown KL. Resection, rotationplasty, and femoropelvic arthrodesis in severe congenital femoral deficiency. A report of the surgical technique and three cases. *J Bone Joint Surg Am* 2001;83:78; Steel HH. Iliofemoral fusion for proximal femoral focal deficiency. In: Herring JA, Birch JG, eds. *The child with a limb deficiency.* Rosemont, IL: American Academy of Orthopaedic Surgeons, 1998:99.

157. McCollough NC. Non-standard prosthetic applications for juvenile amputees. *Interclin Inform Bull* 1963;2:7.

158. Kruger L. Lower limb deficiencies/surgical management. In: Bowker JH, Michael JW, eds. *Atlas of limb prosthetics: surgical, prosthetic, and rehabilitation principles.* St. Louis, MO: Mosby, 1992:759.

159. Bochmann D. Prostheses for the limb-deficient child. In: Kostuik J, Gillespie R, eds. *Amputation surgery and rehabilitation: the Toronto experience.* New York: Churchill Livingstone, 1981:293.

## Congenital Deficiencies of the Upper Extremity

160. Marquardt E. The multiple limb deficient child. In: Bowker JH, Michael JW, eds. *Atlas of limb prosthetics: surgical, prosthetic, and rehabilitation principles.* St Louis, MO: Mosby, 1992:839.

161. Scotland T, Galway H. A long-term review of children with congenital and acquired upper limb deficiency. *J Bone Joint Surg Br* 1983;65:346.

162. Brooks M, Shaperman J. Infant prosthetic fitting: a study of results. *Am J Occup Ther* 1965;19:329.

163. Sorbye R. Upper extremity amputees: Swedish experiences concerning children. In: Atkins DJ, Meier RHI, eds. *Comprehensive management of the upper-limb amputee,* Berlin: Springer-Verlag, 1989:235.

164. Hubbard SA, Kurtz I, Heim W. Powered prosthetic intervention in upper extremity deficiency. In: Herring JA, Birch JG, eds. *The child with a limb deficiency,* Rosemont, IL: American Academy of Orthopaedic Surgeons, 1998:426.

165. Patton JG. Developmental approach to pediatric prosthetic evaluation and training. In: Atkins DJ, Meier RHI, eds. *Comprehensive management of the upper limb amputee,* Berlin: Springer-Verlag, 1991:137.

166. Patton JG. Upper-limb prosthetic components for children and teenagers. In: Atkins DJ, Meier RHI, eds. *Comprehensive management of the upper limb amputee.* Berlin: Springer-Verlag, 1991:99.

167. Muilenburg A, LeBlanc M. Body-powered upper-limb components. In: Atkins K, Meier RHI, eds. *Comprehensive management of the upper-limb amputee,* Berlin: Springer-Verlag, 1988:28.

168. Scott RN. Biomedical engineering in upper-limb prosthetics. In: Atkins DJ, Meier RHI, eds. *Comprehensive management of the upper-limb amputee,* Berlin: Springer-Verlag, 1988:173.

## Acquired Deficiencies

169. Letts M, Davidson D. Epidemiology and prevention of traumatic amputations in children. In: Herring JA, Birch JG, eds. *The child with a limb deficiency.* Rosemont, IL: American Academy of Orthopaedic Surgeons, 1989:235.

170. Trautwein LC, Smith DG, Rivara FP. Pediatric amputation injuries: etiology, cost, and outcome. *J Trauma* 1996;41:831.

## Prosthetics

171. Quigley MJ. Prosthetic management: overview, methods, and materials. In: Bowker JH, Michael JW, eds. *Atlas of limb prosthetics: surgical, prosthetic, and rehabilitation principles.* St. Louis, MO: Mosby, 1992:67.

172. Steele A. A survey of clinical CAD/CAM use. *J Prosthet Orthot* 1994;6:42.

173. Michael JW. Reflections on CAD/CAM in prosthetics and orthotics. *J Prosthet Orthot* 1989;1:116.

174. Sutherland DH. *The development of mature walking.* Oxford: MacKeith Press, 1988.

175. Keen M. Early development and attainment of normal mature gait. *J Prosthet Orthot* 1993;5:34.

176. Pritham C. Workshop on teaching material for above-knee variants. *J Prosthet Orthot* 1989;1:50.

177. Gottschalk F, Stills S, McClellan B, et al. Does socket conuration influence the position of the femur in above-knee amputation? *J Prosthet Orthot* 1990;2:94.

178. Michael JW. Prosthetic knee mechanisms. *Phys Med Rehabil State Art Rev* 1994;8:147.

179. Gard S, Childress D, Uellendahl J. The influence of four-bar linkage knees on prosthetic swing-phase floor clearance. *J Prosthet Orthot* 1996;8:34.

180. Michael JW. Options meet varying needs. *Motion* 1997;7:34.

181. Barth D, Schumacher L, Thomas S. Gait analysis and energy cost of below knee amputees wearing six different prosthetic feet. *J Prosthet Orthot* 1991;4:63.

182. Cummings K, Kapp S. Lower limb pediatric prosthetics: general considerations and philosophy. *J Prosthet Orthot* 1991;4:196.

183. Neilson DH, Shurr DG, Golden JC, et al. Comparison of energy cost and gait efficiency during ambulation in below-knee amputees using different prosthetic feet—a preliminary report. *J Prosthet Orthot* 1988;1:24.

184. Letts M, Pyper A. The modified Chopart's amputation. *Clin Orthop* 1990;256:44.

185. Coutler-O'Berry C. Physical therapy management in children with lower extremity limb deficiencies. In: Herring JA, Birch JG, eds. *The child with a limb deficiency.* Rosemont, IL: American Academy of Orthopaedic Surgeons, 1998:319.

## Role of the Physical/Occupational Therapist

186. Effgen SK. The educational environment. In: Campbell SK, Vanderlinden DW, Palisano RJ, eds. *Physical therapy for children,* 2nd ed. Philadelphia, PA: WB Saunders, 2000.

## Adaptations for Activities and Sports

187. Radocy B. Upper-limb prosthetic adaptations for sports and recreation. In: Bowker JH, Michael JW, eds. *Atlas of limb prosthetics: surgical, prosthetic, and rehabilitation principles.* St. Louis, MO: Mosby-Year Book, 1992:325.

188. Michael JW, Gailey RS, Bowker JH. New developments in recreational prostheses and adaptive devices for the amputee. *Clin Orthop* 1990;256:64.

189. Anderson TF. Aspects of sports and recreation for the child with a limb deficiency. In: Herring JA, Birch JG, eds. *The child with a limb deficiency.* Rosemont, IL: American Academy of Orthopaedic Surgeons, 1998:345.

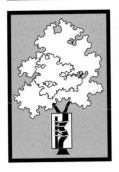

# 32

# Sports Medicine in the Growing Child

*R. Baxter Willis*

## INTRODUCTION

### Risks of Injury During Sports Participation

It is estimated that approximately 30 million children and young adults between the ages of 6 and 21 years engage in sports programs that are held outside of school, and 3.5 million boys and 2 million girls participate in school sports programs (1).

Parents want to know if the benefits of the sports activities warrant the risks involved, so an understanding of sport-specific risks is crucial to provide a comprehensive approach to address this concern.

With appropriate surveillance studies of each sport, specific risks and patterns of injury associated with different sports can be determined and compared. From this data, it may be possible to develop specific interventions designed to reduce the frequency of injuries.

### Epidemiology of Athletic Injuries in Children

What are the facts? What do we know about sports injuries in children?

First, there are sport-specific data which identify the risk of injury to participants for most sports (2–5). These studies, one from the National Athletic Trainers Association and one from the Athletic Health Care System (Seattle) studied injury patterns among children participating in high-school sports.

The data are remarkably consistent and reveal that girls' cross-country has the highest frequency of injury, followed by football, wrestling, girls' soccer, and boys' cross-country (Table 32.1). Of all the injuries reported, approximately 70% to 80% are minor (time loss of 5 to 7 days from participating in the involved sport), whereas 4% to 8% result in a time loss of greater than 3 weeks from participating in the involved sport (4) (Table 32.2).

Injuries to the upper extremity occur more frequently in younger children, due to falls, whereas lower-extremity injuries occur more frequently in older children and adolescents (1,4).

The most comprehensive statistics on children's recreational injuries are available from the United States Consumer Product Safety Commission (CPSC). The CPSC operates the National Electronic Injury Surveillance System (NEISS) whereby data are gathered from the emergency departments of 100 hospitals throughout the United States. These data are then used in conjunction with other models involving the relation between emergency room visits and the number of injuries treated outside hospital emergency rooms to arrive at an estimate of the number of injuries treated for each specific age-group in hospital emergency rooms, doctors offices, clinics, and ambulatory centers. In the year 2000, eight of the most common recreational activities accounted for 2.24 million medically treated injuries of the musculoskeletal system in children from 5 years to 14 years of age (6,7). The cost to society of these injuries, estimated using an "Injury Cost Model," was $33 billion (6,7).

Injury surveillance identifies specific risks for specific sports and may lead to injury prevention by mandatory changes in equipment. Face masks and helmets used in hockey, shin guards used in soccer, and helmets used in baseball are examples of equipment modification put into place after injury surveillance rates indicated the need for change.

## TABLE 32.1
### ALL-SPORTS INJURY DATA ANALYSIS: FALL 1979 THROUGH SPRING 1992

| Rank[a] | Sport | Season | Total Athletes | Injury Rate/100 Athletes/ Season | Injury Rate/1000 Athletic Exposures | Significant[b] Injury Rate/ 1000 Athletic Exposures | Major Injury Rate/1000 Athletic Exposures[c] | Percent of Different Athletes Injured |
|---|---|---|---|---|---|---|---|---|
| 1 | Girls' cross-country | Fall | 1299 | 61.4 | 17.3 | 3.3 | 0.9 | 33.1 |
| 2 | Football | Fall | 8560 | 58.8 | 12.7 | 3.1 | 0.9 | 36.7 |
| 3 | Wrestling | Winter | 3624 | 49.7 | 11.8 | 2.6 | 1.0 | 32.1 |
| 4 | Girls' soccer | Fall | 3186 | 43.7 | 11.6 | 2.9 | 0.7 | 31.6 |
| 5 | Boys' cross-country | Fall | 2481 | 38.7 | 10.5 | 2.3 | 0.5 | 24.6 |
| 6 | Girls' gymnastics | Winter | 1082 | 38.9 | 10.0 | 2.3 | 0.7 | 26.2 |
| 7 | Boys' soccer | Spring | 3848 | 36.4 | 9.5 | 2.1 | 0.4 | 25.2 |
| 8 | Girls' basketball | Winter | 3634 | 34.5 | 7.1 | 1.7 | 0.5 | 24.2 |
| 9 | Girls' track | Spring | 3543 | 24.8 | 6.2 | 1.6 | 0.3 | 18.0 |
| 10 | Boys' basketball | Winter | 3874 | 29.2 | 5.5 | 1.3 | 0.3 | 22.9 |
| 11 | Volleyball | Fall | 3444 | 19.9 | 5.4 | 1.1 | 0.3 | 16.1 |
| 12 | Softball | Spring | 2957 | 18.3 | 4.8 | 1.2 | 0.3 | 14.8 |
| 13 | Boys' track | Spring | 4425 | 17.3 | 4.4 | 1.1 | 0.3 | 13.6 |
| 14 | Baseball | Spring | 3397 | 17.1 | 4.2 | 1.0 | 0.3 | 14.4 |
| 15 | Fast pitch | Spring | 134 | 11.9 | 2.4 | 1.2 | 0.6 | 11.9 |
| 16 | Coed swimming | Winter | 4004 | 8.3 | 2.2 | 0.5 | 0.0 | 6.4 |
| 17 | Coed tennis | Fall/Spring | 4096 | 7.0 | 1.9 | 0.4 | 0.1 | 5.8 |
| 18 | Coed golf | Fall/Spring | 2170 | 1.4 | 0.8 | 0.0 | 0.0 | 1.3 |
| Combined totals | | | 59,758 | 30.6 | 7.6 | 1.8 | 0.5 | 21.1 |

[a] Ranking based on injury rate/1000 athletic exposures.
[b] Significant injuries are defined as five or more consecutive games and/or practices in which the athlete was not at full participation.
[c] Major injuries are defined as 15 or more consecutive games and/or practices in which the athlete was not at full participation.

## TABLE 32.2
### ALL INJURY DATA CLASSIFIED ACCORDING TO AFFECTED BODY PART

| Body Part | Number | Percentage | Game (%) | Practice (%) | Length of Time Lost from Sport) | | | |
|---|---|---|---|---|---|---|---|---|
| | | | | | 1 Day | 2–4 Days | 5–15 Days | >15 |
| Ankle | 1937 | 22.8 | 30.8 | 69.2 | 31.5 | 37.4 | 24.3 | NA |
| Knee | 1415 | 16.7 | 26.6 | 73.4 | 31.7 | 31.8 | 23.8 | 1 |
| Hand, wrist, elbow | 1126 | 13.3 | 29.5 | 70.5 | 43.9 | 27.7 | 19.7 | NA |
| Shin, calf | 829 | 9.8 | 20.3 | 79.7 | 33.5 | 36.3 | 21.1 | NA |
| Thigh, groin | 623 | 7.3 | 15.6 | 84.4 | 32.6 | 43.2 | 22.0 | NA |
| Head, neck, collarbone | 618 | 7.3 | 42.4 | 57.6 | 51.3 | 31.9 | 12.9 | NA |
| Shoulder | 517 | 6.1 | 31.8 | 68.2 | 33.7 | 35.2 | 22.4 | NA |
| Foot | 485 | 5.7 | 17.8 | 82.2 | 36.1 | 36.2 | 21.9 | NA |
| Back | 484 | 5.7 | 25.3 | 74.7 | 32.0 | 38.4 | 20.5 | NA |
| Hip | 234 | 2.8 | 24.2 | 75.8 | 37.6 | 37.2 | 18.8 | NA |
| Hamstring | 211 | 2.5 | 22.4 | 77.6 | 27.5 | 40.3 | 25.1 | NA |
| Totals/average | 8479 | 100 | 27.2 | 72.8 | 35.4 | 35.0 | 21.7 | |

Despite the injuries seen in a sports medicine clinic, the benefits, both physical and psychosocial, of participation in any particular sport outweigh the risks of significant injury, and parents should be advised of both the recognized benefits as well as the sport-specific risks, in order to make an informed decision regarding their child's participation.

## Injury Prevention

Prevention strategies of sports-related injuries in both children and adults generally lag behind injury management strategies. As participation in recreational and scholastic sports increases, there is a desire to examine strategies of injury prevention to lower the risk of injury.

Injury-prevention strategies include a thorough preparticipation physical evaluation to identify medical problems such as asthma or diabetes mellitus that affect training or participation and previous significant injuries such as fractures and sprains that should be assessed before clearing the athlete to participate (8).

As part of the preparticipation physical, an assessment of general health, physical fitness, strength, flexibility, and joint stability and alignment should be performed (9).

A certain level of fitness should be attained before preseason practice begins, and is the responsibility of the coach, parent, and athlete. As well as general aerobic fitness, sport-specific conditioning is recommended to prevent sport-specific injuries. Athletes involved in throwing sports should work on strengthening and stretching exercises for the shoulder girdle and upper extremity (10). Controversy exists as to the benefit of stretching programs in the prevention of muscle-tendon strains or apophysitis. There are no studies that have proven the efficacy of stretching in reducing the incidence of injury, but most coaches, trainers, and sports medicine personnel continue to advocate their use (8).

Probably the most important individual in ensuring injury prevention is the coach. The coach should be qualified in sport-specific methods of training, injury prevention, injury recognition, and proper rehabilitation of the injured athlete before return to participation. An understanding and knowledgeable coach can make a lasting impression on the athlete, especially at the youth level.

Strength training for specific sports is permissible without any concern for overuse injury or effect on growth, as long as the program is supervised and submaximal weights are employed.

## Principles of Rehabilitation

Rehabilitation is a process in which a series of structured activities enables an athlete to return to normal activity or function.

Although the physician will make the diagnosis and assess the functional limitations of the injury, physical therapy is actively involved in the rehabilitation process to enable the athletes to resume their previous level of activity.

The physician should supervise the rehabilitation process and determine when joint functions, muscle strength, and sport-specific functions are restored (11).

For minimal injuries such as minor contusions and sprains, the need for supervised rehabilitation is questionable. However, for major joint injuries such as significant ligament sprains, fractures, and significant resistant overuse syndromes, physical therapy will usually aid the athlete to a speedier return to activity and may also prevent further or repetitive injuries (12).

The phases of rehabilitation include the initial period of acute care when the limb is put at relative rest, and pain and inflammation are controlled by ice, elevation, and compression (11–13). The next phase, or intermediate phase, is aimed at the resolution of pain and restoration of joint motion, flexibility, and strength.

Later care involves progressive strengthening, functional and sport-specific drills, as well as proprioceptive training.

Finally, a maintenance program to prevent further injury is instituted.

Various modalities aid in this process.

### Physical Modalities

**Cold.** For acute injuries, ice should be applied to decrease pain and swelling, blood flow, and muscle spasm. It is the agent of choice for nearly all acute injuries and even overuse injuries.

**Heat.** Heat is employed less commonly; it reduces pain and spasm and increases blood flow and soft-tissue relaxation. It has a limited role in acute injuries or overuse syndromes when swelling and inflammation are present.

**Therapeutic Exercises.** Once swelling and muscle spasm subside, therapeutic exercise is initiated to improve joint range of motion and to stretch and strengthen muscles.

Joint mobilization is best accomplished by active mobilization in which the athlete moves the injured joint. Passive mobilization utilizes another individual, usually a therapist, to move the patient's contracted joint. This technique is often complicated by exacerbation of the injury, tearing or stretching of soft tissues, and hemorrhage, and should only be done by an experienced therapist when active mobilization has failed (11–13).

Active-assist mobilization is a combination of the two methods and has limited indications in the young athlete.

**Stretching Techniques.** Stretching techniques are designed to restore flexibility after an injury. Static stretching employs techniques in which the involved or target muscle is stretched or maintained for approximately 20 seconds. It is safer than ballistic stretching in which sudden bounces or joint motions are permitted. Ballistic stretching can cause activation of the stretch reflex and cause muscle-tendinous strain and is not recommended after acute injuries.

***Strengthening.*** Strengthening is an important part of the rehabilitation program and includes isometric, isotonic, isokinetic, concentric and eccentric, closed kinetic chain, and functional exercises.

*Isometric.* The muscle contracts without changing length. Isometric exercises are most important in the early phase of rehabilitation after injury because the injured joint or muscle is not moved. The exercises are simple to perform and do not require specialized equipment. To the patient's relief, isometric exercises are relatively painless.

*Isotonic.* Isotonic exercise involves the contraction of muscle against fixed resistance while the joint moves through its arc of motion. Examples are free weights and weight machines. Isotonic exercises are initiated after pain and swelling subside and joint motion is restored. Motor performance is superior following isotonic exercise compared to isometric exercise.

*Isokinetic.* Isokinetic exercises replicate the speed of muscle contraction during specific activities and are usually provided by specific and expensive therapeutic machines. The exercises are performed at a constant velocity.

*Concentric and Eccentric.* Concentric exercises involve the contraction of a muscle during exercise (e.g., biceps curl). Eccentric exercises involve lengthening of the muscle while opposing gravity (e.g., elbow extension with free weights after biceps curl). Significant increase of muscle strength occurs with eccentric exercise (11,12). Eccentric conditioning is introduced during the latter stages of rehabilitation.

*Closed or Open Chain Kinetic Exercises.* Closed chain kinetic exercise fixes a body part while performing work (for example, foot on floor while performing squats) whereas open chain kinetic exercises do not fix the body part (e.g., leg lift). Closed chain exercise improves agonist and antagonist muscle contraction (13). These exercises are performed in the later stages of rehabilitation because they may cause pain.

*Functional Exercise.* Functional exercises reproduce patterns of movement involved in a specific sport and involve the integration of several muscle groups working together. This is the final step in the rehabilitation process before the athlete returns to the sporting activity.

### Therapeutic Electrical Modalities

**Electrogalvanic Stimulation.** Electrogalvanic stimulation (EGS) causes small muscle contractions which may reduce swelling and muscle atrophy (11,12,13).

**Transcutaneous Nerve Stimulation.** Transcutaneous nerve stimulation (TNS) employs electrical stimulation to block pain impulses from the site of injury or site of surgery (11,12,13).

There is no objective evidence of the benefits of these two modalities in the treatment of athletic injuries in the child (11,12,13). Most sports injuries in the skeletally immature are amenable to nonoperative management. Not all injuries require supervised rehabilitation, but it has been shown to lessen recovery time and decrease reinjury rates.

## Performance-Enhancing Substances

Widespread publicity about performance-enhancing drugs and the perception of societal reward for exceptional athletic success are the major reasons why young athletes consider the use of these substances (14).

Anabolic steroids in particular are under increasing scrutiny by international athletic organizations as well as the press in an attempt to publicize their role in the performance of elite athletes.

If used in conjunction with a strength training program and proper diet, anabolic steroids have been shown to increase muscle size and strength; but there is little, if any, evidence that their use resulted in improved performance or increased aerobic capacity (14–16).

Reports of steroid use for the last 10 to 20 years indicate patterns of use in up to 10% to 15% of boys and up to 2% to 4% of girls among high-school students (17). Anabolic steroid use is determined by a complex set of factors that includes potential beneficial effects of anabolic steroids, dissatisfaction with current body size and strength, a peer group involved in their use, and a tendency toward risk-taking behavior (14–17).

Anabolic steroids are available in oral and injectable forms. The oral form is metabolized in the liver and converted to testosterone. The injectable form is directly absorbed into the circulation and is therefore less hepatotoxic than the oral form (16).

### Adverse Effects

The adverse effects of anabolic steroids are well known, significant, and affect virtually every organ system (15,16).

For the skeletally immature athlete, premature epiphyseal closure has been documented with intake of a single cycle of anabolic steroids (14–16). In addition, strains and ruptures of the tendons have been noted in young individuals without any predisposing tendonitis (15,16).

Effects on the hepatobiliary system include transient elevation of liver enzymes, blood-filled cysts in the liver which may rupture and cause fatal hemorrhage, and benign and malignant neoplasms (15).

Anabolic steroids cause an elevation of blood pressure (reversible) and an increase in total cholesterol with a reduction in high-density lipoproteins (16,17). Prolonged use may lead to arteriosclerotic heart disease and cardiomyopathy (16,17).

Men taking anabolic steroids may experience acne, male pattern baldness, priapism, impotence, gynecomastia, and testicular atrophy (14–17). Women may develop masculinization including hirsutism, deepening of the voice, and baldness (14–16).

Aggression, emotional instability, and even psychosis have been reported (15,16).

To effect a change in behavior, stiff penalties and peer pressure to avoid cheating are probably necessary. Imparting proper and current medical knowledge without the use of scare tactics may help. Encouragement and availability of proper programs in strength training, conditioning, proper nutrition, and acquisition of sporting skills is probably the best deterrent.

## Strength Training in the Pediatric Population

Weight training or strength training by children or growing adolescents is a controversial topic. The controversy exists because of the belief that weight training causes damage to the physes or joints and the perceived association of weight training with performance-enhancing drugs. Both are enough to cause parents to question the potential benefits of weight training against its perceived risks to their child.

A number of studies have shown that children and adolescents can increase strength up to 40% with a low risk of injury (18–20). In girls and prepubescent boys, it is postulated that a gain in strength occurs due to enhanced recruitment of motor units rather than muscular hypertrophy (18–20).

Specific injuries have been reported in association with weight lifting in children, including distal radius and ulnar fractures, distal radial epiphyseal fractures, patellofemoral pain, clavicular osteolysis, pelvic apophyseal fractures, and meniscal tears (19,21–23). In adolescents, lumbosacral injuries such as disc herniation, spondylolysis, and spondylolisthesis are common injuries (24). Power lifting and Olympic-style weight lifting are *not* recommended for the skeletally immature (18). However, there are no deleterious consequences to a well-supervised program of weight training in the growing youth, provided the movements are done in a slow, controlled fashion with submaximal weights (25,26).

# ACUTE INJURIES

## Acute Patellar Dislocation

Patellar dislocations may be classified as acute, recurrent, or habitual. Acute dislocations tend to occur in adolescent, high-level athletes, whereas recurrent instability occurs in individuals with well-known anatomic variants such as ligamentous laxity, patella alta, and genu valgum (27). Even with acute patellar dislocations there is commonly an underlying anatomical abnormality that predisposes to the dislocation. The common age for acute patellar dislocation is from 14 to 20 years (27–29).

### Anatomy

Understanding the pathology of patellar dislocation requires an understanding of the anatomy of the extensor mechanism of the knee. There are three distinct layers around the patellofemoral joint as part of the extensor mechanism. The superficial layer involves the fascia overlying the sartorius muscle. The second layer comprises the patellar retinaculum and the medial patellofemoral ligament. The final layer comprises the medial collateral ligament and the joint capsule (30,31).

The most important stabilizing structure of the patella is the medial patellofemoral ligament. It arises from the adductor tubercle and inserts along the medial patellar border on its superior two thirds. The medial patellofemoral ligament varies widely in size, shape, and strength, and provides from 50% to 80% of the restraining force to lateral displacement (32–38).

### Mechanism of Injury

The most common mechanism is an indirect force applied to the knee. The foot is planted, knee flexed and in valgus, and an internal rotation moment applied to the femur (39). Patellar dislocation is commonly associated with this mechanism of injury in basketball, football, baseball, gymnastics, and also in falls (29).

Less frequently, direct forces applied to the medial side of the patella or to the lateral side of the knee with a valgus force may cause patellar dislocation (40).

### History and Physical Examination

The patient usually describes a twisting injury with a mechanism not unlike that for an anterior cruciate ligament (ACL) tear. The patient may describe something moving out of position in the knee and then popping back into place. The knee quickly becomes swollen and the child is reluctant to move it.

On physical examination, the patella is almost always reduced or relocated. In the rare instance where it has not reduced, the child's knee is usually still flexed. The patella may be palpated on the lateral aspect of the lateral femoral condyle. If the knee is passively extended and a gentle medial force applied to the patella, the patella should reduce very easily. A large, tense hemarthrosis accompanies an acute patellar dislocation. Plain radiographs, specifically anteroposterior, lateral, and Merchant view (also known as *skyline views*) should be carefully evaluated for patellar reduction, lateral tilt, and osteochondral fracture. The Merchant view is an axial view of the patellofemoral joint with the knee flexed to a consistent 35 to 45 degrees (41) (Fig. 32.1).

The mechanism of injury for an acute patellar dislocation is similar to an ACL tear, and careful examination to rule out the latter must always be performed.

### Treatment

If the patella is still acutely dislocated, reduction should be accomplished promptly with the use of appropriate sedation

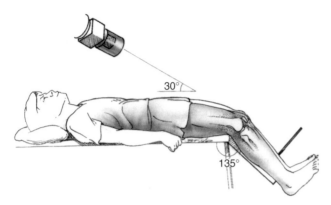

**Figure 32.1** Tangential x-ray view for evaluating the patellofemoral joint. Merchant view allows the quadriceps mechanism to relax. The patella is not artificially held reduced in the distal femoral groove.

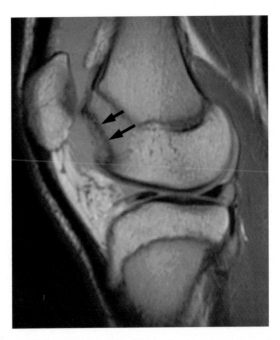

**Figure 32.2** Lateral image of knee [magnetic resonance imaging (MRI)] with large osteochondral defect of lateral femoral condyle after acute patellar dislocation. Arrows (*solid black*) point to defect in lateral femoral condyle.

if required. If the patella cannot be relocated with the patient supine, reduction can be facilitated by placing the patient prone. This allows the hamstrings to relax and with gentle extension of the knee, the patella will reduce.

Treatment following an acute patellar dislocation depends on the presence or absence of an osteochondral fracture. The incidence of osteochondral fracture following patellar dislocation ranges from 5% to 50% (42–45). If an osteochondral fracture is detected, a knee arthroscopy is recommended to visualize the fragment and to determine if the fragment should be replaced or excised. If the fragment is greater than 2 cm and has a significant bony component, fixation should be performed with any number of fixation techniques: low-profile cannulated screws countersunk to avoid abrasion, Herbert screws countersunk in the articular cartilage, or bioabsorbable pins or screws (39). In most cases, the fragment is smaller than 2 cm in diameter and should be excised. If significant anatomic abnormalities also exist, consideration of surgical correction at the time of treatment of the osteochondral fracture should be considered (42,43).

Treatment of acute patellar dislocations without osteochondral fracture involves brief immobilization, then vigorous rehabilitation. The principles of rehabilitation have been elucidated previously and are aimed at resolving the hemarthrosis, reducing the pain, improving the range of motion, and increasing the strength of both the quadriceps and hamstrings (29,38,40).

Once the injured knee has been rehabilitated, return to sports is permitted. There should be no effusion, full range of motion, and approximately 80% of the strength of the uninjured knee prior to resumption of athletic activities. The use of a patellar stabilization brace is recommended during sports.

### Author's Preferred Recommendations

The following reduction of an acute patellar dislocation is imperative to obtain appropriate radiographs to rule out an osteochondral fracture. If symptoms persist, magnetic resonance imaging (MRI) may be helpful in visualizing a chondral or osteochondral defect (Fig. 32.2). If no fracture is detected, rehabilitation is begun. If an osteochondral fracture is detected, a knee arthroscopy determines whether it should be excised (if the fragment is less than 2 cm with very little subchondral bone) or replaced (if the fragment greater than 2 cm with significant subchondral bone). Replacement is accomplished by an arthrotomy with the use of small cannulated screws countersunk to the level of the subchondral component. Acute repair of medial structures including medial patellofemoral ligament and patellar retinaculum is carried out, and usually a lateral retinacular release is done at the same time. The knee is immobilized for approximately 10 to 14 days in a soft dressing and knee immobilizer, followed by vigorous rehabilitation.

There are proponents of acute surgical repair in the absence of osteochondral fracture (42,43,46), but I prefer nonsurgical treatment because 50% to 60% of patients older than 10 years will not experience a recurrence (44,45).

## Recurrent Patellar Dislocation

### Clinical Features

Children with recurrent patellar instability have one or several features which predispose to the recurrence. Anatomic factors include an increased Q angle, increased femoral tibial valgus, excessive external tibial torsion, femoral condylar dysplasia, patella alta, and generalized ligamentous laxity (27–29,39,47–49). The Q angle is the angle formed by a long axis drawn along the quadriceps mechanism from the anterior superior iliac spine (ASIS) to the midaxis of the knee joint subtended by a long axis drawn along the patellar tendon. A normal Q angle is 10 degrees or less (Fig. 32.3A–C). Children with recurrent patellar instability exhibit a positive apprehension test. Apprehension is produced when an attempt is made to displace the patella laterally with the knee flexed approximately 30 degrees.

### Surgical Management

Surgery is indicated when a patient has had three or four recurrences of patellar dislocation and the instability affects his or her lifestyle. Correction of the anatomic variants is crucial for the long-term outcome.

Surgery may entail soft-tissue surgery around the patella, including lateral retinacular release, reconstruction of the medial patellofemoral ligament (MPFL), vastus medialis advancement with medial reefing, or semitendinosis tenodesis.

Lateral retinacular release alone for patellar instability is rarely indicated. There are isolated reports of its success in the treatment of recurrent patellar dislocation, but its exact role in this condition remains to be determined (50,51). Excessive lateral retinacular release combined with aggressive medial reefing may result in iatrogenic medial subluxation, and must be avoided (33,52,53). Lateral retinacular release usually must be combined with reconstruction of the MPFL or by vastus medialis advancement.

Reconstruction of the MPFL has become popular in acute or early recurrent dislocation (33,39). If the natural tissue is found to be deficient, the MPFL should be reconstructed using a free hamstring graft, usually the semitendinosus (33). The graft is anchored by suture anchors at the adductor tubercle and to the medial superior border of the patella.

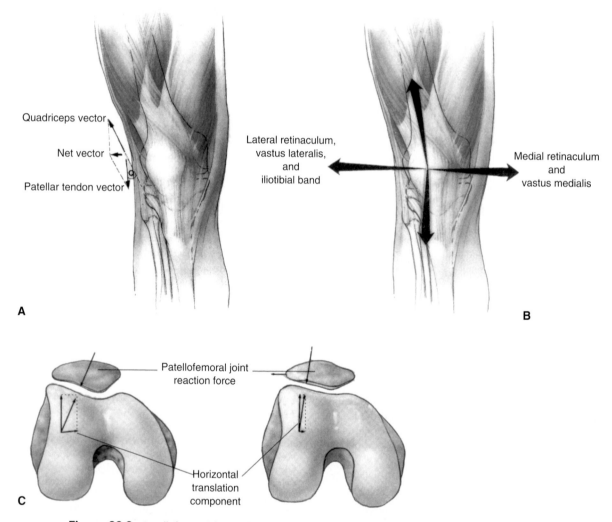

**Figure 32.3** Patellofemoral biomechanics. **A:** The Q angle relates the direction of pull of the quadriceps mechanism to that of the patellar tendon. These are the two most powerful forces exerted on the patella. Their vector sum is directed laterally. **B:** There are additional soft tissue forces applied to the patella. **C:** The laterally directed net vector is opposed by the patellofemoral articulation. If the groove is shallow, there is less potential resistance to horizontal translation than in knees with a deeper femoral groove. The dysplastic patellofemoral articulation results in less resistance to lateral translation, and therefore greater sheer forces on the articular surface.

In the situation of more chronic recurrent dislocations, a vastus medialis obliquus (VMO) advancement distally and laterally with medial reefing will correct the medial deficiency (54–56). In a child 12 years or younger, the medial reefing may be augmented by the semitendinosus tenodesis described by Galeazzi (57,58). This graft reproduces the vector of the patellotibial ligament. It is employed when there is persistent instability after already performing a lateral release and MPFL reconstruction or VMO advancement (Fig. 32.4).

If there is an excessive Q angle, distal realignment is advocated as well. If the individual is a skeletally mature youth, the tibial tubercle is osteotomized and shifted medially without distal transfer (Elmslie-Trillat procedure) (59) (Fig. 32.5A,B). A modification of the Elmslie-Trillat procedure is the Fulkerson procedure (60), in which a more generous osteotomy of the anterior tibial tubercle is performed and the tubercle transferred anteriorly and medially (Fig. 32.5C). This procedure is primarily reserved for patellofemoral pain in adults and is not recommended for instability in adolescents or young adults.

In the immature child with an excessive Q angle and open tibial tubercle apophysis, osteotomy is contraindicated because of the potential for growth arrest and genu recurvatum. In these cases, the patellar tendon may be split, and the lateral half delivered beneath the medial portion of the patellar tendon and sutured to the periosteum of the proximal tibia medially by direct suture or by suture anchors (61) (Fig. 32.6). Acceptable results can

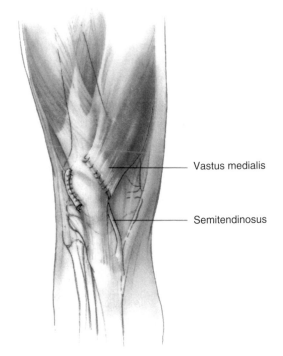

Vastus medialis

Semitendinosus

**Figure 32.4** The Galeazzi procedure transfers the semitendinosus to the inferior pole of the patella. From there, it courses through a drill hole placed obliquely through the patella, exiting the superior lateral aspect. The tendon is then sutured to the soft tissues. This provides a medial tether and effectively alters the net vector of the patellar tendon toward the medial side. Typically, the vastus medialis is advanced approximately one-third the width of the patella.

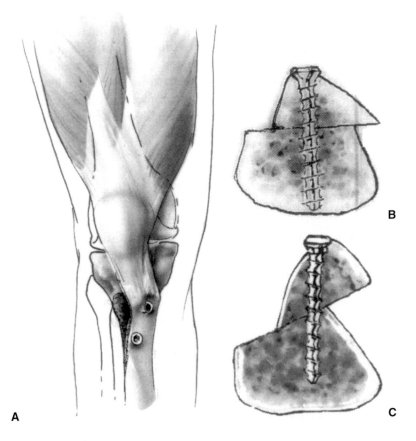

**Figure 32.5** **A,B:** The Elmslie-Trillat technique shifts the tibial tubercle medially. The tubercle stays in the same plane. **C:** The Fulkerson modification involves an oblique cut that results in anterior translation as the tubercle is moved medially. This reduces the patellofemoral contact forces while shifting the pull of the patella medially.

A

B

C

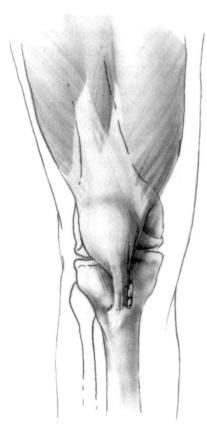

**Figure 32.6** The Roux-Goldthwait procedure splits the patellar tendon. The lateral half is transferred beneath the medial side and sutured to the periosteum along the metaphysis. This redirects the patellar tendon vector more medially.

be expected in up to 90% of cases employing the Roux-Goldthwait procedure (61).

Rehabilitation following a patellar stabilization procedure is very important. It is crucial to move the knee early, and immobilization in a removable knee immobilizer for 3 to 4 weeks is sufficient for healing. Active range of motion and strengthening are essential parts of the rehabilitation program and a resumption of sports activity can be anticipated in 4 to 6 months.

### Author's Preferred Method

The critical steps in correcting recurrent patellar instability include a thorough analysis of anatomic factors preoperatively, and intraoperative evaluation of the reconstruction. I employ a stepwise surgical protocol that almost always involves a lateral retinacular release and medial VMO advancement. If the Q angle is within normal limits and the patella is stable, there is no need for further surgery. It is imperative that the knee is put through flexion and extension to ensure normal patellar tracking and to ensure the VMO advancement is not too ambitious, in which case it will limit flexion. Reconstruction of the medial patellofemoral ligament by means of an autogenous hamstring graft is an option in the adolescent who is

nearing or has attained skeletal maturity (33). The graft is double stranded and attached by means of suture anchors to the medial superior portion of the patella and to the adductor tubercle area of the femur.

If the Q angle is excessive, distal realignment is performed; the Roux-Goldthwait procedure is used for the skeletally immature patients up to 14 years of age, and the Elmslie-Trillat procedure for patients older than 14 years.

If the patella is still unstable, the final surgical procedure is the addition of the semitendinosus tenodesis of the patella.

## Meniscal Injuries in Children

With Fairbanks' (62) classic article of 1948, the deleterious late effects of partial or total meniscectomy, namely, degenerative joint disease, in children and adolescents were amplified. Other authors have provided similar evidence with long-term results after meniscectomy in children and adolescents (63–69). Therefore, preservation of the meniscus, either partially or in its entirety, is a principle of treatment of a torn meniscus in a young patient.

### Embryology and Development

The menisci have developed their mature anatomic relations by approximately 3 months of gestation (70). The menisci have a blood supply which arises from the periphery, but extends throughout the meniscus during intrauterine development. By approximately 1 year of age the central third is avascular, and by the age of 10 years the adult vascular pattern prevails (71). Arnoczky's classical vascular injection studies revealed that the peripheral 10% to 30% of the medial meniscus and the outer 10% to 25% of the lateral meniscus have a vascular supply (72) (Fig. 32.7). Branches of the superior, inferior, medial, and lateral geniculate

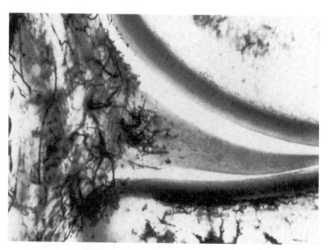

**Figure 32.7** Vascularity of the human meniscus, as seen in a frontal section of the medial compartment of the knee. Branching vessels from the perimeniscal capillary plexus penetrate the capsular third of the adult meniscus. (From Maffuli N, Testa V, Vapasso G. Mediopatellar synovial plica of the knee in athletes: results of arthroscopic treatment. *Med Sci Sports Exerc* 1993;25(9):985.)

arteries form a peripheral vascular plexus. Therefore tears in the peripheral zone (so-called red-red zone) are capable of healing and form the basis for the meniscal repair or suturing techniques that should always be considered in children.

Menisci are made predominantly of Type I collagen, and the fibers are oriented in a circumferential pattern. There are additional radial, oblique, and vertically oriented fibers, which resist hoop stresses (73,74).

The medial meniscus is firmly attached peripherally, and there is normally approximately 2 to 3 mm of posterior translation as the knee flexes. Contrast this with the more unstable lateral meniscus, with up to 10 to 11 mm of posterior translation, and the reasons for fewer lateral meniscal tears become more apparent (73,74).

### Discoid Meniscus

One of the causes of intraarticular knee pathology in the child is the discoid meniscus. Almost always involving the lateral meniscus, this abnormality can cause a loud "snapping" sensation. The incidence of this condition has been reported to be as high as 3% to 5%, higher in the Asian population, and it occurs bilaterally in up to 20% of cases (75–78).

This condition is a congenital or embryonic abnormality, but there is no accepted explanation for its development. The lateral meniscus does not acquire a discoid shape in its embryologic development, and this condition appears to be an anatomic variant (70,71). Discoid menisci are more prone to tears because of increased mechanical stress transmitted to their larger surface area, and because of hypermobility (75,79–81).

### Classification by Watanabe.

The most widely accepted classification is that of Watanabe who described three distinct types (82). Type I discoid menisci cover the entire tibial plateau and have intact peripheral attachments (Fig. 32.8), Type II cover up to 80% of the plateau surface (Fig. 32.9), and Type III have a thick posterior horn, cover 75% to 80% of the plateau surface, and have abnormal peripheral attachments (Fig. 32.10).

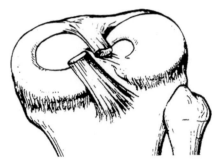

**Figure 32.9** Type II discoid meniscus covering 80% of lateral tibial plateau with intact peripheral attachments.

*Clinical Features.* The clinical presentation of a child with this condition depends on the type of discoid meniscus. The discoid meniscus with deficient peripheral attachments (Type III) presents in a young child of 2 to 3 years of age as a "snapping knee syndrome." As the knee is brought from flexion into full extension, a painless, palpable, and audible snap occurs. The child may also have painless giving way resulting in unexplained falls. Type I and Type II discoid menisci do not usually present until the child or adolescent actually tears the discoid meniscus, which is prone to happen due to its large surface area. These patients have joint-line pain and tenderness, and have an effusion. Catching, locking, and giving way are also suggestive of tears in a discoid meniscus if the location is lateral. This typically occurs in the middle of the child's 2nd decade of life as the child approaches skeletal maturity, or in early adulthood. In other respects Type I and Type II discoid menisci are asymptomatic.

*Imaging Studies.* Plain radiographs may reveal a widened lateral joint space with squaring of the lateral femoral condyle.

MRI is the most useful imaging modality for making the diagnosis. Criteria to define a discoid meniscus include a transverse meniscal diameter of more than 20% of the tibial width on transverse images, or a transverse meniscal diameter of more than 15 mm and continuity between anterior and posterior horns on three or more successive sagittal images (83). MRI can detect tears within a discoid

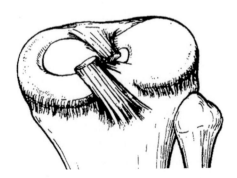

**Figure 32.8** Type I discoid meniscus covering entire lateral tibial plateau and with intact meniscotibial ligaments.

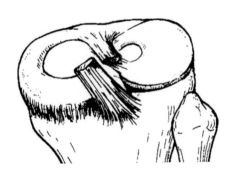

**Figure 32.10** Type III discoid meniscus covering 75% to 80% of lateral tibial plateau with deficient peripheral attachments.

meniscus, but is not sensitive enough to detect subtle peripheral detachments. MRI has a high positive predictive value for discoid menisci, but a low sensitivity (83,84). In other words, a discoid meniscus will be present in almost all cases when picked up by MRI, but MRI will miss many cases of discoid meniscus.

**Treatment.** Treatment of a discoid meniscus depends on whether the patient is symptomatic or not. For stable, asymptomatic discoid menisci detected by MRI or at arthroscopy, no treatment is indicated or recommended. For the patient with symptoms strongly suggestive of a torn discoid meniscus but not detected by MRI, arthroscopic examination is warranted.

If symptoms exist, treatment depends on whether the discoid meniscus is stable or unstable. If the discoid meniscus is stable, "saucerization" of the central portion by arthroscopic or open technique is indicated (75,85–90). In a young child with the complete variety, it is often difficult to visualize the portion of the meniscus to be resected arthroscopically. It may be safer for the inexperienced arthroscopist to do a mini arthrotomy to visualize the central portion of meniscus to be resected as well as the stable peripheral rim. A peripheral rim of 6 to 8 mm of meniscus should be left.

By arthroscopic technique, small pediatric basket punches, scissor punches, and biters are employed with the knee in flexion. Small arthroscopic shavers complete the saucerization technique with the knee flexed and in the "figure 4" position.

Following saucerization, it is important to assess the peripheral stability. This is best accomplished by arthroscopic technique. If peripheral detachment or instability is encountered, meniscal suturing is indicated. The suture technique is best accomplished by an inside-out technique and open incision posterolaterally to identify and protect the common peroneal nerve when the sutures are tied (85).

The repair should be protected by non–weight bearing and restricted range of motion for approximately 4 weeks. This may best be accomplished by a bent-knee cast in very young children who cannot cooperate with crutches or other measures.

Published results of meniscal suturing of unstable discoid menisci are limited, but good results have been reported in up to 75% of cases in a few selected series (80–82). In addition, there is very little information as to the long-term results of saucerization technique, especially as it relates to the incidence or prevention of degenerative changes in the knee (75,87). Long-term studies will be needed to delineate and provide evidence of the efficacy of the treatment.

### Meniscal Tears

As a general rule, meniscal tears in children and adolescents are rare. They are more commonly seen in conjunction with an ACL tear or if the meniscus is abnormal in shape (i.e.,

discoid). They are extremely rare in children younger than 10 years if the meniscus is normal in size and shape (91).

The incidence of meniscal injuries increases with age. Most meniscal injuries are longitudinal in children and adolescents, with medial meniscal tears being more prevalent than lateral meniscal tears. Approximately 30% of meniscal tears in patients younger than 20 years are repairable, and two-thirds of repairable tears of the meniscus are seen in conjunction with ACL tears (92).

Meniscal injury in children and adolescents occurs in sports that involve twisting or pivoting motion, such as basketball, soccer, and football (91,93). Symptoms include pain along the joint line, swelling, giving way, and locking. On physical examination, joint line tenderness and an associated effusion are the most common findings. Differential diagnosis should include: osteochondritis dissecans (OCD), osteochondral fracture, patellofemoral pain and instability, tibial eminence fracture, and even popliteal or patellar tendonitis or synovial plica.

**Diagnostic Imaging.** Plain radiographs should always be taken to rule out other conditions such as tibial eminence fracture, osteochondral fracture, or OCD. The gold standard for delineation of meniscal pathology by imaging is MRI, although normal signal changes in the posterior horn of both the medial and lateral meniscus often result in false-positive reports (83,84,94,95). These signal changes probably represent persistent vascular developmental changes and are normal variants in children and adolescents. MRI is not a fail-safe tool with absolute accuracy and should not be ordered as a screening test for intraarticular pathology.

**Treatment.** Most symptomatic meniscal tears in children require treatment because they are usually large and often associated with ACL pathology (73,75,96). Meniscal suturing is the procedure of choice for most tears in the red-red zone or red-white zone, but must be accompanied by ligament reconstruction or protection of the knee by bracing if the ACL is torn (73,96,97). Meniscal stabilization alone in an ACL-deficient knee will most likely fail. ACL reconstruction techniques are discussed separately.

Because of the long-term deleterious consequences of partial or complete meniscectomy, meniscal stabilization is recommended. For middle-third (red-white zone) and outer-third (red-red zone) tears, there is sufficient healing potential to warrant repair. The most common technique of meniscal repair involves an inside-out technique with sutures passed through cannulae (Fig. 32.11). Care must be taken to avoid neurovascular structures, specifically, the saphenous vein and nerve medially and the peroneal nerve laterally. It is recommended that small skin incisions be made to identify the sutures and ensure that the sutures are tied at the capsule, avoiding any neurovascular structure.

Recently, bioabsorbable devices have been employed in adults to repair certain types of tears, thereby avoiding the

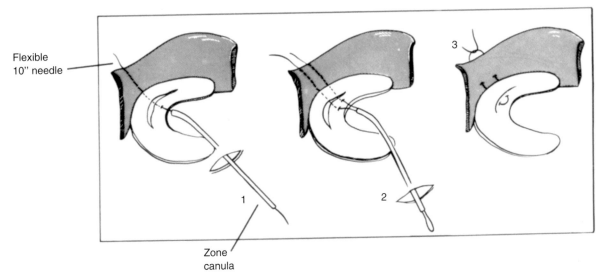

**Figure 32.11** Diagram illustrating inside-out technique of meniscal suturing. *(1)* Suture passed through tear and outside knee. *(2)* Second suture passed. *(3)* Suture tied to approximate edges of meniscal tear.

potential problems of sutures. These devices are inserted as an all-inside device and are most often employed for small posterior horn tears. There are few, if any, reports of their use in children or adolescents, and they are not recommended for widespread use.

Following surgical repair, protected weight bearing and knee motion are an important adjunct to the surgical repair of the meniscal tear. Range of motion is restricted from 0 to 45 degrees for the first 2 weeks, and flexion is restricted to less than 90 degrees for the first 6 weeks. The patient is permitted only toe-touch weight bearing for the first 6 weeks. Because most skeletally immature patients undergoing meniscal repair also undergo an ACL reconstruction, this protocol has become part of the rehabilitation following ACL reconstruction.

The overall results of meniscal repair in skeletally immature patients are excellent, regardless of the necessity for concomitant ACL reconstruction (98). Noyes and Barber-Westin reported a success rate of 75% in patients younger than 20 years who underwent repairs extending into the avascular zone (99,100). In a group of patients 20 years or younger who underwent isolated meniscal repair, Johnson et al. (101) reported healing in 76% of the patients at 10-year follow-up.

Factors associated with a successful meniscal healing after repair include concomitant ACL reconstruction, younger age of patients, peripheral tears in the vascular zone, small-sized tears (<2.5 cm), and time lapse from injury to surgery of less than 8 weeks (63,64,73,92,96,100,102–104).

## Tibial Eminence Fractures

Avulsion fractures of the tibial eminence were first described by Poncet in 1875, and controversy still exists as to the mechanism of injury and appropriate treatment plan (105).

The peak age for this injury is between 8 and 14 years of age. Classically, it occurred after a fall from a bicycle (106), but with increasing participation in competitive sports, these injuries are now often associated with various sporting activities. The mechanism involved is usually a hyperflexion or hyperextension force, with or without the combination of varus or valgus, and a rotational moment about the knee (107–109).

The mechanism of injury involves stretching or attenuation of the ACL, as shown experimentally by Noyes et al. (110), before the fracture of the eminence. The residual sagittal laxity observed in many of these patients is no doubt due to the in-substance elongation of the ACL (107,111–113).

### Classification

The Meyers and McKeever (114) classification is still the most widely accepted classification scheme (Fig. 32.12A–C). Type I fractures are minimally displaced, Type II are elevated anteriorly but remain intact posteriorly through a hinge of bone and/or cartilage (trap-door configuration), and Type III are completely displaced and separated. Type IV fractures are displaced and comminuted.

### Treatment

Treatment is based on the displacement of the fragment and the ability of the surgeon to reduce it by knee extension. The position of immobilization varies from surgeon to surgeon and is based on the tension placed on the ACL in varying degrees of flexion. The ligament is under increased tension at 0 degrees (posterolateral bundle) and at 45 degrees flexion or greater (anteromedial bundle) (115). As a consequence, a position from 10 to 30 degrees flexion has been recommended, but the most important aspect is to reduce the fragment into its bed. In a recent study, Kocher et al. (116) found a 26% incidence of medial meniscus entrapment in Type II injuries and a 65% incidence in Type

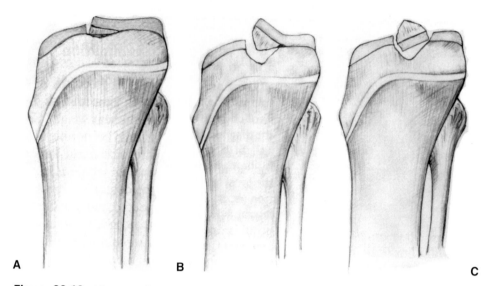

**Figure 32.12**  Meyers and McKeever classification of tibial eminence fractures. **A:** Type I, no or very minimal displacement. **B:** Type II, displaced but with intact posterior hinge. **C:** Type III, totally displaced eminence fracture.

III injuries. Therefore, in order to remove the incarcerated meniscus and allow for anatomic reduction, arthroscopic or open reduction should be considered for Type III fractures and for Type II fractures that do not reduce in extension. Numerous fixation methods have proved effective, including various suture techniques, cannulated screws, and more recently, bioabsorbable fixation pins (117). The exact technique depends on the particular fracture pattern and the surgeon's experience with a particular technique. If the surgeon is unable to fix the fragment by the arthroscopic technique, a small arthrotomy is performed with reduction of the fracture and fixation by one of several available methods.

### Author's Preferred Method

Type I injuries can be managed in full extension in a cylinder cast for approximately 4 to 6 weeks. In Type II and Type III injuries, an attempt is made to reduce the fragment closed by fully extending the knee. If the patient resists the extension maneuver, aspiration of the hemarthrosis and injection with local anesthetic (5 to 10 mL of 0.25% bupivicaine hydrochloride, Abbott Laboratories) may facilitate the reduction.

If the fragment will not reduce or the knee cannot be brought into full extension, I perform an arthroscopy with thorough irrigation and joint lavage. Blocks to reduction of the eminence fragment (meniscus or intermeniscal ligament) are removed and fixation, usually with a small, 1 4.0-mm cannulated screw, is performed (Fig. 32.13A–C)

### Postreduction Rehabilitation

The knee should be immobilized for 3 to 4 weeks if closed methods are employed. Active range-of-motion exercises and strengthening should begin immediately after cast removal.

If internal fixation is employed and the fixation is stable, early range of motion and strengthening is begun, but protective weight bearing is enforced for approximately 6 weeks.

Return to sports is permitted after full range of motion is regained and most of the strength restored, which often takes 3 to 4 months.

The results of treatment of tibial eminence fractures are generally excellent if the fragment is reduced. Some sagittal plane instability is a common feature after treatment, but this objective finding does not correlate with subjective symptoms in most patients (75,105,107,111–113,117). The core of treatment remains reduction of the fragment by closed means, open reduction, or arthroscopic technique.

## Anterior Cruciate Ligament Injury

### Introduction

ACL injury in the skeletally immature athlete has always been considered a relatively rare occurrence. Increased participation in organized sports, especially by girls, and recent improvements in diagnostic ability, including specialized imaging techniques such as MRI, are responsible for the reported increase in incidence of this injury (118–125). Expectations from family and coaches about full return to athletic activities by the injured child are based on well-publicized reports of similar injuries in elite athletes. The decision about treatment of an ACL disruption in the skeletally immature child should only be made after all the risks and benefits of each treatment option are analyzed, including nonoperative management with modification of the athlete's activities.

### Incidence

The true incidence of ACL injury in both adults and children is unknown. In a series of 1000 ACL injuries treated at

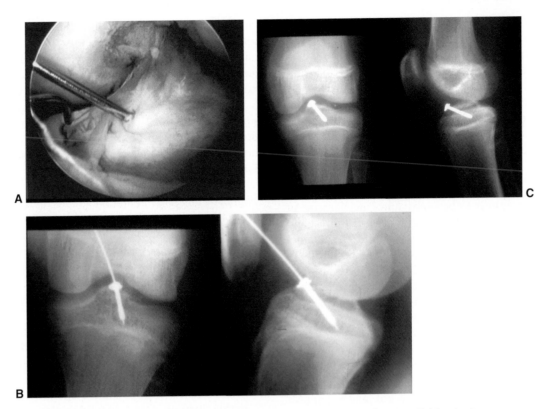

**Figure 32.13** **A:** Arthroscopic image of displaced tibial eminence fracture. Guide wire is transfixing eminence in place prior to insertion of cannulated screw. **B:** Screw and washer have been introduced over guide wire to hold the reduced eminence fracture. Note screw stops short of proximal tibial physis. **C:** Final intraoperative x-rays: Screw provides enough stability to allow early range of motion (2 to 3 weeks after surgery).

the Cleveland Clinic, five patients were younger than 12 years (125). A recent study of insurance claims by players in youth soccer leagues in the United States revealed approximately 550 claims for ACL injury (both sexes) out of a total of 8215 claims. The total number insured during the period was approximately 6 million, giving an incidence of approximately 0.01% (126). Girls in this age group are two to nine times more likely to disrupt their ACL than boys (127).

### Anatomy of the Anterior Cruciate Ligament

The ACL originates from the lateral aspect of the intercondylar notch of the femur posteriorly and inserts on the tibia at the anterior aspect of the tibial eminence. It comprises of two distinct bundles, an anteromedial and a posterolateral, whose function is to provide anteroposterior stability throughout the range of knee flexion and extension. In extension, the posterolateral bundle lengthens and the anteromedial bundle shortens. In flexion the posterolateral bundle shortens and the anteromedial bundle lengthens. The primary function of the ACL is to prevent excessive anterior translation of the tibia, but it also aids in preventing hyperextension, excessive varus and valgus, and internal rotation of the tibia (115,128–134).

The ACL is covered with a synovial reflection. Its blood supply is from branches of the inferior medial and inferior lateral genicular arteries, through the infrapatellar fat pad, and posteriorly near its origin from branches of the middle genicular artery (135).

### Developmental Considerations

Several studies have examined the gender disparity rate of ACL ligament injuries (136). Femoral notch morphology has revealed a narrower femoral notch in women (136), but other factors have been implicated, including differences in strength and conditioning, especially proprioceptive training (136,137), increased joint laxity (137), differences in limb alignment (136,137), and hormonal factors (138). The reasons for the disparity in incidence are probably multifactorial (135).

### Natural History of Anterior Cruciate Ligament Injury

The natural history of untreated ACL injury is well documented in adults. Chronic ACL deficiency leads to intraarticular damage including meniscal tear and chondral damage, especially if the individual continues to participate in physically demanding sports involving change of direction or rapid deceleration (139–141).

However, little is known about the natural history of untreated ACL injury in the skeletally immature. It is assumed that similar deleterious intraarticular pathology ensues if knee stability is not obtained and there is no modification of the patient's activities. Graf et al. (142), McCarroll et al. (122), and Angel and Hall (118) have all reported on the high incidence of continuing symptoms, meniscal tears, and inability to resume preinjury activity levels. Recent studies have revealed a significant incidence of meniscal tears, osteochondral lesions, and degenerative changes in skeletally immature patients not undergoing ACL reconstruction (143,144).

### Clinical Evaluation

**History.** There appear to be two distinct mechanisms of ACL injury in the skeletally immature patient—direct and indirect. In the younger child, direct trauma to the anterior aspect of the knee is not uncommon and may result in an ACL tear. In older children, as in adults, indirect injury by a twisting motion is the most common mechanism. The injury is commonly seen in participants of sports such as basketball, soccer, football, gymnastics, hockey, and volleyball.

The patient describes a characteristic "pop" at the time of injury. Almost always, the foot is planted or fixed and the deforming force (often rotatory) gets applied to the knee. An effusion usually develops quickly, but may not appear for several hours and is a strong indicator of significant intraarticular pathology. Stanitski et al. (123) found that 47% of patients aged 7 to 12 years with a traumatic effusion had an ACL disruption, and the percentage increased to 65% if the patients were aged 13 to 18 years.

**Physical Examination.** Physical examination is extremely important in evaluating for an ACL tear. The presence or absence of an effusion or any loss of motion is an important finding. In almost all acute ACL tears, an effusion will be present due to a hemarthrosis. Loss of extension may be due to impingement at the torn tibial stump of the ACL. The Lachman test is performed with the knee in 20 to 30 degrees of flexion and an anteriorly directed force applied to the tibia while the femur is stabilized. Side to side difference and the presence or absence of a firm end point are evaluated. The same test is performed with the knee flexed to 90 degrees (anterior drawer test) if it is not too painful for the patient. In addition, the pivot shift test is performed, although the patient in the acute situation will often not permit it. As the knee is brought from flexion of 45 to 60 degrees to full flexion, a slight valgus and anterior force is applied to the tibia. As the knee comes into full extension, a positive test occurs when the tibia subluxates anteriorly on the femur, indicating a torn ACL. As the knee is flexed, the tibia reduces. This physical finding is easier to elicit in the patient with a chronic ACL-deficient knee.

The examination should include specific evaluation for injuries to the medial collateral, lateral collateral, and posterior cruciate ligaments, because there may be associated ligamentous disruptions. In the case of a very unstable knee (multiplanar instability) in extension, careful evaluation of the vascularity and neurologic status of the limb is mandatory. Multiplanar instability is often indicative of a knee dislocation or distal femoral physeal injury in which acute or delayed vascular impairment may occur.

Examination of the knee in the first few days after injury is often difficult due to pain, swelling, and muscle spasm. After 2 to 3 weeks of rest, ice, and gentle range of motion, the patient should be reexamined, as the physical examination is often easier to perform then.

**Diagnostic Imaging.** Plain radiographs of the knee should be obtained of all patients with suspected knee ligament injury. Evaluation of the radiographs should be made for bony avulsions, osteochondral fractures, physeal fractures, and patellar dislocation or subluxation as well as for degree of physeal closure.

The indicators for an MRI examination remain controversial. It should not be done as a routine screening tool because of its high rate of false-positive readings for meniscal tear as well as its excessive cost. It is indicated in the patient who fails to improve range of motion and has a persistent effusion after conventional therapy, or in whom the physical examination is difficult to interpret.

In this situation, MRI is helpful in diagnosing meniscal tears and osteochondral lesions, which may affect the decision regarding surgery (Fig. 32.14A,B). If the patient has clinical evidence of a torn ACL alone, an MRI is not indicated.

### Treatment

**Special Considerations in the Growing Child.** Treatment recommendations in skeletally immature patients differ from their adult counterparts because of concern regarding future skeletal growth. The treating orthopaedist must be aware of the unique features of the growing child and the potential for growth arrest associated with conventional surgical techniques. As a consequence, each patient must be assessed individually to arrive at the decision for surgical reconstruction based on the child's activity level, the parents expectations, and the child's potential for further growth. There is no need for urgent surgical reconstruction as the incidence of arthrofibrosis is markedly increased in the acute situation.

**Nonsurgical Treatment.** Initially, all patients undergo a rehabilitation program designed to restore the patient's range of motion and muscle strength. The rehabilitation program may take from 6 weeks to 3 months (135).

If the child is younger than 10 years, an attempt to brace the child's knee with an appropriate ACL brace should be recommended. This facet of treatment should be undertaken by a certified orthotist, and the brace will have to be custom-made for the child. Cost for an ACL brace varies from $500 to $1500. The child is allowed to resume limited participation in sports using the brace, which is designed to

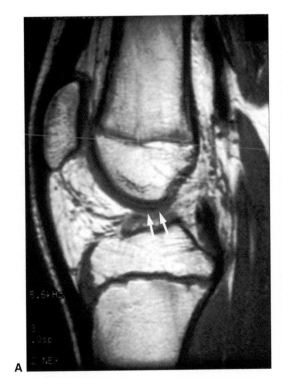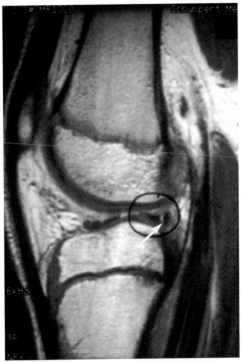

**Figure 32.14** Magnetic resonance imaging (MRI) of a skeletally immature individual with disruption of anterior cruciate ligament (*white arrows*) **(A)**, and peripheral separation of lateral meniscus (*white arrow and black circle*) **(B)**.

prevent anterior subluxation of the tibia with change of direction or stopping.

If the child does not experience instability or episodes of giving way while using the brace, full sports participation is permitted. A frank discussion of the potential risks of continued instability, namely, meniscal tears and chondral damage, should be undertaken with the parents, and recommendations may be made for modification of sports activity to decrease the exposure of the child athlete to potential instability episodes.

Unfortunately, bracing is not effective for every child with an ACL tear. If the child continues to experience episodes of giving way or instability when using the brace, the risk of meniscal tear and chrondral damage increases. If instability in the brace persists or there are signs of meniscal tear, surgery is recommended to stabilize the knee joint.

*Operative Treatment.* Extraarticular reconstructions have been proposed as a temporizing procedure in the skeletally immature patient (145,146). However, the inability of these procedures to control instability, because of their nonanatomic location, results in certain failure.

In the growing child, the treating surgeon must be aware of the potential for growth arrest, the isometry of the graft with various techniques, and the specific properties of different grafts. Stadelmaier et al. (147) and Guzzanti et al. (148) have shown that continuing growth occurs in experimental animals if a tendinous graft is employed through a small, centrally placed drill hole traversing the physis.

Edwards et al. (149) have reported growth changes in experimental animals with a small, centrally placed tendon graft to an "over-the-top" position on the femur when excessive tension was applied to the graft.

The over-the-top position means that the graft is passed through the intercondylar notch of the femur, through the posterior capsule, and "over the top" of the lateral femoral condyle where it is attached to bone by staples, a screw with a special spiked washer, or sutures.

Several authors have reported successful management of ACL-deficient knees in children, employing hamstring tendon grafts through a small central drill hole in the proximal tibial physis, various techniques for the femoral fixation including attachment via an over-the-top position (150,151), and drill holes exiting distal to the distal femoral physis or even through small drill holes through the distal femoral physis (152).

Employing the Tanner staging criteria (153), Dorizas and Stanitski (135) have employed a unique classification system for ACL reconstruction in the skeletally immature patient. Physis-sparing techniques that provide a ligamentous reconstruction while avoiding both the proximal tibial physis and distal femoral physis are used in young children (Tanner stage 0-1) (153) (Fig. 32.15). Critics of this technique remark on the lack of anatomically correct orientation of this graft and therefore the inability to restore isometry and normal knee kinematics.

Partial physis-sparing techniques involve a small 6- to 8-mm drill hole, vertically oriented through the proximal

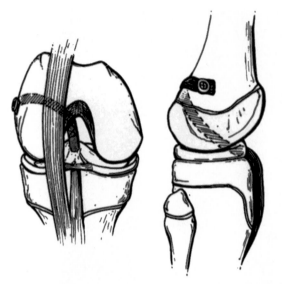

**Figure 32.15** Physis-sparing technique of anterior cruciate ligament (ACL) reconstruction. ACL reconstruction employing patellar tendon graft. The graft is passed behind the intermeniscal ligament to an "over-the-top" position on the distal femur. No violation of either the proximal tibial or distal femoral physis occurs.

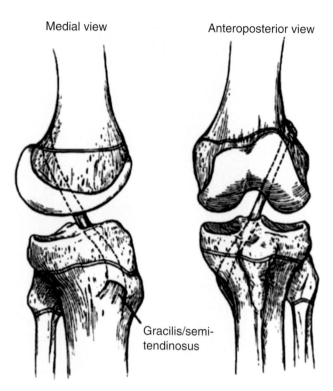

Medial view    Anteroposterior view

Gracilis/semi-tendinosus

**Figure 32.16** Anterior cruciate ligament (ACL) reconstruction using autogenous hamstring graft through tibial drill hole crossing proximal tibial physis to an over-the-top position on the distal femur. Hamstring graft is passed through the posterior knee capsule over the top of the lateral femoral condyle to a position on the distal femoral metaphysis where it is anchored with staples and/or sutures.

tibial physis, and placement of the soft tissue hamstring graft posterolaterally through the intercondylar notch to the lateral femoral metaphysis (over-the-top position) (150,151). This technique is employed in children who are Tanner stage 2 (Fig. 32.16).

Complete transphyseal techniques are similar to reconstructions in the case of adults, but may employ smaller drill holes and avoid any hardware crossing the physis (Fig. 32.17). Advantages of this technique are improved graft fixation and graft isometry (152). Excellent results are reported in adolescents close to maturity (152) (Fig. 32.18A,B). Variations of this technique include the use of Achilles tendon or patellar tendon allograft (154).

Transphyseal techniques can safely be employed in children with 1 year or less of growth remaining as determined by a wrist x-rays and the Greulich and Pyle atlas (Fig. 32.19A,B).

*Rehabilitation.* The success of surgery is partially dependent on the patient's compliance with a strict rehabilitation protocol. There are standard ACL reconstruction protocols that restore range of motion and strength and allow the graft to incorporate and mature. Return to preinjury sports usually takes 6 months following surgery and should not occur sooner.

*Recommendations.* For the child younger than 12 years, significant growth from the distal femoral physis and proximal tibial physis may be disturbed with conventional ACL reconstruction techniques. A trial of bracing is warranted in this age group in an attempt to control their instability and to wait until the child is near skeletal maturity. Full

sports participation is permitted if the brace successfully controls episodes of instability and giving way. If the brace is unsuccessful, a frank discussion regarding discontinuing sports or modifying activities should be undertaken with the child and the parents.

If the child and parents insist on continued athletic participation and understand the potential risks of growth disturbance, surgery should be a consideration.

For the child who has not been helped by bracing and is predicted to have at least 2 years of growth remaining (11 to 12 years of age in girls, 13 to 14 years of age in boys), I favor a partial transphyseal reconstruction employing several strands of hamstring tendon. The tibial drill hole should be 6 to 8 mm in diameter (larger hole for older children) and oriented more vertically than that in a standard ACL reconstruction in an adult. Rather than employing a femoral tunnel, I favor placement of the graft to an over-the-top position. The graft should not be tensioned as much as it is in the adult.

For the child with a torn ACL who is nearing skeletal maturity as demonstrated by bone age (13 years of age in girls and 15 in boys), I favor a complete transphyseal reconstruction (Fig. 32.17, 32.18A,B).

Treatment recommendations are summarized in Figure 32.20.

Medial view          Anteroposterior view

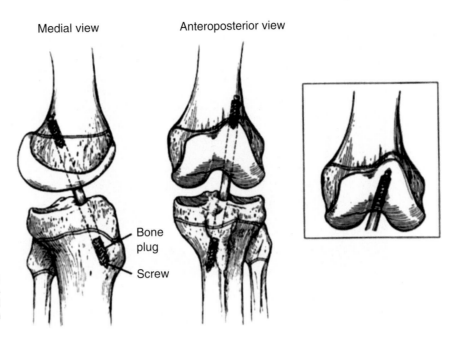

Bone
plug

Screw

**Figure 32.17** Diagram of transphyseal anterior cruciate ligament (ACL) reconstruction. Note vertical orientation of drill holes; fixation should not encroach on either physis.

## Osteochondritis Dissecans

OCD is a developmental condition of the joint in which the articular cartilage and underlying bone are involved. Originally described by Paget (155) as "quiet necrosis," the condition remains an enigma as to etiology, pathogenesis, prognosis, and treatment. Juvenile osteochondritis dissecans (JOCD) has a much better prognosis than its adult counterpart and will be the focus of this discussion. It is a lesion of the articular cartilage and subchondral bone before closure of the growth plate and was originally described by Roberts (156).

### Etiology

The exact etiology of this unusual condition is unknown; it is probably multifactorial (156–163). Proposed causative factors include mechanics (trauma), ischemia, and heredity (161–166).

Langenskiöld (167) demonstrated that removal and replacement of a portion of articular cartilage of the distal femur in rabbits produced a lesion similar to OCD in humans. Biomechanical studies using finite element analysis have demonstrated that stresses are greatest in the subchondral bone of the medial femoral condyle and are maximal at 60 degrees of flexion (168).

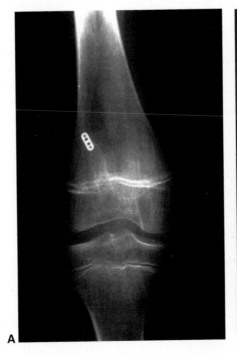
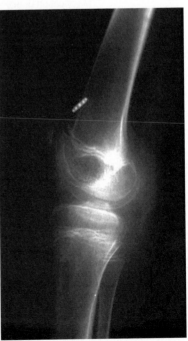

**Figure 32.18  A:** Anteroposterior radiograph of skeletally immature child who underwent transphyseal anterior cruciate ligament reconstruction utilizing autogenous hamstring tendon. Note vertical orientation of drill holes in proximal tibia and distal femur. **B:** Lateral radiograph of same patient.

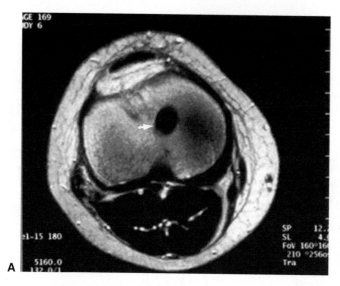
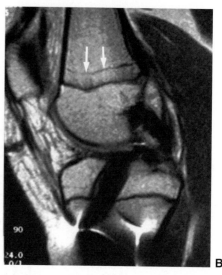

**Figure 32.19**   **A:** Magnetic resonance imaging (MRI) (axial) showing small, centrally placed drill hole in proximal tibia (*white arrow*). **B:** Lateral MRI image of same patient showing graft filling tibial tunnel. Note growth arrest lines on distal femur proximal to distal femoral physis (*white arrows*) indicating continued growth.

Mechanisms which have been shown to cause osteochondral fractures are similar to forces responsible for causing JOCD and include impaction of a tibial spine, direct impaction forces resulting in a "bone bruise,"

```
                Anterior cruciate ligament tear
                          in child
                             │
                             ↓
                Vigorous rehabilitation Bracing
                   Modification of activities
                       ↙              ↘
               No symptoms           Symptoms
                    ↓              ↙          ↘
            Skeletal maturity  Skeletal age   Skeletal age
                ↙     ↘          ♀ <13          ♀ ≥13
    Accommodation  Transphyseal   ♂ <14          ♂ ≥14
     of lifestyle  reconstruction    ↓              ↓
                              Small central drill  Transphyseal
                              hole through         reconstruction
                              proximal tibial physis
                              to over-the-top position
                              on femur or physeal
                              sparing surgery
```

**Figure 32.20**   Algorithm for treatment of anterior cruciate ligament (ACL) tear in children.

joint compression forces, and rotational injury patterns (169–173). In addition, Smillie (174) has suggested that the juvenile form may be caused by a disturbance in ossification of the epiphysis itself, resulting in the separation of small islands of bone from the main bony epiphysis.

Green and Banks (159), in their classic article, noted that the basic process in OCD was aseptic necrosis involving the subchondral bone. However, most other histologic studies of OCD do not reveal ischemic changes, but a reparative process at the interface between the fibrocartilage and the bone (175–177). With the advent of MRI to evaluate OCD lesions of the knee, it is apparent that ischemic changes of bone are rare.

A few articles, including those of Mubarak and Carroll (164) and another by Ribbing (178), discuss the familial nature of the lesion indicating an autosomal dominant inheritance pattern. However, most other large series refute the hereditary nature of the lesion (179).

The condition is most likely caused by multiple factors, including repetitive mechanical trauma or stress, in highly active children and adolescents (180).

### Symptoms and Signs

Nonspecific knee pain is the chief complaint in most children. The pain is activity-related, and its location is nonspecific. The patient may have complaints of giving way, locking, or swelling. In a large multicenter study carried out by Hefti et al. (181), 32% of patients had no or minor pain at presentation.

Tenderness may be elicited with deep palpation over the involved femoral condyle. A positive Wilson test occurs with the knee flexed 90 degrees and internally rotated. As the knee is extended, the patient complains of pain that is relieved by external rotation. The knee examination of patients with JOCD is notoriously poor for detecting the presence of this disorder (182).

## Imaging

Patients suspected of having JOCD should have routine radiographs including a "tunnel view," which is the best view for seeing the lesion in the classic location on the lateral aspect and posterior two-thirds of the medial femoral condyle.

MRI is a useful adjunct to determine the extent of articular cartilage involvement and the stability of the lesion (183–189) (Fig. 32.21A,B). A high-intensity signal on T2-weighted images between the lesion and the surrounding subchondral bone means that synovial fluid from the joint is present between the lesion and underlying subchondral bone, implying instability of the lesion (188). In children, the signal may represent a line of healing vascular granulation tissue, but it is pathognomonic of instability in the adult variety of OCD (189). MRI with gadolinium enhancement improves the ability to assess lesion stability, and MRI arthrography with gadolinium allows for virtually 100% ability to assess stability (190).

## Natural History

The true natural history of OCD is not known, but a large multicenter European study has given clues (181). In this study, patients with JOCD (patients with open physes) did better than adults; 22% of these patients with JOCD had abnormal knees at follow-up, whereas 42% of adults with OCD had abnormal knees.

The outcome of JOCD is significantly better in lesions that are stable at the time of presentation and in the classic location as opposed to any other location. Patients who were less active had a better result at follow-up than did active athletes. Patients with stable lesions at diagnosis did better with conservative (nonoperative) treatment than did those with surgery, regardless of the type of nonoperative treatment. Conversely, patients with unstable lesions did better with surgery than did those with nonoperative treatment. There was no superior method of fixation or resurfacing, as the numbers in these groups were too small for statistical analysis.

## Treatment Recommendations

The prognosis for JOCD is considerably better than the prognosis in its adult counterpart. The goals of treatment in JOCD include preservation of articular cartilage and stability of the lesion.

***Nonsurgical Treatment.*** In the child with open growth plates and a "stable" lesion, a period of nonoperative treatment is indicated. This usually involves immobilization in a non–weight-bearing cylinder cast for 6 to 10 weeks. It is of interest that in the European multicenter study, the results of all conservative treatment methods, including cast immobilization, bracing, physiotherapy, and non–weight-bearing were the same (181). Refraining from sports for 3 to 6 months is probably efficacious in children and adolescents with OCD lesions (156,183,185).

Plain radiographs are employed to evaluate bridging of bone across the lesion; JOCD lesions heal in an average of 4 to 5 months (160,191,192).

In summary, patients with JOCD lesions should undergo a period of nonoperative treatment including non–weight bearing for 6 to 10 weeks. Uncooperative patients should be managed in a cylinder cast. Refraining from sports for up to 6 months is advisable to allow lesions to heal.

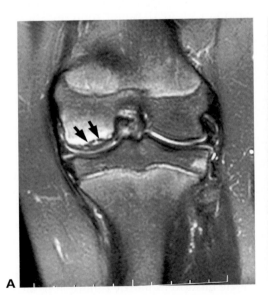 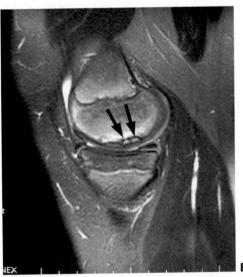

**Figure 32.21   A:** Magnetic resonance image (MRI) of a knee demonstrating osteochondritis dissecans lesion (*black arrows*) in the classical location (lateral aspect of medial femoral condyle). The lesion appears to be stable, with an intact articular surface. **B:** Lateral image of same knee (*black arrows* outline lesion).

*Surgical Treatment.* If the lesion fails to heal after nonoperative treatment of 6 months, or if the lesion is unstable, arthroscopic evaluation and treatment are indicated. Guhl classified lesions arthroscopically as (a) intact lesion, (b) early separated lesion, (c) partially detached lesion, (d) salvageable craters and loose bodies and (f) unsalvageable craters and loose bodies (193).

Intact lesions are usually drilled in a transarticular or retrograde manner to promote healing. The theory is that vascular ingrowth occurs in the small channels created by the K-wires or drill. Excellent results have been reported by several authors using the transarticular drilling technique (160,190,191). Some authors prefer not to violate the articular surface and use an extraarticular drilling method with or without bone graft to stimulate healing (185,193,194). Hefti's multicenter study was more discouraging than these studies (181). In a subgroup of 58 patients demonstrating marked sclerosis, little benefit or healing was noted.

In the situation of early separation or partial detachment, internal fixation of the lesion is indicated (181,191). This can be accomplished by two or more divergent K-wires, by the use of Herbert or other small fragment screws in which the heads of the screws are countersunk below the articular surface, by bioabsorbable pins or screws, or even autogenous bone pegs (195–198).

Postoperatively, the patient remains non–weight bearing for 6 to 8 weeks after fixation. It is imperative to schedule a second-look arthroscopy to see if the fixation is raised before the resumption of weight bearing. If the screw heads are too prominent, they are turned in further to prevent articular cartilage erosion.

If the lesion is partially detached, the bed should be freshened down to bleeding bone. The bed may require a small amount of bone grafting before the OCD lesion is replaced and fixed. It is important to achieve articular congruity at the completion of the fixation procedure (189). The patient is kept non–weight bearing for 6 to 8 weeks and on occasion rearthroscopy of the knee is performed to evaluate if the screw heads are raised and need to be countersunk further or eventually removed when the lesion is definitely healed.

For unsalvageable craters and loose bodies, the loose body or bodies are removed, and the edges of the articular cartilage trimmed. Fragment excision alone appears to have poor long-term results, although in the short-term knee function may be excellent. In the European Pediatric Orthopaedic Society study, Hefti et al. (181) reported 48% poor results after fragment excision alone. Because of the poor results, they recommended some technique to restore the articular surface. Anderson and Pagnani (199) also reported a preponderance of poor results in young patients at follow-up an average of 5 years after fragment excision.

The restoration of the articular surface may be accomplished by microfracture technique or drilling (200,201), osteochondral allografts (202–207), mosaicplasty, or autologous chondrocyte regeneration (208,209). These techniques need further refinement and development before they can be widely recommended for use in children and adolescents.

Treatment recommendations are summarized in Figure 32.22.

## Quadriceps Contusion

Blunt trauma to the anterior thigh is not an uncommon injury that occurs when playing football, hockey, and even non-contact sports such as soccer or basketball. If the force is severe enough, it will result in muscle hemorrhage, followed by the formation of granulation tissue over the course of the next few weeks, which can mature into a dense collagenous scar and lead to significant disability (210). It is therefore important to recognize this injury early to prevent long-term problems.

In the early stages of hemorrhage, significant bleeding may occur. It is accompanied by thigh swelling, pain, and loss of knee flexion.

Radiographs of the femur, including hip and knee, should be taken to rule out fracture and epiphyseal separation. The differential diagnosis should also include osteomyelitis and tumor (osteosarcoma or Ewing sarcoma), which can be ruled out with a careful history and normal laboratory workup.

Initial treatment consists of rest, ice, compression, and elevation (RICE). The knee and thigh may be further protected by employing a knee immobilizer and crutches. When the pain and muscle spasm subside, gentle active range of motion is begun. Passive stretching to increase knee flexion is not permitted and will exacerbate bleeding and formation of scar tissue. Progressive strengthening and exercise are permitted after 90 degrees of knee flexion is obtained. Moderate–to–severe contusions take from 4 to 6 weeks, on an average, to heal before return to sports participation (211–213). Minor contusions take considerably less time.

A careful evaluation of the athlete is performed before allowing full participation in sports. Knee motion of at least 120 degrees, at least 80% strength of the opposite leg, and functional agility are required (211–213). Special thigh guards can be employed to protect from further injury.

Complications of quadriceps contusion include the very rare situation of compartment syndrome of the thigh and myositis ossificans.

Anterior compartment syndrome of the thigh is usually manifested by severe thigh swelling and pain after a significant contusion, and has also been described after relatively minor trauma in a patient with a bleeding disorder. Like its counterpart in the arm or leg, it demands fasciotomy to prevent muscle necrosis (214).

Myositis ossificans traumatica is a complication after severe quadriceps muscle contusion or after reinjury and occurs in up to 20% of quadriceps contusions (211).

Radiographically, flocculated densities appear at 2 to 4 weeks postinjury within the muscle mass, and periosteal

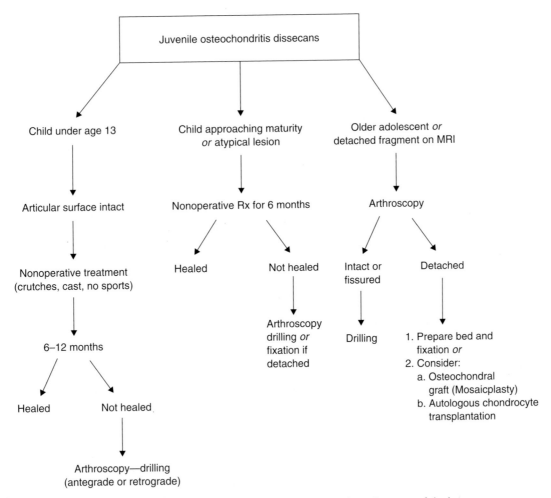

**Figure 32.22**  Algorithm for treatment of juvenile osteochondritis dissecans of the knee.

new bone may also be seen. By 3 to 6 months, the bony changes stabilize (214,215).

Despite these radiographic changes, the athlete often exhibits no functional deficit. No treatment is required if the patient is functioning well, and full participation in sports is permitted.

Loss of knee flexion and pain may rarely occur, in which case surgical excision should be undertaken, but only after the myositis has matured, which usually takes 6 months. Plain radiographs on a sequential basis will provide evidence that the lesion is mature and not continuing to ossify. A bone scan may be helpful in showing the lesion to be relatively quiescent in its uptake of radionucleotide, which is suggestive of maturity of the lesion. Nonsteroid antiinflammatory drugs (NSAIDs) may be used before and after excision of the myositis ossificans to prevent recurrence, but there is no evidence that NSAIDs are beneficial in this clinical situation.

## Ankle Sprains

In the adult population, ankle sprains comprise 25% of athletic injuries (216–218). Younger children are more likely to suffer an injury to the distal fibular physis, whereas ankle sprains are more common in adolescents.

### Mechanism of Injury

Almost all ankle sprains are caused by a plantar flexion and inversion injury. The lateral ligaments; namely, the anterior talofibular ligament, calcaneofibular ligament, and posterior talofibular ligament are injured in that sequence.

With the ankle in plantar flexion and inversion, the effect of bony stability is minimized and the lateral ligaments become the primary lateral stabilizers, with the anterior talofibular becoming the most important (216).

The differentiation between physeal injury (fracture) and ligamentous injury is made primarily on the basis of the anatomical location of the pain and tenderness. If the maximal tenderness is directly over the distal fibula, a fracture or physeal injury is suspected and x-rays are taken. If the maximal tenderness is directly over the anterior talofibular ligament or calcaneofibular ligament, there is little need for x-rays (217). If there is excessive swelling and it is difficult to determine the exact area of maximal tenderness, one should err on the side of caution and obtain three views of the ankle—anteroposterior, lateral, and mortise.

### Classification and Management

Ligament injuries are classified according to severity and disruption of the anatomic structure of the ligaments (219). Grade I sprains (mild) have no appreciable disruption of tissue and there is minimal loss of function. Grade I sprains involve the anterior talofibular ligament only. Grade II sprains (moderate) have some disruption of tissue and partial loss of function with involvement of the anterior talofibular and calcaneofibular ligaments. Grade III sprains (severe) have significant or complete disruption of tissue with involvement of all the lateral ligaments and even the deltoid medially. There is marked loss of function. The type of sprain is best determined by the anatomic location of the pain and swelling and the degree of disability of the patient.

Grade III sprains and interosseous ligament injuries are more prone to develop osteochondral fractures and chronic instability. The diagnosis of interosseous ligament injury is based largely on the mechanism of the injury, the physical findings, and in rare instances radiographic findings.

Interosseous ligament injuries are universally seen in conjunction with a deltoid ligament injury. They are seen when the mechanism of injury is pronation–abduction, pronation–external rotation, and supination–external rotation of the foot. If the syndesmosis is significantly disrupted, squeezing the fibula and tibia together proximally will cause pain distally at the site of the syndesmosis in the ankle. In addition, increased side-to-side mobility of the talus in the ankle mortise when the distal leg is grasped is indicative of a syndesmosis injury. Plain radiographs that show widening of the syndesmosis width greater than 5 mm are indicative of a syndesmosis rupture.

### Rehabilitation of Patients with Ankle Sprains

Rehabilitation after an acute ankle sprain is divided into three phases. Phase I consists of rest and protection (brace, cast, splint, crutches, and ice wrap); control of swelling (ice, compression, and elevation), and early weight bearing. Phase II is aimed at reducing residual swelling and restoring range of motion of the ankle as well as strength, followed by low-impact aerobic training. The final phase (Phase III) includes proprioceptive exercises and sports-specific skills such as running, cutting, and jumping, with a gradual return to sports. With the return to sports, the athlete may benefit from an ankle stabilization brace or taping, although there is no evidence that they prevent further injury (220).

Chronic ankle instability in skeletally immature athletes is distinctly uncommon. A careful clinical and radiographic examination of the ankle and hindfoot is mandatory in patients with continuing symptoms. It is important to differentiate between functional instability and mechanical instability in the patient who complains of giving way after an ankle sprain. Functional instability is a subjective feeling of giving way during physical activity, occurring in up to 50% of patients following an ankle sprain. Its exact mechanism is unclear, but it is thought to be due to a disorder of proprioception, muscle control, and ligamentous stability. Functional instability is best managed with proprioceptive training (ankle tilt board), muscular strengthening, and the use of ankle taping or bracing for athletic activities.

Mechanical instability indicates incompetence of the stabilizing ligaments of the ankle and is demonstrated clinically by the ankle drawer test and talar tilt stress radiographs. A side-to-side difference of 10 mm or more of anterior talar translation and a talar tilt of 9 degrees or more on stress radiographs is highly suggestive of mechanical instability (221).

In addition to chronic ankle instability, the differential diagnosis includes tarsal coalition and osteochondral fracture or OCD of the talar dome.

In the rare case of chronic ankle instability in the young athlete, ligamentous reconstruction may be necessary. A variety of options exist to reconstruct the anterior talofibular ligament and calcaneofibular ligament, among them the Evans procedure (222), Watson-Jones technique (223), and the Chrisman-Snook modification of the Elmslie procedure (224). The most widely used reconstruction method is the Bröstrom repair, a direct repair and imbrication of the anterior talofibular and calcaneofibular ligaments (225). Biomechanical and clinical data support this anatomic reconstruction method (226,227).

## Avulsion Fractures of the Pelvis

Avulsion fractures of the pelvis are not uncommon injuries seen in adolescents and young adults. Avulsion fractures occur primarily between the ages of 14 and 25 years and account for approximately 15% of pelvic fractures in children (228–230).

### Etiology

The usual mechanism is a sudden and forceful concentric or eccentric muscle contraction, which occurs with rapid acceleration or deceleration.

This mechanism is commonly seen in particular sporting activities such as sprinting and jumping sports, as well as soccer and football (228). The same mechanism that would cause a muscle or tendon strain in an adult may cause an apophyseal avulsion in an adolescent.

### Clinical Features

The common avulsions are from the ASIS due to violent contraction of the sartorius as seen in jumping or running, from the anterior inferior iliac spine (AIIS) due to overpull of the straight head of the rectus femoris, and from the ischial tuberosity due to forceful contraction of the hamstrings (Fig. 32.23). Avulsions of the AIIS are often seen in participants of sports involving kicking action, and avulsions of the ischial tuberosity are seen in gymnasts and hurdlers.

The ischial tuberosity appears at 15 years of age and may not unite until 25 years of age, making ischial avulsions possible even in early adulthood (230).

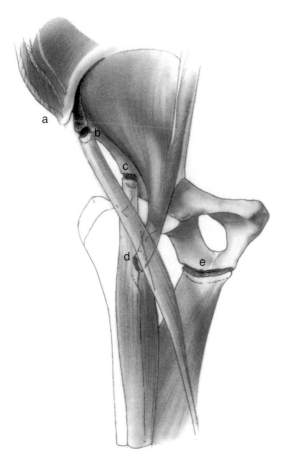

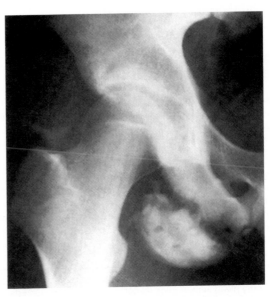

**Figure 32.24** Anteroposterior radiograph of right hip demonstrating how avulsion fracture of ischium may be mistaken for neoplasm or infection.

**Figure 32.23** Avulsion fractures of the growing pelvis result from traction injuries where major muscle groups insert into or originate from apophyses about the pelvis. The abdominal and trunk muscles insert into the iliac apophysis (*a*). The sartorius originates from the anterior superior iliac apophysis (*b*). The direct head of the rectus femoris originates from the anterior inferior iliac apophysis (*c*). The iliopsoas inserts into the lesser trochanteric apophysis (*d*). The hamstrings originate from the ischial apophysis (*e*).

With all apophyseal avulsions, there may be a history of antecedent prodromal pain signifying apophysitis before the avulsion. Athletes with avulsions present with local pain, swelling, and tenderness confined to the avulsed area. Pain is reproduced by active or passive stretch of the involved muscle.

### Radiographic Features

Plain radiographs are usually sufficient to identify the area of avulsion. Special views to place the ASIS or AIIS in profile may help in delineating the avulsion. If the lesion is acute, the diagnosis is usually straightforward.

However, if the patient is seen several weeks after the inciting event, the radiographs may be misinterpreted as showing a neoplasm or infection. A careful history and normal laboratory values aid in making the correct diagnosis (Fig. 32.24).

### Treatment

The recommended treatment of patients with pelvic avulsion fractures has generally been rest, followed by a specific rehabilitation program. Metzmaker and Pappas (231) outlined a five-stage rehabilitation program that consists of rest to relax the involved muscle groups as well as ice wrap and analgesics, initiation of gentle active and passive motion, resistance exercises after 75% of motion is regained, stretching and strengthening exercises with an emphasis on sports-specific exercises, and finally return to competitive sports.

Surgical intervention with attempts at open reduction and internal fixation have been recommended for isolated incidents, but there appears to be no superiority of operative intervention over conservative management (231).

Patients should be advised that the wait for return to competitive athletics may be prolonged. The earliest that such a return can be expected is 6 weeks, but it is not uncommon for complaints to persist for up to 4 to 6 months (228,232).

## Dislocations of the Shoulder (Glenohumeral Joint)

### Incidence

Dislocations of the glenohumeral joint in the young athlete are extremely rare. Overall, the incidence in children younger than 12 years represents less than 5% of all glenohumeral dislocations (233–238).

### Anatomic Considerations

The shoulder joint is inherently unstable, with a relatively large humeral head articulating with a small, shallow, glenoid fossa. The average vertical dimension of the adult humeral head is 48 mm with an average transverse diameter of 45 mm. The glenoid fossa, on the other hand, measures 35 mm in its vertical dimension and 25 mm in its transverse dimension (239). As a consequence, the range of motion in

## TABLE 32.3

### CLASSIFICATION OF DISLOCATION OF THE GLENOHUMERAL JOINT IN CHILDREN

**Traumatic Dislocation**

As result of true traumatic force, proximal humerus may displace anteriorly, posteriorly, or inferiorly

May occur at birth or later as a result of injury to brachial plexus or central nervous system

**Atraumatic Dislocation—Voluntary or Involuntary**

Occurs in a number of nontraumatic causes

Congenital abnormalities or deficiencies

Hereditary joint laxity problems such as Ehlers-Danlos syndrome

Developmental joint laxity problems

Emotional and psychiatric disturbances

Other

From Dameron TB, Rockwood CA. Part 2. Subluxations and dislocations of the glenohumeral joint. In: Rockwood CA, Green DP, eds. *Fractures*, 2nd ed., Vol. 3. Philadelphia, PA: JB Lippincott Co, 1984, with permission.

each direction is accomplished at the expense of stability of the joint. Although still considered a ball and socket joint, the shoulder joint is similar to a golf ball on a tee (239).

### Mechanism of Injury

Traumatic dislocations in children occur with the same mechanisms as those seen in adults, including significant falls on to an outstretched hand and forced abduction and external rotation injuries during contact sports.

### Classification

The most widely used classification system is the Rockwood classification (240). There are two broad categories, namely, traumatic or atraumatic (Table 32.3). Of 44 cases studied by Dameron and Rockwood, 8 were traumatic and 36 were atraumatic.

### Clinical Features

*Acute Dislocation.* A child with a traumatic anterior dislocation presents with the arm held in slight abduction and external rotation. With traumatic posterior dislocations, the arm is held adducted and in marked internal rotation. With either dislocation, the normal rounded contour of the shoulder is lost, and any attempt to move the shoulder either actively or passively is extremely painful. The humeral head may be palpated anteriorly in the subcoracoid position with anterior dislocation or posteriorly with posterior dislocations.

A careful history and physical examination are vital in the diagnosis of recurrent shoulder instability, especially in the young athlete. Assessments of active and passive range of motion, strength of the shoulder girdle and upper arm musculature, as well as examination of the cervical spine should be performed.

Specific tests for impingement in the terminal 10 to 15 degrees of passive forward flexion are noted. Most important for the assessment of instability are the evaluation of translation of the humeral head on the glenoid and apprehension and relocation testing.

*Recurrent Dislocation.* Glenohumeral stability may be assessed with the patient in the sitting or supine position. The sitting position requires a relaxed cooperative patient, but the supine position is usually preferred, especially with provocative tests for dislocation.

Translation of the humeral head is first evaluated with the shoulder in the neutral position, in external rotation for anterior inferior testing, and in flexion and internal rotation for posterior inferior translation. The amount of translation in each direction is quantified and compared to the healthy shoulder (Fig. 32.25). A grading system has been employed as shown in Table 32.4 (241).

### Provocative Tests

These are often referred to as *apprehension tests* and reproduce the mechanism of instability (dislocation) that the patient recognizes.

The anterior apprehension test is performed by abducting and externally rotating the shoulder 90 degrees in each direction. As more force is gently applied, the athlete will

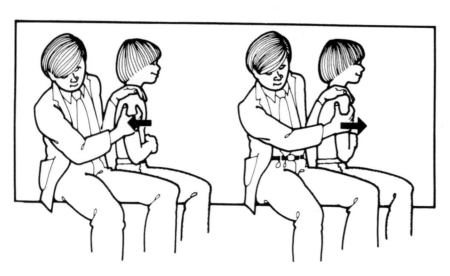

**Figure 32.25** The drawer test for anteroposterior instability of the glenohumeral joint. The examiner, seated next to the patient, uses one hand to grasp the humeral head to translate it anteriorly and posteriorly, while stabilizing the scapula with the opposite hand and forearm. (Modified from Curtis RJ Jr, Rockwood CA. Fractures and dislocations of the shoulder in children. In: Rockwood CA Jr, Matsen FA III, eds. *The shoulder.* WB Saunders, Philadelphia, PA. 1990:991, with permission.)

## TABLE 32.4

### GRADING OF GLENOHUMERAL STABILITY BASED ON TRANSLATION OF THE HUMERAL HEAD

| Grade | Description |
|-------|-------------|
| 1 | No increase in translation |
| 2 | Translation to the glenoid rim |
| 3 | Translation on to the glenoid rim with spontaneous reduction (subluxation) |
| 4 | Translation beyond the glenoid rim (dislocation) |

From Pagnani MJ, Galinat BJ, Warren RF. *Glenohumeral instability in: Orthopaedic sports medicine. Principles and practice.* WB Saunders Co. Philadelphia. 1994:580–623, with permission.

become apprehensive of an impending dislocation and either adduct and internally rotate the shoulder or demonstrate their concern by changing facial expression or by making a sound.

For the posterior apprehension test, the shoulder is flexed to 90 degrees and internally rotated with a posterior force applied to the shoulder joint through the upper extremity.

Relocation tests are performed to validate the examiner's suspicions of shoulder instability, and are best performed with the patient in the supine position. After the anterior apprehension test has been performed, a hand is placed anteriorly over the upper humerus and a posteriorly directed force is applied while again performing the apprehension test. If positive, the relocation test should relieve the patient's apprehension and can be verified by removing the posterior force to see if the apprehension returns.

The posterior relocation test is accomplished in the opposite manner, with a hand held over the posterior aspect of the upper humerus (applying an anteriorly directed force) while the posterior apprehension test is performed.

Inferior or multidirectional instability is evaluated by the sulcus test (Fig. 32.26). With the patient sitting, the humerus is grasped distally just above the elbow, and an inferiorly directed force is applied while stabilizing the scapula. A dimple or gap will appear over the lateral shoulder as the humeral head is translated inferiorly. The sulcus sign is pathognomonic of multidirectional instability (240).

To assess for generalized ligamentous laxity, which is often seen in multidirectional and voluntary dislocations, a number of clinical tests should be quickly assessed, including thumb-to-forearm abduction, hyperextension of metacarpal phalangeal joints (5th finger greater than 90 degrees), elbow hyperextension greater than 10 degrees, knee hyperextension greater than 10 degrees, and palms to floor with knees extended (242). If the athlete has two or more of these signs, the diagnosis and implications of generalized ligamentous laxity should be considered. Surgery is generally contraindicated in this group of patients.

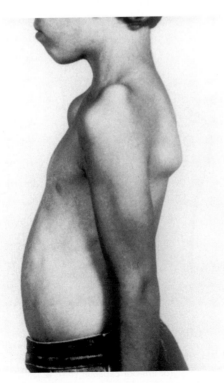
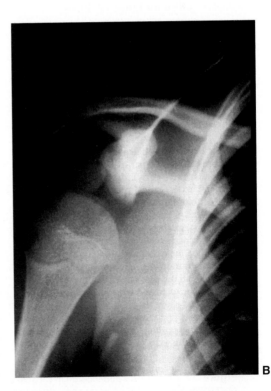

**Figure 32.26**  **A:** A patient with voluntary, atraumatic instability of left shoulder demonstrating "sulcus" sign. **B:** Anteroposterior view of the shoulder, demonstrating inferior subluxation of humeral head.

### Treatment Recommendations

***Nonsurgical.*** Prereduction films should be taken in most patients to confirm the direction of dislocation and to rule out fracture. However, the diagnosis of anterior dislocation is readily apparent with the arm held in slight abduction and external rotation with the humeral head palpable anteriorly. If the treating physician is experienced in diagnosis and management, reduction of the dislocation without prior x-rays is permitted. On the playing field this is accomplished by gentle traction on the arm in slight abduction, forward flexion, and internal rotation prior to the onset of muscle spasm.

In the emergency room, reduction is best accomplished by appropriate sedation and placing the patient prone with the arm hanging free and 5 to 10 lb (2–5 Kg) of weight attached to the upper extremity.

Therapy should be aimed at restoration of motion and then a specific strengthening program. The athlete should work vigorously on the anterior rotator cuff (supraspinatus and subscapularis) as well as the periscapular muscles following an anterior dislocation. In the rare case of a posterior dislocation, the posterior rotator cuff muscles or external rotators (infraspinatus and teres minor) should be isolated and strengthened. Four specific exercises have been shown to strengthen glenohumeral muscles (243):

1. "Press-up" exercise. In seated position, the patient lifts his or her body from a chair by placing the hands on the chair and extending the upper extremities.
2. Elevation of the arm in the sagittal plane.
3. Elevation of the arm in the scapular plane with the arm internally rotated and thumbs pointing down.

4. Horizontal adduction from the prone position with the arm externally rotated.

***Surgical.*** The redislocation rate after the initial event is 80% to 85% in patients younger than 20 years (232–238,244). The high rate of redislocation has prompted some surgeons to recommend surgical repair of the Bankart lesion by arthroscopic technique immediately after the initial dislocation (238–246). This approach should be reserved for high-demand athletes until such time as the evidence of the benefits of early surgical stabilization is verified.

However, once the diagnosis of recurrent glenohumeral instability has been made, recommendations regarding surgical stabilization are strongly advocated in younger patients. The decision regarding surgical intervention is usually made after two or three dislocations and the patient's and family's expressed desire to resume an active lifestyle without the feeling of shoulder instability.

### Complications

***Recurrence.*** In almost all cases of recurrent shoulder dislocation, the instability is due to the so-called Bankart lesion, or avulsion of the capsule and/or labrum from the anterior glenoid. Surgery, be it arthroscopic or open technique, is aimed at restoration or repair of this anterior capsulolabral complex to eliminate the Bankart lesion (245–247).

For the young athlete with recurrent *traumatic* multidirectional instability, an arthroscopic or open capsular shift is recommended (Fig. 32.27). Careful preoperative evaluation of these patients is necessary to differentiate them from the atraumatic group. In the latter group, surgery is usually doomed to failure (240,241).

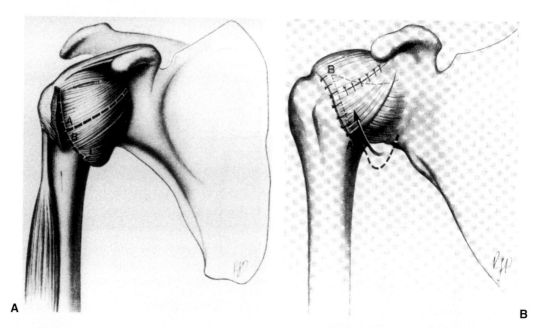

A                                          B

**Figure 32.27  A:** T-shaped incision in capsule in preparation for inferior capsular shift. **B:** Diagram of capsule after inferior capsular shift. After preparing the posterior, inferior, and anterior humeral neck, the lower flap is brought upward, reducing the joint volume and eliminating redundant capsule. The upper flap is sutured over the lower one for further reinforcement. (From Neer CS. *Shoulder Reconstruction.* Philadelphia: WB Saunders, 1990, with permission.)

Atraumatic dislocation is divided into voluntary dislocation, in which the patient learns to voluntarily subluxate or dislocate the glenohumeral joint and involuntary dislocation, in which the dislocation occurs with a specific event such as carrying heavy weight. Involuntary atraumatic dislocation is often seen in association with generalized ligamentous laxity in connective tissue disorders such as Ehlers-Danlos or Marfan syndromes (240).

On the other hand, voluntary dislocation of the glenohumeral joint is encountered in patients with a high incidence of psychological or even psychiatric disorder (248,249). Surgery should never be contemplated in this specific subset of patients, but psychological support and rehabilitation will often help (240,248,249).

Surgery in the involuntary atraumatic group should only be contemplated after failure of a vigorous muscle-strengthening program involving all the muscle groups of the shoulder for at least 6 to 12 months. The rare patient who fails this program may be a candidate for an inferior capsular shift procedure, but the failure rate will still be high due to the association with ligamentous laxity (240,241).

A small group of athletes taking part in sports with a high demand for throwing will complain of pain and decreased ability to throw. On examination, the athlete demonstrates signs of rotator cuff impingement and inflammation, with pain and weakness on resisted supination testing. There are subtle signs of glenohumeral instability upon translation testing and provocative maneuvers. These patients respond well to rest, cessation of throwing, and NSAIDs for 2 to 4 weeks, followed by a vigorous rehabilitation program once the pain has resolved. Specific strengthening of the rotator cuff and scapular stabilizers is employed and also an examination of the throwing mechanics of these athletes. Results with these nonoperative regimes are encouraging (238,250–254).

# NEUROLOGIC INJURY

Injury to the axillary nerve is not uncommon following traumatic or anterior dislocation, and musculocutaneous nerve injury has also been reported (239,240). In both cases, these injuries are almost all traction neuropraxias and will resolve spontaneously.

In the case of open surgical approaches, knowledge of the anatomic location, course, and direction of these nerves is essential to prevent iatrogenic injury (254–257).

# OVERUSE INJURIES

## Anterior Knee Pain in Adolescents

Anterior knee pain is a common entity seen in the adolescent, both the competitive athlete and nonathlete. Anterior knee pain can occur as the result of a number of musculoskeletal conditions and can prove challenging for the orthopaedist to sort out. These conditions may include "chondromalacia patellae" or idiopathic anterior knee pain, Osgood-Schlatter syndrome, Sinding-Larsen-Johansson syndrome, synovial plica, or patellar or quadriceps tendinitis.

Anterior knee pain in adolescents is usually caused by repetitive overload conditions rather than a specific traumatic event.

### Differential Diagnosis

Any child or adolescent with anterior knee pain must have a careful hip examination to rule out referred pain from hip pathology such as slipped capital femoral epiphysis or Legg-Calvé-Perthes disease. In particular, any loss of hip motion or an abnormal gait demands careful clinical and radiographic evaluation of the hip.

### Osgood-Schlatter Syndrome

Osgood-Schlatter syndrome or disease (OSD) is a traction apophysitis of the tibial tubercle. This is an entity that is common in athletes between 10 and 15 years of age, particularly in those involved in jumping sports. Osgood-Schlatter syndrome is historically more prevalent in boys, but occurs with some frequency in girls as well.

The cause of OSD is repetitive traction on the secondary ossification center of the tibial tuberosity. It probably represents a true avulsion or stress fracture of the tibial tuberosity ossification center. Some authors have postulated that OSD occurs more frequently in patients with patella alta (258), while others have postulated the exact opposite as a contributing factor, namely, patella infera or baja (259).

**Clinical Features.** Symptoms vary widely in adolescents with this condition. In the acute phase, pain and tenderness directly over the tibial tubercle are noted. After the acute phase heals, the pain and tenderness subside, and the only positive physical finding may be an anterior mass. Pain in this phase occurs usually after physical activity.

**Radiographic Features.** The diagnosis is almost always a clinical one, and x-rays merely confirm what is already known from history and physical examination. If the condition is bilateral, plain radiographs are not necessary. However, in unilateral cases, x-rays should be ordered to rule out other pathology such as tumor or infection.

Plain radiographs (true lateral view of knee with leg internally rotated 10 to 20 degrees to place the tibial tubercle in profile) usually show fragmentation of the tubercle or a loose ossicle separate from the underlying tuberosity. Further investigations such as MRI, CAT scans, or ultrasound are not necessary (Fig. 32.28).

**Natural History.** In a study of 50 adults who had OSD in childhood, 76% had no symptoms or any limitation of function, 60% had pain when kneeling, and most noted the presence of a prominent tibial tubercle (259). Osgood-Schlatter disease has been noted to be a predisposing factor

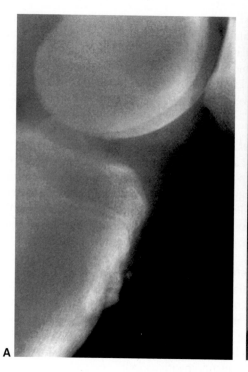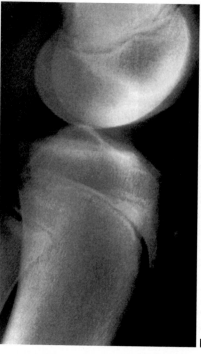

A

B

**Figure 32.28** Osgood-Schlatter disease. **A:** Typical radiographic findings include a prominence of the tibial tubercle with irregularity of the bone at the insertion of the patellar tendon. **B:** In some cases, a separate ossicle may form and not unite. If persistently symptomatic, this ossicle may require excision.

in cases of tibial tubercle fracture, but no direct cause-and-effect relation has been demonstrated (260–262).

### Treatment

*Nonsurgical.* The treatment of OSD in the growing child is always nonoperative. Time, rest, and occasional immobilization usually result in marked improvement of symptoms (263–267). Activity should be limited until the pain resolves and the athlete demonstrates a full painless range of knee motion. Use of ice wraps can help the acute situation and NSAIDs may relieve some of the pain. After the acute phase, a maintenance program of stretching, especially of the quadriceps, and strengthening of the quadriceps and hamstrings may help the athlete.

*Surgical.* If the patient is skeletally mature and still symptomatic, excision of the loose ossicle resolves the symptoms in most cases (268,269).

### Sinding-Larsen-Johansson Syndrome

Sinding-Larsen-Johansson (SLJ) syndrome is a condition similar to Osgood-Schlatter disease, but affecting only the proximal attachment of the patellar tendon to the inferior pole of the patella. It typically affects children at a slightly younger age than is the case with OSD; namely, 10 to 12 years.

Patients present with point tenderness at the inferior pole of the patella. Radiographs may show calcification at the inferior pole (Fig. 32.29). The condition is thought to be due to repetitive tensile stress at the junction of the tendon and bone (270,271).

Treatment is similar to that for OSD. Little is known of the natural history of SLJ syndrome. Most patients respond to rest and NSAIDs (272).

There is little, if any, evidence of the benefits of NSAIDs for the osteochondroses. In almost all cases where they are administered, cessation of physical activity may be just as important in relieving the symptoms. However, their use seems justified, given the inflammatory nature of these conditions.

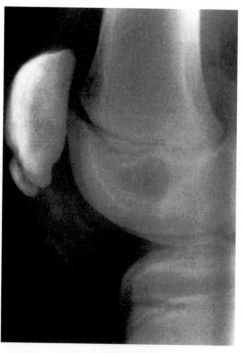

**Figure 32.29** Sinding-Larsen-Johannson disease. The lateral radiograph best demonstrates the irregularity at the inferior pole of the patella.

### Synovial Plica Syndrome

Synovial plica are normal synovial folds within the knee joint that can cause knee pain. With trauma or repetitive motion, the plicae may hypertrophy, causing pain and signs of intraarticular pathology (273–277).

**Clinical Features.** The most common plica to cause symptoms is the medial patellar plica, which anatomically runs from the superior medial pole of the patella or midpatella to the medial patellar fat pad (276). Other plicae which have been described are the suprapatellar, lateral, and infrapatellar plicae (277) (Fig. 32.30).

Most plicae are asymptomatic, but occasionally this condition is a true symptomatic entity. The patient complains of anterior or anteromedial knee pain, often after repetitive activities such as running, jumping, or squatting. The athlete may complain of a popping or snapping sensation with their knee in midflexion. Giving way may also be a symptom.

Physical examination usually reveals tenderness directly over the plica as it comes over the medial femoral condyle to the infrapatellar fat pad, and possibly a palpable snapping sensation as the knee is flexed from 30 to 60 degrees of flexion while the patient is weight bearing or standing. In some cases, synovial plicae are associated with signs of lateral patellar instability.

**Radiographic Features.** Plain radiographs are normal, and other imaging studies have not proven to be of value. This syndrome is a clinical diagnosis of exclusion after other causes of knee pain and popping have been ruled out.

**Pathoanatomy.** Symptomatic plicae demonstrate hypertrophy and inflammation which lead to thickening and eventual fibrosis. With significant fibrosis, changes in the articular surface and even subchondral bone may occur (278).

### Treatment Recommendations

*Nonsurgical.* Treatment should consist of nonoperative therapy including rest, ice wrap, NSAIDs, and a gradual strengthening program, especially of the quadriceps and hamstrings, avoiding terminal extension if pain is reproduced (279).

*Surgical.* Rarely, symptoms will fail to resolve after months of nonoperative treatment. Arthroscopic resection of the plica is indicated in those rare cases, with excellent results expected in 90% of cases (275,280–288). Simple division of the plica has been associated with recurrence and is not recommended. At the time of surgical resection, the joint is thoroughly examined for other causes of internal derangement such as meniscal tear or patellar maltracking.

### Hoffa Syndrome

Originally described by Hoffa in 1904 (289), very little is known about this condition in children or adolescents. Anatomic studies of the fat pad have revealed a densely innervated tissue, and because of its anatomic location, its role as a possible cause of anterior knee pain is debated (290–294). It has been mentioned as a source of pain or pathology in conjunction with other entities such as patellar tendinitis, meniscal tear, ACL disruption and reconstruction, impingement after intramedullary nail placement, and tibial osteotomy (278,294).

Symptoms are similar to those in patients with patellar tendinitis or SLJ syndrome. In the latter condition, maximal tenderness is at the inferior pole of the patella. In Hoffa syndrome, the maximal area of tenderness is at the anterior joint line on either side and deep to the patellar tendon.

Management is nonsurgical and consists of rest, ice, and NSAIDs. A diagnostic intraarticular local anesthetic injection directly into the fat pad may be of help in those patients whose symptoms fail to resolve. There is little information as to the efficacy of surgical management for this condition (295). Because such doubt exists as to the validity of the diagnosis, surgical recommendations as a treatment option cannot be made (296).

### Idiopathic Anterior Knee Pain

Physicians and surgeons are generally unwilling to admit that a patient's complaints defy a plausible explanation. However, anterior knee pain in children and adolescents can exist in the absence of positive physical findings for any of the pathologic conditions causing knee pain. In that case, the term "idiopathic anterior knee pain" is used (296,297).

These patients typically complain of anterior knee pain with insidious onset. The pain is often bilateral, more commonly worse in one knee. The pain is made worse with physical activity such as running, jumping, squatting, going up and down stairs, or after prolonged sitting with the knee in flexed position.

Physical examination may reveal so-called "miserable malalignment" including excessive internal femoral torsion, external tibial torsion, mild genu valgum with medial deviation of the patella, and a tendency to pes planus or

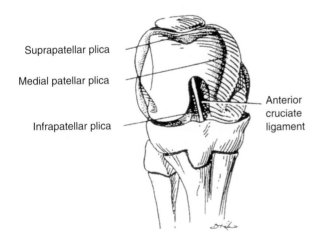

**Figure 32.30** Plicae of the knee. The suprapatellar (superior) plica, the medial plica, which is the one most commonly symptomatic, and the inferior plica (ligamentum mucosum), which overlies the anterior cruciate ligament.

Suprapatellar plica

Medial patellar plica

Infrapatellar plica

Anterior cruciate ligament

foot pronation. Patients typically point to the entire anterior aspect of the knee as the location of the pain. The patients usually do not have an effusion and have a full range of motion. The patella may be hypermobile and have some evidence of maltracking, but without signs of patellar subluxation or dislocation. There may be atrophy of the quadriceps and patellar crepitus with flexion and extension of the knee or a patellar compression test.

Examination of patellar tracking should include assessment of the Q angle, lateral tilt, and lateral tracking.

**Radiographic Assessment.** Plain radiographs including an anteroposterior, lateral, notch view, and Merchant view should be taken (Fig. 32.1). In most cases, the plain radiographs are normal. Unless the clinical diagnosis is suggestive of another pathology, there is no indication to proceed to other imaging studies such as MRI.

**Treatment and Prognosis.** Historically, the term "chondromalacia patellae" has been used to describe this entity (298). "Chondromalacia patellae" implies changes in the articulation between the patella and femoral sulcus, including softening, fibrillation, or erosion of the articular surface. In children and adolescents with idiopathic anterior knee pain, however, the articular surface is often normal. Articular cartilage has no sensory nerve endings, and with the lack of articular cartilage changes in these patients, the source of the pain is not definite. Therefore, one should avoid the use of the term "chondromalacia patellae" in the case of patients with idiopathic anterior knee pain.

In what should be a classic article, Sandow and Goodfellow reported on the natural history of untreated anterior knee pain in adolescent girls followed up for 2 to 8 years (299). The symptoms of most of these patients resolved over time or were significantly improved.

Treatment should be almost exclusively nonsurgical and consist of activity modification, flexibility exercises of the quadriceps and hamstrings, strengthening exercises of the same muscle groups, and the use of other modalities such as ice, heat, ultrasound, and transcutaneous electrical muscle stimulation (299–306). Some patients will benefit from foot orthotics, especially if pes planus is a component of the problem. Knee orthotics such as a patellar stabilization brace or patellar sleeve or strap may also be beneficial.

In summary, idiopathic anterior knee pain in adolescents is commonly referred to as a "headache of the knee" (299). The orthopaedist must assume the role of the "knee psychiatrist" when treating these patients, with a careful and complete clinical history and physical examination, and almost evangelical enthusiasm for nonoperative treatment. It is essential that the patient and his or her family understand that the course of symptoms may be prolonged, but with growth and maturation, activity modification, and an organized rehabilitation program, there is excellent prognosis for return to physical activities and improvement in symptoms (296).

### Popliteal Cysts

Popliteal or Baker cysts are a common entity seen in young children. The common presentation is the discovery of an asymptomatic mass by the mother of the affected child on the posteromedial aspect of the knee at the popliteal crease. The age at presentation is usually 4 to 8 years. Pain is an uncommon feature. There is usually no associated intraarticular pathology in children with this symptom (75).

Plain radiographs demonstrate no bony abnormality. Transillumination of the cyst or ultrasound can document the cystic nature of the lesion and rule out solid soft-tissue lesions such as rhabdomyosarcoma. MRI is only indicated when a cystic lesion is not identified on ultrasound (83).

Anatomically, the cyst arises from the posterior aspect of the knee joint itself, between the medial head of the gastrocnemius and the semimembranosus. Although it may be firmly attached to the fascia of the medial gastrocnemius, it almost always communicates with the knee joint. Spontaneous resolution of popliteal cysts tends to occur, but this often takes up to 12 to 24 months (75).

Surgical excision is rarely indicated and should probably be considered only in cases where rapid enlargement has occurred or pain is a major feature. Recurrence rates are significant after surgery, and the treatment of choice should be watchful waiting and parental reassurance.

## Shin Splints

"Shin splints" is an outdated term which is applied to virtually every type of lower leg pain as a result of overuse. A more appropriate term is shin pain.

### Definition

Shin pain refers to a condition that produces pain and discomfort in the leg due to repetitive running or hiking (307). The condition is limited to musculotendinous inflammations and diagnosis should exclude stress fractures and ischemic disorders. Nevertheless stress fracture and chronic exertional compartment syndrome are part of the differential diagnosis of leg pain in the running athlete.

### Etiology

The etiology of shin splints has been variously reported in the literature. The pain is usually appreciated on the posteromedial border of the tibia from an area approximately 4 cm above the ankle to a more proximal level approximately 10 to 12 cm proximal. It was felt that symptoms were due to an inflammation and overload of the posterior tibial tendon (308,309). Drez (310) has used the term "medial tibial stress syndrome" to describe this pain. Postmortem studies have demonstrated that the site of pain along the posteromedial border of the tibia corresponds to the medial origin of the soleus muscle (311).

## Clinical Features

The physical examination consistently demonstrates tenderness along the posteromedial border of the tibia, centered at the junction of the proximal two-thirds and distal one-third. There is no pain along the subcutaneous border of the tibia, and active and passive motion of the foot and ankle are usually negative. Active resistant plantar flexion and toe raises may elicit the pain.

## Radiographic Features

Routine x-rays are usually interpreted as normal, but there may be hypertrophy of the posterior tibial cortex with subperiosteal lucency or scalloping. Faint periosteal new bone may be present.

## Other Imaging Modalities

Evaluation of troublesome shin pain may include a bone scan. In medial tibial stress syndrome, there is increased uptake in a longitudinal pattern along the posteromedial tibial cortex at the exact site of pain and tenderness (312,313). Tibial stress fractures demonstrate a transverse pattern of increased uptake (312,313).

## Differential Diagnosis

Shin pain in the adolescent athlete can be due to a multitude of causes and should be evaluated for a specific diagnosis. Possible causes of shin pain include medial tibial stress syndrome, stress fracture, exertional compartment syndrome, benign or malignant tumor, infection, and other rare causes.

## Natural History of Medial Tibial Stress Syndrome

Medial tibial stress syndrome is associated with a sudden increase in athletic activity, especially running (314). A study at the U.S. Naval Academy demonstrated that inactive recruits were twice as likely to develop symptoms as were recruits who had been actively training (315). In the same study, rest was shown to be the most important element of treatment.

## Treatment Recommendations

*Nonsurgical.* With rare exceptions, most patients respond to nonsurgical treatment. Rest or restriction of causative factors is the most important modality and is usually combined with ice, NSAIDs, stretching of lower leg muscle groups, and the use of foot orthotics.

It has been demonstrated that patients with medial tibial stress syndrome have a higher incidence of forefoot pronation (314–316). Foot orthotics designed to control or elevate the medial ray of the foot may prove to be beneficial.

Stretching of the gastrocnemius soleus complex has merit because tight heel cords have been shown to be more prevalent in patients with shin splints (310,315).

Most patients show some improvement in symptoms 7 to 10 days after cessation of activity, but recurrence is a common problem, especially if the athlete returns to the preinjury activity level too quickly. A gradual return to full exercise over 6 weeks is recommended.

*Surgical.* In cases of resistant medial tibial stress syndrome after 6 to 12 months of nonsurgical management, surgery in the form of release of the investing fascia overlying the medial soleus (the soleus bridge) and division of the medial soleus origin and periosteum may be indicated (308,315). Surgery in adults has been performed with success, but is rarely indicated in the growing child.

## Chronic Exertional Compartment Syndrome

### Definition

Chronic exertional compartment syndrome is also called *exercise-induced compartment syndrome*; it is characterized by increased intracompartmental pressure that is sufficient to cause pain in the leg and is usually precipitated by running (316).

### Etiology

With exercise and muscle contraction, significant elevations of intracompartmental pressure, up to 80 mm Hg, occur (317,318). Muscle weight and size increase up to 20% during exercise and, because of the unyielding compartment space, lead to increased pressure that eventually exceeds the capillary filling pressure, causing ischemia and pain (318). The ischemia is never severe enough to cause muscle necrosis in exertional compartment syndrome. Indeed, other studies have cast doubt on the ischemic theory of causation (319).

### Clinical Features

The typical presentation is an individual who develops leg pain in one of the muscle groups of the lower leg after training, usually running. The pain is initially dull and may persist after training has ended. Paraesthesia on the plantar aspect of the foot or the dorsum of the foot indicate involvement of the deep posterior compartment or anterior compartment respectively. These are the two most frequent compartments involved (316,317,320,321).

The physical examination is often normal in the patient at rest. Examination of the foot and entire limb for mechanical axis deviations and rotational abnormalities should be performed.

### Diagnostic Studies

If there is a high index of suspicion of exertional compartment syndrome, pressure measurements using either a slit catheter or wick catheter should be performed to evaluate compartment pressure both at rest and after exercise (317,318,322–325).

Pedowitz et al.(325) developed the following criteria:

1. Pre-exercise pressure greater than 15 mm Hg.
2. A 1-minute postexercise pressure of greater than 30 mm Hg.
3. A 5-minute postexercise pressure in excess of 20 mm Hg.

Other studies employed as alternatives to compartment pressure testing, including MRI, near infrared spectroscopy, and thallium-201 single photon emission computed tomography scans, have been inconclusive (326,327).

### Natural History

Unfortunately, conservative treatment methods for exercise-induced compartment syndrome, including the use of orthotics, NSAIDs, activity modification, and physical therapy modalities have been shown to be unsuccessful in cases where pressure measurements have been obtained (315,317,320,321). These studies were performed only in adults.

### Treatment Recommendations

**Surgical.** Fasciotomy of the affected compartment is the treatment of choice (315,317,321,328). Pressure measurements of all four compartments should be conducted prior to surgery, as more than one compartment may be involved. The tibialis posterior may reside in a separate, deep posterior compartment, and careful evaluation should be undertaken after decompression (319,329).

Options for fasciotomy include (a) fibulectomy (324); (b) perifibular fasciotomy; (324) and (c) double incision fasciotomy (328).

**Author's Preferred Recommendations.** I prefer to use multiple, limited, skin incisions for obvious cosmetic reasons. The fascia between the skin bridges must be divided to ensure that the compartment is adequately released. In release of the anterior and lateral compartments, care must be taken to protect the superficial peroneal nerve. Visualization and protection of the saphenous vein and nerve must be done with release of the superficial and deep posterior compartments. The skin is closed primarily, unlike an acute compartment syndrome.

Postoperatively, the patient is kept on crutches for 3 to 4 days, but allowed ambulation and early range of motion of adjacent joints. Strengthening is commenced when the wounds are healed, and the patient can be expected to return gradually to running after 3 to 4 weeks.

Approximately 90% of patients with chronic compartment syndrome are significantly improved with fasciotomy (315,321,329). Recurrence of the symptoms has been reported to be 3.4% in a large series (315). Preoperative evaluation including compartment pressure monitoring is essential prior to surgical intervention.

## Trochanteric Bursitis

### Iliotibial Band Syndrome

In the skeletally immature athlete, trochanteric bursitis is invariably associated with iliotibial band tendonitis or "snapping hip syndrome." Clinically, there is tenderness directly over and distal to the greater trochanter. Pain is accentuated with adduction and external rotation of the hip. The patient can often voluntarily reproduce the snapping with a trick maneuver. Occasionally the pain may also be experienced just above and at the knee on the lateral epicondyle. Associated factors which may contribute to this condition include a broad pelvis, leg-length discrepancy, and excessive pronation of the foot (330).

**Treatment.** This is a condition which generally resolves with nonsurgical treatment (330). Treatment is aimed at stretching the iliotibial band and decreasing the inflammation with NSAIDs. In extreme cases or cases which fail to resolve, local corticosteroid injection into the iliotibial band and greater trochanteric bursa may be indicated.

*Surgery.* Rarely, if nonsurgical methods fail to resolve the symptoms, operative release or lengthening of the iliotibial band may be required (330).

## Stress Fractures

The incidence of stress fractures in children and adolescents has increased in concert with the increase in their participation in organized sports, especially sports involving running (331). Stress fracture should be included in the differential diagnosis of the child with overuse injury and pain.

Stress fractures result from repetitive physical stress that disrupts the normal bone-remodeling mechanism. This stress is below the threshold needed to cause an acute fracture, but is sufficient to interrupt the balance between bone formation and resorption. Physical training, especially after prolonged inactivity, results in stimulation of osteoblastic activity. At the same time there is a concurrent stimulation of bone resorption (osteoclastic activity), and it is believed that stress fractures occur early in this remodeling period when the bone is weakened by osteoclastic resorption (332).

The bones most commonly affected by stress fractures are the proximal tibia, femoral neck, femoral diaphysis or distal femoral metaphysis, medial malleolus, and metatarsals.

### Classification

There are two types of stress fractures. Fatigue fractures are fractures due to an abnormal stress applied to a normal bone. Insufficiency fractures occur when normal stress is applied to abnormal or pathologic bone such as in children with osteogenesis imperfecta, spina bifida, cerebral palsy, or rickets, or in some patients on long-term steroids. Micheli has noted the infrequency of fatigue or stress fractures in children involved in free play (333). Stress fractures almost always occur in children and adolescents involved in strenuous repetitive activities such as running, jumping, or dance (333,334).

### Incidence

The incidence of stress fractures in children and adolescents is not known, but it is generally accepted that the incidence is increasing due to their increased participation in organized sports. A study of Israeli military recruits found that the incidence of stress fracture in recruits younger than twenty years was ten times greater than recruits who were 21 to 26 years of age (335).

### Risk Factors

A number of factors that seem to have a correlation with stress fractures have been elucidated (336–338). In studies undertaken of military recruits, it was seen that those recruits with foot deformity such as pes planus or pes cavus had a higher incidence of stress fracture (332,334,339–341). Those recruits who were not physically fit and had smaller thigh muscle mass were more prone to develop stress fractures (336). In addition, smaller bone diameter, especially of the femur and tibia, was associated with a higher incidence (340). Women with a lower bone mineral density (BMD), with low body fat, or amenorrhea were more likely to develop stress fractures (337,340).

A triad of risk factors was identified in adolescents with stress injury, namely, the combination of muscle weakness, muscle tightness, and ligamentous laxity (340). These effects were magnified if the adolescents also had increased body weight and height, any malalignment of the lower extremities, and were involved in sports that demanded bursts of explosive strength (340).

### Differential Diagnosis

The main concern in diagnosis is differentiating a stress fracture from a malignant bone tumor, especially with some periosteal new bone formation. In addition, the physician must rule out other conditions such as benign tumors (osteoid osteoma), infection, inflammatory arthritis, or soft-tissue injury.

### Clinical Features

A careful and detailed history is important in differentiating stress fracture from these other conditions. A history of repetitive physical activity such as running, jumping, or dancing, causing pain during the activity and relief with rest, should arouse a high index of suspicion (333,334). Night pain is not common in stress fracture, but is common in osteoid osteoma or malignant bone tumors (osteogenic and Ewing sarcoma).

The physical examination should include an evaluation of the foot and ankle, lower leg, and entire lower extremity alignment. Stress fractures occur more commonly in athletes with foot abnormalities such as pes cavus and pes planus (334,339–341).

In addition, an evaluation of muscle strength, muscle tightness or flexibility, and ligamentous laxity should be part of the physical examination (339).

### Imaging Studies

Imaging studies for stress fracture may include plain radiographs with emphasis on bony detail, radionucleotide bone scans, or, more recently, MRI.

Plain radiographs may be negative for several weeks following the onset of symptoms. Until resorption and the proliferative healing response occur in trabecular bone, the x-ray films will appear to be normal. In metaphyseal bone this may take from 10 to 21 days (342) (Fig. 32.31).

The periosteal new bone is usually very localized in stress fractures, especially in the metaphyseal region, whereas malignant bone tumors have a more widespread periosteal reaction with lamination and permeative patchy destruction of the metaphyseal bone. However, distinguishing a stress fracture from a malignant bone tumor may be very difficult.

Bone scans have been very useful in the diagnosis of stress fracture (342,343). However, they are sometimes not as sensitive in ruling out osteomyelitis or neoplastic processes.

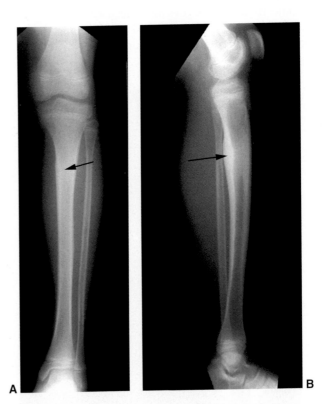

**Figure 32.31  A:** Anteroposterior radiograph of adolescent cross-country runner with pain in proximal tibia for 3 months. Reactive new bone medially (*black arrow*) is suggestive of stress fracture. **B.** Lateral radiograph of same patient. *Arrow* points to area of new bone formation posteriorly.

MRI has proven to be a very useful and sensitive tool, especially in the patient in whom the history and plain radiographs are inconclusive (344,345). MRI can distinguish stress fracture from both osteomyelitis and malignant bone neoplasm in most cases (Fig. 32.32).

In stress fracture, MRI shows bandlike areas of very low signal intensity in the intramedullary area, continuous with the cortical bone. On $T_1$ images, there is decreased signal intensity in the marrow (345).

### Treatment

Treatment of stress fracture in the child or adolescent depends on the site of the injury, the severity of symptoms, and the patient's age (333,346,347).

The most important aspect of treatment in young patients is to modify or eliminate the activities that caused the stress fracture. This may require cast immobilization or off-the-counter orthotics for 4 to 6 weeks to allow sufficient bone deposition to occur.

In most children, stress fractures respond well to this conservative treatment regimen.

***Surgical Treatment.*** There are some anatomical areas that are prone to prolonged symptoms or even nonunion. These include stress fractures of the femoral neck, tibial diaphysis, medial malleolus, and tarsal navicular (334).

Stress fractures of the femoral neck are especially problematic. If the fracture goes on to displacement, risk or the complication of avascular necrosis (AVN) is high and has prompted the recommendation for internal fixation (348).

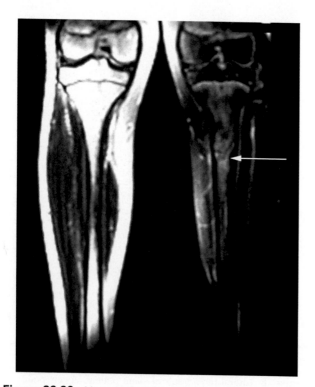

**Figure 32.32** Magnetic resonance imaging (MRI) of the same patient as in Figure 32.31. *Arrow* points to fracture line.

Micheli recommends the use of a hip spica cast in noncompliant young children, but internal fixation may be the conservative treatment of choice in an active adolescent (347).

In contrast to the more common proximal metaphyseal stress fracture, which almost always heals uneventfully (346,347), diaphyseal tibial stress fractures are prone to prolonged symptoms and delayed union (349). In the case of delayed union, a patellar–tendon–bearing (PTB) cast or commercial orthosis should be employed for 4 to 6 months before surgery is considered. If nonunion exists in the skeletally mature adolescent, options to treat the nonunion include the use of an intramedullary nail with or without bone grafting and fibular osteotomy (350). In the skeletally immature individual with a dipahyseal tibial stress fracture that fails to heal after 6 months of nonoperative treatment, operative treatment is indicated. Excision of the fibrous nonunion and autogenous bone grafting from the iliac crest, with possible fibular osteotomy, has been employed successfully in this rare situation (350).

For medial malleolar stress fractures in young athletes, open reduction and internal fixation is recommended to facilitate early healing and recovery (351).

In the case of nonunion of tarsal navicular stress fractures, excision of the nonunion site and autogenous bone grafting has been recommended (352,353).

### Return to Sports

The most important issue for athletes is the decision on when they can return to sports. This is a complex decision which involves healing of the stress fracture clinically, as evidenced by loss of pain, healing of the stress fracture as indicated on radiographs, and modification or elimination of inciting causes and training methods.

## Sever Disease

### Definition

Sever calcaneal apophysitis is a self-limited inflammatory condition of the os calcis in growing children.

### Clinical Features

The typical child with Sever disease is from 9 to 14 years of age and involved in running sports (354). The condition is bilateral in most cases and presents as diffuse pain and tenderness over the prominence of the heel rather than exclusively on the plantar aspect as is seen in plantar fasciitis (355).

### Natural History

Originally described by James Sever (356) in 1912, the condition is presumed to be an inflammatory condition of the calcaneal apophysis. Radiographs are normal, and the condition in all cases improves over time.

### Treatment

With rest, activity modification, and passage of time, the condition always resolves (354–356). Ice, oral NSAIDs, stretching exercise of the Achilles tendon and plantar fascia, and heel pads or inserts may offer some relief from the discomfort (354–356). Cast immobilization may rarely be necessary for the patient with severe, incapacitating symptoms (355). Reassurance and time are the basis of treatment of this common condition.

## Stress Physeal Reactions

Repetitive stress in the upper extremity may lead to a specific stress reaction in the physis. This reaction is not uncommonly seen in the distal radial physis of skeletally immature gymnasts who load their wrists with significant compressive forces while participating in vault and floor exercises (Fig. 32.33). Radiographically the stress reaction is noted as a radiolucency and irregularity on the metaphyseal side of the physis, similar to the radiolucency seen in the medial aspect of the proximal tibia in adolescent tibia vara and in the femoral neck in patients with slipped capital femoral epiphysis.

Caine et al. (357) found radiographic abnormalities in the distal radius in up to 85% of competitive gymnasts who were skeletally immature. The same study found an increased incidence of positive ulnar variance in the wrists of nonelite gymnasts (357). The hypothesis of the study was that repetitive compressive forces to the distal radius led to premature growth arrest resulting in a positive ulnar variance. Positive ulnar variance has been associated with secondary wrist problems including tears of the triangular fibrocartilage complex (TFCC) and ulnar impingement syndrome.

Athletes involved in throwing sports can develop the same symptoms and radiographic abnormalities in the proximal humerus. This condition is commonly seen in Little League pitchers (358) (Fig. 32.34).

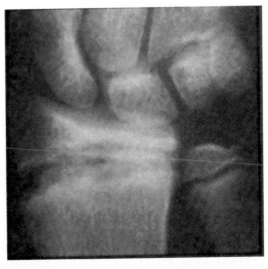

**Figure 32.33** Anteroposterior radiograph of wrist of gymnast with 3-month history of wrist pain. Note radiolucency on metaphyseal side of growth plate (physis) indicative of stress physeal reaction.

Treatment of these overuse stress reactions is centered on the discontinuation of the offending force or modification of activities until the symptoms of pain subside. Baseball pitchers may need to refrain from pitching for 2 to 3 months until the pain that accompanies the throwing motion totally subsides.

Gymnasts with symptomatic radial physeal stress reaction should refrain from loading their wrists for up to 2 to 3 months to allow the reactive changes to heal.

Strengthening exercises to specifically strengthen the wrist flexors should be undertaken in gymnasts, and taping or bracing to limit wrist dorsiflexion may help prevent recurrence.

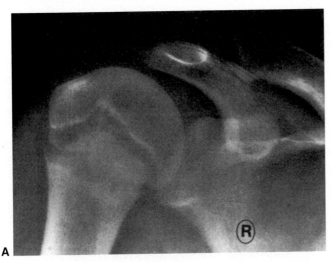
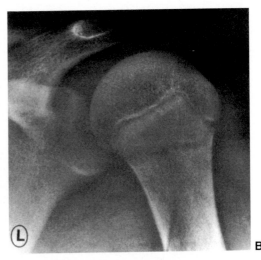

**Figure 32.34** Radiographs of the proximal humerus in a 14-year-old, right-handed baseball pitcher with shoulder pain that progressed over the final few weeks of the season. **A:** Widening and irregularity of the physeal plate are present in the right shoulder. **B:** Radiograph of the left shoulder is provided for comparison.

With rest and refraining from the inciting or offending exercise, the radiographic changes seen at the physis and metaphysis will resolve.

## Elbow Problems in the Throwing Athlete

The elbow of the immature athlete is susceptible to injury when the athlete throws too frequently or uses a style that puts too much stress on the elbow joint.

During the throwing motion, a significant valgus moment is applied to the elbow joint (359). This valgus moment results in excessive tensile or distraction forces on the medial aspect of the joint (medial epicondyle and ulnar collateral ligaments) and excessive compressive forces on the lateral aspect of the joint (radiocapitellar joint) (360,361) (Fig. 32.35).

Safety guidelines published in *USA Baseball News* recommended limits of 52 ± 15 pitches per game for 8- to 10-year-olds, 68 ± 18 for 11- to 12-year-olds and 76 ± 16 for 13- to 14-year-olds (362–364). Studies have also shown that side-arm throwing results in markedly increased elbow pathology in the throwing athlete and should be forbidden for the child athlete involved in throwing sports (365).

"Little League elbow" is the term used to describe all the facets of overuse injury in the young throwing athlete. The term was originally proposed in 1960 and encompasses a spectrum of conditions including medial epicondyle apophysitis, capitellar OCD, radial head deformation, olecranon apophysitis, and flexion contracture (363).

### Pathophysiology

Risk factors that cause elbow problems in the young athlete involved in throwing sports have been studied extensively in recent years. Factors responsible include: age of the pitcher, skeletal maturity, tissue strength, muscle strength, level of conditioning, throwing speed and style, types of pitches thrown, number of pitches per outing, and number of outings per season (362–364).

In a study that analyzed elbow and shoulder problems in the young throwing athlete, 47% of pitchers complained of shoulder or elbow pain, and 68% of the elbow pains were medial (362,365). Twenty-eight percent of the pitchers complained of elbow pain specifically, and throwing split finger pitches or sliders increased the incidence of elbow complaints (365).

### Medial Epicondyle Apophysitis

The muscle, tendon, and bone of the medial epicondyle resist traction forces better than the apophyseal cartilage. These repetitive stresses cause microfractures in the apophyseal cartilage not unlike those seen in Osgood-Schlatter syndrome. The apophysis is seen to widen on x-ray films and may eventually fail catastrophically, resulting in a medial epicondyle avulsion, especially in a throwing athlete.

On examination, point tenderness over the medial epicondyle is elicited. The pain may also be increased if a valgus stress is applied to the elbow or if resisted wrist flexion or pronation is tested.

### Treatment

Treatment for most of the overuse injuries in the skeletally immature athlete is rest and avoidance of the offending activity, and the elbow is no exception. Rest, ice, and the use of acetaminophen or NSAIDs should result in improvement of symptoms. If the athlete develops a true avulsion of the medial epicondyle, treatment should consist of cast immobilization if the apophysis is displaced 5 mm or less, or surgical fixation of the medial epicondyle if displaced more than 5 mm in a throwing athlete or gymnast. Fixation should be accomplished with a small cannulated screw, which allows early range of motion and prevents elbow stiffness.

The screw does not need to pass through the opposite cortex. A fully threaded screw with washer is employed to provide enough stability to allow early range of motion. The epicondyle is positioned without removal of physeal cartilage. The screw is not routinely removed unless it becomes prominent and symptomatic to the patient.

## Capitellar Osteochondritis Dissecans

JOCD of the elbow should be differentiated from juvenile osteochondroses of the capitellum or "Panner Disease" (366,367). Originally described by Panner (367) as a posttraumatic AVN, the juvenile form occurs in children who

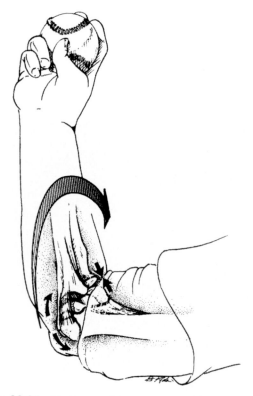

**Figure 32.35** Pitching produces a valgus moment (*large curved arrow*) at the elbow. There are compressive forces (*straight arrows*) across the radiocapitellar joint, and tension (*curved arrows*) across the medial epicondyle and medial collateral ligament.

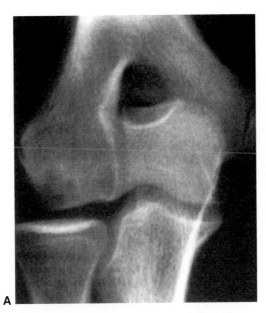

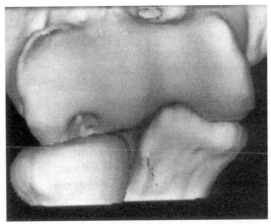

**Figure 32.36** Osteochondral lesion of the capitellum in a 15-year-old baseball player with a painful elbow. **A:** The subchondral plate of the capitellum appears intact. Subchondral cysts are present. **B:** The computed tomography scan with three-dimensional reconstruction demonstrates the bony defect of the capitellum, including loss of the subchondral plate in that area.

are younger than 10 years; it is atraumatic and probably due to variation in ossification rather than typical OCD. It is self-limited and resolves spontaneously (366).

True OCD is thought to be due to excessive compression forces on the lateral side of the joint (radiocapitellar joint) during the throwing motion, resulting in microfractures, edema, AVN, and potential loose body formation (368–370).

Pain on the lateral aspect of the joint during throwing, and tenderness of the radiocapitellar joint to palpation lead to the diagnosis. With progression of the disease, pain on forced flexion, a flexion contracture, and snapping and locking from joint incongruity and loose bodies may occur (Fig. 32.36).

### Treatment

Treatment in the young patient is controversial, but lesions shown on magnetic resonance imaging (MRI) to be stable respond favorably to prolonged rest and cessation of throwing. The lesions may take up to 12 months to heal. MRI is helpful for visualizing any disruption in the integrity of the articular cartilage (fluid behind lesion) and helps direct surgical management. If the lesion is stable, drilling of the involved fragment may promote vascular ingrowth and healing of the lesion. If the lesion is unstable, the base should be freshened and fixed with pins, screws, or bioabsorbable nails. Small, unstable lesions or loose bodies are removed.

Rehabilitation is begun early to promote restoration of motion and strength. The decision to resume throwing sports is one that should not be made until the lesion is healed and the elbow fully rehabilitated.

The skeletally immature elbow is susceptible to overuse injury due to the forces applied to the elbow during throwing (359–362,364,368–370). When the elbow becomes painful,

coaches, trainers, and medical personnel should advise cessation of throwing. Fortunately, nonoperative treatment is successful in alleviating most of the conditions associated with "Little League elbow," but the athlete, parents, and coaches must be educated as to the reasons for the problem and ways to prevent it from recurring.

This chapter outlines the many potentially acute and overuse injuries that can occur to the skeletally immature athlete. Despite these risks, the beneficial aspects of recreational and organized sports far outweigh the hazards. Most important of all the benefits is the development of an active and healthy lifestyle, which offers countless rewards not only during childhood and adolescence but also in adult life.

## REFERENCES

1. Dyment PG, ed. *Epidemiology and prevention of sports injuries in sports medicine: health care for young athletes.* Elk Grove Village, IL: American Academy of Pediatrics, 1991:146–171.
2. Caine DV, Caine CG, Lindner KJ, eds. *Epidemiology of sports injuries.* Champaign, IL: Human Kinetics, 1996.
3. Powell JW. Epidemiological research for injury prevention programs in sports. In: Mueller FO, Ryan AJ, eds. *Prevention of athletic injuries: the role of the sports medicine team.* Philadelphia, PA: FA Davis Company, 1991:11–25.
4. Rice SG. *Risks of injury during sports participation in care of the young athlete.* Rosemont, IL: American Academy of Pediatrics, AAOS, 2000:9–18.
5. Rice SG. Epidemiology and mechanisms of sports injuries. In: Teitz CC, ed. *Scientific foundations of sports medicine,* Toronto: BC Decker, 1989:3–23.
6. U.S. Product Safety Commission. *NEISS coding manual, 2000: national electronic injury surveillance system.* Washington, DC: U.S. Product Safety Commission, 2000.
7. Purvis JM, Burke RG. Recreational injuries in children: incidence and prevention. *J Am Acad Orthop Surg* 2001;9(6):365–374.
8. Barfield WR, Gross RH. *Injury prevention in care of the young athlete.* In: Sullivan JA, Anderson SJ, eds. Care of the Young Athlete. Rosemont, IL: AAOS, American Academy of Pediatrics, 2000:121–130.

9. Bijur PE, Trumble A, Harel Y, et al. Sports and recreation injuries in U.S. children and athletes. *Arch Pediatr Adolesc Med* 1995;149:1009–1116.
10. Hergenroeder AC. Prevention of sports injuries. *Pediatrics* 1998;101:1057–1063.
11. Anderson S. *Principles of rehabilitation in care of the young athlete*. In Sullivan JA, Anderson SJ, eds. Care of the young Athlete. Rosemont, IL: American Academy of Pediatrics. AAOS, 2000: 267–280.
12. Kibler WB, Lee PA, Herring SA, eds. *Functional rehabilitation of sports and musculoskeletal injuries*. Gaithersburg, MD: Aspen Publishers, 1998.
13. Young JL, Press JM. The physiologic basis of sports rehabilitation. *Phys Med Rehabil Clin N Am* 1994;5:9–36.
14. American Academy of Pediatrics Committee on Sports Medicine and Fitness. Adolescents and anabolic steroids: a subject review. *Pediatrics* 1997;99:904–908.
15. Brower K. Anabolic steroids: addictive, psychiatric and medical consequences. *Am J Addict* 1992;1:100–114.
16. Griesmer BA. *Performance enhancing substances in care of the young athlete*. In Sullivan JA, Anderson SJ, eds. Care of the young Athlete. Rosemont, IL: AAOS and American Academy of Pediatrics, 2000:95–104.
17. Johnson MD. Anabolic steroid use in adolescent athletes. *Pediatr Clin North Am* 1990;37:1111–1123.
18. Sewall L, Micheli LJ. Strength training for children. *J Pediatr Orthop* 1986;6:143–146.
19. Brady TA, Cahill BR, Bodnar LM. Weight training related injuries in the high school athlete. *Am J Sports Med* 1982;10:1–5.
20. Weltman A, Janney C, Rians C. The effect of hydraulic resistant strength training in prepubertal males. *Med Sci Sports Exerc* 1986;18:629–638.
21. Scavenius M, Iversen BF. Non-traumatic clavicular osteolysis in weight lifters. *Am J Sports Med* 1992;20:463–446.
22. Gumbs VL, Segal D, Halligan JB, et al. Bilateral distal radius and ulnar fractures in adolescent weight lifters. *Am J Sports Med* 1982;10:375–375.
23. Ryan JR, Salciccioli GG. Fractures of the distal radial epiphysis in adolescent weight lifters. *Am J Sports Med* 1976;4:26–26.
24. Brown EW, Kimball RG. Medical history associated with adolescent powerlifting. *Pediatrics* 1983;72:636–44.
25. Regwold G. Does lifting weights harm a prepubescent athlete? *Phys Sportsmed* 1982;10:141–144.
26. American Academy of Pediatrics. Committee on sports medicine. Weight training and weight lifting: information for the pediatrician. *Phys Sportsmed* 1983;11:157–161.
27. Atkin DM, Fithian DC, Marangi KS, et al. Characteristics of patients with primary acute lateral patellar dislocation and their recovery within the first 6 months of injury. *Am J Sports Med* 2000;28(4):472–479.
28. Bensahel H, Souchet P, Pennecott GF, et al. The unstable patella in children. *JPO J Pract Orthop (B)* 2000;9(4):265–270.
29. Busch MT. Care of the young athlete. In: Morrissy R, Weinstein S, eds. *Pediatric orthopaedics by Lovell and Winter*. Philadelphia, PA: Lippincott Williams & Wilkins, 2000.
30. Dye SF. The knee as a biologic transmission with an envelope of function: a theory. *Clin Orthop* 1996;325:10–18.
31. Warren LF, Marshall JL. The supporting structures and layers on the medial side of the knee: an anatomical analysis. *J Bone Joint Surg* 1979;61A(1):56–62.
32. Conlan T, Garth WP Jr, Lemons JF. Evaluations of the medial soft-tissue restraints of the extensor mechanism of the knee. *J Bone Joint Surg* 1993;75-A(5):682–693.
33. Drez D Jr, Edwards TB, Williams CS. Results of medial patellofemoral ligament reconstruction in the treatment of patellar dislocation. *Arthroscopy* 2001;17(3):298–306.
34. Rieder B, Marshall JL, Koslin B, et al. The anterior aspect of the knee joint. *J Bone Joint Surg* 1981;63A(3):351–356.
35. Desio SM, Burks RT, Bachus KN. Soft tissue restraints to lateral patellar translation in the human knee. *Am J Sports Med* 1998;26(1):59–65.
36. Hautanaa PV, Fithian DC, Kaufman KR, et al. Medial soft tissue restraints in lateral patellar instability. *Clin Orthop* 1998;349:174–182.
37. Burks RT, Desio SM, Bachus KN, et al. Biomechanical evaluation of lateral patellar dislocations. *Am J Knee Surg* 1998;11(1):24–31.
38. Nomura E. Classification of lesions of the medial patellofemoral ligament in patellar dislocation. *Int Orthop* 1999;23(5):260–263.
39. Hinton RY, Sharma KM. Acute and recurrent patellar instability in the young athlete. *Orthop Clin North Am* 2003;34:385–396.
40. Larsen E, Lauridsen F. Conservative treatment of patellar dislocations. *Clin Orthop Relat Res* 1982;171:131–136.
41. Merchant AC, Mercer RL, Jacobsen RH, et al. Roentgenographic analysis of patellofemoral congruence. *J Bone Joint Surg* 1974;56A:1391–1396.
42. Ahmad CS, Stein BE, Matuz D, et al. Immediate surgical repair of the medial patellar stabilizers for acute patellar dislocation. A review of eight cases. *Am J Sports Med* 2000;28(6):804–810.
43. Nikku R, Nietosvaara Y, Kallio PE, et al. Operative versus closed treatment of primary dislocation of the patella. Similar 2 year results in 125 randomized patients. *Acta Orthop Scand* 1997;68(5):419–423.
44. McManus F, Rang M, Heslin DJ. Acute dislocation of the patella in children: the natural history. *Clin Orthop* 1979;139:88.
45. Hawkins RJ, Bell RH, Annisette G. Acute patellar dislocations. The natural history. *Am J Sports Med* 1986;14(2):117–120.
46. Cash JD, Hughston JC. Treatment of acute patellar dislocation. *Am J Sports Med* 1988;16(3):244–249.
47. Caylor D, Fites R, Worrell TW. The relationship between quadriceps angle and anterior knee syndrome. *J Orthop Sports Phys Ther* 1993;17(1):11–16.
48. Fairbank JC, Pynsent PB, van Poortvliet JA, et al. Mechanical factors in the incidence of knee pain in adolescents and young adults. *J Bone Joint Surg* 1984;66B(5):685–693.
49. Livingston LA, Mandigo JL. Bilateral Q angle asymmetry and anterior knee pain syndrome. *Clin Biomech* 1999;14(1):7–13.
50. Metcalf RW. An arthroscopic method for lateral release of the subluxating or dislocating patella. *Clin Ortho Relat Res* 1982;167:9.
51. Schonholtz GJ, Zahn MG, Magee CM. Lateral retinacular release of the patella. *Arthroscopy* 1987;3:269.
52. Hughston JC, Deese M. Medial subluxation of the patella as a complication of lateral retinacular release. *Am J Sports Med* 1988;16(4):383–388.
53. Nonweiler DE, Delee JC. The diagnosis and treatment of medial subluxation of the patella after lateral retinacular release. *Am J Sports Med* 1994;22(5):680–686.
54. Madigan R, Wissinger HA, Donaldson WF. Preliminary experience with a method of quadricepsplasty in recurrent subluxation of the patella. *J Bone Joint Surg Am* 1975;57:600.
55. Baksi DP. Restoration of dynamic stability of the patella by pes anserinus transposition. *J Bone Joint Surg Br* 1981;63:399.
56. Insall J, Falvo KA, Wise DW. Chondromalacia patellae. *J Bone Joint Surg Am* 1976;58:1.
57. Baker RH, Carroll N, Dewar FP, et al. The semitendinosus tenodesis for recurrent dislocation of the patella. *J Bone Joint Surg Br* 1972;54:103.
58. Letts RM, Davidson D, Beaule P. Semitendinosus tenodesis for repair of recurrent dislocation of the patella in children. *J Pediatr Orthop* 1999;19(6):742–747.
59. Brown DE, Alexander AH, Lichtman DM. The Elmslie-Trillat procedure: evaluation in patellar dislocation and subluxation. *Am J Sports Med* 1984;12:104.
60. Fulkerson JP. Anteromedialization of the tibial tubercle for patellofemoral malalignment. *Clin Orthop* 1983;177:176.
61. Chrisman OD, Snook GA, Wilson TC. A long-term prospective study of the Hauser and Roux Goldthwait procedures for recurrent patellar dislocation. *Clin Orthop* 1979;144:27.
62. Fairbanks TJ. Knee joint changes after meniscectomy. *J Bone Joint Surg* 1948;30B:664–670.
63. Manzione M, Pizzutillo PD, Peoples AB, et al. Meniscectomy in children: a long-term follow-up study. *Am J Sports Med* 1983;11:111–115.
64. Medlar RC, Mandiberg JJ, Lyne ED. Meniscectomies in children – report of long-term results. *Am J Sports Med* 1980;8:87–92.
65. Raber DA, Friederich NF, Buzzi R, et al. Discoid lateral meniscus in children: long-term follow-up after total meniscectomy. *J Bone Joint Surg Am* 1998;8:1579–1586.
66. Rangger C, Klesh T, Gloetzer W, et al. Osteoarthritis after arthroscopic partial meniscectomy. *Am J Sports Med* 1995;23:230–244.

67. Vandermeer R, Cunningham F. Arthroscopic treatment of the discoid lateral meniscus: results of long-term follow-up. *Arthroscopy* 1989;5:101–109.

68. Washington ER, Root L, Lierner U, et al. Discoid lateral meniscus in children: long-term follow-up after excision. *J Bone Joint Surg Am* 1995;77(9):1357–1361.

69. Wroble RR, Henderson RC, Campion ER, et al. Meniscectomy in children and adolescents: a long-term follow-up study. *Clin Orthop* 1992;279:180–189.

70. Kaplan ER. Discoid lateral meniscus of the knee joint. *Bull Hosp Joint Dis* 1955;16:111–124.

71. Clark CR, Ogden JA. Development of the meniscus of the human knee joint: morphological changes and their potential role in childhood meniscal injury. *J Bone Joint Surg Am* 1983; 65:538–547.

72. Arnoczky SP, Warren RF. Microvasculature of the human meniscus. *Am J Sports Med* 1982;2:90–95.

73. Gries PE, Holstrom MC, Burdana DD, et al. Meniscal injury: basic science and evaluation. *J Am Acad Orthop Surg* 2002;10: 168–176.

74. King D. The healing of semilunar cartilage. *J Bone Joint Surg Am* 1936;18:333–342.

75. Kocher MS, Micheli LJ. The pediatric knee: evaluation and treatment. In: Insall JN, Scott WN, eds. *Surgery of the knee*, 3rd ed. New York: Churchill Livingstone, 2001:1356–1397.

76. Dickhaut SC, Delee JC. The discoid lateral meniscus syndrome. *J Bone Joint Surg Am* 1982;64:1068–1073.

77. Jordan M. Lateral meniscus variants: evaluation and treatment. *J Am Acad Orthop Surg* 1996;4:191–200.

78. Aichroth PM, Patel DV, Marx CI. Congenital discoid lateral meniscus in children: a follow-up study and evaluation of management. *J Bone Joint Surg Br* 1991;73:932–939.

79. Nathan PA, Cole SC. Discoid meniscus: a clinical and pathological study. *Clin Orthop* 1969;64:107–113.

80. Woods GW, Whelan JM. Discoid meniscus. *Clin Sports Med* 1990;9(3):695–706.

81. Rosenberg TD, Paulos LE, Parker RD, et al. Discoid lateral meniscus: case report of arthroscopic attachment of a symptomatic Wrisberg-ligament type. *Arthroscopy* 1987;3:277–282.

82. Watanabe M, Takada S, Ikeuchi H. *Atlas of arthroscopy*. Tokyo: Igaku-Shvin, 1969.

83. Kocher MS, DiCanzio J, Zurakowski D, et al. Diagnostic performance of clinical examination and selective magnetic resonance imaging in the evaluation of intra-articular knee disorders in children and adolescents. *Am J Sports Med* 2001;29: 292–296.

84. Stanitski CL. Correlation of arthroscopic and clinical examination with magnetic resonance imaging findings of injured knees in children and adolescents. *Am J Sports Med* 1998;26:2–6.

85. Neuschwander DC, Drez D, Finney TP. Lateral meniscal variant with absence of posterior coronary ligaments. *J Bone Joint Surg Am* 1992;74:1186–1190.

86. Hayashi LK, Yamaga H, Ida K, et al. Arthroscopic meniscectomy for discoid lateral meniscus in children. *J Bone Joint Surg Am* 1988;70:1495–1500.

87. Ikeuchi H. Arthroscopic treatment of lateral discoid meniscus: technique and long-term results. *Clin Orthop* 1982;167:19–28.

88. Fujikawa K, Iseki F, Mikura Y. Partial resection of the discoid meniscus in the child's knee. *J Bone Joint Surg Br* 1981;63:391–395.

89. Ogata K. Arthroscopic technique: two piece excision of discoid meniscus. *Arthroscopy* 1997;13(5):666–670.

90. Datel D, Dimakopoulos P, Penoncourt P. Bucket handle tear of a discoid meniscus: arthroscopic diagnosis and partial excision. *Orthopedics* 1986;9:607–608.

91. Dehaven KE, Linter DM. Athletic injuries: comparison by age, sport, gender. *Am J Sports Med* 1986;14:218–224.

92. Cannon WD, Vittori JM. The incidence of healing in arthroscopic meniscal repairs in the anterior cruciate ligament-reconstructed knee versus stable knees. *Am J Sports Med* 1992;20: 176–181.

93. Busch MT. Meniscal injuries in children and adolescents. *Clin Sports Med* 1990;9:661–680.

94. King SL, Curty HML, Brady O. Magnetic resonance imaging of knee injuries in children. *Pediatr Radiol* 1996;26:287–290.

95. Zobel MS, Borello JA, Siegel MJ, et al. Pediatric knee MR imaging: pattern of injury in the immature skeleton. *Radiology* 1994;190:397–401.

96. Greis PE, Holmstrom MC, Bardana DD, et al. Meniscal injury II: management. *J Am Acad Orthop Surg* 2002;10:177–187.

97. Dehaven KE, Arnoczky SP. Meniscus repair: basic science, indications for repair and open repair. *Instr Course Lect* 1994;43: 65–74.

98. Mintzu CM, Richmond JC, Taylor J. Meniscal repair in the young athlete. *Am J Sports Med* 1998;26:630–633.

99. Noyes FR, Barber-Westin SD. Arthroscopic repair of meniscal tears extending into the avascular zone in patients younger than twenty years of age. *Am J Sports Med* 2002;30:589–600.

100. Rubman MH, Noye FR, Barber-Westin SD. Arthroscopic repair of meniscal tears that extend into the avascular zone: a review of 198 single and complex tears. *Am J Sports Med* 1998;26: 87–95.

101. Johnson MJ, Lucas GL, Dusek JK, et al. Isolated arthroscopic meniscal repair: a long-term outcome study (more than 10 years). *Am J Sports Med* 1999;27:44–49.

102. Busek MS, Noyes FR. Arthroscopic evaluation of meniscal repairs after anterior cruciate ligament reconstruction and immediate motion. *Am J Sports Med* 1991;19:489–494.

103. Tenuta JJ, Arciero RA. Arthroscopic evaluation of meniscal repairs – factors that effect healing. *Am J Sports Med* 1994;24: 797–802.

104. Eggli S. Long-term results of arthroscopic meniscal repair: an analysis of isolated tears. *Am J Sports Med* 1995;23:715–720.

105. Gronkvist H, Hirsch G, Johansson L. Fracture of the anterior tibial spine in children. *J Pediatr Orthop* 1984;4(4):465–468.

106. Tolo V. Fractures and dislocations about the knee. In: Green NE, Swiontkowski MF, eds. *Skeletal trauma in children*. Philadelphia, PA: WB Saunders, 1998:444–447.

107. Willis RB, Blokker C, Stoll TM, et al. Long-term follow-up of anterior tibial eminence fractures. *J Pediatr Orthop* 1993;13(3): 361–364.

108. Mah JY, Otsuka NY, McLean J. An arthroscopic technique for the reduction and fixation of tibial-eminence fractures. *J Pediatr Orthop* 1996;16(1):119–121.

109. Binnet MS, Gurkan I, Yilmaz C, et al. Arthroscopic fixation of intercondylar eminence fractures using a 4-portal technique. *Arthroscopy* 2001;17(5):450–460.

110. Noyes FR, DeLucas JL, Torvik PJ. Biomechanics of anterior cruciate ligament failure: an analysis of strain-rate sensitivity and mechanisms of failure in primates. *J Bone Joint Surg Am* 1974; 56(2):236–253.

111. Janarv PM, Westblad P, Johansson C, et al. Long-term follow-up of anterior tibial spine fractures in children. *J Pediatr Orthop* 1995;15(1):63–68.

112. Smith JB. Knee instability after fractures of the intercondylar eminence of the tibia. *J Pediatr Orthop* 1984;4(4):462–464.

113. Baxter MP, Wiley JJ. Fractures of the tibial spine in children. An evaluation of knee stability. *J Bone Joint Surg Br* 1988;70(2): 228–230.

114. Meyers MH, McKeever FM. Fracture of the intercondylar eminence of the tibia. *J Bone Joint Surg Am* 1970;52(8):1677–1684.

115. Kennedy JC, Weinberg HW, Wilson AS. The anatomy and function of the anterior cruciate ligament as determined by clinical and morphological studies. *J Bone Joint Surg Am* 1974;56: 223–225.

116. Kocher MS, Micheli LJ, Gerbino PG, et al. Tibial eminence fractures in children. Prevalence of meniscal entrapment. *Am J Sports Med* 2003;31(3):404–407.

117. Accousti WK, Willis RB. Tibial eminence fractures. *Orthop Clin North Am* 2003;34:365–375.

118. Angel KR, Hall DJ. Anterior cruciate ligament injury in children and adolescents. *Arthroscopy* 1989;5:197–200.

119. DeLee JC, Curtis R. Anterior cruciate ligament insufficiency in children. *Clin Orthop* 1983;172:112–118.

120. Eskjaer S, Larsen ST. Arthroscopy of the knee in children. *Acta Orthop Scand* 1987;58:273–276.

121. Graf BK, Lange RH, Fujisaki CK, et al. Anterior cruciate ligament tears in skeletally immature patients: meniscal pathology at presentation and after attempted conservative treatment. *Arthroscopy* 1992;8:229–233.

122. McCarroll JR, Tettig AC, Shelbourne KD. Anterior cruciate ligament injuries in the young athlete with open physes. *Am J Sports Med* 1988;16:44–47.

123. Stanitski CL, Harvell JC, Fu F. Observations on acute knee hemarthrosis in children and adolescents. *J Pediatr Orthop* 1993;13:506–510.

124. Steiner ME, Grana WA. The young athlete's knee: recent advances. *Clin Sports Med* 1988;7:527–546.

125. Andrish JT. Anterior cruciate ligament injuries in the skeletally immature patient. *Am J Orthop* 2001;30(2):103–110.

126. Shea K, Pfeiffer R, Wang J, et al. ACL injury in pediatric and adolescent athletes: Differences between males and females. Presented at: *Annual Meeting of Pediatric Orthopaedic Society of North America*. Amelia Island, FL: May 2003.

127. Ireland ML. The female ACL: why is it more prone to injury? *Orthop Clin North Am* 2002;33:637–651.

128. Reiman PR, Jackson DW. Anatomy of the anterior cruciate ligament. In: Jackson DW, Drez D, eds. *The anterior cruciate deficient knee*. St. Louis, MO: CV Mosby Co, 1987:17–26.

129. Ellison AE, Berg EE. Embryology, anatomy and function of the anterior cruciate ligament. *Orthop Clin North Am* 1985;16:3–14.

130. Arnoczky SP. Anatomy of the anterior cruciate ligament. *Clin Orthop* 1983;172:19–25.

131. Girgis FG, Marhall JL, Monajem ARSA. The cruciate ligaments of the knee joint. Anatomical, functional and experimental analysis. *Clin Orthop* 1975;106:216–231.

132. Odensten M, Gillquist J. Functional anatomy of the anterior cruciate ligament and a rationale for reconstruction. *J Bone Joint Surg* 1985;67A:257–262.

133. Smith BA, Livesay GA, Woo SL-Y. Biology and biomechanics of the anterior cruciate ligament. *Clin Sports Med* 1993;12:637–670.

134. Amis AA, Dawkins GPC. Functional anatomy of the anterior cruciate ligament. Fibre bundle actions related to ligament replacements and injuries. *J Bone Joint Surg* 1991;73B:260–267.

135. Dorizas JA, Stanitski CL. Anterior cruciate ligament injury in the skeletally immature. *Orthop Clin North Am* 2003;34:355–363.

136. Arendt E, Dick R. Knee injury patterns among men and women in collegiate basketball and soccer. NCAA data and review of literature. *Am J Sports Med* 1995;23(6):694–701.

137. Medvecky MJ, Bosco J, Sherman OH. Gender disparity of anterior cruciate ligament injury: etiological theories in the female athlete. *Bull Hosp Jt Dis* 2000;59(4):217–226.

138. Slauterbeck JR, Harding DM. Sex hormones and knee ligament injuries in female athletes. *Am J Med Sci* 2001;322(4):196–199.

139. Daniel DM, Stone ML, Dobson BE, et al. Fate of the ACL injured patient. A prospective outcome study. *Am J Sports Med* 1994;22:632–644.

140. Hawkins RJ, Misamore GW, Merritt TR. Follow-up of the acute nonoperated isolated anterior cruciate ligament tear. *Am J Sports Med* 1986;14:205–210.

141. Buckley SL, Barrack RL, Alexander AH. The natural history of conservatively treated partial anterior cruciate ligament tears. *Am J Sports Med* 1989;17:221–225.

142. Graf BK, Lange RH, Fujisaki CK, et al. Anterior cruciate ligament tears in skeletally immature patients: meniscal pathology at presentation and after attempted conservative treatment. *Arthroscopy* 1992;8(2):229–233.

143. Kannus P, Jarvinen M. Knee ligament injuries in adolescents. Eight year follow-up of conservative management. *J Bone Joint Surg Br* 1988;70(5):772–776.

144. Aichroth PM, Datel DV, Zorilla P. The natural history and treatment of rupture of the anterior cruciate ligament in children and adolescents. A prospective review. *J Bone Joint Surg Br* 2002;84(1):38–41.

145. Delee JC, Curtis R. Anterior cruciate ligament insufficiency in children. *Clin Orthop* 1983;172:112–118.

146. Michele LJ, Rask B, Gerberg L. Anterior cruciate ligament reconstruction in patients who are prepubescent. *Clin Orthop* 1999;364:40–47.

147. Stadelmaier DM, Arnoczky SP, Dodds J, et al. The effect of drilling and soft tissue grafting across open growth plates: a histological study. *Am J Sports Med* 1995;23:431–435.

148. Guzzanti V, Falciglia F, Gigante A, et al. The effect of intra-articular ACL reconstruction on the growth plates of rabbits. *J Bone Joint Surg Br* 1994;76(6):960–963.

149. Edwards TB, Greene CC, Baratta RV, et al. The effect of placing a tensioned graft across open growth plates. A gross and histologic analysis. *J Bone Joint Surg Am* 2001;83(5):725–734.

150. Lo IK, Bell D, Fowler PJ. In: WD C, ed. *Anterior cruciate ligament injuries in the skeletally immature patient*. Rosemont, IL, American Academy of Orthopaedic Surgeons, 1998:351–359.

151. Andrews M, Noyes F, Barber-Westin SD. Anterior cruciate ligament allograft reconstruction in the skeletally immature athlete. *Am J Sports Med* 1994;22(1):48–54.

152. McCarroll JR, Rettig AC, Shelbourne KD. Anterior cruciate ligament injuries in the young athlete with open physes. *Am J Sports Med* 1988;16(1):4407.

153. Tanner JM, Davies PS. Clinical longitudinal standards for height and height velocity for North American children. *J Pediatr* 1985;107(3):317–329.

154. Aronowitz ER, Ganley TJ, Goode JR, et al. Anterior cruciate ligament reconstruction in adolescents with open physes. *Am J Sports Med* 2000;28(2):168–175.

155. Paget J. On production of some of the loose bodies in joints. *St Bartholemews Hosp Rep* 1870;6:1.

156. Roberts J. Osteochondritis dissecans. In: Kennedy JC, ed. *The injured adolescent knee*. Baltimore, MD: Williams & Wilkins, 1979.

157. Hughston JC, Hergenroeder PT, Courtenay BG. Osteochondritis dissecans of the femoral condyles. *J Bone Joint Surg Am* 1984; 66(9):1340–1348.

158. Lindholm TS, Osterman K. Treatment of juvenile osteochondritis dissecans in the knee. *Acta Orthop Belg* 1979;45(6):633–640.

159. Green W, Banks H. Osteochondritis dissecans in children. *J Bone Joint Surg Am* 1952;35:26–47.

160. Kocher MS, Micheli LJ, Yaniv M, et al. Functional and radiographic outcome of juvenile osteochondritis dissecans of the knee treated with transarticular arthroscopic drilling. *Am J Sports Med* 2001;29(5):562–566.

161. Cahill B. Treatment of juvenile osteochondritis dissecans and osteochondritis dissecans of the knee. *Clin Sports Med* 1985; 4(2):367–384.

162. Milgram JW. Radiological and pathological manifestations of osteochondritis dissecans of the distal femur. A study of 50 cases. *Radiology* 1978;126(2):305–311.

163. Fairbanks HAT. Osteo-chondritis dissecans. *Br J Surg* 1933;21: 67–82.

164. Mubarak SJ, Carroll NC. Familial osteochondritis dissecans of the knee. *Clin Orthop* 1979;140:131–136.

165. Muburak SJ, Carroll NC. Juvenile osteochondritis dissecans of the knee: etiology. *Clin Orthop* 1981;157:200–211.

166. Clanton TO, DeLee JC. Osteochondritis dissecans. History, pathophysiology and current treatment concepts. *Clin Orthop* 1982;167:50–64.

167. Langenskiold A. Can osteochondritis dissecans arise as a sequel of cartilage fracture in early childhood? *Acta Chir Scand* 1955;109:206.

168. Twyman RS, Desai K, Aichroth PM. Osteochondritis dissecans of the knee: a long-term study. *J Bone Joint Surg Br* 1991;73: 461–464.

169. Fairbanks HT. Osteo-chondritis dissecans. *Br J Surg* 1933;21:67.

170. Kennedy JC, Grainger RW, McGraw RW. Osteochondral fractures of the femoral condyles. *J Bone Joint Surg Br* 1966;48:436.

171. Rosenberg N. Osteochondral fractures of the lateral femoral condyle. *J Bone Joint Surg Am* 1964;46:1013.

172. Smillie IS. *Injuries of the knee joint*. Edinburgh. Churchill Livingstone, 1970.

173. Smillie IS. Ligamentous injury and subluxation of the patella. *J Bone Joint Surg Br* 1959;41:214.

174. Smillie IS. *Osteochondritis dissecans*. Baltimore, MD. Williams & Wilkins, 1960.

175. Chiroff RT, Cooke CP III. Osteochondritis dissecans: a histologic and microradiographic analysis of surgically excised lesions. *J Trauma* 1975;15(8):689–696.

176. Rogers W, Gladstone H. Vascular foramina and arterial supply of the distal end of the femur. *J Bone Joint Surg Am* 1950;32:867–874.

177. Reddy AS. Evaluation of the intraosseous and extraosseus blood supply to the distal femoral condyles. *Am J Sports Med* 1998;26: 415–419.

178. Ribbing S. The hereditary multiple epiphyseal disturbance and its consequences for the aetiologies of local malacias-particularly the osteochondrosis dissecans. *Acta Radiol* 1954;25:296–299.

179. Petrie PW. Aetiology of osteochondritis dissecans. Failure to establish a familial background. *J Bone Joint Surg Br* 1977;59(3): 366–367.

180. Wall E, Von Stein D. Juvenile osteochondritis dissecans. *Orthop Clin North Am* 2003;34:341–353.

181. Hefti F, Beguiristain J, Krauspe R, et al. Osteochondritis dissecans: a multicenter study of the European Pediatric Orthopaedic Society. *J Pediatr Orthop B* 1999;8(4):231–245.

182. Wilson JN. A diagnostic sign in osteochondritis dissecans of the knee. *J Bone Joint Surg Am* 1967;49(3):477–480.

183. De Smet AA, Ilahi OA, Graf BK. Untreated osteochondritis dissecans of the femoral condyle: prediction of patient outcome using radiographic and MR findings. *Skeletal Radiol* 1997;26(8): 463–467.

184. Hinshaw MH, Tuite MJ, De Smet AA. "Dem bones": osteochondral injuries of the knee. *Magn Reson Imaging Clin N Am* 2000; 8(2):335–348.

185. Wall E, Nosir H, Smothers C, et al. Juvenile osteochondritis dissecans of the knee: healing prognosis based on x-ray and gadolinium enhanced MRI. American Society for Sports Medicine-specialty day at the American Academy of Orthopaedic Surgeons Annual Meeting. San Francisco, CA:2001;44.

186. Nawata K, Teshima R, Morio Y, et al. Anomalies of ossification in the posterolateral femoral condyle: assessment by MRI. *Pediatr Radiol* 1999;29(10):781–784.

187. Dipaola JD, Nelson DW, Colville MR. Characterizing osteochondral lesions by magnetic resonance imaging. *Arthroscopy* 1991;7(1):101–104.

188. De Smet AA, Ilahi OA, Graf BK. Reassessment of the MR criteria for stability of osteochondritis dissecans in the knee and ankle. *Skeletal Radiol* 1996;25(2):159–163.

189. O'Connor M, Palaniappan M, Khan N, et al. Osteochondritis dissecans of the knee in children. A comparison of MRI and arthroscopic findings. *J Bone Joint Surg Br* 2002;84(2): 258–262.

190. Kramer J, Stiglbauer R, Engel A, et al. MR contrast arthrography (MRA) in osteochondrosis dissecans. *J Comput Assist Tomogr* 1992;16(2):254–260.

191. Aglietti P, Buzzi R, Bassi PB, et al. Arthroscopic drilling in juvenile osteochondritis dissecans of the medial femoral condyle. *Arthroscopy* 1994;10(3):286–291.

192. Bradley J, Dandy DJ. Results of drilling osteochondritis dissecans before skeletal maturity. *J Bone Joint Surg Br* 1989;71(4):642–644.

193. Guhl JF. Arthroscopic treatment of osteochondritis dissecans. *Clin Orthop* 1982;167:65–74.

194. Anderson AF, Richards DB, Pagnani MJ, et al. Antegrade drilling for osteochondritis dissecans of the knee. *Arthroscopy* 1997; 13(3):319–324.

195. Bruffey J, Mubarak SJ, Chambers HG. Extraarticular drilling on osteochondritis dissecans lesions of the knee in children and adolescents. *Annual Meeting of Pediatric Orthopaedic Society of North America*, Vancouver, 2000:75.

196. Dervin GF, Keene GC, Chissell HR. Biodegradable rods in adult osteochondritis dissecans of the knee. *Clin Orthop* 1998;356: 213–221.

197. Matelic T, Stanitski CL. Operative treatment of osteochondritis dissecans in situ by retrograde pinning. *J Orthop Tech* 1995; 3(1):17–24.

198. Thompson NL. Osteochondritis dissecans and osteochondral fragments managed by Herbert compression screw fixation. *Clin Orthop* 1987;224:71–78.

199. Anderson AF, Pagnani MJ. Osteochondritis dissecans of the femoral condyles. Long-term results of excision of the fragment. *Am J Sports Med* 1997;25(6):830–834.

200. Gill TJ. The treatment of articular cartilage defects using microfracture and debridement. *Am J Knee Surg* 2000;13(1):33–40.

201. Steadman JR, Rodkey WG, Rodrigo JJ. Microfracture: surgical technique and rehabilitation to treat chondral defects. *Clin Orthop* 2001;391(Suppl.):S362–S369.

202. Bugbee WD. Fresh osteochondral allografts. *J Knee Surg* 2002; 15(3):191–195.

203. Mahomed MN, Beaver RJ, Gross AE. The long-term success of fresh, small fragment osteochondral allografts used for intraarticular post-traumatic defects in the knee joint. *Orthopedics* 1992;15(10):1191–1199.

204. Tomford WW, Springfield DS, Mankin HJ. Fresh and frozen articular cartilage allografts. *Orthopedics* 1992;15(10):1183–1188.

205. Convery FR, Meyers MH, Akeson WH. Fresh osteochondral allografting of the femoral condyle. *Clin Orthop* 1991;273: 139–145.

206. Levy A. Osteochondral autograft for the treatment of focal cartilage lesions. *Oper Tech Orthop* 2001;11(2):108–114.

207. Solheim E. Mosaicplasty in articular cartilage injuries of the knee. *Tidsskr Nor Laegeforen* 1999;119(27):4022–4025.

208. Peterson L, Minas T, Brittberg M, et al. Treatment of osteochondritis dissecans of the knee with autologous chondrocyte transplantation: results at two to ten years. *J Bone Joint Surg Am* 2003; 85:17–24.

209. Brittberg M, Faxen E, Peterson L. Carbon fiber scaffolds in the treatment of early knee osteoarthritis: a prospective 4 year follow-up of 37 patients. *Clin Orthop* 1994;307:155–164.

210. Walton M, Rothwell AG. Reactions of thigh tissues of sheep to blunt trauma. *Clin Orthop* 1983;176:273–281.

211. Jackson DW, Feagin JA. Quadriceps contusions in young athletes: relation of severity of injury to treatment and prognosis. *J Bone Joint Surg Am* 1973;55:95–105.

212. Lipscomb AB, Thomas ED, Johnston RK. Treatment of myositis ossificans traumatica in athletes. *Am J Sports Med* 1976;4:111–120.

213. Rothwell AG. Quadriceps hematoma: a prospective clinical study. *Clin Orthop* 1982;171:97–103.

214. An HS, Simpson M, Gale S, et al. Acute anterior compartment syndrome in the thigh: a case report and review of the literature. *Orthop Trauma* 1987;1:180–182.

215. Norman A, Dorfman HD. Juxtacortical circumscribed myositis ossificans: evolution and radiographic features. *Radiology* 1970; 96:301–306.

216. Barker HB, Beynnon BD, Renstrom P. Ankle injury risk factors in sports. *Sports Med* 1997;23:69–74.

217. Anderson SJ, Sullivan JA. *Ankle in care of the young athlete*. Rosemont, IL: AAOS and American Academy of Pediatrics,2000: 413–424.

218. Stiell IG, Greenberg GH, McKnight RD, et al. Decision rules for the use of radiography in acute ankle injuries. Refinement and prospective validation. *JAMA* 1993;269:1127–1132.

219. Dyment PG, ed. *Sports medicine: health care for young athletes*. Elk Grove Village, IL: American Academy of Pediatrics, 1991:216.

220. Anderson SJ. Evaluation and treatment of ankle sprains. *Compr Ther* 1996;22:30–38.

221. Karlsson J, Bergsten T, Lasinger O, et al. Surgical treatment of chronic lateral instability of the ankle. *Am J Sports Med* 1989;17: 268–274.

222. Evans GA, Hardcastle A, Frenyo D. Acute rupture of the lateral ligaments of the ankle. *J Bone Joint Surg Br* 1984;66:209.

223. Younes C, Fowles JV, Fallaha M, et al. Long-term results of surgical reconstruction for chronic lateral instability of the ankle: comparison of Watson-Jones and Evans techniques. *J Trauma* 1988;28:1330–1334.

224. Chrisman OD, Snook GA. Reconstruction of lateral ligament tears of the ankle: an experimental study and clinical evaluation of seven patients treated by a new modification of the Elmslie procedure. *J Bone Joint Surg Am* 1969;51:904–912.

225. Brostrom L. Sprained ankles VI. Surgical treatment of "chronic" ligament ruptures. *Acta Chir Scand* 1966;132:551–565.

226. Gould N, Seligson D, Gassman J. Early and late repair of lateral ligaments of the ankle. *Foot Ankle* 1980;1:84–89.

227. Wilkerson GB, Pinerola JJ, Caturano RW. Invertor versus evertor peak torque and power deficiencies associated with lateral ligament injury. *J Orthop Sports Phys Ther* 1997;26:78–86.

228. Waters PM, Millis M. Hip and pelvic injuries in the young athlete. *Clin Sports Med* 1988;7:513.

229. Watts HG. Fractures of the pelvis in children. *Orthop Clin North Am* 1976;7:615.

230. Canale ST, King RE. Pelvic and hip fractures. In: Rockwood CA Jr, Wilkins KE, King RE, eds. *Fractures in children*. Philadelphia, PA: JB Lippincott Co, 1984.

231. Metzmaker JN, Pappas AM. Avulsion fractures of the pelvis. *Am J Sports Med* 1985;13:349.

232. Schlonsky J, Olix ML. Functional disability following avulsion fracture of the ischial epiphysis. *J Bone Joint Surg Am* 1972;54:641.

233. Rowe CR. Prognosis in dislocations of the shoulder. *J Bone Joint Surg* 1956;38A:957–977.

234. Wagner KT, Lyne ED Jr. Adolescent traumatic dislocations of the shoulder with open epiphyses. *J Pediatr Orthop* 1983;3:61–62.

235. Heck CC. Anterior dislocation of the glenohumeral joint in a child. *J Trauma* 1981;21:174–175.

236. Heolen MA, Burgers AM, Rozing PM. Prognosis of primary anterior shoulder dislocation in young adults. *Arch Orthop Trauma Surg* 1990;110:51–54.

237. Hovelius L. Anterior dislocation of the shoulder in teenagers and young adults. Five-year prognosis. *J Bone Joint Surg* 1987; 69A:393–399.

238. Wasserlauf BL, Paletta GA. Shoulder disorders in the skeletally immature throwing athlete. *Orthop Clin North Am* 2003;34: 427–437.

239. Matsen FA III, Thomas SC, Rockwood CA Jr. Anterior glenohumeral instability. In: Rockwood CA, Matsen FA III, eds. *The shoulder*. Philadelphia, PA: WB Saunders, 1990.

240. Dameron TB, Rockwood CA. Part 2. Subluxations and dislocations of the glenohumeral joint. In: Rockwood CA, Green DP, eds. *Fractures*, 2nd ed., Vol. 3. Philadelphia, PA: JB Lippincott Co, 1984.

241. Pagnani MJ, Galinat BJ, Warren RF. Glenohumeral instability. *Orthopaedic sports medicine. Principles and practice*. Philadelphia, PA: WB Saunders, 1994:580–623.

242. Pasque CB, Maginnis DW, Yurko-Griffin L. *Shoulder in care of the young athlete*. In Sullivan JA, Anderson SJ, eds. Care of the young Athlete. Rosemont, IL: American Academy of Orthopaedic Surgeons, American Academy of Pediatrics, 2000:323–347.

243. Townsend H, Jobe F, Pink M, et al. Electromyographic analysis of the glenohumeral muscles during a baseball rehabilitation program. *Am J Sports Med* 1991;19:264–272.

244. Marans HJ, Angel KR, Schemitsch EH, et al. The fate of traumatic anterior dislocation of the shoulder in children. *J Bone Joint Surg* 1992;74A:1242–1244.

245. Bankart ASB. The pathology and treatment of recurrent dislocation of the shoulder joint. *Br J Surg* 1939;26:23.

246. Koss S, Richmond JC, Woodward JS. Two to five year follow-up of arthroscopic bankart reconstruction using a suture anchor technique. *Am J Sports Med* 1997;25:809–812.

247. Gill TJ, Micheli LJ, Gebhard F, et al. Bankart repair for anterior instability of the shoulder. *J Bone Joint Surg* 1997;25:809–812.

248. Huber H, Gerber C. Voluntary subluxation of the shoulder in children. A long-term follow-up study of 36 shoulders. *J Bone Joint Surg* 1994;76B:118–122.

249. Rowe CR, Pierce DS, Clark JG. Voluntary dislocation of the shoulder: a preliminary report on a clinical, electromyographic and psychiatric study of twenty-six patients. *J Bone Joint Surg* 1973;55A:445–460.

250. Ireland ML, Andrews JR. Shoulder and elbow injuries in the young athlete. *Clin Sports Med* 1988;7:473–494.

251. Ireland ML, Satterwhite YE. Shoulder injuries. In: Andrews JR, Zarins B, Wild KE, eds. *Injuries in baseball*. Philadelphia, PA: Lippincott Williams & Wilkins, 1998:271–281.

252. Kocher MS, Waters PM, Michell LJ. Upper extremity injuries in the paediatric athlete. *Sports Med* 2000;30:117–135.

253. Oberlander MA, Chisar MA, Campbell B. Epidemiology of shoulder injuries in throwing and overhead athletes. *Sports Med Arthrosc Rev* 2000;8:115–123.

254. Patel PR, Warner JJP. Shoulder injuries in the skeletally immature athlete. *Sports Med Arthrosc Rev* 1996;4:99–113.

255. Back FR, O'Brien SJ, Warren RF, et al. An unusual neurological complication of the Bristow procedure: a case report. *J Bone Joint Surg Am* 1988;70:458.

256. Richards RR, Hudson AR, Bertoia JT, et al. Injury to the brachial plexus during putti platt and Bristow procedures: a report of eight cases. *Am J Sports Med* 1987;15:374.

257. Willis RB, Galpin RD. In: Letts RM, ed. *Dislocations of the shoulder in: management of pediatric fractures*. New York: Churchill Livingstone, 1994:159.

258. Aparicio G, Abril JC, Calvo E, et al. Radiologic study of patellar height in Osgood-Schlatter disease. *J Pediatr Orthop* 1997;17(1): 63–66.

259. Lancourt JE, Cristini JA. Patella alta and patella infera. Their etiological role in patellar dislocation, chondromalacia and apophysitis of the tibial tubercle. *J Bone Joint Surg Am* 1975; 57(8):1112–1115.

260. Krause BL, Williams JP, Catterall A. Natural history of Osgood-Schlatter disease. *J Pediatr Orthop* 1990;10(1):65–68.

261. Bolista MJ, Fitch RD. Tibial tubercle avulsions. *J Pediatr Orthop* 1986;6(2):186–192.

262. Chow SP, Lam JJ, Leong JC. Fractures of the tibial tuberosity in Adolescents. *J Bone Joint Surg Am* 1990;72(2):231–234.

263. Ogden JA, Southwick WO. Osgood-Schlatter's disease and tibial tuberosity development. *Clin Orthop* 1976;116:180.

264. Crigler NW, Riddervole HO. Soft tissue changes in x-ray diagnosis of the Osgood-Schlatter lesion. *Va Med* 1982;109:176.

265. Kujala UM, Kvist M, Heinonen O. Osgood-Schlatter's disease in adolescent athletes. *Am J Sports Med* 1985;13:236.

266. Willner P. Osgood-Schlatter's disease: etiology and treatment. *Clin Orthop* 1969;62:178.

267. Bowers KD Jr. Patellar tendon avulsion as a complication of Osgood-Schlatters disease. *Am J Sports Med* 1981;59:56.

268. Mital MA, Matza RA, Cohen J. The so-called unresolved Osgood-Schlatter lesion. *J Bone Joint Surg Am* 1980;62:732.

269. Binazzi R, Felli L, Vaccari V, et al. Surgical treatment of unresolved Osgood-Schlatter lesion. *Clin Orthop* 1993;289: 202–204.

270. Ogden JA, McCarthy SM, Jokl P. The painful bipartite patella. *J Pediatr Orthop* 1982;2(3):263–269.

271. Kay JJ, Freiberger RH. Fragmentation of the lower pole of the patella in spastic lower extremities. *Radiology* 1991;101:97.

272. Medlar RC, Lyne ED. Sinding-Larsen-Johansson disease. Its etiology and natural history. *J Bone Joint Surg Am* 1978; 60(8):113.

273. Dupont JY. Synovial plica of the knee. Controversies and review. *Clin Sports Med* 1997;16(1):87.

274. Apple JS, Martinez S, Hardaker WT, et al. Synovial plicae of the knee. *Skeletal Radiol* 1982;7(4):251.

275. Barber FA. Fenestrated medial patella plica. *Arthroscopy* 1987; 3(4):253.

276. Dandy DJ. Anatomy of the medial suprapatellar plica and medial synovial shelf. *Arthroscopy* 1990;6(2):79.

277. Dupont JY. Role of synovial plicae in pathology of the knee. *Rev Chir Orthop Reparatrice Appar Mot* 1985;71(6):401.

278. Duri ZA, Patel DV, Aichroth PM. The immature athlete. *Clin Sports Med* 2002;21(3):461.

279. Amatuzzi MM, Fazzi A, Varella MH. Pathologic synovial plica of the knee. Results of conservative treatment. *Am J Sports Med* 1990;18(5):466.

280. Ewing JW. Plica: pathologic or not? *J Am Acad Orthop Surg* 1993;1(2):117.

281. Andersen E, Paulsen TD. Plica mediopatellaris-arthroscopic resection under local anaesthesia. *Arch Orthop Trauma Surg* 1986;106(1):18.

282. Flanagan JP, Trakru S, Meyer M, et al. Arthroscopic excision of symptomatic medial plica. A study of 118 knees with 1-4 years follow-up. *Acta Orthop Scand* 1994;65(4):408.

283. Hardaker WT, Whipple TL, Basset FH III. Diagnosis and treatment of the plica syndrome of the knee. *J Bone Joint Surg Am* 1980;62(2):221.

284. Johnson DP, Eastwood DM, Witherow PJ. Symptomatic synovial plicae of the knee. *J Bone Joint Surg Am* 1993;75(10):1485.

285. Maffuli N, Testa V, Vapasso G. Mediopatellar synovial plica of the knee in athletes: results of arthroscopic treatment. *Med Sci Sports Exerc* 1993;25(9):985.

286. Munziger U, Ruckstuhl J, Scherrer H, et al. Internal derangement of the knee joint due to pathologic synovial folds: the mediopatellar plica syndrome. *Clin Orthop* 1981;155:59.

287. Stanitski CL. Knee overuse disorders in the pediatric and adolescent athlete. *Instr Course Lect* 1993;42:483.

288. Patel D. Plica as a cause of anterior knee pain. *Orthop Clin North Am* 1986;17(2):273.

289. Hoffa A. The influence of the adipose tissue with regard to the pathology of the knee joint. *JAMA* 1904;43:795–796.

290. Biedert RM, Sanchis-Alfonso V. Sources of anterior knee pain. *Clin Sports Med* 2002;21(3):335–347.

291. Biedert RM, Lobenhoffer P, Latterman C, et al. Free nerve endings in the medial and posteromedial capsuloligamentous complexes: occurrence and distribution. *Knee Surg Sports Traumatol Arthrosc* 2000;8(2):68–72.

292. Biedert RM, Stauffer E, Friederich NF. Occurrence of free nerve endings in the soft tissue of the knee joint. A histologic investigation. *Am J Sports Med* 1992;20(4):430–433.

293. Kennedy JC, Alexander IJ, Hayes KC. Nerve supply of the human knee and its functional importance. *Am J Sports Med* 1982;10(6):329–335.

294. Duri ZA, Aichroth PM, Dowd G. The fat pad. Clinical observations. *Am J Knee Surg* 1996;9(2):55–66.

295. Ogilvie-Harris DJ, Giddens J. Hoffa's disease: arthroscopic resection of the infrapatellar fat pad. *Arthroscopy* 1994;10(2):184–187.

296. Shea KG, Pfeiffer R, Curtin M. Idiopathic anterior knee pain in adolescents. *Orthop Clin North Am* 2003;34:377–383.

297. Stanitski CL. Patellofemoral mechanism-anterior knee pain. In: Stanitski CL, Delee JC, Drez DJ Jr, eds. *Pediatric and adolescent sports medicine*, Philadelphia, PA: WB Saunders, 1994:335–370.

298. Bentley G. Chondromalacia patellae. *J Bone Joint Surg Am* 1970;52(2):221–231.

299. Sandow MJ, Goodfellow JW. The natural history of anterior knee pain in adolescents. *J Bone Joint Surg Br* 1985;67(1):36–38.

300. Dehaven KE, Dolan WA, Mayer PJ. Chondromalacia patellae in athletes. Clinical presentation and conservative management. *Am J Sports Med* 1979;7(1):5–11.

301. Dehaven KE, Dolan WA, Mayer PJ. Chondromalacia patellae and the painful knee. *Am Fam Physician* 1980;21(1):117–124.

302. Insall JN. Patella pain syndromes and chondromalacia patellae. *Instr Course Lect* 1981;30:342–356.

303. Yates C, Grana WA. Patellofemoral pain-a prospective study. *Orthopedics* 1986;9(5):663–667.

304. Yates CK, Grana WA. Patellofemoral pain in children. *Clin Orthop* 1990;255:36–43.

305. Grelsamer RP. The nonsurgical treatment of patellofemoral disorders. *Oper Tech Sports Med* 1999;7(2):65–68.

306. Bennett JG, Stauber WT. Evaluation and treatment of anterior knee pain using eccentric exercise. *Med Sci Sports Exerc* 1986;18(5):526–530.

307. American Medical Association. *Subcommittee on classification of sports injuries. Standard nomenclature of athletic injuries.* Chicago, IL: American Medical Association, 1966:122–126.

308. Andrish JT, Bergfeld JA, Walheim JA. A prospective study on the management of shin splints. *J Bone Joint Surg Am* 1974;56:1697–1700.

309. Bates P. Shin splints—a literature review. *Br J Sports Med* 1985;13:365–366.

310. Drez D. *Therapeutic modalities for sports injuries.* Chicago, IL: Year Book Medical Publishers, 1989.

311. Holder LE, Michael RH. The specific scintigraphic pattern of "shin splints in the lower leg:" concise communication. *J Nucl Med* 1984;25:865–869.

312. Brill DR. Sports nuclear medicine. Bone imaging for lower extremity pain in athletes. *Clin Nucl Med* 1983;8:101–106.

313. Lieberman CM, Hemingway DL. Scintigraphy of shin splints. *Clin Nucl Med* 1980;5:31.

314. Lehman WL Jr. Overuse syndromes in runners. *Am Fam Physician* 1984;29:157–161.

315. Detmer DE. Chronic shin splints. Classification and management of medial tibial stress syndrome. *Sports Med* 1986;3:436–446.

316. Detmer D, Sharpe K, Sufit R, et al. Chronic compartment syndrome: diagnosis, management and outcomes. *Am J Sports Med* 1985;13(3):162–170.

317. Logan J, Rorabeck C, Castle G. The measurement of dynamic compartment pressure during exercise. *Am J Sports Med* 1983;11(4):220–223.

318. McDermott A, Marble A, Yabsley R, et al. Monitoring dynamic anterior compartment pressures during exercise. *Am J Sports Med* 1982;10(2):83–89.

319. Shah SN, Miller BS, Kuln JE. Chronic exertional compartment syndrome. *Am J Orthop* 2004;32(7):335–341.

320. Fronek J, Mubarek S, Hargens A, et al. Management of chronic exertional anterior compartment syndrome of the lower extremity. *Clin Orthop* 1987;220:217–227.

321. Martins M, Backaert M, Vermant G, et al. Chronic leg pain in athletes due to a recurrent compartment syndrome. *Am J Sports Med* 1984;12(2):148–151.

322. Aubrey B, Sienkiewicz P, Mankin H. Chronic exercise-induced compartment pressure elevation measured with a miniaturized fluid pressure monitor. *Am J Sports Med* 1988;16(6):610–615.

323. Matsen F, Mayo K, Sheridan G, et al. Monitoring of intramuscular pressure. *Surgery* 1976;79(6):702–709.

324. Matsen F, Winquist R, Krugmire R. Diagnosis and management of compartment syndromes. *J Bone Joint Surg* 1980;62A(2):286–291.

325. Pedowitz D, Hargens A, Mubarek S, et al. Modified criteria for the objective diagnosis of chronic compartment syndrome of the leg. *Am J Sports Med* 1990;18(1):35–40.

326. Amendola A, Rorabeck CH, Vellet D, et al. The use of magnetic resonance imaging in exertional compartment syndromes. *Am J Sports Med* 1990;18:29–34.

327. Trease L, van Every B, Bennell K, et al. A prospective blinded evaluation of exersice thallium – 201 SPECT in patients with suspected chronic exertional compartment syndrome of the leg. *Eur J Nucl Med* 2001;28:688–695.

328. Mubarek S, Owen C. Double incision fasciotomy of the leg for decompression in compartment syndromes. *J Bone Joint Surg* 1977;59A:184.

329. Rorabeck C, Fowler P, Nott L. The results of fasciotomy in the management of chronic exertional compartment syndrome. *Am J Sports Med* 1988;16(3):224–227.

330. Zoltan DJ, Clancy WG, Keene JS. A new approach to snapping hip and refractory trochanteric bursitis in athletes. *Am J Sports Med* 1986;14:201.

331. Hogan KA, Gross RH. Overuse injuries in pediatric athletes. *Orthop Clin North Am* 2003;34:405–415.

332. Yeni YN, Fyhrie DP. Fatigue damage-fracture mechanics interaction in cortical bone. *Bone* 2002;30(3):509–514.

333. Micheli LJ. Overuse injuries in children's sports. The growth factor. *Orthop Clin North Am* 1983;14(2):337.

334. Micheli LJ, Fehlandt AF. In: Letts RM, ed. *Stress fractures in: management of pediatric fractures.* New York: Churchill Livingstone, 1994:973.

335. Milgrom C, Finestone A, Shlamkovitch N, et al. Youth is a risk factor for stress fracture. A study of 783 infantry recruits. *J Bone Joint Surg Br* 1994;76(1):20–22.

336. Protzman RR, Griffis CG. Stress fractures in men and women undergoing military training. *J Bone Joint Surg Am* 1977;59:825.

337. Zahger D, Abramovitz A, Zelikovsky L, et al. Stress fractures in female soldiers: an epidemiological investigation of an outbreak. *Mil Med* 1988;153:448.

338. Brudvig TJ, Gudger TD, Obermeyer L. Stress fractures in 295 trainees: a one-year study of the incidence as related to age, sex, and race. *Mil Med* 1983;148:666.

339. Paty JG Jr. Diagnosis and treatment of musculoskeletal running injuries. *Semin Arthritis Rheum* 1988;18:48.

340. Giladi M, Milgrom C, Simkin A, et al. Stress fractures: identifiable risk factors. *Am J Sports Med* 1991;19:647.

341. Lysens RJ, Ostyn MS, Vanden Auweele Y, et al. The accident-prone and overuse-prone profiles of the young athlete. *Am J Sports Med* 1989;17:612.

342. Prather JL, Nusynowitz ML, Snowdy HA, et al. Scintigraphic findings in stress fractures. *J Bone Joint Surg* 1977;59:869.

343. Greaney RB, Gerber FH, Laughlin RL, et al. Distribution and natural history of stress fractures in U.S. Marine recruits. *Radiology* 1983;146:339.

344. Mink JH, Deutsch AL. Occult cartilage and bone injuries of the knee: detection, classification and assessment with MR imaging. *Radiology* 1989;170:823.

345. Lee JK, Yao L. Stress fractures: MR imaging. *Radiology* 1988;169:217.

346. Walter NE, Wold MDP. Stress fractures in young athletes. *Am J Sports Med* 1977;5:165.

347. Micheli LJ. Overuse injuries in children. In: Lovell WW, Winter RB, eds. *Pediatric orthopedics*, 2nd ed. Philadelphia, PA: JB Lippincott Co, 1986:1103.

348. Johansson C, Ekenman I, Tornkvist H, et al. Stress fractures of the femoral neck in athletes: the consequence of a delay in diagnosis. *Am J Sports Med* 1990;18:524.

349. Rettig AC, Shelbourne DK, McCarroll JR, et al. The natural history and treatment of delayed union stress fractures of the anterior cortex of the tibia. *Am J Sports Med* 1988;16:250.

350. Green E, Rogers RA, Lipscomb BA. Nonunions or stress fractures of the tibia. *Am J Sports Med* 1985;13:171.

351. Shelbourne KD, Fisher DA, Rettig AC, et al. Stress fractures of the medial malleolus. *Am J Sports Med* 1988;16:60.

352. Orava S, Hulkko A. Delayed unions and nonunions of stress fractures in athletes. *Am J Sports Med* 1988;16:378.

353. Fitch KD, Blackwell JB, Gilmour WN. Operation for non-union of stress fracture of the tarsal navicular. *J Bone Joint Surg Br* 1989;71:109.

354. McKenzie DC, Taunton JE, Clement DB, et al. Calcaneal epiphysis in adolescent athletes. *Can J Appl Sport Sci* 1981;6:123.

355. Micheli LJ, Ireland ML. Prevention and management of calcaneal apophysitis in children: an overuse syndrome. *J Pediatr Orthop* 1987;7:34.

356. Sever JW. Apophysitis of the os calcis. *NY State Med J* 1912;95:1025–1029.

357. Caine D, Howe W, Ross W, et al. Does repetitive physical loading inhibit radial growth in female gymnasts? *Clin J Sports Med* 1997;7(4):302–308.

358. Hansen NM Jr. Epiphyseal changes in the proximal humerus of an adolescent baseball pitcher. A case report. *Am J Sports Med* 1982;10(6):380–384.

359. Werner S, Fleisig G, Dillman C, et al. Biomechanics of the elbow during baseball pitching. *J Orthop Sports Phys Ther* 1993;17:274–278.

360. Pappas A. Elbow problems associated with baseball during childhood and adolescence. *Clin Orthop* 1982;164:30–41.

361. Fleisig G, Andrews JR, Dillman C, et al. Kinetics of baseball pitching with implications about injury mechanisms. *Am J Sports Med* 1995;23:233–239.

362. Lyman S, Fleisig G, Waterbor J, et al. Longitudinal study of elbow and shoulder pain in youth baseball pitchers. *Med Sci Sports Exerc* 2001;33(1):1803–1810.

363. Andrews J, Fleisig G. How many pitches should I allow my child to throw? *USA Baseball News* 1996;4:5.

364. Gerbino PG. Elbow disorders in throwing athletes. *Orthop Clin North Am* 2003;34:417–426.

365. Lyman S, Fleisig G, Andrews J, et al. Effect of pitch type, pitch count and pitching mechanics on risk of elbow and shoulder pain in youth baseball pitchers. *Am J Sports Med* 2002;30(4):463–468.

366. Laurent L, Lindstrom B. Osteochondrosis of the capitellum of the humeri (Panner's disease). *Acta Orthop Scand* 1956;26:111–119.

367. Panner HA. A peculiar affection of the capitulum humeri resembling Calvé-Perthes disease of the hip. *Acta Radiol* 1929;10:234–242.

368. Morrey B, An K, Stormont T. Force transmission through the radial head. *J Bone Joint Surg Am* 1988;70:250–256.

369. Andrews J. Bony injuries about the elbow in the young throwing athlete. *Instr Course Lect* 1978;34:323–331.

370. Lindholm I, Osterman K, Vankka E. Osteochondritis dissecans of the elbow, ankle and hip. A comparison study. *Clin Orthop* 1980;148:245–253.

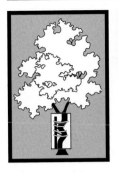

# 33

# Management of Fractures

### *Charles T. Price*  *John M. Flynn*

Injuries of all types are the second leading cause of hospitalization among children younger than 15 years (1). Accidents are the leading cause of death from ages 1 year to 18 years (2). Musculoskeletal trauma, although rarely fatal, accounts for 10% to 25% of all childhood injuries (3). Properly instituted injury prevention programs can be effective in reducing the number and severity of pediatric trauma events (3).

Boys have a 50% risk and girls a 40% risk of incurring a fracture before the age of 18 (4). The fracture rate increases as children grow, with the incidence peaking in early adolescence. New sports and recreational activities such as rollerblading and skateboarding have created new injury patterns, with an increase in the incidence of distal radius fractures (4,5). Fortunately, most fractures are minor. Only 20% require reduction, and greenstick and torus fractures constitute approximately 50% of fractures in children (6,7). Therefore, the management of pediatric fractures is often straightforward, but one must know when to intervene and when to allow nature to take its course. The skeleton of a young child behaves differently than the skeleton of an older child. There are also musculoskeletal differences in biomechanics, anatomy, and physiology between children and adults. It is the purpose of this chapter to highlight the unique aspects of managing fractures in children, and to delineate age-appropriate treatment guidelines.

# GENERAL FEATURES OF FRACTURES IN CHILDREN

## Biomechanical Considerations

The bones of children are less mineralized and have more vascular channels than the bones of adults. This results in a lower modulus of elasticity (8). Therefore, a given stress applied to a specific area of pediatric bone results in more strain than the same stress on the adult bone. Bending strength is lower than in adult bone, but the low modulus of elasticity allows for greater energy absorption before failure. Pediatric bone also has the capacity for plastic deformation in which the bone does not return to its original shape. Microscopic mechanical failure, not evident on routine radiographs, occurs through oblique slip lines or microfractures on the compression side of the bone. This produces no fracture hematoma and minimal periosteal reaction during healing. Plastic deformation results from an applied load after the yield point is reached, but before the breaking point. This partly explains why greenstick fractures can occur when a bending load is applied. Much of the strain energy is dissipated through plastic deformation of the concave cortex, while tension failure occurs on the convex side. This prevents larger, more catastrophic failure from occurring.

In addition to greenstick fractures, children can have torus or "buckle" fractures from compression failure. This usually occurs at the metaphyseal–diaphyseal junction, where the more rigid diaphyseal cortex meets the thinner metaphyseal cortex. The less rigid metaphyseal cortex buckles and deforms without complete failure, creating a relatively stable injury. The rate at which the force is applied also influences the fracture type. Higher load rates more often result in complete fracture (8). Complete fractures display transverse, oblique, or spiral configurations, depending on how the injury force was applied. Comminuted fractures are less common in children than in adults, because pediatric bone can dissipate energy before failure, and its porosity inhibits fracture line propagation. The smaller diameter of pediatric bone also affects its strength compared with adult bone. The polar moment of inertia of a structure, which measures resistance to torque, is proportional to the fourth power of the radius of the structure. Therefore, a relatively small increase in the cortical diameter results in a large increase in a bone's ability to resist torsional load.

The epiphysis also affects the mechanical properties of bone. In young children, the epiphysis is largely cartilaginous and transmits injury forces to the metaphysis. Increasing ossification in the epiphysis occurs with age and imparts more rigidity to the epiphysis. This increased rigidity partially explains why epiphyseal fractures and separations are more commonly seen in older children.

## Anatomic Considerations

Growth plates and their surrounding growth centers are major anatomic features that distinguish children's bones from those of adults. The physis, also called the *growth plate* or the *epiphyseal plate*, is the area of growing cartilage that contributes length to the growing bone. The epiphysis is the region at the end of the bone. The epiphysis forms a secondary center of ossification and determines the shape and size of the articular surface. An apophysis is a secondary growth center at a site of tendon attachment. Apophyses are extraarticular and do not contribute to longitudinal growth. Each of these structures ossifies at predictable times during growth and thus provides information regarding skeletal maturity. Lack of ossification in young children and variable patterns of ossification during growth make the diagnosis of injury an even greater challenge in children than in adults.

Another anatomic characteristic of growing bone is the thick, vascular, and highly osteogenic periosteum. The cambium or osteogenic layer lies directly on the cortex of bone. The outer fibrous layer provides attachment for muscles and ligaments. Between these two layers lie elastic fibers that allow the fibrous layer to be stripped from the bone, leaving the osteogenic layer intact (9). Muscle and periosteum are firmly attached to the bone in only a few places, such as the linea aspera. The periosteum is also firmly attached to the growth plate at the perichondrial ring of LaCroix, which helps stabilize the physis. The thick periosteum in children is rarely torn circumferentially after a fracture and often remains intact on the compression side of the injured bone. This intact periosteal sleeve may then be used as a tension band for fracture reduction and stabilization. Intact periosteum may also prevent soft tissue interposition and facilitate reduction. Conversely, the periosteum itself may become interposed between the fracture fragments, and the longitudinally torn periosteum may interfere with reduction by allowing the bone to "buttonhole" through the periosteal defect.

## Physiologic Considerations

Several authors have noted increased risk of distal radius fracture in children with increased body mass and decreased bone mineral density (10,11). However, this relationship has not been confirmed for fractures at other sites (12). Fracture patterns also vary with age due to changing skeletal maturation.

Fractures in children heal considerably more rapidly than fractures in adults, and nonunion is rare. Most pediatric fractures unite by secondary fracture healing, which occurs without rigid immobilization and involves a combination of intramembranous and endochondral ossification. Fractures cause cellular injury and hematoma formation. Blood, marrow, and necrotic cells release cytokines that stimulate inflammation and the proliferation of stem cells (13). The clot gives rise to platelet-derived growth factor and transforming growth factor $\beta$, leading to general cellular proliferation. Stem cells produce bone morphogenetic proteins that cause cellular differentiation. The exact relation between these factors and other factors involved in the coordination of fracture healing is the subject of ongoing research (14). During the second stage of fracture healing, angiogenesis occurs. This stage of bone healing is facilitated in children by the highly vascular periosteum and preservation of a viable muscle envelope. The periosteum also contributes to bone formation by membranous ossification within 10 to 14 days of injury. Angiogenesis is followed by the formation of soft callus. Low oxygen tension and fracture motion promote cartilage formation as the initial stage of endochondral ossification. This cartilage is subsequently removed and replaced by hard callus with woven bone (9,14). Ultimately, the ossification phase gives way to a more prolonged phase of fracture remodeling.

Remodeling of angulated fractures in children is a well-recognized phenomenon (Fig. 33.1). It is explained in part by the osteogenic potential of the periosteum and the magnitude of the vascular response in children (9). The periosteum is vital to fracture healing and should be preserved as much as possible. Large segments of bone may regenerate and remodel, so long as the periosteal tube is intact. Remodeling at the fracture site occurs by bone resorption on the convexity and deposition on the concavity of the fracture. This phenomenon of "bone drift" is well recognized clinically and has been quantified in the rabbit model (15). However, most of the remodeling occurs by reorientation of the growth plates, with improvement in the overall alignment of the limb. Asymmetric and longitudinal growth of the physis contributes to this remodeling. Therefore, measurement of angular remodeling at the fracture site gives an inadequate picture of the overall limb alignment as remodeling occurs (15,16). Remodeling capacity depends on the number of years of growth remaining, the proximity of the fracture to a rapidly growing physis, the magnitude of angular deformity, and the plane of angulation relative to adjacent joints. Remodeling may continue for 5 to 6 years after fracture, so long as growth occurs during the period of remodeling (16). The rate of remodeling is minimally influenced by age, but the completeness of remodeling may be limited by the number of years of growth remaining (16,17). Fractures in the plane of joint motion and near a rapidly growing physis have the greatest capacity to remodel. Fractures with smaller degrees of malunion are more likely to remodel completely.

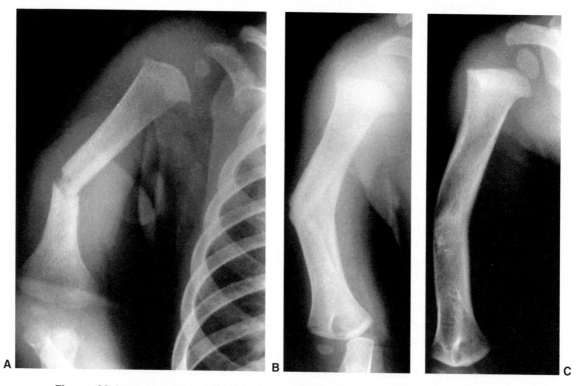

**Figure 33.1** Periosteal bone formation. **A:** Complete fracture of the humeral diaphysis in a 6-month-old child. The periosteum is presumed to be intact on the compression (concave) side. **B:** Four weeks later, the periosteum has formed a complete column of new bone. **C:** Six months after injury, there has been significant remodeling, with a 50% correction of the angular deformity.

Remodeling of rotational deformity has also been noted in children, but this is less predictable than angular remodeling (15,18). It has been postulated that torsional remodeling occurs by helical growth of the physis (15).

Another distinguishing physiologic response to bone healing in children is the potential for growth stimulation after fracture. The age of the patient and the amount of periosteal stripping influence the amount of growth stimulation (9). This phenomenon is most commonly reported after femoral fractures in children between the ages of 3 and 9 years, but it also occurs after other fractures (19–21). The exact mechanism for growth acceleration is unknown, but increased blood flow to the growth plate and release of periosteal tension after fracture are potential causes. Hyperemia as a cause of overgrowth is supported by the observation that growth acceleration may occur with conditions that cause increased vascularity, such as congenital vascular anomalies, inflammatory conditions, and tumoral disorders (19). Transverse sectioning of the periosteum also produces overgrowth. Periosteal stripping or division close to the growth plate increases the effect of transverse periosteal release, but longitudinal incision of the periosteum does not cause growth acceleration (9,22). Hemicircumferential release of the periosteum causes asymmetric growth and subsequent angular deformity (23). This phenomenon is most often seen clinically after fracture of the proximal tibial metaphysis in children, when the medial periosteum is torn transversely while the lateral periosteum remains intact. These findings support the observation that the periosteum acts as a mechanical restraint on epiphyseal growth through its attachments to the perichondrial ring (24). In older children, premature physeal closure has been noted after diaphyseal fracture (25,26). Perhaps the variable growth responses after fracture can be partially explained by differences in periosteal damage or asymmetric hyperemic responses after fracture.

# INJURY TO THE PHYSIS

## Anatomy and Physiology of the Physis

Growth plates are located at the ends of all long bones and contain the cells responsible for bone growth. Longitudinal growth occurs as columns of cartilage form and undergo endochondral ossification. Fracture of the growth plate generally heals within 3 to 4 weeks, because this is a well-vascularized region that is growing rapidly and forming bone at the time of injury.

The development, histology, and physiology of the growth plate are described in greater detail in Chapter 1. Several anatomic features are pertinent for understanding trauma to the growth plate. The germinal zone of cartilage formation is located on the articular side of the physis. This zone consists of resting cells, which initiate the process of long-bone growth by dividing to form the zone of proliferating cartilage. The hypertrophic zone is next. This is a zone of maturation where the chondrocytes begin to enlarge. On the metaphyseal side of this zone, vascular buds grow into the degenerating columns of cartilage and initiate provisional calcification as the chondrocytes degenerate. Remodeling into lamellar bone in the metaphysis rapidly follows provisional calcification.

Fractures through the physis are usually the result of tension or shearing forces. Compressive forces tend to cause fracture through bone. Bright et al. (27), using rapid-loading techniques to simulate *in vivo* forces, demonstrated that the weakest zone is the zone of provisional calcification. However, fracture failure was rarely limited to one zone, and propagating cracks traversed, at least partially, the upper germinal zones in 85% of the animals tested. In younger animals, the fracture was more likely to traverse only the zone between the hypertrophic cells and metaphyseal bone, avoiding the germinal zones. This is clinically relevant because injury to the germinal zone may be more likely in older children and can cause arrest of bone growth.

The perichondrial groove of Ranvier and the perichondrial ring of LaCroix surround each physis circumferentially at the periphery. These structures constitute a separate growth center that provides growth of the physis in width. The groove of Ranvier consists of resting and proliferating cells, whereas the ring of LaCroix consists of cartilage cells that extend toward the metaphysis and become continuous with the metaphyseal periosteum. The groove and ring provide support to the physis and resistance to physeal separation. Additional stability is provided by large and small undulations of the growth plate. The smaller projections are called *mammillary processes*. Larger contours include the lappet formation, which is the overlapping shape of the physis as it cups the metaphysis. The lappet formation is readily appreciated where the anterior portion of the proximal tibial growth plate extends distally as the tibial tuberosity. Muscular, capsular, and ligamentous attachments to the epiphysis may provide additional stability. However, these structures can also transmit force to the growth plate, resulting in characteristic fracture patterns that vary with the specific anatomy of a joint.

The vascularity of the growth plate is essential to its development. There is strict separation of the epiphyseal and metaphyseal circulation, because blood vessels do not cross the growth plate. There are two patterns of blood supply to epiphyses (28). Some epiphyses are completely intracapsular (e.g., the proximal femur and the proximal radius). Blood vessels for these epiphyses must enter the epiphysis around the periphery of the growth plate and through a narrow region between the articular cartilage and the physis. This type of blood supply is very susceptible to damage during physeal separation or occlusion of supporting vessels. The second pattern of epiphyseal blood supply is more common, and is seen in epiphyses that are extracapsular (e.g., the proximal tibia and the distal radius).

Vessels that supply circulation to the epiphysis and the growth plate penetrate directly through the side of the epiphysis where it is covered with periosteum and capsular attachments. Extracapsular epiphyses are less vulnerable to devascularization when physeal separation occurs.

## Clinical Features of Physeal Fractures

Physeal fractures constitute 15% to 30% of all childhood fractures (29). The peak age for injury to the growth plate is early adolescence (11 to 12 years), and physeal fracture is uncommon in children younger than 5 years. Boys are affected twice as often as girls (29,30). Several classification systems have been proposed since Foucher first described different types of physeal fractures in 1863 (30). The most widely used classification of physeal fractures is that described by Salter and Harris (31). There are five types of fractures in this classification. Rang has added a sixth that is commonly recognized (Fig. 33.2) (32).

Type I injury involves a transverse fracture through the entire growth plate without evidence of a metaphyseal fragment. This type of fracture is most commonly seen in infants and young children. The epiphyseal fragment may be nondisplaced or minimally displaced, making diagnosis difficult. Localized swelling and point tenderness may confirm the diagnosis. The prognosis for resumption of growth is excellent with a few notable exceptions, such as physeal separation of the proximal or distal femur. Partial growth arrest may occur with more severe trauma, or when periosteum is entrapped in the physis (33,34).

Type II fractures represent 75% of all physeal fractures. The fracture line passes through a portion of the growth plate and exits through a triangular segment of the metaphysis that remains attached to the intact portion of the growth plate.

The metaphyseal fragment (Thurston Holland fragment) is on the compression side of the fracture. The prognosis for resumption of growth is generally excellent, but the risk of growth disturbance varies with the location of the fracture. Type II fractures of the distal radius rarely lead to physeal closure (35), but type II fractures of the distal femur cause growth disturbance in approximately 50% of patients (36).

Type III injury results when the fracture line traverses a portion of the growth plate, then crosses the epiphysis and the articular surface. The prognosis for resumption of growth is more guarded with this injury, and depends on the vascularity of the physis and damage to the germinal zone. These fractures are more common in older children in whom growth arrest may not be problematic (29). Anatomic reduction is recommended to reduce the risk of growth arrest and to restore the congruity of the articular surface.

Type IV fractures cross all zones of the physis vertically. These fractures are intraarticular and traverse the epiphysis, physis, and metaphysis. In type IV fractures, a relatively small proportion of the physes is affected by injury, yet the risk of growth arrest is high (31). Precise anatomic reduction is recommended to realign the physis and restore the articular surface.

Type V injury results from a crushing force applied to the growth plate. This injury may not be apparent on radiographs because it does not always involve fracture fragment displacement. Growth arrest is common. Crush injury to the germinal physeal cells can occur in combination with other Salter-Harris fracture patterns.

Type VI injury is a peripheral physeal injury at the level of the perichondrial ring (32). This may result from ligamentous avulsion, direct trauma, burn, or other forces. Localized growth arrest may occur and lead to asymmetric growth with angular deformity.

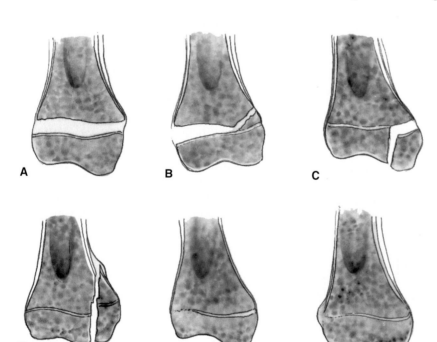

A    B    C

D    E    F

**Figure 33.2** Salter-Harris classification. **A:** Type I is a transepiphyseal separation without evidence of a metaphyseal fragment. **B:** In type II, the fracture line is through the physis, exiting into the metaphysis, leaving a small triangular portion attached to the physeal plate (i.e., Thurston Holland fragment). **C:** The type III fracture is an intraarticular fracture, with the fracture traversing the physis and exiting through the epiphysis. **D:** Type IV describes a vertical fracture line that is intraarticular. It passes through the epiphysis, physis, and metaphysis. **E:** Type V fracture describes a crush injury to the physis that usually is not apparent on initial injury films. **F:** Type VI fracture is a localized injury to a portion of the perichondrial ring. Subsequent healing produces bone formation across the perimeter of the physis, connecting the metaphysis to the epiphysis.

## Physeal Arrest: Pathoanatomy and Diagnosis

Growth arrest after fracture of the growth plate can result from compromised vascularity of the physis, damage to the germinal cells, and bone bridge formation between epiphyseal and metaphyseal bone (37). Destruction of the epiphyseal vasculature leads to central growth arrest followed by complete epiphysiodesis. In contrast, destruction of the metaphyseal vasculature may temporarily interfere with ossification but does not result in growth arrest (38). Direct injury to germinal cells of the growth plate can also lead to physeal arrest, but small areas of physeal damage—less than 7% of the total area—do not usually cause permanent growth disturbance (39,40). Bone bridge formation can also develop after a Salter-Harris type IV fracture when displacement allows the epiphyseal bone to remain in contact with the metaphyseal bone. Peripheral defects result in greater deformities than do central defects of the same size because of their location. Also, small central defects may yield to the force of growth in the remaining viable growth plate.

The size and location of physeal arrest determine the kind of deformity that eventually develops. Complete growth arrest may produce limb-length discrepancy without angular deformity. The amount of discrepancy depends on the growth rate of the affected physis and the age of the child. Contralateral epiphysiodesis should be considered as a treatment option as soon as complete growth arrest is diagnosed. No treatment is required when there is minimal growth remaining or the resultant lower-extremity discrepancy will be less than 2 cm at maturity. Limb lengthening is a treatment option instead of contralateral epiphysiodesis when the projected discrepancy will be greater than 5 cm.

Partial growth arrest is often a more serious problem than complete arrest because partial arrest may result in length discrepancy combined with angular deformity, joint incongruity, or both. Early recognition is desirable to minimize complications. Partial growth arrest can be recognized as early as a few months after fracture, or may take up to 2 years to become evident. A sclerotic bridge of bone or blurring and narrowing of the growth plate is often visible on plain radiographs if the x-ray beam is tangential to the physis. Another early sign of growth disturbance is the development of an oblique growth arrest line (41) (Fig. 33.3). Magnetic resonance imaging (MRI) may also be useful to detect early physeal arrest (42,43).

Three patterns of partial growth arrest have been identified (Fig. 33.4). The most common type is a peripheral bar, which produces an angular deformity. The second type is a central bar, which acts as a central tether and results in tenting of the physis with eventual articular surface distortion. The third pattern of bar formation is referred to as a *linear bar* and involves portions of the central and peripheral physis. This last type is often the result of a Salter-Harris type IV fracture that has healed in a displaced position.

## Treatment of Partial Growth Arrest

There are many treatment options for partial growth-plate damage, depending on the location of the bone bridge, the size of the bar, and the amount of growth remaining. Once identified, partial arrest can be surgically converted to complete arrest to prevent further angulation. This method can also be combined with osteotomy when angular deformity has already developed. Contralateral epiphysiodesis may be performed when the discrepancy is less than 2 cm, or lengthening through the osteotomy site can be performed to equalize limb lengths (44). Bilateral epiphysiodesis with or without osteotomy is particularly appropriate for growth disturbances of slowly growing physes that do not contribute significant length to the limb, such as the distal tibia. This approach can also be utilized instead of bar excision in juvenile patients.

Physeal distraction with disruption of physeal bars has been combined with gradual correction of angular deformity (45). This has been performed for bars that involve as much as 40% of the physis. Recurrence of the bar and growth arrest are common following the procedure, so physeal distraction is recommended only for patients who are near skeletal maturity (45). The authors no longer perform physeal distraction because of limited indications, complications, and pain associated with this technique.

Physeal bar resection is an alternative when less than 50% of the physis is damaged and more than 2 years of growth remain in the affected growth plate. This procedure

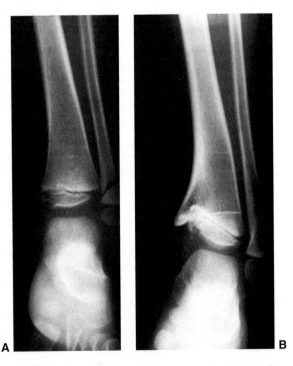

**Figure 33.3** Distal tibial growth arrest. **A:** Distal tibial physeal Salter-Harris type IV injury treated with cast immobilization without reduction. **B:** Two years later, there is varus angulation to the distal tibia from a medial physeal bar. The Harris growth arrest line is not parallel to the distal physis, and does not extend across the entire width of the metaphysis.

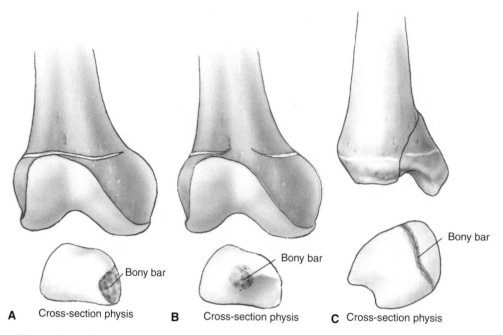

**Figure 33.4**   Growth arrest patterns. **A:** Type I is peripheral growth arrest with a peripheral bony bar. **B:** Type II is central growth arrest with central physeal tethering. The peripheral physis and perichondrial ring are intact. **C:** Type III is combined growth arrest, demonstrating a linear bar involving the peripheral and central portions of the physeal plate. This type of growth arrest is more typical after a Salter-Harris type III or IV fracture.

may eliminate the need for osteotomy if the angular deformity is less than 20 degrees. Success rates are variable, and results are more successful when the bar involves less than 25% of the growth plate (46–48). Before surgical excision, it is necessary to clearly delineate the extent and location of the bar. Plain radiography should be performed with the beam centered on the growth plate and tilted in the same plane as the growth plate. Helical computed tomographic scanning and MRI have largely replaced traditional tomography (49). Three-dimensional reconstruction using these techniques allows accurate identification of the size and location of the bar (50).

Peripheral bone bridges are approached directly, with excision of the overlying periosteum and removal of the abnormal bone until normal physeal cartilage is uncovered. Central bars are approached through a metaphyseal window or through an osteotomy when angular correction is necessary. An alternative approach is to remove a wedge of metaphyseal bone and replace it after the bar resection has been completed (51). The peripheral margins of the physis are carefully preserved. Intraoperative fluoroscopy may help guide the approach to the bone bridge. A linear bar is approached directly where it contacts the periphery of the growth plate. The bone bridge is then resected from one side to the other, creating a tunnel that follows the original fracture line. A high-speed burr, small curettes, and a dental pick facilitate the removal of unwanted bone without damaging the normal physis. Loupe magnification, a headlight, and a dental mirror can facilitate visualization of the normal growth plate. Alternatively, an arthroscope

can be used to verify complete excision. Interposition material is inserted to prevent the bone bridge from recurring. Fat and methylmethacrylate (Cranioplast) are the two most commonly used materials for interposition, but cultured chondrocytes or other biologic tissue may prove useful in the future (52). The material must remain in contact with the physis during further growth. This is accomplished by securing the interposed substance to the epiphysis. Radio-dense markers are usually inserted in the bone to facilitate the measurement of subsequent growth (Fig. 33.5).

The effects of excision on partial growth arrest are difficult to evaluate because there is great variation in location and extent of physeal bars. Also, long-term follow-up is difficult to achieve. Some excellent results have been reported, and partial growth has been restored in many patients (46). Williamson and Staheli (47) noted excellent results in 50% of cases with an average follow-up of 2 years. However, others have reported resumption of growth in only 33% of cases (48). Recurrences and additional surgical procedures are common. This may be because of incomplete resection, reformation of the bar, or migration of the interpositional material (53). Parents should be advised that the results of physeal bar excision are unpredictable. The resected growth plate may grow more slowly than the opposite physis, or premature closure may develop after a period of initial growth.

### Authors' Preferences

Because of the unpredictable results of physeal bar excision, the authors prefer to reserve excision with fat interposition

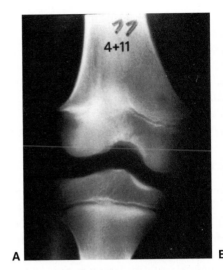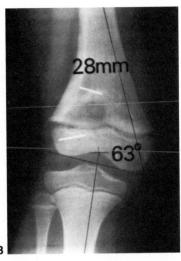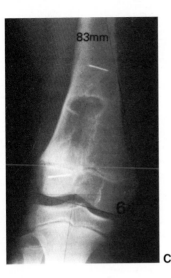

**Figure 33.5** Physeal bar resection. **A:** A distal physeal bar is depicted in this anteroposterior hypocycloidal tomogram. **B:** This condition was treated with bar excision and insertion of Cranioplast. Five months later, the physis remains open, and the two metal markers inserted at the time of surgery are 28 mm apart. There is residual femoral tibial valgus deformity. **C:** Four years later, there has been some improvement in the femoral tibial alignment, and growth of the distal femur has resumed. The markers are 83 mm apart.

for physeal bars that have produced less than 20 degrees of angulation. In addition, the bar should involve less than one-third of the growth plate, and the affected physis should have more than 4 cm of growth remaining. In patients who meet these indications, an osteotomy or lengthening may be avoided or postponed.

When less than 4 cm of growth remains in the physis, the authors prefer bilateral complete epiphysiodesis prior to the development of a discrepancy of more than 2 cm or a symptomatic angular deformity. When deformity is already present without significant discrepancy, as in the ankle region, then osteotomy with bilateral epiphysiodesis is preferred. Growth contribution from the distal tibia and fibula rarely warrants physeal bar excision after 10 years of age. In cases of physeal bars involving more than one-third of the growth plate, and where more than 4 cm of growth is remaining, the authors prefer to perform complete arrest of the growth plate, osteotomy, and lengthening. The involved extremity may be overlengthened to accommodate growth of the opposite limb, or bilateral epiphysiodesis can be performed to limit the amount of lengthening that is required.

# INITIAL MANAGEMENT CONSIDERATIONS

## Multiple Trauma Evaluation and Management

Accidents and injuries are the leading cause of death from ages 1 to 18 years. Deaths from accidental injury in this age group exceed the total number of deaths from the next nine causes combined (3). Death from trauma is most often attributable to head injury, but preventable deaths still

occur. These are most often caused by airway obstruction, pneumothorax, and hemorrhage (54,55). Children respond differently to trauma than adults. The child's vascular system can maintain systolic blood pressure for a prolonged period in the presence of significant hypovolemia. Tachycardia may be the only sign of impending hypovolemic shock, which can occur precipitously. Hypothermia poses a greater problem for children because they have a higher ratio of surface area to body weight than adults. The child also has greater capacity to recover from neurologic injury and hypoxia. For these reasons, all children should be treated aggressively, with the expectation of survival and recovery of function. The optimal timing of fracture management is uncertain, although early fracture stabilization may facilitate patient care (56). Several scoring systems have been developed to predict outcome and assess the need for transport to major trauma centers. The Glasgow Coma Scale is helpful in assessing cortical brain function (57) (Table 33.1). Sequential assessment can help detect worsening or recovery from brain injury. A child with a Glasgow Coma Scale score lower than 8 has a significantly worse prognosis for survival. The score obtained at 72 hours after injury is more predictive of permanent impairment (58). The Pediatric Trauma Score is an effective triage tool and a reliable predictor of injury severity, although it gives an open metacarpal fracture the same weight as an open femur fracture (59) (Table 33.2).

Initial treatment consists of airway management, fluid resuscitation, and blood replacement. Systematic, multidisciplinary management of all organ systems is essential. Musculoskeletal injuries are common in the severely traumatized child and may be initially overlooked. Children with multiple injuries should be treated as though they have a cervical spine injury until this can be ruled out

## TABLE 33.1
### GLASGOW COMA SCALE

| Variable | Score |
|---|---|
| **Opening of the eyes** | |
| Spontaneously | 4 |
| To speech | 3 |
| To pain | 2 |
| None | 1 |
| **Best verbal response** | |
| Oriented | 5 |
| Confused | 4 |
| Inappropriate words | 3 |
| Incomprehensible sounds | 2 |
| None | 1 |
| **Best motor response** | |
| Spontaneous (obedience to commands) | 6 |
| Localization of pain | 5 |
| Withdrawal | 4 |
| Abnormal flexion to pain | 3 |
| Abnormal extension to pain | 2 |
| None | 1 |

The Glasgow Coma Scale is used to measure level of consciousness. A score of <8 carries a worse prognosis for survival.

clinically or radiographically. Regional examination of the spine, pelvis, shoulders, and extremities should be complete, especially if the child cannot communicate.

Management of fractures may need to be altered from conventional methods to meet the general needs of the patient. The Mangled Extremity Severity Score (MESS) may be used in children to assist the physician with immediate management decisions (60). Armstrong and Smith (61) have recommended the following principles for children with major trauma:

1. Make sure that any child with a major long-bone fracture does not have any other significant injuries.
2. Early treatment of the fractures should be compatible with the general care of the patient.

3. Fracture care should consider the need for early mobilization of the child.
4. Care of fractures should facilitate the management of associated soft tissue injuries.
5. The initial method of fracture management should be the definitive method, whenever possible.
6. Fracture care must be carefully individualized.
7. Treat all children as though they are going to survive.

## Open Fractures

Open fractures result from high-energy trauma or penetrating wounds. The tibia is the most commonly involved site in children and adults. Open tibial fractures are discussed in the section on tibial fractures. The femur, forearm, humerus, and other bones may also sustain open injuries.

The traditional classification system of Gustilo (modified by Mendoza) (62) is illustrated in Table 33.3. This classification system is appropriate for children as well as adults, and provides a method of assessment for purposes of management and prognosis.

Management of all open fractures requires prompt initiation of antibiotic and tetanus prophylaxis. Surgical irrigation and debridement of open fractures should be performed to minimize the subsequent risk of infection. Surgical intervention within 6 hours has been the standard recommendation (63). However, moderate delay of surgical management for lesser grades of open fracture may not be associated with an increased infection rate when antibiotics are administered early (64,65). At the time of surgery all necrotic or devitalized material is removed. Debridement of devitalized bone is not necessary in children if the bone is clean and can be adequately covered with soft tissue (66). Bone should be stabilized to create optimal conditions for soft tissue recovery. Cultures can be obtained, but their value for subsequent management is questionable (67). Partial wound closure over a drain is acceptable for clean Type I and Type II injuries (68,69). Antibiotics are generally used for 72 hours. Cephalosporins are used for Type I injury, and an aminoglycoside is added for Type II

## TABLE 33.2
### PEDIATRIC TRAUMA SCORE

| Variable | +2 | +1 | −1 |
|---|---|---|---|
| Weight (kg) | >20 | 10–20 | <10 |
| Airway patency | Normal | Maintained | Unmaintained |
| Systolic blood pressure (mm Hg) | >90 | 50–90 | <50 |
| Neurologic | Awake | Obtunded | Comatose |
| Open wound | None | Minor | Major |
| Skeletal trauma | None | Closed | Open or multiple |

The Pediatric Trauma Score is a reliable predictor of injury severity. Each variable is given one of the three scores. The scores are totaled (range, −6 to +12). A total of ≤8 indicates potentially important trauma. From Tepas J, Mollitt D, Talbert J, et al. The Pediatric Trauma Score as a predictor of injury severity in the injured child. *J Pediatr Surg* 1987;22:14.

## TABLE 33.3

### CLASSIFICATION OF OPEN FRACTURES

| Wound Type | External Wound Size | Fracture Pattern | Soft Tissue Damage |
|---|---|---|---|
| Type I | <2 cm | Simple | Minimal muscle contusion |
| Type II | 2–10 cm | Simple; minimal comminution | Mild muscle damage; no crush |
| Type IIIA | Extensive or gunshot wound | Comminuted or segmental fracture | Adequate local soft tissue coverage |
| Type IIIB | Extensive or crush injury | Extensive periosteal stripping; bone loss | Incomplete coverage; exposed bone |
| Type IIIC | Same as above | Same as above | Neurovascular injury |

From Gustillo R, Mendoza R, Williams D. Problems in the management of type III (severe) open fractures: a new classification. *J Trauma* 1984;24:742, with permission.

or Type III injury. Patients with open wounds are returned to the operating room in 48 to 72 hours for repeat irrigation, debridement, and possible delayed primary closure or flap coverage. Early soft tissue coverage is advantageous and may require local or free-flap reconstruction (69). Vacuum-assisted closure (VAC) aids considerably in wound management and can decrease the need for tissue transfers in pediatric patients (70).

Open fractures in children share many of the same complications reported in the literature for open fractures in adults. These fractures take longer to heal and have more complications than closed injuries (71,72). However, the overall complication rates in children are lower than those in adults with similar injuries (72,73). This is especially true for children younger than 12 years (72,73).

### Compartment Syndromes

Compartment syndrome develops when there is an increase of interstitial pressure in a closed osteofascial compartment, resulting in inadequate circulation to the nerves and muscles of that compartment. There is little documentation of the incidence of compartment syndrome, but it has been reported in numerous anatomic regions, including the abdomen. Increased intracompartmental pressure may develop after athletic exertion, relatively minor injuries, and major trauma (74).

Increased tissue pressure in a confined space leads to obstruction of venous outflow from the compartment. This contributes to further swelling and increased pressure. When the pressure increases above the arteriolar circulatory pressure to muscle and nerve, ischemia will occur, leading to irreversible damage to the contents of the compartment. Muscle and nerve damage commences as soon as 4 to 6 hours after the onset of abnormal pressures.

Pain that is out of proportion to the injury should alert the clinician to the possibility of impending or established compartment syndrome. Excessive pain requiring increased medication is often the earliest symptom (75). This is rapidly

followed by clinical findings that include sensory changes associated with nerve ischemia within the compartment, excessive pain with passive movement of the muscles within the compartment, and loss of active movement of those muscles. Distal pulses and peripheral capillary refill are unreliable indicators of compartment syndrome. Peripheral circulation may be normal because major arterial blood flow through the compartment is preserved in the presence of increased pressures, which eliminate microvascular perfusion to the muscles and nerves within the compartment. The injured extremity should not be elevated when compartment syndrome is suspected because this maneuver reduces mean arterial pressure, causing a reduction in perfusion that leads to further ischemia.

The diagnosis of acute compartment syndrome is based on signs and symptoms which may be difficult to assess accurately in children. For this reason children may have more advanced signs of compartment syndrome at the time of definitive diagnosis. Tissue pressure measurements should be obtained whenever the diagnosis is in doubt (76) (Fig. 33.6). The pressure threshold for fasciotomy is

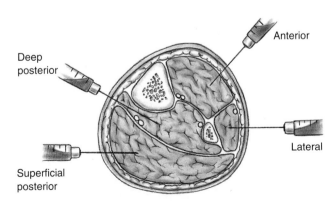

**Figure 33.6** Orientation and entry points for measurement of compartment pressures. (From Gulli B, Templeman D. Compartment syndrome of the lower extremity. *Orthop Clin North Am* 1994;25: 677, with permission.)

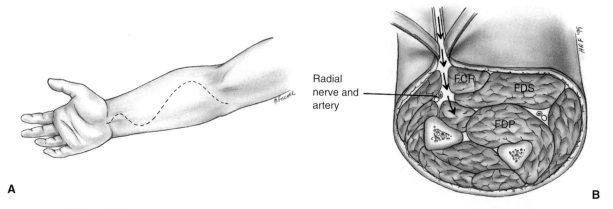

**Figure 33.7** The Henry approach is used for decompression of the volar forearm compartments. **A:** Skin incision crosses the elbow crease and enters the palm along the thenar eminence. **B:** The superficial fascia is divided. The deep compartment is approached by retracting the flexor carpi radialis (*FCR*) to the ulnar side. The superficial radial nerve and brachioradialis are retracted radially. *FDP,* flexor digitorum profundus; *FDS,* flexor digitorum sublimus.

not clearly established. Mubarak and Owen (77) recommend fasciotomy if compartment pressure exceeds 30 mm Hg. Others recommend fasciotomy if the pressure is greater than 35 to 40 mm Hg or within 30 mm Hg of the patient's diastolic pressure (76).

Fasciotomy of the forearm can be accomplished by the volar Henry approach or the volar ulnar approach (78). It is essential to decompress the deep flexor compartment in addition to the superficial flexor compartment muscles (Figs. 33.7 and 33.8). Fasciotomy of the leg can be performed by a single-incision or double-incision technique (76) (Fig. 33.9). The two-incision technique facilitates decompression of the deep posterior compartment. The fibula should be left intact. Devitalized muscle is debrided when necessary, but extensive debridement is usually performed 36 to 72 hours later, when muscle viability is more readily determined. Approaches for foot compartment syndromes are discussed in the section on metatarsal fractures.

## Anesthesia and Analgesia for Emergency Department Management

Numerous techniques have been used to provide sedation and pain relief for outpatient fracture management (79–85). These can be categorized into three groups: blocks, sedation, and dissociative anesthesia (82). When sedation or dissociative anesthesia is used, it is advisable to follow the guidelines for monitoring and management that have been established by the American Academy of Pediatrics (86).

### Blocks

Local and regional blocks include hematoma blocks, nerve blocks, and intravenous regional anesthesia. Hematoma blocks are particularly useful for distal radius fractures. After appropriate skin preparation, a needle is inserted into the fracture hematoma. The hematoma is aspirated, and 3 to 10 mL of 1% or 2% lidocaine (maximum dose is 3 to 5 mg per kilogram of body weight) is injected into the

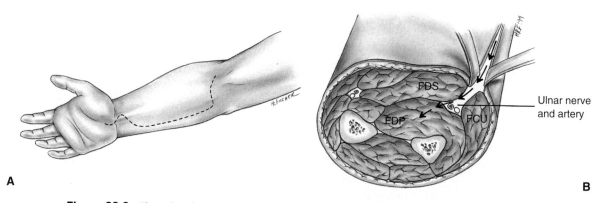

**Figure 33.8** The volar ulnar approach (modified McConnell exposure) is more direct for decompressing the forearm compartments. **A:** Skin incision extends along the ulnar side of the forearm. **B:** The ulnar nerve and artery are retracted to expose the deep flexor compartment. *FDP,* flexor digitorum profundus; *FDS,* flexor digitorum sublimus; *FCU,* flexor carpi ulnaris.

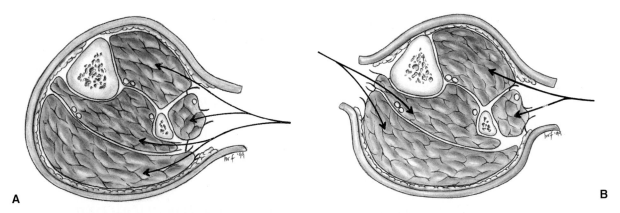

**Figure 33.9** **A:** Single-incision fasciotomy may be used to decompress all four compartments of the leg. Excision of the fibula is not necessary. **B:** Double-incision fasciotomy allows a more direct approach to the deep posterior compartment of the leg. (From Gulli B, Templeman D. Compartment syndrome of the lower extremity. *Orthop Clin North Am* 1994;25:677, with permission.)

fracture site. Volume of injection should be less than 10 mL because hematoma block can increase carpal tunnel pressure and increase the risk of neurologic complications (87). It is the author's opinion that the technique of hematoma block is often difficult when the hematoma is small, as in greenstick fractures, or when the fracture hematoma has already coagulated.

Intravenous regional anesthesia, or Bier block, has been reported to be successful by several authors (81,88). The primary site of the nerve block is thought to be small, peripheral nerve branches. For this reason, it is suggested that nerve blockade is better achieved with a larger volume of dilute anesthetic (81). Intravenous access is obtained in a vein of the dorsum of the hand of the injured extremity. It is not necessary to have additional intravenous access to the opposite extremity (82). The arm is then exsanguinated by elevation, or by gentle application of an elastic bandage. A single blood pressure cuff or tourniquet is then rapidly inflated above the elbow to 100 mm Hg greater than systolic blood pressure. The cuff may be taped to avoid Velcro failure, and the inflation tube may be cross-clamped to prevent premature cuff deflation. Two cuffs may be used to minimize tourniquet discomfort, but this is not usually necessary for fracture reductions. Lidocaine, diluted with normal saline to a 0.125% solution, is then administered in a dose of 1 to 1.5 mg per kilogram of body weight (81). The tourniquet should be kept inflated for at least 20 minutes to permit the lidocaine to become fixed to the tissue, thereby minimizing the risk of lidocaine toxicity after the cuff is deflated. This method has proven most effective for forearm fractures and less effective for supracondylar, finger, and hand fractures (88).

Ulnar nerve block at the elbow, median nerve block at the wrist, or digital blocks can be useful for reduction of certain hand and finger fractures and dislocations. Axillary block has proved to be a safe technique for a variety of upper-extremity fractures in children (89). In most children, the axillary sheath is superficial and the pulse is more easily identified than in adults, who generally have more

subcutaneous fat. Intravenous access in the uninjured extremity is recommended and can be used to administer low-level sedation before axillary block. The arm is abducted and externally rotated to a 90 degree–90 degree ("90–90") position; 1% plain lidocaine is used at a dose of 3 to 5 mg per kilogram of body weight. Cramer et al. (89) recommend the transarterial method of administration. A 23-gauge butterfly needle is inserted through the axillary artery during continuous aspiration. Approximately two-thirds of the lidocaine is slowly injected into the sheath on the opposite side of the artery. Periodic aspiration is performed to minimize the risk of intraarterial injection. The needle is withdrawn just to the superficial side of the sheath, and the remaining lidocaine is injected. This anesthetic technique provides prolonged pain relief for complex manipulations but requires considerable cooperation from the patient.

### Sedation

Conscious sedation is defined as a level of consciousness that maintains protective reflexes and retains the patient's ability to maintain an airway independently. During conscious sedation, the patient can respond appropriately to verbal commands or physical stimulation. Deep sedation is defined as a more profound state of unconsciousness, accompanied by partial or complete loss of protective reflexes and inability to respond purposefully to verbal or physical stimuli. The American Academy of Pediatrics has developed specific guidelines for monitoring and managing pediatric sedation (86). These guidelines state that the risks of deep sedation may be indistinguishable from those of general anesthesia. When the guidelines are followed, the risk of adverse events can be reduced. Administration of chloral hydrate was associated with higher risk, but the effects of nothing by mouth (NPO) status are not statistically significant (90).

Narcotics and benzodiazepines are widely available agents for intravenous sedation. Narcotics provide analgesia, whereas benzodiazepines are primarily sedatives. These drugs act synergistically to induce controlled sedation and analgesia. Intravenous access and continuous monitoring of pulse and oxygen saturation are advised. Respiratory rate and blood pressure should be monitored periodically. An emergency cart with resuscitation equipment should be immediately available. Nasal oxygen and personnel skilled in airway management increase the level of safety.

Numerous medications and combinations of medications have been used (82) (Table 33.4). Varela et al. (85) reported satisfactory pain relief in 98% of patients who were sedated by titrating meperidine (Demerol) and midazolam (Versed). The target doses were 2 and 0.1 mg per kilogram of body weight for meperidine and midazolam, respectively. Meperidine is less potent than morphine, but it has a slightly faster onset and some euphoric properties (82). Fentanyl, a potent narcotic, is sometimes used as a substitute for meperidine because it reaches peak analgesia within 2 to 3 minutes and has a shorter duration of action than meperidine. Hypoxemia and apnea are not uncommon after sedation with midazolam and fentanyl. Monitoring of oxygen saturation is essential because hypoxemia can occur in the absence of apnea. If respiratory depression occurs, reversal agents should be administered. Naloxone is used to reverse the narcotic effect, and the benzodiazepine is reversed with flumazenil (82).

### Dissociative Anesthesia

Ketamine has gained popularity as a useful drug for emergency department use (83). It induces a trancelike state that combines sedation, analgesia, and amnesia with little cardiovascular depression. It has been suggested that protective orotracheal reflexes are preserved, but respiratory depression is dose-related (91,92). The intramuscular or intravenous route may be used to administer ketamine. The intravenous route permits titration and more rapid onset of action, with quicker recovery. The target intravenous dose is 1 to 2 mg per kilogram of body weight. The intramuscular dose is 4 mg/kg, and a repeat dose may be given after 10 to 15 minutes if necessary. Ketamine increases upper-airway secretions, so atropine or glycopyrrolate are recommended before sedation. Emergence hallucinations are more common in children older than 10 years. Therefore, ketamine may be a less desirable choice in older children. When ketamine is used in older children, low-dose midazolam (0.05 mg/kg) can reduce the risk of emergence reactions (84).

## INJURIES OF THE SHOULDER AND HUMERUS

The clavicle, scapula, and humerus articulate to form the shoulder. The clavicle is flat laterally, triangular medially, and has a double curve that is convex anteriorly in the medial third and convex posteriorly in the lateral third. The scapula is a large, flat, triangular bone that is connected to the trunk by muscles only. The spine arises from the dorsal surface of the scapula and forms the acromion laterally. The coracoid process arises from the anterior surface. The clavicle and scapula are attached at the acromioclavicular joint and held in place by the coracoclavicular ligaments. The clavicle connects the shoulder girdle to the axial skeleton at the sternoclavicular joint. This joint is very mobile and allows the clavicle to move through an arc of 60 degrees and accommodate a wide range of scapular rotation. The shoulder girdle articulates with the humerus through the glenohumeral joint. This joint is a ball-and-socket joint that is supported primarily by the articular capsule and surrounding muscle. Thus, the shoulder mechanism functions as a universal joint, allowing freedom of motion in all planes.

---

### TABLE 33.4
### MEDICATIONS MOST COMMONLY USED FOR SEDATION IN PEDIATRIC FRACTURE REDUCTION

| Medication | Dosage | Comments |
| --- | --- | --- |
| Midazolam (Versed) | 0.05–0.2 mg/kg i.v. | Benzodiazepine |
| Meperidine (Demerol) | 1.0–2.0 mg/kg i.v. | Narcotic |
| Fentanyl | 1.0–5.0 $\mu$g/kg i.v. | Potent, rapid-onset narcotic |
| Ketamine | 1.0–2.0 mg/kg i.v.; 3.0–4.0 mg/kg i.m. | Manage emergence reactions with small doses of midazolam |
| Naloxone (Narcan) | 1.0–2.0 $\mu$g/kg i.v. | Narcotic-reversal agent |
| Flumazenil (Romazicon) | 5.0–10.0 $\mu$g/kg i.v. (maximum, 0.2 mg) | Benzodiazepine-reversal agent |
| Atropine | 0.01 mg/kg i.v. or i.m. (maximum, 0.5 mg) | Antisialagogue |
| Glycopyrrolate | 4.0–10.0 $\mu$g/kg i.v. or i.m. (maximum, 0.25 mg) | Antisialagogue |

i.m., intramuscular; i.v., intravenous.
Adapted from McCarty E, Mencio G, Green N. Anesthesia and analgesia for the ambulatory management of fractures in children. *J Am Acad Orthop Surg* 1999;7:81, with permission.

Fractures around the shoulder are generally easy to treat and rarely require reduction or surgical stabilization. The wide range of motion in this region contributes to rapid remodeling and accommodates modest residual deformity.

## Shoulder Injuries in Infants

Difficult birth can result in injury to the infant's shoulder (93). The most common injuries are fracture of the clavicle and brachial plexus palsy. The differential diagnosis should also include proximal humeral physeal separation, septic arthritis of the shoulder, osteomyelitis, and nonaccidental injuries. Lack of arm movement in the neonatal period is the most common clinical finding for each of these problems. Pain, swelling, and crepitus may be noted when fracture has occurred. Often, fracture of the clavicle at birth is undetected until swelling subsides and the firm mass of healing callus is noticed in the midshaft of the clavicle. Parental reassurance and gentle handling are all that are required for managing fracture of the clavicle at birth. Clavicle fracture is occasionally confused with congenital pseudarthrosis of the clavicle. Pseudarthrosis can be distinguished from fracture of the clavicle at birth by the absence of pain and by radiographic features of established pseudarthrosis.

Neonatal trauma may also result in Salter-Harris type I physeal separation of the proximal humerus. This injury may be difficult to diagnose radiographically because the proximal humeral epiphysis does not ossify until 3 to 6 months of age. Ultrasonography, MRI, or joint aspiration may facilitate diagnosis in questionable cases. Closed reduction is not indicated because healing is rapid and remodeling is certain. Immobilization for 2 to 3 weeks provides comfort and allows union to occur.

## Clavicle Injuries

### Clavicle Diaphysis Fracture

The clavicle is frequently fractured in children, and the most common portion injured is the shaft. The mechanism of injury is usually a fall on the shoulder or excessive lateral compression of the shoulder girdle. The subclavian vessels, brachial plexus, and apex of the lung lie beneath the clavicle but are rarely injured at the time of fracture.

Treatment of clavicle shaft fractures in children and adolescents is supportive; reduction is not attempted, except for fractures with extreme displacement. Both a figure-eight harness and a sling may be used initially to provide comfort. After a few days the sling and harness may be discontinued. Sports are avoided for approximately 8 weeks. Uneventful, rapid healing is the rule, although displaced fractures may heal with a visible subcutaneous prominence. Parents should be advised that, regardless of alignment, healing will produce a bump that will remodel over the course of several months. Indications for surgery are rare but include open fractures, severe displacement with the bone end impaled through the trapezius, and irreducible tenting of the skin by the bone fragments. Even in these severe cases internal fixation is rarely required. Nonunion after clavicle fracture has been reported in adolescents, but it responds to bone grafting and plating (94).

### Medial Clavicle Fracture and Sternoclavicular Separation

The medial clavicular ossification center appears at approximately 17 years of age, but the physis does not close until 20 to 25 years of age (95). Therefore, displacements of the medial end of the clavicle are usually physeal separations that mimic sternoclavicular dislocation (96). These are Salter-Harris type I or II injuries, although the epiphyseal fragment is not visualized well on radiographs. The direction of displacement can be anterior or posterior. Posterior displacement by fracture or dislocation can cause dysphagia or respiratory compromise, especially when the child's head and neck are extended. Apical lordotic radiographs are helpful, but computed tomography (CT) scans best visualize the deformity (Fig. 33.10).

Treatment of posterior displacement by closed reduction is often unsuccessful, or results in recurrent displacement (97,98). Posterior displacements are reduced under general anesthesia for complete relaxation. The reduction maneuver entails hyperextension of the clavicle combined with longitudinal arm traction. It may also be necessary to capture the medial clavicle with a percutaneous towel clip and then pull in an anterolateral direction. Ligamentous repair and stabilization with a figure-eight nonabsorbable suture is recommended following reduction (97,98). A shoulder immobilizer or figure-eight harness is used for immobilization postoperatively. Anteriorly displaced epiphyseal separations are less stable, and partial redisplacement may occur. However, remanipulation or surgical treatment may be unnecessary because fracture remodeling will occur.

### Lateral Clavicle Fracture and Acromioclavicular Separation

The mechanism of injury to the distal clavicle is similar to adult acromioclavicular separation. A fall onto the point of the shoulder drives the acromion and scapula distally. This results in distal clavicular physeal separation. This is because the distal epiphysis of the clavicle remains a cartilaginous cap until the age of 20 years or older (95), whereas the acromioclavicular and coracoclavicular ligaments are firmly attached to the thick periosteum of the clavicle. Typically, the lateral metaphysis displaces through the injured dorsal periosteum, leaving the ligaments intact and the epiphyseal end of the clavicle reduced in the acromioclavicular joint (99) (Fig. 33.11). Because these injuries represent physeal disruption with herniation of bone from the periosteal tube, tremendous potential for healing and remodeling exists.

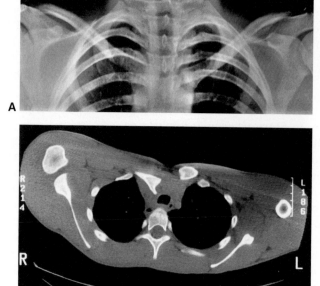

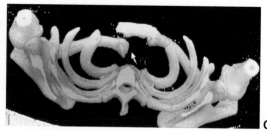

**Figure 33.10** Sternoclavicular separation. This 14-year-old boy sustained an injury to the right clavicle during a wrestling match when his shoulder was compressed against his chest wall. He complained of shortness of breath, especially when he extended his neck. **A:** The anteroposterior radiograph demonstrates asymmetry of the sternal position of the clavicle. **B:** The computed tomographic scan demonstrates posterior displacement of the medial end of the right clavicle, which is near the trachea (*arrow*). **C:** A three-dimensional reconstruction, with a cephalic projection, demonstrates the posterior and midline displacement of the clavicle.

Treatment of most distal clavicle fractures consists of support with a sling or shoulder immobilizer for 3 weeks. Reduction and fixation are unnecessary, except for the rare instance in which the clavicle is severely displaced in an older adolescent (100).

True acromioclavicular separation is very rare before the age of 16. Fracture or physeal separation of the distal clavicle is more common, and has been called *pseudodislocation of the acromioclavicular joint* (101). Tenderness over the acromioclavicular joint and prominence of the lateral end of the clavicle are present with fracture, physeal separation, and joint separation. Radiographs demonstrate increased distance between the coracoid process and the clavicle, compared with the opposite side. The MRI can distinguish among these three similar injuries, but it is rarely necessary because the treatments are similar. When true joint separation occurs, the injury may be a sprain, subluxation, or dislocation. These have been classified as grades I to III, depending on the severity of injury to the acromioclavicular and coracoclavicular ligaments (102).

Treatment of all grades of separation is usually conservative, without attempting reduction. Therefore, it is unnecessary to determine the degree of separation by stress radiography with handheld weights. A sling or shoulder immobilizer is used for 3 weeks, followed by a graduated exercise program. Even in competitive athletes, shoulder strength and range of motion are not impaired after rehabilitation (103–105). In complete separations (type III), the clavicle remains prominent but is usually asymptomatic. The occasional patient who develops late symptoms of pain and stiffness may be relieved by resection of the distal clavicle (104).

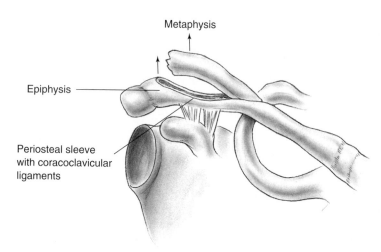

Metaphysis

Epiphysis

Periosteal sleeve with coracoclavicular ligaments

**Figure 33.11** Lateral clavicle fracture-separation. The swelling and dorsal prominence of the clavicle may suggest an acromioclavicular separation. However, the distal epiphysis of the clavicle and acromioclavicular joint remain reduced. New bone forms from the periosteum, with subsequent remodeling of the prominence. (From Ogden J. Distal clavicular physeal injury. *Clin Orthop* 1984;188:68, with permission.)

## Scapular Fracture

Fracture of the scapula, although rare in children, should be suspected whenever there is shoulder tenderness or swelling after trauma. These fractures are usually the result of a severe, direct blow of high energy. Therefore, initial evaluation should include a diligent search for more serious chest injuries, such as rib fractures, pulmonary or cardiac contusion, and injury to the mediastinum. Fractures of the scapula can involve the body, glenoid, or acromion. Avulsion fractures of the scapula have also been reported, and are a result of indirect trauma (106). The CT scan is quite helpful for evaluating scapular fractures and associated injuries.

Treatment of most scapular fractures consists of immobilization with a sling and swathe, followed by early shoulder motion after pain has subsided. The scapular body is encased in thick muscles, so displacement is rare and well tolerated after healing (100). Fractures of the acromion or coracoid require surgery only when severely displaced. Glenoid fractures are the most likely to require reduction and internal fixation. Intraarticular fractures with more than 3 mm of displacement should be restored to anatomic positions. Large glenoid rim fractures can be associated with traumatic dislocations. An anterior approach is recommended for anterior glenoid fractures, and a posterior approach is used for scapular neck and glenoid fossa fractures (107).

## Shoulder Dislocation

Less than 2% of glenohumeral dislocations occur in patients younger than 10 years (108). Atraumatic shoulder dislocations and chronic shoulder instability are discussed elsewhere in this book. Traumatic shoulder dislocation in the adolescent age group is more common. Approximately 20% of all shoulder dislocations occur in persons between the ages of 10 and 20 years. Most displace anteriorly and produce a detachment of the anteroinferior capsule from the glenoid neck (i.e., Bankart lesion).

Treatment of traumatic shoulder dislocation in children and adolescents is nonsurgical, with gentle closed reduction. This is accomplished by providing adequate pain relief, muscle relaxation, and gravity-assisted arm traction in the prone position. An alternative method is the modified Hippocratic method in which traction is applied to the arm while countertraction is applied using a folded sheet around the torso. After reduction, a shoulder immobilizer or sling is used for 2 to 3 weeks before initiating shoulder muscle strengthening. The most frequent complication is recurrent dislocation, which has an incidence between 60% and 85%, usually within 2 years of the primary dislocation (109,110). Posterior dislocations of the shoulder may also recur and require surgical stabilization in children (111). A more detailed discussion of this injury and its treatment is found elsewhere in Chapter 32.

## Proximal Humerus Fractures

Proximal humeral growth accounts for 80% of the length of the humerus. The proximal humeral physis is an undulating structure that forms a tentlike peak in the posteromedial humerus quadrant, near the center of the humeral head. The glenohumeral joint capsule extends to the metaphysis medially. Therefore, a portion of the metaphysis is intracapsular. The proximal humeral physis remains open in girls until 14 to 17 years of age and in boys until 16 to 18 years of age.

Mechanisms of injury that would produce a shoulder dislocation in adults usually result in a proximal humeral fracture in children and adolescents. These are usually Salter-Harris type II epiphyseal separations or metaphyseal fractures. Metaphyseal fractures are more common before the age of 10, and epiphyseal separations are more common in adolescents. The distal fragment usually displaces in the anterior direction, because the periosteum is thinner and weaker in this region. Posteriorly, the periosteal sleeve is thicker and remains intact. The proximal fragment is flexed and externally rotated because of the pull of the rotator cuff, whereas the distal fragment is displaced proximally because of the pull of the deltoid muscle. Adduction of the distal fragment is caused by the pectoralis major muscle. The long head of the biceps may be interposed between the fracture fragments and may further impede reduction (112). Remarkably, this is a relatively benign injury because of the rapid rate of remodeling with growth and the wide range of shoulder motion (113,114).

Most of these fractures are minimally displaced or minimally angulated. They are managed in a shoulder immobilizer for 3 to 4 weeks, followed by range-of-motion exercises and gradually increased activity.

Severely displaced fractures pose a greater dilemma for the treating physician. The alarming radiographic appearance invites overtreatment. These fractures are difficult to reduce and almost impossible to maintain in a reduced position by closed methods. Traction and cast immobilization are not recommended because these techniques are inconvenient, cumbersome, and have not been shown to improve results. Current options for management include immobilization without attempting reduction, and reduction under anesthesia with percutaneous pinning. Authors who have studied these options have concluded that most severely displaced fractures should be treated by sling and swathe immobilization (113–115). Complete displacement, 3 cm overriding, and 60 degrees of angulation may be accepted in patients who are more than 2 years from skeletal maturity. Up to 45 degrees of angulation can be accepted until physeal closure (112) (Fig. 33.12). Closed or open reduction under anesthesia with percutaneous pinning may be indicated for fractures with a greater amount of deformity, open fractures, vascular injuries, and severe displacement (100) (Fig. 33.13), or in situations in which tenting could lead to skin breakdown.

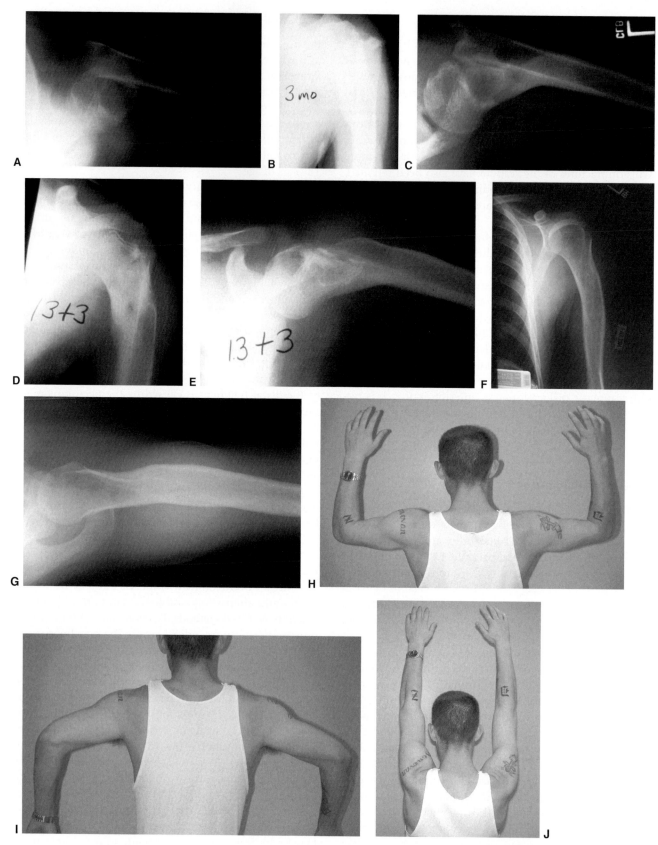

**Figure 33.12** Proximal humeral fracture-separation in a boy aged 12 years, 3 months. **A:** The initial fracture displacement was treated with sling and swath. **B,C:** Three months after injury, healing and early remodeling are evident. **D,E:** One year after injury, remodeling continues. **F,G:** Four years after injury, remodeling is complete. **H–J:** The patient has recovered full range of motion, but has a 1 cm arm-length discrepancy.

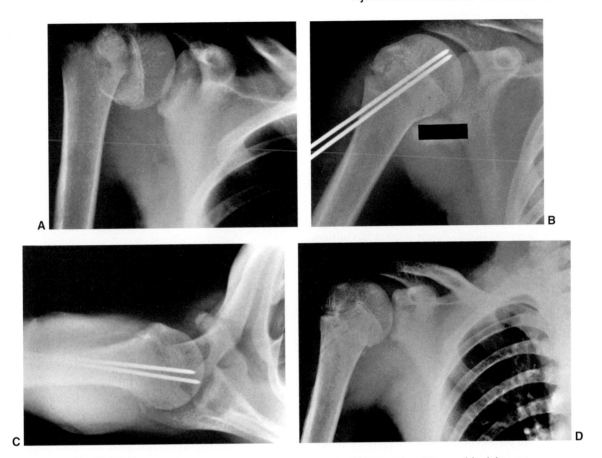

**Figure 33.13**   Salter-Harris type II fracture of the proximal humerus in a 15-year-old adolescent. **A:** Displaced fracture with 70 degrees of angulation. The proximal fragment is abducted and externally rotated, because of the rotator cuff attachments. The shaft is displaced proximally by the pull of the deltoid muscle, and is generally adducted by the action of the pectoralis muscle. The distal fragment is also internally rotated if the arm is placed in a sling. **B,C:** Anteroposterior and lateral radiographs after closed reduction and percutaneous pinning. The arm is externally rotated and abducted with longitudinal traction to achieve this position. **D:** Final alignment after removal of the pins 4 weeks later.

## Humeral Shaft Fracture

Fractures of the humeral shaft may occur at birth because of difficult delivery. Other humeral shaft fractures in children younger than 3 years are often the result of nonaccidental injury (116). In any instance of delay in seeking medical attention, inconsistent history of injury, or evidence of concurrent injuries, there is an increased likelihood of inflicted trauma. However, there is no particular pattern of fracture that is diagnostic of child abuse. Fractures seen in older children are usually the result of blunt trauma. The radial nerve is susceptible to injury, because it is fixed by the intramuscular septum as it passes lateral to the humerus at the junction of the middle and distal thirds. The prognosis for radial nerve recovery is excellent. Nerve injury with closed fractures of the humerus should be observed for 3 months before considering intervention.

Closed management is recommended for most humeral shaft fractures. Infants may be treated with gentle positioning and a small coaptation splint, or the arm may be splinted in extension, using a tongue blade and tape. Healing is prompt in infants and young children. It is the authors' opinion that up to 45 degrees of angulation can be accepted in children younger than 3 years. Older children may be treated with a coaptation splint and a sling to maintain alignment of the arm. A hanging arm cast or collar and cuff may also be used, but a U-slab coaptation splint allows better pain relief and control of the fracture. Occasionally, an abduction splint or pillow is necessary to control varus alignment. In older children and adolescents, complete displacement and 2 cm of shortening are acceptable. In the proximal shaft, one can accept 25 to 30 degrees of angulation. Fracture deformity closer to the elbow is more visible. Up to 20 degrees of angulation is acceptable in the middle third and 15 degrees in the distal third of the humeral shaft (117). Greater degrees of deformity are usually unacceptable cosmetically, although they may remodel without causing functional problems. Indications for surgery include open fractures, multiple injuries, and ipsilateral forearm fractures in adolescents (i.e., "floating elbow"). Fixation techniques include the use of flexible intramedullary nails, antegrade insertion of a Rush rod, and compression plating. Open or comminuted fractures can be stabilized with an external fixator until union is complete or until fracture stability and wound healing permit converting to splint immobilization.

# FRACTURES AND DISLOCATIONS AROUND THE ELBOW

It is wise to assume the worst when evaluating the child with an elbow injury. Only full range of motion, complete absence of swelling, and normal radiographs warrant the diagnosis of elbow sprain or contusion. Any swelling or restriction of movement necessitates thorough evaluation, sometimes with comparison radiographs of the opposite elbow whenever there is doubt regarding normal anatomy. Small fractures that appear to be avulsions should be accurately diagnosed, because they may indicate a major injury. Arthrography, ultrasonography, and MRI have been used to successfully diagnose occult elbow trauma in children (118–120). These techniques should be considered whenever there is doubt regarding the diagnosis.

Precisely defining the fracture patterns is a challenge in young children because of the large cartilage composition of the distal humerus. There are also multiple ossification centers that appear at different ages (Fig. 33.14). The capitellum is the first to appear, at 6 months of age, followed by the radial head and the medial epicondyle at 5 years of age. The trochlea ossifies at 7 years, and the lateral epicondyle and olecranon appear at 9 and 11 years of age, respectively. The lateral epicondyle, trochlea, and capitellum coalesce to form a single epiphysis by 12 years of age. Ossification centers are intraarticular except for the medial and lateral epicondyles.

The elbow is a complex joint, and it has three major articulations: the radiohumeral, ulnohumeral, and radioulnar joints. There are two fat pads: one in the olecranon fossa posteriorly, and the other in the coronoid fossa anteriorly. Displacement of the posterior fat pad may be visible on radiographs after elbow trauma. This is a reliable indication of

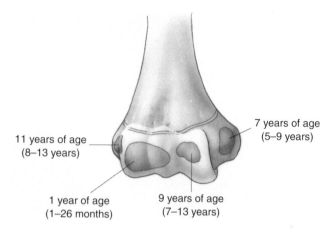

**Figure 33.14** Ossification of the secondary centers of the distal humerus. The average ages are specified, and the age ranges are indicated. The ossification ranges are earlier for girls than for boys. The lateral epicondyle, capitellum, and trochlea coalesce between 10 and 12 years of age, subsequently fusing to the distal humerus between 13 and 16 years of age. This is about the time that the medial epicondyle fuses to the proximal humerus.

intraarticular effusion (121). The anterior fat pad is sometimes seen under normal conditions, and does not necessarily indicate joint effusion. Most of the distal humerus has good collateral circulation, with most of the intraosseous blood supply entering posteriorly. Caution should be exercised to avoid disrupting this posterior blood supply during surgical exposure of fractures (122). The trochlea and medial condyle are particularly vulnerable to avascular necrosis because they are perfused by sets of nonanastomotic nutrient vessels that enter the bone posteriorly and medially (123).

The clinical carrying angle of the normal elbow is a slight valgus alignment, averaging approximately 7 degrees.

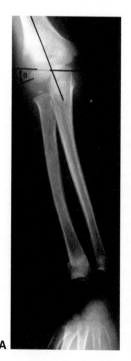

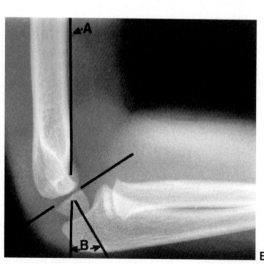

**Figure 33.15** Radiographic lines of the distal humerus. **A:** The Baumann angle is formed between the capitellar physeal line and a line perpendicular to the long axis of the humerus. As this angle becomes smaller, more elbow varus will occur. This angle should be compared with that of the contralateral, uninjured elbow with a similar anteroposterior view of the distal humerus. **B:** Line A is the anterior humeral line, which atypically passes through the middle of the capitellum. Angle B demonstrates the anterior angulation of the capitellum relative to the humeral shaft. This is approximately 30 degrees. As angle B becomes smaller, the fracture site is moved into extension. Fracture alignment with the capitellum behind the anterior humeral line produces a hyperextension deformity and a loss of elbow flexion.

There are several helpful radiographic lines and angles that can be measured to determine if there is adequate postinjury alignment; a comparison view of the other elbow may be valuable as a reference (Fig. 33.15). All measurements are subject to the inaccuracies caused by elbow positioning, and this should be kept in mind when making clinical decisions. The Baumann angle is used to assess the varus attitude of the distal humerus, usually after a supracondylar elbow fracture. It is the angle formed between the capitellar physeal line and a line perpendicular to the long axis of the humerus. This angle normally should be within 5 to 8 degrees of the same angle in the contralateral elbow. An anteroposterior view of the distal humerus, positioned parallel to the radiographic plate, is necessary to reduce the variation of the Baumann angle that occurs when the arm is rotated. Ten degrees of rotation produces a 6-degree change in the angle (124). Another measure of coronal alignment is the medial epicondylar epiphyseal angle. This angle is measured between the long axis of the humerus and a line through the medial epicondylar physis (125). It has the advantage of being reliably measured while the elbow is held in flexion (i.e., Jones view), as during the reduction process. The medial epicondylar epiphyseal line ranges from 25 to 46 degrees. This angle is not reliable for children younger than 3 years or older than 10 (125). Sagittal alignment may be determined by the lateral capitellar angle, which indicates the normal forward-flexed position of the capitellum. This angle averages 30 to 40 degrees. The anterior humeral line offers a similar means to assess the position of the capitellum and is measured on a true lateral radiographic projection. A line along the anterior humeral cortex should pass through the center of the capitellum.

## Supracondylar Fracture

This is the most common elbow fracture. The usual mechanism of injury is a hyperextension load on the elbow from falling on the outstretched arm. The distal fragment displaces posteriorly (i.e., extension) in more than 95% of fractures. The medial and lateral columns of the distal humerus are connected by a very thin area of bone between the olecranon fossa posteriorly and the coronoid fossa anteriorly. The central thinning and the surrounding narrow columns predispose this area to fracture. As the elbow is forced into hyperextension, the olecranon impinges in the fossa, serving as the fulcrum for the fracture. The collateral ligaments and the anterior joint capsule also resist hyperextension, transmitting the stress to the distal humerus and initiating the fracture (126) (Fig. 33.16). Flexion type supracondylar fractures result from a direct fall onto the flexed elbow.

The classification system most commonly used is that of Gartland, who described three stages of displacement (127): type I, nondisplaced or minimally displaced; type II, angulated with moderate disruption but with a portion of the cortex maintaining end-to-end contact; and type III, completely displaced. Supracondylar fractures with medial

impaction may appear to be nondisplaced but may result in cubitus varus attributable to unacceptable angulation (128). After complete fracture, a small amount of rotational malalignment allows tilting of the fragments because of the thin cross-sectional area in the supracondylar region. This may also lead to malunion with cubitus varus or, less commonly, cubitus valgus.

Associated injuries include nerve injuries, vascular injuries, and other fractures of the upper extremity,

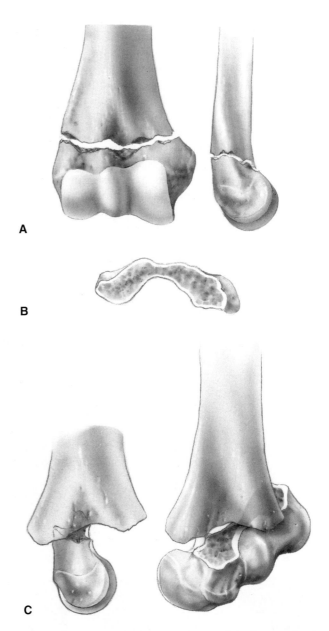

**A**

**B**

**C**

**Figure 33.16** **A:** The typical orientation of the fracture line in the supracondylar fracture. Sagittal rotation of the distal fragment generally results in posterior angulation, although, less commonly, it can be flexed. **B:** The cross-sectional area through the fracture demonstrates the thin cross-sectional area of the supracondylar region. **C:** Any horizontal rotation tilts the distal fragment. Typically, medial tilting occurs, producing cubitus varus. The lateral projection readily demonstrates this horizontal rotation, producing a fishtail deformity. In this instance, the distal portion of the proximal fragment is obliquely profiled, although there is a true lateral view of the distal humeral fragment.

including the ipsilateral forearm. The incidence of nerve injury is approximately 15%; most often, nerve injury is a neuropraxia that resolves spontaneously within 4 months. The nerve that gets injured is related to the position of the displaced fragment (129). Median nerve injuries, including injury to the anterior interosseous nerve, are more common with posterolateral displacement of the distal fragment. Radial nerve injuries are seen more often with posteromedial displacement.

### Treatment

Nondisplaced or minimally displaced fractures may be treated with an above-elbow cast for 3 weeks. Any medial buckling or impaction of the medial metaphysis may indicate a fracture that requires reduction. This fracture is a diagnostic trap, because the collapse of the medial column may be very subtle (Fig. 33.17). The Baumann angle, or the medial epicondylar epiphyseal angle, should be carefully measured bilaterally; more than 10 degrees of varus impaction warrants closed reduction and percutaneous pinning (CRPP). It is difficult to maintain the reduction by cast immobilization alone, and residual deformity will not remodel (128).

Type II supracondylar fractures are usually extension injuries, with an intact or nondisplaced posterior cortex. Type II fractures, in which the capitellum is posterior to the anterior humeral line, have an unacceptable amount of extension. Many of these are stable after closed reduction and casting in 90 to 100 degrees of flexion (130). When more than 100 degrees of flexion is required for maintenance of reduction, percutaneous pinning is recommended, with immobilization in less than 90 degrees of flexion (131). Weekly follow-up for 2 weeks is recommended following closed management to diagnose and treat any loss of reduction.

Type III supracondylar fractures are completely displaced. Treatment begins with a complete assessment of perfusion and nerve function. Neurovascular problems are frequent, and fracture management may be altered if neurovascular compromise is present. In the absence of neurovascular compromise, displaced fractures can be splinted and managed safely in a delayed manner as long as the child is closely monitored (132,133). Primary CRPP is the preferred treatment for type III injuries (134) (Fig. 33.18). Displaced supracondylar fractures treated by closed reduction and casting have a higher incidence of residual deformity than those treated with reduction and pinning (134). Closed reduction and casting also has a higher risk of Volkmann ischemic contracture than treatment with early pinning (134).

*In vitro* biomechanical studies have concluded that crossed-pin fixation is more stable than parallel lateral pin configurations (135). However, divergent lateral pins have similar stability compared to crossed pins (136). Clinical

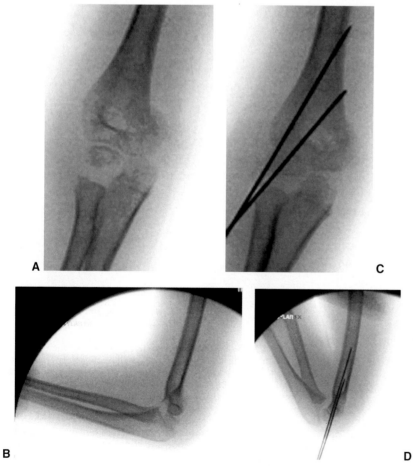

**Figure 33.17** Type II supracondylar humerus fracture with medial impaction and varus alignment. **A,B:** Anteroposterior and lateral views of a type II supracondylar humerus fracture with medial impaction. Note that although there is little displacement on the lateral view, the Baumann angle is 0 degrees on the anteroposterior. **C,D:** Anteroposterior and lateral intraoperative views of the distal humerus after the impacted fracture was reduced and fixed with divergent lateral pins. Note that on the anteroposterior, the Baumann angle is restored, and on the lateral, the anterior humeral line intersects the capitellum. The reduction was maintained during the postoperative period.

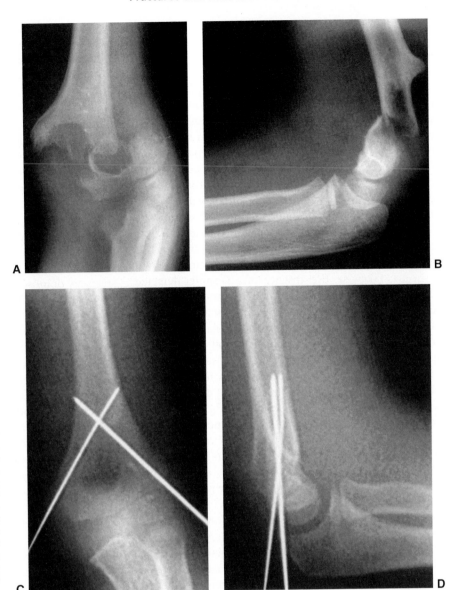

**Figure 33.18** Type III supracondylar humerus fracture. **A:** This type III fracture demonstrates lateral displacement. **B:** The lateral projection also shows flexion of the distal fragment. The treatment of this less common position is the same as that for extension fractures. The posterior periosteum is torn, and hyperflexion of the elbow will excessively forward-flex the distal fragment. The elbow is best pinned at slightly less than 90 degrees of flexion, because it is technically difficult to pin the elbow in extension. **C** and **D:** Anteroposterior and lateral postreduction and pinning films.

experience has demonstrated that two or three laterally placed pins are sufficient for stabilization (137). The authors prefer laterally placed pins without a medial pin except in unusual circumstances. When a medial pin is used, one should be aware that extreme elbow flexion could result in ulnar nerve subluxation from its groove and increase the risk of damage during pinning. When possible, it is advisable to place the lateral pin first to provide provisional stability so that the medial pin can be inserted with the elbow in less than full flexion, placing the ulnar nerve farther posterior. It is also advisable to make a small incision over the medial epicondyle and dissect with a hemostat, so that the medial pin can be placed directly on the bone. Anatomic alignment is preferred, but this may be difficult to achieve in some cases. When the quality of reduction is in doubt, comparison radiographs of the opposite elbow can be obtained intraoperatively. The Baumann angle should be within 5 to 8 degrees of the

angle on the contralateral side. As long as fixation is secure, it is the author's opinion that one may accept up to one-third translation of the distal fragment, 30 degrees of malrotation, and 20 degrees of extension after pinning (capitellum anterior to the anterior humeral line). Initial immobilization should be in a nonconstrictive splint or cast with the elbow in less than 90 degrees of flexion. The authors prefer a cast that has been bivalved and spread with the elbow in approximately 70 degrees of flexion. Oral analgesics are usually sufficient for pain relief. The need for intravenous narcotics may indicate ischemia. Immobilization is continued for 3 to 4 weeks, at which time the pins are removed and active range of motion is initiated.

The rare irreducible fracture may be managed with open reduction through a medial approach, adding a lateral incision, if necessary. An anterior surgical interval can also be used, and is recommended if the neurovascular structures need to be exposed. The posterior approach should be used cautiously because it disrupts any remaining intact soft tissue and may disrupt the primary vascular supply to the distal humeral fragment (122,123).

### Complications

In the event of a pulseless extremity, prompt reduction of the supracondylar fracture usually restores arterial flow (138,139) (Fig. 33.19). Complete vascular disruption is uncommon, because the thick local muscle envelope protects the artery. Vascular evaluation after reduction requires differentiation of the pulseless extremity that is pink and viable from one that is cold and pale with vascular insufficiency. The child who has a well-perfused hand but an absent radial pulse after satisfactory closed reduction does not necessarily require routine exploration of the brachial artery (129,138,140,141). The pulse usually returns within 48 hours. Likewise, the absence of a Doppler-detected pulse at the wrist is not an absolute indication for arterial exploration. The collateral circulation is vast and often provides enough distal perfusion despite brachial artery occlusion. When the hand is warm and normal in color with brisk capillary refill and normal oxygen saturation, the authors recommend careful observation with noncircumferential immobilization and less than 70 degrees elbow flexion. There is no convincing evidence of a clinical problem with cold intolerance or exercise-induced muscle fatigue for the hand surviving on collateral vascularity, but long-term studies addressing the problem are lacking (141).

For persistent true vascular insufficiency (e.g., avascular, cold, pale hand), especially if there is nerve palsy or inadequate reduction, anterior open reduction is recommended. Frequently, the neurovascular bundle is found kinked at the fracture site, and liberation of the artery restores the pulse. There may also be evidence of brachial artery injury. Vascular reconstruction should be performed if the vessel does not respond to local measures (e.g., release of tether, adventitia stripping, lidocaine, papaverine) and the hand remains avascular. The fracture should be stabilized before vascular repair. After reconstruction, there is a significant rate of asymptomatic reocclusion and residual stenosis, although the hand remains well perfused (141).

Nerve injury associated with supracondylar fracture rarely requires exploration (Fig. 33.20). Patients with preoperative nerve injury should undergo reduction and fixation as described. Exploration of the nerve is not necessary when the reduction is anatomic. However, failure to obtain anatomic reduction may indicate that the nerve is interposed at the fracture site, and exploration may be indicated.

Postoperative neurologic deficit that was not noted preoperatively may represent a preexisting nerve deficit that was undetected at the time of the initial examination or an iatrogenic injury sustained during reduction. Median and radial nerve injuries are more frequently seen because of the initial trauma and may be observed when the reduction is anatomic. Postoperative ulnar nerve deficits are more often iatrogenic and usually result from placement of the medial pin (129,142,143). Recommendations for management of this complication vary from observation to exploration. When iatrogenic ulnar neuropathy is suspected, it is the authors' opinion that the medial pin should be removed without exploration. Spontaneous recovery of most neural injuries following elbow fracture is expected within 2 to 6 months. If there has been no recovery of function by 4 to 6 months after injury, then exploration is indicated. The results of late neurolysis or repair are usually favorable in children (144).

Cubitus varus is the most common late complication of supracondylar fracture. This deformity represents fracture malunion and rarely results from partial growth arrest of the medial condylar growth plate. Malunion may be avoided by careful attention to anatomic reduction and secure fixation at the time of initial management. Cubitus varus is generally considered a cosmetically acceptable deformity, but increased risk of lateral condyle fracture, tardy ulnar palsy, and posterior shoulder instability has also been reported (145–147). Osteotomy to correct deformity may be performed at any age, but complications are not uncommon (148). Full-length radiographs of both arms are recommended preoperatively for accurate planning. Simple uniplanar closing wedge osteotomies have the lowest complication rates, but lateral condylar prominence may compromise the cosmetic result in patients older than 12 years (148,149). When osteotomy is required in older patients, the authors translate the distal fragment medially to avoid lateral prominence.

## Floating Elbow

Simultaneous ipsilateral supracondylar and forearm fractures have been termed *floating elbow*. These injuries often

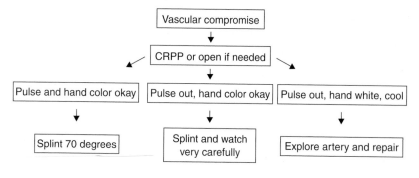

**Figure 33.19** Management of a supracondylar humerus fracture with vascular compromise. This algorithm shows management of a supracondylar humerus fracture associated with vascular compromise. *CRPP*, closed reduction percutaneous pinning.

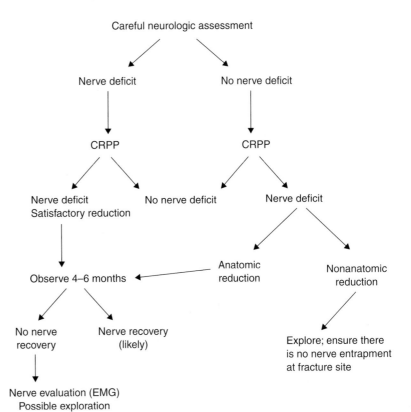

**Figure 33.20** Management strategy with supracondylar humerus fracture and neurologic deficit. *CRPP*, closed reduction percutaneous pinning; *EMG*, electromyogram.

result from high-energy trauma. Increased risks of compartment syndrome and secondary displacement of the forearm fracture have been reported (150–152). Percutaneous pinning of both the supracondylar and forearm fractures is recommended if the forearm fracture requires reduction (150,152,153). This allows less constrictive immobilization and reduces the risk of redisplacement.

## T-condylar Fracture

The T-condylar fracture is a variation of the supracondylar fracture. The mechanism of injury is axial impaction with resultant intraarticular fracture. This injury occurs predominantly in adolescents around the time of physeal closure, but it can also occur in younger children. The capitellum and trochlea usually are separated from each other, and the two are separated from the proximal humerus.

Treatment of displaced fractures should be aimed at restoring the anatomic alignment of the articular surface. Closed reduction and percutaneous fixation has been reported, with transcondylar fixation followed by pinning or flexible nailing of the supracondylar component of the fracture (154,155). When open reduction is necessary, a posterior approach is recommended. This can be accomplished by splitting the triceps, reflecting a distally based tongue of triceps, or by olecranon osteotomy (156,157). Comminution of the articular surface is rare in children, so the triceps-splitting approach is usually adequate without olecranon osteotomy. Extensive dissection of the fragments

should be avoided to minimize the risk of avascular necrosis of the trochlea. Transverse fixation of the trochlea to the capitellum is performed first, and this unit is secured to the distal humerus with sufficiently strong crossed pins or cancellous screws. Alternatively, 2.5-mm reconstruction plates are applied to the medial and lateral columns of the distal humerus. When open reduction is performed, internal fixation should be stable. This allows motion during the early postoperative period (156,158). The recommended period of immobilization should be 3 weeks or less. The authors prefer rigid internal fixation with early motion in patients who are near skeletal maturity.

## Fracture-separation of the Distal Humeral Physis

Fracture-separation of the distal humeral physis is seen primarily in infants and young children. The mechanism of injury involves rotatory shear forces, resulting in a Salter-Harris type I or type II fracture pattern. Abuse should be suspected (159). This injury may present a diagnostic challenge because of the lack of ossification of the distal humerus in young children. Diagnosis of this fracture should be considered in any young child with significant soft tissue swelling and crepitus on elbow motion. This fracture is most often confused with elbow dislocation and lateral condyle fracture. Elbow dislocation is rare in young children; the forearm is displaced laterally and the long axis of the radius is lateral to the capitellum. A lateral condyle fracture in a 2- to 3-year-old child may be confused with transphyseal separation, especially if there is joint subluxation. However, the subluxation associated with lateral condyle fracture is in the lateral direction, whereas distal humeral physeal separations usually displace in a medial direction (Fig. 33.21). Arthrography, MRI, or ultrasonography can help confirm the diagnosis of separation of the entire distal humeral physis. Arthrography is a helpful adjunct at the time of definitive treatment to confirm the quality of fracture reduction (Fig. 33.22).

Treatment and complications are similar to those for supracondylar fractures. Closed reduction and plaster immobilization frequently lead to cubitus varus that does not resolve (146,159). Therefore, fixation with two small-diameter, laterally placed pins is recommended after reduction. Fractures diagnosed after 7 to 10 days should not be manipulated because healing is rapid and growth arrest may result from vigorous attempts at reduction. For fractures with late presentation, it is better to wait and perform supracondylar osteotomy for residual deformity.

## Lateral Condyle Fracture

Fracture of the lateral condyle is the second most common elbow fracture in children. This injury is usually the result of a varus force on the supinated forearm, in which the extensor longus and brevis muscles avulse the condylar

fragment. The peak age range for this injury is 5 to 10 years, but it is often seen in older or younger children.

This is a complex fracture because it involves the physis and the articular surface. It is a Salter-Harris type IV injury in most cases, but a significant portion of the fragment is unossified, especially in children younger than 5 years. Growth disturbance is more common than is generally recognized (160). Fortunately, growth disturbances are usually minor because the distal humerus only contributes 2 to 3 mm of longitudinal growth per year in children older than 7 years (161). The injury is identified by a thin lateral metaphyseal rim of bone, but the fracture line may continue through unossified cartilage, across the physis, and into the elbow joint. An oblique radiograph of the internally rotated distal humerus usually provides the best view of this fracture.

The fracture line may take several paths through the unossified cartilage of the distal humerus. The Milch classification is unreliable and has limited clinical usefulness (160,162). Postmortem studies by Jakob et al. identified three stages of lateral condylar displacement (163) (Fig. 33.23). These stages provide a useful classification for lateral condyle fractures. This classification, on the basis of the observations of Jakob et al., is more useful than the Milch classification with regard to treatment choices. Stage I has an intact cartilage hinge. This fracture pattern is inherently stable. Stage II is a complete but minimally displaced fracture with disruption of the articular cartilage hinge.

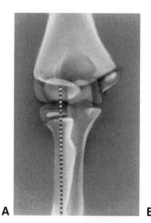
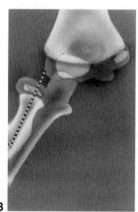
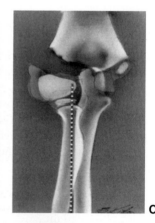

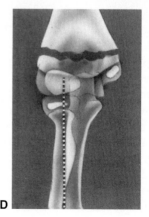
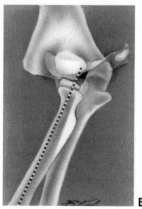

**Figure 33.21 A:** Normal elbow demonstrating the alignment of the radius with the capitellum. **B:** In a dislocation of the elbow, there is disruption of the radiocapitellar alignment. Most dislocations are posterolateral. **C:** In a displaced lateral condyle fracture, there is again disruption of the radial capitellar alignment. **D:** Supracondylar elbow fracture, in which the radius and capitellum remain aligned, despite displacement of the distal humeral fragment. **E:** Fracture-separation of the distal humeral physis. The radiocapitellar relation is preserved, and typically the distal segment is posteromedially displaced. (Adapted from DeLee J, Wilkins K, Rogers L, et al. Fracture separation of the distal humeral epiphysis. *J Bone Joint Surg Am* 1980;62:46, with permission.)

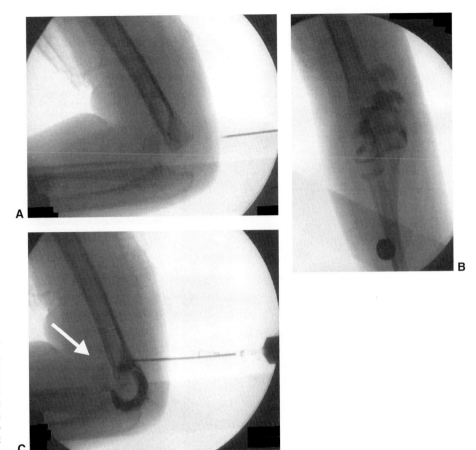

**Figure 33.22** Arthrogram technique. Although many are trained to use the lateral radiocapitellar joint as the entry point for an elbow arthrogram, the olecranon fossa approach is easier and more reliable on the swollen elbow of a small child. This 6-year-old child presented with distal humeral fracture. The surgeon could not distinguish a distal humeral physeal fracture versus a lateral condyle fracture. In the operating room, 5 mL of radiographic dye was injected into the olecranon fossa. **A:** Lateral image, just prior to injection. **B,C:** Anteroposterior and lateral image after injection. The distal humerus was clearly delineated as intact, while a lateral condyle fracture fragment (*arrow*) can be seen anteriorly.

This fracture may displace further and lead to nonunion. Stage III has major rotational displacement with loss of soft tissue stability. Severely displaced fractures lead to symptomatic malunion or nonunion unless they are reduced and stabilized.

Determining the exact location and extent of the fracture line may be difficult. When the fracture gap is equal medially and laterally along the fracture line, there is a very high risk of displacement due to absence of a cartilage hinge (164). Fractures with initial displacement of 3 mm or more also tend to displace further and have a higher incidence of nonunion (165). MRI has been recommended when there is doubt about the presence of an intact cartilage hinge (166). However, the present authors

prefer to assess fracture stability in questionable cases by radiographic follow-up weekly for 2 weeks. It is often necessary to remove the cast to obtain adequate anteroposterior, internally rotated oblique, and lateral radiographs of the distal humerus (Fig. 33.24). Gentle cast removal and radiography will not cause displacement if the fracture is inherently stable.

Treatment depends on the degree of displacement and the assessment of fragment stability. Fractures with initial displacement of 3 mm or more tend to displace further and have a higher incidence of nonunion (165); therefore, it is the authors' preference to pin all fractures that are displaced 3 mm or more. Some lateral condyle fractures that are displaced 3 mm may have an intact cartilage hinge and heal

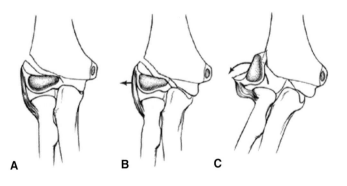

**Figure 33.23** Jakob classification of stages of displacement of a lateral condyle fracture. **A:** Stage I displacement with an intact articular surface. **B:** Stage II displacement. The articular surface is disrupted, but the fracture is minimally displaced. **C:** Stage III displacement with fragment rotated.

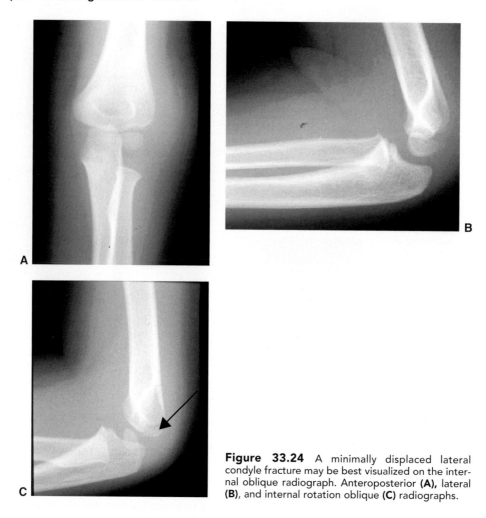

**Figure 33.24** A minimally displaced lateral condyle fracture may be best visualized on the internal oblique radiograph. Anteroposterior **(A)**, lateral **(B)**, and internal rotation oblique **(C)** radiographs.

with cast immobilization (166,167) (Fig. 33.25). Careful follow-up for minimally displaced fractures is essential, so the surgeon should consider pinning minimally displaced fractures when compliance with follow-up is doubtful (168). When initial displacement is 3 mm or less and the patient is reliable, weekly follow-up for 2 weeks with radiographs that are taken without the cast is recommended to determine stability. Any further displacement warrants surgical stabilization. Healing for minimally displaced fractures is complete when bridging callus is identified (usually seen posteriorly on the lateral radiograph). This usually occurs by the fourth week of immobilization, but immobilization for up to 12 weeks may be required in some cases (165).

Closed reduction and percutaneous fixation have been reported for fractures that are separated 3 to 4 mm (169). An arthrogram may provide confirmation of joint surface congruity when closed pinning is performed. However, many of these fractures display rotation of the condylar fragment, which is difficult to correct accurately by closed reduction. Primary open reduction with restoration of articular congruity is preferred in most cases requiring surgery. In severe cases, the condylar fragment may be rotated 180 degrees. A standard lateral approach is utilized between the triceps posteriorly and the brachialis/extensor carpi radialis longus anteriorly. Incision of the anterior

joint capsule facilitates exposure. Soft tissue stripping posteriorly should be avoided to reduce the risk of avascular necrosis of the capitellum and trochlea. Stabilization can be achieved with two smooth pins crossing the fracture site and exiting the opposite cortex. The pins and cast are removed 3 to 6 weeks after surgery, depending on the extent of healing seen on postoperative radiographs.

### Complications

Management of the late-presenting lateral condyle malunion is an area of controversy. Minor degrees of malunion are well tolerated. Correction of malunion more than 6 weeks after fracture is difficult (163,170). Remodeling obscures fracture lines and interferes with restoration of anatomic reduction following osteotomy. Excessive stripping of the condyle to facilitate reduction may result in avascular necrosis and greater joint stiffness. Two surgical approaches are described in the literature for management of symptomatic patients with malunion. Supracondylar osteotomy, combined with ulnar nerve transposition, has been performed with satisfactory improvement in function (163). Intraarticular osteotomies, with partial reduction, have also achieved satisfactory results (171).

Nonunion after lateral condyle fracture is seen most often in untreated patients, with displacement of 3 mm or

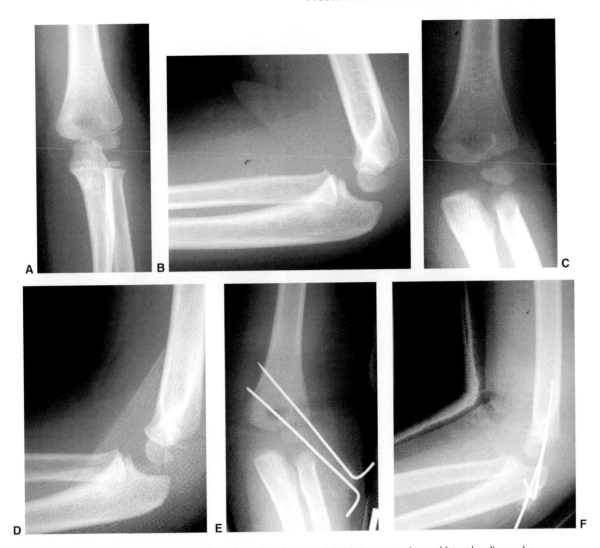

**Figure 33.25**  The drifting lateral condyle fracture. **A,B:** Anteroposterior and lateral radiographs at presentation. This lateral condyle fracture has only approximately 2 mm of displacement on the anteroposterior view. No displacement is noted on the lateral view. The child was placed in a long-arm cast and a follow-up 1 week later was recommended. **C,D:** Anteroposterior and lateral radiographs taken 1 week after injury show further displacement of the lateral condyle fracture with 5 mm of separation of the lateral condyle from the distal humerus. Open reduction and pinning was performed. **E,F:** Radiographs taken in the cast 4 weeks after open reduction and pinning show anatomic alignment and early healing.

more. Delayed union and nonunion has been attributed to fracture instability, exposure to synovial fluid, and decreased vascularity due to the large articular surface of the fracture fragment. Long-term sequelae of nonunion include ulnar neuritis, progressive valgus deformity, and elbow instability with decreased strength. In established nonunions, the lateral condyle fragment should be fixed in a position that preserves the best functional range of motion, realizing that anatomic restoration is not possible (Fig. 33.26) (165,171,172). Bone grafting is recommended to achieve union. Any residual valgus deformity can be corrected with a supracondylar osteotomy. Ulnar nerve transposition may be needed, especially if there are preoperative symptoms (173).

Minor degrees of deformity of the distal humerus are not uncommon following a lateral condyle fracture (160,174). Asymmetric growth of the lateral condyle or

incomplete reduction can produce mild cubitus varus. Fishtail deformity, or deepening of the trochlear groove, may result from central growth arrest or from avascular necrosis. This deformity rarely compromises function, but may predispose to later condylar fracture (160). Dissolution of the medial condyle or the lateral condyle has also been reported following distal humerus fracture in children (175). Corrective osteotomies with nerve decompression or transposition can modify the deformity and symptoms.

## Lateral Epicondyle Fracture

Lateral epicondyle fracture is a rare elbow injury that does not involve the articular surface. This ossification center does not appear until the second decade. This injury is

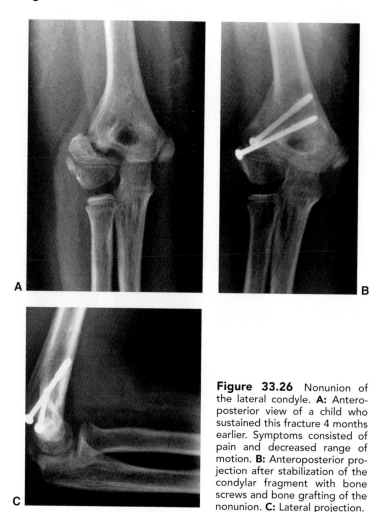

**Figure 33.26** Nonunion of the lateral condyle. **A:** Anteroposterior view of a child who sustained this fracture 4 months earlier. Symptoms consisted of pain and decreased range of motion. **B:** Anteroposterior projection after stabilization of the condylar fragment with bone screws and bone grafting of the nonunion. **C:** Lateral projection.

often misdiagnosed as an avulsion fracture of the lateral condyle. Treatment is usually immobilization followed by early motion, when comfortable. Displacement greater than 5 mm may lead to joint stiffness. If this occurs, early excision of the displaced epicondyle should be considered.

## Medial Epicondyle Fracture

The medial epicondylar apophysis is fractured when a valgus load is applied to the extended elbow. The displacement is encouraged by the pull of the forearm flexor muscle group, which is attached in this region. The medial collateral ligament, which also originates from this apophysis, may play a role in the initial fracture displacement, especially when the fracture is associated with an elbow dislocation. This injury typically occurs in children between the ages of 9 and 14 years, later than the peak age for most other elbow fractures. In younger children, the entire unossified medial condyle may be fractured, giving the appearance of medial epicondylar fracture. Almost 50% of medial epicondyle fractures occur concomitantly with posterolateral elbow dislocation. The medial epicondyle may be trapped in the joint after reduction. When this occurs, the

ulnar nerve may also be in the joint, and vigorous attempts at closed manipulation should be avoided.

### Treatment

There is general agreement that surgical intervention is indicated when the epicondyle is trapped in the joint. Otherwise, management is controversial. There are advocates for the closed treatment of this injury regardless of the magnitude of displacement (176,177). Nonunion is a frequent result of closed management, but many patients are asymptomatic. Valgus instability to stress testing has been suggested as an indication for surgical stabilization (178). However, most fresh medial epicondyle avulsion injuries will demonstrate instability, so most patients will require surgery if this test is used. Late instability after closed management has been reported, but this complication is rare unless the epicondylar fragment has been excised (177,178). Excellent results have also been reported after surgical stabilization of moderately displaced fractures (179). Although nonsurgical management can produce good results, it is the authors' preference to perform open reduction and internal fixation for medial epicondyle fractures when displacement is greater than 5 mm (Fig. 33.27).

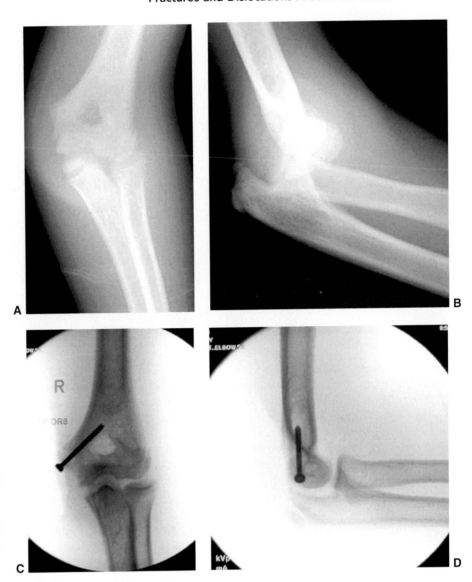

**Figure 33.27** Medial epicondyle fracture with elbow dislocation. **A,B:** Anteroposterior and lateral views of the elbow showing an elbow dislocation with associated medial epicondyle fracture. **C,D:** Intraoperative images after reduction of the elbow dislocation and open reduction of the medial epicondyle fracture with interfragmentary screw fixation.

Surgical intervention for lesser degrees of displacement is also considered for highly competitive gymnasts or throwing athletes who have injured their dominant elbow.

In adolescents, fragment fixation can be accomplished with a cannulated bone screw. When reducing this fracture, it is important to understand that the fragment tends to rotate anteriorly from its posteromedial origin. Stable fixation allows early postoperative range of motion. Preadolescents may require fixation with smooth Kirschner wires and cast immobilization for 3 weeks to minimize the risk of growth arrest of the apophysis.

## Medial Condyle Fracture

Fracture of the medial condyle of the humerus is an unusual injury. Medial condyle fracture may be misdiagnosed as medial epicondyle avulsion in children between the ages of 5 and 7 years, because the epicondylar ossification center is visible on radiographs approximately 2 years before the trochlea ossifies. If a child with an unossified trochlea presents with a swollen elbow, it is important to examine the radiographs for a chip or flake of bone from the metaphysis, which indicates medial condyle fracture. The mechanism of injury is similar to that for medial epicondylar fracture, but medial condyle fracture is a much more serious injury, because it involves the articular surface. If the condyle is displaced more than 2 mm, open reduction and internal fixation is recommended (180).

## Radial Neck Fracture

Fractures of the radial neck are most common in children in the 7- to 12-year age group. Approximately 50% are isolated injuries; associated fractures, most commonly of the proximal ulna, are found in the other 50% (181). Associated injuries should be treated independently as indicated for that particular fracture. Radial neck fractures are predominantly Salter-Harris type I or II injuries. The

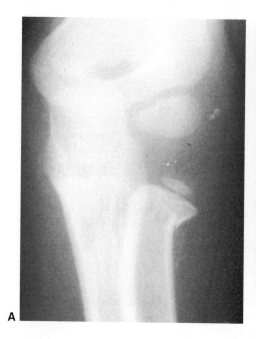
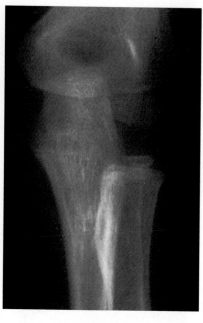

**Figure 33.28** Impacted radial neck fracture in a boy who is 6 years and 5 months old. **A:** Angulation measures 30 degrees. **B:** Nine months later, alignment is normal without treatment. The child regained full range of motion.

radial head is largely cartilaginous and is rarely injured in children. The mechanism of injury is usually valgus stress, with compression of the radial neck from a fall on the extended elbow. Fracture displacement can result in angulation and translation, with or without complete separation of the radial head from the shaft. Angulation after union may remodel, especially in younger children. Union with translation may limit motion because of a cam effect that prevents the radial head from rotating in a circle. Approximately half of the children who sustain fractures of the radial neck will have some permanent limitation of forearm rotation. Factors leading to a poor prognosis are age greater than 10 years, angulation greater than 30 degrees, displacement greater than 3 mm, delayed treatment, associated injuries, and open reduction (182,183).

Treatment depends on the age of the child and the amount of angulation and translation. The plane of maximum angulation can be determined by multiple radiographic views or by fluoroscopy. When angulation is greater than 30 degrees or translation is greater than 3 mm, closed reduction usually should be attempted because anatomic alignment is associated with better outcome. However, closed reduction may fail, and one must decide whether to accept suboptimal alignment or to resort to open reduction, with increased risks in each case. Age is important in this situation (183). For a child younger than 10 years (Fig. 33.28), the authors will accept up to 45 degrees of angulation and 33% translation before resorting to open reduction. In a child older than 10 years, up to 30 degrees of angulation and 3 mm of translation may be accepted.

The manipulation technique for closed reduction consists of traction and varus stress, combined with digital pressure over the radial head. Alternatively, the radial shaft should be forced laterally while the radial head is held in place (Fig. 33.29) (184), or the forearm can be pronated as the elbow is maximally flexed. Wrapping the arm firmly in an Esmarch bandage produces compression and elongation forces, which may also reduce the fracture. Alternatively, a percutaneous pin introduced proximally or a flexible intramedullary wire introduced distally can be used to manipulate and stabilize the proximal fragment (185–187). Open reduction is performed when these methods fail to produce an acceptable reduction. Another indication for open reduction is a displaced Salter-Harris type IV fracture involving more than one-third of the articular surface. Fixation may be achieved with intramedullary fixation from the distal metaphysis (Figs. 33.30 and 33.31) or by distally inserted Kirschner wires placed obliquely across the fracture. A transarticular pin through the humerus should be avoided. Percutaneous fixation is removed in 3 to 4 weeks to begin elbow range of motion. If the metaphyseal fragment is large enough, a minifragment screw can be used instead of Kirschner wires or flexible retrograde nailing.

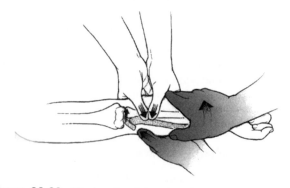

**Figure 33.29** Displaced radial neck reduction technique using manipulation of the proximal radius with the elbow extended and hand supinated. (From Neher CG, Torch MA. New reduction technique for severely displaced pediatric radial neck fractures. *J Pediatr Orthop* 2003;23:626–628.)

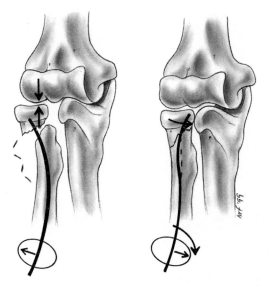

**Figure 33.30** Radial neck fractures may be reduced by introduction of a percutaneous wire from the distal metaphysis. The wire is rotated after it engages the proximal fragment. [From Gonzalez-Herranz P, Alvarez-Romera A, Burgos J, et al. Displaced radial neck fractures in children treated by closed intramedullary pinning (Metaizeau technique). *J Pediatr Orthop* 1997;17(3): 325–331.]

## Complications

Complications of this fracture and its treatment include loss of forearm rotation, radioulnar synostosis, injury to the posterior interosseous nerve, nonunion, premature physeal arrest, and avascular necrosis of the radial head (182,183). These complications are observed without treatment, unless they are progressive or disabling.

## Olecranon Fractures

Olecranon fractures are uncommon in children. In young children, the spongy bone and thick surrounding cartilage often prevent significant displacement. Older children and adolescents are more likely to have displaced fractures and associated injuries. The most common mechanism of olecranon injury is an avulsion or flexion injury that disrupts the posterior periosteum and fractures the cortex (Fig. 33.32). Extension injuries leave the posterior periosteum intact, but often result in angulated fractures and associated fractures attributable to varus or valgus forces acting on the extended elbow. Olecranon fractures may also result from a direct blow that causes comminution but minimal displacement because the periosteum remains intact. Children with osteogenesis imperfecta can present with an olecranon sleeve fracture (Fig. 33.33).

If displacement is minimal, treatment consists of splint or cast immobilization for 2 to 3 weeks. When displacement is greater than 4 mm in metaphyseal bone, or there is a greater than 2 mm joint step-off in the anterior two-thirds of the coronoid fossa, closed reduction is recommended. Open reduction with internal fixation is performed when

closed reduction fails, or when maintenance of reduction is difficult because of fracture instability (188–190). Internal fixation is achieved by standard osteosynthesis, using the AO tension band technique or its modification, which involves placing the distal wire hole anterior to the axis of the intramedullary Kirschner wires (191). This provides additional compression forces across the articular surface of the olecranon (Fig. 33.34). In younger children, heavy nonabsorbable suture may be used in place of the figure-eight wire because healing is rapid. An alternative is to place two divergent compression pins or screws through percutaneous incisions (192).

## Elbow Dislocation

Elbow dislocation is a relatively uncommon injury in young children; the peak incidence is in the second decade of life. Often there is an associated fracture, most commonly of the medial epicondyle, but occasionally of the coronoid process or the radial neck. Elbow dislocation is predominantly a male injury (70%) involving the nondominant arm (60%). The most common pattern is posterolateral displacement of the proximal radius and ulna articulation from the humerus, without disruption of the radioulnar articulation (193).

Reduction is usually achieved by manually applying longitudinal traction, usually in the emergency department, after establishing pain control and muscle relaxation. The surgeon should be aware of possible interposed soft tissue or bony fragments, including the ulnar nerve or medial epicondyle. A posterior splint is applied for 2 weeks; thereafter, elbow range of motion is initiated to minimize the risk of fixed contracture.

### Complications

The most common complication is loss of motion. This can be minimized for stable reductions by initiating early motion 2 weeks after injury (193). Stiffness, in the absence of fracture, usually resolves within 6 to 8 months. The authors recommend avoiding the use of passive stretching devices for at least 4 months. The authors recommend excising associated avulsion fractures if range of motion has not returned to a functional range (30 to 100 degrees) by 6 months after dislocation. When avulsion fractures are absent, surgical release of contracture may be required if the range of motion is less than functional 8 months or more after injury (194,195). Neurapraxia involving the median or ulnar nerves occurs in approximately 10% of dislocations and usually resolves within 3 months.

## Radial Head Dislocation and Nursemaid's Elbow

Traumatic isolated dislocation of the radial head is a rare injury. The radial head dislocates anteriorly. Most of these injuries actually represent occult Monteggia injuries, with

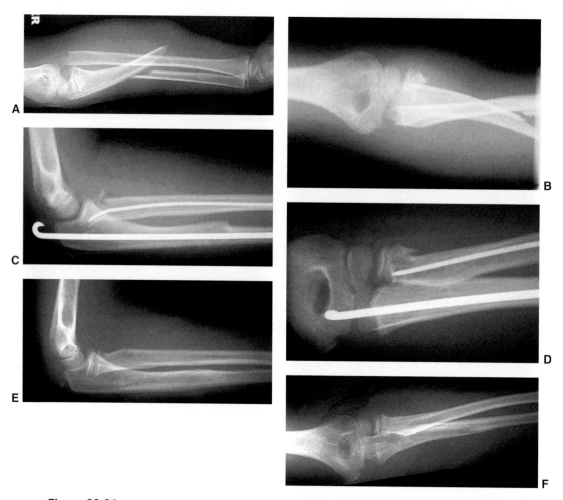

**Figure 33.31**    Monteggia-equivalent fracture treated with intramedullary (IM) reduction and fixation. **A,B:** Anteroposterior and lateral view of a Monteggia-equivalent fracture with a displaced, oblique ulna fracture and completely displaced radial neck fracture, but intact radiocapitellar joint. **C,D:** The ulna was fixed with an IM nail, and the radial neck fracture was reduced and pinned using the Metazeau technique (shown in Fig. 33.30). **E,F:** Late follow-up after implant removal shows good alignment of the ulna and radiocapitellar joint. (Case courtesy of Ken Noonan, MD)

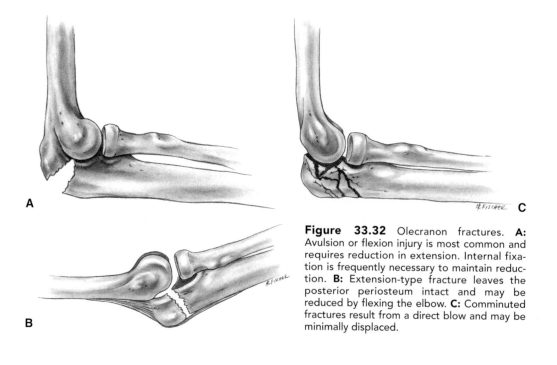

**Figure 33.32** Olecranon fractures. **A:** Avulsion or flexion injury is most common and requires reduction in extension. Internal fixation is frequently necessary to maintain reduction. **B:** Extension-type fracture leaves the posterior periosteum intact and may be reduced by flexing the elbow. **C:** Comminuted fractures result from a direct blow and may be minimally displaced.

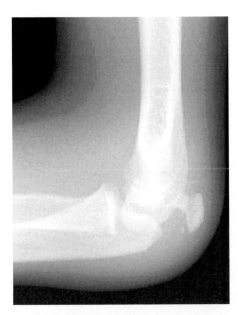

**Figure 33.33** Olecranon sleeve fracture. This lateral radiograph taken at the time of injury shows an olecranon sleeve fracture in a 10-year-old child with a mild osteogenesis imperfecta.

plastic deformation of the ulna and anterior dislocation of the radial head (Fig. 33.35). Treatment consists of closed reduction and immobilization, with the elbow in flexion and supination.

Occasionally, a child with a previously undiagnosed congenital radial head dislocation falls and injures the elbow. Congenital dislocation of the radial head is distinguished from traumatic dislocation by the fact that congenital dislocation is usually in a posterior direction, and the articular surface of the radial head is convex or flat, rather than having the normal concave contour.

Nursemaid's elbow, or pulled elbow, is a very common injury in children between 1 and 4 years of age. Typically, the child is being held by the hand and suddenly falls, or is pulled upward. Pain is variable. The child will not move the arm and will hold it in a slightly flexed and pronated position. Radiographs are not indicated initially and are normal because the injury consists of subluxation of the annular ligament, rather than true joint subluxation (196) (Fig. 33.36). When longitudinal traction is applied to the child's pronated arm, the annular ligament slips off the radius and rides up onto the broader radial head, like a rope that has jumped out of the groove in a pulley wheel. The child is unwilling to move the elbow until the stretched annular ligament is reduced.

Treatment consists of flexing the elbow above 90 degrees, then fully and firmly supinating the forearm. A click or snap is often felt as the ligament snaps back into place. Occasionally, it is necessary to fully pronate, and then supinate, the forearm to achieve reduction. This is especially true for delayed cases. The child should begin to move the arm within a few minutes after reduction. If this is not the case, then radiographs should be obtained to

rule out occult fracture, and the arm may be immobilized in a splint for 2 to 3 days. Normal use of the arm should be expected within 1 day after splint removal. Recurrences are not uncommon but are treated in the same manner as the initial injury. Eventually, children outgrow this condition, and long-term sequelae have not been reported.

## FOREARM AND WRIST FRACTURES

Fractures of the forearm and wrist are common in children, accounting for 30% to 40% of all fractures in children (3,6). There may be an increasing incidence of distal forearm fractures related to increased body mass, decreased bone mineral content, and changing patterns of activity such as rollerblading (5). Most forearm fractures occur in children older than 5 years. The location of the fracture advances distally with increasing age of the child, probably because of the anatomic changes in the metaphyseal-diaphyseal junction that occur with maturity (197). The younger child's radius is more elastic and has a gradual transition of the diameter of the radius from shaft to metaphysis, whereas the transition in diameter is more abrupt at the metaphyseal–diaphyseal junction in the older child. The distal forearm is the site of 70% to 80% of fractures of the radius and ulna. Most of these are nonphyseal. Physeal separations are more likely in early adolescence because of the more adult shape of the radius, which concentrates stress closer to the epiphysis. In 10% to 15% of patients, forearm fractures are associated with elbow fractures. This highlights the importance of a thorough clinical and radiographic examination of the injured extremity.

Anatomically, the forearm is unique. The ulna is a straight bone with a triangular cross section. The radius has a more complex, curved shape with a cylindrical proximal portion, a triangular middle portion, and a flattened distal third. The radius rotates around the ulna during forearm supination and pronation. There are three areas of soft-tissue interconnection between the radius and ulna. Proximally, there is the radioulnar articulation, which is stabilized by the annular ligament. Centrally, the shafts of the two bones are connected by the interosseous membrane, which is wider distally. The fibers run obliquely from the ulna distally to the radius proximally. This helps transmit force to the ulna during load-bearing activities. Distally, the triangular fibrocartilage complex stabilizes the radioulnar joint by means of the ulnar collateral ligament and the volar and dorsal radiocarpal ligaments. The proximal and distal radioulnar joints are most stable in supination, and the interosseous membrane is widest with the forearm in a position of 30 degrees of supination. Because of these interconnections, both bones are usually injured at the time of fracture. When only one bone is broken, there is frequently damage to the proximal or distal radioulnar articulation.

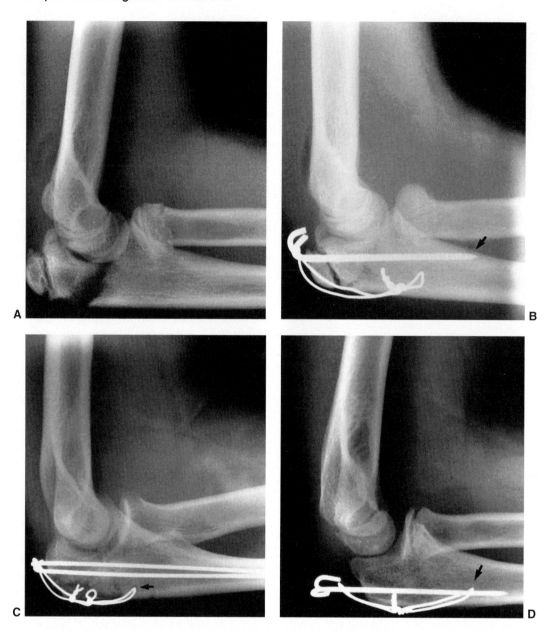

**Figure 33.34** Olecranon fracture. **A:** Lateral projection showing displaced intraarticular olecranon fracture. There is also an impacted radial neck fracture. **B:** Treatment with standard tension band technique. The slight variation from standard fixation is to capture the anterior cortex of the ulna with the Kirschner wires (*arrow*). **C:** Standard AO technique, used in a similar case, with parallel intramedullary Kirschner wires with the tension band transverse hole inferior (*arrow*). **D:** Modified AO technique performed by placing the transverse hole anterior to the Kirschner wires (*arrow*). The compressive force is anterior to the pin, which prevents the articular surface of the semilunar notch from gapping. Ideal joint compressive forces are obtained with placement of the Kirschner wires down the middle axis of the ulna and the transverse hole anterior to this axis.

Forearm and wrist fractures are usually classified into three major categories: fracture-dislocations, fractures of the midshaft, and distal fractures. Fracture-dislocations include the Monteggia and Galeazzi lesions. Midshaft fractures of the radius and ulna tend to follow three injury patterns: plastic deformation, greenstick fracture, and complete fracture. Distal fractures are either metaphyseal fractures or physeal separations. Each type of injury presents unique features with regard to mechanism of injury, recognition, and management.

## Forearm Fracture-dislocations

The combination of forearm fracture with joint dislocation is less common than other types of forearm fractures. Misdiagnosis may result if radiographs of forearm fractures fail to clearly demonstrate the elbow and wrist joints. The peak incidence occurs between 4 and 10 years of age. The Monteggia lesion is more common and involves dislocation of the radial head. The usual mechanism of injury is a fall on the hyperextended arm. The Galeazzi lesion involves

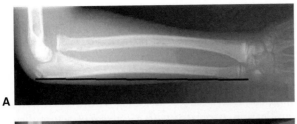

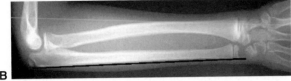

**Figure 33.35** Dislocated radial head with plastic deformation of the ulna. **A:** A 10-year-old boy presented with elbow and forearm pain after a fall. Radiograph shows complete dislocation of the radiocapitellar joint with plastic deformation of the ulna (note the anterior bow of the ulna demonstrated by a line drawn along its subcutaneous border). **B:** Contralateral, uninjured arm. Note the straight subcutaneous border.

fracture of the radius with dislocation of the distal radioulnar joint, or distal ulnar physeal fracture.

### Monteggia Fracture-dislocation

The Monteggia lesion should be suspected with any pediatric forearm fracture, including plastic deformation and minimally angulated greenstick fractures of the ulna. When the posterior border of the ulna deviates from a straight line on a true lateral radiograph, dislocation of the radial head should be suspected (198). A true lateral radiograph of the elbow provides the best assessment of the radiocapitellar joint. In the normal elbow, a line drawn down the long axis of the radial shaft will bisect the capitellum regardless of the position of flexion or extension of the elbow (199) (Fig. 33.37). Congenital dislocation of the radial head is distinguished from traumatic dislocation by the facts that congenital dislocation is usually posterior and the articular surface of the radial head is

convex. In contrast, anterior dislocation of the radial head is common with Monteggia fracture-dislocation (200,201).

Bado devised a classification system of four basic types of injury and several equivalent lesions (201). Type I involves anterior radial head dislocation (i.e., ulnar deformity apex anterior), which accounts for most childhood Monteggia injuries (Fig. 33.38). Type II fracture is the least common and entails posterior or posterolateral radial head dislocation. In type III lesions, the radial head is dislocated laterally, and the ulna fracture is usually in the proximal metaphyseal region. Type III injury accounts for 25% to 30% of pediatric Monteggia injuries. Type IV fracture-dislocations involve anterior dislocation of the radial head, in combination with fracture of the radius and ulna. This may be considered a variant of the type I lesion. There are numerous Monteggia equivalents that represent a multitude of variations. For example, the ulna fracture may be combined with a radial neck fracture rather than a simple radial head dislocation (Fig. 31.31). Segmental fractures and plastic deformation of the ulna are other forms of Monteggia equivalent injury.

Treatment depends on the character of the ulnar fracture because stable, anatomic reduction of the ulna can maintain anatomic reduction of the radial head. Most Monteggia injuries in children younger than 12 years can be managed successfully by closed reduction and above-elbow casting with the elbow in full supination and 90 to 110 degrees of flexion (200,202). Weekly follow-up with good quality elbow radiographs is suggested for 2 to 3 weeks to detect any recurrent radial head subluxation. Transient nerve palsies, most commonly of the posterior interosseous nerve, occur in approximately 10% of patients.

Surgical intervention is indicated when the reduction is unstable. Instability requiring surgical stabilization is more likely when there is an oblique fracture, or very displaced fracture, of the ulna (203). The percutaneous insertion of an ulnar intramedullary pin is a simple and effective way to manage this problem. Alternatively, the ulnar shaft can be plated. On rare occasions, when the radial head is not

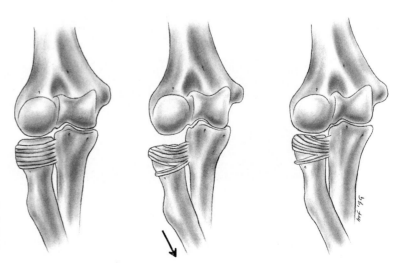

**Figure 33.36** Pulled elbow, or "nursemaid's elbow," occurs as the radial head moves distally. The annular ligament is partially torn and displaced onto the radial head. (From Rang M. *Children's fractures,* 2nd ed. Philadelphia: JB Lippincott, 1983, with permission.)

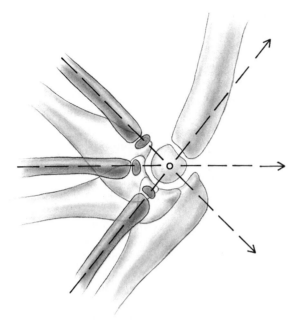

**Figure 33.37**  A true lateral radiograph of the elbow joint allows assessment of the integrity of the radiocapitellar joint. A line drawn down the long axis of the shaft of the radius will bisect the capitellum in all positions of flexion and extension. (From Smith F. Children's elbow injuries: fractures and dislocations. *Clin Orthop* 1967;50:25, with permission.)

reduced after correction of ulnar length and alignment, open examination of the joint is indicated. Interposition of the annular ligament or an intraarticular osteochondral fragment may be found. Transcapitellar pinning of the reduced radial head should be avoided whenever possible.

**Complications.** Delayed diagnosis is the most frequent complication associated with Monteggia fracture-dislocations. Patients presenting less than 3 weeks after injury with persistent dislocation may be treated by closed reduction. If the ulna can be reduced and stabilized, the radial head will usually reduce and remain stable. Open reduction is indicated if closed reduction fails, or when the injury is more than 4 weeks old. Chronic radial head dislocation has been surgically treated by open reduction. Following excision of the interposed fibrocartilaginous mass, the annular ligament can be reconstructed from remnants of the ligament, from a strip of triceps fascia, or from other tissues (204). Corrective osteotomy of the ulna to restore length and alignment has been associated with improved results, with or without annular ligament reconstruction (205,206).

### Galeazzi Fracture-dislocation

The classic Galeazzi lesion is a fracture of the distal third of the radius, without fracture of the ulna, and is associated

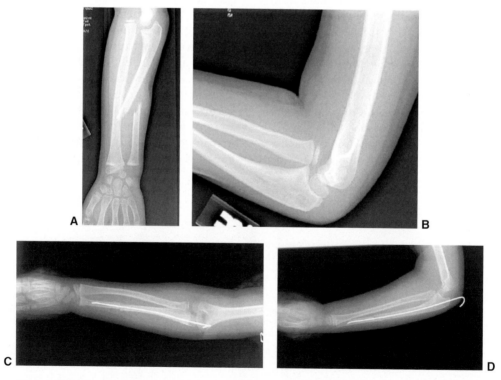

**Figure 33.38**  Type I Monteggia fracture reduced and stabilized with an intramedullary nail in the ulna. **A,B:** Anteroposterior and lateral radiographs of a type I Monteggia fracture with an unstable, widely displaced, oblique fracture of the ulna and an anterior dislocation of the radial head. **C,D:** Anteroposterior and lateral views after closed reduction of the radiocapitellar joint and stabilization of the ulna fracture with a titanium elastic nail.

with dislocation of the distal radioulnar joint. This is an uncommon injury in children. The triangular fibrocartilage complex is disrupted, and the distal ulna is dorsally displaced, as viewed on a lateral radiograph. Injury to the distal radioulnar joint is frequently overlooked, and persistent joint subluxation is responsible for poor long-term results (207). The Galeazzi equivalent injury is more common in children and consists of a fracture of the radius with a physeal fracture of the distal ulna (208). Treatment consists of closed reduction of the radius and ulnar physis with above-elbow casting in full supination. Open reduction may be necessary if the ulna is buttonholed through periosteum, blocking reduction. Occasionally, it is necessary to place a smooth Kirschner wire across the joint or the fracture to maintain reduction. Long-term problems with this injury include premature physeal arrest with ulnar shortening and loss of supination (209).

## Midshaft Forearm Fractures

### Plastic Deformation

Plastic deformation, or traumatic bowing, of the forearm is possible because of the elastic properties of young children's bones. This injury represents a series of microfractures that are not seen on radiographs. Bowing of both bones may occur, but plastic deformation of one bone is often associated with complete or incomplete fracture of the other forearm bone. Swelling and pain are usually less severe with plastic deformation than with complete fractures. This often facilitates examination. Reduction is recommended when deformity is cosmetically unacceptable, or there is greater than 45 degrees loss of forearm rotation. Remodeling capacity of this type of fracture is limited after 6 years of age. In children younger than 6 years, 15 to 20 degrees of angulation can be accepted, but more than 10 degrees angulation in older children may not remodel (210,211).

Treatment of plastic deformation usually requires general anesthesia because a prolonged corrective force must be applied to permanently straighten the bone. The position of immobilization follows the principles outlined in the discussion of greenstick fractures, which follows.

### Greenstick Fractures

A complete fracture of one cortex and plastic deformation of the opposite cortex characterize greenstick fractures. Most greenstick fractures represent a rotational malalignment, in addition to angular deformity (212). Apex-volar

greenstick fracture is the most common type, and results from excessive supination forces applied to the distal segment, combined with axial load. The child presents with the palm facing the apex of the fracture deformity (Fig. 33.39). Apex-dorsal deformity results from excessive pronation force applied to the distal segment; the child presents with the palm facing down, relative to the apex of the fracture deformity (Fig. 33.40). Occasionally, greenstick fractures of the radius and ulna are caused by a direct force producing angular deformity without much malrotation. Reduction is indicated when shaft angulation is greater than 15 degrees in a child younger than 10 years, or greater than 10 degrees in an older child (213,214). Judgment is required because the rotational component of greenstick fracture of the forearm diaphysis does not always correlate with the amount of angulation. Reduction is indicated if forearm deformity was immediately obvious at the time of injury, or when there is rotational deformity of 45 degrees or more in children younger than 10 years, or 30 degrees or more in older children.

Treatment of greenstick fractures requires adequate pain relief for one quick reduction attempt that is usually successful. Reduction is accomplished by reversing the injury mechanism. Apex-volar deformity (apex of fracture in the direction of the palm of the hand) is reduced by pronating the wrist while applying pressure to the volar surface of the forearm. Apex-dorsal deformity (apex of fracture in the direction of the dorsum of the hand) is reduced by supinating the wrist while applying pressure to the dorsal surface of the forearm. Completing the fracture of the opposite cortex is unnecessary, although this facilitates reduction and often occurs during the reduction maneuver. After reduction, the arm is immobilized in a well-molded sugar-tong splint or a bivalved long-arm cast. Three-point pressure is essential for the maintenance of reduction. Weekly follow-up is recommended for 2 to 3 weeks after reduction. It is generally necessary to change the cast for remolding as swelling subsides during this period. Six weeks of immobilization are usually adequate, but refracture is a risk when immobilization is discontinued too soon.

**Complications.** Refracture occurs in 5% to 7% of forearm fractures, but may be more common following greenstick fractures (215). This may be due to impaired healing of the fractured side because the intact cortex reduces micromotion needed for periosteal new bone formation. Lack of compression also leads to gap widening of the fractured

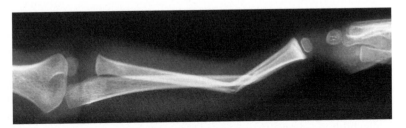

**Figure 33.39** Coupled relation of rotation and angulation. This fracture demonstrates volar angulation. The mechanism of injury was falling on the outstretched hand. When the fractures of the radius and ulna are at different levels, angulation cannot occur without rotation. Note the anteroposterior appearance of the elbow and the lateral projection of the wrist. This deformity is corrected with pronation of the distal fragment.

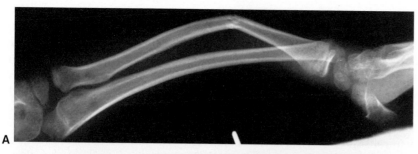

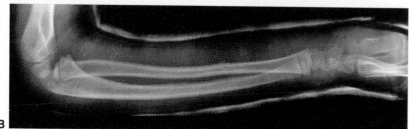

**Figure 33.40** Coupled relation of rotation and angulation. **A:** The radiograph shows deformity with pronation of the distal fragment and dorsal angulation of the radius. The ulna has undergone plastic deformation. When a single bone angulates, it must rotate around the other. **B:** Alignment is restored with supination of the distal fragment. The lateral projections of the elbow and the wrist are now matched.

cortex rather than gap closure. One method to reduce the risk of refracture is to complete the fracture of the intact cortex at the time of reduction. Another option is to use a longer period of immobilization in a cast or removable splint.

### Complete Shaft Fractures

Complete fractures of the forearm result from higher-energy trauma than do greenstick fractures. The proximal segments usually assume a position dictated by muscle forces because the muscle actions are unrestrained by an intact cortex. When the fracture is in the proximal third, the proximal fragment is frequently in supination due to the unrestrained actions of the biceps and supinator muscles. When the fracture is more distal, the pronator teres has a neutralizing effect on the proximal fragment, causing it to assume a position of neutral rotation (212).

Managing these fractures can be troublesome, but nonunions and serious complications are rare regardless of method of management. The principal concerns are the possibilities of residual deformity and loss of forearm rotation. Closed reduction is recommended for low-energy minimally displaced fractures, but intramedullary fixation is an increasingly popular solution for the management of unstable fractures in children older than 8 years.

Guidelines for the closed management of complete forearm fractures are based on the following observations:

1. Younger children with more distal fractures have the best prognosis (213,216,217).
2. Bayonet apposition in the middle and distal third of the shaft does not compromise forearm rotation (218,219).
3. Rotational alignment of the radius is more critical than the rotational alignment of the ulna (212,220). Alignment with 45 degrees of malrotation in the radius can be accepted in younger children (217,218).
4. Midshaft angulation of 15 degrees or less is acceptable in children younger than 8 years (213,221).

5. Midshaft forearm fractures in children older than 8 years should be maintained with 10 degrees or less of angulation (218,222).
6. Residual loss of supination (fixed pronation) is more difficult to accommodate than loss of pronation. When in doubt for complete fractures, immobilize the forearm in neutral or moderate supination (223).
7. Immobilization with the elbow extended may help maintain reduction for proximal-third fractures that are unstable in flexion. Elbow extension also helps maintain reduction for most children younger than 4 years. Incorporate the thumb to avoid cast slippage (224).
8. Gentle molding can make improvements in alignment, either in a new cast or by remanipulation for 1 to 3 weeks after injury (225,226).

When performing closed reduction, pain relief and muscle relaxation are required because more than one attempt may be necessary. Regional (i.e., Bier or axillary block) or general anesthesia is often preferred. The reduction technique typically involves increasing the angular deformity, applying longitudinal traction to lock in place and straighten the fracture, and then correcting any malrotation by supinating or pronating the forearm. If this is unsuccessful, it is often helpful to apply traction by using finger traps for a period of 10 minutes before another attempt is made. Observing the bone widths at the fracture site and matching their contours on radiographs allow assessment of rotational alignment. Comparison radiographs of the opposite extremity, in various degrees of rotation, may also be helpful in determining rotational alignment (217). Alternatively, the position of the bicipital tuberosity may serve as a guide to rotation because the bicipital tuberosity is 180 degrees opposite the radial styloid and thumb (212).

Postreduction casting in an above-elbow cast or splint should maintain a straight lateral border along the ulnar side. A flat interosseous mold along the volar forearm should create an oval shape to the cast. Fracture stability is improved with at least 50% bone apposition. If one bone disengages, shortening may occur, followed by increasing angulation. This may respond to remanipulation or require surgical stabilization. Weekly reevaluation is recommended for the first 3 weeks. Union is usually complete in 6 to 8 weeks. Nonunion is rare, and closed treatment can produce excellent results in more than 95% of patients when the fractures can be maintained within the guidelines stated previously (218,223,227) (Fig. 33.41).

Surgical intervention with internal fixation is indicated for unstable fractures (Fig. 33.42) and when closed management has failed. Internal fixation can also facilitate management and can improve results for refractures with displacement, most open fractures, and unstable floating elbow injuries (152,153,215,228–233). Intramedullary fixation is usually preferred for children and adolescents (234–236). Fixation is achieved by insertion of a small-diameter, flexible pin; a 1.5 to 2.5 mm diameter is sufficient for most cases (234). The ulnar pin can be inserted

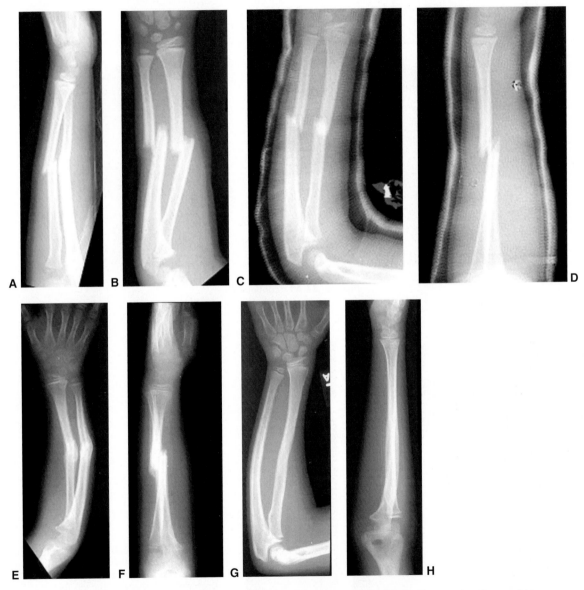

**Figure 33.41**   Malunion and remodeling of a diaphyseal radius and ulna fracture in a 7-year-old boy. **A,B:** Initial anteroposterior and lateral views of the forearm; the completely displaced radius and ulnar fracture were treated with closed reduction and casting. **C,D:** These radiographs were taken 1 week after reduction. There is acceptable angulation of the ulna (approximately 15 degrees) and bayonet apposition of both bones, seen on the lateral view. Note that there is no molding of the cast—in particular, note that the cast lacks a straight ulnar border. **E,F:** These anteroposterior and lateral radiographs of the forearm at the time of cast removal 6 weeks after injury show considerable angulation on the anteroposterior and shortening with bayonet apposition on the lateral. **G,H:** Three years later, there is extensive remodeling, although the ulnar bow persists. **I,J:** Clinical pictures after cast removal show 45 degrees of pronation and supination. **K,L:** Six years after the injury, pronation and supination are symmetric with the uninjured side.

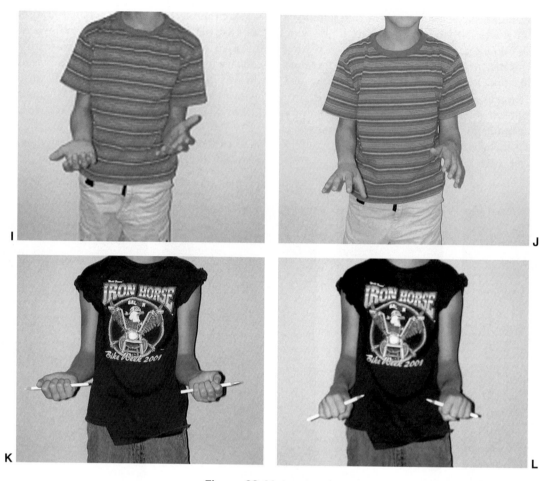

**Figure 33.41** (*continued*)

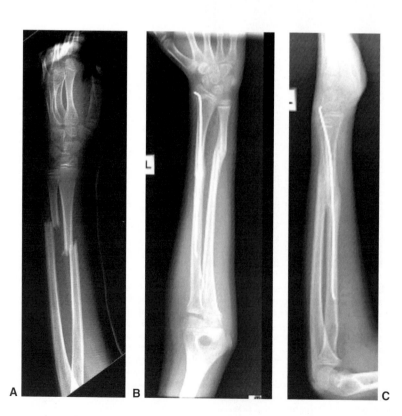

**Figure 33.42** Treatment of a high-energy, unstable radius and ulna fracture with single bone intramedullary fixation of the radius. **A:** Anteroposterior radiograph of the left forearm of a 12-year-old boy who fell 20 ft while skiing. Although this radiograph shows satisfactory bayonet alignment of both the radius and ulna, his fracture was so unstable and his forearm was so swollen that the surgeon opted to use single bone fixation of the radius and a splint rather than closed reduction and a well-molded cast. **B,C:** Anteroposterior and lateral view of the forearm taken 8 weeks after a titanium elastic nail was placed in the radius. Neither fracture site was opened. Both bones have healed in satisfactory alignment.

proximally, just lateral to the tip of the olecranon, or distally in the flare of the ulna. The radial pin is inserted in the distal metaphysis, avoiding penetration of the growth plate. Transphyseal pinning through the distal radius has also been reported without physeal arrest (235,237). When the entry point is metaphyseal, an oblique drill hole is made in the metaphyseal cortex, and the wire is introduced into the medullary canal. Following insertion, the pin is tapped or gently rotated into the medullary canal until it passes the fracture site (Fig. 33.43). Occasionally, it is necessary to perform a limited open reduction at the fracture site to facilitate passage of the wire. Tourniquet time should be kept to a minimum, and multiple attempts at closed pinning should be avoided in order to decrease the risk of compartment syndrome (238). Both bones are usually stabilized, but one is sufficient in some cases (239,240). It is usually best to bend the pins and leave them under the skin for 3 to 5 months because of the possibility of delayed union and also to reduce the risk of refracture (235). Supplemental casting is recommended until union is satisfactory, approximately 6 weeks after fixation.

Plating is rarely used in children and adolescents, but this technique may be indicated for comminuted fractures, or for adolescents who are within 1 year of skeletal maturity. Plating requires more dissection and has the disadvantage that hardware removal may become necessary later, with longer surgical time and the added risk of neurovascular injury and refracture (236,241).

*Complications.* Malunion is the most common complication of closed management, but remodeling may be surprising and function may return to normal despite malunion (218,222,227,242). A 3- to 6-month period of observation is recommended when deformity is less than 20 degrees. Shaft deformities greater than 30 degrees should be corrected as soon as some strength and motion have been regained, usually 2 to 3 months after the initial injury. Deformities between 20 and 30 degrees may require early correction depending on the clinical appearance, the age of the child, and the location of the malunion. Distal

deformity in children younger than 8 years is more likely to remodel (213). Results are better when deformity is corrected within 1 year of the initial injury (243). Intramedullary fixation is usually sufficient for younger children (244). Older children benefit from plate fixation to begin early motion after osteotomy to correct malunion (Fig. 33.44).

Other complications of forearm fractures include refracture, nonunion, compartment syndrome, nerve injuries, and synostosis. Refracture has been addressed as an indication for surgical stabilization when alignment cannot be maintained by closed means. Nonunion often requires surgical intervention, but long-term sequelae are uncommon.

Compartment syndrome of the forearm has been reported in association with floating elbow injuries (151). The risk of compartment syndrome may also be increased when closed intramedullary fixation is difficult and tourniquet time is prolonged (238). Treatment of compartment syndrome is discussed elsewhere in this chapter.

Nerve injuries can occur in association with forearm fractures, but reports of this are uncommon. Nerve entrapment from forearm fracture is rare (245). Management of neurologic deficits following forearm fracture is similar to management for deficits following supracondylar fractures.

Posttraumatic radioulnar synostosis is also rare in children but may occur following closed or open management of forearm fracture. Results of resection are better in adults than in children. However, successful resections have been reported for nonarticular midshaft cross-union (246,247).

## Distal Metaphyseal Fractures of the Radius and Ulna

Distal metaphyseal fractures of the radius and ulna are common. Increased risk of distal radius fracture has been noted in children with decreased bone mineral density and increased body mass (10,11). Fractures of the distal radius and ulna are usually caused by a fall onto the hand with the wrist in a pronated, extended position.

Unicortical fractures (i.e., torus or buckle fractures) are stable injuries that are quite common. Treatment is directed

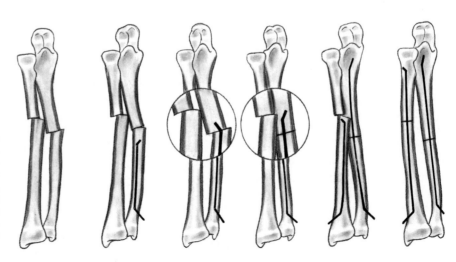

**Figure 33.43** Surgical nailing procedure for flexible intramedullary nails. The ulnar wire can be introduced digitally, as shown, or through the olecranon. (From Verstreken L, Delronge G, Lamoureux J. Shaft forearm fractures in children: intramedullary nailing with immediate motion. A preliminary report. *J Pediatr Orthop* 1988;8:450, with permission.)

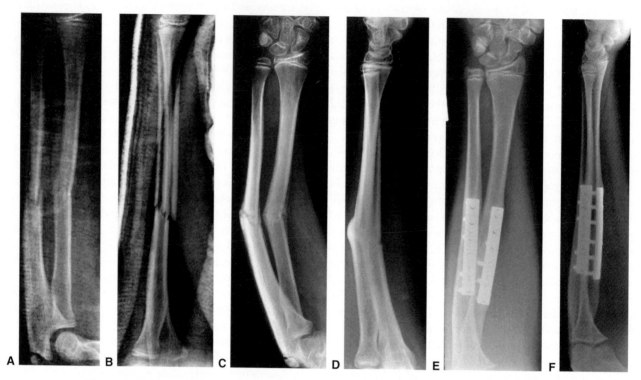

**Figure 33.44** Malunion of the forearm in a 14-year-old child. **A:** Anteroposterior view of the alignment after closed reduction and casting. **B:** The lateral projection shows acceptable alignment. **C:** The anteroposterior projection 12 weeks after treatment shows malunion of the radius and ulna. **D:** A lateral projection shows dorsal angulation. Clinical evaluation demonstrated only 15 degrees of rotation of the forearm. **E:** An anteroposterior projection after osteotomy and internal fixation with 0.35-mm compression plates. **F:** The lateral projection shows restoration of anatomic alignment. The range of motion was improved significantly, with full supination but a loss of the last 20 degrees of pronation.

toward patient comfort and protection of the forearm from further injury. Immobilization with a splint for 3 weeks without further follow-up is sufficient for managing these injuries (248,249). However, torus or unicortical fractures should be differentiated from minimally displaced or angulated bicortical fractures because the latter have a propensity for secondary angulation (250,251). A well-molded cast is recommended for complete fracture. Follow-up radiographs are recommended 1 week after complete bicortical fractures when there is any displacement or angulation greater than 10 degrees (250,251).

Fractures of the distal radial metaphysis have great potential for remodeling because of their proximity to the distal growth plate. Bayonet apposition with 15 degrees of angulation and 1 cm shortening may be accepted until early adolescence (252). Friberg observed that a dorsal tilt up to 20 degrees will remodel so long as there are 2 years of growth remaining (17,253,254). So long as the growth plate remains open, 50% of the remodeling occurs in the first 6 months, and the remaining 50% in the next 18 months (17,253,254). Deformity greater than 20 degrees may also remodel, but this is less predictable, especially in older children. Remodeling capacity is similar for dorsally angulated and palmarly angulated fractures (255). The guidelines for acceptable residual angulation are

age-dependent and serve only as a general indicator of expected results. Immobilization should be attempted to avoid angulation greater than 20 degrees. When malunion occurs, dorsal tilt (apex-volar angulation) of up to 35 degrees can be accepted in children younger than 5 years. This decreases to 25 degrees for children between 5 and 12 years of age. In older children, the dorsal tilt should be controlled at less than 15 degrees to ensure a good outcome. Radial deviation remodels less than angulation in the plane of flexion and extension. Therefore, radial deviation should be kept to less than 15 degrees in children younger than 12 years and to less than 10 degrees in older children (256–258).

Treatment of displaced or angulated fractures consists of closed reduction and immobilization in a plaster cast. In complete fractures, the distal fragment is usually dorsally displaced, but the dorsal periosteum is intact. Reduction may be difficult to achieve but should be attempted initially. The deformity is increased to relax the intact periosteal hinge; longitudinal traction is then applied with digital pressure at the fracture site until length is restored. The angular deformity is then corrected. More reduction force is required if the ulna is intact, and pronating the distal segment during the reduction maneuver may assist in fragment realignment. After reduction, the wrist should be placed in slight palmar flexion and ulnar deviation. The cast is molded with three-point pressure dorsally over the distal fragment, centrally on the volar surface of the forearm, and proximally on the dorsal surface of the forearm. This cast molding technique is designed to counter the tendency for later radial and dorsal fracture displacement. An above-elbow splint or bivalved cast is recommended for immobilization, but it has been demonstrated that a well-molded, below-elbow cast can also effectively stabilize these fractures (259).

Anatomic reduction of a completely displaced, distal-third, metaphyseal fracture may be difficult to achieve by closed manipulation. Displacement and angulation may be accepted so long as alignment is within the described guidelines. However, redisplacement is more common when reduction is incomplete (260). Supination of the forearm has been recommended to reduce the pull of the brachioradialis and thereby reduce the incidence of delayed dorsal angulation (261). Fractures that do not maintain their positions can be remanipulated. Percutaneous pinning has been recommended to avoid repeated manipulation (260,262). A randomized, controlled trial of above-elbow cast management versus the additional insertion of a Kirschner wire determined no significant difference in clinical outcome. However, 21% of patients in the group managed only by cast required remanipulation, compared to none in the group managed with pinning (263). Regardless of method of immobilization, fracture alignment should be monitored closely for the first few weeks after injury. It is the authors' preference to use percutaneous pins when completely displaced distal radius fractures cannot be satisfactorily reduced (guidelines listed previously), or in the rare instance when an ipsilateral supracondylar fracture makes pinning of both injuries the safest treatment (Fig. 33.45). This can be performed by metaphyseal pinning, by transstyloid pinning through the growth plate, or by utilizing the intrafocal leverage technique of Kapandji (264–266) (Fig. 33.46). A modified Kapandji technique for pinning Smith fractures in children utilizes a dorsal entry site with the tip of the pin as a buttress to prevent volar displacement (267).

### Complications

Complications are rare. Significant residual deformity can remodel. Cases with a dorsal tilt of 35 degrees and radial tilt of 15 degrees should be given a chance to remodel before considering osteotomy. Galeazzi-type fracture may also be diagnosed. Galeazzi-type fracture-dislocation should be suspected when an isolated radius fracture is associated with fracture of the ulnar styloid (208). Distal physeal separation of the ulna is uncommon but often leads to premature physeal closure (209).

## Distal Radius Physeal Fracture

Fracture of the growth plate of the distal radius is the second most common physeal injury, with phalangeal fractures being the most common (29). Distal radius physeal fracture accounts for approximately 15% of all forearm fractures, with 70% of these injuries occurring in children older than 10 years (35,197). Eighty percent are Salter-Harris type I or II injuries. More complex injuries are uncommon but have higher rates of premature growth arrest. Anatomic reduction may be required for complex physeal fractures, but anatomic reduction is unnecessary for type I or II physeal injuries of the distal radius because growth usually resumes and provides remodeling. Before 10 years of age, 20 degrees of angulation and 40% of displacement can be accepted without reduction for type II injuries (35).

Treatment guidelines for Salter-Harris fracture types I and II are similar to those previously described for distal radius metaphyseal fracture. Multiple reduction attempts may lead

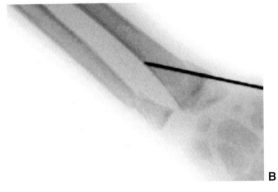
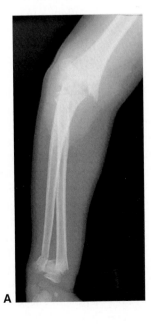

**Figure 33.45** Fixation of a distal radius fracture with an ipsilateral supracondylar fracture. **A:** This anteroposterior radiograph of the forearm and elbow of a 6-year-old boy shows a completely displaced distal radius fracture and a type III supracondylar humerus fracture. The arm was swollen and the hand was perfused, but the radial pulse could not be palpated. Because of the risk of forearm compartment syndrome, the surgeon elected to do closed pinning of both the supracondylar fracture and the distal radius fracture. **B:** Intraoperative image after K-wire fixation was used for the distal radius fracture. After pinning, the arm and elbow were splinted with the elbow in 30 degrees of flexion.

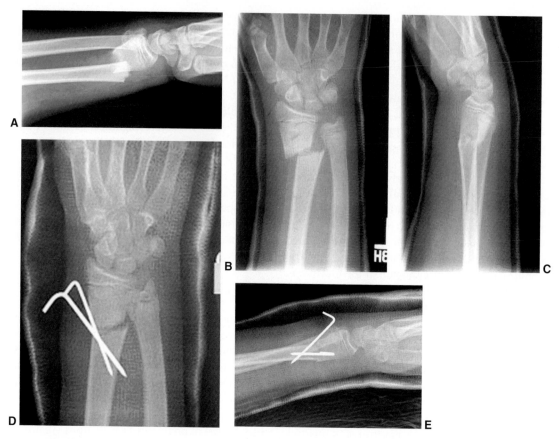

**Figure 33.46**   Kapandji pinning. **A:** Initial radiograph of a displaced distal radius and ulna fractures. **B,C:** Anteroposterior and lateral view of the wrist after best attempt at reduction shows persistent angulation and displacement of the radius. The surgeon chose to do a repeat closed reduction and used the Kapandji pinning technique to reduce and fix the radius fracture. **D,E:** After Kapandji pinning and casting, a satisfactory reduction is maintained.

to growth-plate damage. Two or more attempts have produced growth arrest in slightly more than 25% of these patients (268). Repeat manipulation more than 10 days after injury may further damage the growth plate because physeal healing has already commenced. Cast immobilization can usually be discontinued 4 weeks after injury.

### Complications

Growth arrest after a nondisplaced or minimally displaced fracture is rare, and routine follow-up is not required. However, the authors recommend follow-up 4 to 6 months after complex distal radius and ulna physeal fracture to allow early detection of growth arrest prior to the development of a deformity. If growth arrest occurs, corrective lengthening osteotomy using iliac crest graft has been successful in restoring alignment and function (269,270).

## FRACTURES OF THE THORACIC AND LUMBAR SPINE

### Clinical Features

Spine fractures in children represent 1% to 2% of all pediatric fractures (3). Most of these injuries involve the cervical spine and are discussed in Chapter 21. Causes of spine injury include falls, athletic activities, battering, and trauma due to motor vehicle accidents (271,272). Thoracolumbar spine injuries are less common in children than in adults, but the incidence is difficult to determine. The reported incidence may be too low because some children with trauma severe enough to cause spinal fracture may die from associated injuries (273). Approximately two-thirds of thoracolumbar spine fractures in adults are in the region of T12–L2, but the distribution of pediatric and adolescent spine fractures is more uniform throughout the thoracic and lumbar spine (274).

There is a 50% incidence of associated injuries in children who sustain spine trauma from motor vehicle crashes (271). Complete examination is essential when evaluating a child with multiple injuries because spine fractures are occasionally overlooked (275,276). Examination may reveal tenderness, swelling, ecchymosis, or a palpable defect posteriorly along the spinous processes. A seat belt mark across the abdomen or injury of an abdominal organ should increase the index of suspicion. Any loss of sensory or motor function should be accurately documented.

Spinal cord injury is less frequent in children than in adults. Perhaps this is because the pediatric spine is much more flexible than the adult spine and allows greater deformation without fracture. This increased musculoskeletal elasticity is not shared by the spinal cord and may lead to the occurrence of spinal cord injury without radiographic abnormality (SCIWORA) (277). The disproportionately large head size and other structural features in children place the cervical and upper thoracic region at greatest risk for spinal cord injury. Trauma to the lower thoracic or lumbar spine in children is rarely associated with spinal cord injury. The prognosis for recovery from incomplete neurologic injury is better in children than in adults, but complete lesions rarely improve (271).

Plain radiographs should be obtained when spine trauma is suspected, but these may be difficult to interpret. A CT scan or an MRI or both are indicated for evaluation of most patients when thoracolumbar injuries are suspected or known to be present (276). A CT scan is especially helpful to evaluate the bony structures. Sagittal and coronal reconstruction can be used to evaluate alignment and spinal canal encroachment. MRI is more useful than CT scan to evaluate the spinal cord, intervertebral discs, and other soft tissue structures (276). An MRI is indicated in all cases with neurologic deficit.

## Anatomy and Classification

The thoracic and lumbar vertebrae form three main ossification centers, one each for the left and right sides of the neural arch and one for the body. The junction of the arches with the body occurs at the neurocentral synchondrosis. This junction is visible radiographically until the age of 3 to 6 years. It lies just anterior to the base of the pedicle and can be misinterpreted as a congenital anomaly or fracture in younger children. Secondary centers of ossification occur in flattened, disc-shaped epiphyses superior and inferior to each vertebral body. These centers provide longitudinal growth but do not cover the entire vertebral body (278). Ossification of these growth plates at the age of 7 to 8 years creates the radiographic impression of a groove at the corner of each vertebral body. This groove is circumferential around the upper and lower end plates of each vertebra. The ligaments and discs attach to this groove, which is therefore an apophyseal ring. The ring apophysis develops its own ossification center by the age of 12 to 15 years and fuses with the remainder of the vertebra at skeletal maturity (279).

Classification systems for thoracolumbar spine fractures in children have not been proposed. The three-column theory of Denis (280) allows classification of adult fractures, and also has relevance for the pediatric population. According to this theory, the thoracolumbar spine consists of anterior, middle, and posterior columns. The anterior column includes the anterior longitudinal ligament, the anterior half of the vertebral body, and the anterior portion of the annular ligament. Middle column structures are the posterior half of the vertebral body, the posterior anulus,

and the posterior longitudinal ligament. The posterior column includes the neural arch, the ligamentum flavum, the facet joint capsules, and the interspinous ligament. Spinal stability is primarily dependent on the status of the middle column (281).

Denis (280) applied this three-column theory to classify minor or major thoracolumbar fractures. Minor injuries include isolated fractures of the posterior elements. Major fractures are subdivided into compression fractures, burst fractures, seatbelt-type injuries, and fracture-dislocations. Compression of the anterior column is usually stable and results from axial loading in flexion. Lateral compression fractures of the vertebral body may also occur. Further compression results in a burst fracture that is unstable because the middle column becomes involved. Lap-belt injuries (Chance fractures) are unstable because they disrupt the posterior and middle columns by flexion and distraction forces. Fracture-dislocations usually involve all three columns and result from various combinations of forces.

Certain types of thoracolumbar injuries are unique to children; these include most cases of SCIWORA, posterior limbus or apophyseal fractures, and fractures associated with child abuse.

## Treatment of Thoracolumbar Fractures

Older adolescents sustain injuries similar to those seen in adults and should be managed accordingly (282). Most thoracolumbar spine fractures in children and younger adolescents are minor, stable, and without neurologic deficit. Simple bed rest and gradual resumption of activities are generally sufficient for management of these injuries. In the active athlete with an acute fracture of the pars intraarticularis, a thoracolumbar-sacral orthosis (TLSO) is recommended for 6 to 8 weeks in an attempt to obtain union.

### Compression Fractures

Most compression fractures in children occur in the thoracic spine (Fig. 33.47). Underlying causes of bone fragility, such as leukemia, should be considered when trauma has been minimal. Multiple compression injuries are not uncommon. Remodeling with restoration of anterior vertebral height has been observed in children younger than 13 years (272,274). When wedging of the thoracic or lumbar vertebra is less than 10 degrees, treatment consists of bed rest until the patient is comfortable, then gradual resumption of activities. When wedging is greater than 10 degrees and the Risser sign is less than 3, immobilization in hyperextension is recommended for a period of 2 months, followed by bracing for 1 year or more (272). Surgical stabilization is recommended when compression is greater than 15 degrees, or approximately 50% compression of the anterior vertebra, compared to posterior vertebral height. Surgical stabilization is also recommended when lateral compression is greater than 15 degrees (273,282). The

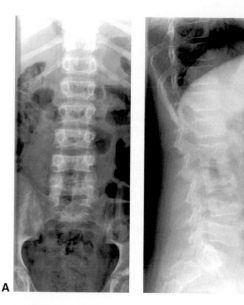

**Figure 33.47** L4 compression fracture. **A:** These anteroposterior **(A)** and lateral **(B)** radiographs were taken after a 13-year-old rear-seat passenger was involved in a motor vehicle accident. There is a 40% compression of L4 (indicated by black arrow). A computed tomography (CT) scan showed no evidence of a burst fracture. He was treated in a thoracolumbar-sacral orthosis (TLSO)

authors follow these guidelines, although prolonged bracing after initial treatment is usually avoided.

### Burst Fractures

Treatment guidelines for burst fractures are similar to those for compression fractures in children and adolescents. These injuries may be managed nonoperatively when the posterior column is intact, deformity is minimal, and there is no neurologic injury (272,283–285). However, progressive kyphosis has been noted in some patients treated nonoperatively (283). Nonsurgical treatment usually consists of hyperextension casting for 2 to 3 months and bracing for an additional 6 to 12 months. Surgical decompression and instrumentation are recommended for patients with greater degrees of deformity or with neurologic compromise (284,285). Posterior distraction and instrumentation may achieve decompression by ligamentotaxis with reduction of the retropulsed fragments (286). Anterior decompression has been recommended in the presence of multiple nerve root paralysis, but the role of anterior decompression and instrumentation remains controversial (287).

### Lap-belt Fractures (Chance-type Fracture)

This flexion-distraction injury has been associated with the use of lap-belt restraints, when the lap belt slides up the torso and rests over the abdomen instead of the proximal thighs and hips (287). The incidence of Chance fractures in children has increased since the introduction of mandatory seat-belt laws. Fortunately, this injury has a better prognosis in children than in adults (288). Neurologic deficits are infrequent, but intraabdominal injury is common and obscures the diagnosis of spine trauma.

This is an unstable injury in most patients. Treatment consists of cast immobilization for 8 to 10 weeks when there is minimal displacement and the fracture line goes through bone. Posterior surgical stabilization is indicated in the presence of displacement, neurologic deficits, or when there is a significant ligamentous disruption. Instrumentation and fusion one level above and one level below the fracture may be required (Fig. 33.48). In some patients one-level posterior fusion is sufficient (275,287). This can be achieved by spinous process wiring and cast immobilization, or by hook/rod and pedicle screw fixation in older children.

### Limbus Fracture (Apophyseal Fracture)

This fracture is typically seen in the adolescent or young adult and presents clinically like a herniated nucleus pulposus. It often results from the patient's lifting a heavy object, but may result from falls or twisting injuries. The patient may describe a "pop" at the time of injury, followed by radiculopathy. Delayed diagnosis is common (289). Takata et al. (290) described four types of growth-plate injuries to the spine. Nonoperative management is rarely successful regardless of the type (284,289). MRI, CT scan, or both should be used to determine the exact location and configuration of the lesion. Surgical excision is then performed by piecemeal excision of the limbus fragment. In order to completely remove bony impingement, the authors recommend laminectomy with direct exposure rather than relying on minimally invasive techniques.

## Complications

Complications of thoracolumbar fractures in children are uncommon unless there is an accompanying neurologic deficit. Inadequate stabilization or late deformity may be problematic when there is an associated neurologic deficit, or after wide laminectomy (291,292). In the absence of spinal cord injury, remodeling is more likely in younger children, particularly when the iliac apophysis is incompletely ossified (Risser sign <3) (272,274). However, remodeling can occur in older children. Spontaneous remodeling and redevelopment of the spinal canal has been observed in adults after burst fractures with canal encroachment (293). End-plate injury has been correlated on MRI with disc degeneration, but back pain is uncommon after spine fractures in children (294).

## PELVIC FRACTURES

### Clinical Features

Fractures of the pelvis are less common in children than in adults (295). The immature pelvis is more malleable than that of an adult, largely because of a greater component of cartilage and the greater flexibility of adjacent joints. This allows greater energy absorption before fracture. The flexibility of the pediatric pelvis also permits single breaks in the

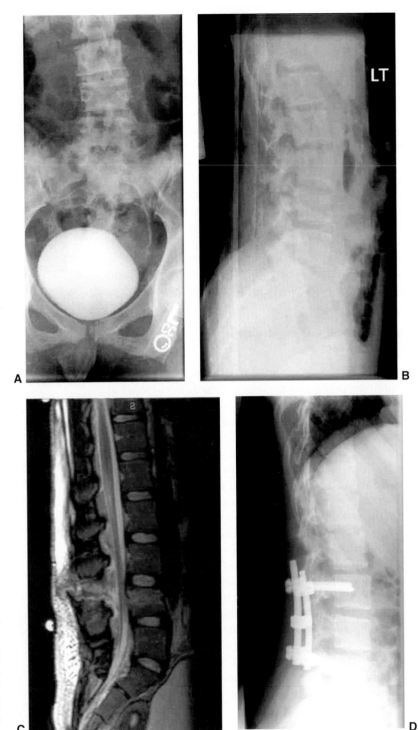

**Figure 33.48** L4 Chance fracture with bony and ligamentous disruption. **A,B:** These antero-posterior and lateral radiographs of the lumbosacral spine were taken upon presentation of a 14-year-old girl who was involved in a high-speed motor vehicle accident. She was a front-seat, restrained passenger. She had no neurologic deficits. An injury at the L4 level was suspected from the radiographs. **C:** This magnetic resonance imaging (MRI) (T2-weighted, sagittal image) shows a fracture of the L-4 vertebral body with complete posterior ligamentous disruption. All posterior tissues were disrupted except the skin and superficial subcutaneous tissue. On the basis of the extent of the posterior ligamentous injury, the surgeon elected to perform a posterior instrumented spinal fusion from L3 to L5. **D:** This lateral radiograph taken 6 months after surgery shows maintenance of alignment at the fracture site and signs of early fusion.

pelvic ring to occur. Avulsion fractures often result from athletic injuries (discussed in Chapter 32). Other types of pelvic fractures in children are often the result of high-energy trauma. Most unstable pelvic fractures are caused when a motor vehicle strikes a pedestrian (296,297). Most pediatric pelvic fractures are stable and minimally displaced.

Approximately 20% of polytraumatized children have pelvic fractures (55), and approximately 60% to 75% of children with pelvic fractures have associated injuries

(296,297). These associated injuries include head injuries, intraabdominal trauma, urologic disruptions, and fractures. Mortality rates are lower in children with pelvic injury than in adults, but death occurs in 3% to 5% of children with juvenile pelvic trauma (295–297). Death is most frequently related to head injury, but exsanguination from fractures or visceral injuries can occur, and the risks of hemorrhage and associated visceral injuries correlate with fracture patterns. Patients with bilateral anterior and posterior fractures are at greatest risk, whereas isolated pubic ramus fractures have the lowest risk of hemorrhage and intraabdominal injury (298,299).

Evaluation includes a careful physical examination for associated injuries, including neurologic deficits. Any laceration should be inspected to determine whether an open fracture has occurred. Rectal examination is indicated to look for hemorrhage signifying bone penetration into the rectum and to verify intact perineal sensation (i.e., sacral plexus function). Pelvic stability should be tested with anterior and lateral compression of the pelvis. Peripheral arterial circulation should also be noted. Plain radiographs are useful for screening but may be difficult to interpret. Pelvic inlet (40 degrees caudal), outlet (40 degrees cephalad), and Judet (45 degrees oblique) views can help define the fracture pattern and the potential involvement of the acetabulum. However, these views have largely been replaced with CT scan, with or without three-dimensional reconstruction.

## Anatomy and Classifications of Pelvic Fractures

The pelvis is formed from three ossification centers: the ischium, the pubis, and the ilium. These come together at the acetabulum to form the triradiate cartilage. Secondary ossification centers can be confused with fractures. These appear at the apophyses in patients between 13 and 16 years of age. The apophyses that are principally associated with avulsion injuries are located on the ischial tuberosity, the anterior inferior iliac spine, and the anterior iliac crest. Secondary centers of ossification can also develop along the pubis and the ischial spine. Several other normal variants can also be confused with fractures. An area of particular confusion is at the junction of the inferior pubic ramus and the ischium. Before ossification, this junction can have the appearance of a fracture, especially when ossification is asymmetric. A swelling may also occur in this area and can simply be observed when asymptomatic.

Several classifications have been proposed for pelvic fractures (300). Plain radiographs allow reliable determination of fracture types, although CT scanning may be helpful in questionable cases or when surgical intervention is anticipated (301). The authors prefer the classification proposed by Watts (302):

1. Avulsions
2. Fractures of the pelvic ring (stable and unstable)
3. Fractures of the acetabulum

Pelvic fracture stability can be subclassified using the AO/ASIF classification of adult pelvic fractures (303). This classification is based on both the mode of injury and the resulting characteristics of the fracture.

### Type A: Stable Injury
Stable injuries include isolated fractures of the pubic ramus (Fig. 33.49) or iliac wing (Fig. 33.50). It should be

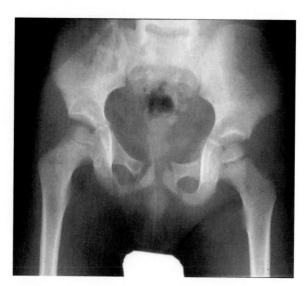

**Figure 33.49** This anteroposterior pelvis radiograph shows typical bilateral pubic rami fractures in a 6-year-old boy hit by a car. He was permitted weight-bearing activities as tolerated with crutches immediately after injury.

noted that, because of the elasticity of the child's pelvis, diastasis of the pubic symphysis can occur in children without instability of the sacroiliac joint posteriorly. In young children, this fracture usually represents separation at the bone-cartilage junction rather than joint disruption.

### Type B: Rotationally Unstable Fractures
This is a pelvic ring disruption that is stable in the vertical plane but unstable in the transverse plane. Mechanisms include lateral compression causing, for instance, pubic and ischial ramus fractures with contralateral sacral fracture.

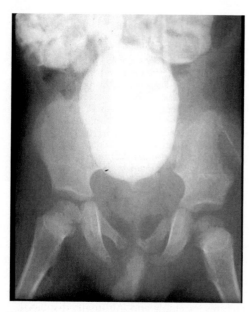

**Figure 33.50** This anteroposterior pelvis radiograph of a 4-year-old child shows a left iliac wing fracture and pubic rami fractures. He was permitted weight-bearing activities as tolerated when comfortable.

Alternatively, anterior compression may cause an "open-book" type of injury with pubic diastasis.

### Type C: Rotationally and Vertically Unstable Fractures

This group includes bilateral pubic rami fractures (straddle injuries), which rarely displace in children; vertical shear fractures through the ipsilateral anterior and posterior pelvic rings; and anterior ring fractures with acetabular disruption.

## Treatment of Pelvic Fractures

### Pelvic Ring Fractures

Most pelvic fractures in children have a favorable result with a minimum of treatment. Stable fractures are managed by bed rest with gradual resumption of weight bearing as tolerated. Unstable pelvic fractures with minimal displacement, which do not involve the acetabulum, can be managed with prolonged bed rest (1 to 2 months). Up to 3 cm displacement may be acceptable in children younger than 10 years, but the acceptable amount of displacement in all age-groups is controversial (304). Careful observation with frequent radiographs is recommended, so that any additional displacement will be recognized and

treated. Union and remodeling occur reliably in younger children in spite of moderate displacement (305,306). Unstable pelvic fractures with greater amounts of displacement, especially in older children, should be reduced with traction or open reduction. The authors recommend reduction of pubic diastasis (open-book) fractures when the diastasis exceeds 3 cm, or when stability is required for urologic reconstruction. Stabilization after reduction can be achieved with external and/or internal fixation for unstable open-book or other type B fractures (300,303) (Fig. 33.51). Type C fractures may require internal fixation of posterior injury, in addition to anterior stabilization with external fixation or other means. Surgical stabilization is also appropriate to reduce retroperitoneal blood loss and to facilitate mobilization of the child who has multiple injuries.

### Acetabular Fractures

Watts classified acetabular fractures into four types (302). This classification has been used to guide treatment (307). Precise restoration of joint congruity is recommended except for stable posterior fracture-dislocations with concentric reductions (Watts type I fractures). Nondisplaced acetabular fractures are managed by closed reduction

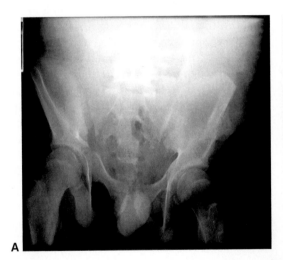

A

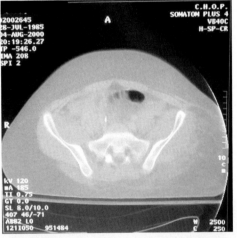

B

C

**Figure 33.51** A rare unstable pediatric pelvic fracture requiring internal fixation. **A:** This pelvic radiograph shows widening of the right sacroiliac joint. **B:** This computed tomography (CT) scan cut confirms disruption of the right sacroiliac joint. **C:** This unstable pelvis was treated with iliac bolt fixation.

(Watts type II fractures). Multiple fragments with instability (Watts type III) are best managed by open reduction with stable internal fixation (303,307). Early motion is also recommended (303). Comminution is often less severe in children than in adults, and the results of surgical management are generally satisfactory. Fractures with central dislocation of the hip have a poor prognosis regardless of surgical or nonsurgical management. Traction may be utilized for these fractures, or surgical management may be attempted when comminution is minimal. Poor results after anatomic reduction may still occur with all types of acetabular fractures due to the magnitude of the initial trauma (308).

Premature closure of the triradiate cartilage is a potential complication that is unique to the immature skeleton (309). Fractures that cause premature closure are usually nondisplaced and do not require open reduction. Children younger than 10 years are at the greatest risk for this complication. Disturbance in growth leads to the development of a shallow acetabulum because the triradiate cartilage is responsible for growth in the height and width of the acetabulum. Hip subluxation may follow, necessitating redirectional pelvic osteotomy.

## Complications

Immediate management of pelvic fractures and associated injuries can be challenging, but long-term complications are rarely attributable to the bony structures. Untreated, severely displaced fractures can result in a limp, rotational deformity, or limb-length discrepancy. Acetabular injuries are at risk for developing traumatic arthritis in spite of anatomic reduction. Premature closure of the triradiate cartilage can be problematic in younger children. However, residual morbidity is more often due to associated injuries, especially traumatic brain injury.

# FRACTURES AND DISLOCATIONS OF THE HIP

## Hip Dislocation

Dislocation of the hip in children is uncommon, representing only 5% of all pediatric dislocations. Most hip dislocations are posterior, but anterior and obturator dislocations can occur (310,311). The mechanism of injury depends somewhat on the age of the child. Hip dislocations in children younger than 10 years are frequently the result of mild trauma because joint laxity is common and the acetabulum is largely cartilaginous (Fig. 33.52) (310). Dislocations in children older than 10 years are more often the result of moderate or severe trauma. Dislocation from moderate trauma may result in spontaneous, incongruous reduction and capsular interposition (312) (Fig. 33.53). This is rare but easily misdiagnosed in children and adolescents. Any suggestion of joint-space widening should be investigated with a CT scan.

### Treatment

Treatment consists of closed reduction with adequate muscle relaxation and analgesia. Early closed reduction within 6 hours of injury is recommended. Reduction is rarely difficult in children, but gentle reduction is especially important in the adolescent age group. Reduction with image guidance should be considered in the adolescent age group because occult epiphyseal injury may be present, and epiphyseal separation can occur during attempted reduction. The reduction technique for posterior dislocation requires hip and knee flexion, usually with adduction of the hip. Longitudinal traction is then applied while an assistant stabilizes the pelvis. The limb is then extended, internally rotated, and abducted. After the hip is reduced, the stable arc of motion should be assessed. Postreduction

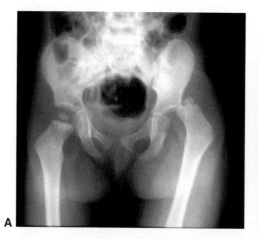
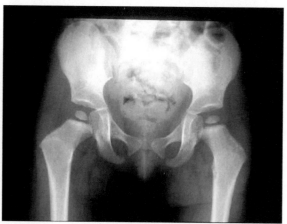

**Figure 33.52**   Traumatic hip dislocation in a 3-year-old boy. **A:** This anteroposterior pelvis radiograph was taken upon presentation of a 3-year-old boy who twisted his leg while running down the stairs. **B:** This anteroposterior pelvis radiograph was taken immediately after closed reduction in the emergency room. On long-term follow-up, there was no avascular necrosis or any other sequelae.

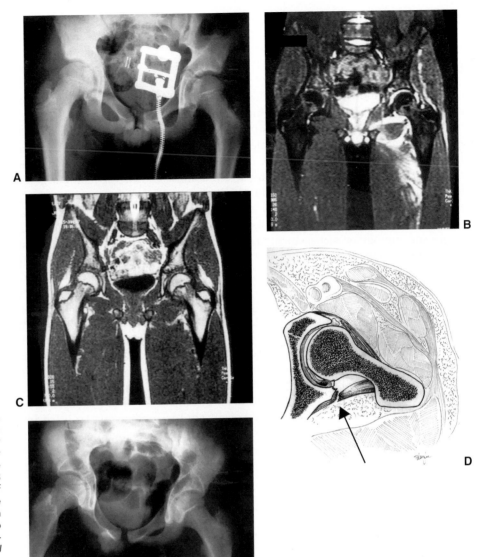

**Figure 33.53** Hip dislocation with entrapped tissue. **A:** Initial anteroposterior pelvis radiograph of a 15-year-old boy following an injury to the left hip in a soccer game. Joint asymmetry was attributed to a joint effusion. **B,C:** A magnetic resonance imaging (MRI) performed 4 days after the injury shows a joint effusion and mild incongruity. Because of persistent symptoms and concerns about interposed tissue, he was taken to the operating room and an arthrotomy was performed through a posterior approach. **D:** This drawing illustrates the intraoperative findings. There was an inverted labrum and capsule trapped in the hip joint (*arrow*). Once this was freed, complete hip joint reduction was achieved. **E:** Anteroposterior pelvis radiograph after surgery shows concentric reduction. The boy was followed up for more than 3 years, and there was no evidence of avascular necrosis or other late sequelae. (From Price CT, Pyevich MT, Knapp DR, et al. Traumatic hip dislocation with spontaneous incomplete reduction: a diagnostic trap. *J Orthop Trauma* 2002;16:730–735, with permission.)

radiographs should include the opposite hip to confirm a concentric reduction with symmetrical joint spaces. A CT scan is recommended after hip reduction in children older than 10 years or in younger children if instability or joint-space widening is noted. A CT scan is not necessary in the younger child with a stable concentric reduction and no evidence of acetabular fracture on plain radiographs. The child younger than 8 years should be immobilized in a spica cast or abduction pillow with strict bed rest for 4 to 6 weeks to reduce the risk of recurrent dislocation. Stable, closed reductions in older children can be managed with activity restriction and decreased weight bearing for 6 weeks to allow capsular healing and reduction of posttraumatic inflammatory response.

The indications for open reduction include unstable closed reduction, nonconcentric reduction, bone or soft tissue fragments within the joint, or a large acetabular rim fragment with instability. Open reduction is recommended from the direction of the dislocation, such as the posterior

interval (i.e., Kocher-Langenbeck approach) for posterior dislocations. Postoperative management after open reduction is the same as that after closed reduction.

### Complications

The reported incidence of avascular necrosis in children is 3% to 10%, approximately half that in adults. The risk of avascular necrosis is diminished when reduction is achieved within 6 hours of injury (310,311). Nerve injury has been reported in 5% of children with hip dislocation, but recovery occurs spontaneously in 60% to 70% of these patients (313). The long-term prognosis for arthritis is related to the severity of the trauma, associated fractures, and treatment delays beyond 24 hours. However, some satisfactory results have been reported when neglected traumatic dislocations have been treated by traction and open reduction (314). Coxa magna in the absence of avascular necrosis has been observed in many children after traumatic hip dislocation. The cause is probably reactive hyperemia secondary to extensive soft tissue injury. Coxa magna does not seem to influence clinical outcome.

## Hip Fractures

Hip fractures in children represent less than 1% of all pediatric fractures (3). In contrast to adult hip fractures, pediatric and adolescent hip fractures are usually the result of high-energy trauma, because considerable force is required to produce a fracture in this age group. The exceptions to this are infants who have been subjected to child abuse, and fracture through a pathologic lesion of the femoral neck (e.g., bone cyst). Complications are frequent and have been reported in 15% to 60% of patients (315,316). Prompt and appropriate management may reduce the risk of subsequent complications.

### Anatomy and Classification

In the infant, the proximal femur is composed of a single large cartilaginous growth plate (317) (Fig. 33.54). The medial portion becomes the epiphyseal center of the femoral head, ossifies at around 4 months of age, and forms the proximal femoral physis. The lateral portion of the proximal femur forms the greater trochanter physis, with ossification of the epiphysis by 4 years of age. Injury to the proximal femur can affect one or both of these centers of growth. The proximal femoral physis is responsible for the metaphyseal growth of the femoral neck and provides approximately 15% of the total length of the femur. The greater trochanter

helps shape the proximal femur, and damage to this apophysis in children younger than 8 to 10 years may produce an elongated, valgus femoral neck (318,319).

The vascular supply of the growing child's proximal femur is jeopardized by these fractures, and the extent of damage greatly affects the final outcome. The dominant arterial source for the femoral head is the lateral epiphyseal vessels, which are the terminal extension of the medial femoral circumflex artery. These posterosuperior and posteroinferior vessels are found at the level of the intertrochanteric groove, where they penetrate the capsule and course along the femoral neck toward the head (320,321) (Fig. 33.55). The lateral circumflex system can supply blood to a portion of the anterior femoral head until 2 to 3 years of age, after which it primarily supplies the metaphysis. In children older than 14 to 18 months, the proximal femoral physeal plate becomes an absolute barrier to the metaphyseal blood supply and prevents direct vascular penetration of the femoral head (320,321). Thus, the epiphyseal and metaphyseal circulation remain separate until complete physeal closure occurs. The vessels of the ligamentum teres do not contribute a significant portion of the blood supply to the femoral head, especially in children younger than 8 years.

It is postulated that some displaced fractures may leave the vascular leash intact but kinked and occluded until realignment is established (322). This has been demonstrated by arteriography before and after reduction of an unstable slipped capital femoral epiphysis (323). Vascular

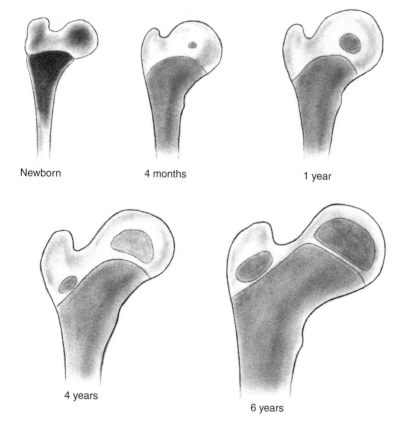

Newborn    4 months    1 year

4 years

6 years

**Figure 33.54** Development of the growth centers in the proximal femur. (From Edgren W. Coxa plana: a clinical and radiological investigation with particular reference to the importance of the metaphyseal changes for the final shape of the proximal part of the femur. *Acta Orthop Scand* 1965;84:24, with permission.)

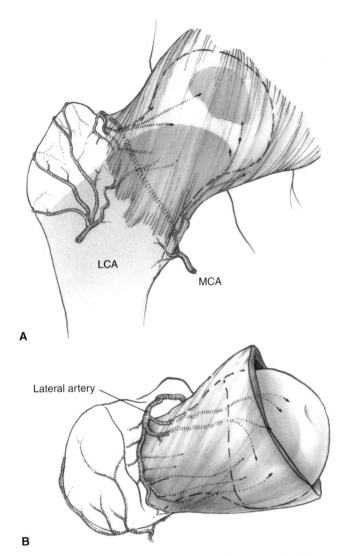

**A**

Lateral artery

**B**

**Figure 33.55** Arterial supply of the developing proximal femur. **A:** The anterior view demonstrates the lateral circumflex artery (*LCA*), which supplies the metaphysis and greater trochanter. The medial circumflex femoral artery (*MCA*) is the dominant vessel to the femoral head. **B:** The superior view shows the lateral ascending artery, which sends numerous epiphyseal and metaphyseal branches (*arrows*) that supply the greatest volume to the femoral head and neck. These ascending cervical branches traverse the articular capsule as the retinacular arteries. The interval between the greater trochanter and the hip capsule is extremely narrow, and is the area where the lateral ascending cervical artery passes. This may be a site of vascular compression or injury.

disruption as a cause of avascular necrosis is supported by the fact that the magnitude of displacement is a prognostic factor for the development of necrosis (324). It has also been suggested that prompt decompression of the intracapsular hematoma contributes to the restoration of normal vascular flow and reduces the incidence of femoral head necrosis (325–328).

A study of nondisplaced hip fractures in adults confirmed high intracapsular pressures with decreased blood flow on bone scan. Following aspiration and fixation, repeat bone scans demonstrated restoration of blood flow (329).

Other studies have also reported high intracapsular pressures that are reduced by joint decompression (329–331). Soto-Hall et al., in 1964, noted that intraarticular pressures increased when intracapsular hip fractures were manipulated by placing the leg in internal rotation and extension (332). The increased joint pressure during reduction of fractures in this position has been confirmed by other authors (329,331). Therefore, it is the present authors' opinion that reduction of intracapsular fractures may improve vascularity by restoring normal arterial position. However, reduction may also lead to increased intracapsular pressure unless the hip is decompressed. Prompt reduction, internal fixation, and decompression are recommended in order to restore circulation in a timely manner. This approach to the management of hip fractures and unstable slipped capital femoral epiphyses in children has been associated with a decreased risk of avascular necrosis (325,327,328,333).

Delbet's classification (Fig. 33.56) offers a useful system for the treatment and prognosis of proximal femur fractures (334). Type I fractures are transphyseal separations. Physeal separation in infants is occasionally seen as a birth fracture or as a result of intentionally inflicted injury. Obstetric fracture-separations have excellent clinical results, without avascular necrosis, although diagnosis and treatment may be delayed (335). Children younger than 2 years with type I fracture also have a good prognosis without surgical management (336). Transepiphyseal separations in older children result from more severe trauma, but separation has been reported during reduction of hip dislocation in the adolescent age group (337). When the epiphyseal fragment is dislocated from the acetabulum, the risk of avascular necrosis approaches 100%. However, the incidence of avascular necrosis is variable when the femoral head remains within the joint (334).

Type II fractures occur in the neck of the femur between the epiphyseal plate and the base of the neck. They constitute approximately 50% of all fractures of the proximal femur (334). Complications are frequent with type II fractures. The incidence of avascular necrosis approaches 50% to 60%, and the nonunion rate is 15%. Premature physeal closure may also occur, but because growth of the proximal femur is approximately 15% of the total limb (338), clinically important leg-length discrepancy is unlikely to occur in older children.

Type III fractures occur in the cervicotrochanteric, or basal neck, region of the femoral neck. This is the second most common type of hip fracture in children. Avascular necrosis occurs in 30% of displaced fractures. Malunion has been reported in 20%, and nonunion occurs in 10%, of these patients. These problems may be lessened by precise fracture reduction, combined with compression across the fracture site by means of cancellous bone screws (i.e., lag technique) (334,339).

Type IV fractures occur in the intertrochanteric region and are associated with the least risk of damage to the femoral head vascular supply. The incidence of avascular

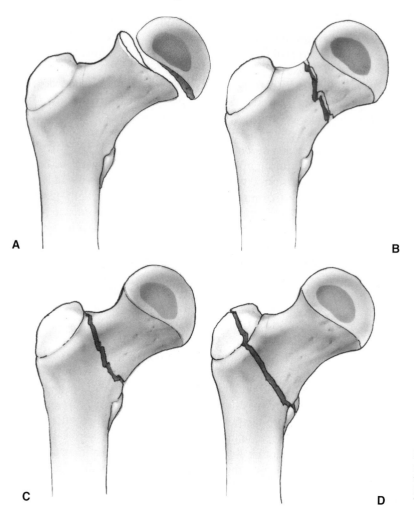

**A**

**B**

**C**

**D**

**Figure 33.56** Delbet's classification for proximal femur fractures. **A:** Type I is a transepiphyseal fracture. **B:** Type II is a transcervical fracture. **C:** Type III is a cervicotrochanteric fracture (basicervical). **D:** Type IV is an intertrochanteric fracture.

necrosis is between 0 and 10%. Varus deformity is the most likely complication, but this may correct with growth in younger children (334,339,340).

### Treatment

Proximal femur fractures should be treated as urgent cases. The risk of avascular necrosis may be minimized with reduction, joint decompression, and stable fixation within 24 hours of injury (316,326,328,341). It is possible that treatment within 6 hours, as is recommended for hip dislocations, would further decrease the incidence of avascular necrosis, but there are no current reports of reduction and decompression within 6 hours. Delay in treatment may be necessary because of associated injuries or other considerations.

*Type I Fractures.* Treatment with closed reduction and casting is appropriate for minimally displaced fractures, and for children younger than 2 years (342). In children aged 2 to 12 years, stabilization of the reduced fracture may be accomplished with two smooth pins supplemented with spica casting. In older children, fixation across the physis is recommended. Open reduction is often necessary

if the epiphysis is dislocated. This is performed through a posterior approach for posterior fracture-dislocations. At the time of open reduction, curettage of the physeal plate has been recommended in an attempt to encourage revascularization of the femoral head (337).

*Type II and Type III Fractures.* If the fracture is definitely stable and nondisplaced, and the patient is younger than 6 years, a spica cast alone can yield good results (343). Displaced fractures can usually be reduced by closed methods, but a small incision to open the hip capsule is recommended because this could decrease the risk of avascular necrosis (325–328). Ng and Cole (326) studied the effect of early hip decompression on the frequency of avascular necrosis. It had no apparent value in type I fractures. For the type II and type III fractures, 41% of 54 patients treated without hip decompression developed avascular necrosis whereas only 8% of 39 patients with hip compression developed avascular necrosis. As previously discussed, prompt reduction, internal fixation, and decompression are recommended by the present authors in an attempt to restore circulation in a timely manner. Fixation is achieved by the percutaneous insertion of two or three cannulated bone screws into the metaphyseal portion of the proximal fragment (Fig. 33.57). If the proximal metaphyseal fragment is too small for secure fixation, smooth pins can be placed across the physis to allow subsequent growth. Stable fixation of the fracture should be given priority over preservation of the proximal femoral physis (334). Spica cast immobilization is used to augment fixation in children, especially when smooth pins have been used. In patients aged 12 years or older, threaded screws may be placed across the physis for better fixation and to avoid the use of a spica cast. Alternatively, a hip screw with a supplemental pin to control rotation may be used in older children. Caution is advised when using compression hip screws in children, because dense bone may generate heat necrosis of the femoral neck during reaming. An

additional smooth pin is recommended to improve rotational stability (Fig. 33.58). Open reduction is occasionally required if suitable alignment is not obtained by closed means. An anterolateral (Watson-Jones) approach is recommended for type II fractures.

*Type IV Fractures.* This fracture does not require prompt stabilization except when surgical fixation improves general management. Nondisplaced fractures in this region can be managed by spica cast immobilization and close follow-up in younger children. Displaced fractures in infants and toddlers may be treated with early closed reduction and casting so long as the neck-shaft angle does not decrease to less than 115 degrees. Displaced fractures in older children

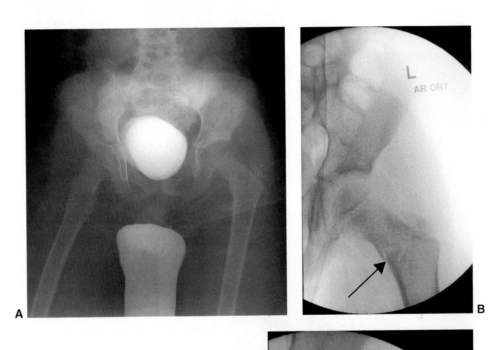

**Figure 33.57** Hip fracture in an 8-year-old boy treated with internal fixation. **A:** Initial radiograph of an 8-year-old boy who fell approximately 50 ft from a ski lift, sustaining a left femoral neck fracture and a pneumothorax. A Delbet type C femoral neck fracture was diagnosed. The surgeon also appreciated that the proximal femur was in varus. **B:** This anteroposterior intraoperative radiograph was taken immediately after closed reduction of the fracture (*arrow*). The neck shaft angle was corrected. **C:** Two screws (7.3 mm and 0.45 mm) were used for internal fixation. In this patient, there was enough room between the fracture and the growth plate, and the physis did not have to be crossed. After fixation, the child was protected in a spica cast for 6 weeks.

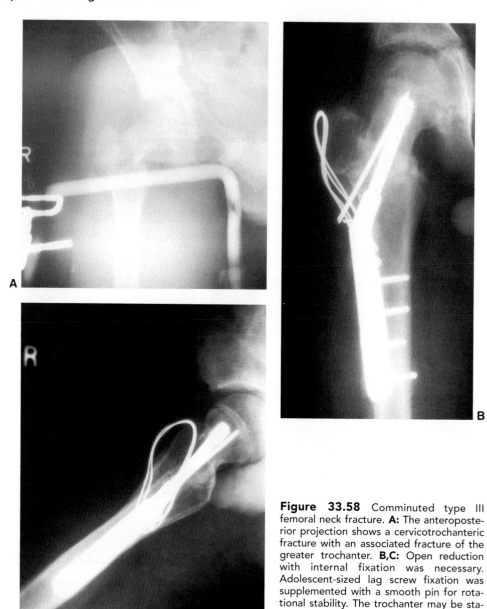

**Figure 33.58** Comminuted type III femoral neck fracture. **A:** The anteroposterior projection shows a cervicotrochanteric fracture with an associated fracture of the greater trochanter. **B,C:** Open reduction with internal fixation was necessary. Adolescent-sized lag screw fixation was supplemented with a smooth pin for rotational stability. The trochanter may be stabilized with Kirschner wires instead of a tension band. Spica cast immobilization is indicated when fixation does not cross the growth plate.

can also be managed by skeletal traction followed by cast immobilization. However, the authors recommend surgical stabilization in children older than 6 years to reduce the risk of malunion and avoid prolonged immobilization. Interfragmentary screws may provide sufficient stability when combined with cast immobilization, but a pediatric-sized hip screw with side plate, or an angled blade plate, is preferred. The physis should be avoided. The femoral neck should be stabilized before reaming, and reaming should be performed slowly to avoid heat necrosis of the cortical bone. Adolescents are treated in the same manner as adults, with stable fixation across the physis using a sliding hip screw or angled blade plate. This avoids the need for a supplemental spica cast for adolescent patients.

### Complications

The most frequent complications after fracture of the proximal femur in children are osteonecrosis of the femoral head, malunion, and nonunion. Other complications include infections, premature closure of the proximal femoral growth plate, and chondrolysis. Exact complication rates are difficult to determine because of changing patterns of treatment. Prompt, accurate reduction, joint decompression, and appropriate internal fixation and immobilization reduce all of these complications (316,326).

Avascular necrosis in children may involve a portion of the femoral head, just the portion of the femoral neck between the fracture and the physis, or the entire femoral neck and head (344). Necrosis of the femoral head occurs in approximately 30% of all hip fractures in children and often leads to poor results (334). Diagnosis of avascularity can be reliably determined by MRI as early as 2 weeks following the fracture (345), or by isotope bone scan 4 months after the fracture. Children with osteonecrosis who are younger than 12 years can be treated with containment, with or without prolonged non–weight-bearing activities. These patients have a possibility of recovering satisfactory function (346,347). The outcome for older children with osteonecrosis of the femoral head is poor. The authors recommend treating adolescents in a manner similar to that for adults, with early detection and core decompression before the occurrence of subchondral fracture (348).

Nonunion occurs in 6% to 10% of pediatric fractures of the proximal femur (334). Treatment is recommended as soon as the diagnosis is established. Subtrochanteric valgus osteotomy is preferred, with bone grafting, internal fixation, and application of a spica cast (334,349). Supplemental vascularized bone grafting with a vascular-pedicle graft from the iliac crest should be considered when there is a large defect in the femoral head or neck (350).

Malunion and coxa vara occur in approximately 20% of reported patients, but this complication has a lower incidence when internal fixation is used (334). Remodeling may occur in younger patients (340). Subtrochanteric osteotomy is recommended for persistent deformity.

# FEMORAL SHAFT FRACTURES

Femoral shaft fractures account for 1% to 2% of all fractures in childhood (3,6). Boys sustain this injury 0.25 times more often than girls. There is a bimodal age distribution, with a peak incidence at 2 to 3 years of age and another peak in adolescence. The cortical thickness of the femur increases rapidly after 5 years of age, and this may explain the decreasing incidence of femur fracture in late childhood. Intentional injury should always be considered in young children, but there are no distinguishing clinical parameters or fracture patterns to help determine which injuries are inflicted and which are accidental (351). In infants younger than 1 year, child abuse has been identified as a cause in 65% of patients when obvious causes such as motor vehicle accidents are eliminated (351). In children aged 1 to 5 years, the incidence of abuse decreases. Children in this toddler age group may sustain fractures with relatively minor trauma from causes such as falling from a low height or tripping while running. In the 4- to 7-year age group, approximately half of the femoral shaft fractures are caused by bicycle accidents. In the adolescent age group, motor vehicle accidents account for most of the femur fractures.

As stated by Mercer Rang (32), "It does not require a physician to diagnose a fractured femur." However, the physician must carefully examine the patient completely. Children and adolescents with femur fracture have a 35%

to 40% incidence of associated injuries. Some of these injuries are occult, such as femoral neck fracture, hip dislocation, ligamentous instability of the knee, and visceral injuries (352,353). Hemodynamic instability or steadily declining hematocrit does not occur because of an isolated, closed femur fracture. Other sources of blood loss must be sought in these patients (353).

## Treatment of Femoral Shaft Fractures

### Principles of Management
A wide variety of management options are currently available for femur fractures in children and adolescents. Each of these options can yield satisfactory results when used properly (354). The surgeon managing femoral fractures in children and adolescents is expected to select and perform the technique that is most appropriate under a variety of circumstances.

The age of the child and the severity of the trauma are the principal determinants of management. Younger children are less likely to require surgical stabilization or prolonged traction. High-energy trauma is more likely to require surgical intervention or prolonged immobilization. At one end of the spectrum there are low-energy injuries in young children that are managed with closed reduction and immediate spica casting (Fig. 33.59). At the other end of the spectrum, high-energy injuries in adolescents are managed with early surgical stabilization. Occasionally, however, infants with severe trauma require surgical stabilization of femoral fractures to facilitate management.

### Anatomical Considerations and Remodeling Potential
Proximal fractures in all age groups are more difficult to control, but residual deformity is better tolerated because of multidirectional hip motion. Deformity is also less obvious with proximal fractures because thick thigh muscles hide residual angulation. Proximal fragments tend to flex, abduct, and externally rotate because of the unopposed action of the iliopsoas, hip abductor, and external rotator muscles. The proximal fragment of a midshaft fracture also tends to flex, abduct, and externally rotate, but the deformity is less extreme because of adductor and hamstring attachments to the proximal fragment. More distal fragments are easier to control and produce little proximal fragment angulation, except for supracondylar fractures, which tend to hyperextend because of the posterior pull of the gastrocnemius muscle on the short distal fragment. Fractures of the distal femur require more precise alignment because the deformity is more visible and remodeling in the coronal plane is limited. Supracondylar fractures of the femur require management that is similar to that for distal femoral physeal separations (355).

Children have remarkable remodeling potential until approximately 10 years of age in girls and 12 years of age in boys. Long-term studies have demonstrated that up to

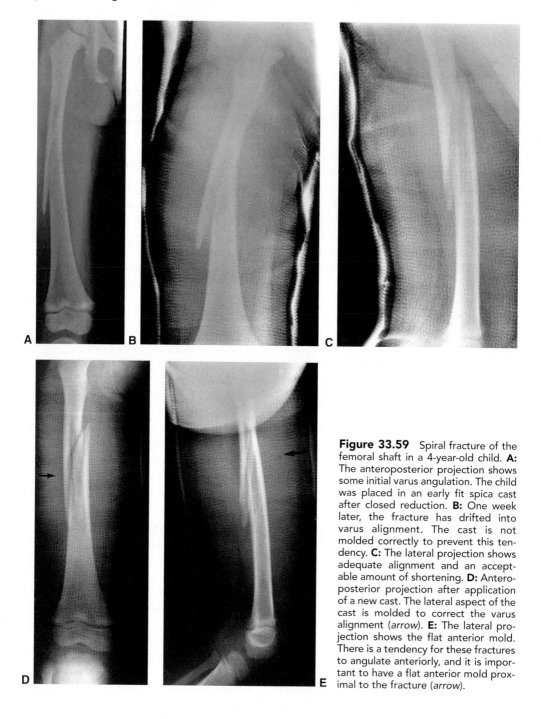

**Figure 33.59** Spiral fracture of the femoral shaft in a 4-year-old child. **A:** The anteroposterior projection shows some initial varus angulation. The child was placed in an early fit spica cast after closed reduction. **B:** One week later, the fracture has drifted into varus alignment. The cast is not molded correctly to prevent this tendency. **C:** The lateral projection shows adequate alignment and an acceptable amount of shortening. **D:** Anteroposterior projection after application of a new cast. The lateral aspect of the cast is molded to correct the varus alignment (*arrow*). **E:** The lateral projection shows the flat anterior mold. There is a tendency for these fractures to angulate anteriorly, and it is important to have a flat anterior mold proximal to the fracture (*arrow*).

25 degrees of midshaft angulation in any plane can be expected to correct satisfactorily in children younger than 13 years (16). Remodeling continues for up to 5 years following fracture. Approximately 25% of remodeling occurs at the fracture site, whereas 75% is attributed to physeal reorientation and longitudinal growth (15,19). Fracture translation may also contribute to realignment of the mechanical axis. Rotational remodeling may also occur, but the precise amount is unpredictable (18,356). Clinically significant rotational deformity is uncommon, even when failure of remodeling has been documented (357,358).

Stimulation of growth after femoral fracture occurs routinely in the 3- to 9-year age group (20,359). Unfortunately, most authors reporting the overgrowth phenomenon do not distinguish between "catch-up growth," which compensates for fracture overriding, and true overgrowth, which results in the fractured femur being longer than normal. Growth stimulation is greater when overriding is greater and may continue for 5 years after fracture. Average total growth stimulation is approximately 1 cm. In a prospective study of children younger than 12 years, Hougaard observed that all fractures of the femur healing with 3 cm or less discrepancy with the contralateral leg spontaneously recovered to less than 2 cm discrepancy (20). Therefore, any femoral fracture that heals in a shortened position should be observed for several years to determine the final outcome (Fig. 33.60). True overgrowth has been reported after reduction with internal fixation, but the risk of overgrowth in this circumstance has not been clearly defined (354). Parents are usually more understanding when the injured femur grows longer than when the femur is allowed to heal in a markedly shortened position.

Special circumstances such as subtrochanteric fractures and floating knee are discussed at the end of this section.

## Management Guidelines by Age

Age or weight is the first determinant of treatment choices. Age is used here with the understanding that the children are of average weight and maturity.

*Infants.* Infants younger than 1 year often sustain femur fractures because of birth trauma or abuse. Osteogenesis imperfecta and other metabolic disorders should also be suspected. Thick periosteum and rapid hematoma consolidation usually prevent worrisome shortening or angulation. Healing is rapid, and remodeling potential is great. One can accept 3 cm of shortening and 30 degrees of angulation in

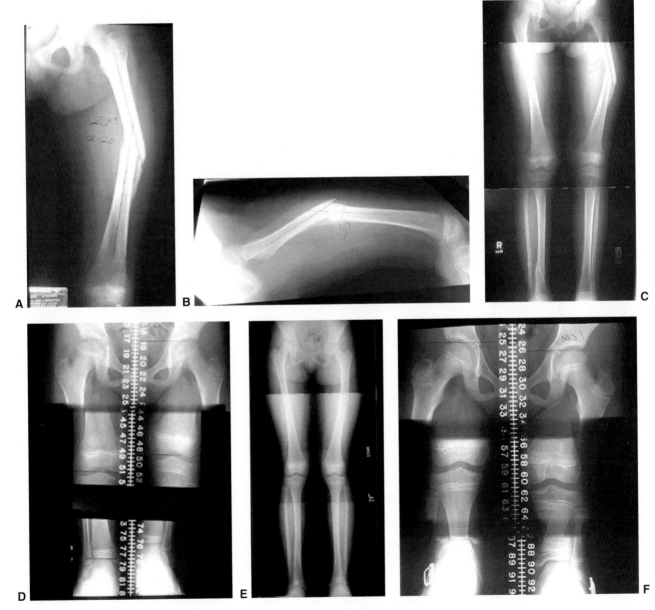

**Figure 33.60** Femoral shaft fracture in a 7-year-old child with varus and flexion malunion. **A,B:** Anteroposterior and lateral radiographs taken 10 weeks after femoral shaft fracture in a 7 + 4-year-old girl. There are 23 degrees of varus malalignment and 35 degrees of flexion. **C,D:** Full-length standing film and scanogram document lower-extremity alignment and a 2-cm leg-length inequality. **E,F:** Twenty months later, remodeling has nearly eliminated the deformity, and the scanogram shows 1 cm discrepancy.

both the coronal and sagittal planes. Infants may be treated with application of a Pavlik harness (best if the infant is 6 months old or younger) or a conventional spica cast (360). Immobilization for 2 to 3 weeks is usually sufficient for infants less than 4 months, and 4 to 6 weeks for infants aged 6 to 12 months.

***Age 1 to 6 Years.*** Isolated femur fractures in children between the ages of 1 and 6 years are usually treated with early spica cast application. All aspects of spica cast treatment are easier for preschool children than for older children (361). Children in this age group also heal rapidly, thus immobilization time is brief. The spica cast may be applied in the emergency department under conscious sedation. Alternatively, splinting is used for comfort until a spica cast can be applied within 48 hours after injury. Alignment in the cast should be as close to normal as possible, but full functional recovery can be expected in this age group if shortening at the time of union is no greater than 3 cm and angulation is less than 20 degrees in any plane. Fractures in the distal third should be angulated no more than 15 degrees.

***Age 6 to 10 Years.*** Children between the ages of 6 and 10 years may be managed by a wide variety of methods, depending on the severity of the fracture and social circumstances. Low-energy injuries without severe displacement or shortening may be managed by early spica cast immobilization (362,363). However, children in the 6- to 10-year age group require a longer period of immobilization than do younger children. This immobilization and

dependency may pose a problem if both parents are working or if the child lives with a single working parent. Surgical stabilization may be beneficial in these and similar social circumstances. High-energy fractures with severe displacement, comminution, or shortening greater than 3 cm require maintenance of length in addition to alignment. This may be achieved by incorporating a traction pin in the spica cast or by traction (Fig. 33.61) for 2 to 3 weeks before cast immobilization to keep the fracture aligned and out to length during the period of early callus formation (364–366). Alternatively, surgical stabilization with internal or external fixation achieves the same objectives and allows early mobilization. Although it has been demonstrated that up to 25 degrees of angulation in any plane will remodel in this age group (17), recommended guidelines for alignment in this age group are up to 15 degrees varus or valgus, 15 degrees of anterior and/or posterior angulation, and up to 20 mm of shortening.

***Age 10 Years to Maturity.*** Children older than 10 years are generally managed by surgical stabilization with internal or external fixation (354). Accurate restoration of length and alignment is desirable in older children because of limited remodeling potential. No more than 10 degrees of varus or valgus, 10 degrees of anterior or posterior angulation, and 15 mm of shortening should be accepted in this age group. Surgical stabilization permits early mobilization and return to school and social activities. Various techniques for stabilization are discussed in the following text. It is generally agreed that rigid, reamed intramedullary nailing through a piriformis fossa should be avoided

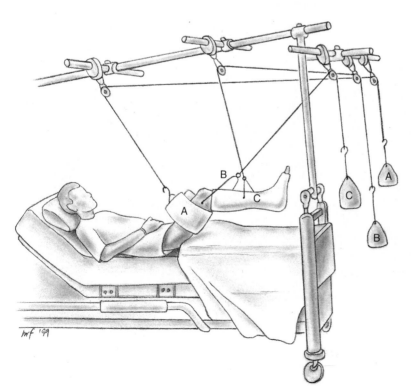

**Figure 33.61** Balanced traction with a distal femoral pin, a thigh sling, and cast suspension of the leg. This is easily converted to 90-90 traction for more proximal fractures. Weight *A* supports the thigh, weight *B* provides traction, and weight *C* supports the leg in a cast.

because of the risk of iatrogenic avascular necrosis of the femoral head (367). The risk of this complication is present as long as the proximal femoral physis remains open.

### Management Techniques
Techniques for management are selected according to the principles and guidelines discussed in the preceding paragraphs.

*Early Fit Spica Cast.* The typical candidate for early cast immobilization is a child younger than 6 years. Children up to 10 years of age may also be treated by early spica casting for low-energy, closed femur fractures that have less than 2 cm overriding at rest (362,363,368). Under anesthesia, gentle longitudinal compression may be applied to verify that the fracture does not shorten more than 3 cm (telescope test) (362). If the fracture shortens more than 3 cm, then surgical stabilization, use of traction, or pins and plaster may be more appropriate than early spica casting. After fracture alignment is obtained, the popliteal area and all bony prominences should be well padded prior to cast application. The authors recommend the 90-90 position with gentle traction on the leg while the hip and knee are held in slight abduction with 90 degrees of flexion at the hip and knee (369,370). Care must be taken to avoid excessive traction in order to avoid peroneal nerve palsy and posterior compartment syndrome of the leg (371,372). Applying the long leg portion of the cast as an initial step may facilitate cast application and maintenance of alignment. After casting, patients are usually discharged within 24 hours. Follow-up visits to monitor alignment are recommended at 1 and 2 weeks after reduction. It is often helpful to tape a paper clip or other small metallic object outside the cast before radiographic examination. This can be used to identify the fracture site if wedging of the cast is required.

*Skeletal Traction.* Skeletal traction is a safe, reliable, and easily instituted form of management for almost any femur fracture in any age group. However, skin traction is sufficient for children of average weight (<80 lb) who are younger than 8 years (364). Traction and casting are rarely the treatment of choice today, however, because excellent results can be obtained from early spica casts in children younger than 6 years, or internal and external fixation in the older child.

There are several ways in which traction can be constructed (373,374). The simplest is the 90-90 position for preadolescents and for managing proximal femur fractures. Adolescents are usually placed in balanced traction with a thigh sling and adjustable knee support to allow 45 degrees of knee flexion. Skeletal traction entails insertion of a pin into the metaphysis of the distal femur, using a medial-to-lateral direction to avoid potential injury to the femoral artery. Local anesthesia and intravenous sedation provide sufficient analgesia for pin insertion. Proximal

tibial pins are avoided due to the risk of growth arrest. However, proximal tibial growth arrest is more likely to result from the mechanism of injury than from pin insertion (375). Optimal femoral pin placement is approximately 2 cm proximal to the distal femoral growth plate and is aligned parallel to the knee joint to reduce the risk of malalignment (376). A traction bow is attached to the pin, and traction is applied. Periodic radiographs are obtained to guide the weight and direction of traction vectors needed to restore alignment. After relative fracture stability has been obtained (17 to 21 days) and callus formation is confirmed on radiographs, a cast is applied for an additional 4 to 8 weeks.

*External Fixation.* The prime indications for external fixation are length-unstable fracture patterns (i.e., significant comminution), some very proximal or distal fractures, or soft tissue damage as in open fractures or burns (Figs. 33.62 and 33.63) (377). Other relative indications include polytrauma, in which the child's general medical condition favors rapid and bloodless stabilization, which is possible with this technique. It may be considered as a form of ambulatory traction enabling the child to be partially weight bearing and independent several days after sustaining the injury. Some authors report few complications with this method, whereas others report many complications (354,378–380).

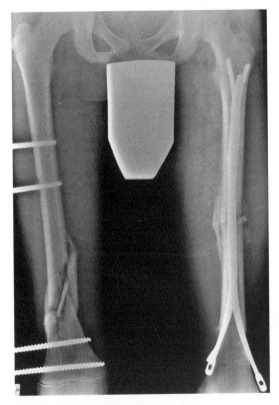

**Figure 33.62**  Bilateral femur fractures. The distal location, proximity to the growth plate, and marked comminution of the right femur fracture are best managed through the application of an external fixator. Although external fixation could have been applied to the contralateral fracture, intramedullary fixation was chosen because of the transverse pattern of the fracture.

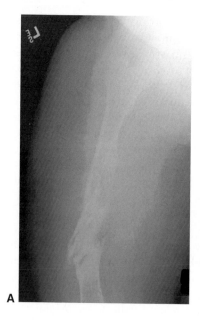
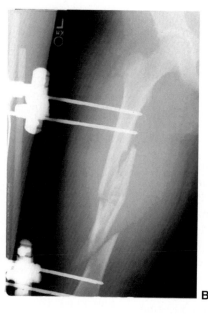

**Figure 33.63** Femur fracture treated with external fixation. **A:** This anteroposterior radiograph of a skeletally immature 13-year-old boy with a comminuted, length-unstable femur fracture. He had other multiple injuries, including an ipsilateral open tibia fracture. **B:** This anteroposterior radiograph was taken immediately after application of external fixator. (Courtesy of Theodore J. Ganley, MD)

The technique involves the sequential insertion of pins above and below the fracture site and attaching them to an external frame. Preferred pin location should be far enough away from the fracture site for the pins to avoid the fracture hematoma. However, the pins should also avoid penetrating the cortex of the femoral neck or the distal femoral physis. Under fluoroscopic guidance, final alignment can be adjusted as the pins are secured to the body of the fixator.

The most frequent problems encountered with the use of external fixation are pin-track infections, delayed union, and refracture after device removal. Pin-track inflammation and superficial infection requiring oral antibiotics are common (379,380). Rarely, deep infection may require intravenous antibiotics or pin removal. In this instance, fixator removal before complete union can be managed by application of a cast. Delayed union and refracture are more frequent with fracture sites that have been opened, or with transverse and short, oblique, midshaft fractures that are anatomically reduced (381,382). Delayed healing has also been associated with excessively rigid constructs, lack of dynamization, and premature removal of the fixation device (380,383). With careful attention to indications, surgical technique, and postoperative management, external fixation may be successfully used to treat pediatric femoral fractures.

*Intramedullary Fixation.* Two devices used for intramedullary fixation are rigid nails and flexible, unreamed nails (384–386). Rigid nails are ideally suited for adults, because they can be locked proximally and distally to control shortening and rotation. However, the use of reamed rigid nails introduced through the piriformis fossa has been associated with avascular necrosis of the femoral head in children and adolescents (367). Rigid nails in children younger than 13 years have also been associated with growth disturbance with femoral neck deformity, including coxa valga and thinning of the femoral neck (387,388). For

these reasons, it is recommended that rigid, reamed nails introduced through the pyriformis fossa should be avoided unless the proximal femoral physis is completely closed.

Flexible or elastic intramedullary nails have the advantage of being applicable to the small, young child without risking damage to the trochanter, the femoral neck, or the vascular supply to the femoral head (389). A transverse or stable fracture pattern is best for this method of internal fixation. Flexible rods are commonly inserted retrograde from the distal femoral metaphysis toward the proximal end of the femur. Two C-shaped nails, one inserted medially and one laterally, usually provide sufficient stability when three-point intramedullary contact is obtained (390,391) (Fig. 33.64). The size of the titanium nail should be approximately 40% of the diameter of the femoral canal at its most narrow point. The authors recommend passing the second nail when the first nail has been inserted just past the fracture site. Other options for insertion include a unilateral approach distally, inserting one C-shaped nail and one S-shaped nail. When the fracture is very distal, nails may be introduced proximally in the region of the greater trochanter. Additional nails may be added for stability. Flexible nails are less stable in heavier, older children, and for comminuted fractures (392). The addition of a cast can supplement unstable internal fixation, but this partially defeats the advantages of surgical stabilization. New types of flexible nails that allow proximal and distal locking are currently being developed to help manage unstable fractures (393).

*Plate Fixation.* Femoral plate fixation has not been widely used for pediatric femur fractures (394). Several authors have reported successful results with conventional compression plating (394,395). Submuscular bridge plating, and subcutaneous, minimally invasive percutaneous osteosynthesis with locking compression plates, are newer techniques that are being utilized for pediatric femur fractures (396,397)

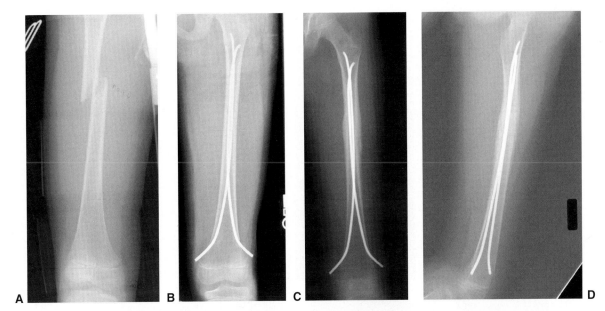

**Figure 33.64** Titanium elastic nail fixation of a midshaft femur fracture in an 11-year-old girl. **A:** Initial radiograph of the short, oblique, midshaft femur fracture. **B:** Anteroposterior radiograph taken immediately after internal fixation with titanium elastic nails. For this patient, the surgeon bent the distal nail away from bone, and this can cause soft tissue irritation. **C,D:** Anteroposterior and lateral radiographs of the femur taken 6 months after internal fixation. There is good healing and maintenance of an anatomic alignment. The nails were removed shortly thereafter.

(Fig. 33.65). Plate fixation may be suitable for comminuted fractures and for fractures that are located in sites difficult to secure with an intramedullary nail or external fixator. The advantages of plate fixation for femur fractures are anatomic reduction and early mobilization. Disadvantages of conventional compression plating include extensive dissection with additional blood loss, device failure, and the risks associated with plate removal. Submuscular bridge plating reduces the amount of dissection required, but subsequent removal through limited incisions may be problematic. Minimally invasive percutaneous osteosynthesis with locking compression plates may avoid these difficulties, but this technique requires advanced technical skill.

## Femoral Fractures in Special Circumstances

Management of pediatric femoral fractures may be altered in complex circumstances as seen in children with head injuries, multiple trauma, open fractures, floating knee, or high subtrochanteric fractures. Children with head injuries or multiple trauma benefit from more aggressive fracture stabilization so that they can be transported and mobilized (55). The general management of open fractures is discussed earlier in this chapter. External fixation is recommended for open fractures with severe soft tissue injury, but grade I and many grade II open femur fractures can be managed in standard fashion after appropriate wound care.

### Floating Knee

Simultaneous ipsilateral fracture of the femur and tibia has been termed the *floating knee* (398–400). This injury pattern

has been classified by Letts et al. (399) (Fig. 33.66). The fracture usually is the result of high-energy trauma. Knee ligament damage occurs in approximately 10% of these patients and is better assessed after fracture stabilization. A juxtaarticular fracture pattern and fractures in children older than 10 years have worse prognoses for early and late problems (398). Surgical stabilization of at least one bone is recommended in most cases (398–400).

### Subtrochanteric Fractures

Subtrochanteric fractures usually result from high-energy trauma. It may be difficult to maintain alignment by closed treatment because the proximal fragment flexes, abducts, and externally rotates. Union in the anatomic position is rarely achieved with closed treatment, but remodeling potential is great in this anatomic region. Fractures that are closer to the greater trochanter and fractures in children older than 8 years more often result in malunion (401,402). Early spica cast application in the "sitting" position may suffice in very young children, but traction in the 90-90 position is frequently necessary until callus formation is visible on radiographs. Alternatively, the authors recommend that children older than 6 years, or younger children with unstable fractures, should be considered for surgical stabilization.

## Complications of Femur Fractures

Malunion, with or without limb-length discrepancy, is the most frequent complication of pediatric femur fractures. Compartment syndrome, neurovascular injuries, nonunion,

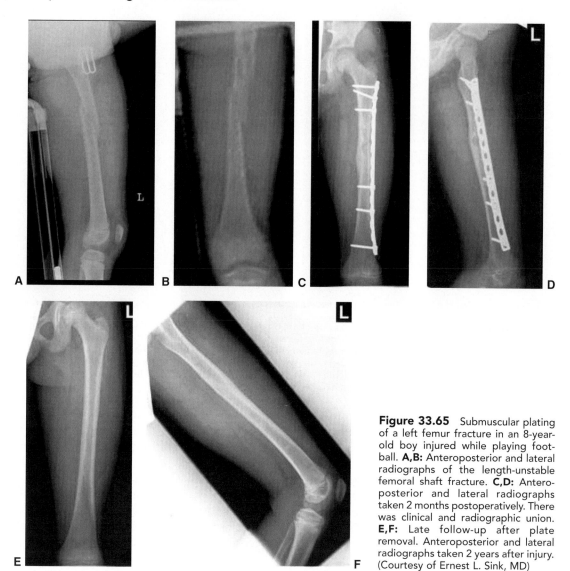

**Figure 33.65** Submuscular plating of a left femur fracture in an 8-year-old boy injured while playing football. **A,B:** Anteroposterior and lateral radiographs of the length-unstable femoral shaft fracture. **C,D:** Anteroposterior and lateral radiographs taken 2 months postoperatively. There was clinical and radiographic union. **E,F:** Late follow-up after plate removal. Anteroposterior and lateral radiographs taken 2 years after injury. (Courtesy of Ernest L. Sink, MD)

and infections may also occur. These latter complications are more frequent after open injuries and are discussed elsewhere. Management principles are similar to those in adults. Malunion and limb-length discrepancy may resolve with remodeling so long as the deformities are within management guidelines discussed previously. Osteotomy is performed to correct persistent deformity in older children, or when remodeling is incomplete in younger children after a period of observation. Persistent limb-length discrepancy is rarely severe and is usually managed by epiphysiodesis of the contralateral extremity at an appropriate age.

# FRACTURES AND DISLOCATIONS AROUND THE KNEE

This section addresses fractures around the knee. Acute patellar dislocations and soft tissue injuries of the juvenile knee are discussed in Chapter 32. Significant trauma to the knee in children usually results in a fracture instead of a ligamentous injury. The attachments of the joint capsule and the surrounding ligaments expose the pediatric knee to certain characteristic avulsions and physeal injuries. The child presenting with an acute hemarthrosis of the knee may have a soft tissue injury, a fracture, or both. Stress views are sometimes useful if there is concern for physeal fracture. MRI has been used to provide additional information, but this modality may be less accurate in children than in adults (403,404). Radiographically silent osteochondral fractures have been noted in 7% to 67% of juvenile patients undergoing arthroscopy for acute hemarthrosis (405,406). However, arthroscopy is rarely necessary for the initial management of acute hemarthrosis in children younger than 13 years. Arthroscopy may be useful in older children when it could lead to definitive management (407,408).

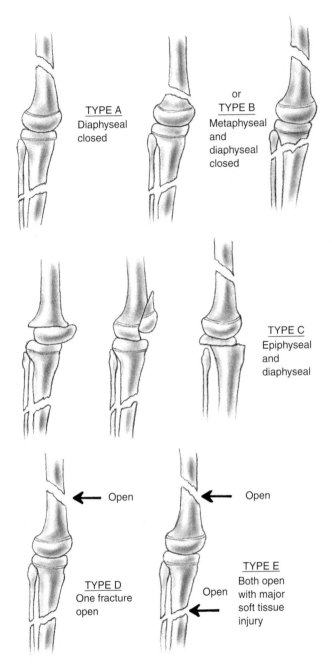

ligamentous injuries on clinical examination. However, careful inspection will reveal that the area of tenderness and swelling is proximal to the joint line. Stress radiographs with the patient sedated can be used to demonstrate the fracture, but these are rarely needed. When the epiphysis is displaced, the direction of displacement reflects the direction of the injuring force. Hyperextension of the knee produces anterior epiphyseal displacement, and valgus or varus stress produces medial or lateral displacement, respectively. Direct impact in the knee-flexed position causes posterior displacement of the femoral epiphysis.

The Salter-Harris type III fracture of the medial femoral condyle usually results from valgus force on the knee. The medial collateral ligament and joint capsule transmit this force to the condyle, producing the fracture. Spontaneous reduction is frequent and may obscure the diagnosis. The Salter-Harris type III injury to the medial condyle may appear innocuous but is often associated with cruciate ligament damage and intraarticular osteochondral fragments (410).

Salter-Harris type I and II fractures account for most of the distal femoral epiphyseal separations, but these injuries are not benign and have a 50% incidence of growth arrest (411–413). It has been observed that growth arrest is closely related to the severity of displacement (411,413).

Fractures in the 2- to 11-year age group are frequently caused by severe trauma and have the greatest likelihood of physeal arrest (413). Fractures in the adolescent age group are often the result of less severe trauma but still have a 50% risk of growth disturbance. Close follow-up is recommended to detect partial or complete growth arrest. In contrast to these fractures in the juvenile and adolescent age groups, distal femoral separations in infants and toddlers have excellent remodeling potential and rarely lead to growth disturbance.

**Figure 33.66**  Classification of the "floating knee" in children. (From Letts M, Vincent N, Gouw G. The "floating knee" in children. *J Bone Joint Surg Br* 1986;68:442, with permission.)

## Distal Femoral Physeal Separations

The distal femoral growth plate has a complex geometric configuration and is securely anchored to the metaphysis. Any fracture at this location, whether displaced or not, confirms considerable trauma. These fractures constitute approximately 5% of all long-bone physeal fractures and 1% to 2% of all fractures in skeletally immature patients (29,409). The diagnosis is easily made except in cases of nondisplaced fractures. Nondisplaced fractures may mimic

### Treatment

Stable, nondisplaced fractures can be immobilized in a long-leg or cylinder cast for 3 to 4 weeks, until the fracture site is nontender. Close follow-up is warranted to detect any tendency toward displacement. Displaced distal femoral physeal separations should be treated with closed reduction under general anesthesia (411). After reduction, fixation is recommended using crossed percutaneous pins to prevent redisplacement while the leg is in a cast. Pins may be placed from distal to proximal (Fig. 33.67); although this means that the pins are within the knee joint, the procedure rarely leads to a secondary joint infection. Alternatively, pins may be placed proximal to distal to avoid traversing the synovium of the knee joint.

If the metaphyseal portion of the Salter-Harris type II metaphyseal fragment is large enough, fixation can be accomplished with percutaneous insertion of one or two cancellous bone screws through this fragment (Fig. 33.68).

Indications for open reduction include entrapped periosteum or muscle blocking reduction, Salter-Harris type III

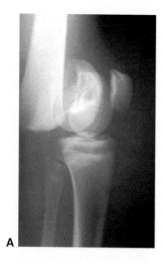
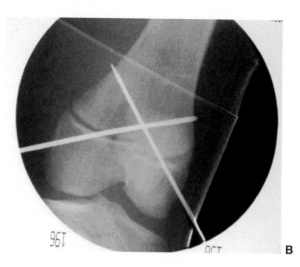

**Figure 33.67** Salter-Harris type I distal femoral fracture. **A:** This lateral radiograph shows a completely displaced Salter-Harris I distal femur fracture in a 12-year-old boy. He had a complete peroneal nerve palsy at presentation. **B:** Intraoperative anteroposterior radiograph after anatomic closed reduction and crossed-pin fixation. Pins were pulled at 4 weeks. He sustained a complete growth arrest of his distal femoral physis, detected approximately 6 months later.

and IV injuries, open injuries, and fractures associated with neurovascular disruption. Salter-Harris type III and IV injuries require precise alignment to restore the articular surface and reduce the risk of growth arrest. Because blocks to reduction are usually on the tension side, the fracture is approached from that side. At least two cannulated screws, 0.65 mm in diameter, are recommended to ensure stability. Cast immobilization is also used for 3 to 4 weeks, especially if there is only sufficient bone for a single screw.

After reduction and fixation, the patient is immobilized in a long-leg or cylinder cast for 3 to 5 weeks. Smooth pins can be removed in the clinic. Gentle range of motion with progressive weight bearing and strengthening is permitted following immobilization. Follow-up consists of evaluation for ligamentous laxity and observation for early signs of growth disturbance. MRI at 3 to 6 months after injury may identify a growth arrest (42,43). Complete closure of the opposite femoral physis should be performed in adolescents when postinjury growth arrest will result in more than 1 cm of limb-length inequality. Management of physeal closure in younger children and management of partial physeal arrest have been discussed in a previous section of this chapter.

## Tibial Spine Fracture

The terms "tibial eminence fracture" and "tibial spine fracture" have been used interchangeably to describe avulsion of the tibial attachment of the anterior cruciate ligament. The tibial eminence consists of two bony spines and is located between the medial and lateral plateaus of the tibia. The anterior cruciate ligament attaches to the medial spine, but nothing attaches to the apex of the lateral spine. Between these spines are the attachments of the menisci. Avulsion of the tibial eminence in children is usually caused by a fall from a bicycle, sporting injuries, or some other indirect trauma to the knee. The typical age range for this injury is 6 to 15 years.

Meyers and McKeever (414) classified this avulsion fracture by degree of displacement:

Type I. Minimally displaced, with only slight elevation of the anterior margin.
Type II. Hinged posteriorly, producing a beak-like appearance on the lateral radiograph.
Type III. Completely displaced and elevated from its bed.

With displacement, the meniscus may become trapped underneath the fragment and interfere with reduction (415). Long-term studies have reported some residual knee laxity despite anatomic reduction with internal fixation (416–418). This would suggest that the fibers of the anterior cruciate ligament are stretched before bone failure. Residual laxity has not led to functional deficits or subjective feelings of knee instability. A more troublesome problem is failure to regain full knee extension. Wiley and Baxter (418) carefully evaluated knee range of motion and determined that 60% of all patients lost more than 10 degrees of extension. This loss of motion was noted in all type III injuries that were treated with closed reduction, and in approximately one-half of the type III injuries treated with open reduction. Long-term functional results are generally excellent except for displaced type III fractures (417–419).

### Treatment

Type I injuries do not require reduction and can be immobilized in a cylinder cast for 4 to 6 weeks. This is followed by range-of-motion exercises, strengthening, and gradual resumption of activities.

Type II fractures may be difficult to distinguish from completely displaced fractures. Aspiration of the joint and injection of local anesthetic facilitates reduction. Reduction is attempted by fully extending the knee and applying an above-knee cast. If radiographs after reduction are inconclusive or demonstrate inadequate reduction, MRI or

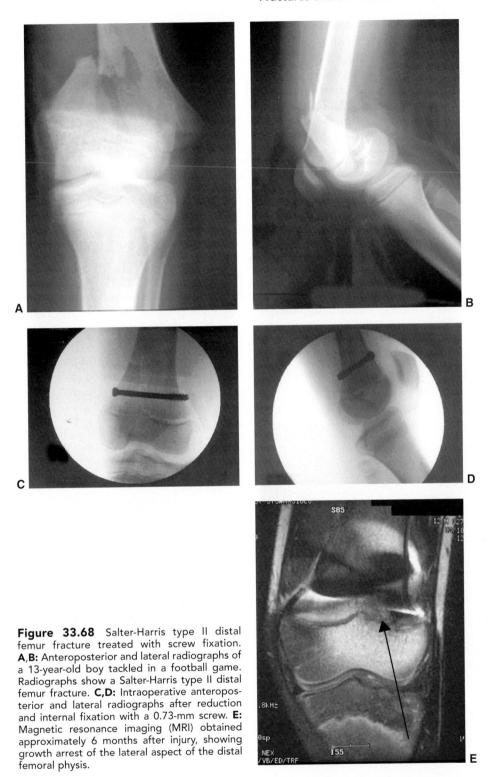

**Figure 33.68** Salter-Harris type II distal femur fracture treated with screw fixation. **A,B:** Anteroposterior and lateral radiographs of a 13-year-old boy tackled in a football game. Radiographs show a Salter-Harris type II distal femur fracture. **C,D:** Intraoperative anteroposterior and lateral radiographs after reduction and internal fixation with a 0.73-mm screw. **E:** Magnetic resonance imaging (MRI) obtained approximately 6 months after injury, showing growth arrest of the lateral aspect of the distal femoral physis.

arthroscopic evaluation may be necessary to determine whether the posterior attachment is disrupted, and whether there is meniscal entrapment. The preferred position of immobilization after reduction is controversial. Some authors recommend immobilization in extension (420,421), whereas others recommend immobilization with 20 to 30 degrees of knee flexion to relieve tension on the anterior

cruciate ligament (421). The present authors recommend immobilization in extension following reduction because loss of extension after union is more problematic than joint instability. Hyperextension should be avoided because this position becomes uncomfortable. When reduction cannot be achieved for type II fractures, open reduction is indicated in a manner similar to that for type III injuries.

Recommended treatment of type III fractures is open or arthroscopic reduction (422). Hallam has performed anatomical and clinical studies that suggest that arthroscopic removal of the entrapped meniscus can be followed by reduction with immobilization in extension (420). However, other authors recommend internal fixation. This can be achieved by using a small intraepiphyseal cancellous screw (423) (Fig. 33.69). Alternatively, sutures or wires can be passed that enter the osteochondral fragment and exit through the periphery of the epiphysis (424,425). When fixation is secure, early mobilization can be initiated to avoid loss of motion.

### Complications

Some loss of motion and ligamentous instability is common after tibial eminence fracture. These problems are usually mild and rarely interfere with function. Arthrofibrosis can also occur following arthroscopic surgical management. Manipulation under anesthesia should be approached with caution due to the risk of distal femoral physeal separation in skeletally immature patients. Occasionally, patients will present late with malunion that limits knee extension. This can be treated with an anterior closing wedge osteotomy and internal fixation (421,426).

## Tibial Tubercle Fracture

The tibial tubercle is the anterior and distal extension of the proximal tibial epiphysis. It develops a secondary ossification center and serves as the insertion site of the patellar tendon. Fracture of the tibial tubercle is an injury of the adolescent knee joint, usually occurring in boys between 13 and 16 years of age (427). During this period of growth, the proximal tibial physis is usually in the process of physiologic closure. The tibial growth plate begins closing centrally, proceeds centrifugally, and finally proceeds distally to include the tubercle. The mechanism of injury for avulsion of the tubercle is forceful quadriceps contraction against resistance (e.g., jumping). There may be a preceding history of Osgood-Schlatter disease (428,429).

Examination reveals swelling, deformity, and tenderness. The ability to perform a straight-leg raise should also be tested. The diagnosis is confirmed on a lateral radiograph by identifying the displaced fragment and a high-riding patella. A classification was proposed by Watson-Jones and modified by Ogden et al. (429) (Fig. 33.70). Type I fracture is through the distal ossification center; type II is at the junction of the tubercle and the tibial ossification centers; and type III involves the articular surface of the tibia. A type

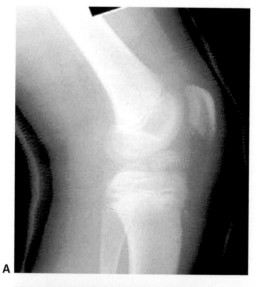

A

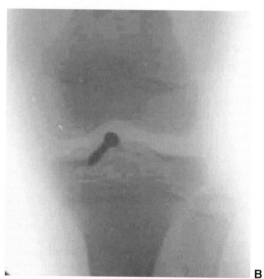

B

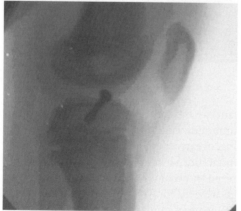

C

**Figure 33.69** Type III tibial eminence fracture fixed with arthroscopic reduction and internal fixation. **A:** Lateral radiograph of a type III tibial eminence fracture that presented after an attempt at closed reduction and casting at another center. The knee was more flexed in the cast than is recommended, and the fracture was still widely displaced. The decision was made to perform arthroscopic reduction and internal fixation. At the time of arthroscopy, the intermeniscal ligament was found trapped between the fragment and the tibia, blocking reduction. **B,C:** Anteroposterior and lateral views from the image intensifier following arthroscopic reduction and screw fixation of the fracture.

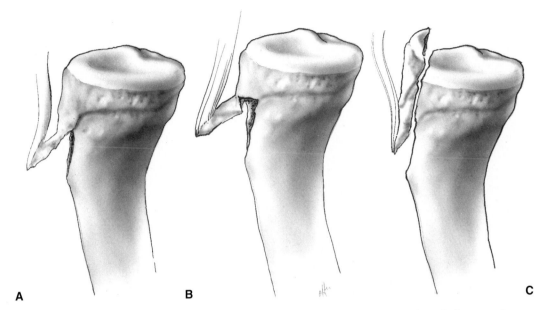

**Figure 33.70** Classification of tibial tuberosity fractures. **A:** Type I fracture through the secondary ossification center. **B:** Type II fracture located at the junction of the primary and secondary ossification centers. Sometimes this fragment is in two pieces. **C:** Type III is an intraarticular fracture (Salter-Harris type III). This can also be a two-part fracture.

IV fracture has been suggested, consisting of avulsion of the entire proximal tibial epiphysis.

### Treatment

Treatment of Type I minimally displaced fractures is non-surgical, but most of the other types require anatomic reduction and internal fixation (427). This can be accomplished by open reduction and insertion of cancellous bone screws (Fig. 33.71). There is usually a large retinacular injury that should be repaired. In younger children with significant growth remaining (an unusual scenario), smooth pins placed obliquely across the fracture can be substituted for screws. This procedure can be supplemented with a tension band suture or wire to the tibial metaphysis if pin fixation is insecure. After knee immobilization for 3 to 4 weeks, active range of motion is begun.

### Complications

Avulsion fractures of the tibial tubercle rarely result in tibial deformity because they occur toward the end of growth. However, several authors have reported acute compartment syndrome of the leg after this injury (430). This may be because the tubercle is near the anterior compartment fascia, and bleeding from the fracture enters this compartment. Pape et al. (430) observed that compartment syndrome may be more frequent in patients who are managed by closed reduction or by percutaneous methods. Bolesta and Fitch (428) recognized this potential complication and performed prophylactic fasciotomy when anterior compartment swelling was present.

Posttraumatic genu recurvatum can occur in younger patients after tibial tubercle avulsion fracture. This is caused by premature arrest of the anterior aspect of the growth plate. Patients with more than 1 year of growth remaining should be observed for development of this deformity. Bilateral proximal tibial epiphysiodesis is generally the preferred procedure when deformity is mild. Greater degrees of deformity may necessitate proximal tibial flexion osteotomy to restore normal alignment (431).

## Patellar Fractures

Patellar fractures are much less common in children than in adults. This may be because the patella is largely cartilaginous until adolescence. The child's patella is also more mobile than the adult's and is subjected to less tensile force during quadriceps contraction. In adolescents the patellar anatomy approaches that of the adult, and the patella is more likely to be damaged by direct trauma. Osteochondral fractures have also been reported in 15% to 70% of children and adolescents sustaining acute patellar dislocations (408).

The diagnosis of patellar fracture may be more difficult in children than in adults. Palpation may reveal a defect, but palpation can be difficult to perform because of pain and tense hemarthrosis. Lack of function and abnormal movement of the extensor mechanism on physical examination are useful indicators of patellar injury. Radiographs can be difficult to interpret. Bipartite patella (i.e., secondary ossification center) may be painful and can be confused with nondisplaced fracture. The characteristic location of a bipartite patella—the superolateral portion of the patella—can be a clue to diagnosis. A fractured patella may be difficult to diagnose accurately due to incomplete

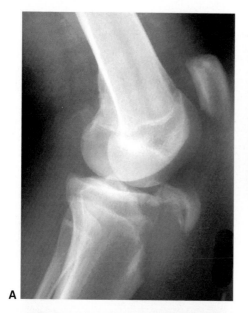

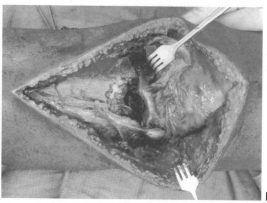

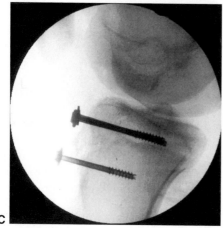

**Figure 33.71** Type III tibial tubercle fracture. **A:** The initial lateral radiograph of a 14-year-old boy who sustained a tibial tubercle fracture after landing from a jump in a basketball game. The radiograph shows complete displacement, with the fracture line extending into the articular surface of the tibial plateau. **B:** Intraoperative photograph showing exposure through a midline anterior knee incision. The typical massive soft tissue injury is illustrated, with tears of the medial and lateral retinacula and stripping of the anterior surface of the tibia. **C:** Lateral image intensifier view taken immediately after open reduction and internal fixation of the fracture.

ossification. The patellar sleeve fracture is a type of patellar fracture that is unique to younger children. The age range for patellar sleeve fracture is 8 to 12 years. This injury consists of an avulsion of the cartilaginous portion of the distal patella from the ossification center (432,433) (Fig. 33.72). Lateral radiographs may demonstrate only patella alta and a very small fragment of bone attached to the distal unossified cartilage. MRI can be diagnostic when there is doubt regarding the nature of the injury.

### Treatment

Treatment of patellar fractures in children is generally the same as for adults (434). The patella is a sesamoid bone that grows by apposition, so growth disturbance is uncommon. Nondisplaced fractures with intact extensor mechanisms may be treated by immobilization in extension for 4 to 6 weeks. Open reduction with internal fixation is indicated for displaced fractures. Stability may be achieved by means of the AO tension band technique with either nonabsorbable suture or wire.

## TIBIAL FRACTURES

Tibial fractures are the most common lower-extremity fracture in children, and account for 10% to 15% of all pediatric fractures (6,409). Many of these are so-called *toddler's fractures,* or low-energy nondisplaced fractures occurring from minor falls or twisting injuries. Motor vehicle accidents and high-energy injuries are more common in older children.

### Proximal Tibial Epiphyseal Fracture

Separation of the proximal tibial epiphysis is uncommon. This is probably because of the supporting ligamentous structures and the shape of the physis. The fibula buttresses the tibia laterally and the physis slopes downward anteriorly in the region of the tibial tubercle. The medial collateral ligament inserts on the metaphysis in addition to the epiphysis. Many of the musculotendinous units that span the knee do not insert on the proximal tibial epiphysis.

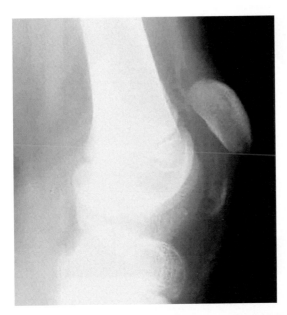

**Figure 33.72**  This lateral radiograph shows a patellar sleeve fracture in a 10-year-old child. Note the patella alta and the small osteochondral fragment 2 cm distal to the inferior pole of the patella.

Therefore, varus and valgus stresses are not transmitted to the tibial epiphysis.

The mechanism of injury to this epiphysis is usually direct force to the knee, as in a fall from a height, lawn mower injuries, or motor vehicle accidents. Hyperextension injuries from sports may also injure this region. Lawn mower injuries are seen in younger children, but most patients with tibial epiphyseal fractures are older than 12 years at the time of injury (435,436). Most proximal epiphyseal injuries are Salter-Harris type II fractures demonstrating posterolateral or posteromedial displacement. These are followed in frequency by type I separations. Hyperextension fractures threaten the popliteal artery because the artery is tethered to the posterior aspect of the tibia by its branches. The posterior branch passes under the arch of the fibers of the soleus muscle, whereas the anterior branch passes into the anterior compartment just distal to the growth plate (Fig. 33.73).

### Treatment

Management consists of closed reduction in most cases. After reduction, percutaneous pinning (Fig. 33.74) or cannulated screw fixation is recommended when the fracture is unstable, when vascular repair is necessary, or when early motion is required. Precise reduction is recommended because future growth may be impaired and residual deformity may not correct spontaneously. Displaced type III and IV fractures are intraarticular injuries. Also, precise reduction and internal fixation is advisable to preserve joint function and reduce the risk of premature physeal closure. These fractures should be followed closely for growth arrest, which occurs in 25% to 33% of patients regardless of the type of physeal separation (436).

### Complications

Vascular compromise requires prompt reduction and stable fixation. If pulses are abnormal, or the foot is cool or discolored, a vascular surgeon should be consulted and the integrity of the vessels evaluated with an angiogram or magnetic resonance angiography (MRA). In the absence of vascular findings, close observation after reduction is imperative. When a period of ischemia has exceeded 4 hours or vascular repair is required, prophylactic fasciotomy is recommended (74). This prevents reperfusion compartment syndrome from developing.

## Proximal Tibial Metaphyseal Fracture (Cozen Fracture)

Metaphyseal fractures of the proximal tibia occur most commonly in children between the ages of 2 and 8 years. The usual mechanism of injury is a valgus force applied to the extended knee producing an incomplete fracture of the tibia, with or without fracture of the fibula. The lateral cortex of the tibia may be buckled, impacted, or may undergo plastic deformation. Pronounced displacement is uncommon except in instances of high-energy trauma. This innocuous-appearing fracture is often in more valgus than one readily appreciates from the initial radiographs. A comparison

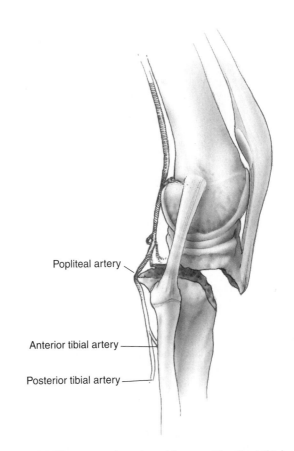

Popliteal artery

Anterior tibial artery

Posterior tibial artery

**Figure 33.73**  Proximal epiphyseal fracture. The distal tibial segment is displaced posteriorly, producing vascular occlusion of the popliteal artery.

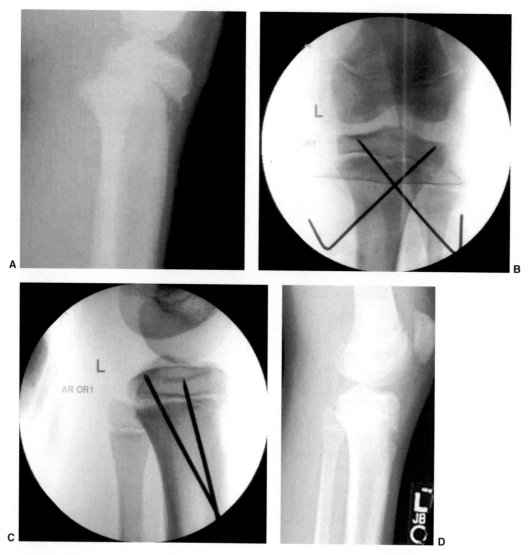

**Figure 33.74** Proximal tibial physeal injury. **A:** This initial lateral radiograph shows a displaced proximal tibial physeal fracture. **B,C:** Intraoperative images after closed reduction and internal fixation with two Kirchner wires. **D:** Lateral radiographs 6 weeks after injury show maintenance of anatomic alignment.

radiograph of the opposite tibia is helpful to determine the true deformity of the injured leg.

### Treatment

Management consists of closed reduction and cast immobilization. Occasionally, open reduction is necessary due to interposed periosteum and pes anserinus. After reduction, the knee is placed in extension. This position allows effective three-point cast molding to generate a varus force. The extension position also facilitates subsequent radiographic interpretation. The authors recommend that reduction should be within 5 degrees of the opposite intact tibia as judged by a line through the physis and a line down the tibial shaft. The cast is maintained until healing is complete, usually 6 weeks. Families should be counseled about the possibility of posttraumatic genu valgum. Displaced proximal tibial fractures in adolescents sometimes require

surgical stabilization to control alignment and expedite mobilization. During the 48 hours after closed reduction and casting, the extremity should be closely monitored for signs of excessive compartment swelling.

### Complications

Progressive valgus deformity of the leg frequently develops in children younger than 10 years who sustain this fracture (437) (Fig. 33.75). Close review of the initial postreduction radiographs occasionally reveals that an incomplete reduction was responsible for at least part of the deformity. However, nondisplaced and anatomically aligned fractures can also develop progressive valgus deformity (437). Increasing angulation begins several weeks after fracture and usually ceases by 12 months after fracture. The cause of this problem remains somewhat obscure, but it probably results from selective overgrowth of the medial tibial

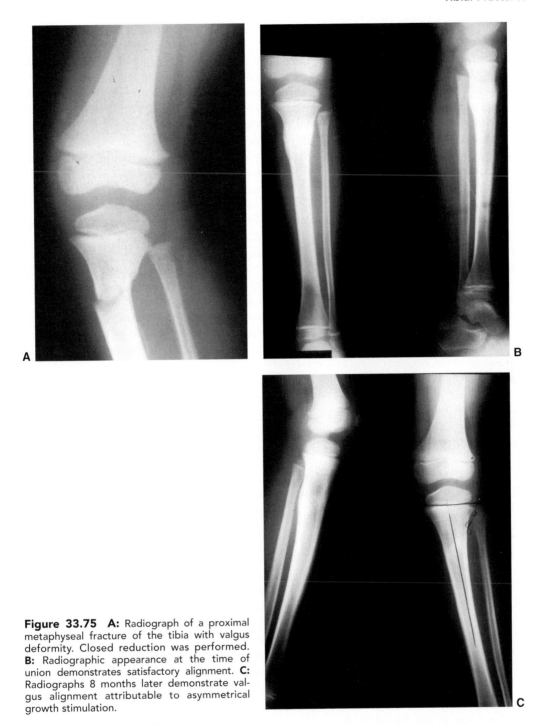

**Figure 33.75** **A:** Radiograph of a proximal metaphyseal fracture of the tibia with valgus deformity. Closed reduction was performed. **B:** Radiographic appearance at the time of union demonstrates satisfactory alignment. **C:** Radiographs 8 months later demonstrate valgus alignment attributable to asymmetrical growth stimulation.

physis (437). Overgrowth of the tibia with tethering by the intact fibula has also been postulated as a possible cause, but progressive valgus deformity can develop even when the fibula is fractured. Treatment of this deformity for children younger than 5 years consists of observation (438). Valgus deformity usually resolves spontaneously in this age group with the development of a slightly S-shaped tibia (438–440). Tibial osteotomy and hemiepiphyseal stapling have been reported for correction of more severe deformities (438,441). In the authors' opinion, osteotomy should be avoided because of the high risk of recurrent deformity

(439). Although rarely indicated, the authors recommend temporary hemiepiphyseal stapling to correct deformity in children older than 5 years who have a deformity greater than 15 degrees.

## Tibial Diaphysis Fractures

Fractures of the shaft of the tibia or fibula account for approximately 4% to 5% of all pediatric fractures (6,409). These fractures generally fall into three categories: (i) nondisplaced, (ii) oblique or spiral, and (iii) transverse and comminuted displaced fractures (442,443). In infants and young children, the tibial shaft is relatively porous and is more likely to bend, buckle, or sustain a nondisplaced spiral fracture than to fracture completely. The surrounding periosteum is strong and imparts stability to the fracture site. This limits displacement and shortening. In contrast, the adolescent tibial shaft is composed of more dense cortical bone and a thinner, weaker periosteum. Fractures in the adolescent age group are more often the result of high-energy trauma and are associated with greater fracture displacement, comminution, and slower healing rates than in younger children.

The remodeling potential of the tibia is limited. Infants and toddlers can correct approximately 50% of residual angulation with growth. In children older than 10 years, only 25% of the axial malalignment improves. Hansen and Grieff (442) reported only 13.5% correction of angular deformity with subsequent growth, but Shannak (443) demonstrated that one-third of children with more than 10 degrees of angulation at healing had persistence of the angulation at final follow-up assessment. In general, varus malalignment seems to remodel more completely than valgus deformity. Although long-term studies show that moderate angulation is well tolerated (444), the authors recommend that attempts should be made to maintain alignment within 10 degrees of angulation in any direction for children older than 6 years and within 15 degrees of angulation for younger children (442–445). Rotational deformity may not remodel, although external rotation deformity is better tolerated than internal rotation deformity (443).

Some shortening at the fracture site can remodel, but the ability to compensate for shortening decreases with age. Children younger than 5 years show the greatest capacity. However, growth acceleration greater than 5 to 7 mm is unusual (446). In a review of 142 tibial fractures, Shannak (443) reported an average of only 4.35 mm of growth acceleration. Comminuted and long spiral fractures displayed the greatest amount of overgrowth, including those that were treated with anatomic reduction and internal or external fixation. Overgrowth is not routinely seen in girls older than 8 years or boys older than 10 years.

### Nondisplaced Fractures of the Tibial Shaft

Nondisplaced tibial fractures are more common in younger children. Toddler's fracture is seen in the 1- to 4-year age group. A mildly traumatic event may have been observed, but often the child presents with an acute limp of unknown cause. Approximately 20% of these acutely limping toddlers have sustained occult fractures, and half of these fractures are in the tibia (447). Low-energy torsional forces, as when the child twists a leg, usually cause these fractures. The child limps or refuses to walk on the affected lower limb. Examination may reveal a point of tenderness or subtle swelling in the distal third of the leg, but often the examination is unremarkable. Radiographs

may show a fracture, but frequently the fracture line is not initially evident. Toddler's fracture is differentiated from pathology of the hip and femur by the child's ability to crawl, in addition to the finding of a normal range of motion of the hip. Infectious processes need to be considered in the differential diagnosis, but these can usually be diagnosed by the presence of fever and laboratory studies demonstrating increased sedimentation rate, C-reactive protein, and leukocyte count. A triphase bone scan may help establish the diagnosis when pain and limp are severe and the workup remains equivocal (448). MRI is more specific but usually requires sedation in these young patients. Treatment is initiated when fracture is suspected, and the diagnosis is usually confirmed 10 to 14 days later, when periosteal new bone has formed.

Treatment of nondisplaced fractures of the tibial shaft in all age groups consists of immobilization in a short-leg cast for distal fractures or long-leg cast for fractures proximal to the midshaft. Immobilization is continued until union has occurred, usually 3 to 4 weeks for toddlers and 6 to 10 weeks for older children.

### Oblique or Spiral Fractures of the Tibial Shaft

Isolated fracture of the tibia with an intact fibula is the most common tibial shaft fracture in the pediatric age group (445,449). A rotational or twisting force results in a spiral or oblique fracture at the junction of the middle and distal thirds of the tibial shaft. The most common mechanism of injury is indirect trauma such as sports accidents or falls. The intact fibula imparts stability, but it may have plastic deformation that interferes with reduction of displaced tibial fractures. The intact fibula may also contribute to the development of varus angulation.

Treatment consists of reduction and immobilization in an above-knee cast, with the knee flexed to 30 degrees and the ankle in 15 degrees of plantar flexion to minimize varus muscle forces and prevent recurvatum (445,449). Unstable, displaced fractures may require surgical stabilization with external fixation or flexible nails (Fig. 33.76). Angulation greater than 10 degrees in any direction should be corrected, except in children younger than 6 years, in whom 15 degrees may be accepted (442–445).

### Transverse and Comminuted Displaced Fractures of the Tibia and Fibula

Complete fractures of the tibia and fibula are more common in older children. These fractures result from high-energy trauma and are frequently unstable. Open fractures of the tibia are not uncommon and account for 4% of all tibial fractures in children and adolescents (450). Soft tissue damage and periosteal stripping predispose to more severe complications such as compartment syndrome, delayed union, and infection. Inherent fracture stability after reduction is variable.

Treatment of closed injuries is similar to that for oblique and spiral fractures. Closed reduction may be easier to

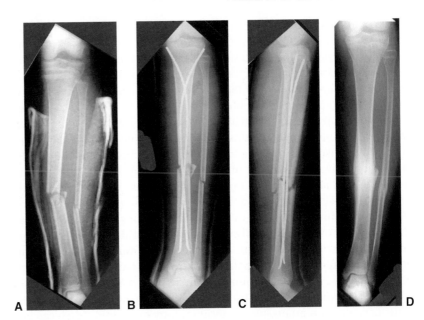

**Figure 33.76** Titanium elastic nail fixation for an unstable tibia fracture in a skeletally immature girl. **A:** This anteroposterior radiograph shows a transverse midshaft tibia and fibula fracture. This was a high-energy, closed injury with possible impending compartment syndrome. The surgeon elected to perform internal fixation. Because the proximal tibial physis was open, titanium elastic nailing was chosen over standard solid tibial nailing. **B,C:** Plain radiographs taken 1 week after internal fixation of the tibia fracture with antegrade titanium elastic nailing. **D:** Anteroposterior radiograph taken 6 months after injury. The fracture is healed in approximately 5 degrees of varus, within the range of a satisfactory result.

achieve when the fibula is fractured, but there is a tendency for the fracture to drift into valgus and procurvatum because of the greater muscle bulk posterolaterally in the leg. An above-knee cast is used for 4 to 8 weeks until initial stability has been achieved. Immobilization may then be continued with a patella-tendon-bearing cast until healing is complete. Final axial alignment should be within 10 degrees in any direction.

Unstable fractures may require surgical stabilization to maintain alignment or facilitate rehabilitation. The techniques for surgical stabilization are similar to the techniques discussed with regard to femur fractures. Fixation techniques include the use of flexible intramedullary nails introduced through the metaphysis, plates and screws, and external fixation. Additional indications for surgical stabilization of tibial fractures include associated head injuries, multiple trauma, floating knee, vascular injury, and open fractures requiring wound access.

### Open Fractures of the Tibia

The general management of open fractures has been discussed earlier in this chapter. Open fractures of the tibia in children are the result of high-energy trauma, with associated injuries in 25% to 50% of these patients (63,450).

**Treatment.** Initial management consists of administration of intravenous antibiotics and tetanus prophylaxis, followed by aggressive wound irrigation and debridement (63,450–452). Surgical intervention within 6 hours has been the standard recommendation (63). However, moderate delay of surgical management for lesser grades of open fracture may not be associated with an increased infection rate when antibiotics are administered early (64,65). Clean, grade I open wounds may be loosely closed over a drain after adequate debridement, but most wounds should be left open with repeated debridement

before soft tissue coverage (451). Debridement of devitalized bone is not necessary in children if the bone is clean and can be adequately covered with soft tissue (66). Surgical stabilization facilitates wound management. External fixation is generally preferred, but satisfactory results have been reported with plates and screws and with flexible intramedullary fixation (63,450–452).

**Complications.** Open fractures in children share many of the same complications reported in the literature for fractures in adults (71,453). Several authors have noted that age is the most significant prognostic indicator (72,452). Children younger than 12 years require less aggressive surgical management, heal faster, have lower infection rates, and have fewer complications than older children. Children older than 12 years have fracture patterns and complications that are similar to those in the adult population. However, limb salvage and reconstruction has a higher rate of success than in the adult population (454).

## FRACTURES OF THE ANKLE

Ankle fractures in children constitute approximately 5% of all pediatric fractures and one out of every six physeal fractures (17%) (3,29). The same mechanisms that produce spiral fractures of the tibial shaft in younger children may produce epiphyseal fractures of the ankle in older children. Tillaux and triplane fractures are specific injuries that occur as the distal tibial growth plate begins to close (455). Tillaux and triplane fractures are referred to as *transitional fractures* because they occur in adolescents during the transition to skeletal maturity.

The ossification centers of the distal tibial and fibular epiphyses appear between the ages of 6 months and 2 years. The medial malleolar extension forms at around 7 to

8 years of age and is complete by the age of 10. Closure of the distal tibial growth plate begins centrally, proceeds medially, and ends on the lateral side. This sequence of closure is responsible for transitional fracture patterns. The fibular physis lies at the level of the talar dome, and closes 1 to 2 years later than the distal tibia.

Ankle motion consists essentially of plantar flexion and dorsiflexion only, rendering this region susceptible to injury from twisting or bending forces. Medial stability is provided by the deep fibers of the deltoid ligament that attach the medial malleolus to the body of the talus. The lateral ligament complex consists of anterior and posterior talofibular ligaments and the calcaneofibular ligament. Strong ligamentous structures also bind the distal tibia to the fibula at the level of the joint. The anterior tibiofibular ligament is important in the pathomechanics of transitional fractures. Ligaments around the ankle principally attach to the epiphyses distal to the level of the growth plate. This anatomic arrangement transmits injury forces to bone and results in physeal fractures in older children and adolescents.

Diagnosis can be difficult in patients with nondisplaced or minimally displaced fractures. This is particularly true for distal fibular physeal separations and Tillaux fractures. Swelling may be minimal. Careful palpation usually reveals that the most tender area is the growth plate rather than the joint or ligaments. Displaced fractures are painful, with visible deformity due to the subcutaneous nature of the ankle joint. The position of the foot relative to the tibia provides evidence of the mechanism of injury and indicates the direction of manipulation required for reduction. Motor, sensory, and vascular assessments should be performed before reduction. Plain radiographs usually confirm the diagnosis and define the fracture pattern. CT scanning, with or without three-dimensional reconstruction, is useful for evaluation and management of transitional fractures. An MRI does not offer great advantage over plain radiography except to evaluate complications such as growth arrest (456).

Malleolar avulsion fractures are more common in younger children, whereas a variety of epiphyseal injuries may be seen in older children. Fractures with syndesmosis disruption are uncommon in children until late adolescence. The most common avulsion injury is avulsion of the tip of the lateral malleolus, followed by separation of the distal fibular physis (457).

## Classifications

Ankle injuries in children have been classified by mechanism of injury, by type of growth-plate injury, and by combinations of both systems (458,459). Classifications based on mechanism of injury have been proposed to help guide reduction, but these classifications have been formulated independently of clinical examination. Also, children rarely have comminution or syndesmosis disruption, which have poor prognoses in adult classification schemes. In children, the steps necessary for reduction are usually evident when the clinical examination of foot position is combined with the radiographic appearance. Classifications have also been proposed that combine mechanism of injury with the type of growth-plate injury, but these classifications can be confusing and difficult to remember. The authors agree with Vahvanen and Aalto (457), who stated: "The simultaneous use of the classifications based on both type of trauma and type of epiphyseal lesion for classifying ankle fractures in children has led to unsatisfactory and unnecessarily complex groupings. In children the mechanism of trauma can often not be identified, and experimental work, such as what Lauge-Hansen did to support the mechanism-of-trauma classification in adults, is lacking in children." Those authors subsequently proposed a simple classification to guide management and predict outcome. According to their system, ankle fractures in children can be classified into two categories (457):

Group I. Low-risk, including avulsion fractures and epiphyseal separations (Salter-Harris types I and II)

Group II. High-risk, including fractures through the epiphyseal plate (Salter-Harris types III, IV, and V) and transitional fractures

In this classification scheme, transitional fractures would be considered high-risk. The present authors prefer to consider transitional fractures as a separate category because of the distinct pathoanatomy of these injuries. Spiegel et al. (460) used a slightly different classification of high-risk and low-risk pediatric ankle fractures, with a third category for transitional fractures.

## Treatment

### Low-risk Fractures

This category includes avulsion fractures that do not involve the growth plate, and all Salter-Harris type I and II physeal injuries. Nondisplaced distal fibular physeal fractures are treated with a weight-bearing short-leg cast for 4 to 6 weeks. Children with nondisplaced, low-risk ankle fractures involving the tibia are placed in a short-leg cast and limited to non–weight-bearing activities for 2 to 3 weeks; they are allowed full weight-bearing activities thereafter. Union occurs at approximately 6 weeks after injury. Follow-up radiographs in the cast are recommended 7 to 10 days after initial treatment to ensure maintenance of alignment.

Displaced low-risk fractures are usually managed by closed reduction (Fig. 33.77). This can be attempted in the emergency room, but complete muscle relaxation may be required for successful manipulation. Following reduction, a residual physeal gap of greater than 3 mm may indicate the presence of entrapped soft tissue. This may lead to a greater risk of physeal closure unless open reduction is performed to remove interposed tissue (34). A flap of

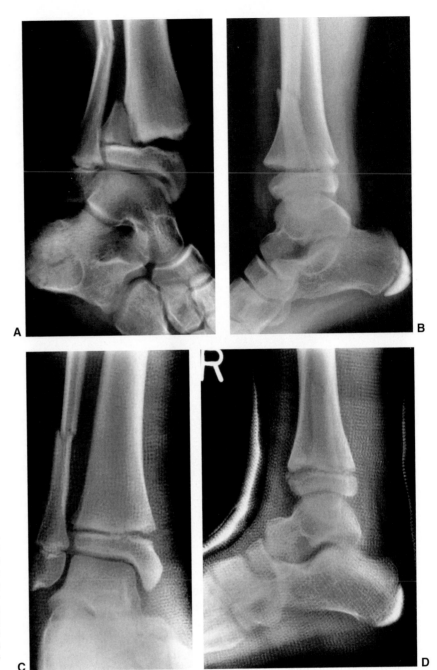

**Figure 33.77** Pronation and external rotation ankle fracture. **A:** This anteroposterior radiograph demonstrates a Salter-Harris type II fracture of the distal tibia. The Thurston Holland fragment is lateral. The fibular fracture is transverse and located well above the fibular physis. **B:** Lateral projection of the same injury. **C:** This fracture was treated with closed reduction and application of an above-knee cast. **D:** A lateral radiograph demonstrates acceptable alignment. This fracture was managed successfully with closed reduction.

periosteum is usually found, but tendons or neurovascular structures can also become interposed. Internal fixation with smooth pins or metaphyseal screws can be used after open reduction, but this is not required if the fracture is stable clinically. Minor amounts of displacement and angulation can be accepted, especially in children younger than 8 years, because these injuries are usually extraarticular and have good prognoses for resumption of growth. Immobilization in an above-knee cast (non–weight-bearing) is recommended for the first 3 weeks after closed reduction. A below-knee, weight-bearing cast is then applied until union is obtained. A total of 6 weeks of immobilization is usually sufficient.

### High-risk Fractures

These fractures include Salter-Harris type III and IV fractures. They are intraarticular, usually with joint instability. Hairline fractures in which the fracture line is 1 mm or less on all views can be managed by immobilization in a long-leg cast. Greater degrees of displacement require accurate reduction. Salter and others (461,462) have noted that reduction of these fractures must be "perfect" to restore the articular surface and minimize the risk of growth arrest. Closed reduction may be attempted for displaced fractures, but is rarely successful. Open reduction is usually performed with fixation using intraepiphyseal smooth Kirschner wires or small, cannulated screws (Fig. 33.78).

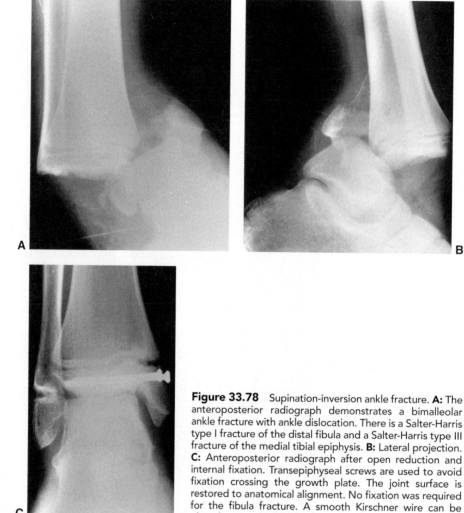

**Figure 33.78** Supination-inversion ankle fracture. **A:** The anteroposterior radiograph demonstrates a bimalleolar ankle fracture with ankle dislocation. There is a Salter-Harris type I fracture of the distal fibula and a Salter-Harris type III fracture of the medial tibial epiphysis. **B:** Lateral projection. **C:** Anteroposterior radiograph after open reduction and internal fixation. Transepiphyseal screws are used to avoid fixation crossing the growth plate. The joint surface is restored to anatomical alignment. No fixation was required for the fibula fracture. A smooth Kirschner wire can be placed across this physis, if needed, for ankle stability.

Lintecum and Blasier (463) described a technique of direct visualization and reduction through an anterior arthrotomy incision. This was accompanied by percutaneous fixation with cannulated screws inserted medially or laterally. Every effort should be made to avoid crossing the growth plate with internal fixation devices. However, restoration of articular integrity is more important than preserving growth at the ankle. The distal tibial and fibular epiphyses contribute only 5 to 7 mm of longitudinal growth per year. When unstable fractures occur in children older than 12 years, it is occasionally advisable to place internal fixation devices across the physis and perform epiphysiodesis to avoid subsequent angular deformity if sufficient growth remains.

### Transitional Fractures

These fractures are also high-risk and include the Tillaux and triplane injuries. These fractures occur as the growth plate is in the process of closing, so growth disturbance is not a concern. Restoration of articular congruity is the objective of treatment.

Tillaux fracture results from an external rotational force, and consists of avulsion of the anterolateral portion of the distal tibial epiphysis by the anterior tibiofibular ligament. This is a biplane Salter-Harris type III injury that can be difficult to detect on plain radiographs. Closed reduction is often successful and is performed by internal rotation and immobilization in an above-knee cast. The quality of reduction should be accurately documented. CT scans are helpful if plain radiographs are inconclusive. Open reduction with internal fixation is indicated when joint surface step-off after closed reduction is greater than 2 mm (455,464) (Fig. 33.79). An anterolateral approach is used, and the fracture is fixed with cancellous screws crossing the physis.

Triplane fracture is also caused by external rotation of the foot. On anteroposterior radiographs it appears as a Salter-Harris type III fracture, but on the lateral projection it appears to be a type II fracture (Fig. 33.80). The triplane fracture may be a two-part or a three-part fracture, but greater degrees of comminution can occur. The CT scans of two-part fractures reveal a single fracture line on the horizontal section through the epiphysis. Three-part fractures

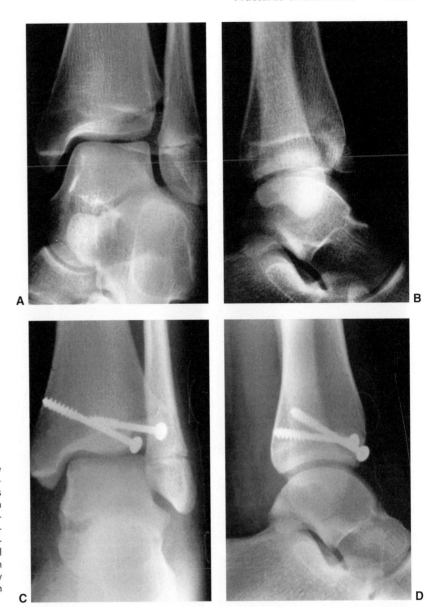

**Figure 33.79** Transitional fracture. **A:** The anteroposterior radiograph shows displacement of the anterolateral distal epiphysis (Tillaux fracture). **B:** The lateral radiograph demonstrates anterior displacement and rotation of the fragment. **C:** Postoperative radiograph after open reduction and internal fixation with cancellous bone screws. **D:** Lateral radiograph. In this instance, the screws can cross the physeal line because this injury occurred in an adolescent after the growth plate had begun physiologic closure.

demonstrate three radiating fracture lines ("Mercedes sign") on the transverse section through the epiphysis. An extraarticular type of triplane fracture can also occur when the fracture line exits through the medial malleolus beyond the articular surface (455). When seen early, initial management consists of attempted closed reduction with internal rotation and application of a long-leg cast. CT scan is recommended to confirm reduction (Fig. 33.81). Open reduction with internal fixation is indicated when joint surface incongruity exceeds 2 mm, when the patient

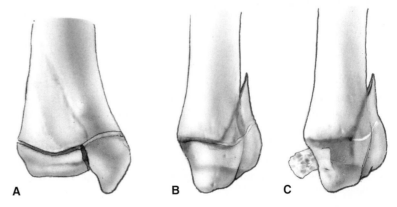

**Figure 33.80** Triplane fracture. **A:** On the anteroposterior radiograph, the fracture appears as a Salter-Harris type III fracture of the distal tibial epiphysis. **B:** On the lateral view, the fracture appears as a Salter-Harris type II fracture of the distal tibia. **C:** In the three-part triplane fracture, the anterolateral epiphyseal fragment is displaced as a separate fragment.

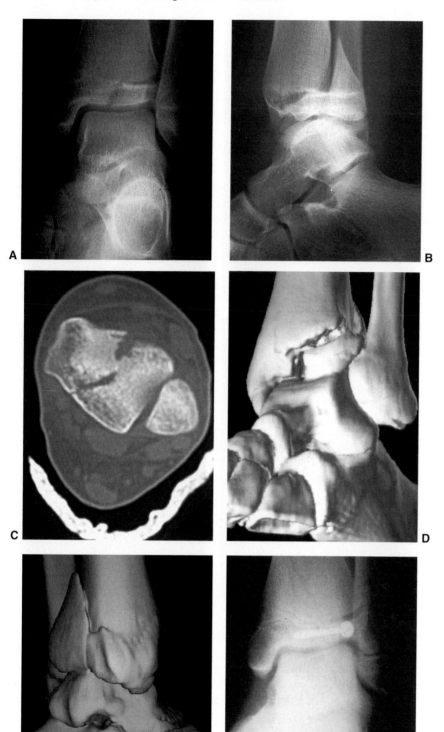

**Figure 33.81** Triplane fracture of the distal tibia in a 12-year-old girl with computed tomography (CT) evaluation. **A:** The anteroposterior radiograph shows a Salter-Harris type III fracture. **B:** The lateral radiograph shows an apparent Salter-Harris type II fracture. This indicates a triplane injury. **C:** CT through the epiphysis confirms a two-part fracture. **D,E:** Three-dimensional reconstruction demonstrates the fracture from the anterolateral and posteromedial views. **F:** Closed reduction was unsuccessful. Arthroscopically assisted open reduction was performed. The fracture was stabilized with a single anterolateral cannulated screw inserted percutaneously.

presents late, or after failed closed reduction (Fig. 33.82) (455,464,465). The anterolateral approach is satisfactory for reduction and fixation of two-part fractures. Three- and four-part fractures generally require anterolateral and posteromedial exposures. In rare circumstances in which articular congruity cannot be assured by direct visual inspection or radiographic evaluation, arthroscope-assisted reduction can be helpful.

## Complications

Complications of pediatric ankle fractures are related to joint incongruity and growth disturbance. Both of these are influenced by the adequacy of reduction. Kling et al. (462) reported that 19 of 20 Salter-Harris type III and IV fractures that were treated with accurate open reduction and internal fixation healed without growth disturbance. In contrast,

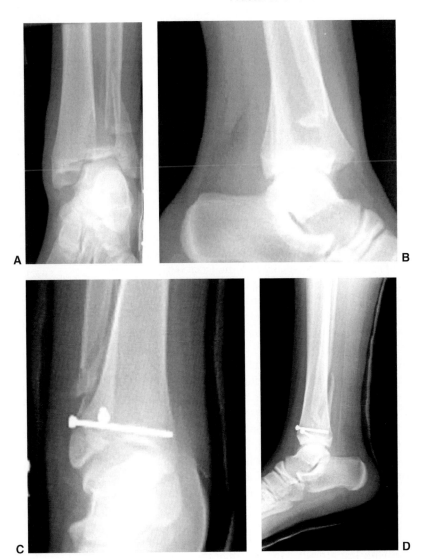

**Figure 33.82** Triplane fracture. **A,B:** Antero-posterior and lateral triplane fracture in a 14-year-old. **C,D:** Anteroposterior and lateral radiograph after closed reduction and internal fixation of the distal tibia. No fixation was chosen for the distal fibula.

five of nine similar fractures that were treated by closed means developed bone bridges. The distal tibia and fibula grow 5 to 7 mm per year. Therefore, leg-length discrepancy is rarely a major problem, except in younger children. The more common problem is angular deformity due to asymmetric growth arrest. Complete epiphysiodesis, with or without contralateral epiphysiodesis, should be considered as soon as growth disturbance is recognized. Other alternatives for management of growth arrest are discussed in the injury to the physis section of this chapter. When ankle deformity has occurred, transphyseal osteotomy is a successful method of correction (466).

Restoration of joint congruity is essential to prevent long-term disability (464,465). It is generally agreed that attempts should be made to reduce the step-off at the articular surface to 2 mm or less (467). The amount of gap that can be accepted without step-off is not clearly defined, but it may be slightly greater than 2 mm. Although every attempt should be made to restore articular surfaces without placing fixation across the physis, it is the authors'

opinion that maintenance of articular integrity is a higher priority than preservation of growth around the ankle.

## FRACTURES OF THE FOOT

Fractures of the metatarsals and phalanges of the toes are common, accounting for 7% to 9% of all pediatric fractures (3,6,29). However, fractures of the tarsal bones are uncommon in children and account for less than 1% of all fractures in childhood. Most of these are nondisplaced and may be an underreported cause of limping in toddlers (468,469). The rarity of fractures of the midfoot and hindfoot is attributed to the fact that the juvenile foot is very flexible, with a large component of cartilage until late adolescence. The ossification center of the medial cuneiform does not appear until 4 years of age. Some of the secondary ossification centers do not appear until 10 years of age or later. Therefore, there are numerous ossification centers in various stages of development. This can make radiographic interpretation difficult. Comparison radiographs of the opposite foot should be obtained when the diagnosis of a fracture is in question. A CT scan or MRI is often helpful to evaluate complex injuries.

## Anatomy

The calcaneus functions posteriorly with the distal first and fifth metatarsals to form a tripod for weight bearing and shock absorption. Ligamentous structures, joint capsules, bone geometry, and dynamic muscular forces maintain longitudinal and transverse arches. The talus is a complex bone that links the tibia to the foot and bears all the forces of body weight. It is composed of three parts: head, neck, and body. The talus is supported by the calcaneus, and the head of the talus articulates with the tarsal navicular bone. The cuboid laterally and the three cuneiforms medially constitute the distal row of tarsal bones.

The talus allows plantar flexion and dorsiflexion through the ankle joint and accommodates pronation-supination motion through the obliquely oriented subtalar joint. This articular function requires the talus to be largely covered with articular cartilage, leaving few avenues of entry for nutrient vessels. Therefore, the talus is particularly susceptible to osteonecrosis after fracture. The navicular is also susceptible to osteonecrosis and lies between the head of the talus and the cuneiforms. Idiopathic or posttraumatic necrosis of the navicular is a self-limited condition without long-term sequelae. However, this condition, also known as *Kohler disease*, can cause pain and have the radiographic appearance of a fracture.

The calcaneus supports the talus with a bony architecture that is much more cancellous and has a thin cortical wall with less articular covering than the talus. The calcaneus has a direct weight-bearing function through the complex subcutaneous septae and the thick skin of the heel pad. Anteriorly, transmission of longitudinal forces is achieved at the calcaneocuboid joint. The calcaneus is susceptible to compression failure and collapse of the outer cortical shell when subjected to direct impact, such as the force sustained in a fall from a height. In addition, the wedge-like lateral process of the talus may be driven into the superior region of the calcaneus between the posterior and middle or anterior surfaces of the subtalar joint. This intraarticular mechanism of injury is seen more often in adults and older adolescents. It results in division of the calcaneus into anterior and posterior fracture fragments.

## Talus Fractures and Dislocations

### Talar Neck Fractures

Fractures of the talar neck are thought to result from forced dorsiflexion. However, there is a 25% to 30% incidence of associated medial malleolar fractures, which suggests a supination component to the deforming force (470). Most talar neck fractures in children are nondisplaced. Most displaced fractures are from high-energy trauma. Displacement jeopardizes the tenuous blood supply of the talus because the neck region is the primary site of vascular penetration into the talus. Fortunately, there are numerous vascular anastomoses within the body of the talus. The principal blood supply penetrates the neck from within the tarsal canal that is formed by the sulcus of the calcaneus and the sulcus of the talus at the base of the neck. The other major blood supply is a deltoid branch from the posterior tibial artery that enters the medial body of the talus along the deltoid ligament (471).

Letts and Gibeault (472) proposed a classification for pediatric fractures of the talus, which is helpful to determine prognosis:

Type I. Minimally displaced fracture of the distal talar neck (the incidence of osteonecrosis is low)

Type II. Minimally displaced fracture of the proximal neck or body (the risk of osteonecrosis is low with this type also)

Type III. Displaced talar neck or body fracture (osteonecrosis is more likely)

Type IV. Talar neck fracture with dislocation of the body fragment (osteonecrosis is expected in these fracture-dislocations)

**Treatment.** Fractures that are minimally angulated (<5 degrees on the anteroposterior view) and displaced less than 2 mm can be managed closed (473). The foot is placed in slight plantar flexion to reverse the mechanism of injury. Immobilization in a non–weight-bearing below-knee cast is continued until union is evident, usually at about 6 weeks. Then a full–weight-bearing cast is used for an additional 4 to 6 weeks. Displaced fractures require open reduction with internal fixation. The anteromedial approach is preferred for fragment reduction. Kirschner wires or cannulated screws can be placed anterior to posterior or retrograde, depending on the location of the fracture (Fig. 33.83). Lag screws are recommended because they may eliminate displacement better than smooth wires (470). Cast immobilization with non–weight-bearing activities is maintained until union is achieved.

Osteonecrosis in children does not usually prevent healing of the fracture, and the long-term outcome may be satisfactory. Prolonged non–weight-bearing in a cast yields the best results when osteonecrosis has developed (473). Subchondral lucency may become visible in the body of the talus 6 to 8 weeks after fracture (Hawkins sign). This sign results from disuse osteopenia, and indicates that the body of the talus is vascularized.

### Osteochondral Fractures of the Talar Dome

Forced supination of the foot, as in a sprained ankle, may produce osteochondral fracture of the medial or lateral margin of the talar body. This lesion should be suspected when a "sprained ankle" does not improve as expected. Medial lesions tend to be posteromedial and result from inversion,

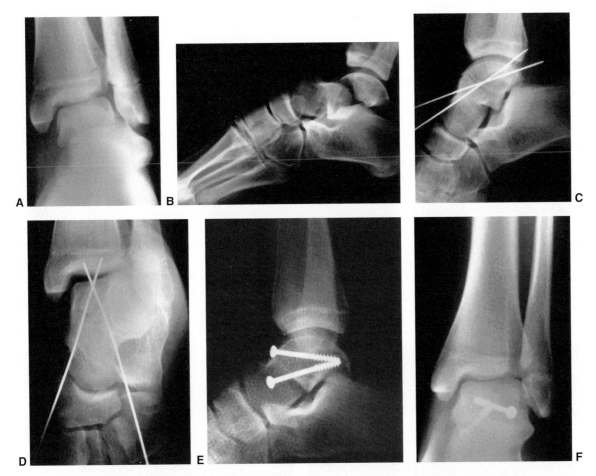

**Figure 33.83** Talus fracture. **A:** Anteroposterior radiograph of the ankle of a 13-year-old gymnast who injured her foot during a dismount. It appears that the head and neck of the talus are displaced laterally toward the fibula. **B:** The lateral projection shows a type III talus fracture with subluxation of the talonavicular joint. **C:** The intraoperative film shows provisional fixation with Kirschner wires. The fracture is reduced with plantar flexion of the foot. **D:** Another intraoperative anteroposterior view shows anatomical alignment of the talar neck with the body. The entry sites for the screws are in the nonarticular portion of the talar neck. **E:** The postoperative film shows cancellous screw placement. **F:** An anteroposterior radiograph shows restoration of the normal alignment of the ankle. Compared with the injury radiograph, there is no longer a prominence of the talar neck laterally.

plantar flexion, and external rotation. Lateral lesions tend to be anterolateral and result from inversion and dorsiflexion. Plain radiographs of the ankle mortise in plantar flexion and dorsiflexion may be necessary to visualize the fracture. A CT scan or MRI is useful in problematic cases.

Initial treatment after diagnosis is non–weight-bearing immobilization for 6 to 8 weeks. Many patients become asymptomatic in spite of persistent defects (474). Drilling and pinning, or removal of the loose fragment, is indicated if symptoms persist after a period of immobilization. This frequently can be accomplished arthroscopically.

### Lateral Process Fracture

Lateral process fractures of the talus may occur in a dorsiflexion-inversion or twisting injury to the foot. These fractures are easily missed because the initial symptoms are similar to those of an ankle sprain (475). A high index of suspicion and good quality anteroposterior radiographs of the talus are required for diagnosis. More commonly, the

patient presents with persistent symptoms after an "ankle sprain" (476). The diagnosis can be made with stress radiographs or CT scanning. Displaced fractures are often associated with other fractures.

Treatment consists of cast immobilization for nondisplaced injuries. When the patient presents late or an acute fracture is displaced, small fragments can be excised, but large fragments should be treated with reduction and internal fixation.

### Calcaneus Fracture

Fractures of the calcaneus may be extraarticular, sparing the subtalar joint, or intraarticular. Extraarticular fractures are more frequent in younger children (75% of cases), whereas intraarticular fractures account for most calcaneus fractures in adolescents and adults. Fracture of the calcaneus may be minimally displaced and can be easily overlooked in children. Delay in diagnosis occurs in 30% to 50% of cases

(477–479). Swelling, pain, or localized tenderness after a fall should alert the clinician to the possibility of calcaneus fracture. Multiple radiographic views are recommended for diagnosis. However, CT scan has evolved as the best method for imaging calcaneal fractures, both for the assessment of displaced fractures and occasionally for the diagnosis of occult fractures.

Schmidt and Weiner (479) classified calcaneal fractures in children as extraarticular, intraarticular, or those with loss of the insertion of the Achilles tendon and significant soft tissue injury (e.g., lawn mower injury). Intraarticular fractures in adults have been further classified by Sanders et al. (480) to help plan surgical management and predict outcome.

### Treatment

Nondisplaced and extraarticular fractures have good prognoses. Closed injuries are usually treated with 4 to 6 weeks of cast immobilization and progressive ambulation as tolerated. Displaced avulsion fracture of the tuberosity of the calcaneus is an extraarticular fracture that requires reduction (481). This may be accomplished by closed reduction using direct pressure over the Achilles insertion while the knee is flexed and the ankle is plantar-flexed to relax the posterior calf muscles. Open reduction with internal fixation is recommended if closed reduction is unsuccessful.

Long-term satisfactory results have been reported in younger children after nonsurgical management of intraarticular calcaneal fractures (482,483). However, open reduction and internal fixation is recommended for most displaced intraarticular fractures (484). The preferred approach is through a lateral, L-shaped incision, lifting the peroneal tendons within their sheath and protecting the sural nerve. The lateral wall of the calcaneus is folded down to reveal the medial side and allow elevation of depressed central fragments. Internal fixation of the posterior facet is achieved by placing subchondral cancellous screws into the medial sustentaculum. The lateral wall is buttressed with an H-shaped or Y-shaped plate (Fig. 33.84). Excessive

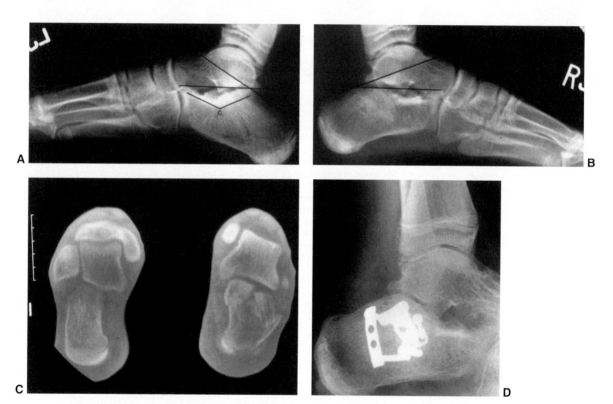

**Figure 33.84**   Calcaneus fracture. This 12-year-old boy injured both feet after jumping off a second-story deck. **A:** The lateral radiograph of his left foot reveals a minimal fracture of the body of the calcaneus. The Bohler angle is subtended by a line connecting the anterior process of the calcaneus to the highest part of the posterior articular surface, intersecting a line along the most superior point of the calcaneal tuberosity. This angle normally is 25 to 40 degrees, and usually is compared with the contralateral side. The crucial angle (c) is directly related to the shape of the overlying lateral process of the talus. In axial compression fractures, the lateral process is driven into the calcaneus, and the crucial angle is distorted. **B:** The radiograph of the more significantly injured right calcaneus shows flattening of the calcaneus, reduction in the Bohler angle, and flattening of the crucial angle. **C:** The computed tomography scan demonstrates displacement of the posterior facet of the calcaneus, with impaction of the lateral fragment and widening of the body of the calcaneus. The lateral wall is fractured. This injury should be treated with open reduction and internal fixation. **D:** After reduction of the posterior facet, a cancellous bone screw is placed through the lateral joint fragment into the sustentacular fragment, securing the subtalar reduction. The lateral wall can be buttressed with a contoured Y-shaped plate or a small H-shaped plate. The Bohler angle and the height of the calcaneus are restored.

comminution of the articular surface precludes this type of surgery (480). Long-term results in children are usually good.

## Midfoot Fractures and Tarsometatarsal Injuries

Injuries to the tarsometatarsal joints and fractures of the cuboid or cuneiform bones are rare in children but can have long-term sequelae (485,486). Fracture of the base of the second metatarsal is usually an indication of associated tarsometatarsal joint injury. These injuries are often misdiagnosed and may occur more commonly than recognized (487) (Fig. 33.85). The mechanism of injury may be direct impact but, more commonly, forced plantar flexion of the forefoot combined with a rotational force produces midfoot injuries (488). Heel-to-toe compression of the foot can also produce these injuries. Dislocations or displaced fractures require closed reduction. Percutaneous pinning and cast immobilization may be necessary to maintain reduction.

## Fractures of the Metatarsals

Metatarsal fractures are common in children, accounting for 5% to 7% of all pediatric fractures (3,6). The second, third, and fourth metatarsals are most commonly injured. The mechanism of injury producing metatarsal fracture is usually direct trauma or crush to the foot. Associated swelling can be significant and may cause compartment syndrome.

Fractures of the base of the fifth metatarsal are usually avulsion injuries. These injuries can cause diagnostic confusion. A transverse fracture at the junction of the metaphysis and diaphysis is called a *Jones fracture*. This fracture has a high incidence of nonunion. An oblique avulsion fracture through the tuberosity of the fifth metatarsal may be confused with the normal secondary ossification center of the apophysis or avulsion of the apophysis. The apophysis does not extend into the joint. Stress fractures may also occur at this location. Prolonged casting is frequently required for fractures at the base of the fifth metatarsal, and healing should be verified before resumption of activities.

Nondisplaced and minimally displaced metatarsal fractures can be immobilized in a below-knee cast for 4 to 6 weeks, with weight bearing as tolerated. Surgical treatment is indicated for open fractures, displaced fractures of the metatarsal heads, and displaced intraarticular fractures (Fig. 33.86). Kirschner wire fixation is usually adequate, but the pinning technique requires securing the metatarsophalangeal joint in a reduced position. If this is not done, extension contracture of the metatarsophalangeal joint can result in development of a prominent and painful metatarsal head. The wires are left in place for 3 to 4 weeks with non–weight-bearing immobilization, followed by weight bearing in a cast until union is complete.

Compartment syndrome of the foot should be considered when severe pain and swelling develop after injury. The inciting trauma is often substantial, such as a foot run over by a car or crushed by a heavy object. Fasciotomy is indicated if compartment syndrome is confirmed. Compartment syndrome of the foot can involve any of the four compartments: medial (i.e., abductor hallucis), central (i.e., flexor brevis, lumbricals, quadratus), lateral, and interosseous (489). Fasciotomy may be performed through a medial approach, with incision from the medial malleolus to the first metatarsal head. The neurovascular bundle

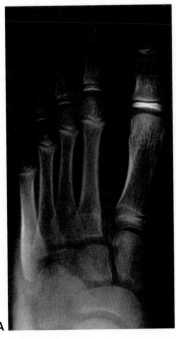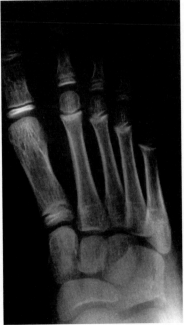

**Figure 33.85** Tarsometatarsal joint injury. A file cabinet landed on the dorsum of this 4-year-old girl's foot. **A:** There is widening between the first and second metatarsals, and a small fragment of bone is seen in the space. This suggests a partial incongruity, with lateral subluxation of the metatarsals. **B:** The contralateral foot shows a normal relation of the tarsometatarsal joint.

A           B

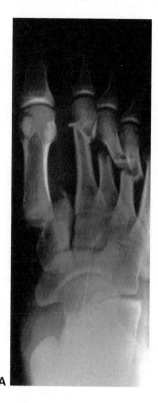
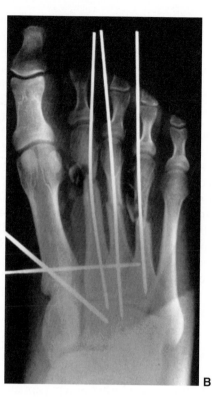

A        B

**Figure 33.86** Tarsometatarsal displacement. **A:** Anteroposterior projection of the foot of a 14-year-old boy who sustained a plantar flexion injury in a motor vehicle crash. There is complete dislocation of the first metatarsal–cuneiform joint and medial displacement. There are fractures of the second, third, and fourth metatarsal shafts. The ipsilateral tibial fracture was treated with intramedullary fixation. The swelling in the foot was attributed to the tibial shaft injury, and diagnosis of the foot injury was delayed. **B:** The postoperative anteroposterior radiograph demonstrates reduction and pinning of the fracture-dislocation.

is identified and released, including the tarsal tunnel. This releases the medial compartment and allows retraction for exposure of the central, lateral, and interosseous compartments from the plantar side. Alternatively, two longitudinal dorsal incisions are centered over the second and fourth metatarsals. Blunt and sharp dissection is performed through each interspace to release all compartments. The dorsal approach can also be combined with a medial incision to release the medial compartment.

## Fractures of the Phalanges

A direct blow usually causes these common injuries. Fractures of the phalanges can be treated with closed management, such as buddy taping and use of a hard-soled shoe. The exception to this is an open fracture, which most often occurs to the proximal phalanx of the great toe and may require open debridement and stabilization with Kirschner wires. The physis of the great toe's proximal phalanx underlies the nail bed and may be injured in the same fashion as a nail bed avulsion of the hand (490). Antibiotics should be prescribed if there is concern about a communicating skin breach. Obvious contamination requires debridement.

## REFERENCES

1. Irwin CJ, Cataldo M, Matheny A Jr, et al. Health consequences of behaviors: injury as a model. *Pediatrics* 1992;90:798.
2. Leading causes of death reports. In: *National conference for injury prevention and control.* Atlanta, GA: Center for Disease Control and Prevention, 2003.
3. Landin LA. Epidemiology of children's fractures. *J Pediatr Orthop* 1997;6B:79.
4. Jones IE, Williams SM, Dow N, et al. How many children remain fracture-free during growth? A longitudinal study of children and adolescents participating in the Dunedin Multidisciplinary Health and Development Study. *Osteoporos Int* 2002;13(12):990–995.
5. Khosla S, Melton LJ III, Dekutoski MB, et al. Incidence of childhood distal forearm fractures over 30 years: a population-based study. *JAMA* 2003;290(11):1479–1485.
6. Worlock P, Stower M. Fracture patterns in Nottingham children. *J Pediatr Orthop* 1986;6B:656–660.
7. Brudvik C, Hove LM. Childhood fractures in Bergen, Norway: identifying high-risk groups and activities. *J Pediatr Orthop* 2003;23(5):629–634.

### General Features of Fractures in Children

8. Currey J, Butler G. The mechanical properties of bone tissue in children. *J Bone Joint Surg* 1975;57A:811.
9. Jacobsen J. Periosteum: its relation to pediatric fractures. *J Pediatr Orthop* 1997;6B:84.
10. Skaggs DL, Loro ML, Pitukcheewanont P, et al. Increased body weight and decreased radial cross-sectional dimensions in girls with forearm fractures. *J Bone Miner Res* 2001;16:1337–1342.
11. Goulding A, Jones IE, Taylor RW, et al. Bone mineral density and body composition in boys with distal forearm fractures: a dual-energy x-ray absorptiometry study. *J Pediatr* 2001;139:509–515.
12. Ma D, Jones G. The association between bone mineral density, metacarpal morphometry, and upper limb fractures in children: a population-based case-control study. *J Clin Endocrinol Metab* 2003;88:1486–1491.
13. Lane J. Breakout session 2: fracture repair process. *Clin Orthop* 1998;355S:354.
14. Lieberman JR, Daluiski A, Einhorn TA. The role of growth factors in the repair of bone: biology and clinical applications. *J Bone Joint Surg* 2002;84A(6):1032–1044.
15. Murray D, Wilson-MacDonald J, Morscher E, et al. Bone growth and remodeling after fracture. *J Bone Joint Surg* 1996;78B:42–50.
16. Wallace MHE. Remodelling of angular deformity after femoral shaft fractures in children. *J Bone Joint Surg* 1992;74B:765.
17. Friberg K. Remodelling after distal forearm fractures in children II: the final orientation of the distal and proximal epiphyseal plates of the radius. *Acta Orthop Scand* 1979;50:731.

18. Hagglund G, Hansson L, Norman O. Correction by growth of rotational deformity after femoral fracture in children. *Acta Orthop Scand* 1983;50:87.

19. Gasco J, de Pablos J. Bone remodeling in malunited fractures in children. Is it reliable? *J Pediatr Orthop B* 1997;6(2):126–132.

20. Hougaard K. Femoral shaft fractures in children: a prospective study of the overgrowth phenomenon. *Injury* 1989;20(3):170–172.

21. Shapiro F. Fractures of the femoral shaft in children. The overgrowth phenomenon. *Acta Orthop Scand* 1981;52(6):649–655.

22. Wilde GP, Baker GC. Circumferential periosteal release in the treatment of children with leg-length inequality. *J Bone Joint Surg Br* 1987;69(5):817–821.

23. Carvell JE. The relationship of the periosteum to angular deformities of long bones. Experimental operations in rabbits. *Clin Orthop* 1983;173:262–274.

24. Houghton GR, Rooker GD. The role of the periosteum in the growth of long bones. An experimental study in the rabbit. *J Bone Joint Surg Br* 1979;61-B(2):218–220.

25. Beals RK. Premature closure of the physis following diaphyseal fractures. *J Pediatr Orthop* 1990;10(6):717–720.

26. Hresko MT, Kasser JR. Physeal arrest about the knee associated with non-physeal fractures in the lower extremity. *J Bone Joint Surg Am* 1989;71(5):698–703.

## Injury to the Physis

27. Bright RW, Burstein AH, Elmore SM. Epiphyseal-plate cartilage. A biomechanical and histological analysis of failure modes. *J Bone Joint Surg Am* 1974;56(4):688–703.

28. Dale GG, Harris WR. Prognosis of epiphysial separation: an experimental study. *J Bone Joint Surg Br* 1958;40-B(1):116–122.

29. Peterson HA, Madhok R, Benson JT, et al. Physeal fractures: part 1. Epidemiology in Olmsted County, Minnesota, 1979–1988. *J Pediatr Orthop* 1994;14(4):423–430.

30. Peterson HA. Physeal fractures: part 3. Classification. *J Pediatr Orthop* 1994;14(4):439–448.

31. Salter R, Harris WR. Injuries involving the epiphyseal plate. *J Bone Joint Surg Am* 1963;45:587.

32. Rang M. *Children's fractures*. Edited. Philadelphia, PA: JB Lippincott Co, 1983.

33. Gruber HE, Phiffer LS, Wattenbarger JM. Physeal fractures, part II: fate of interposed periosteum in a physeal fracture. *J Pediatr Orthop* 2002;22:710–716.

34. Barmada A, Gaynor T, Mubarak SJ. Premature physeal closure following distal tibia physeal fractures: a new radiographic predictor. *J Pediatr Orthop* 2003;23:733–739.

35. Houshian S, Holst AK, Larsen MS, et al. Remodeling of Salter-Harris type II epiphyseal plate injury of the distal radius. *J Pediatr Orthop* 2004;24(5):472–476.

36. Eid AM, Hafez MA. Traumatic injuries of the distal femoral physis. A retrospective study on 151 cases. *Injury* 2002;33:251–255.

37. Wattenbarger JM, Gruber HE, Phieffer LS. Physeal fractures, part I: histologic features of bone, cartilage, and bar formation in a small animal model. *J Pediatr Orthop* 2002;22:703–709.

38. Trueta J. The vascular contribution to osteogenesis. *J Bone Joint Surg Br* 1960;42:571.

39. Janarv PM, Wikstrom B, Hirsch G. The influence of transphyseal drilling and tendon grafting on bone growth: an experimental study in the rabbit. *J Pediatr Orthop* 1998;18(2):149–154.

40. Makela EA, Vainionpaa S, Vihtonen K, et al. The effect of trauma to the lower femoral epiphyseal plate. An experimental study in rabbits. *J Bone Joint Surg Br* 1988;70(2):187–191.

41. Hynes D, O'Brien T. Growth disturbance lines after injury of the distal tibial physis. Their significance in prognosis. *J Bone Joint Surg Br* 1988;70(2):231–233.

42. Gabel GT, Peterson HA, Berquist TH. Premature partial physeal arrest. Diagnosis by magnetic resonance imaging in two cases. *Clin Orthop* 1991;272:242–247.

43. Smith BGRF, Jaramillo D, Shapiro F. Early MR imaging of lower-extremity physeal fracture-separations: a preliminary report. *J Pediatr Orthop* 1994;14(4):526–533.

44. Noonan KJ, Price CT, Sproul JT, et al. Acute correction and distraction osteogenesis for the malaligned and shortened lower extremity. *J Pediatr Orthop* 1998;18(2):178–186.

45. Canadell J, de Pablos J. Correction of angular deformities by physeal distraction. *Clin Orthop* 1992;283:98–105.

46. Peterson HA. Review: partial growth plate arrest and its treatment. *J Pediatr Orthop* 1984;4(2):246–258.

47. Williamson RV, Staheli LT. Partial physeal growth arrest: treatment by bridge resection and fat interposition. *J Pediatr Orthop* 1990;10(6):769–776.

48. Birch JG. Surgical treatment of physeal bar resection. In: Eilert RE, ed. *Instructional course lectures*. Rosemont, IL: American Academy of Orthopaedic Surgeons, 1992:445–450.

49. Borsa JJ, Peterson HA, Ehman RL. MR imaging of physeal bars. *Radiology* 1996;199(3):683–687.

50. Carlson WO, Wenger DR. A mapping method to prepare for surgical excision of a partial physeal arrest. *J Pediatr Orthop* 1984;4(2):232–238.

51. Jackson AM. Excision of the central physeal bar: a modification of Langenskiold's procedure. *J Bone Joint Surg Br* 1993;75(4):664–665.

52. Lee EH, Chen F, Chan J, et al. Treatment of growth arrest by transfer of cultured chondrocytes into physeal defects. *J Pediatr Orthop* 1998;18(2):155–160.

53. Hasler CC, Foster BK. Secondary tethers after physeal bar excision. *Clin Orthop* 2002;405:242–249.

## Initial Management Considerations

54. Ismail N, Bellemare JF, Mollitt DL, et al. Death from pelvic fracture: children are different. *J Pediatr Surg* 1996;31(1):82–85.

55. Loder RT. Pediatric polytrauma: orthopaedic care and hospital course. *J Orthop Trauma* 1987;1(1):48–54.

56. Moulton SL. Early management of the child with multiple injuries. *Clin Orthop* 2000;376:6–14.

57. Teasdale G, Jennett B. Assessment of coma and impaired consciousness. A practical scale. *Lancet* 1974;2(7872):81–84.

58. Michaud LJ, Rivara FP, Grady MS, et al. Predictors of survival and severity of disability after severe brain injury in children. *Neurosurgery* 1992;31(2):254–264.

59. Letts M, Davidson D, Lapner P. Multiple trauma in children: predicting outcome and long-term results. *Can J Surg* 2002;45:126–131.

60. Fagelman MF, Epps HR, Rang M. Mangled extremity severity score in children. *J Pediatr Orthop* 2002;22:182–184.

61. Armstrong P, Smith J. Initial management of the multiply injured child. In: Letts RM, ed. *Management of pediatric fractures*. New York: Churchill Livingstone, 1994:27.

62. Gustilo R, Mendoza R, Williams D. Problems in the management of type III (severe) open fractures: a new classification. *J Trauma* 1984;24:742.

63. Kreder HJ, Armstrong P. A review of open tibia fractures in children. *J Pediatr Orthop* 1995;15(4):482–488.

64. Harley BJ, Beaupre LA, Jones CA, et al. The effect of time to definitive treatment on the rate of nonunion and infection in open fractures. *J Orthop Trauma* 2002;16:484–490.

65. Skaggs DL, Kautz SM, Kay RM, et al. Effect of delay of surgical treatment on infection in open fractures in children. *J Pediatr Orthop* 2000;20:19–22.

66. Bartlett ICS, Weiner LS, Yang EC. Treatment of type II and type III open tibia fractures in children. *J Pediatr Orthop* 1997;11:357–362.

67. Lee J. Efficacy of cultures in the management of open fractures. *Clin Orthop* 1997;339:71–75.

68. Patzakis MJ, Wilkins J. Factors influencing infection rate in open fracture wounds. *Clin Orthop* 1989;243:36–40.

69. Fischer MD, Gustilo RB, Varecka TF. The timing of flap coverage, bone-grafting, and intramedullary nailing in patients who have a fracture of the tibial shaft with extensive soft-tissue injury. *J Bone Joint Surg Am* 1991;73(9):1316–1322.

70. Mooney JF III, Argenta LC, Marks MW, et al. Treatment of soft tissue defects in pediatric patients using the VAC system. *Clin Orthop* 2000;376:26–31.

71. Hope PG, Cole WG. Open fractures of the tibia in children. *J Bone Joint Surg Br* 1992;74(4):546–553.

72. Blasier RD, Barnes CL. Age as a prognostic factor in open tibial fractures in children. *Clin Orthop* 1996;331:261–264.

73. Jones BG, Duncan RD. Open tibial fractures in children under 13 years of age: 10 years experience. *Trauma* 2003;34:776–780.

74. Mubarak SJ, Carroll NC. Volkmann's contracture in children: aetiology and prevention. *J Bone Joint Surg Br* 1979;61-B(3):285–293.

75. Bae DS, Kadiyala RK, Waters PM. Acute compartment syndrome in children: contemporary diagnosis, treatment, and outcome. *J Pediatr Orthop* 2003;21:680–688.

76. Gulli B, Templeman D. Compartment syndrome of the lower extremity. *Orthop Clin North Am* 1994;25(4):677–684.

77. Mubarak S, Owen C. Double-incision fasciotomy of the leg for decompression in compartment syndromes. *J Bone Joint Surg Am* 1977;59:184.

78. Willis RB, Rorabeck CH. Treatment of compartment syndrome in children. *Orthop Clin North Am* 1990;21(2):401–412.

79. Case RD. Haematoma block—a safe method of reducing Colles' fractures. *Injury* 1985;16(7):469–470.

80. Evans JK, Buckley SL, Alexander AH, et al. Analgesia for the reduction of fractures in children: a comparison of nitrous oxide with intramuscular sedation. *J Pediatr Orthop* 1995;15(1):73–77.

81. Juliano PJ, Mazur JM, Cummings RJ, et al. Low-dose lidocaine intravenous regional anesthesia for forearm fractures in children. *J Pediatr Orthop* 1992;12(5):633–635.

82. McCarty EC, Mencio GA, Green NE. Anesthesia and analgesia for the ambulatory management of fractures in children. *J Am Acad Orthop Surg* 1999;7(2):81–91.

83. McCarty EC, Mencio GA, Walker LA, et al. Ketamine sedation for the reduction of children's fractures in the emergency department. *J Bone Joint Surg* 2000;82A:912–918.

84. Proudfoot J. Analgesia, anesthesia, and conscious sedation. *Emerg Med Clin North Am* 1995;13(2):357–379.

85. Varela CD, Lorfing KC, Schmidt TL. Intravenous sedation for the closed reduction of fractures in children. *J Bone Joint Surg Am* 1995;77(3):340–345.

86. American Academy of Pediatrics Committee on Drugs. Guidelines for monitoring and management of pediatric patients during and after sedation for diagnostic and therapeutic procedures. *Pediatrics* 1992;89(6 Pt 1):1110–1115.

87. Kongsholm J, Olerud C. Neurological complications of dynamic reduction of Colles' fractures without anesthesia compared with traditional manipulation after local infiltration anesthesia. *J Orthop Trauma* 1987;1(1):43–47.

88. Bolte RG, Stevens PM, Scott SM, et al. Mini-dose Bier block intravenous regional anesthesia in the emergency department treatment of pediatric upper-extremity injuries. *J Pediatr Orthop* 1994;14(4):534–537.

89. Cramer KE, Glasson S, Mencio G, et al. Reduction of forearm fractures in children using axillary block anesthesia. *J Orthop Trauma* 1995;9(5):407–410.

90. Hoffman GM, Nowakowski R, Troshynski TJ, et al. Risk reduction in pediatric procedural sedation by application of an American Academy of Pediatrics/American Society of Anesthesiologists process model. *Pediatrics* 2002;109:236–243.

91. Green SM, Nakamura R, Johnson NE. Ketamine sedation for pediatric procedures: part 1, a prospective series. *Ann Emerg Med* 1990;19(9):1024–1032.

92. Green SM, Johnson NE. Ketamine sedation for pediatric procedures: part 2, review and implications. *Ann Emerg Med* 1990;19(9):1033–1046.

## Injuries of the Shoulder and Humerus

93. McBride MT, Hennrikus WL, Mologne TS. Newborn clavicle fractures. *Orthopedics* 1998;21(3):317–319; discussion 319–320.

94. Manske DJ, Szabo RM. The operative treatment of mid-shaft clavicular non-unions. *J Bone Joint Surg Am* 1985;67(9):1367–1371.

95. Ogden JA, Conlogue GJ, Bronson ML. Radiology of postnatal skeletal development. III. The clavicle. *Skeletal Radiol* 1979;4(4):196–203.

96. Denham R, Dingley A. Epiphyseal separation of the medial end of the clavicle. *J Bone Joint Surg Am* 1967;49:1179.

97. Waters PM, Bae DS, Kadiyala RK. Short-term outcomes after surgical treatment of traumatic posterior sternoclavicular fracture-dislocations in children and adolescents. *J Pediatr Orthop* 2003;23:464–469.

98. Goldfarb CA, Bassett GS, Sullivan S, et al. Retrosternal displacement after physeal fracture of the medial clavicle in children. *J Bone Joint Surg* 2001;83B:1168–1172.

99. Ogden JA. Distal clavicular physeal injury. *Clin Orthop* 1984;188:68–73.

100. Curtis RJ Jr. Operative management of children's fractures of the shoulder region. *Orthop Clin North Am* 1990;21(2):315–324.

101. Black GB, McPherson JA, Reed MH. Traumatic pseudodislocation of the acromioclavicular joint in children. A fifteen year review. *Am J Sports Med* 1991;19(6):644–646.

102. Allman FL Jr. Fractures and ligamentous injuries of the clavicle and its articulation. *J Bone Joint Surg Am* 1967;49(4):774–784.

103. MacDonald PB, Alexander MJ, Frejuk J, et al. Comprehensive functional analysis of shoulders following complete acromioclavicular separation. *Am J Sports Med* 1988;16(5):475–480.

104. Taft TN, Wilson FC, Oglesby JW. Dislocation of the acromioclavicular joint. An end-result study. *J Bone Joint Surg Am* 1987;69(7):1045–1051.

105. Walsh WM, Peterson DA, Shelton G, et al. Shoulder strength following acromioclavicular injury. *Am J Sports Med* 1985;13(3):153–158.

106. Goss TP. The scapula: coracoid, acromial, and avulsion fractures. *Am J Orthop* 1996;25(2):106–115.

107. Hardegger FH, Simpson LA, Weber BG. The operative treatment of scapular fractures. *J Bone Joint Surg Br* 1984;66(5):725–731.

108. Rowe CR. Prognosis in dislocations of the shoulder. *J Bone Joint Surg Am* 1956;38-A(5):957–977.

109. Hoelen MA, Burgers AM, Rozing PM. Prognosis of primary anterior shoulder dislocation in young adults. *Arch Orthop Trauma Surg* 1990;110(1):51–54.

110. Hovelius L. Anterior dislocation of the shoulder in teen-agers and young adults. Five-year prognosis. *J Bone Joint Surg Am* 1987;69(3):393–399.

111. Kawam M, Sinclair J, Letts M. Recurrent posterior shoulder dislocation in children: the results of surgical management. *J Pediatr Orthop* 1997;17(4):533–538.

112. Dobb MB, Luhmann SL, Gordon JE, et al. Severely displaced proximal humeral epiphyseal fractures. *J Pediatr Orthop* 2003;23:208–215.

113. Baxter MP, Wiley JJ. Fractures of the proximal humeral epiphysis. Their influence on humeral growth. *J Bone Joint Surg Br* 1986;68(4):570–573.

114. Beringer DC, Weiner DS, Noble JS, et al. Severely displaced proximal humeral epiphyseal fractures: a follow-up study. *J Pediatr Orthop* 1998;18(1):31–37.

115. Larsen CF, Kiaer T, Lindquest S. Fractures of the proximal humerus in children. Nine-year follow-up of 64 unoperated cases. *Acta Orthop Scand* 1990;61:255–257.

116. Shaw BA, Murphy KM, Shaw A, et al. Humerus shaft fractures in young children: accident or abuse? *J Pediatr Orthop* 1997;17(3):293–297.

117. Beaty JH. Fractures of the proximal humerus and shaft in children. *Instr Course Lect* 1992;41:369–372.

## Fractures and Dislocations Around the Elbow

118. Akbarnia BA, Silberstein MJ, Rende RJ, et al. Arthrography in the diagnosis of fractures of the distal end of the humerus in infants. *J Bone Joint Surg Am* 1986;68(4):599–602.

119. Davidson RS, Markowitz RI, Dormans J, et al. Ultrasonographic evaluation of the elbow in infants and young children after suspected trauma. *J Bone Joint Surg* 1994;76A(12):1804–1813.

120. Greenberg D, Jones J, Zink W, et al. Anatomy and pathology of the pediatric elbow using magnetic resonance imaging. *Contemp Orthop* 1989;19:345.

121. Skaggs DL, Mirzayan R. The posterior fat pad sign in association with occult fracture of the elbow in children. *J Bone Joint Surg* 1999;81A:1429–1433.

122. Gennari JM, Merrot T, Piclet B, et al. Anterior approach versus posterior approach to surgical treatment of children's supracondylar fractures: comparative study of thirty cases in each series. *J Pediatr Orthop B* 1998;7:307.

123. Morrissy RT, Wilkins KE. Deformity following distal humeral fracture in childhood. *J Bone Joint Surg Am* 1984;66(4):557–562.

124. Camp J, Ishizue K, Gomez M, et al. Alteration of Baumann's angle by humeral position: implications for treatment of supracondylar humerus fractures. *J Pediatr Orthop* 1993;13(4):521–525.

125. Biyani A, Gupta SP, Sharma JC. Determination of medial epicondylar epiphyseal angle for supracondylar humeral fractures in children. *J Pediatr Orthop* 1993;13(1):94–97.

126. Abraham E, Powers T, Witt P, et al. Experimental hyperextension supracondylar fractures in monkeys. *Clin Orthop* 1982;(171): 309–318.

127. Gartland JJ. Management of supracondylar fractures of the humerus in children. *Surg Gynecol Obstet* 1959;109(2):145–154.

128. DeBoeck H, De Smet P, Penders W, et al. Supracondylar elbow fractures with impaction of the medial condyle in children. *J Pediatr Orthop* 1995;15:444.

129. Campbell CC, Waters PM, Emans JB, et al. Neurovascular injury and displacement in type III supracondylar humerus fractures. *J Pediatr Orthop* 1995;15(1):47–52.

130. Parikh SN, Wall EJ, Foad S, et al. Displaced type II extension supracondylar humerus fractures: do they all need pinning? *J Pediatr Orthop* 2004;24(4):380–384.

131. Battaglia TC, Armstrong DG, Schwend RM. Factors affecting forearm compartment pressures in children with supracondylar fractures. *J Pediatr Orthop* 2002;22:431–439.

132. Green NE. Overnight delay in the reduction of supracondylar fractures of the humerus in children. *J Bone Joint Surg* 2001;83A: 321–322.

133. Iyengar SR, Hoffinger SA, Townsend DR. Early vs. delayed reduction and pinning of type III displaced supracondylar fractures of the humerus in children: a comparative study. *J Orthop Trauma* 1999;13:51–55.

134. Pirone AM, Graham HK, Krajbich JI. Management of displaced extension-type supracondylar fractures of the humerus in children. *J Bone Joint Surg Am* 1988;70(5):641–650.

135. Zionts LE, McKellop HA, Hathaway R. Torsional strength of pin configurations used to fix supracondylar fractures of the humerus in children. *J Bone Joint Surg Am* 1994;76(2):253–256.

136. Lee SS, Hahar AT, Miesen BS, et al. Displaced pediatric supracondylar humerus fractures: biomechanical analysis of percutaneous pinning techniques. *J Pediatr Orthop* 2002;22:440–443.

137. Skaggs DL, Cluck MW, Mostofi A, et al. Lateral-entry pin fixation in the management of supracondylar fractures in children. *J Bone Joint Surg* 2004;86A:702–707.

138. Garbuz DS, Leitch K, Wright JG. The treatment of supracondylar fractures in children with an absent radial pulse. *J Pediatr Orthop* 1996;16(5):594–596.

139. Shaw BA, Kasser JR, Emans JB, et al. Management of vascular injuries in displaced supracondylar humerus fractures without arteriography. *J Orthop Trauma* 1990;4(1):25–29.

140. Flynn JC, Matthews JG, Benoit RL. Blind pinning of displaced supracondylar fractures of the humerus in children. Sixteen years' experience with long-term follow-up. *J Bone Joint Surg Am* 1974;56(2):263–272.

141. Sabharwal S, Tredwell SJ, Beauchamp RD, et al. Management of pulseless pink hand in pediatric supracondylar fractures of humerus. *J Pediatr Orthop* 1997;17(3):303–310.

142. Royce RO, Dutkowsky JP, Kasser JR, et al. Neurologic complications after K-wire fixation of supracondylar humerus fractures in children. *J Pediatr Orthop* 1991;11(2):191–194.

143. Rasool MN. Ulnar nerve injury after K-wire fixation of supracondylar humerus fractures in children. *J Pediatr Orthop* 1998; 18(5):686–690.

144. Amillo S, Mora G. Surgical management of neural injuries associated with elbow fractures in children. *J Pediatr Orthop* 1999; 19:573–577.

145. Gurkan I, Bayrakci K, Tasbas B, et al. Posterior instability of the shoulder after supracondylar fractures recovered with cubitus varus deformity. *J Pediatr Orthop* 2002;22:198–202.

146. Abe M, Ishizu T, Nagaoka T, et al. Epiphyseal separation of the distal end of the humeral epiphysis: a follow-up note. *J Pediatr Orthop* 1995;15(4):426–434.

147. Davids JR, Maguire MF, Mubarak SJ, et al. Lateral condylar fracture of the humerus following posttraumatic cubitus varus. *J Pediatr Orthop* 1994;14(4):466–470.

148. Voss FR, Kasser JR, Trepman E, et al. Uniplanar supracondylar humeral osteotomy with preset Kirschner wires for posttraumatic cubitus varus. *J Pediatr Orthop* 1994;14(4):471–478.

149. Wong HK, Lee EH, Balasubramaniam P. The lateral condylar prominence: a complication of supracondylar osteotomy for cubitus varus. *J Bone Joint Surg* 1990;72B:859–861.

150. Ring D, Waters PM, Hotchkiss RN, et al. Pediatric floating elbow. *J Pediatr Orthop* 2001;21:456–459.

151. Blakemore LC, Cooperman DR, Thompson GH, et al. Compartment syndrome in ipsilateral humerus and forearm fractures in children. *Clin Orthop* 2000;376:33–38.

152. Roposch A, Reis M, Molina M, et al. Supracondylar fractures of the humerus associated with ipsilateral forearm fractures in children: a report of forty-seven cases. *J Pediatr Orthop* 2001;21: 307–312.

153. Tabak AY, Celebi L, Murath HH, et al. Closed reduction and percutaneous fixation of supracondylar fracture of the humerus and ipsilateral fracture of the forearm in children. *J Bone Joint Surg Br* 2003;85(8):1169–1172.

154. Ruiz AL, Kealey WDC, Cowie HG. Percutaneous pin fixation of intercondylar fractures in young children. *J Pediatr Orthop* 2001;10: 211–213.

155. Kanellopoulos AD, Yiannakopoulous CK. Closed reduction and percutaneous stabilization of pediatric T-condylar fractures of the humerus. *J Pediatr Orthop* 2004;24:13–16.

156. Re PR, Waters PM, Hresko T. T-condylar fractures of the distal humerus in children and adolescents. *J Pediatr Orthop* 1999; 19(3):313–318.

157. McKee MD, Kim J, Kebaish K, et al. Functional outcomes after open supracondylar fractures of the humerus. *J Bone Joint Surg* 2000;82B:646–651.

158. Jarvis JG, D'Astous JL. The pediatric T-supracondylar fracture. *J Pediatr Orthop* 1984;4(6):697–699.

159. DeLee JC, Wilkins KE, Rogers LF, et al. Fracture-separation of the distal humeral epiphysis. *J Bone Joint Surg Am* 1980;62(1): 46–51.

160. Skak SV, Olsen SD, Smaabrekke A. Deformity after fracture of the lateral humeral condyle in children. *J Pediatr Orthop* 2001;10B: 142–152.

161. Pritchett JW. Growth and predictions of growth of the upper extremity. *J Bone Joint Surg* 1988;70A:520–525.

162. Mirsky EC, Karas EH, Weiner LS. Lateral condyle fractures in children: evaluation of classification and treatment. *J Orthop Trauma* 1997;11(2):117–120.

163. Jakob R, Fowles JV, Rang M, et al. Observations concerning fractures of the lateral humeral condyle in children. *J Bone Joint Surg* 1975;57B:430–436.

164. Thonell S, Mortensson W, Thomasson B. Prediction of the stability of minimally displaced fractures of the lateral humeral condyle. *Acta Radiol* 1988;29(3):367–370.

165. Flynn JC, Richards JF Jr, Saltzman RI. Prevention and treatment of non-union of slightly displaced fractures of the lateral humeral condyle in children. An end-result study. *J Bone Joint Surg Am* 1975;57(8):1087–1092.

166. Horn BD, Herman MJ, Crisci K, et al. Fractures of the lateral humeral condyle: role of the cartilage hinge in fracture stability. *J Pediatr Orthop* 2002;22:8–11.

167. Ippolito E, Tudisco C, Farsetti P, et al. Fracture of the humeral condyles in children: 49 cases evaluated after 18–45 years. *Acta Orthop Scand* 1996;67(2):173–178.

168. Launay F, Leet AI, Jacopin S, et al. Lateral humeral condyle fractures in children: a comparison of two approaches to treatment. *J Pediatr Orthop* 2004;24(4):385–391.

169. Mintzer CM, Waters PM, Brown DJ, et al. Percutaneous pinning in the treatment of displaced lateral condyle fractures. *J Pediatr Orthop* 1994;14(4):462–465.

170. Dhillon KS, Sengupta S, Singh BJ. Delayed management of fracture of the lateral humeral condyle in children. *Acta Orthop Scand* 1988;59(4):419–424.

171. Wattenbarger JM, Gerardi DO, Johnston CE. Late open reduction internal fixation of lateral condyle fractures. *J Pediatr Orthop* 2002;22:394–398.

172. Flynn JC. Nonunion of slightly displaced fractures of the lateral humeral condyle in children: an update. *J Pediatr Orthop* 1989; 9(6):691–696.

173. Masada K, Kawai H, Kawabata H, et al. Osteosynthesis for old, established non-union of the lateral condyle of the humerus. *J Bone Joint Surg* 1990;72A:33–40.

174. Badelon O, Bensahel H, Mazda K, et al. Lateral humeral condylar fractures in children: a report of 47 cases. *J Pediatr Orthop* 1988;8(1):31–34.

175. Nwakama AC, Peterson HA, Shaughnessy WJ. Fishtail deformity following fracture of the distal humerus in children: historical review, case presentations, discussion of etiology, and thoughts on treatment. *J Pediatr Orthop* 2000;9B:309–318.

176. Josefsson PO, Danielsson LG. Epicondylar elbow fracture in children. 35-year follow-up of 56 unreduced cases. *Acta Orthop Scand* 1986;57(4):313–315.

177. Farsetti P, Potenza V, Caterini R, et al. Long-term results of treatment of fractures of the medial epicondyle in children. *J Bone Joint Surg* 2001;83A:1299–1305.

178. Woods GW, Tullos HS. Elbow instability and medial epicondyle fractures. *Am J Sports Med* 1977;5(1):23–30.

179. Dunn P, Ravn P, Hansen L, et al. Osteosynthesis of medial humeral epicondyle fractures in children: 8-year follow-up of 33 cases. *Acta Orthop Scand* 1994;654:439.

180. Leet AI, Young C, Hoffer MM. Medial condyle fractures of the humerus in children. *J Pediatr Orthop* 2002;22:2–7.

181. Evans M, Graham H. Radial neck fracture in children: a management algorithm. *J Pediatr Orthop B* 1999;8:93.

182. D'Souza S, Vaishya MS, Klenerman L. Management of radial neck fractures in children: a retrospective analysis of one hundred patients. *J Pediatr Orthop* 1993;13:232–238.

183. Vocke AK, Von Laer L. Displaced fractures of the radial neck in children: long-term results and prognosis of conservative treatment. *J Pediatr Orthop* 1998;7B:217–222.

184. Neher CG, Torch MA. New reduction technique for severely displaced pediatric radial neck fractures. *J Pediatr Orthop* 2003;23:626–628.

185. Evans MC, Graham HK. Radial neck fractures in children: a management algorithm. *J Pediatr Orthop* 1999;8:93–99.

186. Gonzalez-Herranz P, Alvarez-Romera A, Burgos J, et al. Displaced radial neck fractures in children treated by closed intramedullary pinning (Metaizeau technique). *J Pediatr Orthop* 1997;17(3):325–331.

187. Stiefel D, Meuli M, Altermatt S. Fractures of the neck of the radius in children: early experience with intramedullary pinning. *J Bone Joint Surg* 2001;83B:536–541.

188. Evans MC, Graham HK. Olecranon fractures in children; Part I: a clinical review; Part II: a new classification and management algorithm. *J Pediatr Orthop* 1999;19:559–569.

189. Gaddy BC, Strecker WB, Schoenecker PL. Surgical treatment of displaced olecranon fractures in children. *J Pediatr Orthop* 1997;17(3):321–324.

190. Graves SC, Canale ST. Fractures of the olecranon in children: long-term follow-up. *J Pediatr Orthop* 1993;13:239–241.

191. Rowland SA, Burkhart SS. Tension band wiring of olecranon fractures. A modification of the AO technique. *Clin Orthop* 1992;277:238–242.

192. Gicquel P, Giacomelli M-C, Karger C, et al. Surgical technique and preliminary results of a new fixation concept for olecranon fractures in children. *J Pediatr Orthop* 2003;23:398–401.

193. Carlioz H, Abols Y. Posterior dislocation of the elbow in children. *J Pediatr Orthop* 1984;4(1):8–12.

194. Bae DS, Waters PM. Surgical treatment of posttraumatic elbow contracture in adolescents. *J Pediatr Orthop* 2001;21:580–584.

195. Wu CC. Posttraumatic contracture of elbow treated with intraarticular technique. *Arch Orthop Trauma Surg* 2003;123:494–500.

196. Salter RB, Zaltz C. Anatomic investigations of the mechanism of injury and pathologic anatomy of "pulled elbow" in young children. *Clin Orthop* 1971;77:134–143.

## Forearm and Wrist Fractures

197. Tredwell SJ, Van Peteghem K, Clough M. Pattern of forearm fractures in children. *J Pediatr Orthop* 1984;4(5):604–608.

198. Lincoln TL, Mubarak SJ. "Isolated" traumatic radial-head dislocation. *J Pediatr Orthop* 1994;14:454–457.

199. Smith FM. Children's elbow injuries: fractures and dislocations. *Clin Orthop* 1967;50:7–30.

200. Letts M, Locht R, Wiens J. Monteggia fracture-dislocations in children. *J Bone Joint Surg Br* 1985;67(5):724–727.

201. Bado JL. The Monteggia lesion. *Clin Orthop* 1967;50:71–86.

202. Wiley JJ, Galey JP. Monteggia injuries in children. *J Bone Joint Surg* 1985;67B:728–731.

203. Ring D, Waters PM. Operative fixation of Monteggia fractures in children. *J Bone Joint Surg Br* 1996;78(5):734–739.

204. Seel MJ, Peterson HA. Management of chronic posttraumatic radial head dislocation in children. *J Pediatr Orthop* 1999;19(3):306–312.

205. Horii E, Nakamura R, Koh S, et al. Surgical treatment for chronic radial head dislocation. *J Bone Joint Surg* 2002;84A:1183–1188.

206. Inoue G, Shionoya K. Corrective ulnar osteotomy for malunited anterior Monteggia lesions in children. *Acta Orthop Scand* 1998;69(1):73–76.

207. Walsh HP, McLaren CA, Owen R. Galeazzi fractures in children. *J Bone Joint Surg Br* 1987;69(5):730–733.

208. Letts M, Rowhani N. Galeazzi-equivalent injuries of the wrist in children. *J Pediatr Orthop* 1993;13(5):561–566.

209. Ray TD, Tessler RH, Dell PC. Traumatic ulnar physeal arrest after distal forearm fractures in children. *J Pediatr Orthop* 1996;16(2):195–200.

210. Sanders WE, Heckman JD. Traumatic plastic deformation of the radius and ulna. A closed method of correction of deformity. *Clin Orthop* 1984;188:58–67.

211. Vorlat P, De Boeck H. Bowing fractures of the forearm in children: a long-term followup. *Clin Orthop* 2003;413:233–237.

212. Evans E. Fractures of the radius and ulna. *J Bone Joint Surg Br* 1951;33:548–561.

213. Johari AN, Sinha M. Remodeling of forearm fractures in children. *J Pediatr Orthop* 1999;8:84–87.

214. Tarr RR, Garfinkel AI, Sarmiento A. The effects of angular and rotational deformities of both bones of the forearm. *J Bone Joint Surg* 1984;66A:65–70.

215. Schwartz N, Pienaar S, Schwarz AF, et al. Refracture of the forearm in children. *J Bone Joint Surg* 1996;78B:740–744.

216. Younger AS, Tredwell SJ, Mackenzie WG, et al. Accurate prediction of outcome after pediatric forearm fracture. *J Pediatr Orthop* 1994;14(2):200–206.

217. Creasman C, Zaleske DJ, Ehrlich MG. Analyzing forearm fractures in children. The more subtle signs of impending problems. *Clin Orthop* 1984;188:40–53.

218. Price CT, Scott DS, Kurzner ME, et al. Malunited forearm fractures in children. *J Pediatr Orthop* 1990;10:705–712.

219. McHenry TP, Pierce WA, Lais RL, et al. Effect of displacement of ulna-shaft fractures on forearm rotation: a cadaveric model. *Am J Orthop* 2002;31:420–424.

220. Tynan M, Fornalski S, McMahon PJ, et al. The effects of ulnar axial malalignment on supination and pronation. *J Bone Joint Surg* 2000;82A:1726–1731.

221. Sarmiento A, Ebramzadeh E, Brys D, et al. Angular deformities and forearm function. *J Orthop Res* 1992;10(1):121–133.

222. Daruwalla JS. A study of radioulnar movements following fractures of the forearm in children. *Clin Orthop* 1979;139:114–120.

223. Carey PJ, Alburger PD, Betz RR, et al. Both-bone forearm fractures in children. *Orthopedics* 1992;15(9):1015–1019.

224. Walker JL, Rang M. Forearm fractures in children: cast treatment with the elbow extended. *J Bone Joint Surg* 1991;73B:299–301.

225. Chan C, Meads B, Nicol R. Remanipulation of forearm fractures in children. *N Z Med J* 1977;110:249.

226. Voto SJ, Weiner DS, Leighley B. Redisplacement after closed reduction of forearm fractures in children. *J Pediatr Orthop* 1990;10(1):79–84.

227. Fuller DJ, McCullough CJ. Malunited fractures of the forearm in children. *J Bone Joint Surg Br* 1982;64(3):364–367.

228. Thompson GH, Wilber JH, Marcus RE. Internal fixation of fractures in children and adolescents. A comparative analysis. *Clin Orthop* 1984;188:10–20.

229. Luhmann SJ, Schootman M, Schoenecker PL, et al. Complications and outcomes of open pediatric forearm fractures. *J Pediatr Orthop* 2004;24:1–6.

230. Greenbaum B, Zionts LE, Ebramzadeh E. Open fractures of the forearm in children. *J Orthop Trauma* 2001;15:111–118.

231. Luhman SJ, Schootman M, Schoenecker PL, et al. Complications and outcomes of open pediatric forearm fractures. *J Pediatr Orthop* 2004;24:1–6.

232. Stanitski CL, Micheli LJ. Simultaneous ipsilateral fractures of the arm and forearm in children. *Clin Orthop* 1980;153:218–222.

233. Harrington P, Sharif I, Fogarty EE, et al. Management of the floating elbow injury in children. *Arch Orthop Trauma Surg* 2000;120:205–208.

234. Verstreken L, Delronge G, Lamoureux J. Shaft forearm fractures in children: intramedullary nailing with immediate motion: a preliminary report. *J Pediatr Orthop* 1988;8(4):450–453.

235. Shoemaker SD, Comstock CP, Mubarak SJ, et al. Intramedullary Kirshner wire fixation of open or unstable forearm fractures in children. *J Pediatr Orthop* 1999;19:329–337.

236. Van der Reis WL, Otsuka NY, Moroz P, et al. Intramedullary nailing versus plate fixation for unstable forearm fractures in children. *J Pediatr Orthop* 1998;18:9–13.

237. Yung PSH, Lam CY, Ng BKW, et al. Percutaneous transphyseal intramedullary Kirschner wire pinning: a safe and effective procedure for treatment of displaced diaphyseal forearm fracture in children. *J Pediatr Orthop* 2004;24:7–12.

238. Yuan PS, Pring ME, Gaynor TP, et al. Compartment syndrome following intramedullary fixation of pediatric forearm fractures. *J Pediatr Orthop* 2004;24(4):370–375.

239. Flynn JM, Waters PM. Single-bone fixation of both-bone forearm fractures. *J Pediatr Orthop* 1996;16(5):655–659.

240. Kirkos JM, Beslikas T, Kapras EA, et al. Surgical treatment of unstable diaphyseal both-bone forearm fractures in children with single fixation of the radius. *Injury* 2000;31:591–596.

241. Deluca PA, Lindsey RW, Ruwe PA. Refracture of bones of the forearm after the removal of compression plates. *J Bone Joint Surg Am* 1988;70(9):1372–1376.

242. Hogstrom H, Nilsson BE, Willner S. Correction with growth following diaphyseal forearm fracture. *Acta Orthop Scand* 1976;47(3):299–303.

243. Trousdale RT, Linscheid RL. Operative treatment of malunited fractures of the forearm. *J Bone Joint Surg* 1995;77A:894–902.

244. Blackburn N, Ziv I, Rang M. Correction of the malunited forearm fracture. *Clin Orthop* 1984;188:54–57.

245. Gainor BJ, Olson S. Combined entrapment of the median and anterior interosseous nerves in a pediatric both-bone forearm fracture. *J Orthop Trauma* 1990;4:197–199.

246. Vince KG, Miller JE. Cross-union complicating fracture of the forearm: part 2: children. *J Bone Joint Surg* 1987;69A:654–661.

247. Aner A, Singer M, Feldbrin Z, et al. Surgical treatment of post-traumatic radioulnar synostosis in children. *J Pediatr Orthop* 2002;22:598–600.

248. Davidson JS, Brown DJ, Barnes SN, et al. Simple treatment for torus fractures of the distal radius. *J Bone Joint Surg* 2001;83B:1173–1175.

249. Mbubaegbu CE, Munshi NI, Currie L. Audit of patient satisfaction with self-removable soft cast for greenstick fractures of the distal radius. *J Clin Eff* 1997;2:14–15.

250. Green JS, Williams SC, Finlay D, et al. Distal forearm fractures in children:the role of radiographs during follow up. *Injury* 1998;29(4):309–312.

251. Schranz PJ, Fagg PS. Undisplaced fractures of the distal third of the radius in children: an innocent fracture? *Injury* 1992;23(3):165–167.

252. Do T, Strub WM, Foad SL, et al. Reduction versus remodeling in pediatric distal radius fractures: a preliminary cost analysis. *J Pediatr Orthop* 2003;12B:109–115.

253. Friberg K. Remodelling after distal forearm fractures in children I: the effect of residual angulation on the spatial orientation of the epiphyseal plates. *Acta Orthop Scand* 1979;50:537.

254. Friberg K. Remodelling after distal forearm fractures in children III: correction of residual angulation in fractures of the radius. *Acta Orthop Scand* 1979;50:741.

255. Zimmerman R, Gschwentner M, Pechlaner S, et al. Remodeling capacity and functional outcome of palmarly versus dorsally displaced pediatric radius fractures in the distal one-third. *Arch Orthop Trauma Surg* 2004;124:42–48.

256. Roy DR. Completely displaced distal radius fractures with intact ulnas in children. *Orthopedics* 1989;12(8):1089–1092.

257. Mani GV, Hui PW, Cheng JC. Translation of the radius as a predictor of outcome in distal radial fractures of children. *J Bone Joint Surg Br* 1993;75(5):808–811.

258. Roberts JA. Angulation of the radius in children's fractures. *J Bone Joint Surg Br* 1986;68(5):751–754.

259. Chess DG, Hyndman JC, Leahey JL, et al. Short arm plaster cast for distal pediatric forearm fractures. *J Pediatr Orthop* 1994;14(2):211–213.

260. Proctor MT, Moore DJ, Paterson JM. Redisplacement after manipulation of distal radial fractures in children. *J Bone Joint Surg* 1993;75B:453–454.

261. Gupta RP, Danielsson LG. Dorsally angulated solitary metaphyseal greenstick fractures in the distal radius: results after immobilization in pronated, neutral, and supinated position. *J Pediatr Orthop* 1990;10(1):90–92.

262. Choi KY, Chan WS, Lam TP, et al. Percutaneous Kirschner-wire pinning for severely displaced distal radial fractures in children. *J Bone Joint Surg* 1995;77B:797–801.

263. McLauchlan GJ, Cowan B, Annan IH, et al. Management of completely displaced metaphyseal fractures of the distal radius in children: a prospective randomised control trial. *J Bone Joint Surg* 2002;84B:413–417.

264. Stoffelen DVC, Broos PL. Kapandji pinning or closed reduction for extra-articular distal radius fractures. *J Trauma* 1998;45:753–757.

265. Silverman AT, Paksima DO. Biplanar Kapandji intrafocal pinning of distal radius fractures. *Am J Orthop* 2004;33:40–41.

266. Yung PSH, Lam CY, Ng BKW, et al. Percutaneous transphyseal intramedullary Kirschner wire pinning: a safe and effective procedure for treatment of displaced diaphyseal forearm fractures in children. *J Pediatr Orthop* 2004;24:7–12.

267. Guichet J-M, Moller C-C, Dautel G, et al. A modified Kapandji procedure for Smith's fracture in children. *J Bone Joint Surg* 1997;79B:734–737.

268. Lee BS, Esterhai JL Jr, Das M. Fracture of the distal radial epiphysis. Characteristics and surgical treatment of premature, post-traumatic epiphyseal closure. *Clin Orthop* 1984;185:90–96.

269. Hove LM, Engesaeter LB. Corrective osteotomies after injuries of the distal radial physis in children. *J Hand Surg [Br]* 1997;22(6):699–704.

270. Zehntner MK, Jakob RP, McGanity PL. Growth disturbance of the distal radial epiphysis after trauma: operative treatment by corrective radial osteotomy. *J Pediatr Orthop* 1990;10(3):411–415.

## Fractures of the Thoracic and Lumbar Spine

271. McPhee IB. Spinal fractures and dislocations in children and adolescents. *Spine* 1981;6(6):533–537.

272. Pouliquen JC, Kassis B, Glorion C, et al. Vertebral growth after thoracic or lumbar fracture of the spine in children. *J Pediatr Orthop* 1997;17(1):115–120.

273. Aufdermaur M. Spinal injuries in juveniles. Necropsy findings in twelve cases. *J Bone Joint Surg Br* 1974;56B(3):513–519.

274. Magnus KK, Anders M, Ralph H, et al. A modeling capacity of vertebral fractures exists during growth—an up to 47-year follow-up. *Spine* 2003;28(18):2087–2092.

275. Gumley G, Taylor TK, Ryan MD. Distraction fractures of the lumbar spine. *J Bone Joint Surg Br* 1982;64(5):520–525.

276. Spivak JM, Vaccaro AR, Cotler JM. Thoracolumbar spine trauma: I. Evaluation and classification. *J Am Acad Orthop Surg* 1995;3(6):345–352.

277. Bosch PP, Voght MT, Ward WT. Pediatric spinal cord injury without radiographic abnormality (SCIWORA): the absence of occult instability and the lack of indication for bracing. *Spine* 2002;27:2788–2800.

278. Bick E, Copel J. Longitudinal growth of the human vertebra. *J Bone Joint Surg Am* 1950;32:803.

279. Bick E, Copel J. The ring apophysis of the human vertebra. *J Bone Joint Surg Am* 1951;33:783.

280. Denis F. The three column spine and its significance in the classification of acute thoracolumbar spinal injuries. *Spine* 1983;8(8):817–831.

281. Bucholz RW, Gill K. Classification of injuries to the thoracolumbar spine. *Orthop Clin North Am* 1986;17(1):67–73.

282. Spivak JM, Vaccaro AR, Cotler JM. Thoracolumbar spine trauma: II. Principles of management. *J Am Acad Orthop Surg* 1995;3(6):353–360.

283. LaLonde F, Letts M, Yang JP, et al. An analysis of burst fractures of the spine in adolescents. *Am J Orthop* 2001;30:115–120.

284. Crawford AH. Operative treatment of spine fractures in children. *Orthop Clin North Am* 1990;21(2):325–339.
285. Andreychik DA, Alander DH, Senica KM, et al. Burst fractures of the second through fifth lumbar vertebrae. Clinical and radiographic results. *J Bone Joint Surg Am* 1996;78(8):1156–1166.
286. Kim NH, Lee HM, Chun IM. Neurologic injury and recovery in patients with burst fracture of the thoracolumbar spine. *Spine* 1999;24(3):290–293; discussion 294.
287. Voss L, Cole PA, D'Amato C. Pediatric Chance fractures from lapbelts: unique case report of three in one accident. *J Orthop Trauma* 1996;10(6):421–428.
288. Glassman SD, Johnson JR, Holt RT. Seatbelt injuries in children. *J Trauma* 1992;33(6):882–886.
289. Epstein NE, Epstein JA. Limbus lumbar vertebral fractures in 27 adolescents and adults. *Spine* 1991;16(8):962–966.
290. Takata K, Inoue S, Takahashi K, et al. Fracture of the posterior margin of a lumbar vertebral body. *J Bone Joint Surg Am* 1988;70(4):589–594.
291. Altiok H, Mekhail A, Vogel LC, et al. Issues in surgical treatment of thoraco-lumbar injuries associated with spinal cord injuries in children and adolescents. *Am J Orthop* 2002;31:647–651.
292. Mayfield JK, Erkkila JC, Winter RB. Spine deformity subsequent to acquired childhood spinal cord injury. *J Bone Joint Surg Am* 1981;63(9):1401–1411.
293. DeKlerk L, Fontijne Q, Stijnen T, et al. Spontaneous remodeling of the spinal canal after conservative management of thoracolumbar burst fractures. *Spine* 1998;23:1057.
294. Kerulla LI, Serlo WS, Tervonen OA, et al. Post-traumatic findings of the spine after earlier vertebral fracture in young patients. *Spine* 2000;25:1104–1108.

## Pelvic Fractures

295. Demetriades D, Karaiskakis M, Velmahos GC, et al. Pelvic fractures in pediatric and adult trauma patients: are they different injuries? *J Trauma* 2003;54:1146–1151.
296. Silber JS, Flynn JM, Koffler KM, et al. Analysis of the cause, classification, and associated injuries of 166 consecutive pediatric pelvic fractures. *J Pediatr Orthop* 2001;21:446–450.
297. Chia JPY, Holland AJA, Little D, et al. Pelvic fractures and associated injuries in children. *J Trauma* 2004;56:83–88.
298. McIntyre RC Jr, Bensard DD, Moore EE, et al. Pelvic fracture geometry predicts risk of life-threatening hemorrhage in children. *J Trauma* 1993;35(3):423–429.
299. Bond SJ, Gotschall CS, Eichelberger MR. Predictors of abdominal injury in children with pelvic fracture. *J Trauma* 1991;31(8):1169–1173.
300. Torode I, Zieg D. Pelvic fractures in children. *J Pediatr Orthop* 1985;5(1):76–84.
301. Silber JS, Flynn JS, Katz MA, et al. Role of computed tomography in classification and management of pediatric pelvic fractures. *J Pediatr Orthop* 2001;21:148–151.
302. Watts HG. Fractures of the pelvis in children. *Orthop Clin North Am* 1976;7(3):615–624.
303. Rieger H, Bruge E. Fractures of the pelvis in children. *Clin Orthop* 1997;336:226–239.
304. Blasier RD, McAtee J, White R, et al. Disruption of the pelvic ring in pediatric patients. *Clin Orthop Relat Res* 2000;376:87–95.
305. Musemeche CA, Fischer RP, Cotler HB, et al. Selective management of pediatric pelvic fractures: a conservative approach. *J Pediatr Surg* 1987;22(6):538–540.
306. Lane-O'Kelly A, Fogarty E, Dowling F. The pelvic fracture in childhood: a report supporting nonoperative management. *Injury* 1995;26(5):327–329.
307. Heeg M, de Ridder VA, Tornetta P, et al. Acetabular fractures in children and adolescents. *Clin Orthop Relat Res* 2000;376:80–86.
308. Heeg M, Klasen HJ, Visser JD. Acetabular fractures in children and adolescents. *J Bone Joint Surg Br* 1989;71(3):418–421.
309. Bucholz RW, Ezaki M, Ogden JA. Injury to the acetabular triradiate physeal cartilage. *J Bone Joint Surg Am* 1982;64(4):600–609.

## Fractures and Dislocations of the Hip

310. Offierski CM. Traumatic dislocation of the hip in children. *J Bone Joint Surg* 1981;63-B(2):194–197.
311. Mehlman CT, Hubbard GW, Crawford AH, et al. Traumatic hip dislocation in children. *Clin Orthop* 2000;376:68–79.
312. Price CT, Pyevich MT, Knapp DR, et al. Traumatic hip dislocation with spontaneous incomplete reduction: a diagnostic trap. *J Orthop Trauma* 2002;16:730–735.
313. Cornwall R, Radomisli TE. Nerve injury in traumatic dislocation of the hip. *Clin Orthop* 2000;377:84–91.
314. Kumar S, Jain AK. Open reduction of late unreduced traumatic posterior hip dislocation in 12 children. *Acta Orthop Scand* 1999;70:599–602.
315. Bagatur AE, Zorer G. Complications associated with surgically treated hip fractures in children. *J Pediatr Orthop* 2002;11:219–228.
316. Flynn JM, Wong KL, Yeh GL, et al. Displaced fractures of the hip in children: management by early operation and immobilisation in a hip spica cast. *J Bone Joint Surg* 2002;84B:108–112.
317. Edgren W. Coxa plana. A clinical and radiological investigation with particular reference to the importance of the metaphyseal changes for the final shape of the proximal part of the femur. *Acta Orthop Scand* 1965;(Suppl. 84):1–129.
318. Gage JR, Cary JM. The effects of trochanteric epiphyseodesis on growth of the proximal end of the femur following necrosis of the capital femoral epiphysis. *J Bone Joint Surg* 1980;62A:785–794.
319. Raney EM, Ogden JA, Grogan DP. Premature greater trochanteric epiphysiodesis secondary to intramedullary femoral rodding. *J Pediatr Orthop* 1993;13(4):516–520.
320. Chung SM. The arterial supply of the developing proximal end of the human femur. *J Bone Joint Surg Am* 1976;58(7):961–970.
321. Ogden JA. Changing patterns of proximal femoral vascularity. *J Bone Joint Surg Am* 1974;56(5):941–950.
322. Swiontkowski MF, Winquist RA. Displaced hip fractures in children and adolescents. *J Trauma* 1986;26(4):384–388.
323. Maeda S, Kita A, Funayama K, et al. Vascular supply to slipped capital femoral epiphysis. *J Pediatr Orthop* 2001;21(5):664–667.
324. Lam SF. Fractures of the neck of the femur in children. *J Bone Joint Surg Am* 1971;53(6):1165–1179.
325. Cheng JC, Tang N. Decompression and stable internal fixation of femoral neck fractures in children can affect the outcome. *J Pediatr Orthop* 1999;19(3):338–343.
326. Ng GP, Cole WG. Effect of early hip decompression on the frequency of avascular necrosis in children with fractures of the neck of the femur. *Injury* 1996;27(6):419–421.
327. Song KS, Kim YS, Sohn SW, et al. Arthrotomy and open reduction of the displaced fracture of the femoral neck in children. *J Pediatr Orthop* 2001;10B:205–210.
328. Bohler J. Hip fracture in children. *Clin Orthop Relat Res* 1981;161:339–341.
329. Stromqvist B, Nilsson LT, Egund N, et al. Intracapsular pressures in undisplaced fractures of the femoral neck. *J Bone Joint Surg Br* 1988;70(2):192–194.
330. Crawfurd EJ, Emery RJ, Hansell DM, et al. Capsular distension and intracapsular pressure in subcapital fractures of the femur. *J Bone Joint Surg Br* 1988;70(2):195–198.
331. Maruenda JI, Barrios C, Gomar-Sancho F. Intracapsular hip pressure after femoral neck fracture. *Clin Orthop* 1997;340:172–180.
332. Soto-Hall R, Johnson LH, Johnson RA. Variations in the intra-articular pressure of the hip joint in injury and disease. A probable factor in avascular necrosis. *J Bone Joint Surg Am* 1964;46:509–516.
333. Gordon JE, Abrahams MS, Dobbs MB, et al. Early reduction, arthrotomy, and cannulated screw fixation in unstable slipped capital femoral epiphysis treatment. *J Pediatr Orthop* 2002;22(3):352–358.
334. Hughes LO, Beaty JH. Fractures of the head and neck of the femur in children. *J Bone Joint Surg Am* 1994;76(2):283–292.
335. Theodorou SD, Ierodiaconou MN, Mitsou A. Obstetrical fracture-separation of the upper femoral epiphysis. *Acta Orthop Scand* 1982;53(2):239–243.
336. Forlin E, Guille JT, Kumar SJ, et al. Transepiphyseal fractures of the neck of the femur in very young children. *J Pediatr Orthop* 1992;12:164–168.
337. Odent T, Glorion C, Pannier S, et al. Traumatic dislocation of the hip with separation of the capital epiphysis. *Acta Orthop Scand* 2003;74:49–52.
338. Dimeglio A. Growth in pediatric orthopedics. In: Morrissy, ed. *Lovell and Winter's pediatric orthopedics.* Philadelphia, PA: Lippincott.

339. Azouz EM, Karamitsos C, Reed MH, et al. Types and complications of femoral neck fractures in children. *Pediatr Radiol* 1993; 23(6):415–420.

340. DeLuca FN, Keck C. Traumatic coxa vara. A case report of spontaneous correction in a child. *Clin Orthop* 1976;(116):125–128.

341. Cheng JC, Cheung SS. Modified functional bracing in the ambulatory treatment of femoral shaft fractures in children. *J Pediatr Orthop* 1989;9(4):457–462.

342. Forlin E, Guille JT, Kumar SJ, et al. Transepiphyseal fractures of the neck of the femur in very young children. *J Pediatr Orthop* 1992;12(2):164–168.

343. Davison BL, Weinstein SL. Hip fractures in children: a long-term follow-up study. *J Pediatr Orthop* 1992;12(3):355–358.

344. Ratliff AHC. Fractures of the neck of the femur in children. *J Bone Joint Surg* 1962;44B:528–542.

345. Asnis SE, Gould ES, Bansal M, et al. Magnetic resonance imaging of the hip after displaced femoral neck fractures. *Clin Orthop* 1994;298:191–198.

346. Canale ST, Bourland WL. Fracture of the neck and intertrochanteric region of the femur in children. *J Bone Joint Surg Am* 1977;59(4):431–443.

347. Ovesen O, Arreskov J, Bellstrom T. Hip fractures in children. A long-term follow up of 17 cases. *Orthopedics* 1989;12(3):361–367.

348. Hungerford DS. Which primary total hip replacement? *J Bone Joint Surg Br* 1997;79(5):880.

349. Huang CH. Treatment of neglected femoral neck fractures in young adults. *Clin Orthop* 1986;206:117–126.

350. Leung PC, Chow YY. Reconstruction of proximal femoral defects with a vascular-pedicled graft. *J Bone Joint Surg Br* 1984; 66(1):33–37.

## Femoral Shaft Fractures

351. Gross RH, Stranger M. Causative factors responsible for femoral fractures in infants and young children. *J Pediatr Orthop* 1983; 3(3):341–343.

352. Buckley SL, Sturm PF, Tosi LL, et al. Ligamentous instability of the knee in children sustaining fractures of the femur: a prospective study with knee examination under anesthesia. *J Pediatr Orthop* 1996;16(2):206–209.

353. Lynch JM, Gardner MJ, Gains B. Hemodynamic significance of pediatric femur fractures. *J Pediatr Surg* 1996;31(10):1358–1361.

354. Stans AA, Morrissy RT, Renwick SE. Femoral shaft fracture treatment in patients age 6 to 16 years. *J Pediatr Orthop* 1999;19: 222–228.

355. Smith NC, Parker D, McNicol D. Supracondylar fractures of the femur in children. *J Pediatr Orthop* 2001;21:600–603.

356. Brouwer J, Molenaar C, Van Linge B. Rotational deformities after femoral shaft fractures in childhood: a retrospective study 27–32 years after the accident. *Acta Orthop Scand* 1981;302:27.

357. Benum P, Ertresvag K, Hoiseti K. Torsion deformities after traction treatment of femoral fractures in children. *Acta Orthop Scand* 1979;50:87.

358. Davids JR. Rotational deformity and remodeling after fracture of the femur in children. *Clin Orthop* 1994;302:27–35.

359. Corry I, Nicol R. Limb length after fracture of the femoral shaft in children. *J Pediatr Orthop* 1995;15:217.

360. Podeszwa DA, Mooney JF III, Cramer KE, et al. Comparison of Pavlik harness application and immediate spica casting for femur fractures in infants. *J Pediatr Orthop* 2004;24(5):460–462.

361. Hughes BF, Sponseller PD, Thompson JD. Pediatric femur fractures: effects of spica cast treatment on family and community. *J Pediatr Orthop* 1995;15(4):457–460.

362. Buehler KC, Thompson JD, Sponseller PD, et al. A prospective study of early spica casting outcomes in the treatment of femoral shaft fractures in children. *J Pediatr Orthop* 1995;15(1):30–35.

363. Irani RN, Nicholson JT, Chung SM. Long-term results in the treatment of femoral-shaft fractures in young children by immediate spica immobilization. *J Bone Joint Surg Am* 1976;58(7): 945–951.

364. Dwyer AJ, Mam MK, John B, et al. Femoral shaft fractures in children—a comparison of treatment. *Int Orthop* 2003;27: 141–144.

365. Gracilla RV, Diaz HM, Penaranda NR, et al. Traction spica cast for femoral-shaft fractures in children. *Int Orthop* 2003;27:145–148.

366. Curtis JF, Killian JT, Alonso JE. Improved treatment of femoral shaft fractures in children utilizing the pontoon spica cast: a long-term follow-up. *J Pediatr Orthop* 1995;15(1):36–40.

367. Mileski RA, Garvin KL, Huurman WW. Avascular necrosis of the femoral head after closed intramedullary shortening in an adolescent. *J Pediatr Orthop* 1995;15(1):24–26.

368. Weiss AP, Schenck RC, Sponseller PD, et al. Peroneal nerve palsy after early cast application for femoral fractures in children. *J Pediatr Orthop* 1992;12:25–28.

369. Czertak DJ, Hennrikus WL. The treatment of pediatric femur fractures with early 90–90 spica casting. *J Pediatr Orthop* 1999;19: 229–232.

370. Illgen R II, Rodgers WB, Hresko MT, et al. Femur fractures in children: treatment with early sitting spica casting. *J Pediatr Orthop* 1998;18(4):481–487.

371. Weiss AP, Schenck RC, Sponseller PD, et al. Peroneal nerve palsy after early cast application for femoral fractures in children. *J Pediatr Orthop* 1992;12:25–28.

372. Large TM, Frick SL. Compartment syndrome of the leg after treatment of a femoral fracture with early sitting spica cast. *J Bone Joint Surg* 2003;85A:2207–2210.

373. Ryan JR. 90–90 skeletal femoral traction for femoral shaft fractures in children. *J Trauma* 1981;21(1):46–48.

374. Woolson ST, Meeks LW. A method of balanced skeletal traction for femoral fractures. *J Bone Joint Surg Am* 1974;56(6): 1288–1289.

375. Bowler JR, Mubarak SJ, Wenger DR. Tibial physeal closure and genu recurvatum after femoral fracture: occurrence without a tibial traction pin. *J Pediatr Orthop* 1990;10(5):653–657.

376. Aronson DD, Singer RM, Higgins RF. Skeletal traction for fractures of the femoral shaft in children. A long-term study. *J Bone Joint Surg Am* 1987;69(9):1435–1439.

377. Bar-On E, Sagiv S, Porat S. External fixation or flexible intramedullary nailing for femoral shaft fractures in children. A prospective, randomised study. *J Bone Joint Surg Br* 1997;79(6): 975–978.

378. Hedin H, Hjorth K, Rehnberg L, et al. External fixation of displaced femoral shaft fractures in children: a consecutive study of 98 fractures. *J Orthop Trauma* 2003;17:250–256.

379. Blasier RD, Aronson J, Tursky EA. External fixation of pediatric femur fractures. *J Pediatr Orthop* 1997;17(3):342–346.

380. Gregory P, Pevny T, Teague D. Early complications with external fixation of pediatric femoral shaft fractures. *J Orthop Trauma* 1996;10(3):191–198.

381. Kesemenli CC, Subasi M, Arslan H, et al. Is external fixation in pediatric femoral fractures a risk factor for refracture? *J Pediatr Orthop* 2004;24:17–20.

382. Mendelow M, Kanellopoulos A, Mencio G, et al. External fixation of pediatric femur fractures. *Orthop Trans* 1997;21:185.

383. Green S. Failure to obtain union. In: Green S, ed. *Complications of external skeletal fixation*. Springfield, IL: Charles C Thomas Publisher, 1981.

384. Beaty JH, Austin SM, Warner WC, et al. Interlocking intramedullary nailing of femoral-shaft fractures in adolescents: preliminary results and complications. *J Pediatr Orthop* 1994; 14(2):178–183.

385. Levy J, Ward WT. Pediatric femur fractures: an overview of treatment. *Orthopedics* 1993;16(2):183–190.

386. Gregory P, Sullivan JA, Herndon W. Adolescent femoral shaft fractures: rigid versus flexible nails. *Orthopedics* 1995;18:645.

387. Gonzalez-Herranz P, Burgos-Flores J, Rapariz JM, et al. Intramedullary nailing of the femur in children. Effects on its proximal end. *J Bone Joint Surg Br* 1995;77(2):262–266.

388. Skak S, Overgaard S, Nielsen J, et al. Internal fixation of femoral shaft fractures in children and adolescents: a ten- to twenty-one-year follow-up of 52 fractures. *J Pediatr Orthop B* 1996;5:195.

389. Flynn JM, Luedtke LM, Ganley TJ, et al. Comparison of titanium elastic nails with traction and a spica cast to treat femoral fractures in children. *J Bone Joint Surg* 2004;86A:770–777.

390. Heinrich SD, Drvaric D, Darr K, et al. Stabilization of pediatric diaphyseal femur fractures with flexible intramedullary nails (a technique paper). *J Orthop Trauma* 1992;6(4):452–459.

391. Mazda K, Khairouni A, Pennecot G, et al. Closed flexible intramedullary nailing of the femoral shaft fractures in children. *J Pediatr Orthop B* 1997;6:198.

392. Flynn JM, Luedtke L, Ganley TJ, et al. Titanium elastic nails for pediatric femur fractures: lessons from the learning curve. *Am J Orthop* 2002;31:71–74.

393. Linhart WE, Roposch A. Elastic stable intramedullary nailing for unstable femoral fractures in children: preliminary results with a new method. *J Trauma* 1999;47:372–378.

394. Ward WT, Levy J, Kaye A. Compression plating for child and adolescent femur fractures. *J Pediatr Orthop* 1992;12(5):626–632.

395. Caird MS, Mueller KA, Puryear A, et al. Compression plating of pediatric femoral shaft fractures. *J Pediatr Orthop* 2003;23:448–452.

396. Agus H, Kalenderer O, Eryanilmaz G, et al. Biological internal fixation of comminuted femur shaft fractures by bridge plating in children. *J Pediatr Orthop* 2003;23:184–189.

397. Wagner M. General principles for the clinical use of the LCP. *Injury* 2003;34(Suppl. 2B):31–42.

398. Bohn WW, Durbin RA. Ipsilateral fractures of the femur and tibia in children and adolescents. *J Bone Joint Surg Am* 1991;73(3):429–439.

399. Letts M, Vincent N, Gouw G. The "floating knee" in children. *J Bone Joint Surg Br* 1986;68(3):442–446.

400. Arslan H, Kapukaya A, Kesemenli C, et al. Floating knee in children. *J Pediatr Orthop* 2003;23:458–463.

401. Lane J, Hensinger R, Graham T, et al. Evaluation and management of pediatric subtrochanteric femur fractures. *Orthop Trans* 1990;14:688.

402. Theologis TN, Cole WG. Management of subtrochanteric fractures of the femur in children. *J Pediatr Orthop* 1998;18(1):22–25.

## Fractures and Dislocations Around the Knee

403. McDermott MJ, Bathgate B, Gillingham BL, et al. Correlation of MRI and arthroscopic diagnosis of knee pathology in children and adolescents. *J Pediatr Orthop* 1998;18(5):675–678.

404. Stanitski C. Correlation of arthroscopic and clinical examinations with magnetic resonance imaging findings of the injured knees in children and adolescents. *Am J Sports Med* 1998;26:2.

405. Stanitski CL, Harvell JC, Fu F. Observations on acute knee hemarthrosis in children and adolescents. *J Pediatr Orthop* 1993;13(4):506–510.

406. Matelic T, Aronsson D, Boyd D, et al. Acute hemarthrosis of the knee in children. *Am J Sports Med* 1995;23:668.

407. Wessel LM, Scholz S, Rusch M. Characteristic patterns and management of intra-articular knee lesions in different pediatric age groups. *J Pediatr Orthop* 2001;21:14–19.

408. Luhmann SJ. Acute traumatic knee effusion in children and adolescents. *J Pediatr Orthop* 2003;23:199–202.

409. Mann DC, Rajmaira S. Distribution of physeal and nonphyseal fractures in 2,650 long-bone fractures in children aged 0–16 years. *J Pediatr Orthop* 1990;10(6):713–716.

410. Torg JS, Pavlov H, Morris VB. Salter-Harris type-III fracture of the medial femoral condyle occurring in the adolescent athlete. *J Bone Joint Surg Am* 1981;63(4):586–591.

411. Thomson JD, Stricker SJ, Williams MM. Fractures of the distal femoral epiphyseal plate. *J Pediatr Orthop* 1995;15(4):474–478.

412. Lombardo SJ, Harvey JP Jr. Fractures of the distal femoral epiphyses. Factors influencing prognosis: a review of thirty-four cases. *J Bone Joint Surg Am* 1977;59(6):742–751.

413. Riseborough EJ, Barrett IR, Shapiro F. Growth disturbances following distal femoral physeal fracture-separations. *J Bone Joint Surg Am* 1983;65(7):885–893.

414. Meyers MH, McKeever KF. Fracture of the intercondylar eminence of the tibia. *J Bone Joint Surg Am* 1959;41-A(2):209–220; discussion 220–222.

415. Kocher MS, Micheli LJ, Gerbino P, et al. Tibial eminence fractures in children: prevalence of meniscal entrapment. *Am J Sports Med* 2003;31:404–407.

416. Kocher MS, Foreman ES, Micheli LJ. Laxity and functional outcome after arthroscopic reduction and internal fixation of displaced tibial spine fractures in children. *Arthroscopy* 2003;19:1085–1090.

417. Janarv PM, Westblad P, Johansson C, et al. Long-term follow-up of anterior tibial spine fractures in children. *J Pediatr Orthop* 1995;15(1):63–68.

418. Wiley JJ, Baxter MP. Tibial spine fractures in children. *Clin Orthop* 1990;255:54–60.

419. Willis RB, Blokker C, Stoll TM, et al. Long-term follow-up of anterior tibial eminence fractures. *J Pediatr Orthop* 1993;13(3):361–364.

420. Hallam PJB, Fazal MA, Ashwood N, et al. An alternative to fixation of displaced fractures of the anterior intercondylar eminence in children. *J Bone Joint Surg* 2002;84B:579–582.

421. Fyfe I, Jackson J. Tibial intercondylar fractures in children: a review of the classification and the treatment of mal-union. *Injury* 1981;13:165.

422. McLennan JG. Lessons learned after second-look arthroscopy in type III fractures of the tibial spine. *J Pediatr Orthop* 1995;15(1):59–62.

423. Davies EM, McLaren MI. Type III tibial spine avulsions treated with arthroscopic Acutrak screw reattachment. *Clin Orthop* 2001;388:205–208.

424. Osti L, Merlo F, Liu SH, et al. A simple modified arthroscopic procedure for fixation of displaced tibial eminence fractures. *Arthroscopy* 2000;16:379–382.

425. Mah JY, Otsuka NY, McLean J. An arthroscopic technique for the reduction and fixation of tibial-eminence fractures. *J Pediatr Orthop* 1996;16(1):119–121.

426. Panni AS, Milano G, Tartarone M, et al. Arthroscopic treatment of malunited and nonunited avulsion fractures of the anterior tibial spine. *Arthroscopy* 1998;14:233–240.

427. Mosier SM, Stanitski CL. Acute tibial tubercle avulsion fractures. *J Pediatr Orthop* 2004;24:181–184.

428. Bolesta MJ, Fitch RD. Tibial tubercle avulsions. *J Pediatr Orthop* 1986;6(2):186–192.

429. Ogden JA, Tross RB, Murphy MJ. Fractures of the tibial tuberosity in adolescents. *J Bone Joint Surg Am* 1980;62(2):205–215.

430. Pape JM, Goulet JA, Hensinger RN. Compartment syndrome complicating tibial tubercle avulsion. *Clin Orthop* 1993;295:201–204.

431. Pappas AM, Anas P, Toczylowski HM. Asymmetrical arrest of the proximal tibial physis and genu recurvatum deformity. *J Bone Joint Surg* 1984;66A:575–581.

432. Grogan DP, Carey TP, Leffers D, et al. Avulsion fractures of the patella. *J Pediatr Orthop* 1990;10(6):721–730.

433. Houghton GR, Ackroyd CE. Sleeve fractures of the patella in children: a report of three cases. *J Bone Joint Surg Br* 1979;61-B(2):165–168.

434. Maguire JK, Canale ST. Fractures of the patella in children and adolescents. *J Pediatr Orthop* 1993;13(5):567–571.

## Tibial Fractures

435. Burkhart SS, Peterson HA. Fractures of the proximal tibial epiphysis. *J Bone Joint Surg Am* 1979;61(7):996–1002.

436. Shelton WR, Canale ST. Fractures of the tibia through the proximal tibial epiphyseal cartilage. *J Bone Joint Surg Am* 1979;61(2):167–173.

437. Ogden JA, Ogden DA, Pugh L, et al. Tibia valga after proximal metaphyseal fractures in childhood: a normal biologic response. *J Pediatr Orthop* 1995;15(4):489–494.

438. Muller I, Muschol M, Mann M, et al. Results of proximal metaphyseal fractures in children. *Arch Orthop Trauma Surg* 2002;122:331–333.

439. McCarthy JJ, Kim DH, Eilert RE. Posttraumatic genu valgum: operative versus nonoperative treatment. *J Pediatr Orthop* 1998;18(4):518–521.

440. Tuten HR, Keeler KA, Gabos PG, et al. Posttraumatic tibia valga in children. A long-term follow-up note. *J Bone Joint Surg Am* 1999;81(6):799–810.

441. Mielke CH, Stevens PM. Hemiepiphyseal stapling for knee deformities in children younger than 10 years: a preliminary report. *J Pediatr Orthop* 1996;16(4):423–429.

442. Hansen B, Grieff J. Fractures of the tibia in children. *Acta Orthop Scand* 1976;47:448.

443. Shannak AO. Tibial fractures in children: follow-up study. *J Pediatr Orthop* 1988;8(3):306–310.

444. Dietz FR, Merchant TC. Indications for osteotomy of the tibia in children. *J Pediatr Orthop* 1990;10(4):486–490.

445. Yang JP, Letts RM. Isolated fractures of the tibia with intact fibula in children: a review of 95 patients. *J Pediatr Orthop* 1997;17(3):347–351.

446. Grieff J, Bergmann F. Growth disturbance following fracture of the tibia in children. *Acta Orthop Scand* 1980;51:315.

447. Oudjhane K, Newman B, Oh K, et al. Occult fractures in preschool children. *J Trauma* 1988;28:858.

448. Aronson J, Garvin K, Seibert J, et al. Efficiency of the bone scan for occult limping toddlers. *J Pediatr Orthop* 1992;12(1):38–44.

449. Briggs TW, Orr MM, Lightowler CD. Isolated tibial fractures in children. *Injury* 1992;23(5):308–310.

450. Irwin A, Gibson P, Ashcroft P. Open fractures of the tibia in children. *Injury* 1995;26:21.

451. Cullen MC, Roy DR, Crawford AH, et al. Open fracture of the tibia in children. *J Bone Joint Surg Am* 1996;78(7):1039–1047.

452. Song KM, Sangeorzan B, Benirschke S, et al. Open fractures of the tibia in children. *J Pediatr Orthop* 1996;16(5):635–639.

453. Buckley SL, Smith G, Sponseller PD, et al. Open fractures of the tibia in children. *J Bone Joint Surg Am* 1990;72(10):1462–1469.

454. Liow RY, Montgomery RJ. Treatment of established and anticipated nonunion of the tibia in childhood. *J Pediatr Orthop* 2002;22:754–760.

## Fractures of the Ankle

455. von Laer L. Classification, diagnosis, and treatment of transitional fractures of the distal part of the tibia. *J Bone Joint Surg Am* 1985;67(5):687–698.

456. Petit P, Panuel M, Faure F, et al. Acute fracture of the distal tibial physis: role of gradient-echo MR imaging versus plain film examination. *Am J Roentgenol* 1996;166:1203.

457. Vahvanen V, Aalto K. Classification of ankle fractures in children. *Arch Orthop Trauma Surg* 1980;97(1):1–5.

458. Dias LS, Tachdjian MO. Physeal injuries of the ankle in children: classification. *Clin Orthop* 1978;136:230–233.

459. Karrholm J, Hansson L, Laurin S. Pronation injuries of the ankle in children. *Acta Orthop Scand* 1983;54:1.

460. Spiegel PG, Cooperman DR, Laros GS. Epiphyseal fractures of the distal ends of the tibia and fibula. A retrospective study of two hundred and thirty-seven cases in children. *J Bone Joint Surg Am* 1978;60(8):1046–1050.

461. Salter R. Injuries of the ankle in children. *Orthop Clin North Am* 1974;5:147.

462. Kling TF Jr, Bright RW, Hensinger RN. Distal tibial physeal fractures in children that may require open reduction. *J Bone Joint Surg Am* 1984;66(5):647–657.

463. Lintecum N, Blasier RD. Direct reduction with indirect fixation of distal tibial physeal fractures: a report of a technique. *J Pediatr Orthop* 1996;16(1):107–112.

464. Rapariz JM, Ocete G, Gonzalez-Herranz P, et al. Distal tibial triplane fractures: long-term follow-up. *J Pediatr Orthop* 1996;16(1):113–118.

465. Ertl JP, Barrack RL, Alexander AH, et al. Triplane fracture of the distal tibial epiphysis. Long-term follow-up. *J Bone Joint Surg Am* 1988;70(7):967–976.

466. Lubicky JP, Altiok H. Transphyseal osteotomy of the distal tibia for correction of varus/valgus deformities of the ankle. *J Pediatr Orthop* 2001;21:80–88.

467. Karrholm J. The triplane fracture: four years of follow-up of 21 cases and review of the literature. *J Pediatr Orthop* 1997;6B:91–102.

## Fractures of the Foot

468. Schindler A, Mason DE, Allington NJ. Occult fracture of the calcaneus in toddlers. *J Pediatr Orthop* 1996;16(2):201–205.

469. Simonian PT, Vahey JW, Rosenbaum DM, et al. Fracture of the cuboid in children. A source of leg symptoms. *J Bone Joint Surg Br* 1995;77(1):104–106.

470. Jensen I, Wester JU, Rasmussen F, et al. Prognosis of fracture of the talus in children. 21 (7–34)-year follow-up of 14 cases. *Acta Orthop Scand* 1994;65(4):398–400.

471. Mulfinger G, Trueta J. The blood supply of the talus. *J Bone Joint Surg Am* 1970;52:160.

472. Letts RM, Gibeault D. Fractures of the neck of the talus in children. *Foot Ankle* 1980;1(2):74–77.

473. Canale ST, Kelly FB Jr. Fractures of the neck of the talus. Long-term evaluation of seventy-one cases. *J Bone Joint Surg Am* 1978;60(2):143–156.

474. Wester JU, Jensen IE, Rasmussen F, et al. Osteochondral lesions of the talar dome in children. A 24 (7–36) year follow-up of 13 cases. *Acta Orthop Scand* 1994;65(1):110–112.

475. Liebner ED, Simanovsky N, Abu-Sneinah K, et al. Fractures of the lateral process of the talus in children. *J Pediatr Orthop* 2001;10B:68–72.

476. Heckman JD, McLean MR. Fractures of the lateral process of the talus. *Clin Orthop* 1985;199:108–113.

477. Inokuchi S, Usami N, Hiraishi E, et al. Calcaneal fractures in children. *J Pediatr Orthop* 1998;18(4):469–474.

478. Schantz K, Rasmussen F. Calcaneus fracture in the child. *Acta Orthop Scand* 1987;58(5):507–509.

479. Schmidt TL, Weiner DS. Calcaneal fractures in children. An evaluation of the nature of the injury in 56 children. *Clin Orthop* 1982;171:150–155.

480. Sanders R, Fortin P, DiPasquale T, et al. Operative treatment in 120 displaced intraarticular calcaneal fractures. Results using a prognostic computed tomography scan classification. *Clin Orthop* 1993;290:87–95.

481. Cole RJ, Brown HP, Stein RE, et al. Avulsion fracture of the tuberosity of the calcaneus in children. A report of four cases and review of the literature. *J Bone Joint Surg Am* 1995;77(10):1568–1571.

482. Ceccarelli F, Faldini C, Piras F, et al. Surgical versus non-surgical treatment of calcaneal fractures in children: a long-term results comparative study. *Foot Ankle* 2000;21:825–832.

483. Schantz K, Rasmussen F. Good prognosis after calcaneal fracture in childhood. *Acta Orthop Scand* 1988;59(5):560–563.

484. Pickle A, Benaroch TE, Guy P, et al. Clinical outcome of pediatric calcaneal fractures treated with open reduction and internal fixation. *J Pediatr Orthop* 2004;24:178–180.

485. Holbein O, Bauer G, Kinzl L. Fracture of the cuboid in children: case report and review of the literature. *J Pediatr Orthop* 1998;18(4):466–468.

486. Wiley JJ. Tarso-metatarsal joint injuries in children. *J Pediatr Orthop* 1981;1(3):255–260.

487. Buoncristiani AM, Manos RE, Mills WJ. Plantar-flexion tarsometatarsal joint injuries in children. *J Pediatr Orthop* 2001;21:324–327.

488. Johnson G. Pediatric Lisfranc injury: "bunk bed" fracture. *Am J Roentgenol* 1981;137:1041.

489. Silas SI, Herzenberg JE, Myerson MS, et al. Compartment syndrome of the foot in children. *J Bone Joint Surg Am* 1995;77(3):356–361.

490. Kensinger DR, Guille JT, Horn BD, et al. The stubbed great toe: importance of early recognition and treatment of open fractures of the distal phalanx. *J Pediatr Orthop* 2001;21:31–34.

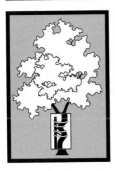

# 34

# The Role
# of the Orthopaedic
# Surgeon in Diagnosing
# Child Abuse

*Tom F. Novacheck*

## DEFINITION

Abuse of dependent children has unfortunately been a part of human social interactions transcending time and cultures. Recorded history indicates that violence toward children has been condoned and even accepted. The nature of the abuse has encompassed a broad spectrum of injuries inflicted on children and the neglect of children by those who are responsible for their well-being. The notion of children's rights is relatively modern. Historically, paternal power was absolute, including the right to abandon, abuse, and even kill one's child. Correction and discipline was limited only by the father's conscience. This right was extended to anyone involved in rearing the child.

Children were considered to be a source of cheap labor during the Industrial Revolution. Reaction to this practice was partly responsible for the development during the 19th century of social groups dedicated to the prevention of child abuse, and many societies began to recognize child abuse as a problem that should not be ignored. The Society for the Prevention of Cruelty to Children was established in the mid-1800s. In 1860, Ambrose Tardieu reported 32 cases with the physical signs that are typical of abuse, which included cutaneous lesions, fractures (before x-ray films were available), subdural hematomas described as "thickening of blood on the surface of the brain," and death. His report also addressed the social aspects of the relationship between the abused and the abuser.

Caffey (1) focused the medical community's attention on this problem with his publication in 1946 describing the association between long-bone fractures and subdural hematomas. In 1962, approximately 100 years after Tardieu's first report, the term "battered child syndrome" was coined by C. Henry Kempe (2). It reported one of the most dramatic manifestations of family violence and implied that children are injured by being struck by or thrown against something. When first described, it was suggested that battered child syndrome "should be considered in any child with a combination of multiple fractures, subdural hematoma, failure to thrive, and soft-tissue swellings or skin bruising; when sudden, unexplained death occurred; and in situations in which the type and degree of injury were inconsistent with the history."

Silverman (3) is recognized as an important figure in formulating the concept of "unrecognized trauma in infants." He advocated the term "syndrome of Ambroise Tardieu" in recognition of the French physician's pioneering work. The "Child Abuse Prevention Act" in 1974 and the subsequent development of state reporting laws in the United States followed the publication of Kempe's and Silverman's articles (4).

Definitions as recent as 1968 were restricted to physical injury inflicted on children by persons caring for them (5). The popular term "battered child" was recognized as inadequate at that time, but it had an impact. Since then, the concept of child abuse has been broadened to include the entire spectrum of childhood injuries including physical and emotional neglect as well as physical, psychological, and sexual abuse. "Manifestations of the Battered-Child Syndrome," by Akbarnia et al., (6) was one of the early reports on this topic in orthopaedic literature. It appeared in the *Journal of Bone and Joint Surgery* in 1974 and alerted orthopaedists to the existence and prevalence of this problem.

Subsequently, this problem came to be referred to as nonaccidental injury (NAI). Defining a condition by what it is not is unsatisfactory. The adoption of this terminology not only requires an acceptable definition of what constitutes an accident, but also suggests that any injury that does not fit that definition is child abuse. In addition, it diminishes the gravity of the active infliction of harm by the abuser and thereby deflects attention from the perpetrator.

Should the definition imply or directly indicate an intent to cause harm? Although the definition must include the fact that the act was willful (otherwise, it would truly be accidental), the assailant may not be aware of the consequences of his or her actions. Therefore, premeditation is not required to diagnose abuse. The type of handling and magnitude of the force involved is on the opposite end of the spectrum of the reasonableness with which parents and caregivers should gently, tenderly, and lovingly care for children. Some understanding of behavior patterns that are typical of those responsible for the care of a child must be considered when determining if an act constitutes abuse. In addition, the definition must be comprehensive to include the spectrum of childhood injuries. Defining it with precision remains a challenge even for experts.

Terms and definitions must not be too restrictive and must be able to encompass the scope of the problems that must be included in the spectrum of child abuse. We recognize today that child abuse fits in the spectrum of family violence (7). Most people now consider abuse 'not as a discrete illness entities or syndromes, but as symptoms of different issues and risks for particular children in individual families' (8).

Childhelp USA, Inc. provides the following definition: "Child abuse consists of any act of commission or omission that endangers or impairs a child's physical or emotional health and development. Child abuse includes any damage done to a child which cannot be reasonably explained and which is often represented by an injury or series of injuries appearing to be nonaccidental in nature" (9). Included are forms of physical, sexual, and emotional abuse as well as neglect. The *Child Abuse Prevention and Treatment Act* (CAPTA) defines child abuse and neglect as "at a minimum, any act or failure to act resulting in imminent risk of serious harm, death, serious physical or emotional harm, sexual abuse, or exploitation of a child by a parent or caretaker who is responsible for the child's welfare."

This chapter will be limited to the discussion of the orthopaedic aspects of this spectrum. Several good reviews of this topic are available, and the reader is referred to them (10,11). The chapter on child abuse in the previous edition of this text is also excellent (4).

## EPIDEMIOLOGY

CAPTA was amended in 1988 to direct the Secretary of the United States Department of Health and Human Services (HHS) to establish a national data collection and analysis program to make available information on child abuse and neglect that is reported at the state level. The department responded by establishing the National Child Abuse and Neglect Data System (NCANDS). NCANDS is a federally sponsored effort that collects and analyzes annual data on child abuse and neglect submitted voluntarily by all the States and the District of Columbia.

The HHS Administration for Children and Families (www.acf.dhhs.gov) releases its most current child abuse statistics, as reported by the states, in April of each year. The statistics reported in the following text were released in April 2004 and represent an analysis of the data for calendar year 2002 (US Department of Health and Human Services, Administration for Children and Families. Child Maltreatment 2004: Reports from the States to the National Child Abuse and Neglect Data System). This was accessed by the present author on November 21, 2004 at http://www.acf.dhhs.gov/programs/cb/stats/ncands/. The results are available in a publication called *Child Maltreatment 2002* (12).

During 2002, an estimated 896,000 children were victims of abuse and neglect (an increase from 826,000 just 2 years earlier). An estimated 2.6 million referrals of abuse or neglect concerning approximately 4.5 million children were received by child protective service agencies. More than two-thirds of those referrals were accepted for investigation or assessment (most others were unsubstantiated).

The maltreatment rate was 12.3 per 1000 children annually, making child abuse more common than developmental dysplasia of the hip and 30 times the incidence of new cases of myelomeningocele. It is widely held that child abuse is significantly underreported (13). The actual incidence of abuse and neglect is estimated to be three times the number that is reported to authorities. All statistics should be considered suspect, as they represent only the tip of the iceberg.

More than half of all reports of alleged child abuse or neglect were made by such professionals as educators, law enforcement and legal personnel, social services personnel, medical personnel, mental health personnel, child daycare providers, and foster care providers. Educators made 16.1% of all reports, whereas law enforcement made 15.7%, and social services personnel made 12.6%. Only 7.8% of reports were made by medical personnel. Such nonprofessionals as friends, neighbors, and relatives submitted approximately 43.6% of reports.

Children of Native Americans, natives of Alaska, and African Americans had the highest rates of victimization. While the rate of white victims of child abuse or neglect was 10.7 per 1000, the rate among Native Americans or natives of Alaska was 21.7 per 1000 children, and for African Americans, it was 20.2 per 1000 children. Half of all victims were white.

Nationally, more than 60% of child victims experienced neglect (including medical neglect), approximately 20% were physically abused, approximately 10% were sexually abused, and 6.5% were emotionally or psychologically maltreated. In 2002, an estimated 1400 children died of abuse or neglect (more than three children per day)—a rate of 1.98 per 100,000 children nationally. This is a significant increase from an estimated 1300 children who died in 2001. Most (84.5%) of the children who die are younger than 6 years. Forty-one percent of the fatalities were in children under the age of 1 year. Three out of four fatalities occur in children younger than 4 years. Abuse of girls is slightly more common than abuse of boys (48% male; 51.5% female; the victim's sex was not reported in 0.5% of cases.) Most victims were abused by a parent (81%), although reported sexual abuse by a parent occurs in the minority. The median age of the perpetrators was 31 years for women and 34 years for men.

One in three abused children is seen by an orthopaedist (14). Fractures are the second most common presentation in child abuse (skin lesions are the most common). More detailed analysis of the nature and frequency of abusive fractures will be provided in the subsequent section on fractures.

Copies of the report and other information about child maltreatment are available at the National Clearinghouse on Child Abuse and Neglect Information at 1-800-394-3366, or http://nccanch.acf.hhs.gov/index.cfm.

## ETIOLOGY

In the early 1980s, Bittner and Newberger (8) promoted the thinking that child abuse is a culmination of a series of stresses that impinge on parents and children. This idea is based on Helfer and Kempe's three elements that contribute to the propensity for abuse: a child with qualities that are provocative; a parent with the psychological predisposition; and a stressful event that triggers a violent reaction (5). In Bittner and Newberger's model, there are social and cultural factors that provide a background in which a family develops. Family stresses (caused by the child, by the parent, and by social/situational factors) provide an environment in which a triggering situation can lead to maltreatment of the child. How the risk for child abuse may operate in any individual family must be assessed clinically. They proposed that the team of clinicians must understand the social, familial, psychological, and physiologic concomitants of child abuse in order to assess the situation and subsequently develop a comprehensive management plan.

Violence as a response to conflict can be socially learned (and unlearned). Wolfner and Gelles (15) regarded it as a constitutional predisposition to violence, the signs of which appear only in the presence of an environmental stressor. This is analogous to someone with a dust allergy who does not respond with an allergic reaction unless placed in a dusty environment.

Several risk factors are commonly identified (Table 34.1). Numerous sources are available and they all generally agree on common predisposing factors (1,2,12,15,16). Care must be taken in interpreting the results, as data gathered

## TABLE 34.1

### RISK FACTORS FOR CHILD ABUSE

Child
  Younger age
  Lower socioeconomic status
  Firstborn
  Unplanned birth
  Premature birth
  Stepchild
  Multiple birth
  Special needs
Abuser
  Younger age
  Single
  Drug-abusing
  Parent who was himself/herself abused
  Unemployed

from different sources will likely lead to different risk profiles, incidence, ratios of physical abuse to sexual abuse to neglect, and so on.

Data gathered from surveys (such as those reported by NCANDS) and reviews of records from medical data gathered through hospital systems will almost certainly differ. Interpreting these data can be misleading and must be done with care. Underreporting in certain segments of the population may also skew the results. Notable areas of concern are risk profiles that identify minorities or ethnic groups and those in the lower socioeconomic class as being more likely to abuse their children.

Identifying the characteristics that are risk factors for child abuse can help society to focus limited resources for its prevention and detection on situations that present a high risk. One might also believe that health care providers with a knowledge of risk factors will pay closer attention to an injured child whose social situation is characterized by numerous risk factors for child abuse. However, because abuse can affect children in all environments, dismissing the injuries of a white child from a more advantaged background as not being caused by abuse, without adequate investigation, is a disservice to that child. Health care providers have a moral and legal obligation to maintain a high index of suspicion to avoid underdiagnosis of vulnerable individuals.

## CLINICAL FEATURES

### History

One hallmark of nonaccidental fractures is lack of a plausible history. This fact emphasizes why orthopaedic expertise regarding fracture mechanisms is required. Understanding the antecedents of the child's injury and assessing the plausibility of the history are two of the initial goals of history taking. For example, the body mass of a child younger than 12 months typically will not generate sufficient force to fracture a normal bone in a fall from a bed, crib, or couch. One must suspect abuse when a nonambulatory child presents with a fracture. Of course, an insufficiency fracture through pathologic bone is another possibility in the differential. Because injuries of any kind are rare in nonabused infants, age is one of the most important factors in making the diagnosis of child abuse.

The interview with the very young child is of course impossible, and even with older children it is typically brief and consists of asking the child how the injury occurred and, in the case of apparent abuse, who inflicted the injury. The interviewer should assess the child's affect and developmental status, and observe the child's verbal and behavioral interactions with family members and other adults. Interviews of caretakers should be more detailed and must be done separately. Thorough medical and developmental histories must be obtained.

Children with disabilities are mistreated more often than healthy developing children. Indications of abuse are the same in both groups. Behavioral indicators in a child with a disability may not be recognized or may be attributed to the underlying condition. Risk factors include increased demands for care, chronic stress on the care providers, parental attachment problems, parental isolation, unrealistic expectations, aggressive behavior in the child, communication limitations leading to decreased ability to report information about the abuse, inability to communicate specific needs resulting in neglect, and increased dependency on many caretakers (17). Children with severe disabilities may be at increased risk of malnutrition and failure to thrive. Malnutrition is sometimes accepted as part of the disability, but it can be viewed as neglect to provide a basic bodily need (18,19). Some children's developmental disorders are due to abuse, for example, shaken baby syndrome can lead to cerebral palsy. There is a lack of adequate studies regarding the incidence and nature of abuse in children with disabilities, but these children certainly represent a vulnerable population. Awareness of the uncommon Munchausen syndrome by proxy (20) will help avoid missing this complicated form of abuse.

The medical component is just a part of the needed response to potential maltreatment. Cooperation and liaison with official community agencies such as the child protection service (CPS), law enforcement, and prosecutors is crucial and legally mandated. Open, good-faith exchange with these agencies is legal and protected. It is not restricted by the Privacy Rule of the Health Insurance Portability Accountability Act (HIPAA).

Someone from the medical care team must thoroughly document a description of the injury. Whether that is the orthopaedist or another member of the health care team depends on the local medical community and the situation of the particular case. Use quotations when possible, identify "players," control information exchange, do not suggest a mechanism of injury, and avoid confrontation, accusation, and prejudicial statements. Document everything including parental behavior and the presence of visitors. The interviewer should keep in mind that questioning does not equal blaming. Immediately address the concern that the injuries may have been inflicted. What has happened cannot be changed, what is happening currently can be stopped, and abuse that could occur in the future can be prevented. The needs of the child and provision of medical care to the child are the primary concerns and should be given priority over the child abuse workup. Family-centered care may have to take a back seat. The parents' right to know needs to be balanced against possible threats (direct or indirect) to the child's safety. Obtaining and documenting adequate information to rule out inflicted injury is crucial, but these efforts are often inadequate. Oral et al. (21) retrospectively reviewed emergency room charts and orthopaedic office notes. In a large percentage of cases, they found that documentation was insufficient to explain the cause of fractures and thereby rule out inflicted trauma. They advocated the use of forms, protocols, and periodic chart review to help ensure compliance (see the section of this chapter entitled "Author's Preferred Treatment").

## Physical Examination

A thorough, multisystem physical examination is required. Again, the environment will determine which professional is primarily responsible for this. If the child is seen in the emergency room of an urban children's hospital, an emergency room physician or pediatrician will be accountable. If it is a more rural or isolated environment, the orthopaedist may need to take a more active role. In addition, the orthopaedist's role will vary depending on whether the cause of the injuries has already been identified as abuse at the time of consultation. If so, the role will be to ensure that all musculoskeletal injuries are found and to document their nature and severity. If abuse is not known or suspected, then only professional awareness and a high degree of suspicion will identify the cause of the injury.

In their review of 371 children, McMahon et al. found that soft-tissue injuries were present in 92% of children suspected of being victims of child abuse (14). A child's age, the pattern and location of soft-tissue injury(s), the number of injuries, and the age of the lesion(s) are all important to consider. The classic soft-tissue lesions such as cigarette burns, bite marks, or multiple linear ecchymoses in the shape of an electrical cord leave little doubt that abuse occurred, but in McMahon's report these were uncommon. Therefore, these findings are quite specific, but not sensitive. The examiner must be careful to identify subtle signs of abuse, because the "classic" findings may be present in only some abused children, typically in the more severe cases.

The typical physical findings of acute fractures include pain on movement of the injured extremity, swelling at the fracture site, and deformity. Dos Santos et al. (22) found that less swelling was present on presentation in children with long bone fractures caused by abuse than similar fractures that occurred because of accidents. The history and the reported time when the injury occurred are often unreliable in cases of child abuse. Frequently, delays in seeking care for these children allow resolution of these acute signs and symptoms. The absence of the typical acute findings of fractures in abused children is one of the reasons that screening for fractures in suspected cases of abuse includes skeletal surveys and bone scans (see the section in this chapter entitled "Other Imaging Studies").

Any soft-tissue injury in a child younger than 9 months is suspicious and indicates possible abuse. Soft-tissue injuries of the head and face are much more common in abused children and are rare in the absence of abuse. Ecchymoses are common, but may not be of the suspicious pattern (14). Soft-tissue injuries are less common after accidental injury, but do occur frequently in approximately 37% of cases (23). Therefore, the mere presence of a soft-tissue injury does not clearly imply that the injury was a result of abusive force. Location is important, because toddlers commonly have bruises over the shins, knees, elbows, and brow. They may have a few old cuts or scars around the eyes or cheekbones because of normal collisions. However, bruising of the buttocks, perineum, trunk, back of the legs, and especially the head or neck suggests inflicted trauma.

Just as it can be important to identify the telltale signs of multiple fractures in various stages of healing, the same is true for skin lesions. Wilson (24) has suggested the following guidelines for estimating the age of a bruise from its color: from 0 to 3 days after injury, a bruise usually is red, blue, or purple; from 3 to 7 days, it is green or green-yellow; and from 8 to 28 days, it is yellow or yellow-brown.

Burn injuries are common and are seen in 10% of abused children (4). These lesions can be scalding injuries, cigarette burns, or burns caused by flames. Burns are most common among children between birth and 2 years of age (14). The pattern of deliberate immersion burns often is symmetric, with sharp lines between the burned and unburned skin. Accidental scald burns usually are distributed asymmetrically (25).

Photographs of any unusual findings from head to toe can be invaluable in cases of child abuse. It is best to obtain more than one view, with different lighting. Many centers have protocols in place for obtaining satisfactory and complete photographs.

Abusive head trauma is the most common cause of death due to child abuse. Caffey's (1) classic article in 1946 reported the association between long-bone fractures and subdural hematomas. Typically, one of two histories is provided: (i) a fall from a short height or a similar minor, blunt traumatic episode is described, or (ii) the baby is brought for medical attention due to the development of symptoms including poor feeding, irritability, vomiting, seizures, lethargy, breathing difficulties, and unresponsiveness (26). The head is the most vulnerable part of the body for accidental injury and child abuse because of its relatively large size, the weak neck muscles, and the less dense bone with open sutures in younger children. The type of skull fracture is not specific for identifying cases of child abuse, as similar fractures may occur in different settings (27).

Abdominal trauma is the second leading cause of death due to child abuse. Essentially, all the injuries that are known to be caused by blunt trauma can be seen in victims of child abuse. Death due to child abuse can be caused by internal hemorrhage because of the rupture of abdominal organs after punches or kicks. The death rate from these injuries can be high and is attributable to both the severity of the trauma and the delay in diagnosis. Delays can result from lack of timely diagnosis in the emergency room or delays on the part of the abuser in seeking medical attention for the child. Hematuria can be one sign of blunt internal injury. It is often the recognition of other signs of abuse, however, along with a high index of suspicion for associated abdominal trauma, that is required to identify this potentially life-threatening type of injury.

Ocular injuries in cases of abuse include retinal and conjunctival hemorrhage and orbital swelling. Retinal hemorrhages in infancy are almost invariably caused by shaking and are seen in shaken baby syndrome (28).

## RADIOGRAPHIC FEATURES

Diagnosing abuse would be relatively easy for orthopaedists if all abusive fractures had a typical appearance. Although there are some patterns of fractures that are distinctive, many of the patterns are also seen in cases of accidental trauma (Table 34.2). There is some debate as to which patterns are most common. Loder and Bookout (29) noted that suspicious fracture patterns include metaphyseal corner fractures, lower extremity fractures in non-ambulatory children, bilateral acute fractures, rib fractures, spine fractures, and physeal fractures in young children. Kleinman (13) stated that the most likely fracture in an abused infant is a long bone metaphyseal lesion, followed by rib, skull, and long bone shaft fractures. Kleinman et al. subsequently reported on the challenges of dating the characteristic metaphyseal fracture (30). Blakemore et al. (31) reported that single, fresh, long bone diaphyseal fractures are most common. It is likely that there is a sampling bias that explains some of these discrepancies, but different standards for radiographic technique and the frequency with which skeletal surveys, follow-up skeletal surveys, and bone scans are done may also lead to variations in the reported rates (13).

Classic fracture patterns should be easy to recognize as being inflicted by abusive trauma. Metaphyseal "bucket-handle" or "corner" fractures often form the basis for the diagnosis of abuse (Fig. 34.1) and are considered pathognomonic

| TABLE 34.2 |
| --- |
| **SPECIFICITY OF RADIOLOGIC FINDINGS** |

**High Specificity**
  Classic metaphyseal lesions
  Rib fractures, especially posterior
  Scapular fractures
  Spinous process fractures
  Sternal fractures

**Moderate Specificity**
  Multiple fractures, especially bilateral
  Fractures of different ages
  Epiphyseal separations
  Vertebral body fractures and subluxations
  Digital fractures
  Complex skull fractures

**Common, but low specificity**
  Subperiosteal new bone formation
  Clavicular fractures
  Long bone shaft fractures
  Linear skull fractures

Highest specificity applies to infants.
From Kleinman PK. *Diagnostic imaging of child abuse*, 2nd ed. St. Louis, MO: Mosby, 1998:9.

for abusive trauma. They have highly distinctive radiographic characteristics (32) that result from the isolation of a mineralized disc (or a part thereof) that can be seen radiographically. Depending on its size and the orientation and angle of the radiograph, one will see a bucket-handle lesion, corner fracture, or metaphyseal lucency. The metaphyseal lesion may be difficult to identify on plain radiographs. High-detail imaging may be needed. Kleinman (13) prefers the term *classic metaphyseal lesion* (CML) to describe this type of injury because it represents a radiologic alteration that most

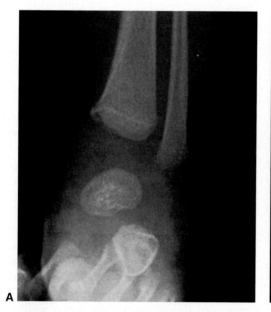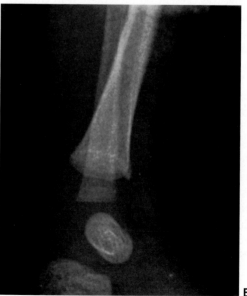

**Figure 34.1**  Classic metaphyseal lesion of the distal tibia in a 2-week-old infant. **A:** Anteroposterior ankle. **B:** Lateral ankle. This finding is pathognomonic for child abuse.

closely satisfies the need for an objective finding that "regardless of history in an otherwise normal patient, can be viewed as a highly specific inflicted injury." He states that it is rarely seen as an isolated finding in a healthy infant for whom a plausible accidental event is available to explain the injury, and it is invariably due to severe indirect forces. Most injuries due to child abuse "occur by indirect forces which develop as the child is grabbed by an extremity, shaken, slammed, or hurled into a solid object" (13). They occur because of avulsive forces applied to the periosteal attachment to the surface of the metaphysis. The periosteum serves as the anchor for the epiphyseal cartilage to the metaphysis. Failure of the bone in this area results in a corner fracture. The bucket-handle fracture results from the same type of indirect force, but represents a separation of a crescentic fragment from the zone of provisional calcification that is tipped into an oblique plane (33).

Skull fractures are not uncommon in children. They can be difficult to diagnose due to the various sutures, synchondroses, and fissures that may be present throughout the development of a child. Diagnosing these variants as a fracture is a common pitfall. Fractures appear as radiolucent, sharply etched lines that may or may not branch but finally taper and become indistinct. Sutures, on the other hand, have a serpiginous appearance, symmetry, sclerotic edges, and typical anatomic positions (34). Vascular markings are more linear, have a near constant anatomic branching pattern, and involve only the inner table. Other radiographic views or computed tomography (CT) scan of the head can assist in cases that are confusing. As mentioned previously, the type of skull fracture is not specific for identifying child abuse. Similar fractures can occur in different settings (27).

Complex skull fractures and rib fractures (especially multiple rib fractures in children younger than 2 years ) are highly suggestive of intentional injury (Figs. 34.2 and 34.3). The amount of force required to inflict them makes these injuries very unlikely to be accidental. Rib fractures (especially posterior) may be difficult to detect, but are

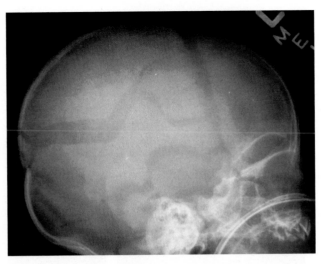

**Figure 34.2** Acute skull fracture in a 5-month-old abused child. This fracture could be consistent with accidental injury if there were a documented history of significant trauma (a fall or auto accident).

not uncommon in children who are abused. In a study of 62 children younger than 3 years with rib fractures (316 collectively), the finding of a rib fracture had a positive predictive value of 95% for the diagnosis of abuse. The positive predictive value rose to 100% after the exclusion of children with a defined history of accident or disease (35).

The most difficult task of the orthopaedist and the radiologist arises when the radiographic appearance of a fracture resulting from abuse is not characteristic. Many of the fracture patterns caused by abuse can also be seen after accidental trauma (Fig. 34.4). In this situation, making the correct diagnosis is more difficult. In such cases, age is one of the most important factors in differentiating accidental from abusive trauma (31,36). Some fractures that would not raise suspicion in ambulatory children (because they are common and accidental) do not occur in infants unless excessive force is applied and therefore are highly suspicious for abuse in this age-group. For example, a spiral fracture of

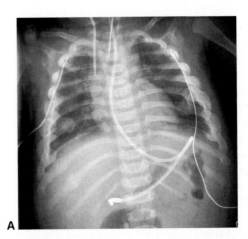 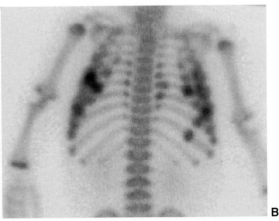

**Figure 34.3** Multiple healing rib fractures seen on chest x-ray film (CXR) **(A)** and on bone scan **(B)** in the same child as in Figure 34.2. The findings of multiple healing rib fractures (including posterior) and the acute skull fracture (Fig. 34.2) clearly indicate child abuse.

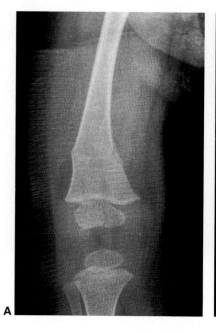
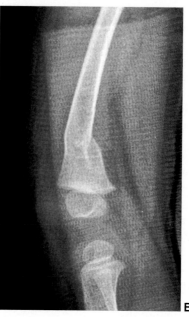

**Figure 34.4** Metaphyseal fracture of distal femur in a 13-month-old child. **A:** Anteroposterior view. **B:** Lateral view. Was this fracture caused by abuse, or was it accidental? This fracture pattern could be seen in either situation. If the child were 4 months old, the fracture would be very suspicious for abuse. At 13 months of age, and if the child is ambulatory, it could be accidental.

the humerus in a young child is particularly indicative for abuse. Strait et al. (37) reported that abuse was rare (1 of 99 cases) in children older than 15 months presenting with humeral fractures, but these fractures in 9 of 25 children younger than 15 months were diagnosed as having been caused by abuse.

Likewise, single diaphyseal spiral fractures of the tibia or femur are common accidental injuries in toddlers, but are suspicious if the child is preambulatory (31). There is no diaphyseal fracture pattern that is specific for abuse. Twisting injury to an extremity causes spiral fractures. In the ambulatory child, the twists associated with falls while walking, running, climbing, or falling down stairs are sufficient to cause fractures (38). It is impossible for a preambulatory child, however, to sustain this level of trauma unless it is applied to him/her directly. Transverse or oblique long bone fractures, on the other hand, are more common with abusive injury than are spiral fractures. The peak incidence of pediatric femur fractures is between 2 and 3 years of age (39). Femur fractures can result from low-energy falls and are two to three times more common in boys than in girls (40). King et al. (41) found that approximately half of the 189 abused children in their retrospective study had a single fracture and that a transverse fracture was the most common type (as was the case for the child illustrated in Fig. 34.4).

Rex and Kay (42) found that the vast majority (13 of 14) of nonaccidental femur fractures occurred in children younger than 1 year. Comparing them with 33 femoral fractures known to be caused by accident, the authors concluded that there is no specific radiographic site or fracture pattern that allows differentiation between accidental and nonaccidental femoral fractures. Blakemore et al. (31) also felt that age is the most important factor in diagnosing abuse, because isolated femur fractures are commonly seen in children who are 1 to 5 years of age. Some authors would suggest that the incidence of long-bone fractures

caused by abuse in ambulatory children is relatively low (31,36). Dalton et al. (43) recommended that because 31% of 138 femoral fractures in children younger than 3 years were due to abuse, and only 10% (one third of the total abuse cases) were identified as abuse at admission, a high index of suspicion must be maintained even in the ambulatory child. They recommended that although the "cause of isolated shaft fractures in young children is low, the clinician should still have a high degree of vigilance and have the circumstance investigated when the history and physical findings are disturbing." Only 18% of 34 humerus shaft fractures in children younger than 3 years were classified as probably caused by abuse in the review by Shaw et al. (44). The history and physical findings (not the fracture pattern itself) were critical in establishing cause. Neither age nor fracture pattern is pathognomonic of abuse, so suspicion should remain high.

It is interesting to note that only 5 of the 42 children included in Blakemore's study (31) had skeletal surveys. In addition, for any fracture to be categorized as abuse, its cause had to be confirmed at a legal hearing. Therefore, interpretation of the scope of the results of this study seems to be limited, because inclusion in the category of abuse was quite restricted (some abused children may have been placed in the accidental injury group) and screening for fractures was not highly sensitive (some fractures may have been missed). Maintaining a high degree of suspicion may even uncover abuse when an isolated long bone fracture in an infant caused by a legitimate injury mechanism is investigated further (45). In the review by Strait et al. (37), 18.5% of 124 humerus fractures were indeterminate in children younger than 15 months.

Schwend et al. (36) pointed out that isolated fractures of the femur are analogous to the toddler's fracture of the tibia. Like other authors, they concluded that the ability to walk was the strongest predictor of abuse. Ten (42%) of 24 children not old enough to walk had been abused, whereas only 3 of 115 toddlers had been. Although child protective services were frequently consulted, the authors felt that it may have been unnecessary in 42% to 63% of cases. They felt that unless other evidence of abuse such as an inconsistent history, bruises, or other fractures was present, abuse was very unlikely in the child old enough to walk.

It is important to note that fractures are not uncommon, but occur in the minority of abused children. Only 17% of the 904 abused children in the report of Merten et al. (46) had fractures. McMahon et al. (14) in their review of 371 abused children found that most did not show the classic signs of child abuse that we, as orthopaedists, expect to see. Although only 9% had fractures identifiable on x-ray film, 92% had soft-tissue injuries (ecchymosis was most common). The metaphyseal lesion was not seen, and long bone fractures tended to be diaphyseal. Although the McMahon article is very enlightening regarding abused children who do not present with the classic findings, only 10% of the children included in the report actually had radiographs taken! One can only speculate as to the number and type of fractures that may have been found if full skeletal surveys had been performed. The rate of fractures reported by different authors depends on the source of the information (social service agencies vs. orthopaedists offices vs. emergency rooms, etc.) and the methods employed to identify fractures. Because neglect is the most common form of abuse, and neglected children do not commonly have fractures, it is likely that few victims of abuse have fractures. However, orthopaedists are typically not involved in many cases of neglect; therefore, from our vantage point, it can be presumed that a substantial percentage of the young patients we see with fractures have been abused. Approximately 30% of fractures in children younger than 3 years (27) and 56% of fractures in children younger than 1 year have been found to be nonaccidental (16). Although corner fractures, fractures at different stages of healing, and injuries at multiple sites may be more specific, the clinician must remember that all types of fractures at all locations can be seen in children who have been abused (Table 34.2).

Because the identification of fractures in various stages of healing can be important in identifying abuse, it is extremely

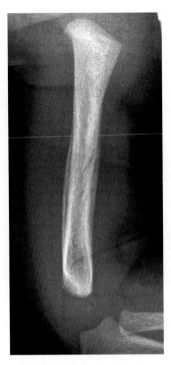

**Figure 34.5** Subperiosteal new bone formation (SPNBF). Lateral x-ray film of the humerus showing a healing fracture and typical SPNBF in an 11-week-old infant. Although this fracture pattern itself is not very troubling, the finding of a long bone fracture in an infant is very suspicious for abusive trauma.

important to be able to identify the ages of fractures based on their radiographic appearance (47,48) (Table 34.3). Soft-tissue swelling may be the only radiographic finding for recent fractures. The orthopaedist is accustomed to identifying this finding on x-ray films of acute fractures. Because care for abused children is frequently delayed, this finding may be absent on the initial radiographs. The earliest sign of bone healing is subperiosteal new bone formation (SPNBF). SPNBF will not be seen until at least 5 days after injury. This finding has low specificity as there are multiple etiologies (see "Differential Diagnosis" section), and it must be distinguished from the many other conditions that can lead to this radiographic appearance. Indistinctness of the fracture line is the next finding that helps to date the fracture between approximately 10 days to 2 weeks (Fig. 34.5). Soft callous formation and

---

**TABLE 34.3**

**TIMETABLE OF RADIOLOGIC CHANGES IN CHILDREN'S FRACTURES[a]**

| Category | Early | Peak | Late |
|---|---|---|---|
| 1. Resolution of soft tissues | 2–5 d | 4–10 d | 10–21 d |
| 2. SPNBF | 4–10 d | 10–14 d | 14–21 d |
| 3. Loss of fracture line definition | 10–14 d | 14–21 d | — |
| 4. Soft callus formation | 10–14 d | 14–21 d | — |
| 5. Hard callus formation | 14–21 d | 21–42 d | 42–90 d |
| 6. Remodeling | 3 mo | 1 yr | 2 yr to physeal closure |

SPNBF, Subperiosteal new bone formation.
[a]Repetitive injures may prolong categories 1, 2, 5, and 6.
From Kleinman PK. *Diagnostic imaging of child abuse*, 2nd ed. St. Louis, MO: Mosby, 1998:176.

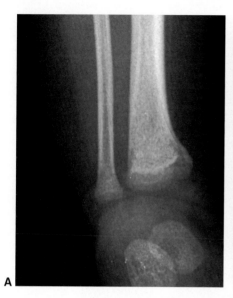

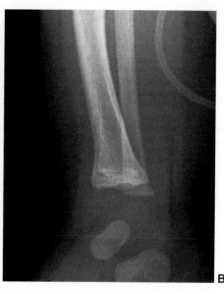

**Figure 34.6** Healing classic metaphyseal lesion (CML). **A:** Antero-posterior view. **B:** Lateral view. This is the same patient who also had the humeral shaft fracture shown in Figure 34.5. This fracture pattern along with the findings in Figure 34.5 clearly indicates that these fractures were caused by abuse.

indistinctness of the fracture line date fractures to similar ages—between 2 and 3 weeks. Numerous factors (age of the child, mechanism of injury, fracture stability, and fracture location) determine whether either or both are seen. The subsequent stages of hard callous formation and remodeling are even more variable, but are typically distinct from the early findings. It would likely be impossible to distinguish a fracture that is 4 weeks old from one that is 6 weeks old. Subsequent growth that separates a physeal fracture from the physis (Salter-Harris growth arrest line) helps identify older fractures (Fig. 34.6). One should remember that not all fractures heal at the same rate. For example, an ulnar diaphyseal fracture will heal more slowly than a coexisting distal radial metaphyseal fracture (a common combination seen when both bones of the forearm fracture). During healing they can have the radiographic appearance of fractures of different ages. One should be aware of such possibilities.

## OTHER IMAGING STUDIES

The rationale for obtaining skeletal surveys and bone scans is that many fractures from abuse are not apparent on physical examination. Accurate diagnosis of abusive injury can be reached in most cases by careful appraisal of the social and family history, combined with painstaking clinical radiographic and other imaging evaluations.

The skeletal survey is the method of choice for global skeletal imaging to assess suspected abuse (49). It is necessary for two primary reasons. As mentioned, the typical physical findings of fractures (pain with movement of the injured extremity, swelling at the fracture site, and deformity) may be absent in abused children (22). In addition, identifying multiple fractures can be crucial to the diagnosis of child abuse. The additional information may prove invaluable during a subsequent investigation and prosecution. American Academy of Pediatrics guidelines state that a skeletal survey should be mandatory in all cases of suspected physical abuse in children younger than 2 years (49). In children older than 5 years, skeletal survey and bone scan have little value as screening tools. Injuries in children in the 2 to 5 year age-group should be handled individually (Table 34.4).

The specific views that are recommended to be included vary from one source to another, but the American College of Radiology has published standards for skeletal survey imaging in cases of suspected abuse (50) (Table 34.5). Additional views may be included in some hospitals. For example at one of the local hospitals in the author's community, lateral views of both arms and lower extremities, five views of the skull (anteroposterior, both laterals, Towne, Waters), and cone down views of tibia and fibula, with internal rotation if the child is ambulatory, are included in the routine skeletal survey to assess child abuse. "Babygrams" do not provide sufficient radiographic detail. They are inadequate for screening for abuse and should not be accepted.

### TABLE 34.4

**IMAGING RECOMMENDATIONS FOR SKELETAL INJURY IN CHILDREN IN DIFFERENT AGE GROUPS**

0–12 mo
    Skeletal survey[a]
    Follow-up skeletal survey (2 wk)
12 mo–2 yr
    Skeletal survey or scintigraphy
2–5 yr
    Skeletal survey or scintigraphy in selected cases where physical abuse is strongly suspected
5 yr and older
    Radiographs of individual sites of injury suspected on clinical grounds

[a]Scintigraphy added in selected cases—see discussion in text.
From Kleinman PK. *Diagnostic imaging of child abuse*, 2nd ed. St. Louis, MO: Mosby, 1998:240.

## TABLE 34.5

### STANDARD SKELETAL SURVEY

Appendicular skeleton
    Humeri (AP)
    Forearms (AP)
    Hands (oblique PA)
    Femurs (AP)
    Lower legs (AP)
    Feet (AP)

Axial skeleton
    Thorax (AP and lateral)
    Pelvis (AP; including mid and lower lumbar spine)
    Lumbar spine (lateral)
    Cervical spine (lateral)
    Skull (frontal and lateral)

AP, anteroposterior; PA, posterolateral.

Quality and adequacy of the skeletal survey images must be assured by a radiologist. With the trend to convert to digital radiographic techniques, digital image quality must be comparable to high-detail film screen radiography before it replaces the standard techniques.

There has been some disagreement regarding the role of skeletal survey versus bone scan in screening for child abuse. Bone scans are particularly sensitive for detecting rib fractures, subtle shaft fractures, and early periosteal elevation (51). Bone scans can help identify unsuspected sites of skeletal injury or occult or subtle lesions seen on plain radiographs. The bone scan can be negative acutely. There is also concern that the bone scan may miss subtle spine fractures and CMLs due to the typical increased level of activity seen at the growth plate on bone scans. Both fulfill the need for screening children who are too young to localize pain for the examiner. Bone scans lack specificity, are more expensive, and expose the child to a radionuclide. Any lesions identified on the bone scan must be followed up with radiographs. Conventional radiographs have the advantages that they are easy to perform, can be interpreted in minutes, can differentiate from other pathologies such as tumor and infection, can show different stages of healing, and are less expensive. Both modalities are felt to be sensitive. The specificity is high for skeletal survey and low for bone scintigraphy.

In their review of 261 suspected victims of abuse, Sty and Starshak (52) found that radiographs were positive in 105 cases and false-negative in 32. Bone scans were positive in 120 and false-negative in 2. The authors concluded that scintigraphy should be the screening procedure of choice in cases of suspected abuse. Mandelstam et al. (53) found that 20% of children with inflicted injuries were identified on bone scan only. Like other authors, they also found that the CML can be missed on bone scan (only 35% were identified). The authors concluded that neither a bone scan nor a skeletal survey is ideal, but they provide complementary information to one another. Therefore, they recommended that both studies be done in suspected cases of physical abuse. Flynn et al. (40) suggest a bone scan when abuse is suspected and the skeletal survey is negative or equivocal. Follow-up skeletal survey 2 weeks later has been shown to increase the diagnostic yield and should be considered when abuse is strongly suspected, but not confirmed initially (54). The American Academy of Pediatrics Section on Radiology states that if the child is in a safe environment, a follow-up skeletal survey in 2 weeks could be considered instead of initial bone scan. Bone scan does not obviate the need for a second skeletal survey (49).

Imaging of suspected physeal fractures may not be adequate with plain radiographs, particularly in cases of nonossified epiphyses. The proximal femur and the elbow are common examples. Repeat close-up views in proper alignment that are centered over the physis in question may be sufficient when coupled with a good knowledge of normal anatomy and consideration of comparison views to the contralateral side. If not, ultrasonography, magnetic resonance imaging (MRI), or arthrography can be considered for further imaging of these challenging anatomical areas.

Cranial CT scan, MRI, or both must be done in infants and children with suspected intracranial injury. These studies are not considered standard components of the evaluation in all suspected abuse cases. They should be considered for a child younger than 1 year who presents with a history of serious trauma, brutality, or shaking, or a child who presents with serious bruising or trauma, abdominal trauma, or a positive skeletal survey (34). CT scan of the head may not clearly document subdural bleeding, but it does provide diagnostic and clinical information needed for immediate management of the child. CT scan is better than MRI for evaluation of acute hemorrhage and can detect cranial and facial fractures. Delayed MRI (5 to 7 days) is recommended because acute hemorrhage may not be detected initially. It offers very high sensitivity and specificity in subacute and chronic situations. In a few days, hemorrhagic areas become bright on T2-weighted images as fresh blood turns to methemoglobin.

It is well known that a high percentage of children with spinal injury resulting in paralysis will have negative radiographs [spinal cord injury without radiographic abnormality (SCIWORA)]. MRI of the spine is the imaging modality of choice. Thoracoabdominal trauma can be evaluated with a CT scan if the child is stable. Evaluation and management are similar to those in cases of accidental trauma.

## OTHER DIAGNOSTIC STUDIES

Bleeding abnormalities must be ruled out if a child presents with any signs of bruising, so coagulation studies must be obtained.

If there is a history or suspicion of shaking, an ophthalmology consultation must be obtained. Shaking is a key element in creating hemorrhagic retinopathy (28). Certain patterns of hemorrhagic retinopathy are particularly indicative of shaking, with a very narrow differential diagnosis.

# DIFFERENTIAL DIAGNOSIS

Normal variants, accidental and obstetric trauma, osteogenesis imperfecta (OI), and several less common skeletal diseases must be considered in the differential diagnosis of fractures caused by abuse. The skeletal diseases in the differential for child abuse are listed in Table 34.6. They receive little or no mention in this text as they are listed in the table, and more information is available in the excellent work by Brill et al. (55). The more common challenge that the orthopaedist will face is distinguishing abusive injuries from accidental and obstetric trauma, normal variants, and OI.

## Normal Variants

Nutrient canals can be seen as an oblique radiolucency that extends from the cortical surface to the endosteal margin. They result from vessels that course through dense cortical bone. Normal metaphyseal variants, including beaking, step-offs, and spurs, must be distinguished from the CML (56). The absence of a fracture line or its presence

bilaterally can help differentiate these from abuse. The typical finding of metaphyseal beaking of the proximal tibia in toddlers (Fig. 34.7) could be mistaken for the CML of child abuse, especially during healing (Fig. 34.6B). Physiologic SPNBF is a recognized normal variant in the long bones of infants between 1 and 6 months of age and most commonly involves the femur, humerus, and tibia (Fig. 34.8). It is not uncommon and has been reported to be present 30% to 50% of the time (57). It is radiographically indistinguishable from other conditions that cause SPNBF, such as diaphyseal fractures, osteomyelitis, and congenital syphilis.

## Accidental Injury

Given the previous discussion regarding the nonspecific radiographic appearance of long-bone fracture patterns, it should be clear that differentiating accidental from abusive trauma represents the most common challenge for the orthopaedist. Falling down the stairs or from a height can result in fracture patterns that are similar to fractures caused by abuse. Parents and caretakers may not be

## TABLE 34.6

### DIFFERENTIAL DIAGNOSIS OF SKELETAL DISEASES

| Disease | Shaft Fracture | Subperiosteal New Bone | Metaphyseal Irregularity | Generalized Osteopenia | Comments |
|---|---|---|---|---|---|
| Congenital indifference to pain | + | + | + | − | Normal neurologic examination results except for lack of pain and occasional temperature sensation |
| Myelodysplasia | + | + | + | − | Spinal dysraphism |
| Osteomyelitis | − | + | + | − | Often multifocal in infancy |
| Congenital syphilis | − | + | + | − | — |
| Rickets | + | + | + | + | Insufficiency fractures |
| Scurvy | − | + | + | + + | — |
| Vitamin A intoxication | − | + | − | − | Increased intracranial pressure |
| Caffey disease | − | + + | − | − | Mandible usually involved |
| Leukemia | − | + | − | + | Bone changes extremely variable |
| Prostaglandin E$_1$ therapy | − | + | − | − | — |
| Methotrexate therapy | + | − | ± | + + | Unlikely to occur with current regimens |
| Menkes syndrome | − | + | + | ± | Wormian bones, low serum copper, bladder diverticula, tortuous vessels |
| Copper deficiency | + | + | + | + + | Low birth weight, total parental nutrition, anemia, neutropenia |
| Metaphyseal and spondylometaphyseal dysplasias | − | − | + | − | Short stature |

From Kleinman PK. *Diagnostic imaging of child abuse*, 2nd ed. St. Louis, MO: Mosby, 1998:79.

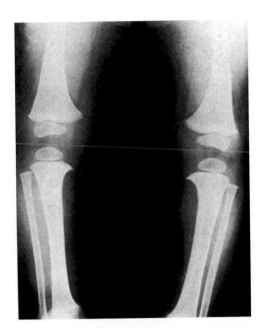

**Figure 34.7** Normal metaphyseal beaking of the proximal tibia in a toddler. (From Keats TE, *Atlas of normal roentgen variants that may simulate disease* 6th ed. St. Louis: Mosby Year Book, 1996:564.)

aware of the risks associated with a child's attainment of new developmental milestones (climbing up on objects, climbing down stairs, falling down). As mentioned earlier, age and attainment of toddlerhood is a primary consideration when trying to determine whether a fracture was accidental or not (31,36–38,40,42–44). The amount of soft-tissue swelling may be a helpful sign. Dos Santos et al. (22) found that less swelling was present initially in long bone fractures caused by abuse than similar fractures that were accidental. The authors concluded that the history and the time of the injury may not be reliable in suspected cases of abuse.

One of the "classic" findings of child abuse is skull and multiple rib fractures. Even this constellation of findings is not specific for abuse, as injuries due to motor vehicle accidents can result in the same findings (27).

## Osteogenesis Imperfecta

Differentiating child abuse from OI is one of the most classic differential diagnostic challenges that the orthopaedist and radiologist can face. Claiming that their child has OI can be a common defense used by an abusive family in legal defenses. The classification of Sillence (58,59) is well known. For the purposes of this discussion, only a brief summary will be offered. The reader is referred for further details of this condition to Chapter 8. OI is a rare disorder of type I collagen (incidence of approximately 1 in 25,000 live births). OI type I is mild and is typically distinguished by distinctly blue sclerae (however, some children with OI type I do not have blue sclerae). OI type II is lethal in the perinatal period. OI type III is severe and causes progressive deformity. OI type IV is typically a milder form, with normal sclerae. Of the two subtypes, type IVA has no dentinogenesis imperfecta. OI is either dominantly inherited or occurs sporadically as a consequence of a new mutation. However, mosaicism has been reported and could explain the occurrence of more than one affected child to apparently "unaffected" parents. The only types that represent a practical differential challenge of abuse are the unusual type I OI without blue sclerae and type IVA OI.

Certainly biochemical analysis of type I collagen can be instrumental in confirming cases of OI when abuse is otherwise considered to be the cause (60). If testing is indicated, a skin biopsy for cultured dermal fibroblasts can detect approximately 85% of OI cases. Collagen analysis to exclude type IV OI is recommended *only* in rare cases in

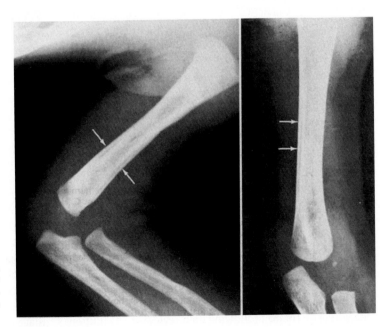

**Figure 34.8** Normal subperiosteal new bone formation (SPNBF) in an infant with no history of trauma or fracture. (From Keats TE, *Atlas of normal roentgen variants that may simulate disease* 6th ed. St. Louis: Mosby Year Book, 1996:422.)

which the diagnosis of child abuse remains in doubt after thorough evaluation by clinicians in consultation with experienced radiologists (61). When faced with making this distinction, clinicians can rely on several helpful points (40). Child abuse is much more common than OI (3 in 100 vs. 1 in 25,000). Typically, a family history is present in OI. Common abusive injuries (skull and rib fractures, subdural hematomas, retinal hemorrhages, and metaphyseal corner fractures) are not associated with OI. Although normal infants younger than 4 months may have blue sclerae, they do not have the dental findings, osteopenia, or wormian bones on skull radiographs seen in children with OI. If there is a reliable reporter and a history of multiple fractures with minimal trauma, OI is likely. Smith offered these guidelines (62):

1. In suspicious circumstances, suspect child abuse.
2. Consider collagen testing if
   a. bruises or burns are not seen
   b. the reported injury seems too minor to have caused a fracture
   c. fractures occur in different environments

When the diagnosis is uncertain, children are typically placed in protective custody. In such an environment, a child with OI type IVA will still fracture. The fractures will likely cease to occur in the abused child. Children with OI can also be victims of abuse (63). Collagen synthesis testing is rarely required to rule out OI, as the diagnosis would have already been strongly suspected in most cases (64).

The reliability of bone mineral density (BMD) measurements to differentiate between abuse and OI is unknown, as values for BMD are not available for either typically developing children younger than 2 years or for children with OI.

## Obstetric Trauma

Obstetric trauma is less common now with modern delivery techniques. Clavicular fractures are most common and occur not only with difficult deliveries but also with uneventful deliveries of large babies. They can be associated with brachial plexus palsies. Some are only noted incidentally on subsequent x-ray films, so they may be more common than reported in the literature. Humerus fractures occur with breech deliveries and have become much less common with the increased utilization of cesarean section. Sonography can help with identification of proximal humeral physeal fractures. Absence of SPNBF at 11 days of age is compelling evidence against a birth injury (65). Subdural hematoma can be caused by obstetric trauma. Evaluation of obstetric injuries has provided useful insight into the biomechanics and imaging characteristics of inflicted skeletal injuries.

## Temporary Brittle Bone Disease

"Temporary brittle bone disease" is a condition proposed by Paterson et al. (66,67) following their review of 39 children younger than 1 year with fractures. They felt that these infants had a "self-limiting variant of OI" due to a transient defect in collagen formation. Since its introduction in 1990, this condition has stirred intense controversy. A number of medical authors and legal proceedings have challenged the findings of this paper. It has been pointed out that none of the authors was a radiologist, thereby bringing into question the accuracy of their findings. Most of the radiographic features of this condition are the same as those seen in child abuse (68). Paterson et al. (66,67) reported that some fractures developed after hospitalization. Although they concluded that this was consistent with the transient osteopenic state, it is well documented that some abusive fractures occurring before hospitalization become evident only on follow-up studies. Ablin and Sane (61) stated that "until clinical research scientifically establishes the existence of temporary brittle bone disease, it should remain strictly a hypothetical entity and not an acceptable medical diagnosis," and Albin states, it "remains a medical hypothesis lacking the support of sound scientific data" (69). Legal proceedings involving testimony by Paterson have cast doubts on his findings. The possibility of temporary brittle bone disease may "compromise or obstruct protection of a child" and that by being aware of and referring others to relevant law reports, pediatricians can help keep the issues in perspective (70).

Copper deficiency has similarly been implicated as the cause of fractures. Chapman and Hall (68) indicated that there were approximately 20 cases reported in the world literature, and fractures as late sequelae of copper deficiency have never been reported. British courts have sought to define what is acceptable opinion versus untried hypothesis. "Untested and unacceptable views should not be put forward—advice American courts should take note of in this age of 'pseudoscience' in the courtroom" (70).

## PATHOANATOMY

Except for CML, the pathoanatomy of musculoskeletal injury caused by abuse is the same as traumatic fractures and soft-tissue injuries due to other causes. The pathoanatomy of the CML is pathognomonic for abuse. It has been described in detail by Kleinman et al. (32) in a classic article that received the Society for Pediatric Radiology John Caffey Award. The authors studied four children who died because of their injuries. The histopathology of their lesions was correlated with fracture patterns on pre- and postmortem radiographs and anatomy from autopsy specimens. The CML is due to a series of subepiphyseal planar fractures through the most immature part of the metaphyseal bone. The separation occurs in the region of transition from the zone of calcified cartilage to the primary spongiosa. If the injury extends to the periphery of the bone, it undermines and isolates a peripheral fragment of bone encompassing the periosteal collar. The periosteum serves as the anchor for the epiphyseal cartilage to the metaphysis. The CML occurs because of avulsive forces applied to the periosteal attachment to the surface of the metaphysis. The result is the isolation of a mineralized disc (or a part thereof) that can be seen radiographically.

A subsequent study of the pathology of healing CMLs by the same senior author (33) documents thickening of the zone of hypertrophic cartilage, with some cases showing extension of the growth plate into the metaphysis. Because estimating the age of CMLs is difficult, the authors suggested that the extent of healing may be helpful in dating these fractures.

## NATURAL HISTORY

Abused children have a substantial risk of repeated abuse and death. It is accepted and well known that a high percentage of children will be reinjured and some will die if they are returned to the abusive environment. Therefore, abuse must be diagnosed, and either some intervention or removal of the child from the abusive environment must be enforced.

## TREATMENT RECOMMENDATIONS

Making the diagnosis of child abuse can be one of the trickiest aspects of managing this condition. Kleinman writes that, as with other clinical situations, "the most effective approach to diagnosis is one based on thoughtful and measured acquisition of data that is carefully analyzed in the light of one's knowledge and experience" (13). Managing fractures due to abuse is typically not difficult or challenging. Identifying all fractures, making the diagnosis, and instituting the process to protect the child from reinjury are the challenging aspects of child abuse.

To see a vulnerable child who has been abused may not be easy. To feel angry is human. As professionals, controlling our emotional response is essential in carrying out our responsibility to care for and protect the child. Particularly in cases that are less clear, the physician should try to form a relationship with the family which will foster their participation in the subsequent diagnostic and therapeutic workup. One must also explain the case report and aspects of the protective service process to the family.

In each case, the physician should determine the level of ongoing risk. Banaszkiewicz et al. (71) advise that all children younger than 1 year with a fracture be admitted to the hospital and referred to a pediatrician for child protection assessment. Management should be multidisciplinary, with the key being recognition because of the risk to the abused child (11). Such teams and resources are available in most, if not all, institutions. The importance of diagnosing abuse and intervening on behalf of the vulnerable child cannot be overemphasized.

Anxiety regarding subsequent legal actions may be one of the potential disincentives for a practitioner to initiate an investigation or to make the diagnosis. Advance preparation and knowledge about the process may help minimize this potential disincentive. Physicians have certain rights that they should expect to be able to exercise when they testify (72).

- The right not to know
- The right to understand the question
- The right to ask for a question to be repeated
- The right not to be confused
- The right to refresh one's memory
- The right to ask if a factual statement or an opinion is being requested.

What might an orthopaedist be asked in court? The common possibilities include (40):

- Factual information about the child's fractures
- Possible mechanism of injury
- Amount of force/energy needed to cause the fractures
- Dating fractures
- Judge information based on reasonable medical certainty
- Potential for future fractures

Akbarnia and Campbell's (4) chapter on child abuse in the previous edition of this book has an extensive section on medicolegal issues for the orthopaedist. It is excellent and recommended for the reader interested in more information. Further insights to diffuse these concerns are addressed in the following text.

## AUTHOR'S PREFERRED RECOMMENDATIONS

As orthopaedists, it goes without saying that we see many fractures. We should ask ourselves if we recognize abusive fractures when we see them. The reported maltreatment rate is 1% to 1.5% annually. Given the widely held belief that child abuse is significantly underreported, this incidence is likely to be lower than the actual rate of occurrence. Fractures are the second most common presentation in child abuse. These statistics should cause us to pause and wonder whether we recognize the etiology of abusive fractures often enough. Some are obvious; diagnosing the rest is where the challenge lies.

It seems that to make the diagnosis of child abuse, it is essential for the orthopaedist to consider two key issues. The first is that we must have a *high index of suspicion*. Without it, we will not recognize abuse often enough. Many of us also care for children with disabilities, and must remember that they are particularly vulnerable. Not only are they at increased risk of physical injury; medical neglect in the form of lack of provision of adequate nutrition by the caregiver is not uncommon. We should recognize this when it is present, and ask our pediatrician colleagues to assess and intervene.

The second is that we must *avoid the disincentive to become involved*. We must be wary of this lurking danger. The time involved and anxiety regarding the legal rigmarole may insidiously erode our willingness to report suspicious fractures and institute the process. The clinician may also feel psychosocial pressure to not report cases that are of concern. We may want to avoid putting a family through the embarrassment of filing a report and completing an investigation. Methods to minimize these disincentives are addressed later in this section.

On the other hand, one must also be careful to avoid becoming overzealous. One must remember that ambulatory status is a very strong predictor of likely abuse. Child Protective Services may be consulted unnecessarily in some cases (36). Unless other evidence of abuse such as an inconsistent story, bruises, or other fractures is present, abuse of the toddler (who might, for example, have a toddler's fracture of the tibia) is much less likely than abuse of the infant. Of course, there are enthusiasts on both sides. Physicians and other professionals practicing in this field may seek to simplify matters, taking extreme positions that reflect either an overly passionate approach to diagnosing abuse or an unwillingness to consider abuse in all but the most flagrant cases. Financial rewards for legal counsel may increase the zealousness with which cases are pursued.

Knowledge and resources are key elements in providing effective and safe care. The following resources are those that I have found to be particularly useful. Paul Kleinman's multiauthored book *Diagnostic Imaging of Child Abuse 2nd ed.* (13) is an essential reference for all centers. Dr. Kleinman is a radiologist with a worldwide reputation for his expertise in the field of child abuse. During his career, he has been active in research and education.

A handy, two-page summary handout was prepared under the auspices of the Pediatric Orthopaedic Society of North America Trauma Committee (Chairman: Peter Pizzutillo, M.D.) in 2002 (40). It is a very useful, quick-glance guide that is also handy for residents' education. It is available by emailing John M. Flynn, M.D. at the Children's Hospital of Philadelphia—Flynnj@email.CHOP.edu.

The Quarterly (Robert M. Reece, M.D., Editor) (www.quarterlyupdate.org) contains reviews of recent peer-reviewed articles on the diagnosis, prevention, and treatment of child abuse and neglect. Medical, legal, mental health, and social work professionals known for their expertise and experience summarize the articles which are chosen from more than 1000 medical journals. The reviewers offer opinions about the validity and significance of the research findings.

Table 34.7 covers points to remember and recommendations that will hopefully help the orthopaedist avoid pitfalls.

We all have a legal and moral obligation to protect children. For the physician not to report child abuse because

---

**TABLE 34.7**

**AVOIDING PITFALLS**

**Remember**

- We have a legal and moral obligation to identify and report abuse.
- Age is a strong predictor of child abuse.
- Not all fractures heal at the same rate. Fractures that may appear to be at different stages of healing may not be of different ages (some fractures, even forearm fractures, heal at different rates and may produce the radiographic appearance of fractures of different ages).
- There is no uncertainty regarding the cause of the CML. It is pathognomonic for abuse.
- There is no evidence that "temporary brittle bone disease" exists.
- Bone scans and skeletal surveys are complementary, not mutually exclusive studies.
- A bone scan is especially useful for subtle rib fractures, but it is not a stand-alone test.
- A bone scan can be negative acutely and has a high false-negative rate for the CML.
- The skeletal survey should be read by the radiologist before the child leaves the radiography department.
- The skeletal survey should be standardized and read by a pediatric radiologist to increase sensitivity.

**Recommendations**

- Use protocols
  - for obtaining the history and physical exam as well as photographs
  - for ordering other studies such as the CT scan, skeletal survey, and MRI
  - for techniques for each of these tests
  - for ordering consults.
- Have a low threshold for brain MRI.
- Head CT scans are not always completely satisfactory.
- Delay a few days for hemorrhagic areas to turn to methemoglobin (lights up on T2-weighted images). In Minnesota, children can be held for 72 hr, so obtaining this should be easy.
- Repeat the complete skeletal survey 2 weeks later.
- Do not accept babygrams. They are too insensitive.
- Consider accessing the resources available at a referral center.

CML, classic metaphyseal lesion; CT, computed tomography; MRI, magnetic resonance imaging.

"child protective services is unlikely to do anything" is a self-fulfilling prophecy and should not happen (72). Consulting the physicians and staff of referral centers that specialize in the management of child maltreatment removes at least some of the disincentive to reporting. Many physicians are uncomfortable in the courtroom. Much of the legal work can be handled by expert physicians who work in referral centers. In this case, the orthopaedist may not be needed as often in court. If disincentives are removed, we can be appropriately suspicious. The radiologist and members of the referral center staff can be more objective and more detached from psychological pressures to not report. These centers are typically referred to as children's advocacy centers [the local center in my community is the Midwest Children's Resource Center (MCRC) in St. Paul, Minnesota, United States]. They typically utilize the multidisciplinary team (MDT) approach for the treatment or prevention of child abuse and neglect in their respective communities. Many provide 24-hour coordination of suspected child abuse and neglect (SCAN) cases, integrating hospital services with outside community agencies. They can formulate and provide many of the necessary protocols mentioned in the preceding text. They partner pediatric subspecialty consultants (hospital MDTs) with providers in the community (community MDTs). A hospital MDT includes physicians, nurses, social workers, and risk managers. A community MDT includes law enforcement, child protection investigators, and county attorneys. Child abuse consultants provide expertise in diagnosis of inflicted trauma. The medical care team is therefore more free to first and foremost provide medical care.

The staff of the center can provide professional consultation for case reviews, telephone consultation, and expert testimony. They are also active in education for both health care and community providers, often supporting combined, multidisciplinary interaction and education. They typically offer both medical and psychological assessments. The National Association of Children's Hospitals and Related Institutions (NACHRI) is considering designating qualifying programs as centers of excellence. They provide training supported by a national grant from the Department of Justice. The American Academy of Pediatrics Section on Child Abuse and Neglect (SOCAN) maintains a listing of these centers across the United States and Canada. This can be accessed at www.aap.org/sections/scan/ and the link "State Child Abuse Programs." Numerous policy statements are available on this website as well.

A more recent development has been the inclusion of law enforcement to the teams at referral centers. Those in law enforcement add expertise in acquisition of information and the ability to evaluate and photograph the scene of the injury. They can provide an evaluation and report on conditions in the home, the number of calls for domestic disputes that have been made, and whether there is any prior history of intervention. The initial report to the appropriate police department is oral and is followed by a written report.

The International Society for Prevention of Child Abuse and Neglect (ISPCAN) (www.ispcan.org) was organized to support individuals and organizations working to protect children from abuse and neglect worldwide. Founded in 1977, it is the only multidisciplinary international organization that brings together a worldwide cross section of committed professionals to work toward the prevention and treatment of child abuse, neglect, and exploitation globally. ISPCAN's mission is "to prevent cruelty to children in every nation, in every form: physical abuse, sexual abuse, neglect, street children, child fatalities, child prostitution, children of war, emotional abuse, and child labor. ISPCAN is committed to increasing public awareness of all forms of violence against children, developing activities to prevent such violence, and promoting the rights of children in all regions of the world." The organization's journal, *Child Abuse and Neglect: The International Journal* is published by Elsevier Science (www.elsevier.com). ISPCAN partners with numerous national organizations such as American Professional Society on the Abuse of Children (APSAC) in the United States.

Children's advocacy centers may be accessed for consultation only, or one may consider referring a child to a tertiary referral center for assessment and management. These referrals may be helpful because such centers have the equipment and expertise to perform the necessary studies and interpret them appropriately. Although it is impractical to restrict evaluations to specialized centers, the scope of services they offer may be helpful to the orthopaedist. Alternatively, developing connections to access the consultative services of a pediatric radiologist with expertise in the field could be valuable to the orthopaedist without ready access to a specialized center in his or her local area.

# REFERENCES

### Definition

1. Caffey J. Multiple fractures in the long bones of infants suffering from chronic subdural hematoma. *AJR Am J Roentgenol* 1946;56:163–173.
2. Kempe CH, Silverman FN, Steele BF, et al. The battered-child syndrome. *JAMA* 1962;181:17–24.
3. Silverman FN. Unrecognized trauma in infants, the battered child syndrome, and the syndrome of Ambroise Tardieu. *Radiology* 1972;104:337–353.
4. Akbarnia BA, Campbell RM. The role of the orthopaedic surgeon in child abuse. In: Morrissy RT, Weinstein SL, eds. *Lovell and winter's pediatric orthopaedics*, 5th ed. Philadelphia, PA: Lippincott Williams & Wilkins, 2000:1424–1443.
5. Helfer RE, Kempe CH. *The battered child.* Chicago, IL: University of Chicago Press, 1968.
6. Akbarnia BA, Torg JS, Kirkpatrick J, et al. Manifestations of the battered-child syndrome. *J Bone Joint Surg* 1974;6A:1159–1166.
7. Zillmer DA, Bynum DK, Kocher MS, et al. Family violence for the orthopaedic surgeon. *Instr Course Lect* 2002;52:791–802.
8. Bittner S, Newberger EH. Pediatric understanding of child abuse and neglect. *Pediatr Rev* 1981;2(7):197–207.
9. Child abuse definitions, www.childhelpusa.org, accessed December 8, 2004.
10. Beaty JH. Orthopedic aspects of child abuse. *Curr Opin Pediatr* 1997;9:100–103.
11. Kocher MS, Kasser JR. Orthopaedic aspects of child abuse. *J Am Acad Orthop Surg* 2000;8(1):10–20.

## Epidemiology

12. National Center on Child Abuse and Neglect. *Child maltreatment 2004, reports from the states to the National Center on Child Abuse and Neglect*. Washington, DC: National Center on Child Abuse and Neglect, 2004.
13. Kleinman PK. *Diagnostic imaging of child abuse*, 2nd ed. St. Louis, MO: Mosby, 1998.
14. McMahon P, Grossman W, Gaffney M, et al. Soft-tissue injury as an indication of child abuse. *J Bone Joint Surg* 1995;77A: 1179–1183.

## Etiology

15. Wolfner GD, Gelles RJ. A profile of violence toward children: a national study. *Child Abuse Negl* 1993;17:197–212.
16. Akbarnia BA, Akbarnia NO. The role of orthopaedist in child abuse and neglect. *Orthop Clin North Am* 1976;7:733–742.

## Clinical Features

17. American Academy of Pediatrics Committee on Child Abuse and Neglect and Committee on Children with Disabilities. Assessment of maltreatment of children with disabilities. *Pediatrics* 2001; 108(2):508–512.
18. Alexander RC, Sherbondy AL. Child abuse and developmental disabilities. In: Wolraich ML, ed. *Disorders of development and learning: a practical guide to assessment and management*. St Louis, MO: Mosby–Year Book, 1996.
19. Benedict MI, White RB, Wulff LM, et al. Reported maltreatment in children with multiple disabilities. *Child Abuse Negl* 1990;14: 207–217.
20. Rosenberg DA. Web of deceit: a literature review of Munchausen syndrome by proxy. *Child Abuse Negl* 1987;2:547–563.
21. Oral R, Blum KL, Johnson C. Fractures in young children: are physicians in the emergency department and orthopedic clinics adequately screening for possible abuse? *Pediatr Emerg Care* 2003;19(3):148–153.
22. Dos Santos LM, Stewart G, Meert K, et al. Soft tissue swelling with fractures: abuse versus nonintentional. *Pediatr Emerg Care* 1995;11(4):215–216.
23. Robertson DM, Barbor P, Hull D. Unusual injury? Recent injury in normal children and children with suspected non-accidental injury. *Br Med J* 1982;285:1399–1401.
24. Wilson EF. Estimation of the age of cutaneous contusions in child abuse. *Pediatrics* 1977;60:750.
25. Lenoski EF, Hunter KA. Patterns of inflicted burns. *J Trauma* 1977;17:842.
26. Duhaime AC, Partington MD. Overview and clinical presentation of inflicted head injury in infants. In: Adelson PD, Partington MD, guest eds. *Neurosurgery clinics of North America*. Philadelphia, PA: WB Saunders, 2002;13(2):149–154.
27. Kowal-Vern A, Paxton TP, Ros SP, et al. Fractures in the under-3-year old age cohort. *Clin Pediatr (Phila)* 1992;31:653–659.
28. Levin AV. Ophthalmology of shaken baby syndrome. In: Adelson PD, Partington MD, guest eds. *Neurosurgery clinics of North America*. Philadelphia, PA: WB Saunders, 2002;13(2):201–211.

## Radiographic Features

29. Loder RT, Bookout C. Fracture patterns in battered children. *J Orthop Trauma* 1991;5:428–433.
30. Kleinman PK, Marks SC, Spevak MR, et al. Extension of growth-plate cartilage into the metaphysis: a sign of healing fracture in abused infants. *AJR Am J Roentgenol* 1991;156:775–779.
31. Blakemore LC, Loder RT, Hensinger RN. Role of intentional abuse in children 1 to 5 years old with isolated femoral shaft fractures. *J Pediatr Orthop* 1996;16(5):585–588.
32. Kleinman PK, Marks SC, Blackbourne B. The metaphyseal lesion in abused infants: a radiologic-histopathologic study. *AJR Am J Roentgenol* 1986;146(5):895–905.
33. Kleinman PK, Marks SC Jr. Relationship of the subperiosteal bone collar to metaphyseal lesions in abused infants. *J Bone Joint Surg Am* 1995;77:1471–1476.
34. Rustamzadeh E, Truwit CL, Lam CH. Radiology of nonaccidental trauma. In: Adelson PD, Partington MD, eds. *Neurosurgery clinics of North America*. Philadelphia, PA: WB Saunders, 2002;13(2): 183–199.

35. Barsness KA, Char E, Bensard DD, et al. The positive predictive value of rib fractures as an indicator of nonaccidental trauma in children. *J Trauma* 2003;54:1107–1110.
36. Schwend RM, Werth C, Johnston A. Femur shaft fractures in toddlers and young children: rarely from child abuse. *J Pediatr Orthop* 2000;40(4):475–481.
37. Strait RT, Siegel RM, Shapiro RA. Humeral fractures without obvious etiologies in children less than 3 years of age. When is it abuse? *Pediatrics* 1995;96:667–671.
38. Thomas SA, Rosenfield NS, Leventhal JM, et al. Long-bone fractures in young children: distinguishing accidental injuries from child abuse. *Pediatrics* 1991;88(3):471–476.
39. Hedlund R, Lindren U. The incidence of femoral shaft fractures in children and adolescents. *J Pediatr Orthop* 1986;6:47–50.
40. Flynn the POSNA Trauma Committee, 2002 Chairman: Peter Pizzutillo, MD, John M. Flynn, MD at the Children's Hospital of Philadelphia, Flynnj@email.CHOP.edu.
41. King JD, Diefendorf D, Apthorp J, et al. Analysis of 429 fractures in 189 battered children. *J Pediatr Orthop* 1988;8(5):585–589.
42. Rex C, Kay PR. Features of femoral fractures in nonaccidental injury. *J Pediatr Orthop* 2000;20(3):411–413.
43. Dalton HJ, Slovis T, Helfer RE, et al. Undiagnosed abuse in children younger than 3 years with femoral fracture. *Am J Dis Child* 1990;144:875–878.
44. Shaw BA, Murphy KM, Shaw A, et al. Humerus shaft fractures in young children: accident or abuse? *J Pediatr Orthop* 1997;17(3): 293–297.
45. Swischuk LE. Supracondylar femoral fracture in an infant. *Pediatr Emerg Care* 2003;19(2):104–107.
46. Merten DF, Radkowski MA, Leonidas JC. The abused child: a radiological reappraisal. *Radiology* 1987;146:377–381.
47. Campbell RM. Child abuse. In: Beaty JH, Kasser JR, eds. *Rockwood and Wilkins' fractures in children*, 5th ed. Philadelphia, PA: Lippincott Williams & Wilkins, 2001:241–266.
48. O'Connor JF, Cohen J. Dating fractures. In: Kleinman PK, ed. *Diagnostic imaging of child abuse*, 2nd ed. St. Louis, MO: Mosby, 1998:168–177.

## Other Imaging Studies

49. American Academy of Pediatrics Section on Radiology. Diagnostic imaging of child abuse. *Pediatrics* 2000;105(6):1345–1348.
50. American College of Radiology. Imaging of the child with suspected physical abuse. *American college of radiology appropriateness criteria for imaging and treatment decisions*. Reston, VA: American College of Radiology, 1995:PD-5.1–PD-5.6.
51. Conway JJ, Collins M, Tanz RR, et al. The role of bone scintigraphy in detecting child abuse. *Semin Nucl Med* 1993;23:321–333.
52. Sty JR, Starshak RJ. The role of bone scintigraphy in the evaluation of the suspected abused child. *Radiology* 1983;146:369–375.
53. Mandelstam SA, Cook D, Fitzgerald M, et al. Complementary use of radiological skeletal survey and bone scintigraphy in detection of bony injuries in suspected child abuse. *Arch Dis Child* 2003;88:387–389.
54. Kleinman PK, Nimkin K, Spevak MR, et al. Follow-up skeletal surveys in suspected child abuse. *Am J Radiol* 1996;167:893–896.

## Differential Diagnosis

55. Brill PW, Winchester P, Kleinman PK. Differential diagnosis I: diseases simulating abuse. In: Kleinman PK, ed. *Diagnostic imaging of child abuse*, 2nd ed. St. Louis, MO: Mosby, 1998:178–196.
56. Kleinman PK, Kwon DS. Differential diagnosis IV: normal variants. In: Kleinman PK, ed. *Diagnostic imaging of child abuse*, 2nd ed. St. Louis, MO: Mosby, 1998:225–236.
57. Kwon DS, Spevak MR, Kleinman PK, et al. Subperiosteal new bone formation in the sudden infant death syndrome. *Radiology* 1997;205:495.
58. Sillence DO, Senn A, Danks DM. Genetic heterogeneity in osteogenesis imperfecta. *J Med Ethics* 1979;16:101–116.
59. Sillence D. Osteogenesis imperfecta: an expanding panorama of variants. *Clin Orthop* 1981;159:11–25.
60. Gahagan S, Rimsza ME. Child abuse or osteogenesis imperfecta: how can we tell? *Pediatrics* 1991;88(5):987–992.
61. Ablin DS, Sane SM. Non-accidental injury: confusion with temporary brittle bone disease and mild osteogenesis imperfecta. *Pediatr Radiol* 1997;27:111–113.

62. Smith R. Osteogenesis imperfecta, non-accidental injury, and temporary brittle bone disease. *Arch Dis Child* 1995;72:169–176.

63. Knight DJ, Bennet GC. Non-accidental injury in osteogenesis imperfecta: a case report. *J Pediatr Orthop* 1990;10:542–544.

64. Steiner RD, Pepin M, Byers PH. Studies of collagen synthesis and structure in the differentiation of child abuse from osteogenesis imperfecta. *J Pediatr* 1996;128:542–547.

65. Cumming WA. Neonatal skeletal fractures: birth trauma or child abuse? *J Can Assoc Radiol* 1979;30:30–33.

66. Paterson CR, Burns J, McAllion SJ. Osteogenesis imperfecta: The distinction from child abuse and the recognition of a variant form. *Am J Med Genet* 1993;45:187–192.

67. Paterson CR, Burns J, McAllion SJ. Osteogenesis imperfecta variant vs. child abuse (reply). *Am J Med Genet* 1995;56:117–118.

68. Chapman S, Hall CM. Non-accidental injury or brittle bones. *Pediatr Radiol* 1997;27:106–110.

69. Ablin DS. Osteogenesis imperfecta: a review. *Can Assoc Radiol J* 1998;49:110–123.

70. Lynch MA. A judicial comment on temporary brittle bone disease. *Arch Dis Child* 1995;73:379.

## Treatment Recommendations

71. Banaszkiewicz PA, Scotland TR, Myerscough EJ. Fractures in children younger than age 1 year: importance of collaboration with child protection services. *J Pediatr Orthop* 2002;22(6):740–744.

72. Krugman RD, Bross DC. Medicolegal aspects of child abuse and neglect. In: Adelson PD, Partington MD, guest eds. *Neurosurgery clinics of North America*. Philadelphia, PA: WB Saunders, 2002;13(2):243–246.

# Subject Index